D1256144

OCCUPATIONAL SKIN DISEASE

OCCUPATIONAL SKIN DISEASE

3rd EDITION

Robert M. Adams, M.D.

Clinical Professor of Dermatology, Emeritus

Stanford University School of Medicine

Stanford, California

W.B. Saunders Company

A Division of Harcourt Brace and Company

Philadelphia London Toronto Montreal Sydney Tokyo

W.B. SAUNDERS COMPANY
A Division of Harcourt Brace & Company

The Curtis Center
Independence Square West
Philadelphia, Pennsylvania 19106

Library of Congress Cataloging-in-Publication Data

Occupational skin disease / [edited by] Robert M. Adams.—3rd ed.

p.   cm.

Includes bibliographical references.

ISBN 0–7216–7037–7

1. Occupational dermatitis.   2. Skin—Diseases.   3. Occupational
    diseases.   4. Dermatotoxicology.   I. Adams, Robert M.
    [DNLM: 1. Dermatitis, Occupational.   WR 600 01552 1999]

RL241.027 1999   616.5—dc21

DNLM/DLC   98–25698

OCCUPATIONAL SKIN DISEASE   ISBN 0–7216–7037–7

Printed in the United States of America

Last digit is the print number: 9   8   7   6   5   4   3   2   1

To my dear wife Lorene who makes it
possible for me to do what I do

Contributors

Robert M. Adams, M.D.
Clinical Professor of Dermatology, Emeritus,
Stanford University School of Medicine,
Stanford, California
*Contact Dermatitis Due to Irritation: Cement
Burns, Dermatitis Due to Fibrous Glass, Chronic
Hypertrophic Dermatosis of the Palms;
Occupational Skin Cancer; Diagnostic Patch-
Testing; Prevention, Treatment, Rehabilitation, and
Plant Inspection; Metals; Paints, Varnishes, and
Lacquers; Solvents; Job Descriptions with Their
Irritants and Allergens*

Armando Ancona, M.D.
Associate Professor of Dermatology, Medical
Faculty, National Autonomous University of
Mexico; Head, Contact and Occupational
Dermatoses Unit, Department of Dermatology,
National Medical Center, Instituto Mexicano del
Seguro Social, Mexico City, Mexico
Biological Causes

Klaus E. Andersen, M.D., Ph.D.
Professor, Department of Dermatology, Odense
University Hospital, Odense, Denmark
Systemic Toxicity from Percutaneous Absorption

Donald V. Belsito, M.D.
Professor of Medicine (Dermatology), University
of Kansas School of Medicine; Director of
Division of Dermatology, University of Kansas
Medical Center, Kansas City, Kansas
*Allergic Contact Dermatitis: Immunological
Aspects*

Bert Björkner, M.D., Ph.D.
Professor, Lund University; Senior
Dermatologist, Department of Occupational and
Environmental Dermatology, University Hospital,
Malmö, Sweden
Plastic Materials

**Desmond Burrows, M.D., F.R.C.P.,
F.D.C.Ped, F.R.C.P.**
Consultant Dermatologist, Royal Victoria
Hospital; Honorary Lecturer, Queens University,
Belfast, Ireland
Metals

Richard Cohen, M.D., M.P.H.
Clinical Professor, Division of Occupational and
Environmental Medicine, University of
California, San Francisco Medical School, San
Francisco, California
Physical Causes: Radiation Effects, Radiation

A. Dooms-Goossens, R.Pharm, Ph.D.
Dermatology, Contact Allergy, Magistral
Preparations Skin Care; Faculty of Medicine
(Leuven), Faculty of Pharmacy (Leuven and
Antwerp); Contact Allergy Unit, Department of
Dermatology, University Hospital, Catholic
University Leuven, Leuven, Belgium
Corticosteroids

P. Elsner, M.D.
Professor of Dermatology, University of Jena
Medical School; Chairman, Department of
Dermatology, Friedrich Schiller University, Jena,
Germany
*Contact Dermatitis Due to Irritation: Clinical
Appearance, Predisposing Factors, and Therapy*

Edward A. Emmett, M.D.
Professor of Medicine, Director, Center for
Occupational and Environmental Health Policy
and Practice, Jefferson Medical College of
Thomas Jefferson University, Philadelphia,
Pennsylvania
Phototoxicity and Photosensitivity Reactions

John H. Epstein, M.D.
Clinical Professor of Dermatology, University of
California, San Francisco, School of Medicine,
San Francisco, California
Occupational Skin Cancer

Torkel Fischer, M.D.
Professor, National Institute for Working Life,
Solna; Department of Dermatology, Karolinska
Hospital, Stockholm, Sweden
*Diagnostic Patch-Testing; Paints, Varnishes, and
Lacquers*

Alexander A. Fisher, M.D.
Clinical Professor of Dermatology, New York
University School of Medicine, New York, New
York
*Contact Dermatitis Due to Irritation: Ethylene
Oxide Burns; Contact Urticaria*

G. N. Flint, B.Sc., F.R.S.C., F.I.M.
Consultant to the Nickel Development Institute,
Environmental Matters, London, England
Metals

Joseph F. Fowler, Jr., M.D.
Associate Clinical Professor of Dermatology and
Director, Occupational Dermatology and Patch-
Testing, University of Louisville School of
Medicine, Louisville, Kentucky
Acne, Folliculitis, and Chloracne

Susanne Freeman, M.D., F.A.C.D.
Lecturer in Dermatology, University of New
South Wales; Visiting Medical Officer
(Dermatologist), St. Vincent's Hospital; Head,
Contact Dermatitis Clinic, Skin and Cancer
Foundation, Sydney; Skin and Cancer
Foundation, Darlinghurst, Sydney, Australia
Diagnosis and Differential Diagnosis

Gary R. Fujimoto, M.D.
Chairman, Department of Occupational
Medicine, Palo Alto Medical Foundation, Palo
Alto; Clinical Professor, Stanford University
School of Medicine, Stanford, California
Semiconductor Industry

Gerald A. Gellin, M.D., F.A.C.P.
Clinical Professor of Dermatology, University of
California, San Francisco, School of Medicine;
Chief, Division of Dermatology, California
Pacific Medical Center, San Francisco, California
*Contact Dermatitis Due to Irritation: Pigmentary
Changes*

Lee H. Grafton, M.D.
Chief Resident, Dermatology, Louisiana State
University Medical Center, New Orleans,
Louisiana
Pesticides and Other Agricultural Chemicals

Jere D. Guin, M.D.
Professor Emeritus of Dermatology, University of
Arkansas for Medical Sciences, Little Rock,
Arkansas
Natural and Synthetic Rubber

Curt Hamann, M.D.
President and Chief Executive Officer, Smart
Practice, Phoenix, Arizona
Natural and Synthetic Rubber

Jon M. Hanifin, M.D.
Professor of Dermatology, Oregon Health
Sciences University School of Medicine;
Privileges, University Hospital, Portland, Oregon
Atopy and Atopic Dermatitis

Daniel J. Hogan, M.D.
Chief of Dermatology, Professor of Medicine and
Pediatrics, Louisiana State University School of
Medicine in Shreveport, Shreveport, Louisiana
Pesticides and Other Agricultural Chemicals

**D. Linn Holness, M.D., M.H.Sc.,
F.R.C.P.C.**
Associate Professor and Director, Division of
Occupational Medicine, Departments of Medicine
and Public Health Science, University of Toronto
Faculty of Medicine; Chief, Department of
Occupational and Environmental Health, St.
Michael's Hospital, Toronto, Ontario, Canada
*Industrial Processes Commonly Associated with
Skin Disease*

D. Iliev, M.D.
Resident, Department of Dermatology, Ernst von
Bergmann Hospital, Potsdam, Germany
*Contact Dermatitis Due to Irritation: Clinical
Appearance, Predisposing Factors, and Therapy*

Lasse Kanerva, M.D., Ph.D.
Chief, Section of Dermatology, Finnish Institute
of Occupational Health, Helsinki, Finland
*Physical Causes and Radiation Effects: Physical
Causes*

Joseph LaDou, M.D.
Division of Occupational and Environmental
Medicine, University of California, San
Francisco, School of Medicine, San Francisco,
California
Workers' Compensation

Yung-Hian Leow, M.D.
Dermatologist, National Skin Centre, Singapore
Contact Urticaria

Hon-Wing Leung, Ph.D.
Director of Toxicology, Union Carbide Corp.,
Danbury, Connecticut
Health Risk Assessment

James G. Marks, Jr., M.D.
Professor of Medicine, Head, Section of
Dermatology, Pennsylvania State University
College of Medicine, Hershey, Pennsylvania
Cosmetics; Plants and Woods

Martha J. Maso, M.D., M.P.H.
Associate in Clinical Dermatology, Presbyterian
Hospital, New York, New York; Assistant
Attending, Pascack Valley Hospital, Westwood,
New Jersey
Occupational Nail Disorders

C. G. Toby Mathias, M.D.
Clinical Professor, Department of Environmental
Health; Associate Clinical Professor, Department
of Dermatology; University of Cincinnati College
of Medicine; Staff Dermatologist, Group Health
Associates, Cincinnati, Ohio
Soaps and Detergents

M. Matura, M.D., Ph.D.
Dermatologist, Department of Dermatology,
Central Military Hospital, Budapest, Hungary
Corticosteroids

Linda Morse, M.D.
Assistant Clinical Professor of Medicine,
University of California, San Francisco, School
of Medicine; Assistant Chief, Occupational
Health Services, Kaiser-Permanente, San
Francisco, California
*Occupational and Environmental Connective
Tissue Disorders*

Enrique A. Mullins, M.D.
Assistant Professor, Head of the Orient Division,
Department of Dermatology, Faculty of
Medicine, University of Chile; Dermatologist,
Staff Member of the Department of Dermatology,
Hospital del Salvador, Santiago, Chile
The Computer

James R. Nethercott, M.D.
Professor, Department of Dermatology,
Epidemiology, and Preventive Medicine,
University of Maryland School of Medicine;
Attending Physician, Johns Hopkins Hospital,
and University of Maryland Medical System,
Baltimore, Maryland
*Industrial Processes Commonly Associated with
Skin Disease*

Alice Ormsby, M.D.
Associate in Dermatology, University of
Washington School of Medicine; Clinical

Dermatology, Virginia-Mason Medical Center,
Seattle, Washington
Occupational Skin Cancer

Dennis Paustenbach, Ph.D.
Adjunct Professor, University of California,
Irvine, College of Medicine; Adjunct Professor,
University of Massachusetts, Worcester; Group
Vice-President (Health Sciences), Exponent
Corp., Menlo Park, California
Health Risk Assessment

Julie A. Rothrock, M.S.
Senior Environmental Scientist, Exponent Corp.,
Boston, Massachusetts
Health Risk Assessment

**R.J.G. Rycroft, M.D., F.R.C.P., F.F.O.M.,
D.I.H.**
Honorary Senior Lecturer and Consultant
Dermatologist, St. John's Institute of
Dermatology, St. Thomas's Hospital, London,
U.K.
Petroleum and Petroleum Derivatives

Richard K. Scher, M.D., F.A.C.P.
Professor of Clinical Dermatology, Columbia
University, College of Physicians and Surgeons;
Attending in Dermatology, Presbyterian Hospital,
New York, New York
Occupational Nail Disorders

Elizabeth F. Sherertz, M.D.
Professor and Vice Chair, Department of
Dermatology, Bowman Gray School of Medicine
of Wake Forest University, Winston-Salem,
North Carolina
*Allergic Contact Dermatitis: General Principles
and Causes*

Kim M. Sullivan, B.A. (Education)
Vice President of Operations, Smart Practice,
Associate Director of Clinical Research, Phoenix,
Arizona
Natural and Synthetic Rubber

James S. Taylor, M.D.
Head, Section of Industrial Dermatology, The
Cleveland Clinic Foundation, Cleveland, Ohio
Contact Urticaria

Abba I. Terr, M.D.
Clinical Professor of Medicine, Stanford
University School of Medicine; Director, Allergy
Clinic, Stanford University Medical Center,
Stanford, California
Multiple Chemical Sensitivities

Michael V. Vance, M.D.
Paradise Valley, Arizona
Contact Dermatitis Due to Irritation: Hydrofluoric Acid Burns

J. E. Wahlberg, M.D.
Professor, National Institute for Working Life;
Karolinska Hospital, Stockholm, Sweden
Solvents

W. Wigger-Alberti, M.D.
Resident, University of Jena Medical School;
Resident, Department of Dermatology, Friedrich Schiller University, Jena, Germany
Contact Dermatitis Due to Irritation: Clinical Appearance, Predisposing Factors, and Therapy

Kathryn A. Zug, M.D.
Assistant Professor of Medicine (Dermatology), Dartmouth Medical School, Hanover;
Clinical Staff Dermatologist, Dartmouth-Hitchcock Medical Center, Lebanon, New Hampshire
Plants and Woods

Foreword

It was a significant honor for me to be asked to follow the forewords of Dr. Alexander A. Fisher in 1983 and Dr. Etain Cronin in 1990 with this foreword in 1999. I welcome you with great pleasure to this remarkable third edition of Dr. Robert M. Adams' textbook of *Occupational Skin Disease*. The startling increase in the size of this work from the 477 pages in its first edition is a testament to the importance of occupational skin diseases and the intensity with which they have been studied in the past 16 years.

This book is absolutely fresh and fully encyclopedic. There are brand new chapters and eager new contributors who present complete rewrites of the previous edition's chapters. American dermatologists with interest in occupational skin disease have viewed this book as a national treasure. Now, even more than in the second edition, it is internationally authored, although never lacking the application of Dr. Adams' personal knowledge, writings, and oversight.

As in previous editions, the reader's expectation that the most current studies are reviewed and cited is met. Tables are complete and useful for both research and patient care. The unique Appendix at the book's end, tying job descriptions with their irritants and allergens, is better than ever.

Dr. Adams' joy in working with patients with contact dermatitis in his own practice and in working with residents' studying contact dermatitis at Stanford University Medical School led him to form the American Contact Dermatitis Society with several colleagues and to serve as its president for 2 years. He is the founding editor of the society's journal, the *American Journal of Contact Dermatitis,* which thrives today as a means to present the most current studies of contact dermatitis.

This book really is a remarkable labor of love. How fortunate we are that dermatology has Dr. Adams, an individual with the knowledge to provide us with this reliable resource that we can use to help our patients, teach our students, and interest our colleagues in the study of occupational skin disease.

FRANCES J. STORRS, M.D.
Professor Emerita
Department of Dermatology
Oregon Health Sciences University
Portland, Oregon

Preface

Occupational Skin Disease, 3rd edition, is a complete rewriting of the two previous editions. Much of the information in the other editions has been retained, but all of it has been re-examined and brought to as current a level as possible. Forty-nine experts, with national and worldwide reputations, have contributed their knowledge to this edition. Three new chapters have been added, examining subjects of current interest and importance: multiple chemical sensitivities, risk assessments, and corticosteroid reactions. The appendix on irritants and allergens found in 100 occupations is expanded and up-to-date, with hundreds of new references.

Since 1982, when the first edition of Occupational Skin Disease was published, there has occurred a marked increase in the recognition and importance of the workplace in the development of skin disease. Family physicians and internists, as well as dermatologists throughout the world, have taken part in the endeavor to add to this knowledge. In the United States, the Occupational Safety and Health Act and Freedom of Information legislation have contributed significantly to the ability of physicians to recognize the causes of occupational diseases. At the same time, awareness of these problems by industry has also increased, frequently leading to measures to minimize the development and harmful long-range effects of work-related skin disease. The utilization of patch-testing and other methods of evaluation has also contributed to greater awareness. The creation of national and international societies devoted entirely to the study and dissemination of knowledge about contact dermatitis and contact allergens has also taken place. These groups have caused an expansion of our knowledge as well as a greater participation by physicians—not only dermatologists but also allergists and occupational physicians—and by related industry personnel.

ROBERT M. ADAMS, M.D.
San Mateo, California

Preface

Acknowledgments

This edition of *Occupational Skin Disease* has been truly a labor of love. I wish to acknowledge with gratitude each of the contributors, whose knowledge, generosity, and conscientiousness made this work possible. I want also to thank the personnel of W.B. Saunders Company, Judith Fletcher, Linda Garber, and Donna Morrissey among others, for their care, attention, and considerable talent in composing this book. It has been a great pleasure to work with them. Finally, I want to thank my wife, Lorene, for her patience, help, understanding, and encouragement during this endeavor.

Contents

Contact Dermatitis Due to Irritation

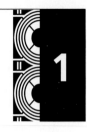

Clinical Appearance, Predisposing Factors, ■ and Therapy

W. WIGGER-ALBERTI, M.D.
D. ILIEV, M.D.
P. ELSNER, M.D.

Irritant contact dermatitis (ICD) that has been defined as "a nonimmunologic local inflammatory reaction characterized by erythema, edema, or corrosion following single or repeated application of a chemical substance to an identical cutaneous site"[1] is a frequent and important condition in general and occupational dermatology and causes economic damage to workers, companies, and social security systems worldwide. The perception that ICD is more trivial than the more intellectually appealing problem of allergic sensitization has recently changed dramatically. In Germany, skin diseases are the second most frequent occupational disease following musculoskeletal disorders, and most occupational dermatoses are cases of contact dermatitis. Among these, ICD is probably more frequent than allergic contact dermatitis (ACD), although reliable data are still very limited.

In contrast to ACD, ICD is defined as being the result of a primarily unspecific damage to the skin. It is not a clinical entity, but rather a spectrum of diseases. The clinical aspect of ICD is determined by the dose-effect relationship.[2] The morphology of acute ICD shows erythema, edema, vesicles that may coalesce, bullae, and oozing. Necrosis and ulceration are only seen with primary irritants. The clinical features of chronic ICD include redness, lichenification, excoriations, scaling, and hyperkeratosis. Any skin site can be affected; however, the sites most frequently affected by ICD are the hands, as they are the human "tools" that most interact with the environment and have intensive contact with irritants. Spilling of fluids may irritate the forearms or other body sites, especially when fluids soak through work clothes. Airborne ICD develops in irritant-exposed sensitive skin, mostly the face and especially the periorbital region.[3, 4] Dooms-Goossens et al.[3] presented a compilation of substances that caused irritant airborne contact dermatitis (Table 1–1). Irritant dermatitis caused by dust may mimic textile dermatitis, with lesions most prominent in sites with close skin-garment contact, such as the axilla, the gluteal region, or the thighs.

CLINICAL TYPES OF IRRITANT CONTACT DERMATITIS

Clinical manifestations of the ICD syndromes are modified by external factors (type of irritant [Table 1–2], exposure, environmental factors such as mechanical pressure, temperature, and humidity) and depend on predisposing characteristics of the individual[5] (age, sex, ethnic origin, pre-existing skin disease, especially atopic skin diathesis, and anatomical region exposed[6]). For instance, elderly people are not only affected more often by contact dermatitis because of their lower epidermal barrier, but also show more severe symptoms of this disease.[2, 7]

Environmental influences, such as low ambient humidity and cold, are important factors in decreasing the water content of the stratum corneum.[8] Cold alone may also reduce the plasticity

TABLE 1–1 • Irritants that Cause Airborne Irritant Contact Dermatitis

Acids and alkalis
Aluminum
Ammonia
Anhydrous calcium sulfate
Arsenic
Bromacetoxy-2-butene
Calcium silicate
Cement
Diallylglycol carbonate monomer
Dichlorvos
Domestic products (e.g., cleaning products)
Epoxy resins
Formaldehyde
Fiberglass
Hexanediol diacrylate
Industrial solvents
Metallic oxide powders (slag)
Paper, carbonless copy paper
Phenol formaldehyde resins
Phenol vapors
Quinine dust
Sawdust from toxic woods
Sewage sludge
Silver
Sodium sesquicarbonate (trona)
Urea-formaldehyde insulation foam
Wood dust

From Dooms-Goossens AE, Debusschere KM, Gevers DM, et al. Contact dermatitis caused by airborne agents. A review and case reports. *J Am Acad Dermatol* 1986; 15:1–10.

of the horny layer, with consequent cracking of the stratum corneum. Occlusion increases the water content of the stratum corneum, with consequent enhanced percutaneous absorption of water-soluble substances.

Several different types of ICD have been described[9, 10]:

- Acute
- Acute delayed
- Irritant reaction
- Cumulative
- Traumiterative
- Exsiccation eczematid
- Traumatic
- Pustular and acneiform
- Nonerythematous
- Subjective

Acute ICD

Acute ICD develops when the skin is exposed to a potent irritant. Usually this happens as an accident at work or in special emergency situations. The irritant reaction reaches its peak quickly and

then starts to heal; this is called the *decrescendo phenomenon*. Because the lag time is short (usually minutes to hours after exposure) and the associations between exposure and skin symptoms are usually clear, the diagnosis is easy in most cases. It may become difficult when the patient was unaware of an exposure. Acute ACD also has to be considered in the differential diagnosis. It is caused by a delayed sensitization reaction and requires 24 to 48 hours after allergen contact for symptoms to appear. This type of contact dermatitis is characterized by the *crescendo phenomenon* (i.e., a transient increase of signs and symptoms despite removal of the allergen). The clinical appearance of acute ICD is highly variable, and it may even be indistinguishable from the allergic type.

There are numerous reports in the literature of even experienced dermatologists being misled into an initial assumption of ACD that later, after a careful workup, turned out to be "only irritation."[11] Furthermore, the combination of allergic and irritant dermatitis is frequent (e.g., "blackspot poison ivy dermatitis"[12] as an acute ICD superimposed on an ACD.

Symptoms of acute irritant dermatitis are burning, stinging, and soreness of the skin. Signs include erythema, edema, bullae, and possibly necrosis (Fig. 1–1). These lesions are restricted to the area where the irritant or toxicant damaged the tissue. Borders are mostly sharply demarcated, and the asymmetrical patterns of lesions hints at an exogenous cause. The prognosis of this type is good.[13] The most frequent potent irritants leading to ICD are acids and alkaline solutions (Fig. 1–2).[14] A typical accident situation is chemical burning in construction workers[15] when alkaline concrete fluid soaks through garments or spills into work boots.

Chemical burns by fluoric acid are the most dangerous of all injuries caused by acids and need

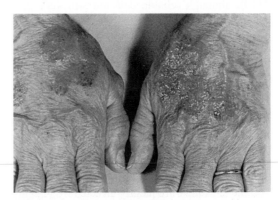

FIGURE 1–1 • Sharply demarcated lesions caused by an alkaline solution.

TABLE 1–2 • Irritants and Their Mode of Action

Substance	Mechanisms of Toxicity
Detergents	Solubilization and/or organization of barrier lipids and natural moisturizing factors in the stratum corneum
	Protein denaturation
	Membrane toxicity
Acids	Protein denaturation
	Cytotoxicity
Alkalines	Barrier lipid denaturation
	Cytotoxicity through cell swelling
Oils	Disorganization of barrier lipids
Organic solvents	Solubilization of barrier lipids
	Membrane toxicity
Oxidants	Cytotoxicity
Reducing agents	Keratolysis
Water	If barrier is disrupted, cytotoxicity through swelling of viable epidermal cells

From Eisner P. Irritant dermatitis in the workplace. *Dermatol Clin* 1994; 12:461–467.

special treatment. Even substances thought to be less toxic, such as N-methyl-2-pyrrolidone, may cause acute ICD.[16]

Acute Delayed ICD

Acute delayed ICD is characteristic for certain irritants, such as anthralin, that elicit a retarded inflammatory response (Table 1–3). Clinically, acute delayed ICD resembles acute ICD. The visible inflammation is not seen until 8 to 24 hours or more after exposure.[16] Delayed irritation may be more common than generally thought thus far. Other substances causing acute delayed ICD include benzalkonium chloride and tretinoin. Irritant patch-test reactions to benzalkonium chloride may be papular and increase in intensity with time, thus imitating ACD. On the normal skin surrounding psoriatic plaques, dithranol causes redness and edema, which may become very severe on the legs because of venous stasis. Irritation due to tretinoin develops after a few days and is characterized by mild to fiery redness followed by desquamation or large flakes of stratum corneum. The symptoms are burning rather than itching. The skin becomes sensitive to touch and to water.[11]

Irritant Reaction ICD

Irritant reaction ICD is a type of subclinical irritant dermatitis in individuals exposed to wet work, such as hairdressers or metal workers, in their first months of training. This diagnosis is made if the clinical picture is monomorphic rather than polymorphic and is characterized by one or more of the following signs: scaling, redness, vesicles, pustules, and erosions.[11]

On the hands it often begins under rings and then may spread over the fingers to the hands and the forearms. It usually affects the dorsum of the

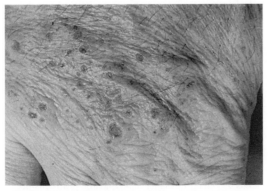

FIGURE 1–2 • Multiple necrotic lesions on the hand caused by cement.

 TABLE 1–3 • Chemicals Inducing Delayed Acute Chemical Irritation

Anthralin
Bis(2-chloroethyl)sulfide
Butanedioldiacrylate
Dichloro(2-chlorovinyl)arsine
Epichlorhydrin
Ethylene oxide
Hydrofluoric acid
Hexanediol diacrylate
Hydroxypropyl acrylate
Podophylline
Propane sulfone

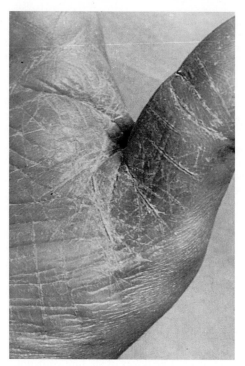

FIGURE 1–3 • Scaling and fissuring by cumulative contact dermatitis caused by soaps and detergents.

hands and fingers, but irritants can also cause eczema of the palmar sides of the fingers and the hands (Fig. 1–3).

This distribution occurs in caterers and is described as *dyshidrotic eczema*. It has been reported in metal workers with an ICD from cooling lubricants.[17] Frequently, this condition heals spontaneously, resulting in hardening of the skin; sometimes it progresses to cumulative irritant dermatitis.

Cumulative ICD

According to Malten[18] (Fig. 1–4), cumulative ICD is a consequence of multiple subthreshold damages to the skin if the time between the insults is too short for complete restoration of skin barrier function. It may be the result of too frequent repetition of one impairing factor, but is more commonly the result of a variety of stimuli, each beginning to be active before recovery from the foregoing stimuli has been competed. Clinical symptoms will develop only when the damage exceeds a certain "manifestation threshold," which is individually determined. Persons with sensitive skin are characterized by a decreased threshold or an increased restoration time leading to earlier development of clinical irritant dermatitis. The threshold is not a fixed value for an individual, but it may decrease with the disease. This explains why in patients with cumulative ICD even limited irritant exposure may perpetuate the condition. Cumulative ICD is not linked to exposure to a potent irritant, but to exposure to weak irritants. Very often, this exposure occurs not only at work but also in private life (Fig. 1–5). Because the link between exposure and disease is often not obvious to the patient, diagnosis may be delayed considerably. This is one of the reasons for the rather doubtful prognosis of this disease.[19]

Symptoms of chronic irritant dermatitis are itching and pain due to cracking of hyperkeratotic skin. Signs include dryness, erythema, and vesicles, but mainly lichenification, hyperkeratosis (Fig. 1–6), and chapping. In contrast to acute irritant dermatitis, the lesions are less sharply demarcated. Xerotic dermatitis is the most frequent type of cumulative toxic dermatitis.[14]

Many bioassays have been proposed for the purpose of identifying sensitive skin. A 24-hour

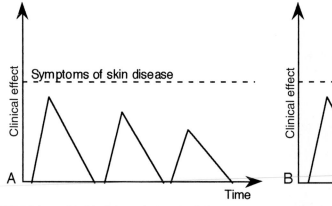

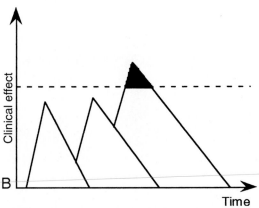

FIGURE 1–4 • Model of the pathogenesis of chronic irritant dermatitis according to Malten.[18] A, Subliminal irritants do not lead to clinical irritant dermatitis if they are far enough apart for restoration of skin barrier function. B, When the same irritants follow each other closely, or when the irritant threshold is reduced, irritant dermatitis develops.

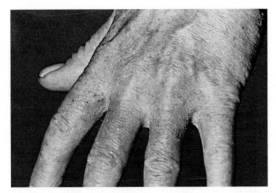

FIGURE 1–5 • Chronic irritant dermatitis due to wet work, sometimes called "housewives' hands."

patch test with sodium lauryl sulfate and repetitive patch test, such as the 21-day cumulative irritation assay, the chamber scarification test, and the soap chamber test, have been used.[20]

Traumiterative ICD

In contrast to cumulative ICD resulting from a too early repetition of exposures differing in type, traumiterative ICD is a result of too early repetition of just one type of load.[22] Nevertheless, these two types are very similar clinically.

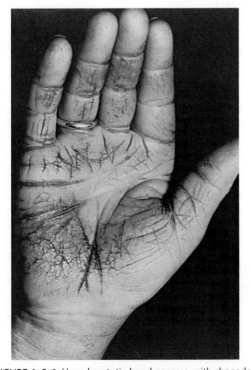

FIGURE 1–6 • Hyperkeratotic hand eczema with rhagades.

Exsiccation Eczematid

Exsiccation eczematid is a special variant of ICD that is seen mainly in elderly individuals with a history of frequent showering and bathing without remoisturizing their skin. Patients suffer from intensive itching, and their skin appears dry with ichthyosiform scaling. The condition mainly occurs during the winter months, when humidity is low.

Traumatic ICD

Traumatic ICD may develop after acute skin trauma, such as burns, lacerations, and acute ICD. Patients should also be asked whether they have cleansed the skin with strong soaps or detergents. The syndrome is characterized by eczematous lesions and delayed healing. This eczematous condition persists for a considerable time, with a minimum of 6 weeks.[11]

The most common location is the hands. In a fully developed case, redness, infiltration, and scaling with fissuring is seen all over the affected areas.

Pustular and Acneiform ICD

Pustular and acneiform ICD is a result of exposure to certain irritants, such as croton oil, mineral oils, tars, greases, and naphthalenes. This syndrome must always be considered in conditions in which acneiform lesions develop outside the typical acne age. Those most affected are patients with seborrhea, macroporous skin conditions, and prior acne vulgaris, as well as atopics. The pustules are sterile and transient; however, subcorneal pustular eruption may also be a manifestation of allergy to trichloroethylene, which has to be considered as a differential diagnosis in patients with appropriate history.[22]

Nonerythematous ICD

Nonerythematous ICD may be defined as a subclinical form of ICD with early stages of skin irritation characterized only by changes in the stratum corneum barrier function without a clinical correlate.[23–25]

Subjective ICD

Subjective or sensory ICD is characterized by the lack of clinical signs. Sick individuals report a stinging or burning feeling after contact with certain chemicals, such as lactic acid, which is also a model irritant for this type of nonvisible cutaneous

irritation. This reaction may be reliably reproduced in a double-blinded exposure test. Important
parameters are the quality and the concentration
of the exposing agent. Also, neural pathways are
considered to be responsible.

IRRITATION OR ALLERGY?

The distinction between ICD and ACD has become increasingly blurred. Despite their different
pathogeneses, ACD and ICD, especially of the
chronic type, show a remarkable similarity with
respect to clinical appearance, histology, and im-
munohistology.[2–5] It is apparent that some of the
same inflammatory immune mechanisms are operating for both ACD and ICD. The epidermal
and dermal cell activity that produces the cascade
of inflammation appears to be similar and applicable to both irritants and allergens. A review of all
of the comparative studies that suggest these two
entities are more alike than they are not has recently been presented by Gaspari[26] (Table 1–4).
Frequently, even therapy is similar.[27, 28] Additionally, the concept that irritants are thought to cause
symptoms and signs within minutes to hours
whereas allergens take days has been disqualified
for one of the most widely studied irritants.
Twenty-four hours of occlusion of sodium lauryl
sufate clearly resulted in more signs of inflammation at 48 hours, a time course more characteristic
of allergic reactions.[29]

EPIDEMIOLOGY

While population-based epidemiological studies
on the frequency of ICD are rare, there is
agreement that irritant dermatitis is more frequent
than ACD, although ACD tends to have more
severe consequences for the patient. Coenraads
and Smit[30] reviewed international prevalence studies for eczema due to all causes conducted with
general populations in five countries (England,
the Netherlands, Norway, Sweden, and the United
States). They showed point prevalence rates of 1.7
to 6.3% and 1- to 3-year prevalence rates of 6.2
to 10.6%.

In a questionnaire study performed by Meding[31]
and Meding and Swanbeck[32] on a random sample
of 20,000 individuals from the Swedish city of
Gothenburg, 11.8% reported having had hand eczema within the previous 12 months (period prevalence), whereas 5.4% suffered from hand eczema
at the time of investigation (point prevalence).
The period prevalence was higher in women
(14.6%) than in men (8.8%). The prevalence of
hand eczema in the population working full-time
(10.3%) was lower than in the general population.
However, in the subgroup doing medical and nursing work the 1-year prevalence of hand eczema
was 15.9%, and in the population doing service
work it was 15.4%. The occurrence of irritant
dermatitis was significantly increased in women
exposed to water and detergents and in men exposed to oils and solvents, whereas the occurrence
of allergic dermatitis was not significantly influenced by these exposures.

The perception that ICD is more frequent than
ACD in the occupational setting is supported by
data from Singapore. Of 557 patients with occupational dermatoses, 55.7% (310) had ICD, 38.6%
(215) had ACD, and 5.7% (32) had noncontact
dermatitis.[33] However, the incidence rates of selected occupations according to the diagnosis of
ICD and ACD in a population-based study in
North Bavaria showed different preferences for
ICD or ACD due to different occupational
groups.[34] Because cases of ICD tend to be less
severe and chronic than those of ACD, the latter
may outnumber the former in specialized occupational dermatology clinics.[35]

RISK FACTORS

A number of individual factors for irritant dermatitis have been identified. Although occupational
irritant hand dermatitis is more frequent in females,[31] no sex difference of irritant reactivity
could be established experimentally.[36] It is suspected that increased exposure to irritants at home
accounts for the higher prevalence in females.

This is supported by the observation that caring
for children under the age of 4 years and the lack
of a dishwashing machine significantly increased
the risk of contracting hand eczema in a population of female hospital workers.[37] Irritant reactivity
declines with increasing age. This is true not only
for acute but also for cumulative irritant dermatitis.[38] Atopy is probably the best established risk
factor for irritant hand dermatitis.[32, 39] It has to be
stressed, however, that respiratory manifestations
of atopy seem to be less predictive of irritant
reactivity than skin manifestation. At the level of
the individual, there remains considerable uncertainty in the prediction of irritant reactivity. As
was shown in a Swedish study, about 25% of the
atopics in extreme risk occupations, such as ladies' hairdressers and nursing assistants, did not
develop hand eczema.[40]

The incidence of ICD correlates with irritant
exposure of the workers in a given profession.[41]
Some high-risk occupations are caterers,[42–44] build-

TABLE 1–4 · Comparison of Irritant and Allergic Contact Dermatitis

	Irritant	Allergic
Clinical morphology	Dermatitis can be similar to ACD	Dermatitis can be similar to ICD Kinetics of resolution may be slower than ICD during patch testing
Histology	Spongiosis, exocytosis, dermal edema, and a mononuclear infiltrate; occasionally, neutrophil-rich infiltrates	Same as ICD; neutrophils usually less prominent
Immunochemistry T cells	Predominantly CD4+ T cells; some CD8+ T cells; activated state indicated by IL-2 receptor expression	Predominantly CD4+ T cells; some CD8+ T cells; activated state indicated by IL-2 receptor expression
Frequency of hapten-specific T cells in infiltrate	Not known	Estimated to be approximately 1%
Langerhans' cells number	No consistent changes	Decreased then recovery
Morphology	Alterations noted, but are highly dependent on chemical	Alterations noted, particularly with high doses of hapten
Accessory molecules		
HLA-DR	Increased	Increased
ICAM-1	Increased	Increased
B7-1	Increased	Increased
Cytokine profiles		
TNF-α	Increased	Increased
IFN-γ	Increased	Increased
GM-CSF	Increased	Increased
IL-1α, β	Not detected	Increased
IP-10	Not detected	Increased
MIP-2	Not detected	Increased
IL-4	Not detected	Increased at 24 hr, absent by 48 hr
Transgenic mice		
Overexpression of		
B7-1 by keratinocytes	Increased	Increased
ICAM-1 by keratinocytes	Increased	Increased
Knockout mice that lack		
TNF-α RI	Not tested	Increased
CD4	Decreased	Decreased
CD8	Decreased	Decreased
CD28	Decreased	Decreased

From Gaspari AA. The role of keratinocytes in the pathophysiology of contact dermatitis. *Immun Allergy Clin* 1997; 17:377–405.

ing workers,[45] furniture industry workers,[46] hospital workers[47, 48] (nurses,[49] cleaners,[50] kitchen workers), hairdressers,[51, 52] chemical industry workers,[53] dry cleaners,[54] metal workers,[55–59] and warehouse workers.[60] Generally, occupations involving "wet work" are especially prone to irritant dermatitis.

DIAGNOSIS

Irritant contact dermatitis has to be diagnosed by excluding other causes for the dermatitis. Al-though this is more easily done on the basis of signs and symptoms for acute ICD, it is usually more difficult for cumulative irritant dermatitis. Allergic contact dermatitis, which tends to show spreading papules and vesicles, is the most important diagnosis to be excluded. It is hard to differentiate in the chronic state. Irritant dermatitis may be diagnosed if patch tests remain negative, if there is an exposure to irritants, and if the disease develops and heals, depending on the frequency and intensity of this exposure.

Because cumulative ICD may become chronic

TABLE 1-5 • Noninvasive Bioengineering Methods for Characterization of Skin Properties in Occupational Dermatology

Skin Property	Possible Significances in Occupational Dermatology	Measured Parameters	Principle of Measurement	Device
Barrier function of stratum corneum	Prediction of eczema risk, detection of a subclinical eczema, therapy control	Transepidermal water loss (TEWL)	Measurement of air moisture gradient in defined distance to the skin	Evaporimeter, Tewameter
Skin moisture	Prediction of eczema risk, detection of a subclinical eczema, therapy control	Conductivity	Measurement of conductance between two electrodes	Skicon
		Capacity	Measurement of capacity between two electrodes	Corneometer
Acid mantle of the skin	Buffer capacitance against alkali substances (prediction of eczema risk), detection of a subclinical eczema, therapy control	Skin surface pH	Hydrogen ion activity at a pH electrode	pH Meter
Skin blood flow	Tolerance to temperature, detection of a subclinical eczema	Capillary erythrocyte flow	Wavelength shift of reflected light because of the Doppler effect	Laser Doppler velocimeter
Skin roughness	Prediction of eczema risk, detection of a subclinical eczema, therapy control	Adhesional and glide friction	Measurement of the power necessary to move an object on the skin surface	Frictionmeter
	Prediction of eczema risk, detection of a subclinical eczema, therapy control	Deviation of elevations and grooves from the mean	Mechanically or laser-controlled profilometry of a skin surface replica	Profilometer, visiometer
Stratum corneum cohesion	Mechanical resistance	Corneocyte cohesion	Measurement of the power	Cohesiometer
Skin color	Objectivation of erythema and pigmentations as proof of eczema and light-induced changes	Light reflection	Measurement of reflection of a defined light flash with a photo element	Tristimulus colorimeter, spectrophotometer
Skin thickness	Quantification of eczema-induced lichenifications	Distance between skin surface and coriumsubcutis border	Reflection of a high frequency ultrasound signal at the skin surface and at the acoustic border between corium and subcutis	A scan or C scan ultrasound

From Iliev D, Hinnen U, Elsner P. Skin bioengineering methods in occupational dermatology. In: Elsner P, Barel AO, Berardesca E, Gaberd B, Serup J, eds. Skin Bioengineering Techniques and Applications in Dermatology and Cosmetology. Basel: Karger; 1988:145–150.

in a later stage, the relation between exposure and disease tends to weaken. Histological examination of a biopsy specimen cannot differentiate between chronic irritant and allergic or atopic dermatitis. However, chronic ICD differs morphologically from acute ICD.[61] Immunohistological staining has not shown any significant differences in the inflammatory infiltrate of chronic irritant and allergic dermatitis.[62] Whereas a biopsy specimen may be helpful to exclude palmar psoriasis, psoriasis can usually be excluded or confirmed on clinical grounds that consider sharply demarcated hyperkeratotic or pustular lesions in contrast to the fuzzy borders of eczema while searching for other features such as nail and scalp involvement.

The new bioengineering techniques such as measuring transepidermal water loss as an indicator of epidermal barrier function are well suited to detect minute epidermal barrier impairment earlier than clinical examinations and to assess the grade of dermatitis quantitatively, but they are not useful in making a safe differential diagnosis between ACD and ICD. Rather, they offer the possibility to evaluate inflammation parameters such as redness, scaling, and infiltration objectively and to quantify these reactions. In Table 1–5 an overview of biophysical measurements is given that can be used to characterize functional and morphological properties of irritated skin.

TREATMENT AND PROGNOSIS

Avoiding the irritant(s) remains the basis of treating occupational ICD. This is achieved through technical measures (exchange of working substances, encapsulation of irritating fluids), individual skin protection (gloves, protective suits, protective creams), and, if necessary, sick leave until the epidermal barrier has completely regenerated, which may be a lengthy process, especially in cumulative irritant dermatitis.

The use of topical corticosteroids in the successful treatment of ACD has been questioned in irritant dermatitis.[63] They may be effective in chronic, hyperkeratotic irritant dermatitis, but their prolonged use may lead to epidermal atrophy and consequently increased irritant sensitivity. Other therapeutic options in irritant dermatitis include topical tars and phototherapy (UVB or PUVA). In difficult cases of chronic irritant hand dermatitis, radiation may be indicated.[64] Bacterial superinfection may be a complication of contact dermatitis; it is treated with topical or systemic antibiotics. Potential irritants not even in the worksite but also in the home environment, such as irritant cleansing products, must be identified and whenever possible eliminated.[65]

Prognosis for acute ICD is good if irritant contact is avoided. Cumulative irritant dermatitis, however, has a doubtful prognosis. In a recent survey, it was stressed that the prognoses of occupational and nonoccupational contact dermatitis, ICD, and ACD are similar and that a job change does not affect the course of the disease.[36] However, Goh[66] concluded that most studies appear to indicate that patients with ICD have a poorer prognosis than those with ACD. A reason could be that in allergic dermatitis a specific causative allergen can be identified and avoided and the cause of ICD is often unknown. Well-known factors that cause a poor prognosis of ICD are the existence of atopic dermatitis[67, 68] or what Wall and Gebauer[68a] termed *persistent post occupational dermatitis*. In our experience, cutting fluid dermatitis in metal workers took up to several years to heal despite job change and avoidance of irritants. This stresses the importance of early intervention in irritant dermatitis before it reaches the chronic stage.

Ethylene Oxide Burns ■

A.A. FISHER, M.D.

By volume ethylene oxide (EO) is one of the most widely used chemical compounds in the United States. Much of it used for medical sterilization. The petroluem derivative also is used to make ethylene glycol, from which automobile antifreeze and polyester clothing fibers are manufactured.

In hospitals, EO gas sterilizers are used to clean certain delicate medical devices that cannot be put in a steam autoclave or dunked in a sterilizing solution. Some sterilizers are small table-top models. Other hospital ones are larger, and really large EO gas sterilizers are used by the manufacturers of medical devices. The machines also are used in research laboratories and medical, dental, and veterinarian clinics.

In the food industry, EO is used as a fumigant where spices, copra, and black walnuts are stored. It also is registered with the U.S. Environmental Protection Agency for use as a fumigant on objects such as furs, leather, books, and jet aircraft.

LaDage[70] reported a severe facial irritation from excess EO in anesthesia masks. Hanifin[71] described six cases of contact dermatitis that were traced to EO residue in prepacked nitrofurzone dressings. Ippen and Mathies[72] observed three workers who suffered from third-degree burns of the hands, forehead, axillae, periumbilical region, and genitalia after cleaning a storage container that had traces of EO. These authors suggest that, if an industrial case is seen, immediate treatment should be to rinse the affected area with water under great pressure such as may be obtained from a hose. Contaminated garments should also be cleaned thoroughly. However, if water under pressure is not available, Taylor[73] states that liquid EO spilled directly on the skin should be allowed to vaporize before being washed with water. All clothing contaminated with liquid EO should be removed at once, especially shoes and gloves, and washed immediately with large quantities of water.

Biro et al.[74] and Fisher[75] reported that 19 hospitalized women suffered postoperatively from severe burns of the buttocks and back from contact with reusable surgical gowns and drapes that had been sterilized with EO and not properly aerated. Initially, an "epidemic" of bullous impetigo was suspected. Severe irritant reactions to detergents and antiseptics were also considered. The burned skin resembled a localized form of Lyell's disease. Testing samples of reusable gowns that had been worn by the patients showed that the amount of EO residue varied from 3,600 to 10,800 ppm. The safe level for EO gas recommended by both Health Industries Associated and the Z-79 Committee of New York Mt. Sinai Hospital is 200 ppm (maximum). The levels of residual EO in the implicated gowns were thus determined to be 16 to 50 times the safe level for skin contact.

Ethylene oxide burns are most likely to occur when EO is held in close contact with the skin, as happened with the hospital patients (Fig. 1–7), or when gloves or shoes are contaminated with EO.

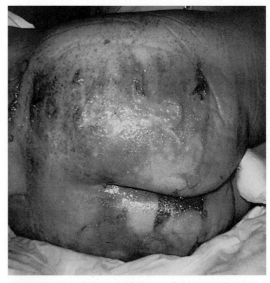

FIGURE 1–7 ● Ethylene oxide burn of the buttocks in a hospital patient caused by contact with a surgical sheet incompletely aerated after sterilization with EO. (Courtesy of A.A. Fisher, M.D.)

Cement Burns ■

ROBERT M. ADAMS, M.D.

Although most cases of cement dermatitis are due to the alkalinity and abrasive quality of cement, severe burns can result from contact with wet cement. When water is added to dry cement, highly alkaline calcium oxide is formed, the mixture reaching a pH of nearly 13. Those affected with cement burns are mostly persons working on projects at home or inexperienced and inadequately trained workers. The burns and ensuing ulcerations result either from kneeling in the wet cement[76, 77] or from spilling it into boots or gloves where, with the fabric, it acts as a compress.[78–80] Because of its alkalinity and weight, wet cement is especially irritating under these conditions. Burns of the hands also occur from working concrete by hand without protection.[81] Workers often delay removing contaminated boots and gloves because of a desire to finish the job before the concrete hardens (Fig. 1–8).[76]

Initially the worker experiences a burning discomfort while in contact with the cement, and a dusky erythema appears soon after contact ceases and the skin is cleaned. Because the immediate symptoms are often quite mild, the worker may not change boots and socks when the spillage occurs or may find it impractical to change until much later in the day.[82] Within 12 to 24 hours, however, necrotic ulcers appear, which are often deep and, on healing, leave disfiguring scars. Complete healing may be delayed for 8 to 10 weeks. Calcium oxide and hydroxide appear to be the principal causes of these burns.[83]

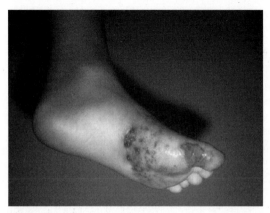

FIGURE 1–8 • Cement burn of the foot from wet cement spilled into the shoe during the spreading of concrete. (Courtesy of A.A. Fisher, M.D.)

Dermatitis Due to Fibrous Glass ■

ROBERT M. ADAMS, M.D.

Fibrous glass is a manufactured fiber made from silicon dioxide with various metals and other elements. It is extruded in a molten state into fibers that solidify without crystallization.

Because exposed workers experience the sudden onset of severe itching, they often become very apprehensive, especially about any potential harmful effects. In addition to itching, fibrous glass dermatitis includes folliculitis with excoria-tions, especially on arms, face, neck, and sometimes the legs (Fig. 1–9). Paronychia is common.[84] In some cases the eruption becomes widespread, and from repeated scratching and rubbing the picture may suggest nummular eczema or contact dermatitis. Burning of the eyes, sore throat, and cough are common complaints; wearing contact lenses may become impossible.[85] Curiously, not all workers similarly exposed are affected. The dermatitis increases in warm, humid climates but also occurs commonly in winter, especially when the relative humidity is low.[86]

For most workers, the symptoms disappear within a week or two, but a small number must leave work because of discomfort and sometimes from unwarranted concerns regarding possible systemic effects. Eventually, many workers appear to become "hardened" and continue working with little difficulty.[87] In individuals with dermographism, however, the urticarial symptoms may become severe and necessitate a job change.

Diagnosis can sometimes be accomplished by placing skin scrapings on a slide, adding a drop or two of 20% potassium hydroxide, and examining the specimen under the low power of a light microscope.[88] Strands of glass fiber may be seen, but frequently they cannot, and the diagnosis must be made solely from the history and clinical appearance.[86]

Ninety percent of fibrous glass manufactured in the United States has a fiber diameter greater than 3.5 μm. It is these fibers that cause irritation of tissues. Fibers with a diameter of less than 3.5 μm, used only since the late 1960s, are thought to be harmless.[89] The tissue reaction to glass fibers is entirely mechanical and transient; the pathological tissue response is not granulomatous, as from asbestos,[90] but eczematous, with spongiosis and a perivascular mononuclear infiltrate, with microtrauma at the surface.[91] The fibers are neither carcinogenic[92, 93] nor allergenic.[84] Allergic contact dermatitis, however, may result from resins used to impregnate the fibers to make insulation material, pipes, conveyor belts, and the like.[94]

Treatment consists of removal from the causative environment, which may be only temporary,

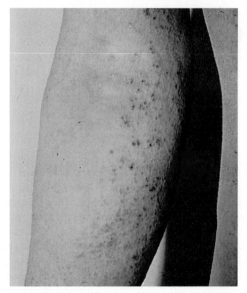

FIGURE 1–9 • Dermatitis due to fibrous glass is highly pruritic, in some respects resembling scabies. The symptoms usually subside in a few days, however, unless secondary infection develops.

as many patients are able to return later to the identical exposure conditions without recurrence. Adhesive tape such as Scotch tape or plumbers' duct tape, applied directly to the affected areas, may remove the fibers from the skin.[95] Other preventive measures include application of a mild dusting powder prior to exposure (D. J. Birmingham, personal communication, 1978).

Protective clothing should be loose fitting and changed daily. Showering at the workplace is essential. Workers should not use air hoses or brooms to remove fibers from each other, as the fibers may then further penetrate the skin.[86]

Chronic Hypertrophic Dermatosis ■ of the Palms

ROBERT M. ADAMS, M.D.

This condition occurs mostly in elderly or older workers, usually male, is manifested by a sharply marginated, hyperkeratotic dermatitis of the palms (Fig. 1–10), and has been termed *chronic hyperkeratotic dermatosis of the palms* by Hersle and Mobacken.[96] These patients usually have worked with their hands for years, often handling metal

and metal parts, with constant friction and pressure. The hyperkeratotic lesions are especially prone to develop painful, bleeding fissures.

The condition is usually diagnosed as psoriasis, but personal and family histories fail to confirm this, and evidence of psoriasis is not present elsewhere, including the nails. They also are not atopics, nor is there evidence of fungal infection. The biopsy material is not psoriasiform, and on biopsy shows only marked hyperkeratosis, with elongated rete and numerous mononuclear cells infiltrating the epidermis, as well as spongiosis.

Treatment has a minimal effect on the course, and even after leaving work the condition remains essentially unchanged. Hard manual work over many years seems to be the activator, which can be considered similar to the gradual destruction of joints of athletes, dancers, and so forth after many years of hard, repeated trauma.

The condition is fairly common, but its importance as a disabling condition in older men (and sometimes women) has not been sufficiently recognized. In contrast to psoriasis, the condition improves only slightly on leaving work, and retirement from the workplace is usually required.

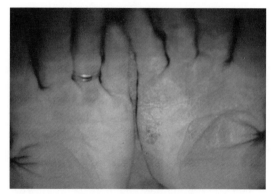

FIGURE 1–10 ● Chronic hypertrophic dermatosis of the hands resembles, but is unrelated to, psoriasis. Affected workers are often near retirement, having worked for years in jobs in which hand friction and pressure are integral and persistent aspects of the job.

Hydrofluoric Acid Burns ■

MICHAEL V. VANCE, M.D.

Hydrofluoric acid (HF), the inorganic acid of fluorine, is used in the etching of glass, metal, and stone as the only inorganic acid capable of dissolving silicon. It is widely used in the electronics and semiconductor industries and is also a common constituent of commercial and household rust, stain, and scale removers.

Hydrofluoric acid produces relatively little topical acid burn contact with skin, primarily owing to its limited dissociation constant (K = 3.53 $\times$ 10^{-4}). However, this chemical property also allows it to penetrate intact skin, and subsequent dissociation into free hydrogen ion and free fluoride ion will occur in deeper tissues. While the hydrogen ion may produce some typical acid injury, the free fluoride ion is responsible for most of the tissue destruction on HF exposures.

Fluoride ion is an extremely cytotoxic agent. It complexes with bivalent cations, particularly calcium and magnesium, to form insoluble fluoride salts, and it interferes with a variety of cellular enzyme systems.[97] Enzyme interference inhibits cellular respiration and membrane activity, resulting in cellular injury and death.[98]

CLINICAL PRESENTATION

Patients with an acute exposure to HF may present a difficult diagnostic problem for the physician. First, patients may not even know that the product they have been using contains HF, as product labels may be incomplete or the fine print illegible even to the visually unimpaired. Second, patients may have been exposed to HF inadvertently because of unrecognized HF contamination of materials and worksites. Third, the typical signs and symptoms of an acute HF injury may be delayed for many hours after an exposure, and patients may not make the connection between the two events even if the HF exposure was recognized.

The onset of symptoms of acute HF exposure is dependent on the concentration of acid and the duration of exposure. Highly concentrated (70%) HF may contain enough hydrogen ions to produce some burning sensation on the the skin and may provide some warning of an acute exposure. However, lower concentrations of HF (especially concentrations less than 10%) will not produce any symptoms at the time of contact, and delayed onset of symptoms to 10 to 12 hours is not unusual.

The initial presenting complaint of acute HF injury is pain. This is usually described as an initial "tingling" sensation, which progresses to a "burning" pain, and ultimately the typical deep, throbbing, excruciating pain of HF injury. It is extremely important to recognize that this pain may be present in the absence of any visible signs of injury at the site, and any patient presenting with such complaints should be suspect for HF exposure.

Visible evidence of HF burns also follows a fairly characteristic pattern. The burn site initially becomes erythematous and may be somewhat edematous. As tissue injury progresses, the site assumes a pale, blanched appearance. This may be followed by development of local vesiculation and frank tissue necrosis (Fig. 1–11). Fluoride may penetrate into underlying bone, and demineralization may ensue. This destructive process may progress over several days in inadequately treated patients, resulting in the development of deep ulceration and extensive tissue loss, including entire digits (Fig. 1–12).[99]

PATIENT MANAGEMENT

The initial step in management of an acute HF exposure is thorough skin decontamination with a water flush. This should be accomplished as soon as an HF exposure is recognized. However, the delayed presentation of most patients with HF burns makes it unlikely that significant amounts of HF still remain on the surface of the skin.

A popular first aid measure for known or sus-

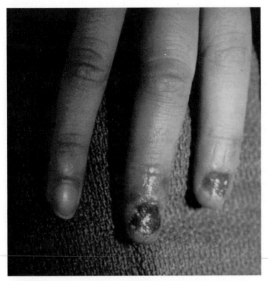

FIGURE 1–11 ● The site of an HF burn is swollen, pale, and extremely painful and soon becomes necrotic.

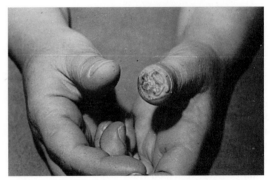

FIGURE 1–12 ● If not promptly and adequately treated, HF acid burns may result in loss of part of a digit.

pected HF burns is the use of topical soaks, creams, and ointments. These usually contain calcium gluconate, magnesium oxide, and a quaternary ammonium salt (benzalkonium or benethonium chloride). In addition, concentrated aloe gel, vitamins A and D, and even magnesium hydroxide antacid preparations have been tested.[100, 101] These are intended to form insoluble complexes with any surface fluoride ion to prevent penetration into tissue, thereby minimizing or preventing deep cellular injury. These topical preparations probably are of some benefit if applied *immediately* after initial decontamination of a known, recognized exposure.[100–102] However, they are of no use after the fluoride has penetrated into the deeper layers of the skin and subcutaneous tissue, which is the usual case by the time a patient presents with progressive pain and other symptoms of deeper tissue injury.

At best, topical therapies in treating a late or relatively early-presenting patient with an HF exposure will provide the patient with something to do (massaging the solution/cream/gel into the affected area) while being transported to or awaiting definitive treatment. At worst, reliance on topical therapies will delay definitive treatment and allow greater tissue injury to develop.[99]

Definitive treatment of acute HF burns involves the administration of calcium gluconate into the tissue affected by the exposure. In soft tissues with sufficient loose tissue space for injection of a volume of fluid, this is easily accomplished by the direct injection of a 10% calcium gluconate solution at the burn site. A small, 3-gauge needle should be used to minimize patient discomfort and mechanical tissue damage, and care should be taken to infiltrate into, around, and beneath the burn area as completely as possible. Another alternative to large, soft-tissue HF burns on extremities is the use of the classic Bier's block[103] method with the intravenous infusion of calcium gluconate following exsanguination of the affected extremity,[104] although preliminary studies suggest that this method is more effective for soft tissue exposures, as opposed to digital exposures.[105]

In loading the local tissue with calcium the mechanism of fluoride injury is terminated and even reversed by the precipitation of free fluoride and replenishment of decreased tissue calcium levels. It should be emphasized that only calcium gluconate should be used for local infiltration, because calcium chloride produces direct injury when injected into tissues.[106]

Digital HF burns deserve special consideration. Fingertip burns are particularly painful owing to the rich sensory nerve supply and are particularly difficult to infiltrate with calcium gluconate for the same reason. In addition, only small amounts of calcium gluconate may be injected directly into the fingertips because of limited space for introduction of additional fluid volume in an end-arterial circulation region, and repeated injections are frequently necessary to neutralize all the fluoride present. Finally, HF may penetrate beneath the fingernails, and the nails must be removed prior to injecting calcium gluconate directly into the nail bed to avoid the unbearable pain associated with administering even a minimal volume of fluid into the closed space between the nail plate and the distal phalanx.[100, 106]

An alternative to direct injection of calcium gluconate into digital HF burns is the infusion of calcium gluconate into the arterial supply of the involved digit(s). This technique involves insertion of an indwelling arterial catheter into the radial or brachial artery of the involved extremity and slowly infusing a dilute solution of calcium gluconate via an infusion pump. This allows the calcium to be delivered to the affected tissues through the vascular supply and avoids the mechanical problems associated with the pain and tissue distention associated with direct injection.[99, 107]

DISPOSITION

Patients with HF burns require much closer follow up than patients with virtually any other kind of corrosive injury. Repeated calcium infiltrations or infusions are frequently required, and lesions that demonstrate vesiculation or necrosis prior to or despite adequate treatment should be referred for wound care. In addition, extensive HF exposures should be carefully monitored for the possibility of fluoride absorption systemically, as fatal fluoride poisoning has been reported with as little as 5% total body surface area burns with HF.[108]

Pigmentary Changes ■

GERALD A. GELLIN, M. D.

The pigmentation of the skin may be increased or decreased by exposure to physical or chemical agents.[109] Such insults to the skin may lead to either hyper- or hypopigmentation in the same individual. Inflammation is the usual antecedent event. However, the inflammation may be subclinical and inapparent.

TERMINOLOGY

Melanosis and *melanoderma* are terms to denote hyperpigmentation. *Leukoderma* defines the pigment loss acquired from an environmental irritation or injury to the skin. *Vitiligo* is an improper term to apply to occupationally induced depig-

mentation. It is better reserved for idiopathic or hereditary acquired leukoderma, which may be associated with autoimmune or endocrine abnormalities.[110, 111]

Dyschromia is an altered state of the skin wherein there are areas of increased and decreased pigmentation in the same site or contiguous areas.

OCCUPATIONAL MELANOSIS (MELANODERMA)

Physical Causes

Such events as blunt trauma, solitary or repeated, can increase the pigmentation. Friction, chemical

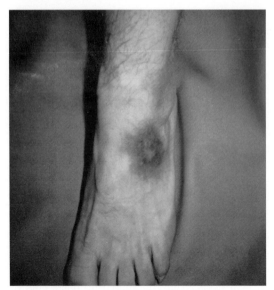

FIGURE 1–13 • Hyperpigmentation following chronic irritation from friction and pressure of a climbing apparatus. Patient is a 52-year-old telephone company worker.

and thermal burns (Fig. 1–13), and artificial or natural ultraviolet light (sun exposure) may also darken the skin (Fig. 1–14).[112]

Chemical Causes

Coal tar, pitch, asphalt, creosote, and other derivatives of the distillation of coal can produce melanosis (as well as other cutaneous effects such as photosensitivity, folliculitis, acne, and epithelial hyperplasia such as warts, keratoses, and malignancies).[113]

Psoralens, found in various fruits and vegetables, can cause phytophotodermatitis and hyperpigmentation. The chemicals that produce irritant or allergic contact dermatitis can lead to postinflammatory hyperpigmentation.

OCCUPATIONAL LEUKODERMA

Physical Causes

Chemical and thermal burns (Fig. 1–15), ionizing radiation (x-ray–induced radiodermatitis and necrosis), and blunt or repeated trauma to the skin may produce hypo- or depigmentation.

Chemical Causes

Alkylphenols (phenols and catechols) may irritate or depigment directly exposed skin.[114] At times, distant, untouched areas of skin subsequently depigment.[115] Monobenzyl ether of hydroquinone and hydroquinone per se are major causes.[109] Related alkyl phenols that have been proved to depigment the skin are *p*-tertiary butyl phenol and *p*-tertiary butyl catechol (Fig. 1–16).[116, 117] Chemicals that induce irritant or allergic contact dermatitis can induce temporary or long-standing leukodema (Fig. 1–17). Rhus dermatitis (poison ivy, poison oak, and poison sumac), the most common cause of allergic contact dermatitis in the United States, may lead to leukoderma.[118]

The first report of occupationally acquired leukoderma was 60 years ago.[119] The chemical was monobenzyl ether of hydroquinone, an antioxidant in synthetic rubber. The industrial uses of the chemical antioxidants that have been imputed as causes of leukoderma include the manufacture of insecticides, paints, plastics, and synthetic rubber. They may be found in lubricating and motor oils, photographic chemicals, germicides and disinfectants, detergents, deodorants, and inks.[120–125]

Outbreaks of occupational leukoderma have been reported from many countries.[126] In addition to hydroquinone and monobenzyl ether of hydro-

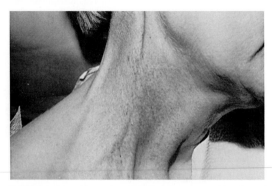

FIGURE 1–14 • Hyperpigmentation from a combination of sunlight and application of a perfume or cologne containing large amounts of psoralens.

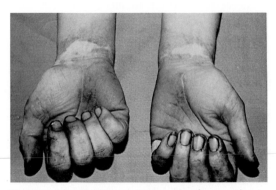

FIGURE 1–15 • Depigmentation resulting from a solvent-induced chemical burn.

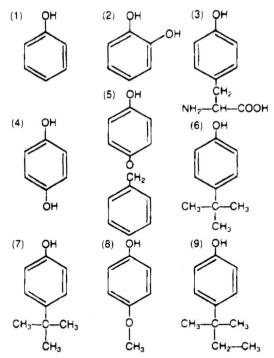

FIGURE 1–16 • Selected phenolic compounds, including potent depigmenters: (1) phenol; (2) catechol; (3) tyrosine; (4) hydroquinone; (5) monobenzyl ether of hydroquinone; (6) *p*-tertiary butyl phenol; (7) *p*-tertiary butyl catechol; (8) monomethyl ether of hydroquinone (4-hydroxyanisole); and (9) *p*-tertiary amyl phenol.

quinone, *p*-tertiary butylphenol and *p*-tertiary amylphenol are the major causes. Phenolics such as *p*-phenylphenol, octyl phenol, and nonylphenol have been associated with pigment loss.[127–129]

Investigative studies have been performed on a variety of animal models. The earliest study was by Oettel in 1936.[122] Brown cats were fed hydroquinone. Body hair lightened. Other animals chal-

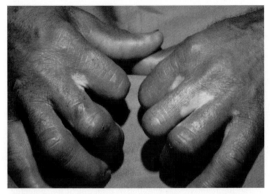

FIGURE 1–17 • Depigmentation of the hands of an auto assembler. Differentiation from idiopathic vitiligo is important and at times difficult.

lenged experimentally with depigmenting chemicals were rabbits, black goldfish, brown and black guinea pigs, and brown mice.[116, 130, 131]

The depigmenting action of industrial chemicals has been demonstrated throughout the world (Table 1–6).[126, 132] Chemically induced leukoderma is an accepted and bona fide industrially acquired condition.[121] In vitro studies have confirmed the melanocytotoxicity of certain alkyl phenols.[116, 133–135]

CLINICAL PICTURE

The pattern of chemically induced leukoderma is indistinguishable from that of vitiligo.[136] The latter affects about 1% of the general population.[110] Proven cases of industrially related leukoderma are much less common. Invariably, the hands, wrists, and forearms are affected. Symmetry is usual. Depigmentation may appear in distant body sites not in direct contact with the chemical cause (e.g., axillae, genitalia, and the torso). Loss of scalp hair color or eye color has not been reported. Antecedent or concurrent contact dermatitis is often reported, but not always observed.[114]

The minimum time for skin to depigment has been 2 to 4 weeks. The pigment loss may take up to 6 months of repeated contact (in laboratory animals) to become visible.[137] Many exposed workers do not depigment, indicating host factors of susceptibility. Why this resistance to depigmentation exists for many, if not most, exposed workers is unknown.

DIAGNOSIS

The appearance of leukoderma on the hands of workers, especially if there are multiple workers engaged in the same job, should raise the suspicion of an industrial cause. The chemical identity of work chemicals should be obtained. If the chemical is an alkyl phenol, as cited in Table 1–7, a presumptive diagnosis of chemical leukoderma

TABLE 1–6 • **Industrial Exposures to Depigmenting Chemicals**

Manufacture of insecticides, paints, plastics, and synthetic rubber
Lubricating and motor oils
Photographic chemicals
Germicides and disinfectants
Detergents and deodorants
Inks

TABLE 1–7 • Chemicals Causing Leukoderma

Hydroquinone
Monobenzyl ether of hydroquinone
Monomethyl ether of hydroquinone
(*p*-methoxyphenol of *p*-hydroxyanisole)
p-Tertiary butyl phenol
p-Tertiary butyl catechol
p-Tertiary amylphenol
p-Isopropyl catechol
p-Octylphenol
p-Nonylphenol
p-Phenylphenol
p-Cresol

can be made. Patch testing may indicate simultaneously acquired allergic hypersensitivity as well as a depigmenting action. This has been demonstrated with *p*-tertiary butyl catechol.[115] A positive patch-test site depigmented within a few weeks, remaining leukodermatous for several months. When dealing with a previously unreported (but suspected) depigmenting chemical, animal studies should be performed. Black guinea pigs and brown mice are useful test animals.

MECHANISM OF ACTION

The specific site of damage is the melanocyte. Depigmenting chemicals produce structural changes in these cells, leading to cell distortion and death.[133, 134] Chemical interaction with the enzyme tyrosinase has been considered. It is probably relevant that alkyl phenols are chemically similar to tyrosine, the building block of melanin. Another mechanism reported is the formation of semiquinone free radicals in the melanocytes, leading to lipid peroxidation and destruction of lipoprotein membranes of the melanocyte.[138]

TREATMENT

There is no reliably effective treatment to reverse melanoderma or leukoderma. Partial and gradual restitution of the altered state of pigmentation may take months or years. If at all possible, the inciting cause should be removed from the worker's environment. Cosmetic camouflage may provide benefit for persons with leukoderma or dyschromia. It is important that depigmented skin be protected from ultraviolet light in the sunburn range.

References

1. Mathias CGT, Maibach HI. Dermatotoxicology monographs I. Cutaneous irritation: Factors influencing the response to irritants. *Clin Toxicol* 1978; 13:333–346.
2. Patil S, Maibach HI. Effect of age and sex on the elicitation of irritant contact dermatitis. *Contact Dermatitis* 1994; 30:257–264.
3. Dooms-Goossens AE, Debusschere KM, Gevers DM, et al. Contact dermatitis caused by airborne agents. A review and case reports. *J Am Acad Dermatol* 1986; 15:1–10.
4. Lachapelle JM. Industrial airborne irritant or allergic contact dermatitis. *Contact Dermatitis* 1986; 14:137–145.
5. Pinnagoda J, Tupker RA, Smit JA, Coenraads PJ, Nater JP. The intra- and inter-individual variability and reliability of transepidermal water loss measurements. *Contact Dermatitis* 1989; 21:255–259.
6. Emtestam L, Ollmar S. Electrical impedance index in human skin: Measurements after occlusion in 5 anatomical regions and in mild irritant contact dermatitis. *Contact Dermatitis* 1993; 28:104–108.
7. Ghadially R, Brown BE, Sequeira-Martin SM, Feingold KR, Elias PM. The aged epidermal permeability barrier. Structural, functional, and lipid biochemical abnormalities in humans and a senescent murine model. *J Clin Invest* 1995; 95:2281–2290.
8. Mozzanica N. Pathogenetic aspects of allergic and irritant contact dermatitis. *Clin Dermatol* 1992; 10:115–121.
9. Berardesca E, Distante F. Mechanisms of skin irritation. In: Elsner P, Maibach HI eds. *Irritant Dermatitis: New Clinical and Experimental Aspects*. Basel: Karger; 1995:1–8.
10. Iliev D, Elsner P. Clinical irritant contact dermatitis syndromes. *Immun Allergy Clin* 1997; 17:365–375.
11. Frosch PJ. Cutaneous irritation. In: Rycroft RJG, Menné T, Frosch PJ, eds. *Textbook of Contact Dermatitis*. Berlin: Springer; 1995:28–61.
12. Hurwitz RM, Rivera HP, Guin JD. Black-spot poison ivy dermatitis. An acute irritant contact dermatitis superimposed upon an allergic contact dermatitis. *Am J Dermatopathol* 1984; 6:319–322.
13. Elsner P. Irritant dermatitis in the workplace. *Dermatol Clin* 1994; 12:461–467.
14. Eichmann A, Amgwerd D. Toxische Kontaktdermatitis. *Schweiz Rundsch Med Prax* 1992; 19:615–617.
15. Skogstad M, Levy F. Occupational irritant contact dermatitis and fungal infection in construction workers. *Contact Dermatitis* 1994; 31:28–30.
16. Malten KE, den Arend JA, Wiggers RE. Delayed irritation: Hexanediol diacrylate and butanediol diacrylate. *Contact Dermatitis* 1979; 3:178–184.
17. Cronin E. Hand eczema. In: Rycroft RJG, Menné T, Frosch PJ, eds. *Textbook of Contact Dermatitis*. Berlin: Springer; 1995:207–218.
18. Malten KE. Thoughts on irritant contact dermatitis. *Contact Dermatitis* 1981; 7:238–247.
19. Elsner P, Maibach HI. Irritant and allergic contact dermatitis. In: Elsner P, Martius J, eds. *Vulvovaginitis*. New York: Marcel Dekker; 1993:61–82.
20. Lee CH, Maibach HI. Study of cumulative irritant contact dermatitis in man utilizing open application on subclinically irritated skin. *Contact Dermatitis* 1994; 30:271–275.
21. Malten KE, den Arend JA. Irritant contact dermatitis: Traumiterative and cumulative impairment by cosmetics, climate, and other daily loads. *Derm Beruf Umwelt* 1985; 33:125–132.
22. Goh CL. Noneczematous contact reactions. In: Rycroft

RJG, Menné T, Frosch PJ, eds. *Textbook of Contact Dermatitis*. Berlin: Springer; 1995:221–236.

23. Berardesca E, Maibach HI. Racial differences in sodium lauryl sulphate induced cutaneous irritation: Black and white. *Contact Dermatitis* 1988; 18:65–70.
24. van der Valk PGM, Nater JP, Bleumink E. Vulnerability of the skin to surfactants in different groups of eczema patients and controls as measured by water vapour loss. *Clin Exp Dermatol* 1985; 10:98–103.
25. Lammintausta K, Maibach HI, Wilson D. Mechanisms of subjective (sensory) irritation. Propensity to non-immunologic contact urticaria and objective irritation in stingers. *Derm Beruf Umwelt* 1988; 36:45–49.
26. Gaspari AA. The role of keratinocytes in the pathophysiology of contact dermatitis. *Immun Allergy Clin* 1997; 17:377–405.
27. Binnick AN. Allergic and irritant contact dermatitis. *Compr Ther* 1981; 1:17–21.
28. Lauerma AI, Stein BD, Homey B, Lee CH, Bloom E, Maibach HI. Topical FK506: Suppression of allergic and irritant contact dermatitis in the guinea pig. *Arch Dermatol Res* 1994; 286:337–340.
29. Rietschel RL. Comparison of allergic and irritant dermatitis. *Immun Allergy Clin* 1997; 17:359–364.
30. Coenraads PJ, Smit J. Epidemiology. In: Rycroft RJG, Menné T, Frosch PJ eds. *Textbook of Contact Dermatitis*. Berlin: Springer; 1995:133–150.
31. Meding B. Epidemiology of hand eczema in an industrial city. *Acta Derm Venereol (Stockh)* 1990; 153[suppl]:1–43.
32. Meding B, Swanbeck G. Occupational hand eczema in an industrial city. *Contact Dermatitis* 1990; 22:13–23.
33. Goh C. Occupational skin disease in Singapore: Epidemiology & causative agents. *Ann Acad Med Singapore* 1987; 16(2):303–305.
34. Diepgen TL, Coenraads PJ. What can we learn from epidemiological studies on irritant contact dermatitis? In: Elsner P, Maibach HI, eds. *Irritant Dermatitis: New Clinical and Experimental Aspects*. Basel: Karger; 1995:18–27.
35. Kanerva L, Estlander T, Jolanki R. Occupational skin disease in Finland. An analysis of 10 years of statistics from an occupational dermatology clinic. *Int Arch Occup Environ Health* 1988; 60:89–94.
36. Hogan DJ, Dannaker CJ, Maibach HI. The prognosis of contact dermatitis. *J Am Acad Dermatol* 1990; 23:300–307.
37. Nilsson E. Individual and environmental risk factors for hand eczema in hospital workers. *Acta Derm Venereol (Stockh)* 1986; 128[suppl]:1–63.
38. Suter-Widmer J, Elsner P. Age and irritation. In: van der Valk PGM, Maibach HI, eds. *The Irritant Contact Dermatitis Syndrome*. Boca Raton: CRC Press; 1994:257–261.
39. Lammintausta K, Maibach HI, Wilson D. Irritant reactivity in males and females. *Contact Dermatitis* 1987; 17:276–280.
40. Rystedt I. Work-related hand eczema in atopics. *Contact Dermatitis* 1985; 12:164–171.
41. Goldner R. Work-related irritant contact dermatitis. *Occup Med* 1994; 9:37–44.
42. Cronin E. Dermatitis of the hands in caterers. *Contact Dermatitis* 1987; 17:265–269.
43. Wood BP, Greig DE. Catering industry. *Clin Dermatol* 1997; 15:567–571.
44. Cleenewerck MB, Martin P. Irritants: Food. In: van der Valk PGM, Maibach HI, eds. *The Irritant Contact Dermatitis Syndrome*. New York: CRC Press; 1996:157–184.
45. Avnstorp C. Irritant cement eczema. In: van der Valk PGM, Maibach HI, eds. *The Irritant Contact Dermatitis Syndrome*. New York: CRC Press; 1996:111–119.

46. Gan SL, Goh CL, Lee CS. Occupational dermatitis among sanders in the furniture industry. *Contact Dermatitis* 1987; 17:237–240.
47. Gawkrodger DJ, Lloyd MH, Hunter JA. Occupational skin disease in hospital cleaning and kitchen workers. *Contact Dermatitis* 1986; 15:132–135.
48. Wrangsjö K, Meding B. Hospital workers. *Clin Dermatol* 1997; 15:573–578.
49. Kassis V, Vedel P, Darre E. Contact dermatitis to methyl methacrylate. *Contact Dermatitis* 1984; 11:26–28.
50. Singgih SI, Lantingha H, Nater JP, Woest TE, Kruyt-Gaspersz JA. Occupational hand dermatoses in hospital cleaning personnel. *Contact Dermatitis* 1986; 14:14–19.
51. van der Walle HB, Brunsveld VM. Dermatitis in hairdressers. I: The experience of the past 4 years. *Contact Dermatitis* 1994; 30:217–221.
52. Uter W, Gefeller O, Schwanitz HJ. Occupational dermatitis in hairdressing apprentices. In: Elsner P, Maibach HI, eds. *Irritant Dermatitis: New Clinical and Experimental Aspects*. Basel: Karger; 1995:49–55.
53. Conde Salazar L, Gomez J, Meza B, Guimaraens D. Artefactual irritant contact dermatitis. *Contact Dermatitis* 1993; 28:246.
54. Aoki T, Kageyama R. Three cases of dry cleaning dermatitis. *Nippon Hifuka Gakkai Zasshi* 1989; 9:1035–1038.
55. de Boer EM, van Ketel WG, Bruynzeel DP. Dermatoses in metal workers I: Irritant contact dermatitis. *Contact Dermatitis* 1989; 20:212–218.
56. Foulds IS, Koh D. Dermatitis from metalworking fluids. *Clin Exp Dermatol* 1990; 15:157–162.
57. Goh CL, Yuen R. A study of occupational skin disease in the metal industry (1986–1990). *Ann Acad Med Singapore* 1994; 23:639–644.
58. Rycroft RJG. Metal working industry. *Clin Dermatol* 1997; 15:565–566.
59. Wigger-Alberti W, Hinnen U, Elsner P. Predictive testing of metalworking fluids: A comparison of 2 cumulative human irritation models and correlation to epidemiological data. *Contact Dermatitis* 1997; 36:14–20.
60. Ashworth J, Rycroft RJG, Waddy RS. Irritant contact dermatitis in warehouse employees. *Occup Med* 1993; 43:32–34.
61. Willis CM. The histopathology of irritant contact dermatitis. In: van der Valk PGM, Maibach HI, eds. *The Irritant Contact Dermatitis Syndrome*. New York: CRC Press; 1996:291–303.
62. Brasch L, Burgard J, Sterry W. Common pathogenetic pathways in allergic and irritant contact dermatitis. *J Invest Dermatol* 1992; 98:166–170.
63. van der Valk PGM, Maibach HI. Do topical corticosteroids modulate skin irritation in human beings? Assessment by transepidermal water loss and visual scoring. *J Am Acad Dermatol* 1989; 21:519–522.
64. Goldschmidt H, Panizzon RG. *Radiation Therapy of Benign Tumors, Hyperplasias, and Dermatoses*. Berlin: Springer; 1991.
65. Frosch PJ. Irritant contact dermatitis. In: Frosch PJ, Dooms-Goossens A, Lachapelle JM, Rycroft RJG, Scheper RJ, eds. *Current Topics in Contact Dermatitis*. Berlin: Springer; 1989:385–403.
66. Goh CL. Prognosis of contact and occupational dermatitis. *Clin Dermatol* 1997; 15:655–659.
67. Hogan DJ. The prognosis of irritant contact dermatitis. In: van der Valk PGM, Maibach HI, eds. *The Irritant Contact Dermatitis Syndrome*. New York: CRC Press; 1996:9–15.
68. Seidenari S. Skin sensitivity, interindividual factors: Atopy. In: van der Valk PGM, Maibach HI, eds. *The Irritant Contact Dermatitis Syndrome*. New York: CRC Press; 1996:267–277.

68a. Wall L, Gebauer K. A follow-up study of occupational skin disease in Western Australia. *Contact Dermatitis* 1991; 524:241–243.

69. Iliev D, Hinnen U, Elsner P. Skin bioengineering methods in occupational dermatology. In: Elsner P, Barel AO, Berardesca E, Gaberd B, Serup J, eds. *Skin Bioengineering Techniques and Applications in Dermatology and Cosmetology.* Basel: Karger; 1998:145–150.

70. LaDage LH. Facial irritation from ethylene oxide sterilization of anesthesia mask. *Plast Reconstr Surg* 1970; 45:179.

71. Hanifin JM. Ethylene oxide dermatitis *JAMA* 1971; 217:215.

72. Ippen H, Mathies V. Die protrahierte Verätzung. *Berufsdermatosen* 1970; 18:144.

73. Taylor JS. Dermatologic hazards from ethylene oxide. *Cutis* 1977; 19:189.

74. Biro L, Fisher AA, Price E. Ethylene oxide burns, a hospital outbreak involving 19 women. *Arch Dermatol* 1974; 110:924.

75. Fisher AA. Post-operative ethylene oxide dermatitis. *Cutis* 1973; 12:177.

76. Rowe RJ, William GH. Severe reaction to cement. *Arch Environ Health* 1963; 7:709–711.

77. Fisher AA. Cement burns resulting in necrotic ulcers due to kneeling. *Cutis* 1979; 23:272.

78. Morris GE. The primary irritant nature of cement. *Arch Environ Health* 1960; 1:301.

79. Vickers HR, Edwards DSH. Cement burns. *Contact Dermatitis* 1976; 2:73–78.

80. Skiendzielewsky JJ. Cement burns. *Ann Emerg Med* 1980; 9:316–318.

81. McGeown G. Cement burns of the hand. *Contact Dermatitis* 1984; 10:246.

82. Buckley DB. Skin burns due to wet cement. *Contact Dermatitis* 1982; 8:407–409.

83. Hannuksela M, Suhonen R, Karvonen J. Caustic ulcers caused by cement. *Br J Dermatol* 1976; 95:547–549.

84. Sulzberger MB, Baer RL. The effects of fiber glass on animal and human skin. *Ind Med Surg* 1942; 11:482–484.

85. Verbeck SJA, Buise-van Unnik EMM, et al. Itching in office workers from glass fibres. *Contact Dermatitis* 1981; 7:354.

86. Possick PA, Gellin GA, Key MM. Fibrous glass dermatitis. *Am Ind Hyg Assoc J* 1970; 31:12–15.

87. Bjornberg A, Lowhagen GB, Tendberg JE. Skin reactivity in workers with and without itching from occupational exposure to glass fibres. *Acta Derm Venereol* 1979; 59:49.

88. Fisher BK, Warkentin JD. Fiber glass dermatitis. *Arch Dermatol* 1969; 99:717–719.

89. Heisel EB, Hunt FE. Further studies in cutaneous reactions to glass fibers. *Arch Environ Health* 1968; 17:705–711.

90. NIOSH: *A Recommended Standard for Occupational Exposure to Fibrous Glass.* Cincinnati: U.S. Department of Health, Education and Welfare, Public Health Service; 1977.

91. Cuypers JMC, Hoedemaeker PHJ, Nater JP, et al. The histopathology of fiberglass dermatitis in relation to von Hebra's concept of eczema. *Contact Dermatitis* 1975; 1:88–95.

92. Enterline PE. The health of retired fibrous glass workers. *Arch Environ Health* 1975; 30:113–116.

93. Milne J. Are glass fibers carcinogenic to man? A critical appraisal. *Br J Ind Med* 1976; 33:47–48.

94. Conde-Salazar L, Guimaraena D, Romero LV, et al. Occupational dermatitis from glass fiber. *Contact Dermatitis* 1985; 13:195–196.

95. Deeken JH. Tape treatment for fiberglass splinters. *Arch Dermatol* 1978; 114:623.

96. Hersle K, Mobacken H. Hyperkeratotic palmar dermatosis of the palms. *Br J Dermatol* 1982; 107:195.

97. Kono K, Yoshida Y, Harada A. An experimental study on the biochemical consequences of hydrofluoric acid burns. *Bull Osaka Med Sch* 1982; 28:124–133.

98. McIvor ME. Fluoride-induced sudden death. *Md State Med J* 1984; 33:536–537.

99. Vance MV, Curry SC, Kunkel DB, Ryan PJ, Ruggeri SB. Digital hydrofluoric acid burns: Treatment with intraarterial calcium infusion. *Ann Emerg Med* 1986; 15:890–896.

100. Bracken WM, Cuppage F, McLaury RL, Kirwin C, Klassen CD. Comparative effectiveness of topical treatments for hydrofluoric acid burns. *J Occup Med* 1985; 27:733–39.

101. Burkhart KK, Brent J, Kirk MA, Baker DC, Kulig KW. Comparison of topical magnesium and calcium treatment for dermal hydrofluoric acid burns. *Ann Emerg Med* 1994; 24:9–13.

102. Dunn BJ, MacKinnon MA, Knowlden NF, et al. Topical treatments for hydrofluoric acid dermal burns. *J Occup Environ Med* 1996;38:507–514.

103. Bier A. *Arch Klin Chir* 1908; 86:1007. *Trans Surv Anesth* 1967; 11:294.

104. Henry JA, Hla KK. Intravenous regional calcium perfusion for hydrofluoric acid burns. *Clin Toxicol* 1992; 30:203–207.

105. Graudins A, Burns MJ, Aaron CK. Regional intravenous infusion of calcium gluconate for hydrofluoric acid burns of the upper extremity. *Ann Emerg Med* 1997; 30:604–607.

106. Trevino MA, Hermann GH, Sprout WL. Treatment of severe hydrofluoric acid exposures. *J Occup Med* 1983; 25:861–863.

107. Koehnlein HE, Achinger R. A new method of treatment of hydrofluoric acid burns of the extremities. *Chir Plast* 1982; 6:297–305.

108. Mayer TD, Gross PL. Fatal systemic fluoriosis due to hydrofluoric acid burns. *Ann Emerg Med* 1985; 14:149–153.

109. Schwartz L. Occupational pigmentary changes in the skin. *Arch Dermatol Syphilol* 1947; 56:592–600.

110. Lerner AB. On the etiology of vitiligo and gray hair. *Am J Med* 1971; 51:141–147.

111. Lerner AB, Nordlund JJ. Vitiligo. What is it? Is it important? *JAMA* 1978; 239:1183–1187.

112. Fountain RB. Occupational melanoderma. *Br J Dermatol* 1967; 79:59–60.

113. Hunter D. *Diseases of Occupations.* London: The English Universities Press; 1975:780.

114. Gellin GA. Pigment responses: Occupational disorders of pigmentation. In: Maibach HI, ed. *Occupational and Industrial Dermatology,* 2nd ed. Chicago: Year Book Medical Publishers; 1987:134–141.

115. Gellin GA, Possick PA, Davis IH. Occupational depigmentation due to 4-tertiary butyl catechol (TBC). *J Occup Med* 1970; 12:386–389.

116. Gellin GA, Maibach HI. Detection of environmental depigmenting chemicals. In: Marzulli FN, Maibach HI, eds. *Dermatotoxicology,* 3rd ed. New York: Hemisphere Publishing Corporation; 1987:497–513.

117. Kahn G. Depigmentation caused by phenolic detergent germicides. *Arch Dermatol* 1970; 102:177–180.

118. McCarthy L, McCarthy LK. Leukoderma following dermatitis venenata. *Arch Dermatol Syphilol* 1925; 12:356–359.

119. Oliver EA, Schwartz B, Warren LH. Occupational leukoderma: Preliminary report. *JAMA* 1939; 113:927–928.

120. Bentley-Phillips B. Occupational leukoderma following misuse of a disinfectant. *S Afr Med J* 1974; 48:810.

121. Calnan CD, Cooke MA. Leucoderma in industry. *J Soc Occup Med* 1974; 24:59–61.

122. Gellin GA, Maibach HI, Misiaszek MH, et al. Detection of environmental depigmenting substances. *Contact Dermatitis* 1979; 5:201–213.

123. Fisher AA. Differential diagnosis of idiopathic vitiligo. Part III: Occupational leukoderma. *Cutis* 1994; 53:278–280.

124. Rietschel RL, Fowler JF Jr. Contact leukoderma (vitiligo): Hyperpigmentation and discolorations from contactnats. In: Fisher AA, ed. *Contact Dermatitis*, 4th ed. Baltimore: Williams and Wilkins; 1995:765–777.

125. Bajaj AK, Gupta SC, Chatterjee AK. Footwear depigmentation. *Contact Dermatitis* 1996; 35:117–118.

126. Malten KE, Seutter E, Hara I, Nakajima T. Occupational vitiligo due to paratertiary butylphenol and homologues. *Trans St Johns Hosp Dermatol Soc* 1971; 57:115–134.

127. Ortonne J-P, Mosher DB, Fitzpatrick TB. Chemical hypomelanosis. In: Ortonne J-P, Mosher DB, eds. *Vitiligo and Other Hypomelanoses of Hair and Skin*. New York: Plenum Medical Book Co; 1983:479–508.

128. Tosti A, Gaddoni G, Piraccini BM, deMaria P. Occupational leukoderma due to phenolic compounds in the ceramics industry. *Contact Dermatitis* 1991;25:67–68.

129. Hogan DJ, Tangiertsampan C. The less common occupational dermatoses. *Occup Med* 1992; 7:385–401.

130. Bleehen SS, Pathak MA, Hori Y, Fitzpatrick TB. Depigmentation of skin with 4-isopropyl catechol, mercapto-amines, and other compounds. *J Invest Dermatol* 1968; 30:103–117.

131. Menter JM, Etemade AA, Chapman W, et al. In vivo depigmentation by hydroxybenzene derivatives. *Melanoma Res* 1993; 3:443–449.

132. Stevenson CJ. Occupational vitiligo: Clinical and epidermiological aspects. *Br J Dermatol* 1981; 105[suppl 21]:51–56.

133. Fukuyama K, Gellin GA, Nishimura M, et al. Occupational leukoderma morphological and biological studies of 4-tertiary butyl catechol depigmentation. In: Kligman AM, Leyden JJ, eds. *Safety and Efficacy of Topical Drugs and Cosmetics*. New York: Grune & Stratton; 1982:135–155.

134. Jimbow K, Obata H, Pathak MA, Fitzpatrick TB. Mechanism of depigmentation by hydroquinone. *J Invest Dermatol* 1974; 62:436–449.

135. McGuire J, Hendee J. Biochemical basis of depigmentation of skin by phenolic germicides. *J Invest Dermatol* 1971; 57:256–261.

136. Nordlung JJ. Vitiligo. In: Thierss BH, Dobson RL, eds. *Pathogenesis of Skin Disease*. New York: Churchill Livingstone; 1986:99–127.

137. Gellin GA, Possick PA, Perone VB. Depigmentation from 4-tertiary butyl catechol—An experimental study. *J Invest Dermatol* 1970; 55:190–197.

138. Rily PA. Acquired hypomelanosis. *Br J Dermatol* 1971; 84:290–293.

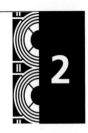

Allergic Contact Dermatitis

General Principles and Causes ■

ELIZABETH F. SHERERTZ, M.D.

With increasing attention to environmental control of irritants through modifications of industrial processes and use of personal protective equipment, the relative proportion of allergic contact dermatitis (ACD) causing significant occupational skin disease may be increasing. Previous estimates of 25% of instances of occupational skin disease being ACD have recently been challenged by studies in some work populations in whom it could be demonstrated that 40% of work-related dermatoses were ACD.[1,2] Further, in some types of occupational ACD, such as with metal allergy or allergy to biocides in oil and cutting fluids, an earlier confirmed diagnosis of ACD was associated with an improved prognosis.[3–5] This underscores the importance of considering allergy as well as irritant factors early in the diagnosis and outlining avoidance management for the affected employee.

Allergic contact dermatitis is a type IV, delayed, or cell-mediated classification of immunological reaction (see "Immunologic Aspects").[6,7] The term "hypersensitivity" is misleading in the medicolegal context of workers' compensation because to lawyers and employers, "hypersensitivity" may imply an individual predisposition not related to the specific workplace. The immunological use of the phrase "delayed contact hypersensitivity" refers to a unique cell-mediated immunological reaction to a specific allergen (substance). If exposure to that specific allergen is most likely to occur in the occupational setting, then the resulting dermatitis is considered to be work-related. Most contact allergens produce a sensitizing allergic reaction in only a small percentage of exposed individuals, and numerous factors may contribute to the development of a delayed contact hypersen-

sitivity (Table 2–1). By far, the most important host factor is recent or present skin damage (trauma, irritation) at the site of contact of the potential allergen.[8–10] This may explain some circumstances in which an employee with no change in exposures after months to years "suddenly" develops an allergic contact dermatitis.[11,12]

It is difficult to predict the contact allergenicity of a substance in a real-use industrial setting. Conditions present when assessing sensitization may not predict the potential for contact allergy to develop under different exposure conditions because of the interplay of the factors listed in Table 2–1.[13–16] These factors may also explain

 TABLE 2–1 • Factors That May Influence the Development of Allergic Contact Sensitization

Allergen Factors
Physicochemical nature of the substance
Dosage and concentration
Site and route of exposure
Number and frequency of exposures
Vehicle delivering allergen to the skin
Occlusion of the allergen against the skin

Environmental Factors
Temperature
Humidity

Host Factors
Recent or current skin damage
  Clinical—trauma, irritant dermatitis, other dermatoses
  Subclinical—recent dermatitis (within the past 3–4 months)

some of the nuances in the clinical appearance of contact dermatitis, as described below.

CLINICAL APPEARANCE

It is difficult and often impossible to make a clinical diagnosis of allergic vs. irritant contact dermatitis based on cutaneous lesion morphology.[17–19] The classifications of acute, subacute, and chronic dermatitis are of generic usefulness in describing the skin's appearance, but they do not necessarily correlate directly with new, recent, or chronic exposure to a substance, again because of the interplay of factors. The stage at which an employee seeks medical attention also varies.

Acute contact dermatitis is characterized by erythema, papules, and vesicles. The appearance of small (1–3 mm) vesicles, and occasionally bullae, is a hallmark of allergic contact dermatitis. On palmar or plantar surfaces, the thick stratum corneum may obscure the vesiculation, whereas at other sites (such as forearm, eyelids, face), the edema, vesicles, and subsequent oozing of serous fluid may be dramatic. Itching is often intense in acute dermatitis, especially at bedtime, and may disrupt sleep (Fig. 2–1).

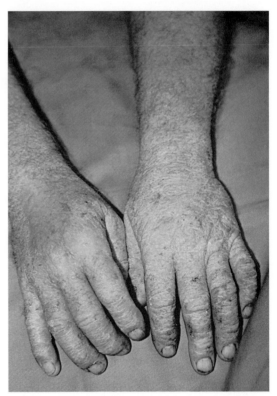

FIGURE 2–2 ● Chronic, and in places subacute, allergic contact dermatitis to 0-phenylphenol in a coolant. The dermatitis had recurred for many years but cleared completely within 6 weeks after removal of the allergen from his work environment.

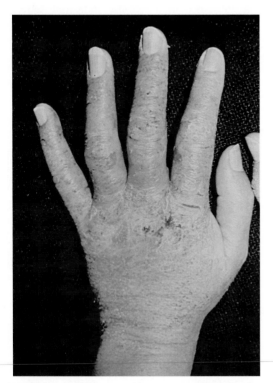

FIGURE 2–1 ● Hairdresser with severe, recurring allergic contact dermatitis to glyceryl monothioglycolate used in "acid perms." (Courtesy of Frances J. Storrs, M.D.)

With strong sensitizers or if a large area of skin surface has been exposed to an allergen, acute dermatitis initially may appear urticarial or erythema multiforme-like, may develop as an acute exfoliative dermatitis with blisters, or may appear as a chemical burn.

Subacute contact dermatitis is also characterized by erythema and itching, but vesicles give way to secondary fine peeling or scale and reactive epidermal thickening. Temporary hypopigmentation may occur because of increased epidermal turnover. Itching often continues, and scratching causes small excoriations which may be punctate or linear. These superficial erosions may be accompanied by linear fissures at sites of mechanical trauma, especially on the hands.

Chronic contact dermatitis may be minimally inflamed and is usually characterized by thickened skin that is scaling or shiny on the surface, again with cracking and fissuring at sites where the skin is stretched by motion (Fig. 2–2). Burning or stinging within the fissures is frequently a complaint at this stage, more so than itching.

A particular patient's allergic contact dermatitis

does not necessarily go through each of these clinical stages; a case varies according to concomitant contact with irritants, secondary bacterial infection, and concentration or frequency of allergen exposure. Over-the-counter or prescribed topical therapy may also modify the classic clinical appearance, as can occlusion.

The distribution of the dermatitis often provides a useful clinical hint about the nature of the contact exposure, but even this may not be as clearcut as one might expect. With direct skin exposure in an allergic patient, the dermatitis is limited primarily to the site of exposure (Fig. 2–3). On the hands (e.g., glove allergy), there is usually a symmetrical eruption involving both hands. The occlusive fit of the glove, the presence of skin damage on one hand more than on the other and variation in the mechanical use of the hand (being right-handed vs. left-handed) may contribute to an asymmetrical eruption or to the initial occurrence on one hand, followed by what is perceived to be spread to the other.[20–22]

Airborne exposure to an allergen (gaseous, vapor, or particulate) generally causes dermatitis at exposed sites like the face, neck, and arms. The scalp, if not covered with hair or a hat, could be involved, as can the eyelids. Areas under clothing are usually less involved, but that may depend on the fit of the clothing, on the amount of sweating, and on mechanical factors (e.g., sawdust could accumulate around a waistline).

Certain potential allergens are immunologically activated by light, resulting in dermatitis that occurs in areas of contact that are exposed to light. The classic distribution of a photocontact derma-

titis involves the face, sparing the shaded areas of the upper eyelids, the upper lip, and the submental areas of the chin. The dorsal surfaces of the hands and extensor surfaces of the arms (if short sleeves are worn) would be more involved in dermatitis if the allergen contacts those sites, as those parts of the upper extremity receive more light.

Spread of the dermatitis beyond obvious sites of contact can be difficult to explain. Allergen in contact with the hands can be spread to other sites by inadvertent touching, especially around the neck and face, and dermatitis (usually less severe) may then occur at those distant sites. Protective equipment may be incomplete so that skin contact could occur on the wrist between a glove and a sleeve, for example. Different penetration characteristics of the skin according to body site can also explain unusual distributions, because the sites of greatest exposure may not always be the sites of greatest involvement (e.g., the thick skin of the palms vs. the thinner stratum corneum of the sides and dorsal surface of the fingers). Once a contact allergy develops, if the skin is exposed to other sources of the same or of a crossreacting allergen, they will evoke a dermatitic response. For example, if a person develops delayed contact hypersensitivity to thiuram in a rubber glove and then uses a rubber condom or a rubber makeup sponge or rubber shoe insoles containing thiuram, a dermatitis would occur on the genital area, face, or feet, respectively, as well as on the hands. This apparent spread can make it difficult to convince an employer or others that the exposure to gloves in the workplace is the original cause of such a peculiar distribution.

The phenomenon of excitable skin, or an id reaction, is another potential explanation for the spread of a dermatitis beyond the initial exposure sites.[23] This nonspecific inflammatory reaction at unexposed sites is most likely to occur with an acute vesicular dermatitis and is characterized by diffuse erythematous papulovesicles that are intensely pruritic and that can become generalized. Acute contact dermatitis on the feet or on the legs is especially likely to produce a concomitant id reaction on the hands and arms, and it may look like a primary vesicular contact dermatitis at those sites as well.

Another cause of a widespread, generalized reaction is the systemic (oral or parenteral) administration of an allergen or crossreacting substance after an initial sensitizing exposure occurred through exogenous skin contact.[24] One example is sulfonamide administration to a person such as a hairdresser who is allergic to paraphenylenediamine.

Mucous membranes (conjunctiva and oral and

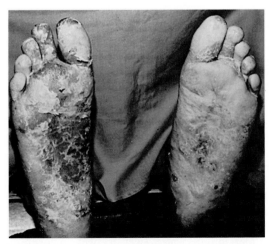

FIGURE 2–3 • Wearing, in workboots, an insole that contained the rubber additive ethylbutyl thiourea caused this severe, disabling dermatitis that remained undiagnosed for many months.

genital mucosa) are often spared clinical evidence of dermatitis despite known contact. This is probably because of reduced allergen recognition at those sites. So, for example, an allergen in an eyedrop would be more likely to cause dermatitis on the eyelids and cheek than to cause conjunctival erythema.

DIFFERENTIAL DIAGNOSIS

Some of the major considerations in the clinical differential diagnosis of allergic contact dermatitis may at times be coexistent with ACD, so it is helpful to sort out the contributing factors rather than to assume there is only one possible diagnosis. Table 2–2 offers a handy list of considerations to refer to when evaluating a patient with a dermatitis. The additional diseases to consider are determined by the clinical appearance at the time of evaluation (i.e., acute or chronic) and include the following:

- Psoriasis,
- Pustular eruptions—psoriasis, acne mechanica (Fig. 2–4),
- Id reaction to primary dermatophyte infection of the feet,
- Drug eruptions,
- Insect bites or infestations,
- Primary vesicular bullous dermatoses, such as dermatitis herpetiformis, miliaria, porphyria cutanea tarda, and
- Primary papulosquamous dermatoses, including pityriasis rosea and lichen planus.

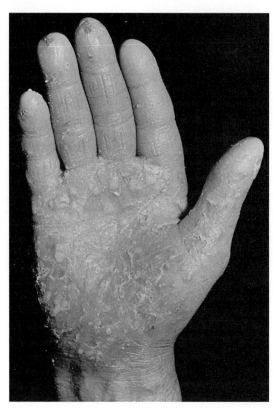

FIGURE 2–4 • Pustular eruptions of the palms are extremely recalcitrant to therapy and can sometimes be confused with allergic contact dermatitis.

Patient history, clinical experience in dermatologic diagnosis, cultures and, occasionally, skin biopsy can be helpful in clarifying another diagnosis. Patch testing is the most important confirmatory diagnostic procedure for ACD; it can be superimposed on any of the above diagnoses. Also, establishing another diagnosis does not rule out an occupational aggravating factor, as noted in other chapters (5–11).[25, 26] Likewise, if an employee has a known contact allergy, one should not assume that a subsequent dermatitis is necessarily caused by that specific allergen.

PREDISPOSING FACTORS

The predisposing factors in the development of an allergic contact dermatitis are summarized in Table 2–1.[27, 28] Damage resulting from intermittent immersion in water (wet-dry-wet exposures), sweating, pressure, and or friction (including repetitive motion trauma to the skin) is the most common cause of irritant contact dermatitis. This

TABLE 2–2 • "AIAIU"
Considerations for Dermatitis Diagnosis

One or more of the following may be involved:
A = Atopic dermatitis
I = Irritant contact dermatitis (chemical, mechanical, low humidity)
A = Allergic (delayed-type) contact dermatitis
I = Infection
Bacterial: primarily *Staphylococcus aureus* and/or Group A beta-hemolytic *Streptococcus*
Fungal: dermatophyte or *Candida* sp.
Viral: Herpes simplex > Herpes zoster
U = Urticaria from contact exposure
Nonimmunologic, including dermatographism
Immunologic, especially immediate
Contact hypersensitivity to latex or other plant or animal proteins

damage may be subclinical or frank irritant-contact dermatitis. Numerous studies have indicated this in both clinical and artificial circumstances.[29-34] Even skin that has apparently healed of trauma or dermatitis, based on clinical appearance, may be more susceptible to an allergic sensitization if the exposure circumstances are right.[35-39]

References

1. Nethercott JR, Holness DL. Occupational allergic contact dermatitis. *Clin Rev Allergy* 1989;7:399–415.
2. Rosen RH, Freeman S. Occupational contact dermatitis in New South Wales. *Austr J Dermatol* 1992;33:1–11.
3. Holness DL, Nethercott JR. Is a worker's understanding of their diagnosis an important determinant of outcome in occupational contact dermatitis? *Contact Dermatitis* 1991;25:296–301.
4. Mackey SA, Marks JG. Dermatitis in machinists: a retrospective study. *Am J Contact Derm* 1993;4:22–26.
5. Halbert AR, Gebauer KA, Wall LM. Prognosis of occupational chromate dermatitis. *Contact Dermatitis* 1992;27:214–219.
6. Baer RL. Allergic eczematous contact dermatitis. In: Baer RL, Witten VH, eds. *Yearbook of Dermatology, 1956–1957.* Chicago: Year Book Medical Publishers; 1957:11.
7. Katz SI. Mechanisms involved in allergic contact dermatitis. *J Allergy Clin Immunol* 1990;86:670–672.
8. Burckhardt W. Cutaneous resistance to alkalis, acids, and commercial solvents. In: Lowenthal LJA, ed. *The Eczemas.* London: Livingstone; 1954.
9. Epstein WL, Kligman AM. Some factors affecting the reaction of allergic contact dermatitis. *J Invest Dermatol* 1959;33:231–243.
10. Magnusson B, Kligman AM. Factors influencing allergic contact desensitization. In: Marzulli F, Maibach HI, eds. *Dermatotoxicology and Pharmacology.* New York: John Wiley & Sons; 1977:289.
11. Malten KE. Thoughts on irritant contact dermatitis. *Contact Dermatitis* 1981;7:238–247.
12. Mathias CGT. Contact dermatitis from use or misuse of soaps, detergents, and cleansers in the workplace. *Occup Med* 1986;1:205–218.
13. Shmunes E. Predisposing factors in occupational skin diseases. *Dermatol Clin* 1988;6:7–13.
14. Moon KC, Maibach HI. Percutaneous absorption in diseased skin. In: Menné T, Maibach HI, eds. *Exogenous Dermatoses: Environmental Dermatitis.* Boca Raton, Fla.: CRC Press; 1990:217–226.
15. Basketter DA, Griffiths HA, Wang XM, Wilhelm KP, McFadden J. Individual, ethnic and seasonal variability in irritant susceptibility of skin: the implications for a predictive human patch test. *Contact Dermatitis* 1996;35:208–213.
16. Upadhye MR, Maibach HI. Influence of area of application of allergen on sensitization in contact dermatitis. *Contact Dermatitis* 1992;27:281–286.
17. Holness DL, Nethercott JR. Comparison of occupational and nonoccupational contact dermatitis. *Am J Contact Derm* 1994;5:207–212.
18. Paul MA, Fleischer AB Jr, Sherertz EF. Patients benefit

19. Conde-Salazar L, Baz M, Guimaraens D, Cannaro A. Contact dermatitis in hairdressers: patch test results in 379 hairdressers (1980–1993). *Am J Contact Derm* 1995;6:19–23.
20. Ramsing DW, Agner T. Effect of glove occlusion on human skin: short-term experimental exposure. *Contact Dermatitis* 1996;34:1–5.
21. Lynfield YL, Winiger M, Frank L. Allergic contact dermatitis on the palms. *J Invest Dermatol* 1968; 51:494–496.
22. Birmingham DJ. Prolonged and recurrent occupational dermatitis: some whys and wherefores. *Occup Med* 1986;1:349–356.
23. Polak L, Turk JL. The flare-up of previous test sites of contact sensitivity and the development of a generalized rash. *Clin Exp Immunol* 1968;3:253–262.
24. Veien NK, Menné T, Maibach HI. Systemically induced allergic contact dermatitis. In: Menné T, Maibach HI, eds. *Exogenous Dermatoses: Environmental Dermatitis.* Boca Raton, Fla.: CRC Press; 1990:267–282.
25. Sherertz EF, Zanolli MD. Occupational allergic contact and frictional dermatitis leading to plaques of psoriasis: a challenge in diagnosis. *Am J Contact Derm* 1991;2:52–55.
26. Heidenheim M, Jemec GBE. Concomitant psoriasis and allergic contact dermatitis: coexistent interrelated clinical entities. *Am J Contact Derm* 1991;2:175–180.
27. Walker FB, Smith PD, Maibach HI. Genetic factors in human allergic contact dermatitis. *Int Arch Allergy Immunol* 1967;32:453–462.
28. Kwangsukstith C, Maibach HI. Effect of age and sex on the induction and elicitation of allergic contact dermatitis. *Contact Dermatitis* 1995;33:289–298.
29. Grunewald AM, Gloor M, Gehring W, Kleesz P. Damage to the skin by repetitive washing. *Contact Dermatitis* 1995;32:225–232.
30. Allenby CF, Basketter DA. An arm immersion model of compromised skin: influence of minimal eliciting patch test concentrations of nickel. *Contact Dermatitis* 1993;28:129–133.
31. McLelland J, Shuster S, Matthews JNS. Irritants increase the response to an allergen in allergic contact dermatitis. *Arch Dermatol* 1991;127:1016–1019.
32. Klas PA, Corey G, Storrs FJ, Chan SC, Hanifin JM. Allergic and irritant patch test reactions and atopic disease. *Contact Dermatitis* 1996;34:121–124.
33. Lammintausta K, Maibach HI. Irritation insights: epidemiology and experimental status. In: Menné T, Maibach HI, eds. *Exogenous Dermatoses: Environmental Dermatitis.* Boca Raton, Fla.: CRC Press; 1990:179–186.
34. Dahl MV. Chronic irritant contact dermatitis: mechanisms, variables, and differentiation from other forms of contact dermatitis. *Adv Dermatol* 1988;3:261–276.
35. Hogan DJ, Dannaker CJ, Maibach HI. The prognosis of contact dermatitis. *J Am Acad Dermatol* 1990;23:300–307.
36. Effendy I, Loeffler H, Maibach HI. Baseline transepidermal water loss in patients with acute and healed irritant contact dermatitis. *Contact Dermatitis* 1995;33:371–374.
37. Widmer J, Eisner P, Burg G. Skin irritant reactivity following experimental cumulative irritant contact dermatitis. *Contact Dermatitis* 1994;30:35–39.
38. Tur E, Eshkol Z, Brenner S, Maibach HI. Cumulative effect of subthreshold concentrations of irritants in humans. *Am J Contact Derm* 1995;6:216–220.
39. Chia SE, Goh CL. Prognosis of occupational dermatitis in Singapore workers. *Am J Contact Derm* 1991;2:105–109.

Immunological Aspects ■

DONALD V. BELSITO, M.D.

The development of allergic contact dermatitis (ACD) involves the exposure of a genetically susceptible host to critical levels of allergen. Subsequently, the allergen is processed by antigen-presenting cells and presented to T cells. Finally, the skin is invaded by allergen-specific T cells and other nonspecific inflammatory cells. During the past several decades, much has been learned about the molecular processes that are involved in and that control the above sequence of events (Fig. 2–5).

THE ALLERGENS

Most environmental allergens are haptens—small (< 500 daltons) electrophilic molecules that covalently bind to carrier proteins.[1] The major exception to such covalent bonding occurs among the metallic salts (for example, nickel and cobalt), which are thought to intercollate with proteins

as cobalt complexes with vitamin B_{12}.[2] Not all electrophilic, protein-binding substances are haptens.[3] The determinants of antigenicity are multifactorial, including the type of binding that the hapten undergoes with the carrier and the final three-dimensional configuration of the conjugate.[4] Additionally, the carrier for the hapten is vitally important; potent contact sensitizers, when complexed to nonimmunogenic carriers, induce tolerance rather than sensitization.[5] HLA-DR or class II antigens on the surface of the antigen-presenting cells act as the binding site (carrier) for contact allergens.[6]

ANTIGEN PROCESSING AND PRESENTATION

The antigen-presenting cells within the skin are the suprabasilar, epidermal Langerhans cells (LCs), which are bone marrow-derived dendritic

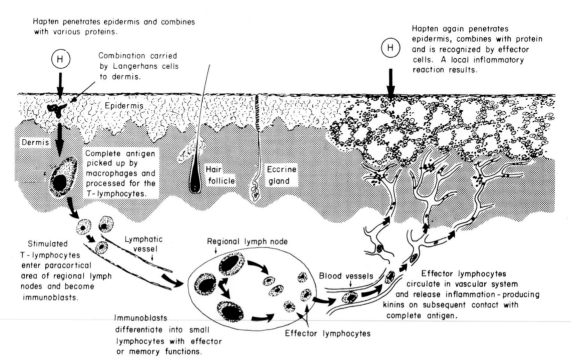

FIGURE 2–5 ● A simplified scheme showing the development of allergic contact dermatitis.

TABLE 2–3 • Accessory Molecules Facilitating Langerhans Cell–T Cell Interaction

Accessory Molecules On			
Langerhans Cell	T Cell	Effect	Reference
ICAM-1	LFA-1	Enhances T-cell response	Kuhlman et al.[14]
LFA-3	CD2	Lowers antigen dose/response	Prens et al.[15]
B7	CD28	Stabilizes mRNA for IL-2	Lindsley et al.[17]

cells.[7] Under normal circumstances, LCs are the only epidermal cells that constitutively express the immune-associated class II (Ia or HLA-DR) antigens. Depending upon the allergen, LCs can either directly bind the hapten or "process" it into a complete antigen.[8] Antigen processing by LCs involves ingestion by pinocytosis, followed by nonlysosomal degradation of the allergen into peptides that are bound to HLA-DR and recycled onto the cell surface.[9] ATPase on the surface of LCs, which is endocytosed with antigen, aids degradation by driving an acidifying proton pump.[10]

During antigen processing, LCs undergo phenotypic changes that facilitate their subsequent presentation of antigen to T cells. The acquisition of these accessory molecules (Table 2–3) on the surface of LCs is regulated by cytokines. In experimental models, it has been shown that interleukin (IL)-1β is secreted by LCs within 15 minutes of contact with an allergen.[11] In autocrine fashion, IL-1β upregulates intercellular adhesion molecule (ICAM)-1 (CD54), B7-2 (CD86), and CD40 on LCs.[12] Subsequently, the interaction between CD40 on LCs and its ligand (CD40-L) on T cells further stimulates production of ICAM-1 and B7-2, as well as lymphocyte function-associated antigen (LFA)-3 (CD58) on LCs.[13] These accessory molecules provide important secondary signals that enhance antigen presentation via interaction with their corresponding ligands on T cells: ICAM-1 with LFA-1,[14] LFA-3 with CD2,[15] and B7-2 with CD28.[16] The mechanisms by which these molecular interactions facilitate T-cell responses are currently being evaluated. Regarding

the interaction between B7 and CD28, data suggest that it stimulates T cells by stabilizing mRNA for IL-2.[17] Furthermore, the interaction between B7 and CD28 appears to be crucial to the induction of sensitization; in the absence of CD28, tolerance, rather than sensitization, is induced.[18]

For sensitization to occur, antigen-primed LCs must interact with CD4+ T cells (T-helper cells) with specific receptors for class II antigen and the contact allergen. The antigen receptor on a T cell consists of the transducing protein CD3, which is found on all T cells, coupled with Ti, a heterodimeric protein with a variable region, which acts as an additional antigen-binding site.[19] Stimulation of these CD4+ helper T cells is MHC-restricted in that the antigen must be presented in association with class II molecules on the antigen-presenting cell.[20] In fact, CD4 is itself an additional recognition site on T cells for class II molecules.[21] Following the initial activation of the receptor complex, crosslinking of CD3 with CD4 occurs and further enhances the responsiveness of T cells.[22]

During initial sensitization, antigen-bearing LCs interact with CD4+ T cells that have not been previously exposed to the allergen. These virgin T cells, which express L-selectin (an adhesion molecule that targets them to peripheral lymph nodes), and the appropriate antigen receptor (CD3-Ti) are CD45RA+[23, 24] and are also called T_H0 cells. As outlined in Table 2–4, appropriate presentation of antigen by LCs in the presence of various regulatory factors—including the LC-derived cytokines IL-1β,[11] IL-6,[25] IL-12,[26] and transforming growth factor (TGF)β[27]—results in the

TABLE 2–4 • Cytokine-Regulated T-Cell Development During Antigen Presentation

Cytokine	Effect	Reference
IL-12	Directs differentiation of T_H0 to T_H1	Dilulio et al.[37]
TGF-β	Phenotypic conversion: CD45RA to CD45 RO	Picker et al.[28]
IL-1	Activates T cells to secrete IL-2 and express IL-2R	Luqman et al.[29] Holsti, Raulet[31]
IL-6	Synergizes with TGF-β and IL-1 in their above activities	Picker et al.[28] Holsti, Raulet[31]

clonal expansion of antigen-specific T cells.[28] In the ensuing immune response, IL-1 (previously known as lymphocyte-activating factor) activates T cells to synthesize and release IL-2 (previously called T-cell growth factor).[29] IL-6 functions as a second signal for production of IL-2,[30] which classically has been thought to be responsible for driving the efferent, or response, phase of cell-mediated reactions. In conjunction with IL-1 and IL-6,[31] IL-2 induces its own receptor (IL-2R) on T cells.[32] Although initially produced by antigen-specific CD4+ cells, IL-2 acts nonspecifically to stimulate T cells with and without specific antigen receptors, causing them to proliferate, to express DR antigens (which are absent in the resting state), and to secrete IL-2, interferon (IFN)-γ and other cytokines.[33–35]

Under the influence of IL-6 and TGF-β, the expanding population of antigen-specific T cells undergoes phenotypic conversion from CD45RA+ virgin cells to CD45RO+ memory/effector cells,[23] which express the newly acquired "skin-homing" antigens, common leukocyte antigen (CLA) and very late antigen (VLA)-4.[28, 36] In addition, under the influence of IL-12, these T_H0 cells differentiate into T_H1-like memory cells,[37] the classic effector cells for ACD. T_H1 cells preferentially secrete IL-2 and IFN-γ, among other cytokines. In contrast, T_H2 cells, which secrete IL-4 and IL-10 and represent another mature T_H subtype important in the regulation of IgE synthesis, develop from T_H0 following different stimuli. Although the notion that T_H1 and T_H2 cells subserve well-differentiated immunologic functions has in vitro support, the in vivo immune response to contact allergens is more complex.[38, 39] Although both T_H1 and T_H2 cells may be involved in ACD, IL-12 seems crucial to the initial response, as neutralization of IL-12 in vivo not only prevents the induction of ACD but also induces hapten-specific tolerance.[40]

The processing and presentation of the antigen are referred to as the afferent phase of ACD. Whether this occurs in the draining lymph nodes or in the skin is controversial. Studies have shown that antigen-bearing LCs migrate to the lymph nodes following immunological stimulation of the epidermis.[41, 42] The controlled migration of LCs from epidermis to draining lymph node is the subject of much interest. Recent data suggest that tumor necrosis factor (TNF)-α, by regulating the expression of adhesion molecules or by other mechanisms, is critical to LC migration.[43] Among the adhesion molecules that control LC migration are sialyl Lewis x and E-cadherin. Sialyl Lewis x (a selectin) is upregulated on LCs during allergic reactions at the same time as E-selectin (a ligand for sialyl Lewis x) is upregulated on endothelial cells.[44] In addition, the expression of E-cadherin (an adhesion molecule for keratinocytes (KCs) is downregulated on LCs following cutaneous application of antigens.[45] This downregulation of E-cadherin, together with increased expression of sialyl Lewis x, may be the critical factors for LC migration.

LCs clearly migrate out of the skin following antigen challenge, but the clinical expression of ACD is cutaneous, not nodal. Therefore, it seems likely that both peripheral and central presentation of allergen occur. Indeed, Frey and Wenk[46] demonstrated that sensitization requires only intact lymphatic pathways, whereas elicitation of the allergy requires only intact blood vessels. These observations suggest the following mechanism: At the time of initial antigen exposure, antigen-bearing LCs, some of which remain in the skin and some of which migrate to lymph nodes, are statistically more likely to appose the small number of virgin T cells bearing specific antigen receptors in the lymph nodes. However, upon reexposure, there is an increased likelihood that these T cells will encounter the allergen within the skin before, or concurrently with, LC migration to the draining lymph nodes, because memory T cells are more numerous and more "skin-homing" after the primary exposure.

CUTANEOUS RESPONSE

In the efferent phase, inflammatory cells invade the skin. The mechanisms by which memory T cells and other inflammatory cells are attracted to the site of contact with the allergen are now being defined (Table 2–5). As mentioned, the CD45RO+ memory T cells constitutively express CLA. CLA interacts with E-selectin, its ligand, which is induced on vascular endothelium by TNF-α.[47] As a result of this interaction, memory T cells circulating past activated endothelial cells begin to roll slowly along the endothelial cell surface.[48] After they roll, firm adhesion of leukocytes to endothelium and migration of leukocytes through the endothelial gaps are mediated by the interactions between vascular cell adhesion molecules (VCAM)-1 and ICAM-1 (endothelial proteins with immunoglobulin domains) and VLA-4 (a β_1 integrin) as well as by the interaction between LFA-1 (a β_2 integrin) and lymphocytes.[49, 50] Following their exit into the dermis, these LFA-1+ T cells migrate toward epidermal cells that have been induced to express ICAM-1.[51] This hypothesized mechanism of T-cell homing to skin is supported by phenotypic studies of early patch-test reactions that reveal significant upregulation of

TABLE 2–5 • The Vascular Addressins and T-Cell Adhesion Molecules Responsible for Recruiting Memory T Cells to the Skin

Endothelial Cell	T Cell	Effect	Reference
E-selectin	CLA	T cells roll along endothelium	Lawrence, Springer[48]
VCAM-1	VLA-4	T cells firmly adhere to endothelial cells	Elices[49]
ICAM-1	LFA-1	T-cell diapedesis	Dustin, Springer[50]

VCAM-1 and E-selectin within 8 hours of antigen application.[52]

The induction and kinetic expression of both endothelial and epithelial adhesion molecules by cytokines have been well studied. Upon stimulation of endothelium with TNF-α or IL-1, E-selectin[53] and VCAM-1[54] are synthesized in, and expressed on, the endothelial cell membrane within several hours. In contrast, endothelial ICAM-1 is enhanced only after T cells have already attached to the endothelial surfaces, suggesting that upregulation of ICAM-1 is under the influence of IFN-γ secreted by activated T cells.[55] In addition, as the allergic reaction progresses, increasing amounts of ICAM-1 are expressed on epidermal cells (primarily KCs) between 48 and 96 hours after antigen challenge.[56] Given the temporal correlation between this expression of ICAM-1 on KCs and the migration of LFA-1⁺ T cells into the epidermis, it is likely that epithelial expression of ICAM-1 depends not only on epidermal cell-derived IL-1 and TNF-α (cytokines known to be upregulated in LCs and/or KCs within 15 minutes following antigen application), but also on T-cell-derived IFN-γ. Finally, some allergens (e.g., urushiol) directly induce ICAM-1 on KCs by activation of protein kinase C.[57] This might account, at least in part, for the frequency and intensity of reactions induced by exposure to urushiol. For most allergens, however, cytokine-coordinated expression of adhesion molecules on vascular endothelial cells and on epithelial cells results in the directed migration of skin-homing memory T cells to the challenged site.

Although the regulation of endothelial cells by adhesion molecules could be influenced by epidermal cytokines, mast cells are more likely to be the principal regulators of endothelial E-selectin and VCAM-1, especially given their perivascular location and their content of preformed TNF-α.[58] In humans[59] and rodents,[60] mast cells are activated during ACD, presumably by a T-cell-derived antigen-binding factor that reportedly causes release of serotonin from mast cells approximately 2 hours after antigenic challenge.[61] Pharmacologic blockade of serotonin prevents the delayed (24 to 48 hours) ACD reaction.[62] Serotonin and other vasoactive amines are likely to be important regulators of ACD because they induce endothelial gaps that permit the ingress and egress of effector cells. Thus, the observed peaks of mast cell degranulation at 1 to 4 hours and at 12 hours following antigen challenge closely correspond with the influx of inflammatory cells, which begins as early as 2 to 4 hours and is maximal at 24 hours.[60]

In addition to mast cells, nerve fibers also appear to regulate the allergic response. Indeed, one of the more exciting findings of the past decade has been the observation that nerve fibers directly impinge on LCs.[63] Given the known role of neurochemicals in vascular reactivity and inflammation,[64] a number of laboratories have been studying the effect of neuropeptides, principally substance P (SP) and calcitonin gene-related peptide (CGRP), on ACD. Release of SP from nerve fibers upregulates ACD at least in part by enhancing secretion of TNF-α from mast cells[65] and monocytes[66] and by enhancing the synthesis and secretion of IL-2 and expression of its receptor.[67] In contrast, CGRP inhibits antigen presentation and T-cell proliferation, possibly by stimulating production of KC-derived IL-10, which results in decreased expression of B7-2.[68]

The end result of this exquisitely orchestrated interplay of cytokines and adhesion molecules is, for most allergens, the entrance into the skin of CD45RO⁺ memory T cells secreting IL-2 and IFN-γ. IFN-γ (immune interferon) further amplifies the immune response; it activates cytotoxic T cells, natural killer cells, and macrophages.[69] IFN-γ also enhances the expression of class II antigens on LCs[70] and KCs,[71] but the functional in vivo significance of this action is unclear; in vitro, upregulation of HLA-DR on antigen-presenting cells improves their functioning.[72] In addition, IFN-γ results in the expression of interferon-inducible protein-10 (IP-10) on KCs,[11] which adds to the recruitment of monocytes and macrophages.[73] Other cytokines, especially IL-1 and TNF-α, stimulate production of monocyte chemoattractant-1 (MCA-1),[74] monocyte chemotactic, and activating factor (MCAF)[75] and of macrophage inflammatory protein (MIP)-2 by KCs.[11] Thus, monocytes and macrophages are nonspecifically recruited to the site of contact with the allergen. It is this collection of lymphohistiocytic cells, along with their chemical mediators, that is responsible for the epidermal spongiosis (intercellular edema) and dermal infiltrate that are the histological hallmarks of ACD. Thus, although ACD is driven by a specific allergen, the final clinical response is antigen-nonspecific.

HYPOSENSITIZATION AND TOLERANCE INDUCTION

Although the possibility of hyposensitizing patients with occupational ACD has intrigued dermatologists, it is not a viable alternative. Despite the early encouraging work of Schamberg[76] and Strickler[77] who used *Toxicodendron* antigen to desensitize the rhus-allergic individual, such hyposensitization therapy has never been demonstrated to be effective. In his exhaustive study, Kligman[78] concluded that "complete desensitization of the highly sensitive subject by oral or intramuscular administration is impossible." In this and other studies,[79] multiple treatments with Toxicodendron oleoresin resulted in a temporary lessening of the allergic response's intensity, but not in its ablation.

In the absence of effective hyposensitization, one theoretical possibility for prevention of occupational ACD is the induction of tolerance to known occupational allergens before employment. When an antigen to which an individual has not yet been sensitized is administered either systemically[80] or topically to areas deficient in functional Langerhans cells,[81] long-lived tolerance rather than sensitization ensues. As previously mentioned, other mechanisms for inducing tolerance include use of antibodies directed against B7/CD28[18] and interference with the production and function of IL-12[41] at the time of initial sensitization. However, the ethics and scientific wisdom of tolerance induction are debatable. Because allergic reactions to apparently innocuous materials such as nickel persist in the human genome, one must question whether there is a selective advantage to the trait. It is possible that the antigenic moieties of simple chemicals may be similar to more complex viruses and malignancies. Hence, the risk of tolerance induction to a contact allergen could potentially outweigh the benefit. Clearly, much more needs to be known not only about the nature of the antigenic moiety, but also about the entire process of ACD. At this time, once acquired, ACD remains "incurable."

References

1. Landsteiner K, Chase MW. Studies on the sensitization of animals with simple chemical compounds, IX. Skin sensitization induced by injection of conjugates. *J Exp Med* 1941;73:431–438.
2. Dupuis G, Benezra C. *Allergic Contact Dermatitis to Simple Chemicals: A Molecular Approach*. New York: Marcel Dekker; 1982:52–66, 83.
3. Sommer G, Parker D, Turk JL. Epicutaneous induction of hyporeactivity in contact sensitization: demonstration of suppressor cells induced by contact with 2,4-dinitrothiocyanatebenzene. *Immunology* 1975;29:517–525.
4. Parker D, Long PV, Turk JL. A comparison of the conjugation of DNTB and other dinitrobenzenes with free protein radicals and their ability to sensitize or tolerize. *J Invest Dermatol* 1983;81:198–201.
5. Katz DH, Davie JM, Paul WE, et al. Carrier function in anti-hapten antibody responses, Vol. 4. Experimental conditions for the induction of hapten-specific tolerance or for the stimulation of anti-hapten anamnestic responses by "non-immunogenic" hapten polypeptide conjugates. *J Exp Med* 1971;134:201–223.
6. Nalefski EA, Rao, A. Nature of the ligand recognized by a hapten- and carrier-specific, MHC-restricted T cell receptor. *J Immunol* 1993;150:3806–3816.
7. Katz SI, Tamaki K, Sachs DH. Epidermal Langerhans cells are derived from cells originating in bone marrow. *Nature (London)* 1979;282:324–326.
8. Mommaas AM, Mulder AA, Out CJ, et al. Distribution of HLA class II molecules in epidermal Langerhans cells in situ. *Eur J Immunol* 1995;25:520–525.
9. Sallusto F, Cella M, Danieli C, et al. Dendritic cells use macropinocytosis and the mannose receptor to concentrate macromolecules in the major histocompatibility complex class II compartment: downregulation by cytokines and bacterial products. *J Exp Med* 1995;182:389–400.
10. Girolomoni G, Stone DK, Bergstresser PR, et al. Vacuolar acidification and bafilomycin-sensitive proton translocating ATPase in human epidermal Langerhans cells. *J Invest Dermatol* 1991;96:735–741.
11. Enk AH, Katz SI. Early molecular events in the induction phase of contact sensitivity. *Proc Natl Acad Sci USA* 1992;89:1398–1402.
12. Ozawa H, Nakagawa S, Tagami H, et al. Interleukin-1 beta and granulocyte-macrophage colony-stimulating factor mediate Langerhans cell maturation differently. *J Invest Dermatol* 1996;106:441–445.
13. Péguet-Navarro J, Dalbiez-Gauthier C, Moulon C, et al. Functional expression of CD40 antigen on human epidermal Langerhans cells. *J Immunol* 1995;155:4241–4247.
14. Kuhlman P, Moy VT, Lollo BA, et al. The accessory function of murine intercellular adhesion molecule-1 in T lymphocyte activation: contributions of adhesion and co-activation. *J Immunol* 1991;146:1773–1782.
15. Prens EP, Benne K, vanJoost T, et al. Differential role of lymphocyte function-associated antigens in the activation of nickel-specific peripheral blood T lymphocytes. *J Invest Dermatol* 1991;97:885–891.
16. Rattis F-M, Péguet-Navarro J, Staquet MJ, et al. Expression and function of B7-1 (CD80) and B7-2 (CD86) on human epidermal Langerhans cells. *Eur J Immunol* 1996;26:449–453.
17. Linsley PS, Brady W, Grosmaire L, et al. Binding of the B cell activation antigen B7 to CD28 costimulates T cell proliferation and interleukin 2 mRNA accumulation. *J Exp Med* 1991;173:721–731.
18. Kalish RS, Wood JA. Introduction of hapten-specific tolerance of human CD8+ urushiol (poison ivy)-reactive T lymphocytes. *J Invest Dermatol* 1997;108:253–257.
19. Reinherz EL, Meuer SC, Schlossman SF. The delineation of antigen receptors on human T lymphocytes. *Immunol Today* 1983;4:5–9.

20. Schwartz RH. T lymphocyte recognition of antigen in association with gene products of the major histocompatibility complex. *Annu Rev Immunol* 1985;3:237–261.

21. Swain SL. T cell subsets and the recognition of MHC class. *Immunol Rev* 1983;74:129–142.

22. Anderson P, Blue ML, Morimoto C, et al. Cross-linking of T3 (CD3) with T4 (CD4) enhances the proliferation of resting T lymphocytes. *J Immunol* 1987;139:678–682.

23. Ferrer JM, Plaza A, Kreisler M, et al. Differential interleukin secretion by *in vitro* activated human CD45RA and CD45RO CD4+ T cell subsets. *Cell Immunol* 1992;141:10–20.

24. Dearman RJ, Basketter DA, Coleman JW, et al. The cellular and molecular basis for divergent allergic responses to chemicals. *Chem Biol Interactions* 1992;84:1–10.

25. Cumberbatch M, Dearman RJ, Kimber I. Constitutive and inducible expression of interleukin-6 by Langerhans cells and lymph node dendritic cells. *Immunology* 1996;87:513–518.

26. Kang K, Kubin M, Cooper KD, et al. IL-12 synthesis by human Langerhans cells. *J Immunol* 1996;156:1402–1407.

27. Gruschwitz MS, Hornstein OP. Expression of transforming growth factor type beta on human epidermal dendritic cells. *J Invest Dermatol* 1992;99:114–116.

28. Picker LJ, Treer JR, Ferguson-Darnell B, et al. Control of lymphocyte recirculation in man, II. Differential regulation of the cutaneous lymphocyte-associated antigen, a tissue-selective homing receptor for skin-homing T cells. *J Immunol* 1993;150:1122–1136.

29. Luqman M, Greenbaum L, Lu D, et al. Differential effect of interleukin 1 on naive and memory CD4+ T cells. *Eur J Immunol* 1992;22:95–100.

30. Garman RD, Jacobs KA, Clark SC, et al. B cell stimulatory factor-2 (β2 interferon) functions as a second signal for interleukin 2 production by mature murine T cells. *Proc Natl Acad Sci USA* 1987;84:7629–7633.

31. Holsti MA, Raulet DH. IL-6 and IL-1 synergize to stimulate IL-2 production and proliferation of peripheral T cells. *J Immunol* 1989;143:2514–2519.

32. Malek TR, Ashwell JD. Interleukin 2 upregulates expression of its receptor on a T cell clone. *J Exp Med* 1985;161:1575–1580.

33. Chang TW, Testa D, Kung PC, et al. Cellular origin and interactions involved in gamma-interferon production induced by OKT3 monoclonal antibody. *J Immunol* 1982;128:585–589.

34. Ko HS, Fu SM, Winchester RJ, et al. Ia determinants on stimulated human T lymphocytes: occurrence on mitogen- and antigen-activated T cells. *J Exp Med* 1979;150:246–255.

35. Vilcek J, Henriksen-Destefano D, Siegel D, et al. Regulation of IFN-gamma induction in human peripheral blood cells by exogenous and endogenously produced interleukin 2. *J Immunol* 1985;135:1851–1856.

36. Horgan KJ, Luce GE, Tanaka Y, et al. Differential expression of VLA-α4 and VLA-β1 discriminates multiple subsets of CD4+CD45RO+ "Memory" T cells. *J Immunol* 1992;149:4082–4087.

37. Dilulio NA, Xu H, Fairchild RL. Diversion of CD4+ T cell development from regulatory T helper to effector T helper cells alters the contact hypersensitivity response. *Eur J Immunol* 1996;26:2606–2612.

38. Müller KM, Rocken M, Carlberg C, et al. The induction and functions of murine T-helper cell subsets. *J Invest Dermatol* 1995;105:8S–13S.

39. Picker LJ, Singh MK, Zdraveski Z, et al. Direct demonstration of cytokine synthesis heterogeneity among human memory/effector T cells by flow cytometry. *Blood* 1995;86:1408–1419.

40. Riemann H, Schwarz A, Grabbe S, et al. Neutralizaton of IL-12 *in vivo* prevents induction of contact hypersensitivity and induces hapten-specific tolerance. *J Immunol* 1996;156:1799–1803.

41. Silberberg-Sinakin I, Thorbecke GJ, Baer RL, et al. Antigen-bearing Langerhans cells in skin, dermal lymphatics and in lymph nodes. *Cell Immunol* 1976;25:137–151.

42. Macatonia SE, Edwards AJ, Knight SC. Dendritic cells and the initiation of contact sensitivity to fluorescein isothiocyanate. *Immunology* 1986;59:509–514.

43. Wang B, Kondo S, Shivji GM, et al. Tumour necrosis factor receptor II (p75) signalling is required for the migration of Langerhans' cells. *Immunology* 1996;88:284–288.

44. Ross EL, Barker JN, Allen MH, et al. Langerhans' cell expression of the selectin ligand, sialyl Lewis X. *Immunology* 1994;81:303–308.

45. Schwarzenberger K, Udey MC. Contact allergens and epidermal proinflammatory cytokines modulate Langerhans cell E-cadherin expression *in situ*. *J Invest Dermatol* 1996;106:553–558.

46. Frey JR, Wenk P. Experimental studies on the pathogenesis of contact eczema in the guinea pig. *Int Arch Allergy Appl Immunol* 1957;11:81–100.

47. Bevilacqua MP. Endothelial-leukocyte adhesion molecules. *Annu Rev Immunol* 1993;11:767–804.

48. Lawrence MB, Springer TA. Leukocytes roll on a selectin at physiologic flow rates: distinction from and prerequisite for adhesion through integrins. *Cell* 1991;65:859–873.

49. Elices MJ, Osborn L, Takada Y, et al. VCAM-1 on activated endothelium interacts with the leukocyte integrin VLA-4 at a site distinct from the VLA-4/fibronectin binding site. *Cell* 1990;60:577–584.

50. Dustin ML, Springer TA. Lymphocyte function-associated antigen-1 (LFA-1) interaction with intercellular adhesion molecule-1 (ICAM-1) is one of at least three mechanisms for lymphocyte adhesion to cultured endothelial cells. *J Cell Biol* 1988;107:321–331.

51. Garioch JJ, Mackie RM, Campbell I, et al. Keratinocyte expression of intercellular adhesion molecule 1 (ICAM-1) correlated with infiltration of lymphocyte function associated antigen 1 (LFA-1) positive cells in evolving allergic contact dermatitis reactions. *Histopathology* 1991;19:351–354.

52. Brasch J, Sterry W. Expression of adhesion molecules in early allergic patch test reactions. *Dermatology* 1992;185:12–17.

53. Bevilacqua MP, Pober JS, Mendrick DL, et al. Identification of an inducible endothelial-leukocyte adhesion molecule. *Proc Natl Acad Sci USA* 1987;84:9238–9242.

54. Osborn L, Hession C, Tizard R, et al. Direct expression cloning of vascular cell adhesion molecule 1, a cytokine-induced endothelial protein that binds to lymphocytes. *Cell* 1989;59:1203–1211.

55. Dustin ML, Rothlein R, Bhan AK, et al. Induction by IL1 and interferon-gamma: tissue distribution, biochemistry, and function of a natural adherence molecule (ICAM-1). *J Immunol* 1986;137:245–254.

56. Lewis RE, Buchsbaum M, Whitaker D, et al. Intercellular adhesion molecule expression in the evolving human cutaneous delayed hypersensitivity reaction. *J Invest Dermatol* 1989;93:672–677.

57. Griffiths CEM, Nickoloff BJ. Keratinocyte intercellular adhesion molecule-1 (ICAM-1) expression precedes dermal T lymphocytic infiltration in allergic contact dermatitis (*Rhus* dermatitis). *Am J Pathol* 1989;135:1045–1053.

58. Groves RW, Allen MH, Ross EL, et al. Tumour necrosis factor alpha is pro-inflammatory in normal human skin and modulates cutaneous adhesion molecule expression. *Br J Dermatol* 1995;132:345–352.

59. Waldorf HA, Walsh LJ, Schechter NM, et al. Early cellular events in evolving cutaneous delayed hypersensitivity in humans. *Am J Pathol* 1991;138:477–486.

60. Kerdel FA, Belsito DV, Scotto-Chinnici R, et al. Mast cell participation during the elicitation of murine allergic contact hypersensitivity. *J Invest Dermatol* 1987;88:686–690.

61. Askenase PW, Rosenstein RW, Ptak W. T cells produce an antigen-binding factor with *in vivo* activity analogous to IgE antibody. *J Exp Med* 1982;157:862–873.

62. Van Loveren H, Askenase PW. Delayed-type hypersensitivity is mediated by a sequence of two different T cell activities. *J Immunol* 1984;133:2397–2401.

63. Hosoi J, Murphy GF, Egan CL, et al. Regulation of Langerhans cell function by nerves containing calcitonin gene-related peptide. *Nature* 1993;363:159–163.

64. Eedy DJ. Neuropeptides in skin. *Br J Dermatol* 1993;128:597–605.

65. Ansel JC, Brown JR, Payan DG, et al. Substance P selectively activates TNF-α gene expression in murine mast cells. *J Immunol* 1993;150:4478–4485.

66. Lee HR, Ho WZ, Douglas SD. Substance P augments tumor necrosis factor release in human monocyte-derived macrophages. *Clin Diagn Lab Immunol* 1994;1:419–423.

67. Calvo CF, Chavanel G, Senik A. Substance P enhances IL-2 expression in activated human T cells. *J Immunol* 1992;148:3498–3504.

68. Fox FE, Kubin M, Cassin M, et al. Calcitonin gene-related peptide inhibits proliferation and antigen presentation by human peripheral blood mononuclear cells: effects on B7, interleukin 10, and interleukin 12. *J Invest Dermatol* 1997;108:43–48.

69. Vilcek J, Gray PW, Rinderknecht E, et al. Interferon-gamma: a lymphokine for all seasons. *Lymphokines* 1985;11:1–32.

70. Belsito DV, Epstein SP, Schultz JM, et al. Enhancement by various cytokines or 2-β-mercaptoethanol of Ia antigen expression on Langerhans cells in skin from normal aged and young mice: effect of cyclosporine A. *J Immunol* 1989;143:1530–1536.

71. Basham TY, Nickoloff BJ, Merigan TC, et al. Recombinant gamma interferon differentially regulated class II antigen expression and biosynthesis on cultured normal human keratinocytes. *J Interferon Res* 1985;5:23–32.

72. Shimada S, Caughman SW, Sharrow SO, et al. Enhanced antigen-presenting capacity of cultured Langerhans cells is associated with markedly increased expression of Ia antigen. *J Immunol* 1987;139:2551–2555.

73. Taub DD, Lloyd AR, Conlon K, et al. Recombinant human interferon-inducible protein 10 is a chemoattractant for human monocytes and T lymphocytes and promotes T cell adhesion to endothelial cells. *J Exp Med* 1993;177:1809–1814.

74. Yu X, Barnhill RL, Graves DT. Expression of monocyte chemoattractant protein-1 in delayed type hypersensitivity reactions in the skin. *Lab Invest* 1994;71:226–235.

75. Kristensen MS, Deleuran BW, Larsen CG, et al. Expression of monocyte chemotactic and activating factor (MCAF) in skin-related cells: a comparative study. *Cytokine* 1993;5:520–524.

76. Schamberg JF. Desensitization of persons against ivy poison. *JAMA* 1919;73:1213.

77. Strickler A. The value of the toxin (antigen) of *Rhus toxicodendron* and *Rhus venenata* in the treatment and desensitization of patients with dermatitis venenata. *JAMA* 1923;80:1588–1590.

78. Kligman AM. Hyposensitization against *Rhus dermatitis*. *Arch Dermatol* 1958;78:47–72.

79. Epstein WL, Baer H, Dawson CR, Khurana RG. Poison oak hyposensitization: evaluation of purified urushiol. *Arch Dermatol* 1974;109:356–360.

80. Chase MW. Inhibition of experimental drug allergy by prior feeding of the sensitizing agent. *Proc Soc Exp Biol Med* 1946;61:257–259.

81. Elmets CA, Bergstresser PR, Tigelaar RE. Analysis of the mechanism of unresponsiveness produced by haptens painted on skin exposed to low-dose ultraviolet radiation. *J Exp Med* 1983;158:781–794.

Physical Causes and Radiation Effects

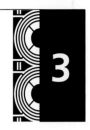

Physical Causes ■

L A S S E K A N E R V A , M . D .

MECHANICAL TRAUMA

An important task of the skin is to resist mechanical trauma. The skin is well adapted to cope with many types of trauma, but excessive friction and microtrauma can result in the formation of various dermatoses. Microtrauma includes a variety of superficial skin injuries: friction, abrasions, pressure, stretching, compressions, and cuts. Mechanical insults to the skin may affect all levels of the skin from the cornified layer through the subcutaneous fat. The time allowed for adaptation determines the reaction of the skin. Slowly increasing pressure or friction induces hyperkeratosis, lichenification, and calluses, while sudden friction can induce blisters. The effects of trauma are modified by humidity, sweating, age, sex, nutritional status, infection, and genetic and racial factors. Women may have thinner skin, containing less collagen, and they may thus be at greater risk for mechanical assaults.[1] Patients with genetic palmoplantar keratoderma develop hyperkeratosis exceptionally easily. Slight trauma induces bulla formation in epidermolysis bullosa patients.

Many cases of trauma are common and accepted as natural occurrences by workers who do not often seek occupational compensation. According to a Finnish study, 6% of occupational dermatoses were caused by mechanical factors.[2] During a 7-year period mechanical causes comprised 139 cases out of a total of 4,320 cases (3%) of occupational skin diseases in Finland.[3] The actual number is probably much higher,[4] but the cases are not reported.

Mechanical insults to the skin can cause a wide variety of clinical manifestations. The clinical picture is then a summation of the various mechanical forces on the skin. Table 3–1 and Figure 3–1 summarize some effects of mechanical trauma on the skin.

The present chapter provides an updated review of previous articles by the authors.[5–8]

 TABLE 3–1 • Skin Manifestations from Mechanical Trauma

Hyperkeratoses/calluses
Fissuring
Lichenification/hyperpigmentation
Blistering/friction injury
Pulpitis
"Black heel"/rupture of capillaries
Increased susceptibility to the effects of chemical irritants and allergens
Increased susceptibility to penetration of bacteria, fungi, viruses, and parasites
Irritant and foreign body reactions to fiberglass, nonabsorbable dusts (asbestos), and metal filings (beryllium)
Tattooing from occupational exposures to metals
Scars and keloids
Cutaneous neoplasms secondary to burns and scars
Cutaneous neoplasms secondary to repeated mechanical trauma
Koebner's phenomenon (psoriasis) from friction
Dermographic urticaria, pressure urticaria, vibratory angioedema
Raynaud's phenomenon ("white/dead" fingers) and sclerodactyly from vibration
Post-traumatic eczema
Chronic hyperkeratotic hand eczema

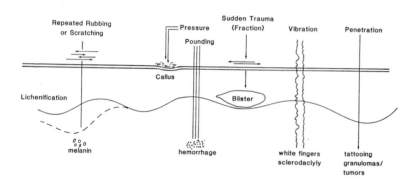

FIGURE 3–1 • A scheme of the effects of mechanical trauma to the skin.

Pressure

Prolonged or excessive pressure may produce erythema, vesicobullae, and necrosis.[8, 9] Pressure intensifies contact dermatitis.[10] Usually pressure is accompanied by friction, and this combination is mainly responsible for the callosities and deformities that constitute most of the so-called stigmata (Table 3–2) peculiar to certain occupations.[11]

Pounding

Pounding may result in rupture of the papillary capillaries. "Black heel" results from pressure and pounding in those sports where repeated jumping and sudden stops or twists of the heel occur, as in basketball, football, squash, lacrosse, track and field, and tennis. Closely aggregated clusters of bluish-black specks occur suddenly at the back or side of the heel, just above the hyperkeratotic edge of the foot.[12] An identical condition occurs on the hands of weight lifters and on the balls of the thumbs of golfers.[13] Black heel has also been reported as a melanocytic hyperplasia without mechanical cause.[14] Different types of dermatological disorders caused by mechanical trauma in athletes have been reviewed by Bergfelt and Taylor[13] and by Powell.[14]

Friction

A moderate degree of friction in everyday life is usually harmless, but excessive friction causes different types of changes in the skin. Intermittent or repeated friction (rubbing, scratching) of low intensity induces lichenification (thickening), frequently accompanied by hyperpigmentation (friction melanosis[15]). With stronger force and pressure, corns and callosities form. In the calluses, the thick horny layer is subject to painful fissures.

Friction can also cause erosions, ulcers, or blisters.[16] Friction blisters are common reactions to mechanical trauma. They seldom present a diagnostic problem, but can help to diagnose an underlying disease. The most important causative component is a shearing force horizontal to the surface; pressure, temperature, stretching, and ischemia do not seem to play a direct role in friction injury.[17] Friction blisters seldom occur on loose skin, which easily stretches.

The literature on the chronic effects of occupational mechanical trauma, including friction, is rather scanty.[4] Menné[18] described a postal worker with palmar dermatitis resulting from constant friction on the palm with a rough-surfaced table top. Menné and Hjorth[19] reported cases of frictional dermatitis in workers handling large quantities of pressure-sensitive carbonless copy paper. As pointed out by Menné,[18] frictional dermatitis is not uncommon, but very little scientific information is available. Storrs[20] reported a case of frictional dermatitis associated with paper work (Fig. 3–2), and Kanerva et al.[21] presented a case of hand dermatitis from telefax paper. Storrs[20] believes that frictional dermatitis seen on the fingertips of secretaries is one variant of the entity of hyperkeratotic hand eczema (see later discussion).

Abrasive Materials

Abrasion is a major and visible damage to the epidermis caused by friction. Abrasions facilitate

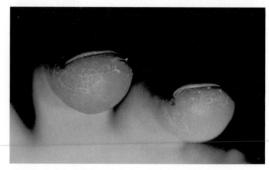

FIGURE 3–2 • Frictional dermatitis associated with paperwork—characteristically scales and fissures and does not vesicate or itch. (Courtesy of F.J. Storrs, M.D.)

TABLE 3–2 • Occupational Marks by Mechanical Trauma

Persons/Activities	Cause	Marks
Asbestos workers (carders, weavers, mattress makers)	Penetration of fibers	Corns, warts on palms
Athletes		
Basketball	Pressure and pounding	Punctate hemorrhages on heels ("black heel," calcaneal petechiae)
	Friction	Blisters
Boxing	Punch	Cauliflower ear
Gymnastics	Friction	Hyperkeratoses, callosities on the hands and feet
Jogging	Friction	Erythema, separation of toenail ("jogger's toe")
		Scaly, hyperkeratotic patches on heel ("runner's bumps")
		Erosions of the nipples ("jogger's nipples")
	Mechanical pressure	Piezogenic papules, multiple small papular projections for the heel margins accentuated by the pressure of standing (herniations of fat into the dermis)
Skiing	Friction	Shin abrasions, erosions, and ulcers ("skier's shins")
Soccer	Pressure on nails	Ingrowing nails. Tender, painful, swollen paronychial tissue; granulation tissue; lateral paronychia
Surfing	Friction	Subcutaneous, nontender masses ("surfer's nodules")
Tennis	Shearing	Splinter hemorrhages of toenails ("tennis toe")
	Pressure and pounding	Painful erythema and swelling of the great toe ("turf toe") (athletes who play on artificial turf surfaces)
Weight lifting	Mechanical pressure, stretching	Striae (consider also anabolic steroid misuse)
Bakers	Pressure on kneading board	Callosities on the palmar and cubital surface of little finger
Band jobbers	Friction of twine dragged through rollers	Excoriations and thickening on the ulnar side of the hands
Bank executives	Rubbing	Lichenification of the elbows
Barbers	Sharp hair penetrates into the skin	Inflamed interdigital papules ("barber's sinus")
Basket makers	Hammering canes with clenched fist	Thickening on the ulnar side of the palms
	Bending and intertwining hard cane	Callosity and broadening on the thumbs
	Innumerable cuts from handling materials	Cicatrices, rhagades on the palmar surface of the fingers and the hands
Blacksmiths	Heat and pressure	Bullae on palms, fingers
Burnishers of metal	Pressure of tools	Multiple callosities on hands
Butchers	Hot water and resin used in depilation of hides	Hyperkeratosis on palms

Table continued on following page

TABLE 3–2 • Occupational Marks by Mechanical Trauma *Continued*

Persons/Activities	Cause	Marks
Carpenters, joiners	Pressure of plane	Thickening, hygromata on thumbs, index fingers
Carpet installers	Pressure and friction	Hyperkeratosis on the knuckles and dorsal aspects of the hands and feet
Cement workers	Burn from occlusion with alkaline cement	Abraded skin, "cement knees"
Cotton mill workers		
Winders	Guiding yarn into clearer slot	Thickening on the right index finger
Doffers	Friction from replacing bobbins	Thickening on the web between the thumb and the forefinger
Cutters of clothing	Pressure of shears	Callosities on thumb, fingers
Cutters of fustian	Pressure of shears	Papilloma on the inner side of the thumb joint
Diamond setters	Pressure	Knuckle pads (on the third finger)
Electricians	Friction and pressure	Lichenification
Engravers	Pressure of engraving tools	Callosities on the palmar surface of the little finger
File cutters	Pressure	Hypertrophy on the right little finger
Fishermen	Handling of cables and ropes wet with salt water, especially if skin is abraded	Dermatitis on hands
Flax hacklers	Pulling flax off pins	Callosities on the right index finger
Flax spinners	Blows from the flyer	Callosities on the hypothenar eminence of the left hand
Foundry workers	Bumping or rubbing	Abrasions
Garment cutters	Rubbing of the scissors	Callosities on the thumb and middle finger
Glove makers	Pressure on knife and scissors	Callosities, deformities on hands and fingers
Grinders of lenses	Friction from abrasives	Thickening on middle finger
Hairdressers	Friction/teasing hair, sharp hair penetrates into skin	Inflamed interdigital papules (corresponds to barber's sinus)
Harp players	Friction from strings	Thickening on fingertips
Hatters		
Felt-hat sizers	Friction and immersion in hot and cold water	Keratosis, rhagades on palmar surface from wrist to fingertips
Plankers	Rolling cylinder with hands	Callosities on thenar eminences, fingers
Straw-hat makers	Picking and plaiting straw	Callosities on palms and fingers
Hod carriers	Weight bearing	Thickening on shoulders
Janitors	Friction and pressure	Lichenification
Lathe workers	Pressure and friction	Bullae, callus on palms
Leather buffers	Pressure and friction	Callosities on thumb
Leather cutters	Friction form tools	Callosities on right index finger
Leather glazers	Friction from tools	Callosities on knuckles
Miners	Friction from tools	Callosities on hands
Coal miners	Impregnation of skin with coal dust	Blue-black tattooing on upper half of the body
Molders	Droppings of molten metal	Scars from burns on dorsum of feet

TABLE 3–2 • Occupational Marks by Mechanical Trauma *Continued*

Persons/Activities	Cause	Marks
Musicians		
Brass instruments (trumpet, trombone, French horn, baritone horn, tuba)	Pressure, friction	Upper lip callus, perioral/lip dermatitis due to mouthpiece irritation or allergy, hand dermatitis from polishing compounds
Cello	Pressure, friction	Left-finger callus, cellist's chest, cellist's knee, cellist's scrotum
Clarinet	Pressure, friction	Lower-lip callus, clarinetist's cheilitis
Flute	Pressure, friction	Flautist's chin
Harp	Pressure, friction	Onycholyysis, subungual hemorrhages, paronychia
Oboe	Pressure, friction	Upper lip callus
Piano	Pressure, friction	Vasospastic white finger disease, paronychia
Recorder	Pressure, friction	Perioral (lip) dermatitis due to irritation or allergy to exotic woods
Saxophone	Pressure	Lower lip callus, cheilitis
Viola	Pressure, friction	Left-finger callus, fiddler's neck, exacerbation of pseudofolliculitis of the beard
Violin	Pressure, friction	Left-finger callus, fiddler's neck, exacerbation of pseudofolliculitis of the beard, Garrod's pads
Paperhangers	Friction and pressure	Lichenification
Plumbers	Friction and pressure	Lichenification
Porters		
Alabaster blocks	Weight bearing, friction	Lichenification
Boxes, cases	Weight bearing, friction	Callosities on shoulders
Timber	Carrying logs	Bullae on hands
Potters	Friction of revolving lathe	Horny thickening, atrophy of skin on left hand
Printers, compositors	Pressure of type	Callosities on fingertips
Shoemakers	Pressure of tools	Callosities on folds of fingers, thigh above patella
Cobblers	Cutting leather	Scars from cuts on right thigh
Stakers, glazers	Pressure	Knuckle pads on the dorsum of the hands
Stenographers	Pressure of pencil	Callosities on the middle finger
Stone workers	Pressure of tools, impregnation with particles	Bullae and tattooing, pigmentation on palms and dorsa of hands
Sugar workers	Manipulating machine cutting cubes	Callosities between fingers
Tile, floor, and linoleum layers	Friction and pressure	Lichenification on knees
Typists	Pressure	Callosities on the thumbs
Washerwomen	Friction against edge of washtub	Callosities on the inner surface of the forearms

Modified from Ronchese F. *Occupational Marks and Other Physical Signs: A Guide to Personal Identification.* New York: Grune & Stratton; 1948.

the entry of allergens and irritants into the skin. Friction and other microtrauma may contribute to irritant and allergic contact dermatitis.

The chamber-scarification test of Frosch and Kligman[22] can be used to study the combined effects of abrasions and mechanical irritants. The skin is scored with a 30-gauge needle in a grid pattern, and the irritant test solution is then applied to the test site. The needle abrades and lacerates the horny layer, and the combined effect of the irritant and mechanical trauma can be investigated. The irritant effects of abrasive materials have been reviewed by Fleming and Bergfelt.[23]

Plants may induce mechanical irritant dermatitis from delicate hairs called *trichromes* or hairs with tiny barbs knowns as *glochids*. Sabra dermatitis is an irritant dermatitis seen in workers who pick the fruit of prickly pears, which possess small barbed bristles.[24] The awns of barley and other cereal grasses may cause a mechanical occupational dermatitis.[24] Dieffenbachia,[25] daffodil *(Narcissus)*, and hyacinth *(Hyacintus)* are plants that possess fine, needle-shaped calcium oxalate crystals.[24] The irritation caused by these plants is thought to be induced by both the mechanical action of the oxalate crystal and the subsequent penetration of a plant enzyme or toxin into the skin.[26] Irritant plants have recently been reviewed by Lovell.[27] Tiny glass needles have been reported to penetrate into the skin of workers in a fluorescent lamp factory.[28]

Abrasive material in occupational settings includes sharp-textured small particles (e.g., machinists may develop irritant dermatitis from metal chips [shavings, swarf] present in cutting fluids).[29] Abrasive mineral dusts have caused dermatitis in miners.[30] Wool and fiberglass textiles may produce an occupational dermatitis through a mechanical irritant effect.[31] Nonoccupational frictional dermatitis has also been reported from artificial fur[32] and pantyhose.[33]

Hyperkeratotic Hand Eczema from Friction and Pressure

Chronic hyperkeratotic dermatitis is chiefly encountered in middle-aged or elderly men. It may be a manifestation of psoriasis.[34] Hersle and Mobacken's 10-year review[35] of 32 cases did not support this view, however. Thirteen of their patients had been engaged in hard manual work. They proposed a real clinical entity of hyperkeratotic hand eczema. Wilkinson[36] suggested that friction and pressure play a determining role in this condition. The condition is severe and accounted for 2.5% of all applications for permanent disability determined in a Danish study.[34] Hyperkeratotic

dermatitis of the palms was recently reviewed by Menné,[37] and he accepted this disease as a separate entity, independent of psoriasis and of mechanical irritation.

Post-Traumatic Eczema

It is known from clinical practice that dermatitis recurs at the site of prior cutaneous trauma. The interval between injury and the development of eczema was considered by Calnan[38] to be about 2 weeks. Wilkinson[39] had a patient who 1 week after a caustic soda burn developed a discoid eczema that persisted for 15 months. Another of his patients developed eczema 3 weeks after an accident, and a year later the eczema spread to other sites. Zuehlke et al.[40] reported 13 patients with predilective development of eczema in previously damaged skin and called it *dermatitis in loco minoris resistentiae*. They adapted the term from *locus minoris resistentiae*, meaning a site of diminished resistance. The skin had mainly been damaged by surgery or burns, and Zuehlke et al.[40] speculated that injury might have caused permanent changes in the skin structures resulting in functional alterations.

Mathias[41] reported 13 similar cases, which he termed *post-traumatic eczema* (Table 3–3). The injuries were mainly of occupational origin. Eczema started within a few weeks after the trauma, and the individual lesions recurred for up to 8 years. The age of the patients ranged between 20 and 55 years, and five had a personal history of atopy. Mathias[41] divided post-traumatic eczema into two types. It may occur in association with an underlying endogenous eczema or as an isolated idiopathic reaction when endogenous eczema is absent. Post-traumatic eczema has to be differentiated from other eczematous and noneczematous disorders such as trauma-induced psoriasis, foreign body reaction, and recurrent herpes simplex precipitated by trauma. Superimposed allergic contact dermatitis from topical preparations used to treat the eczematous skin must be excluded.

When the injury occurs as a result of a job-related accident, it may be covered under state workers' compensation.[41] This has been accepted, for example, in Sweden and Finland for more than 30 years.

Compromised Skin

Bruynzeel and de Boer[42] introduced the term *compromised skin*. The term is explained as follows. Clinically healed skin needs a long period of rest before it no longer reacts with an exacerbation of the dermatitis after minor insults like dish wash-

TABLE 3–3 • Clinical Summary of Cases with Post-Traumatic Eczema

Case No.	Time from Injury to Onset (Weeks)	Occupation	Associated Skin Condition	Injury Type	Site	Time from Onset to Last Follow-Up
1	3	Painter	Stasis dermatitis	Abrasion	Ankle	6 Months
2	4	Wine blender	Atopic dermatitis	Laceration	Finger	10 Months
3	3	Student	Atopic dermatitis	Sunburn	Heels	2 Weeks
4	3	Machinist	Irritant dermatitis	Puncture	Finger	6 Weeks
5	3	Farmer	Obesity	Thermal burn	Both calves	8 Years
6	3	Truck mechanic	None	Abrasion	Shin	8 Years
7	3	Painter	None	Abrasion	Finger	1 Year
8	3	Electrical assembler	Fungal infection on soles, opposite palm	Laceration	Thumb	2 Months
9	3	Machine assembler	None	Laceration	Thumb	3 Months
10	3	Butcher	Bacterial infection	Laceration	Skin, calf	2 Years
11	3	Maintenance mechanic	None	Puncture	Palm	3 Years
12	3	Machine operator	None	Thermal burn	Dorsal hand	7 Months
13	3	Gardner	None	Laceration	Thigh	3 Months

Adapted from Mathias CGT. Post-traumatic eczema. *Dermatol Clin* 1988; 6:35–42.

ing. The skin is still irritable and is apparently not normal because of the previous inflammation. This skin Bruynzeel and de Boer[42] called *compromised*.

Pulpitis

Fingertip eczema, known as *pulpite* in France, localizes to the pulps rather than to the backs of the fingers. Cronin[43] describes pulpitis as a dry, scaly, fissured, painful change on the pulps of the fingers of young women. She finds it common, although seldom reported. It may be endogenous, but is worsened by, for example, domestic work by housewives. Probably mechanical factors are also involved. Burton[44] and Wilkinson[45] recognized two patterns. The first involves preferentially the thumb and forefinger of the masterhand, but all of the fingers may be involved. The second affects the thumb and first two fingers of the masterhand and is usually occupational, caused by repetitive handling of items such as newspapers.[45] Pulpitis responds poorly to all forms of treatment. We have often encountered the same clinical picture in dental personnel with allergic patch-test reactions to acrylate compounds.[46, 47] The pulpitis cases in our patients have healed slowly and have been accompanied by acrylate-induced paresthesias of the fingertips.[46, 47]

The Isomorphic Koebner Response

The presence of certain underlying diseases may result in replication and aggravation of those diseases in the area of injury. Psoriasis and lichen planus are classic examples. The palm of the hand is usually the area of involvement. As examples of psoriatic lesions after trauma from occupation, Samitz[17] mentions palmar psoriasis in seamstresses working in the garment industry, in machinists and lathe workers who have developed lesions from gripping tools, in a pushcart peddler from the cart's hand grips, and in a pharmacist from twirling finger movements while handling bottle caps. Psoriatics should be advised not to enter jobs in which the possibility of mechanical trauma is obvious. The differential diagnoses include noneczematous skin diseases associated with Koebner's phenomenon, foreign body reactions, bacterial infections, herpes simplex recidivans, and a secondary allergic contact dermatitis to topical preparations.[48]

Occupational Marks

Occupational marks represent the effects of a particular occupation on a worker's skin. They are usually calluses or corns that develop in locations subjected to repeated friction, pressure, or other trauma and include discolorations, telangiectases, tattoos, odors, deformities, and other changes. In some occupations, the marks may be quite variable (e.g., musicians).[49] Earlier such marks were common among workers and served to identify many occupations. Today, with increasing automation, less frequent manual operation of tools, better protective clothing, and a shorter work week, occupational marks have become less frequent. They have almost disappeared from many industries, but can probably still be found in less industrialized countries. Table 1–2 lists a large number of occupational marks based on Ronchese's classic and valuable book[11] and articles by Samitz,[17] Harvell and Maibach,[49] Powell[14] and others. Occupational marks must be distinguished from so-called pseudo-occupational marks, such as knuckle pads, knuckle biting, nail biting, cuticle pulling, and trichotillomania.

Occupational Skin Granulomas

Foreign substances penetrating the skin may induce granulomas. Granulomas are palpable nodular lesions varying in size from a few millimeters to centimeters.[50] Foreign body granulomas are caused by substances such as silk, wool, nylon, paraffin, talcum powder, oils, and plants.[26, 50] Young et al.[51] reported a case of a foreign body granuloma induced by graphite fibers in a golf club. Foreign body granulomas have also been reported from barium sulfate contained in the liquid core of golf balls.[52, 53] Allergic granulomas may be caused by contact allergic reactions triggered by exposure to zirconium, beryllium, and tattoo pigments.[54] Milkers' hand, caused by the penetration of cow hairs into the skin during milking, is an occupational skin granuloma. Similar granulomas may be induced in hairdressers from human hair.

Sensitization in Traumatized Skin

It is believed that the majority of the cases of occupational contact allergic sensitivity develop on a preexisting dermatitis caused by irritants, pressure, friction, sweating, and prolonged immersion in water. Some examples are mentioned. Fischer and Rystedt[55] considered that the traumatic frictional effect of grinding and etching was an important factor in the development of cobalt allergy in hard-metal workers. The high incidence of allergic sensitization in hospital cleaning personnel[56] may be due partly to the trauma encountered in this work. Gloves are the most important cause of occupationally induced allergic rubber dermatitis.[57, 58] This might be due to the fact that protective gloves are not taken into use before a preexisting eczema has already developed. Cuts, wounds, and abrasions incurred on the job, while not very serious injuries per se, should be regarded as having greater clinical importance insofar as they increase the likelihood of contact sensitization to allergens.[59] Workers themselves may disregard such traumas as unimportant and unworthy of attention, but later allergic reactions may cause considerable distress and may even require a change of jobs.[59]

Mechanically Induced Epidermal Carcinogenesis

Repeated mechanical injuries are capable of enhancing papillomas and carcinomas in mouse skin.[60] Repeated mechanical trauma at work could predispose to epidermal neoplasms, but this has not been proven.[60] Malignancies occurring in burn scars have been accepted as occupational cancers.[61] About 15% of Canadian farmers with skin cancer reported a past history of trauma or frostbite in the involved area.[62]

Mechanically Induced Urticaria

Urticarias resulting from nonchemical insults are classified as physical urticarias (Table 3–4) and are dealt with later in the chapter. The dermographic urticaria (Fig. 3–3), pressure urticaria, and vibratory angioedema are induced mechanically.

Effects of Mechanical Trauma on Nails

This is discussed in Chapter 9. We recently reported two hairdressers with occupational koilonychia from a combined effect of mechanical trauma and ammonium thiglycolate present in solutions for permanent waves (Fig. 3–4).[63]

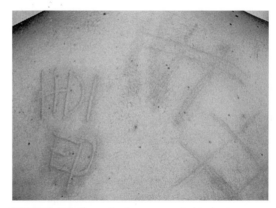

FIGURE 3–3 • The patient was suspected to have an occupational dermatitis from 1,6-hexamethylene diisocyanate (HDI) but turned out to have a severe dermographic urticaria.

Mechanical Acro-Osteolysis

Among many other etiological factors, mechanical trauma may cause acro-osteolysis (see Table 6–6).[64–66]

Choice of Gloves for Protection Against Mechanical Hazards

Gloves give good protection against minor injuries.[67] Leather and textile gloves protect against abrasions, lacerations and cuts, and brief exposure to heat. They also minimize the effects of impacts and protect in welding. Leather gloves can be reinforced by steel staples or studs to improve their cut resistance. Textile gloves can be im-

TABLE 3–4 • Urticarias Induced by Mechanical Insults to the Skin	
Type	**Stimulus**
Dermographism	Stroking, scratching, rubbing
Pressure	Pressure
Vibratory angioedema (nonhereditary)	Vibration
Koebner's phenomenon in chronic idiopathic urticaria	Local pressure
Hereditary angioedema	Local pressure or "knocks"

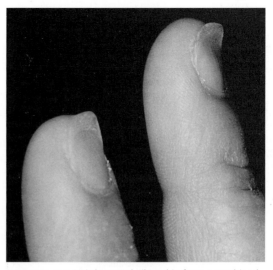

FIGURE 3–4 • Hairdresser's koilonychia from a combined effect of chemicals (thioglycolate in permanent wave solutions) and repeated, low-grade mechanical trauma.

proved by rubber or plastic coatings, which also increase the slip resistance of the grip. Gloves with metal mesh have been developed for meat cutters and slaughterers. Metal-mesh gloves made of welded nickel-plated brass or stainless steel are used in the textile industry.[67] Gloves, such as ones made of polyurethane, may give some protection against vibration, thus reducing the risk of developing Raynaud's phenomenon and the vibration syndrome.[68, 69]

HEAT

Burns

Burns result from exposure to extremes of heat. The lowest temperature at which a burn can occur has been estimated to be 44°C (111°F).[70] Burns may be of industrial, domestic, or environmental origin. Industrial burns are common[71] and may have characteristic occupational patterns. Although in the United States, Great Britain, and many other countries dermatologists rarely treat burns, they frequently are requested to evaluate impairment of patients with healed burns. Scarring and pigmentary alteration are the chief sequelae for consideration. Sometimes scarring is extensive enough to limit joint mobility in addition to producing varying degrees of disfigurement.

Classification of burns is based on the depth of the burn. The depth of skin injury is classified as first, second, or third degree (Table 3–5).[72]

Burns may cause either hyperpigmentation or hypopigmentation. When total loss of pigment occurs, it denotes deeper burns with destruction of melanocytes, and recovery of skin color is doubtful. With more superficial burns, hyperpigmenta-

tion may result, depending on the depth of the burn and the genetic background of the patient. Blacks and other pigmented persons show the greatest hyperpigmentation, which on the face and other exposed areas may be greatly disfiguring. Fading occurs slowly; a final evaluation of permanency should not be made until 18 to 24 months after the burn has completely healed.

Electrical Burns

Electrical burns are of increasing importance with the growth of electrical apparatuses and installations. Out of 290 fatal factory accidents in Great Britain, 21 were due to electric shock. A larger number died from burns with domestic 240 V current.[71] The body lesions are due to heat and direct injury by electricity.[12] High-voltage burns are severe, while low-voltage burns are milder but penetrate more deeply than is apparent following nerves and vessels, extending some distance away from the edge of the visible wound. Late rupture of blood vessels is particularly likely to occur, even as long as 3 weeks after the burn. Electrothermal burns may be caused by grasping a heated electrical element. Burns from cardiac defibrillators have caused local skin ulcers. The depth of an electric flash burn depends on the temperature of the agent and the duration of the contact. Flash burns from atomic explosions were extensive and bizarrely patterned.[12] Campbell and coworkers[73] reported high-voltage electrical injury in two hang-glider pilots from 11,000 V power lines. Magnetic resonance imaging is a new diagnostic aid in the care of high-voltage electrical burns.[74]

Burns from lightning cause a bizarre, superficial erythema that Bartholome et al.[75] considered pa-

TABLE 3–5 • Classification of Burns Based on the Depth of the Burns

Classification of Burns	Surface Appearance	Sensation	Outcome/Prognosis
First degree	Dry, erythematous, no blisters	Painful, hypersensitive	Complete healing within 1 week; no scar
Second degree, superficial	Blisters, red oozing base, good capillary refill, blanching on pressure	Painful, extremely sensitive to pinprick	Complete healing within 3 weeks; may be erythematous early after healing
Second degree, deep	Blisters may be present; pale, indurated areas; some areas red	Some insensitive areas; many areas anesthetic to pinprick	Firm, thick scar with loss of hair follicles, sweat glands, and skin pigmentation; healing may take 1 month
Third degree	Pearly white or brown opaque gray; firm, leathery, dry	No sensation	Total skin loss, includes all appendages; heals by scar formation if small

Adapted from Burke JF, Bondoc CC. Burns: The management and evaluation of the thermally injured patient. In: Fitzpatrick TB, Eisen AZ, Wolff K, et al., eds. *Dermatology in General Medicine,* 4th ed. New York: McGraw-Hill; 1993:1592–1598.

thognomonic. The skin shows numerous erythematous macules arranged in a streaked featherlike or fernlike pattern. Blanching on diascopy does not occur, and in those persons who survive, fading occurs in 24 to 48 hours. The condition is probably due to the transmission of static electricity along the superficial vasculature, similar to that occurring when an electrodessiccating current is used to destroy small angiomas. Lightning injuries are occupational risks of outdoor workers such as railroad and highway construction workers, surveyors, geologists, foresters, and agricultural workers. The heat torch, capable of generating a blast of hot air up to 1,000°F within 1 or 2 minutes, can cause severe burns when operated improperly, especially when used as a hand tool. Considerable ultraviolet light is also emitted.

Chemical Ulcers and Burns

Many chemicals in industry and the home cause burns (Table 3–6). Of 95 chemical burns observed at an English hospital,[71] 39 were caused by acids, 19 by alkalis, and 28 by other inorganic agents. Bruze and Fregert[76] and Holland et al.[77] have reviewed the causes of chemical burns (Table 3–6). A few of the more important causes are mentioned below.

Acids and Alkalis

Potassium hydroxide and sulfuric acid are the most common causes of chemical burns. Strong acids cause necrosis and discolor tissues, while alkalis saponify fats and form proteinates.[12] Concentrated sodium hydroxide is especially hazardous, producing extensive tissue destruction and scarring.

Calcium Salts

Soda ash (calcium carbonate, Ca_2CO_3) is an important commercial alkaline salt that is used to manufacture soap, paper, and glass and in the textile dyeing industry. It combines with perspiration and can cause ulcers.[78] Quicklime, or calcium oxide (CaO), is used in steel manufacture, leather tanning, glass production, and in the production of various calcium products. It also combines with sweat and can cause ulcers.[78]

Cement

Wet cement is highly alkaline and can cause cement burns.[79–81] The common feature is a skin contact of 2 to 6 hours with freshly mixed cement under pressure in the region of the knees ("cement knees" Fig. 3–5; see also next section).[82] Healing occurs spontaneously during several weeks or

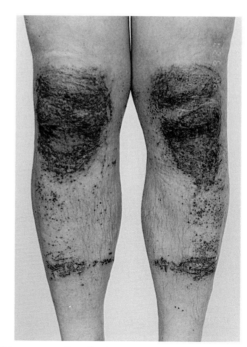

FIGURE 3–5 • Nonallergic cement knees caused by wet cement. (Courtesy of R. Suhonen.)

months. Onuba and Essiet[83] reported two cases of direct thermal burns from *hot* cement powder.

Chromic Acid/Chromates

Chrome ulcers or "chrome holes" are the most common lesions resulting from occupational exposure to chromium. Chromic acid can produce renal failure,[71] and hexavalent chrome or dichromate is also associated with about a 10-fold increase in lung cancer in long-term workers.[84] Chromium dermatoses are dealt with in more detail in Chapter 24.

Ethylene Oxide Burns

Nineteen hospitalized women postoperatively suffered from severe burns of the buttocks and back from contact with reusable surgical gowns and drapes that had been sterilized with ethylene oxide and had not been properly aerated.[85] (See Chapter 1.)

Hydrofluoric Acid

This extremely strong acid is widely used in industry and research. Burns are characterized by intense, often delayed pain and deep tissue necrosis, which progresses for days. Burns due to hydrofluoric acid in concentrations under 30% develop slowly over several hours, becoming more devastating as the fluoride penetrates into subcutaneous tissue. Skin contact should be dealt with

TABLE 3–6 • Agents Causing Chemical Burns

Acids	Alkalis	Miscellaneous	Miscellaneous *Continued*
Acetic	Amines	Acetyl chloride	Glutaraldehyde
Acrylic	Ammonia	Acrolein	Halogenated solvents
Benzoic	Barium hydroxide	Acrylonitril	Hexylresorcinol
Boric	Calcium carbonate	Alkali ethoxides	Iodine
Bromoacetic	Calcium hydroxide	Alkali methoxides	Isocyanates
Chlorosulfuric	Hydrazine	Aluminium bromide	Kerosene fuel
Fluorophosphoric	Lithium hydroxide	Aluminium chloride	Limonene
Fluorosilic	Lye	Aluminium trichloride	Lithium
Fluorosulfonic	Potassium hydroxide	Ammonium difluoride	Lithium chloride
Formic	Sodium carbonate	Ammonium persulfate	Mercury compounds
Fumaric	Sodium hydroxide	Ammonium sulfide	Methylchloroisothiazolinone
Hydrobromic	Sodium metasilicate	Antimone trioxide	Methylenedichloride
Hydrochloric		Aromatic hydrocarbons	Methylisothiazolinone
Hydrofluoric		Arsenic oxides	Morpholine
Lactic		Benzene	Perchloroethylene
Nitric		Benzoyl chloride	Peroxides
Perchloric		Benzoyl chlorodimethyl	Benzoyl
Peroxyacetic		hydantoin	Cumene
Phosphonic		Benzoyl chloroformiate	Cyclohexanone
Phosphoric		Borax	Hydrogen
Phthalic		Boron tribromide	Methylethyl ketone
Picric		Bromine	Potassium
Propionic		Bromotrifluoride	Sodium
Salicylic		Calcium carbide	Tetrahydronaphth
Sulfonic		Cantharides	Phenolic compounds
Sulfuric		Carbon disulfide	Phosphorus
Tartaric		Carbon tetrachloride	Phosphorous bromides
Toluenesulfonic		Chlorobenzene	Phosphorous chlorides
Tungstic		Chlorinated acetophenons (tear gas)	Phosphorous oxychloride
		Chlorinated solvents	Phosphorous oxides
		Chloroform	Piperazine
		Chlorocresols	Potassium
		Chlorophenols	Potassium cyanide
		Chromates	Potassium difluoride
		Chromium oxichloride	Potassium hypochlorite
		Chromium trioxide	Potassium permanganate
		Creosote	Propionic oxide
		Cresolic compounds	Propylene oxide
		Croton aldehyde	Quaternary ammonium compounds
		Dichloroacetyl chloride	Reactive diluents
		Dichromates	Sodium
		Dimethyl acetamide	Sodium borohydride
		Dimethyl formamide	Sodium difluoride
		Dimethyl sulfoxide	Sodium hypochlorite
		Dioxane	Sodium sulfite
		Dipentene	Sodium thiosulfate
		Dithranol	Styrene
		Epichlorohydrine	Sulfur dichloride
		Epoxy reactive diluents	Sulfur dioxide
		Ethylene oxide	Sulfur mustard
		Ferric chloride hexahydrate	Thioglycolates
		Fluorides	Thionyl chloride
		Fluorine	Tributylin oxide
		Fluorosilicate	Trichloroethylene
		Formaldehyde	Turpentine
		Gasoline	White spirit
		Gentian violet	Zinc chloride

The chemicals listed are the most commonly reported causes of chemical burns in industries, hobbies, and households. The list contains strong corrosive substances and also less irritating compounds that require special conditions; for example, occlusion, to give chemical burns.

From Bruze M, Fregert S. Chemical skin burns. In: Menné T, Maibach HI, eds. *Hand Eczema.* Boco Raton, Fla: CRC Press; 1994:21–30.

immediately with abundant washing with water or a saturated solution of sodium bicarbonate. Ten percent calcium gluconate is infiltrated intralesionally. Surgical debridement may be required later as in all chemical burns. (See Chapter 1.)

Phenol

Phenol causes numerous toxic effects. It is rapidly absorbed through intact skin. Local necrosis is proportionate to concentration.

Phosphorus

During the 19th century, poisoning due to white phosphorus (also called *yellow phosphorus*) was one of the chief occupational hazards of the kitchen match industry. Entering the workers' decayed teeth, the phosphorus caused severe damage to deep tissues and bone, a condition known as *phossy jaw*. In addition to its toxic properties, white phosphorus can cause very destructive burns. The small amount used in Napalm B during the Vietnam conflict caused deep, extensive burns on its victims. A curious accompaniment of such injuries, even when only 10 to 15% of the body surface is burned, is sudden and unexplained death. The cause is not understood, but death may result from cardiac arrhythmias secondary to hypocalcemia and hyperphosphatemia.[86] White phosphorus is still used in the manufacture of rat poisons, fireworks, and other incendiaries; in the semiconductor industry; and as an intermediate for the synthesis of other phosphorus compounds.

Potassium Cyanide

Potassium cyanide can cause skin ulcers, which are as indolent as chrome holes.[78]

Miliaria

Miliaria is caused by sweat retention. Heat causes swelling of the keratin within sweat ducts, resulting in poral closure and rupture of the ducts immediately beneath the obstruction. If the obstruction occurs within the stratum corneum, miliaria crystallina (sudamina) results, producing small, clear vesicles that soon rupture, resulting in desquamation. Cutaneous bacteria, particularly staphylococci, play a role in the pathogenesis of miliaria.[87] The skin surface may be faintly erythematous or is not associated with erythema. It is most commonly seen clinically after mild damage to the epidermis such as after sunburn. The condition occurs frequently on the palms and in intertriginous areas. While miliaria crystallina is usually asymptomatic, patients may become concerned when they suddenly notice the entire palm is dequamating.[88] Widespread involvement may in rare cases interfere with thermoregulation.

When closure occurs somewhat deeper in the epidermis, in the granular layer, firm vesicles are formed accompanied by marked pruritus. Called *miliaria rubra*, or *prickly heat*, it is easily confused with contact dermatitis. This condition is more troublesome than miliaria crystallina because the eruption may be quite extensive and accompanied by paroxysms of burning and itching. The lesions are small erythematous macules and vesicles unassociated with follicular openings; a hand lens aids in visualization. The lesions may appear a few days after exposure to a hot, humid environment, but most commonly appear after several months.

The trunk and intertriginous areas are especially involved. The palms and soles are spared. When poral closure is severe, hyperpyrexia and heat exhaustion occur, causing a decrease in work efficiency. The lesions that later develop may be pustular from infiltration of inflammatory cells and may be complicated by secondary bacterial invasion.

If obstruction is deep in the epidermis or in the upper dermis miliaria profunda (mamillaria) results,[89] producing deep-seated asymptomatic vesicles that appear much like gooseflesh, but close examination shows that they spare the follicles. The lesions consist of pale white papules 1 to 3 mm in diameter, which are most prominent on the trunk. Erythema and pruritus are mild or absent. This serious condition is caused by widespread inactivation of sweat glands from prolonged exposure to a hot environment. It usually follows an extended period of miliaria rubra. Heat exhaustion and collapse are common sequelae. A condition called *tropical anhidrotic asthenia* with acute fatigue, nausea, dizziness, palpitations, tachycardia, and malaise has been observed among military personnel during wartime in very hot, humid environments. Tropical anhidrotic asthenia is secondary to widespread miliaria profunda in particularly adverse conditions.[90]

Treatment of miliaria consists of cooling the patient to reduce sweating. Mild, nonocclusive lotions may be used. In miliaria crystallina removal of the damaged area by mechanical means or by natural sloughing stops the process.

In miliaria rubra a week of rest from the inciting factors allows removal of the damaged portion of the epidermis by natural desquamation, while in miliaria profunda rest in cool surroundings for several weeks is needed for complete recovery. Systemic and topical steroids are useless.

Occupations where excessive heat exposure can occur are listed in Table 3–7.

TABLE 3–7 • Workers Potentially Exposed to Excessive Heat

Animal rendering workers
Asphalt workers
Bakers
Bitumen workers
Boiler heaters
Cannery workers
Chemical plant operators working near hot
    containers and furnaces
Cleaners
Coke oven operators
Cooks and other kitchen workers
Firemen
Foundry workers
Glass manufacturing workers
Greenhouse workers
Kiln workers
Maintenance workers in nuclear plants
Miners in deep mines
Outdoor workers during hot weather
Sailors in hot climatic zones
Shipyard workers when cleaning cargo holds
Smelter workers
Steel and metal forgers
Textile manufacturing workers
    (weaving, dyeing)
Tire (rubber) manufacturing workers
Workers wearing tight protective clothing (all
    occupations), e.g., maintenance worker in
    nuclear plants

Erythema Ab Igne

Infrared radiation, composed of wavelengths of 800 to 170,000 nm, results in thermal burns at temperatures over 44°C.[91] Chronic exposure to heat can result in erythema ab igne and skin cancer. Characterized by a mottled, reticulate hyperemia with melanoderma and teleangiectases, erythema ab igne occurs after prolonged exposure to heat (i.e., infrared radiation), which is usually insufficient to produce burn. After months or years of such exposure hyperkeratotic nodules appear along with skin changes resembling those seen in chronic actinic exposure. At one time the condition was common on the anterior legs and inner thighs of women who sat for long periods before an open fire and on the abdomens of patients with chronic abdominal pain who applied heating pads for hours at a time. New cases are now being seen as heating with wood fires has become more common again. A resurgence of the condition in the United States occurs not only in elderly people but also in "impecunious students"[92] because of the high cost of central heating. Heater cushions still cause erythema ab igne.[93] Erythema ab igne

may be a sign leading one to suspect hypothyroidism. It has also been reported as a marker of chronic pancreatitis.[94]

Workers who may develop erythema ab igne include stokers, blacksmiths, glassblowers, foundry workers, bakers (especially those using old-fashioned brick-lined ovens), and cooks and others working over a heat source. Schwartz et al.[78] described the condition in stenographers who sit very close to radiators in cold weather. According to Wilkinson,[12] it also occurs in silversmiths and jewellers. In mentally disturbed patients with thermophilia bizarre areas of erythema ab igne have been encountered.[12]

Infrared Elastosis

Infrared radiation may significantly enhance aging and the carcinogenic effects of ultraviolet radiation.[92, 94] Kligman and Kligman[92] reported a woman who sat under a hood-type hair dryer for 1.5 hours a day for 7 years. She developed pouches of lax, inelastic skin on both cheeks.

Erythermalgia

Erythermalgia is a syndrome of bilateral symmetrical burning and redness of the lower, or sometimes upper, extremities. Symptoms can be initiated by exercise or exposure to heat, while rest and cold bring relief.[95, 96] Primary erythermalgia usually arises in childhood. Secondary erythermalgia develops in adults with or without an underlying disorder. Aspirin has given the best results,[95] but treatment may be difficult, and symptoms may persist throughout life. Secondary erythermalgia can arise as a side effect of drugs, but otherwise the etiology is unknown.[96, 97]

Heat-Induced Carcinomas

After an interval of up to over 30 years, thermal skin injury and erythema ab igne may proceed to cancer.[98] These carcinomas include the Kang cancer of northwest China from sleeping on beds of hot bricks[99] and the Kangri cancer of Kashmir, India. Kangri is an earthenware pot covered with wickerwork in which charcoal is burned. The pots are worn against the body for heat, exposing the skin to temperatures of 65° to 95°C. Burns, scars, ulcerations, and squamous cell cancers can result.[90, 100] Kairo cancer of Japan from carrying metallic benzene-burning flasks for warmth is a similar type of carcinoma. In some parts of India there are cancers of the hard palate due to smoking a local type of cigar, called *chutta*, with the burning end inside the mouth.[90] Over 160 cases of "turf" or "peat fire" cancers arising on erythema ab igne of the lower leg have been reported in rural Irishwomen from standing for long hours in front of open hearths containing burning peat.[95, 101] Basal cell carcinomas have been reported at the site of the cheeks from wearing rimless glasses. Increased temperature due to focusing of sun rays on the cheeks has been considered the cause.[102] Squamous cell carcinomas arising in burn scars are discussed in Chapter 8.

Intertrigo

A macerated, erythematous eruption in body folds—intertrigo—can occur from excessive sweating, especially in obese persons. Rubbing of opposing surfaces in addition to sweat retention are important etiological factors. Secondary bacterial or candidal infection commonly accompanies intertrigo. The groin, axillae, and interdigital areas are favored sites. In particular, the interdigital space between the third and fourth fingers is a common site for intertrigo and secondary candidal infection among cannery workers, bartenders, medical and dental personnel, and others performing wet work for prolonged periods. Cooks, swimming instructors, nurses, and others exposed to moisture are also disposed to this condition.

Heat and Urticaria

Physical exercise plus overheating may result in cholinergic urticaria and in the rare exercise-induced anaphylaxis. Contact with heat can induce heat contact urticaria. The different types of physical urticarias are dealt with in Chapter 6.

Miscellaneous Conditions

Acne vulgaris and rosacea are aggravated by prolonged chronic exposure to heat, especially intense heat from ovens, steam, open furnaces, or heat torches. Herpes simplex may be triggered by sudden blasts of heat. Prolonged exposure to excessive heat also increases irritability, decreases workers' ability to concentrate, and results in a generally lower level of efficiency.

COLD

The ability to work in a cold environment is dependent on the functional integrity of brain and limbs. Cooling the brain leads to confusion and later to incoordination, while cooling the limbs results in numbing and clumsiness, making the performance of intricate tasks difficult.

Everybody reacts to cold, but in addition to the physiological responses to cold, abnormal reactions may occur in some individuals. Chilblains may result from chronic exposure to moderate cold. Cold plays an important role in, for example, Raynaud's phenomenon and cryoglobulinemia, and cold urticaria occurs in 3 to 4% of patients with cryoglobulinemia.[95] Accordingly, cutaneous reactions to cold can be divided into reactions to abnormal cold and abnormal reactions to "normal" cold. The diseases caused or aggravated by cold are listed in Table 3–8.

Cold Injury

There are three stages of freezing cold injury: first, massive vasoconstriction causing a rapid fall in skin temperature; second, the hunting phenomenon, that is, transient cyclic vasodilation by the opening of arteriovenous anastomoses causing a cyclic rise and fall in skin temperature; and third, if cold exposure continues, freezing, as the skin temperature falls to approach ambient temperature.[95, 103]

The events that occur after freezing and nonfreezing cold injury are similar and include arterial and arteriolar vasoconstriction, excessive venular and capillary vasodilation, increased endothelial leakage, erythrostasis, arteriovenous shunting, segmental vascular necrosis, and massive thrombosis.[95]

The degree of cellular injury depends on the minimum temperature; the duration of time at that

 TABLE 3–8 • Diseases Caused or Aggravated by Cold

Reactions to Abnormal Cold
  Cold injury
  Frostbite
  Nonfreezing cold injury
    Immersion or trench foot
    Immersion foot
    Tropical immersion foot

Abnormal Reactions to Cold
  Perniosis
  Pulling-boat hands
  Acrocyanosis
  Erythrocyanosis
  Livedo reticularis
  Cold urticaria
  Cold erythema
  Cold panniculitis
  Sclerema neonatorum
  Subcutaneous fat necrosis of the newborn
  Cryoglobulinemia
  Raynaud's phenomenon

temperature; the cooling rate, with rapid cooling causing more destructive intracellular ice crystal formation and hence more destruction as is obvious from cryotherapy; and rewarming rate. In slow rewarming, intracellular ice crystals become larger and more lethal for the cell. Finally, repeated freeze-thaw cycles lead to greater injury. Different cell types vary in their susceptibility to cold. Melanocytes are very sensitive, and damage occurs at $-4°$ to $-7°C$ (19° to 25°F). Accordingly, cryotherapy causes hypopigmentation.[95]

Frostbite

Frostbite is due to actual freezing of the tissues resulting in ice crystals, usually at temperatures below $-2°C$, causing tissue injury. Frostbite causes impairment of circulation due to slowly progressing vasoconstriction. In its mildest form only redness and pain are present. In more severe cases, tissue destruction and blistering occur, and this may be superficial, full thickness, or involve deep tissues analogous to the burns (see Table 3–5). In its most extreme form gangrene and loss of limb may result. Exposed parts, such as toes, feet, fingers, ears, nose, and cheeks, are most often affected.

As tissue temperature falls, the area becomes numb, and the initial redness is gradually replaced by a white, waxy appearance with blistering and later necrosis. The affected part becomes pain free and the discomfort of cold disappears. In the early stages it is difficult to predict the extent of tissue loss; accurate estimation may not be possible for several weeks.[104] The more superficial the injury, the better the prognosis, especially if infection is absent. Even without loss of tissue, long-term effects include vasomotor instability with Raynaud-like changes, paresthesia, and hyperhidrosis. This is attributed to damage to the blood vessels and sympathetic nerves. Squamous cell carcinoma may arise in the old scars.[105]

In slow rewarming, intracellular ice crystals become larger and more lethal for the cells. Therefore, treatment entails rapidly rewarming the part, for which a whirlpool or waterbath or warm air for 20 minutes (until the most distal part is flushed) is useful. A temperature no higher than blood temperature[106] or 42°C[95] has been recommended. Thereafter, the affected part is rested at usual room temperature. The procedure is painful and causes an increase in erythema and blistering. The pain should be relieved with analgesics. The damaged part should be elevated and blisters left intact. Infection must be treated vigorously. The popular old idea of rubbing the affected part with snow[11] has an adverse, or even disastrous, effect.

Historically, the persons at greatest risk of frostbite have been military personnel. Nearly 200,000 cold casualties occurred during World Wars I and II and the Korean conflict.[106] Today, many cases are associated with alcohol consumption, homelessness in urban centers, and car breakdown.[107] Frostbite also occurs in winter sports; for example, in cross country skiers and backpackers. Workers at risk include oil pipeline workers in northern regions; utility maintenance personnel; sailors, especially those working on icebreakers; fishermen; firefighters; mail delivery persons; rescue personnel; researchers in cold laboratories and Arctic areas; and others who work outdoors in cold regions (Table 3–9).

Immersion Foot/ Nonfreezing Cold Injury

Formerly called *trench foot*, immersion foot results from exposure to cold temperatures above freezing for several days. In the presence of moisture and constrictive clothing, however, continuous exposure for as little as 19 hours may be sufficient.[108] Immersion foot is less severe than frostbite and develops in three stages: initial erythema, edema, and tenderness (stage I); followed within 24 hours by paresthesia, marked edema, numbness, and sometimes bullae (stage II); and progressing to gangrene (stage III). Gangrene does not develop unless there is infection. Convalescence may be prolonged for several weeks or months, during which time there is cold sensitivity, vasomotor instability, hyperemia, and hyperhidrosis. Rest, analgesics, and antibiotics are the mainstays of treatment, which is the same as for frostbite.

During the Korean and Vietnam conflicts thousands of cases occurred, and immersion foot became a major cause of disability. In industries in which workers are required to stand for long peri-

 TABLE 3–9 • Workers Potentially Exposed to Excessive Cold

Cooling room workers
Divers
Dry ice workers
Firefighters
Ice makers
Liquefied gas workers
Outdoor workers during cold weather
Packing house workers
Refrigerated warehouse workers
Refrigeration workers
Winter sports instructors

ods in cold wet mud or water, as when excavating foundations for new construction, immersion-type injuries may be frequent.[78] Street and sewer workers as well as golf caddies walking for hours on wet grass are also at risk.[109] Interestingly, immersion foot can also develop in the tropics (tropical immersion foot; see Table 3–8).

A historical review of nonfreezing frostbites has been published by Francis.[110]

Chilblain (Perniosis)

The mildest form of cold injury, chilblains, or perniosis, occur as an abnormal reaction to cold in the temperate, humid climate of Great Britain and northwestern Europe, where there is a lack of central heating.[95] Chilblains are less often seen in cold climates such as Finland, where well-heated houses and warm clothing are essential. The lesions are reddish blue discolorations that become swollen and boggy, with tense bullae and later ulcerations that may result in scarring. Often, chilblains are superimposed on a background of acrocyanosis or erythrocyanosis. Lesions occur especially on the dorsa of the proximal phalanges of the fingers and toes, heels, lower legs, thighs, nose, and ears. The shiny red plaques itch and burn severely. Chilblains are particularly frequent in children, where they tend to start in the early part of the winter. In adults who work outdoors, chilblains often start in the spring months when the workers are exposed to the combination of cold and light, which might be an aggravating factor.[95] Genetic factors producing vasomotor instability are important.

The most important point in management is prophylaxis with warm housing, warm clothing, and regular exercise. Once chilblains have appeared, treatment is mainly symptomatic with antipruritic local application. Some patients may derive benefit from ultraviolet radiation at the beginning of the winter.[95] This therapy may relieve chronic vasospasm believed to occur in chilblains.[95] Nifedipine may be effective in the treatment of severe recurrent perniosis.[111] In 7 of 10 patients, clearing ranged from 8 days for lesions of the hands to 23 days for foot lesions.[111]

Pulling-Boat Hands

This dermatosis has been described from coastal New England.[112] Erythematous macules and plaques developed on the dorsa of the hands and fingers of instructors and students after 3 to 14 days aboard a pulling boat. Later, small vesicles appeared, accompanied by itching, burning, and tenderness. Subjects had been exposed to high humidity, cool air, and wind, which was considered an ideal setting for the development of this nonfreezing type of dermatosis. Hours of vigorous rowing provided additional repetitive trauma. Some of the patients also had a history of frostbite and Raynaud's phenomenon. This syndrome may be caused by a combination of nonfreezing cold and the mechanical effects of rowing.[112]

Other Reactions to Cold

Cold urticaria and Raynaud's phenomenon are dealt with later in the chapter. The reader interested in other types of abnormal reactions to cold (see Table 3–8) is referred to major text on dermatology, such as the article of Heller Page and Sheer.[95]

LOW HUMIDITY

Low humidity occupational dermatoses are skin conditions caused either entirely or primarily by low relative humidity in the working environment. The importance of low humidity as a primary or contributing factor in the genesis of occupational skin problems has been stressed.[113–116] Low humidity of the air is believed to cause dehydration of the horny layer and thus drying of the skin. Below a water content of 10%, the stratum corneum loses its softness and pliability.[117] The water content of the horny layer remains below 10% when the relative humidity is less than 50%.[115] High temperature and flowing air accentuates the drying of the horny layer. An open-plan office next to or under the ventilation system, where warm, unhumidified air is introduced into the room, is a typical working site, and the risk of low humidity dermatosis is apparent. Low humidity dermatoses are accentuated by small irritant or hygroscopic airborne particles, such as textile particles, dust from ceramics, small particles from paper cutting, and fine angular, hygroscopic particles such as in a soft lens factory.[114, 115] Domestic and general climatic conditions can potentiate low humidity occupational dermatoses: Air-conditioned buildings have a low relative humidity, and, in temperate areas such as Scandinavia, the low humidity/high temperature indoor environment is accompanied by low humidity/low temperature outdoor climate during the winters, which also has a drying effect on the stratum corneum. Some of the occupations in which low humidity dermatoses have been reported are listed in Table 3–10.

These dermatoses are far more distressing than the comparative paucity of physical signs might suggest.[115] Pruritus and burning can be the only

TABLE 3–10 • Reported Low Humidity Risk Occupations

Offices
Soft contact lens factories
Silicon chip factories (semiconductor industry)
Cabin crew of long-distance airplanes
Resident staff in hospitals and hotels
Traveling salesmen (from automobile heaters)

TABLE 3–12 • Classification of Urticarial Reactions to Cold Stimuli

Localized Contact Reactions to Cold
  Immediate cold urticaria
    Idiopathic
    Secondary
  Delayed cold urticaria
  Cold-dependent dermographism (summation
    urticaria)
  Localized cold contact urticaria
  Localized cold reflex urticaria
  Perifollicular cold urticaria
  Familial delayed cold contact urticaria

**Systemic Reactions to Cold (cold air and cold
  water uriticaria)**
  Systemic cold urticaria
  Cold-induced cholinergic urticaria
  Familial cold urticaria (familial polymorphous
    cold eruption)

sign of low humidity. Puffiness of the cheeks and eyelids has been observed. The skin lesions evolve through dryness of the skin to erythema and round or oval patches of eczema. Erythema has been accompanied by urticarial whealing possibly secondary to scratching pruritic skin. In some cases areas covered by clothing have been predominantly involved, while facial itching with diffuse superficial scaling on the cheeks, forehead, and neck have been the main anatomical areas in other instances. Patchy erythema on the shaven face of male employees has been observed. Fair-skinned individuals are at higher risk. Both atopics and nonatopics have been affected.

Differential diagnoses include a wide variety of possibilities that have to be considered, such as inhalable and ingestible allergens, irritant or allergic airborne contact dermatitis, psychological causes, menopausal hot flashes, rosacea, and seborrheic eczema (Tables 3–11 to 3–13).

Another classification is based on the severity of symptoms[167]: type I, localized urticaria and angioedema; type II, systemic reactions with hypotensive symptom; type III, severe systemic reactions with fainting, disorientation, and shock.

From Czarnetzki BM. *Urticaria*. Berlin: Springer-Verlag; 1986; and Henz BM, Zuberbier T, Grabbe J, Monroe E. *Urticaria*. Berlin: Springer-Verlag (in press).

Treatment should include routine use of emollients and increasing the relative humidity to about 50% during the whole low humidity season (Table 3–14).

TABLE 3–11 • Classification, Relative Frequency, and Diagnostic Tests of Physical Urticaria

Type of Urticaria	Relative Frequency (%)	Eliciting Stimulus	Diagnostic Test
Dermographic (tarda)	50	Firm stroking or scratching (rubbing for red dermographism)	Firm stroking of the skin
Cholinergic	30	Physical exercise with overheating, mental stress	Bicycling, running, sauna
Cold	15	Cold contact	Cold objects: ice cube, cold arm bath, cold wind, or cool air
Solar	3	Light of varying wavelengths	Phototest with light of different wavelengths
Pressure	2	Pressure	Locally applied weights
Heat contact	Rare	Contact with heat	Warm bath
Aquagenic	Rare	Contact with water	Bath, compresses
Vibratory angioedema	Rare	Vibration	Vibrating motor
Exercise-induced anaphylaxis	Rare	Exercise after a heavy meal	Exercise
Familial cold urticaria	Rare	Cold wind	Cold wind and subsequent rewarming

Adapted from Czarnetzki BM. *Urticaria*. Berlin: Springer-Verlag; 1986; and Henz BM, Zuberbier T, Grabbe J, Monroe E. *Urticaria*. Berlin: Springer-Verlag (in press).

TABLE 3–13 • Diagnostic Tests To Determine Cold Urticaria

Cold Contact
  Source of cold
    Ice cube in plastic bag
    Crushed ice in plastic bag
    Chlorethyl spray
    Ice-filled copper cylinder
  Exposure time
    3–5 minutes

Cold Water Contact
  Source of cold
    Arm bath, 8°–10°C and 21°C
  Exposure time
    5–15 minutes

Cold Air Contact
  Source of cold
    Cold room 4°C
  Exposure time
    5–10 minutes with light clothing

Further Examinations
  Serologic tests for syphilis, borrelliosis,
    Epstein-Barr virus, HIV
  Serum cryoprotein
  Exclusion of systemic lupus erythematosus,
    hematological and lymphtic diseases,
    tumors
  Omission of suspicious drugs

The observation time after exposure should be 15 minutes for immediate and 8 and 24 hours for delayed reactions.

From Czarnetzki BM. *Urticaria.* Berlin: Springer-Verlag; 1986; and Henz BM, Zuberbier T, Grabbe J, Monroe E. *Urticria.* Berlin: Springer-Verlag (in press).

In some countries patients often complain of skin symptoms from work with visual display terminals.[118, 119] A study from Sweden among 353 routine office workers showed an increased tendency for seborrhoic eczema and nonspecific erythema. Organizational conditions during visual display terminal work, such as high work load and

 TABLE 3–14 • Therapy for Cold Urticaria

Patient education
Therapy of underlying diseases (with antibiotics)
Avoidance of cold exposure
Symptomatic therapy with H_1-antihistamines
Stanozolol/danazole
Sulfones or dapsone
β_2-Sympathomimetics and aminophylline
Induction of cold tolerance
Omission of suspected drugs

inability to take rest breaks, were found to be associated with the reported skin symptoms. A low relative humidity was associated with a diagnosis of seborrhoic eczema. No associations were found between current field levels of electric or magnetic field and skin diseases/signs or reported symptoms.[120]

RAYNAUD'S PHENOMENON (VIBRATION SYNDROME)

Episodic pallor caused by reversible vascular spasm followed by cyanosis and erythema of fingers and toes from exposure to cold, pressure, or emotional stimuli is known as *Raynaud's phenomenon*, first described in 1862. Women are more commonly affected than men, with the onset usually during the twenties and thirties. The fingers are most often affected. The thumbs are sometimes spared. The condition is bilateral and usually symmetrical. It may be mild and occur infrequently or many times a day. In severe cases, late sequelae include telangiectases of the nail fold, thinning and ridging of the nail, and atrophy and sclerosis of the finger (sclerodactyly). Raynaud's phenomenon may be associated with many different pathological conditions. Classification of Raynaud's phenomenon is listed in Table 3–15. When no underlying cause can be found, the term *Raynaud's disease* (primary or idiopathic Raynaud's phenomenon) is used. Secondary Raynaud's disease is associated with a large number of contributing conditions or diseases (Table 3–15). Here, only the occupational causes are dealt with, that is, disorders from physical agents, occupational acro-osteolysis from vinyl chloride manufacture, and scleroderma in workers exposed to silica dust.

Lorigo in 1911 described "vascular spasm" in the hands of pneumatic tool miners, and since then several surveys have confirmed the connection between vibration of hand-held tools and Raynaud's phenomenon.[121, 122] The clinical condition is known under several names, including *occupational Raynaud's phenomenon, dead fingers, white fingers, traumatic vasospastic disease*, and *vibration-induced white finger* (VWF) disease.[69, 123] The workers potentially exposed to hand-arm vibration are those who operate jackhammers, pounding machines, riveting hammers, and hand grinders (Table 3–16). The vasospastic symptoms may be associated with neuromuscular and arthritic symptoms, and even with bone degeneration. The complex of VWF and associated findings in the arterial and other systems has been termed *vibration syndrome* (VS).

TABLE 3–15 • Classification of Raynaud's Phenomenon

Primary Raynaud's Disease Is Raynaud's Phenomenon Without Associated or Contributing Conditions or Diseases

Secondary Raynaud's Disease Is Raynaud's Phenomenon Associated with Contributing Conditions or Diseases
Disorders from physical agents
  After direct trauma
    Occupational
      Vibration-induced white finger (VWF) disease
      Occlusive arterial disease of the hand
      Vasospastic phenomena of pianists and typists
      Meat cutters
      Nonoccupational (injury or operation)
  Frostbite and immersion syndrome
Occupational acro-osteolysis
Scleroderma from silica dust
Collagen-vascular disease
  Scleroderma
  Systemic lupus erythematosus
  Dermatomyositis and polymyositis
  Mixed connective tissue disease
  Rheumatoid arthritis
  Polyarteritis and vasculitis
  Sjögren's syndrome
Obstructive arterial disease
  Buerger's disease
  Arterial embolism
  Thrombosis
Neurogenic disorders
  Thoracic outlet syndrome
  Carpal tunnel syndrome
  Reflex sympathetic dystrophy
  Hemiplegia
  Poliomyelitis
  Multiple sclerosis
  Syringomyelia
Drugs
  Tobacco
  β-Adrenergic blockers
  Ergot preparations
  Methylsergide
  Bleomycin and vinblastine
  Clonidine
  Cyclosporine
  Bromocriptine
Hematological causes
  Cryoproteins
  Cold agglutinins
  Macroglobulins
  Polycythemia
Miscellaneous
  Hypothyroidism
  Neoplasms
  Vasculitis and hepatitis B antigenemia
  Arteriovenous fistula
  Intra-arterial injections

 TABLE 3–16 • Occupational Exposure to Vibration

Chain sawyers
Electrical grinder (rotary, stand, swing grinders)
Metal extrusion operators
Motorcycle speedway riders
Miners (jack leg and hand tools)
Pneumatic tool operators (chippers, staple gun operators, construction workers, and road operation workers)
Saw blade straightener
Ski-doo drivers (e.g., reindeer keepers)
Wood products manufacturing workers

Clinical Manifestations

The early clinical manifestations are mild: slight tingling and numbness, followed later by blanching of the tips of one or two fingers. Numbness and clumsy movement accompany the blanching, lasting for 15 to 60 minutes or longer. All digits may ultimately be involved, often sparing the thumbs. The symptoms may be indistinguishable from other forms of Raynaud's phenomenon, but asymmetry of lesions is relatively common. Onset may be as early as 3 months after beginning the activity, but is more commonly seen after 2 to 3 years. The vascular symptoms of VS seldom cause occupational disability in industrial workers who operate at room temperature. Even those working outdoors in the cold seldom consider the disability great enough to give up their jobs,[123] but those having paresthesias and neuromuscular disturbances such as weakening of grip force might have greater disability. The symptoms and signs associated with VS have been graded clinically by Taylor.[124] Table 3–17 quantifies tingling, numbness, and blanching linked to activities at work, home, and hobbies. It covers stage 0 with no symptoms to stage 4 where VS is so severe that the worker has to change occupations. Vibration syndrome is progressive as long as exposure to vibration continues.

Risk Factors

Vibrations are characterized in terms of frequency (expressed in cycles per second or Hertz [Hz]). Vibration frequencies between 30 and 300 Hz are those most strongly associated with VS. In addition to the physical factors of the vibration, other external and occupational risk factors such as ergonomic, operational, and environmental factors can affect the development of VS (Table 3–18). Experience, training, and exposure to vasoconstricting agents, especially smoking, are important risk

TABLE 3–17 • **Stages of Raynaud's Phenomenon of Occupational Origin**

Stage	Condition of Digits	Work, Social, and Hobby Interference
00 (no vibration exposure)	No signs or symptoms	No complaints; no interference with any activities
0 (vibration exposed)	No signs or symptoms or intermittent tingling and numbness in hands and digits	No complaints; no interference with any activities
1 (vibration exposed)	The subject notices that one or more fingertips go white with or without tingling and/or numbness. First noticed in winter	No complaints; no inteference with any activities
2 (vibration exposed)	The blanching extends beyond the tips in digits with or without tingling and numbness; complaints confined to winter months	No interference at work; interference with outside activities
3 (vibration exposed)	Extensive blanching usually to base of fingers bilaterally; frequent attacks occurring in summer months as well as winter; tingling and/or numbness may be present in addition to blanching	Definite interference at work and in social and hobby pursuits; hobbies given up
4 (vibration exposed)	Extensive blanching; frequent attacks summer and winter; thumbs may now be involved	Because of interference and discomfort, subject changes occupation

Adapted from Wasserman D, ed. *Vibration White-Finger Disease in U.S. Workers Using Pneumatic Chipping and Grinding Hand Tools. I. Epidemiology.* Publ. No. 82–118. Cincinnati: NIOSH; 1982.

factors. However, in the study of Hellstrom and Lange Anderson,[125] there was no significant difference in prevalence of VWF in smokers and nonsmokers. Table 3–14 lists examples of how different risk factors caused by different machine shop tools and jobs have been evaluated in Sweden from a medical insurance point of view.[126] Machine shop tools in group I are not generally considered to cause VS; tools in group II may cause risk, especially if the exposure has been long; and in group III already an exposure time of 30 minutes daily causes high risk of developing VS.

Diagnostic Tests

There is no single test that will accurately assess VS. Objective tests of vibration syndrome should include (1) tests for vibration-induced white finger, (2) tests for peripheral nerves and receptors, (3) vibrotactile sensation tests, and possibly (4) tests for the bones and the joints. Peripheral vascular function tests include plethysmography, arteriography, skin thermography, capillary microscopy, skin and muscular rheography, and cold provocation. Several types of cold provocation tests are in use.[68, 69, 123, 127]

A negative result does not exclude the possibility of Raynaud's phenomenon.[123] The results of the cold provocation test can vary in repeated trials with the same individuals.[123] A cold provocation test combined with the measurement of systolic blood pressure in the finger in strain-gauge plethysmography has been proposed to be more accurate than bare visual inspection.[128] Recording the recovery of skin temperature from the fingers after cooling in water gives the advantage of testing several fingers simultaneously, and the test can be performed under more primitive conditions such as in the workplace.

Other Skin Symptoms from Vibration

Dart[129] has reported a vasomotor disturbance associated with the use of light, high-speed vibrating electric tools of the type widely used in the aircraft industry during World War II. The symptom appeared as pain accompanied by swelling and erythrocyanotic discolorations of the hands. Chilling did not cause blanching. Vibratory angioedema has been known since 1972. A case of occupationally acquired vibration angioedema with secondary carpal tunnel syndrome without Raynaud's phenomenon was reported by Wener et al.[130] in a metal grinder.

Prevention

In the past 20 years there has been a marked improvement in the design of chainsaws (i.e., de-

TABLE 3–18 • Examples of Relative Risk of Developing VS for Different Types of Vibrating Machine Shop Tools.

Machine Type/Job	I	II	III	Comments
Angle grinders		×	×	The grinding disc greatly affects the level
Straight grinders		×		Most
Straight grinders	×			Equipped with file
Surface grinders		×		Auto repair work, for example
Mounted grinders		×	×	Exposure to vibrations in the material
Electric, nonimpact drills	×			Punching holes in wood, plastic, and iron, for example
Air-driven, nonimpact drills		×		Manufacturing
Impact drills and drill hammers				
Fine		×		Electricians, wiring
Coarse			×	Hole drilling during building
Manual rock drills			×	Mining and installation work
Chisel hammer			×	Mostly larger and/ or older; engineering industry, auto repair shops
Chisel hammer		×		Certain more modern constructions, e.g., auto repair shops
Impact chisels			×	Most
		×		Certain more recent constructions
Riveting hammers			×	Older, airplane manufacture, shipyards
Riveting hammers	×	×		New construction, airplane manufacture
Holding-up tool				
Riveting knob			×	Traditional iron piece
Riveting knob	×	×		New construction, finer rivets give the lower values
Wrenches		×		Most, auto repair; larger machines usually cause higher vibration levels
Wrenches	×			Certain tough wrenching tools
Pneumatic drill for breaking up asphalt, etc.			×	Most; lower levels with softer base
Motor saws			×	Older (pre-1968)
Motor saws		×		Newer
Clearing saws		×		Most
Clearing saws	×			With antivibration handle
Circular saws for plate shearing		×		Auto repair work
Stave vibrator		×		Most
Stave vibrator	×			Certain more recent constructions
Control and levers	×			Higher levels achieved in certain farm tractors

I, small risk; II, moderate risk; III, high risk. Modified from Gemne G, Ekenvall L, Hansson JE, et al. Skadlig inverkan av hand-arm-vibrationer—en försäkringsmedicinsk bedömningsmodell. Arbete Hälsa 1986; 2.

creased vibration acceleration and lighter weight). This has resulted in a decline in VS in Great Britain and Scandinavia.[68, 131] Similar progress ought to be achieved with other kinds of vibrating tools.

Treatment

The standard therapies as used for other causes of Raynaud's phenomenon (summarized in Table 3–19) are used.[95] If VS is not in an advanced stage, no treatment other than stopping exposure to vibration is needed. Advice about protection from cold and wearing warm gloves and socks should be given, and smoking should be prohibited. Therapy of more severe cases is far from satisfactory, although a large number of drug therapies have been used successfully in some cases.

TABLE 3–19 • Treatment of Raynaud's Phenomenon

General Measures	Remove cause (drugs, occupation)	Second-Line Drug Therapy	Methyldopa
	Treat underlying disease		Reserpine
	Avoid precipitating factors		Phenoxybenzamine
	Stop smoking		Guanethidine
	Biofeedback		Stanozolol
	Wear gloves		Griseofulvin
First-Line Drug Therapy	Nifedipine		Topical nitroglycerin (adjuvant)
	Diltiazem	Others	Intra-arterial reserpine
	Prazosin		Low-molecular-weight dextran
	Ketanserin		Sympathectomy
	Prostaglandin E$_1$ and		Captopril
	prostaglandin I$_2$ infusions		Plasmapheresis
	Transdermal prostaglandin E$_1$		

From Heller Page E, Shear NH. Disorders due to physical factors. In: Fitzpatrick TB, Eisen AZ, Wolff K, et al., eds. *Dermatology in General Medicine,* 4th ed. New York: McGraw-Hill; 1993:1581–1592.

TABLE 3–20 • Causes of Acro-Osteolysis

Acrodermatitis continua Hallopeau	Pycnodysostosis
Acromegaly	Porphyria
Bureau-Barriere's disease	Psoriatic arthritis
Buerger's disease	Progeria
Carpal tunnel syndrome	Raynaud's disease
Collagen disease	Reiter's disease
Mixed connective tissue disease	Renal osteodystrophy
Polymyositis	Rothmund's disease
Scleroderma	Sarcoidosis
Rheumatoid arthritis	Self-mutilation after spinal cord injury
Sjögren's syndrome	Sezary's syndrome
Congenital insensitivity to pain syndrome	Spine tumors
Diabetic neuropathy	Syringomyelia
Ehlers-Danlos syndrome	Syphilis
Epidermolysis bullosa	Tabes dorsalis
Gout	Thevenard's disease
Hyperparathyroidism	Vascular diseases
Ichthyosiform erythroderma	Ainhum
Infections	Atherosclerosis
Juvenile hyalin fibromatosis	Buerger's disease
Leprosy	Van Bogaert-Hazay syndrome
Metastases	Vinyl chloride disease
Mucopolysaccharidoses	Werner's syndrome
Multicentric reticulohistiocytosis	
Neoplasms	
Nutritional deficiencies	
Pachydermoperiostosis	
Physical injuries	
Burns	
Frostbite	
Fulguration	
Mechanical stress (guitar players)	

From Baran R, Tosti A. Occupational acroosteolysis in a guitar player. *Acta Derm Venereol (Stockh)* 1993;73:64–65.

Occupational Raynaud's Phenomenon from Other Causes than Vibration

Raynaud's phenomenon can arise from repeated occupational trauma (Table 3–15).[69, 132] Included in this group are farmers and mechanics who frequently use tools that require a squeezing action of the hands.[132] Creamery workers or laborers whose hands are subjected to repeated blunt trauma are other examples. Furthermore, workers who hammer can obtain the hypothenar hammer syndrome. Other examples are squeezing as in the obstetrician's use of forceps and the dentist's or carpenter's use of hand tools. Traumatic vasospastic disease can also occur in a variety of other workers such as pianists, typists, riveters, and butchers. A common clinical procedure in dermatology, cryotherapy, may be an occupational hazard for physicians with Raynaud's disease.[133]

Occupational Acro-Osteolysis

First described in the Soviet Union in 1949 and in Romania in 1963,[134, 135] Raynaud's phenomenon with osteolytic bone lesions occurs in workers who manual clean reactor tanks containing monomer of vinyl chloride.[136, 137] The symptom complex consists of Raynaud's phenomenon, scleroderma-tous skin changes, and lytic bone lesions, especially of the fingers.[138] The incidence rate is quite low, occurring in approximately 3% of those cleaning the polyvinyl chloride reactors, which likely indicates individual idiosyncrasy.[139]

Systemic abnormalities may occur, such as hepatomegaly, splenomegaly, thrombocytopenia, pulmonary obstructive defects, and others.[138, 140] Besides those involved in manually cleaning the reactor tanks, other workers may also be affected, such as maintenance workers repairing pipes, valves, and pumps. With engineering modifications, exposure to the monomer of vinyl chloride can be virtually eliminated, and, as a result, this condition is rarely seen today.

Organic solvents and exposure to silica dust have also been reported as causes of sclerodermatous changes.[141, 142] Baran and Tosti[66] reported a case of occupational acro-osteolysis in a guitar player due to mechanical stress on the fingers.[64, 65] They also reviewed the causes of acro-osteolysis, including acro-osteolysis from physical injury (Table 3–20). A familial and idiopathic type of acro-osteolysis also exists.[143]

Scleroderma in workers exposed to silica dust is an occupational disease entity in which Raynaud's phenomenon also plays a prominent role.

Radiation Effects ∎

RICHARD COHEN

The electromagnetic radiation spectrum (in order of decreasing frequency and energy) is composed of ionizing, ultraviolet, visible, infrared, and radio-frequency radiation (Fig. 3–6). Health effects generally are dependent on energy level and dose. However, there are major variations in the type and risk of radiation-induced injury regardless of dose or wave energy along this infinitely wide spectrum owing to differences in skin penetration, absorption, pathophysiology, and radiation physics. Recognition of exposure to all forms of electromagnetic radiation is hampered by the fact that it has little or no warning properties such as odor, sound, or physical movement. Even in the case of heat or light sources, it may not be readily apparent, as in the case of ultraviolet or infrared laser beams.

IONIZING RADIATION

Ionizing radiation is so named because of its intrinsic high energy level, which upon reaction with biological tissues can cause ionization or displacement of atomic particles from their usual location. It occurs both in waveform, such as synthetically generated x-rays or naturally occurring gamma rays, and in particulate form, such as beta, alpha, and other atomic particles. In addition to cosmic radiation, naturally occurring sources are radioactive elements that spontaneously produce both wave and particulate emissions; natural decay results in continuous radioactivity that varies in its health impact owing to individual differences in rate of decay, type of ionizing radiation emitted, and intensity/energy.

FIGURE 3–6 • Electromagnetic spectrum.

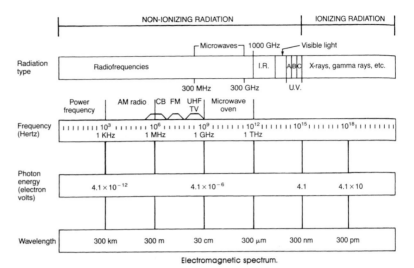

Electromagnetic spectrum.

Ionizing radiation exposures occur in industry through numerous processes, including curing plastics, sterilizing foods and drugs, testing materials, medical and dental radiography and therapy, and operation of high-power electronic equipment, including such consumer products as television sets.

Despite much wider use of ionizing radiation, there is much less exposure today than there was several decades ago, not only because of better construction and shielding of x-ray equipment but also because of less frequent use of x-rays to treat benign conditions. In addition, the public is now more aware of the health risks associated with exposure. Laws against improper use are consequently stronger and better enforced. Nevertheless, the exposure potential has broadened considerably with the newer applications of ionizing radiation in consumer products, in medicine, and in many industrial processes.

ACUTE RADIODERMATITIS

Occupational exposure to ionizing radiation is usually localized. In acute radiodermatitis, exposure of a small area to a single dose of 1,000 roentgens (R)* or more causes a skin reaction that progresses through several stages. Initially there is erythema, edema, and blanching of the skin, which reach a peak at 48 hours following exposure and then rapidly subside. Then, on about the sixth

*Roentgen (R): exposure (dose) at a given point

Gray (Gy): absorbed dose (radiation per unit of mass), 1 Gy = 100 rads

Sievert (Sv): dose equivalent (absorbed dose in terms of estimated biological effect), 1 Sv = 100 rem

to tenth day, the skin again becomes erythematous, with purplish ecchymotic areas that become vesicular and later bullous. The pain is intense and may require narcotics for suppression. This stage continues for 2 or 3 weeks, after which the repair stage occurs. Reepithelialization takes place, but the skin becomes atrophic, hairless, and without functioning sebaceous glands. With large single doses (6,000 R or above), a roentgen ulcer may form 2 or 3 months later. Healing is very slow and usually leaves a disfiguring scar. Very intense acute exposures may entail loss of the epidermis and nail plate within 2 to 3 days, followed by redness and desquamation with intense pain and ulcerations 2 to 3 months or up to a year later. In some cases amputation may be required.[144]

Total-body exposure to 1 Gy of radiation or greater over a brief time produces the acute radiation syndrome. Exposures over 30 Gy are acutely lethal owing to encephalopathy with ataxia, lethargy, tremor, and convulsions. Exposures between 10 and 30 Gy can cause immediate gastrointestinal symptoms, including nausea, vomiting, weakness, diarrhea, and often shock.

Assuming survival, following a latent period of approximately 10 to 14 days fever appears with manifestations of the hematopoietic effects that usually result from exposures in the range of 1 to 10 Gy. At this point hemorrhagic petechiae and ecchymoses develop over the skin, followed by loss of hair. Ulcerations may occur, and the patient becomes extremely ill with great weakness, fever, and bloody diarrhea. Death may result from bone marrow suppression or associated infection. Generally, the greater the exposure the shorter the latent period. Depending on the severity of the exposure, central nervous system or gastrointestinal effects may predominate. Accidents of this type, caused by contamination of wide areas of the workplace, are major medical emergencies often involving several workers.

Acute exposures have also been associated with reproductive effects such as impaired spermatogenesis, embryonic death, abortion, and cessation of menses.

CHRONIC RADIODERMATITIS

With exposure to smaller doses of ionizing radiation (300 to 800 R received daily or weekly over a long period, up to a total dose of 5,000 to 6,000 R), the skin develops an eczematous reaction with intense erythema accompanied by a burning pain and hyperesthesia. Although the epidermis may slough, regrowth occurs gradually within 4 to 6 weeks. Hair is lost slowly, and the sebaceous glands cease activity. The skin becomes hypopigmented and atrophic. After months or years the atrophy increases, and telangiectases appear.

Even with very small doses, such as 50 to 100 R received irregularly over many years, progressive dryness of the skin, loss or scantiness of hair, irregular areas of hyperpigmentation, and signs of premature aging may be seen. Until quite recently these effects were somewhat common among dentists, radiologists, and x-ray technicians, the hands and face being primarily affected. A common sign of chronic x-ray damage of this type is flattening of the epidermal ridges on the fingers. The fingernails are also brittle and easily cracked.

Significant delayed effects following high acute or cumulative ionizing radiation exposures include a variety of cancers (skin, thyroid, liver, bone, and leukemia), in addition to radiodermatitis. Follow-up of atomic bomb survivors indicates that the prevalences of basal cell carcinoma and senile keratosis increase with their ionizing radiation dose.[145] The probability of skin carcinogenesis following ionizing radiation exposure has been estimated at 2×10^{-4}/Sv.[146] With the exception of leukemia, most cancers have been associated with localized organ radioactive exposures, such as thyroid cancer following childhood thymus irradiation. Other high-dose exposure effects include shortening of life, premature aging, and teratogenic and reproductive abnormalities. Low cumulative ionizing radiation dose effects are less clear. Although doses as low as 10 cGY have been associated with significant health effects, their practical significance is unclear owing to the fact that the cumulative lifetime average exposure for an American is approximately 8 to 10 cGy.

ULTRAVIOLET RADIATION

Ultraviolet radiation includes that portion of the electromagnetic spectrum with wavelengths between 100 and 400 nm. Ultraviolet light is divided according to wavelength into the A, B, and C bands, the A band being the longest. The C band represents wavelengths less than 200 nm, which are biologically inactive.

Although the skin is permeable to solar radiation of wavelengths from 290 to 1,000 nm, almost all clinically important reactions take place between 290 and 400 nm. The visible spectrum between 400 and 700 nm has little skin effect, and the chief result of longer wavelengths (700 to 1,000 nm) is heating of the skin. Ultraviolet radiation between 290 and 320 nm is in the peak sunburn spectrum. Almost all this irradiation is absorbed by the upper epidermis; only about 10% reaches the dermis.[147] Melanin provides an effective barrier to the sunburn wavelengths, but longer wavelengths are readily transmitted. Black skin rarely sunburns, but it is as susceptible as white skin to photodynamic effects within the 320 to 400 nm range.

The severity of injury from ultraviolet radiation depends on the intensity of the radiation source, exposure time, wavelength, distance from the source, and other factors. The degree of melanization of the skin and thickness of the stratum corneum are especially important. Time of day, atmospheric conditions, and latitude also influence the reaction. Close to the equator the hazard of sunburn persists throughout the year, but it diminishes during the winter months as one moves farther away. Even during the winter in northern latitudes a blond, light-eyed person is susceptible to the long-term effects of excessive sunlight.

Sunlight is most intense between the hours of 10 am and 3 pm solar time. Fog and clouds screen out the infrared and longer wavelengths, but the shorter, more penetrating ultraviolet light still reaches the skin. Ultraviolet reflections from water, snow, sand, concrete, and metal surfaces also induce damage. Although window glass screens out shorter ultraviolet wavelengths, wavelengths above 320 nm pass through.

Industry uses many artificial sources of ultraviolet radiation. These include carbon arcs, welding and cutting torches, electric arc furnaces, germicidal and black light lamps, and numerous pieces of laboratory equipment. Today, printing inks and dental adhesives may be cured by ultraviolet rays. Commercial tanning booths have become popular and expose workers and customers to the risk of injury from excessive ultraviolet, either accidentally or as part of the procedure. If these persons are also taking medications that increase their susceptibility to ultraviolet light, such as chlorothiazides, phenothiazines, or griseofulvin, burning may result even from normal exposure.

A germicidal ultraviolet bulb installed at a hospital nursing station caused an outbreak of sunburn and conjunctivitis among 58 exposed persons.[148] Erythema and desquamation associated with pruritus developed on the face, neck, arms, and hands. Fortunately, none of the injuries was severe.

Sunburn, polymorphous light eruption, and discoid lupus erythematosus may be seen in welders.[149]

The cutaneous effects of sunlight are either acute or chronic. The acute effect is sunburn, which develops from exposure to radiation between 290 and 320 nm, and ranges from mild erythema to marked blistering. Severe sunburn may be accompanied by chills, fever, nausea, and even shock and circulatory collapse. Within minutes of exposure an initial transient erythema develops, which soon disappears. True erythema begins within 2 to 3 hours, reaches a peak at 24 to 48 hours, and gradually subsides, occasionally with desquamation. Visible darkening of the skin becomes apparent within about 48 hours and increases up to approximately 3 weeks, persisting for several months. If severe blistering occurs, scarring and loss of pigment may result.

An interesting photosensitivity reaction is onycholysis of fingernails and toenails on exposure to sunlight following ingestion of certain drugs. The first drug implicated in this condition was demethylchlortetracycline (Declomycin).[150] Among 27 of 108 ambulatory dermatological patients taking this drug, seven showed onycholysis in addition to an exaggerated sunburn reaction. The distal one-third of the nail becomes loosened from its bed, which is noted approximately 3 weeks after the mild sunburn and is accompanied by burning pain in the fingertips. The condition usually clears in 3 or 4 months. Other drugs that cause photosensitivity may induce similar photo-onycholysis.

The chronic cumulative effects of ultraviolet exposure are premature aging, actinic keratoses, and cutaneous malignancies. Ultraviolet light exaggerates the skin's aging process, producing wrinkling, atrophy, hyperpigmentation, and telangiectases. The shorter wavelengths of the sunburn range are chiefly responsible, but longer wavelengths may also play a role.

Excessive cumulative ultraviolet exposure has been clearly associated with nonmelanotic (basal and squamous cell) skin and lip cancers.[151] It is now accepted that sunlight plays a major role in the development of malignant melanoma, particularly in those persons who have repeated short-term, high-intensity radiation resulting in sunburn.[152] Studies of the relationship between cumulative ultraviolet exposure (nonoccupational or occupational) and malignant melanoma yielded less consistent results.[153]

Photosensitivity reactions to ultraviolet rays may be phototoxic or photoallergic. Systemic medications responsible for these reactions are listed in Table 3–21. Most photosensitive reactions are phototoxic; photoallergic reactions are much less common, affecting only a small percentage of exposed persons. Until recently the most common substances responsible for contact photoallergy were germicidal agents found in soaps and detergents, but perfume ingredients, such as methylcoumarin and certain sunscreen ingredients, appear to have taken their place. Schauder[154] reported a photoallergy in 15 pig breeders due to airborne exposure to olaquindox, a growth promoter.

A number of diseases are associated with photosensitivity. Porphyria includes a group of diseases of which the most important to dermatologists is porphyria cutanea tarda. This is usually associated with chronic alcoholism but may also be induced by inhalation or skin absorption of the polyhalogenated hydrocarbons causing chloracne. Photosensitivity in porphyria cutanea tarda is manifested by blisters and bullae appearing on exposed parts, with skin fragility, hyperpigmentation, hypertrichosis, and scarring. Erythropoietic protoporphyria is an inherited disease in which various degrees of photosensitivity are present. Polymorphous light eruption occurring in outdoor workers such as farm laborers may be very persistent and difficult to treat.

Other diseases in which sunlight and/or ultraviolet light play a causative or aggravating role, but in which no known photosensitizer has been found, include systemic lupus erythematosus, dermatomyositis, pemphigus foliaceus, pellagra, and miscellaneous genetic conditions. Willis[155] and Klein[156] reported exacerbation of cutaneous lupus due to photocopier emissions. The triggering effect of ultraviolet rays on herpes simplex is well

TABLE 3–21 • Systemically Administered Drugs That May Cause Photosensitivity

Amiodarone	Phenothiazines
Griseofulvin	Psoralens
Nalidixic acid	Sulfonamides
Nonsteroidal anti-inflammatory agents	Sulfonylureas
	Tetracyclines
	Thiazides

known; prevention is occasionally possible with the use of sunscreens.

Another dermatitis associated with photosensitivity is actinic reticuloid. Patients with this condition commonly are older with a chronic photosensitivity dermatitis suggesting lymphoma. In the most severe cases, large confluent plaques resembling those of lymphoma are present in sunlight-exposed areas. Histological examination reveals a picture often suggesting mycosis fungoides, with an epidermal mononuclear infiltrated and Pautrier abscesses.[157, 158] Many of these patients have positive patch or photopatch tests to various environmental chemicals.

Brown et al.[159] suggested that fluorescent lighting might maintain the activity of actinic reticuloid. In discussing this report, Harber[160] agreed that urticarial and eczematous reactions may occur on exposure to "daylight" fluorescent tubes. Ultraviolet emission from daylight fluorescent bulbs may aggravate such conditions as rosacea and contact photosensitivity, especially if the exposure is very close to the skin. However, fluorescent lighting is now considered an unlikely cause of malignant melanoma.[161] Workers who require high illumination for close, detailed worked are listed in Table 3–22.

Owing to its inability to significantly penetrate intact skin, the only other target organ for ultraviolet radiation is the eye. Acute intense exposure to wavelengths less than 315 nm can result in photokeratoconjunctivitis ("welder's flash"), the symptoms beginning 6 to 12 hours following exposure. Cataract has been attributed to both photochemical and thermal effects of intense ultraviolet light exposures, usually occurring within 24 hours of exposure. Retinal effects have not been reported, probably owing to the lens-shielding effect, although retinal damage is theoretically possible in aphakic individuals. Cataract following long-term, lower level ultraviolet light exposures has been suggested but not well documented. Pterygium, a benign hyperplasia of the bulbar conjunctiva, is strongly associated with high cumulative sunlight exposure.

TABLE 3–23 • Workers with High Infrared Exposure	
Bakers	Iron workers
Blacksmiths	Kiln operators
Braziers	Lacquer dryers
Chemists	Laser operators
Cloth inspectors	Motion picture machine
Cooks	operators
Electricians	Plasma torch operators
Foundry workers	Skimmers, glass
Furnace workers	Solderers
Gas mantle hardeners	Stationary firefighters
Glassblowers	Steel mill workers
Glass furnace workers	Stokers
Heat treaters	Welders

From Moss E, Murray W, Parr W, et al. Physical hazards. In: Key MM, ed. *Occupational Diseases: A Guide to Their Recognition.* Cincinnati: NIOSH; 1977:478.

INFRARED EXPOSURE

The primary effect of infrared radiation is heating of tissue. Infrared radiation includes that portion of the electromagnetic spectrum with wavelengths between 750 and 3 million nm. However, because water absorbs infrared radiation wavelengths above 2,000 nm, the most biologically active portion of the spectrum falls between 750 and 2,000 nm.

Repeated exposure to infrared rays causes hyperpigmentation and telangiectasis, as seen in erythema ab igne. The ophthalmic reaction is more severe; the shorter wavelengths cause posterior cataracts after several years of exposure. Glassblowers and workers tending furnaces are especially at risk. A latent period of 10 to 15 years is characteristic.[162]

Industrial applications of infrared include drying and baking paints, varnishes, printing inks, and other coatings; dehydrating textiles, paper, and leather; and heat-shrinking processes for assembling plastics to metal surfaces. Workers with potentially high infrared exposure are listed in Table 3–23.

RADIOFREQUENCY AND MICROWAVES

Radiofrequency radiation constitutes the remainder of the electromagnetic spectrum and has the longest wavelengths. In one portion of the radio-

TABLE 3–22 • Workers Requiring High Illumination for Close Work
Draftsmen
Electronic equipment assemblers
Engravers
Jewelers
Quality control inspectors
Watchmakers

From Moss E, Murray W, Parr W, et al. Physical hazards. In: Key MM, ed. *Occupational Diseases: A Guide to Their Recognition.* Cincinnati: NIOSH; 1977:478.

frequency is the microwave spectrum, with wavelengths ranging from 1 mm to 30 cm (frequency 300 MHz to 300 GHz). Radiofrequency and microwave radiation vary in their ability to penetrate intact skin, with microwave penetration/absorption being greatest in the megahertz range and up to 25 GHz.

Microwaves are generated by radiofrequency power tubes, such as magnetrons, klystrons, and amplitrons. In contrast to thermal heating, in which heat spreads inward from the surface, microwaves pass through matter to produce a volume heating effect. All dipolar molecules are activated at the same time, generating heat rapidly throughout the exposed part.

Microwaves are extensively used in industry today because more precise control of heating is possible with great efficiency, with more economical use of plant space, and at a lower cost than with conventional heating. The pharmaceutical industry uses microwaves to dry products, kill and inhibit growth of bacteria, and heat chemicals during processing. As recently as 1970 only commercial cooking used microwave ovens, but they are now standard home kitchen equipment. Microwaves are also used to cure plastics and to dry paint, paper, and printing inks. The military uses microwave generators for navigation, tracking, and communications. Accurate weather forecasting would be impossible without their use.

The danger of microwaves is that they cause internal heating. High-intensity microwave exposures are usually associated with a feel of warmth to the exposed body part, followed by hot burning skin, erythema, blistering, and induration occurring with 24 to 48 hours. More severe microwave oven exposures have caused deep soft tissue injury and neuropathy. Other acute symptoms include headache, watery eyes, irritability, a gritty eye sensation, light-headedness, and nausea.

Other health effects following acute high-intensity microwave exposure may include the development of transient hypertension and psychiatric sequelae, similar to the post-traumatic stress syndrome.

The effects of long-term, low-dose exposure to extremely low-frequency radiofrequencies (outside of the microwave spectrum), known as *magnetic fields*, are being examined because of some studies that have found increased leukemia rates among individuals living in proximity to low-frequency, high-power electrical lines. Other studies have shown increased rates of brain, breast, and other cancers among individuals working in electronics-related occupations. Their significance is unclear because of the inconsistency of results,

lack of a biological mechanism, and possible cofounders.

LASERS

Lasers produce an intense beam of light consisting of a very pure single color. Ultraviolet, visible, or infrared radiation is concentrated in a narrow beam in the plane of polarization and varies in energy level. Because of the focused beam generated, the laser has many and varied uses. The greatest potential worker exposure occurs in the construction industry, where accuracy of alignment is crucial, such as in pipeline and tunnel construction projects, sewer lines, and surveying. Lasers are also used for cutting and drilling hard metals, glass, and diamonds and in many different types of surgery, such as in ophthalmology and dermatology.

Biological effects from low-intensity laser exposure have not been observed. Depending on wavelength, as the laser's energy intensity increases, thermal damage to exposed skin or eyes can result. Because many of the lasers used in industry contain radiation outside the visible light spectrum, potential exposure to the laser beam may not be readily apparent to the worker. Skin effects are due to simple heating and can range from a mild thermal burn to instant necrosis, depending on the power of the laser.

The eye is at greatest risk from lasers, usually from accidental exposure. Cataracts may be induced by ultraviolet light lasers functioning in the 300 to 400 nm rage.[163] Lasers using infrared wavelengths cause skin damage ranging from mild erythema to blistering and necrosis.

VIDEO DISPLAY TERMINALS

Although a variety of health effects, from spontaneous abortions to cataracts, have been attributed to work with video display terminals (VDTs), the only clear and consistent association with their use involves the ergonomics of the operator in relation to the workstation and its design, including the VDT itself. Complaints of neck strain, back pain, tendinitis, and eyestrain have usually been due to disharmony between the position of the operator and the structure and function of the workstation, including the VDT, table, keyboard, and chair. Measurements of radiation emissions from VDTs have shown, in almost all studies, nondetectable levels or levels consistent with background. The only exception to this has been demonstration of increased magnetic fields in very close proximity to the terminal box itself. The levels of magnetic fields to which an operator would be exposed have not been associated with health effects in other literature.

Several studies of skin symptoms and/or effects in VDT operators have been conducted. Findings have been inconsistent, and in many cases positive findings have been related to confounding factors such as ambient humidity, "stress," indoor air quality, and psychosocial factors.[164–166]

References

1. Kligman AM. The chronic effects of repeated mechanical trauma to the skin. *Am J Ind Med* 1985; 8:257–264.
2. Kanerva L, Estlander T, Jolanki R. Occupational skin disease in Finland. An analysis of 10 years of statistics from an occupational dermatology clinic. *Int Arch Occup Environ Health* 1988; 60:89–94.
3. Kanerva L, Jolanki R, Toikkanen J, Tarvainen K, Estlander T. Statistics on occupational dermatoses in Finland. *Curr Probl Dermatol.* 1995; 23:28–40.
4. Susten AS. The chronic effects of mechanical trauma to the skin: A review of the literature. *Am J Ind Med* 1985; 8:281–288.
5. Adams RM. Physical and biologic causes of occupational skin disease: In: Adams RM, ed. *Occupational Skin Disease.* New York: Grune & Stratton; 1983:27–57.
6. Adams RM. Occupational dermatoses and disorders due to chemical agents. In: Fitzpatrick TB, Eisen AZ, Wolff K, et al., eds. *Dermatology in General Medicine,* 4th ed. New York: McGraw-Hill; 1993:1767–1783.
7. Kanerva L. Physical causes of occupational skin disease. Mechanical trauma. In: Adams RM, ed. *Occupational Skin Disease,* 2nd ed. Philadelphia: WB Saunders Co.; 1990:41–65.
8. Kanerva L. Mechanical causes of occupational skin disease. In: van der Valk P, Maibach HI, eds. *The Irritant Contact Dermatitis Syndrome.* Boca Raton: CRC Press, Inc.; 1996:195–204.
9. Gellin GA. Physical and mechanical causes of occupational dermatoses. In: Maibach HI, Gellin GA, eds. *Occupational and Industrial Dermatology,* 2nd ed. Chicago: Year Book Medical Publishers; 1987:88–93.
10. Gollhausen R, Kligman AM. Effects of pressure on contact dermatitis. *Am J Ind Med* 1985; 8:323–328.
11. Ronchese F. *Occupational Marks and Other Physical Signs: A Guide to Personal Identification.* New York: Grune & Stratton; 1948:1–181.
12. Wilkinson DS. Cutaneous reactions to mechanical and thermal injury. In: Rook A, Wilkinson DS, Ebling FJG, et al., eds. *Textbook of Dermatology,* 4th ed. Oxford: Blackwell Scientific Publications; 1986:587–622.
13. Bergfelt WF, Taylor JS. Trauma, sports, and the skin. *Am J Ind Med* 1985; 8:403–413.
14. Powell FC. Sports dermatology. *J Eur Acad Derm Venereol* 1994; 3:1–15.
15. Hayakawa R. Friction melanosis. In: van der Valk P, Maibach HI, eds. *The Irritant Contact Dermatitis Syndrome.* Boca Raton: CRC Press, Inc.; 1996:213–220.
16. Freeman S, Rosen RH. Irritant contact dermatitis resulting from repeated, low-grade frictional trauma. In: van der Valk P, Maibach HI, eds. *The Irritant Contact Dermatitis Syndrome.* Boca Raton: CRC Press; 1996: 205–210.
17. Samitz MH. Repeated mechanical trauma to the skin: Occupational aspects. *Am J Ind Med* 1985; 8:265–271.
18. Menné T. Frictional dermatitis in post office workers. *Contact Dermatitis* 1983; 9:172–173.
19. Menné T, Hjorth N. Frictional contact dermatitis. *Am J Ind Med* 1985; 8:401–402.
20. Storrs FJ. All the things I knew were true about contact dermatitis that arent't. *Cutis* 1994; 52:301–306.
21. Kanerva L, Estlander T, Jolanki R, Henriks-Eckerman M-L. Contact dermatitis from telefax paper. *Contact Dermatitis* 1992; 27:12–15.
22. Frosch PJ, Kligman AM. The chamber-scarification test for irritancy. *Contact Dermatitis* 1976; 2:314–324.
23. Fleming MG, Bergfelt WF. The etiology of irritant contact dermatitis. In: Jackson EM, Goldner R, eds. *Irritant Contact Dermatitis.* New York: Marcel Dekker, Inc.; 1990:41–66.
24. Evans EJ, Schmidt RJ. Plants and plant products that induce contact dermatitis. *Planta Medica* 1980; 38:289–316.
25. Stoner JG, Rasmussen JE. Plant dermatitis. *J Am Acad Dermatol* 1983; 9:1–15.
26. Epstein WL. House and garden plants. In: Jackson EM, Goldner R, eds. *Irritant Contact Dermatitis.* New York: Marcel Dekker, Inc.; 1990:127–165.
27. Lovell CR. Irritant plants. In: van der Valk P, Maibach HI, eds. *The Irritant Contact Dermatitis Syndrome.* Boca Raton: CRC Press, Inc.; 1996:87–94.
28. Grzegorczk L. "Glashände"—ein neues berufsbedingtes Syndrom [Glass hands—a new professional syndrome]. *Derm Beruf Umwelt* 1987; 35:62–62.
29. Fischer T, Rystedt I. Hand eczema among hard-metal workers. *Am J Ind Med* 1985; 8:381–394.
30. Williamson DM. Skin hazards in mining. *Br J Dermatol* 1981; 105 (suppl 21): 41–44.
31. Hatch KL, Maibach HI. Textile fiber dermatitis. *Contact Dermatitis.* 1985; 12:1–11.
32. Paulsen E, Andersen KE. Irritant contact dermatitis of a gardener's hands caused by handling fur-covered plant ornaments. *Am J Contact Dermatitis* 1991; 2:113–116.
33. Gould WM. Friction dermatitis of the thumbs caused by pantyhose. *Arch Dermatol* 1991; 127:1740.
34. Menné T, Bachman E. Permanent disability from skin diseases. *Dermatosen* 1979; 27:37–42.
35. Hersle K, Mobacken H. Hyperkeratotic dermatitis of the palms. *Br J Dermatol* 1982; 107:195–202.
36. Wilkinson DS. Dermatitis from repeated trauma to the skin. *Am J Ind Med* 1985; 8:307–317.
37. Menné T. Hyperkeratotic dermatitis of the palms. In: Menné T, Maibach HI, eds. *Hand Eczema.* Boca Raton: CRC Press; 1994:95–98.
38. Calnan CD. Eczema for me. *Trans St John's Hosp Dermatol Soc* 1968; 54:54–64.
39. Wilkinson DS. Letter to editor. *Contact Dermatitis* 1979; 5:118–119.
40. Zuehlke RL, Rapini RP, Puhl SC, Ray TL. Dermatitis in loco minoris resistentiae. *J Am Acad Dermatol* 1982; 6:1010–1013.
41. Mathias CGT. Post-traumatic eczema. *Dermatol Clin* 1988; 6:35–42.
42. Bruynzeel DP, de Boer EM. Compromised skin. In: van der Valk P, Maibach HI, eds. *The Irritant Contact Dermatitis Syndrome.* Boca Raton: CRC Press, Inc.; 1996:283–287.
43. Cronin E. Hand eczema. In: Rycroft RJG, Menné T, Frosch PJ, eds. *Textbook of Contact Dermatitis,* 2nd ed. Berlin: Springer-Verlag; 1995:207–218.
44. Burton JL. Eczema, lichenification, prurigo and erythroderma. In: Champion RH, Burton JL, Ebling FJG, eds. *Textbook of Dermatology.* London: Blackwell Scientific Publications; 1992:537–588.

45. Wilkinson DS. Introduction, definition, and classification. In: Menné T, Maibach H, eds. *Hand Eczema*. Boca Raton: CRC Press; 1996:1–12.

46. Kanerva L, Estlander T, Jolanki R. Allergic contact dermatitis from dental composite resins due to aromatic epoxy acrylates and aliphatic acrylates. *Contact Dermatitis* 1989; 20:201–211.

47. Kanerva L, Estlander T, Jolanki R, Tarvainen K. Dermatitis from acrylates in dental personnel. In: Menné T, Maibach H, eds. *Hand Eczema*. Boca Raton: CRC Press; 1994:231–254.

48. Andersen KE. Mechanical trauma and hand eczema. In: Menné T, Maibach H, eds. *Hand Eczema*. Boca Raton: CRC Press; 1994:31–34.

49. Harvell J, Maibach HI. Skin disease among musicians. *Med Probl Performing Artists* 1992; 7:114–120.

50. Bigardi AS, Pigatto PD, Moroni P. Occupational skin granulomas. *Clin Dermatol* 1992; 10:219–223.

51. Young PC, Smack DP, Sau P, Johnson FB, James WD. Golf club granuloma. *J Am Acad Dermatol* 1995; 32:1047–1048.

52. Johnson FB, Zimmerman LE. Barium sulfate and zinc sulfide deposits resulting from golf-ball injury to the conjunctiva and eyelid. *Am J Clin Pathol* 1965; 44:533–538.

53. Honda Y, Nishi R. Foreign-body granuloma due to the liquid core of a golf ball. *Jpn J Ophthalmol* 1978; 32:1251–1253.

54. Fisher AA. *Contact Dermatitis*, 2nd ed. Lea & Febiger; 1986.

55. Fischer T, Rystedt I. Cobalt allergy in hard metal workers. *Contact Dermatitis* 1983; 9:115–121.

56. Lammintausta K, Kalimo K, Havu VK. Occurrence of contact allergy and hand eczema in hospital wet work. *Contact Dermatitis* 1982; 8:84–90.

57. Estlander T, Jolanki R, Kanerva L. Dermatitis and urticaria from rubber and plastic gloves. *Contact Dermatitis* 1986; 14:20–25.

58. Estlander T, Jolanki R, Kanerva L. Allergic contact dermatitis from rubber and plastic gloves. In: Mellström G, Wahlberg JE, Maibach HI, eds. *Protective Gloves for Occupational Use*. Boca Raton: CRC Press; 1994:221–239.

59. Meneghini CL. Sensitization in traumatized skin. *Am J Ind Med* 1985; 8:319–321.

60. Argyris TS. Promotion of epidermal carcinogenesis by repeated damage to mouse skin. *Am J Ind Med* 1985; 8:329–337.

61. Epstein JH, Ormsby A, Adams RM. Occupational skin cancer. In: Adams RM, ed. *Occupational Skin Disease*, 2nd ed. Philadelphia: WB Saunders Co.; 1990:136–159.

62. Hogan DJ, Lane P. Dermatologic disorders in agriculture. *Occup Med State Art Rev* 1986; 1:285–300.

63. Alanko K, Kanerva L, Estlander T, Jolanki R, Leino T, Suhonen R, Hairdresser's koilonychia. *Am J Contact Dermatitis* 1997; 8:177–178.

64. Joung RS, Bry K, Ratner H. Selective phalangeal tuft fractures in a guitar player. *Br J Radiol* 1977; 50:147–148.

65. Destouet JM, Murphy WA. Guitar player acro-osteolysis. *Skel Radiol* 1981; 6:275–277.

66. Baran R, Tosti A. Occupational acroosteolysis in a guitar player. *Acta Derm Venereol (Stockh)* 1993; 73:64–65.

67. Estlander T, Jolanki R, Kanerva L. Protective gloves. In: *Hand Eczema*. Menné T, Maibach H, eds. Boca Raton: CRC Press; 1994:311–321.

68. Guignard JC. Evaluation of exposure to vibration. In: Cralley LV, Cralley LJ, eds. *Patty's Industrial Hygiene and Toxicology, vol III, Theory and Rationale of Industrial Hygiene Practice*. New York: Wiley Interscience; 1979.

69. Taylor JS. Vibration syndrome in industry: Dermatological viewpoint. *Am J Ind Med* 1985;8:415–432.

70. Moritz AR, Henriques FC Jr. Studies in thermal injuries. II. The relative importance of time and surface temperature in the causation of cutaneous burns. *Am J Pathol* 1947;23:695–720.

71. Cason JS. *Treatment of Burns*. London: Chapman & Hall; 1981:205–220.

72. Burke JF, Bondoc CC. Burns: The management and evaluation of the thermally injured patient. In: Fitzpatrick TB, Eisen AZ, Wolff K, et al., eds. *Dermatology in General Medicine*, 4th ed. New York: McGraw-Hill; 1993:1592–1598.

73. Campbell DC, Nano T, Pegg SP. Pattern of burn injury in hang-glider pilots. *Burns* 1996;22:328–330.

74. Nettelblad H, Thuomas KA, Sjöberg F. Magnetic resonance imaging: A new diagnostic aid in the care of high-voltage burns. *Burns* 1996;22:117–119.

75. Bartholome CW, Jacoby WD, Ramchand SC. Cutaneous manifestations of lightning injury. *Arch Dermatol* 1975;111:1466–1468.

76. Bruze M, Fregert S. Chemical skin burns. In: Menné T, Maibach HI, eds. *Hand Eczema*. Boca Raton: CRC Press; 1994:21–30.

77. Holland G, York M, Basketter DA. Irritants: Corrosive materials, oxidizing/reducing agents, acids, and alkalis, concentrated salt solutions, etc. In: *The Irritant Contact Dermatitis Syndrome*. van der Valk P, Maibach HI, eds. Boca Raton: CRC Press; 1996:55–64.

78. Schwartz L, Tulipan L, Birmingham DJ. *Occupational Diseases of the Skin*. Philadelphia: Lea & Febiger; 1957.

79. Hannuksela M, Suhonen R, Karvonen J. Caustic ulcers caused by cement. *Br J Dermatol* 1976; 95:547–549.

80. Vickers HR, Edwards DH. Cement burns. *Contact Dermatitis* 1976; 2:73–78.

81. Avnstorp C. Irritant cement eczema. In: van der Valk P, Maibach HI, eds. *The Irritant Contact Dermatitis Syndrome*. Boca Raton: CRC Press, Inc.; 1996:111–119.

82. Suhonen R. Cement knees. *Forum Nordic Derm Venereol* 1997; 2:19.

83. Onuba O, Essiet A. Cement burns of the heels. *Contact Dermatitis* 1986; 14:325–326.

84. Tindall JP: Occupationally related problems of special interest. In: Fitzpatrick TB, Eisen AZ, Wolff K, et al., eds. *Dermatology in General Medicine*, 3rd ed. New York: McGraw-Hill; 1987: 1575–1590.

85. Biro L, Fisher AA, Price E. Ethylene oxide burns. *Arch Dermatol* 1974; 110:924–925.

86. Bowen TE, Whelan TJ, Nelson TG. Sudden death after phosphorous burns: Experimental observations of hypocalcemia and electrocardiographic abnormalities following production of a standard white phosphorous burn. *Ann Surg* 1971; 174:779–784.

87. Mowad CM, McGinley KJ, Foglia A, Leyden JJ. The role of extracellular polysaccharide substance produced by *Staphylococcus epidermidis* in miliaria. *J Am Acad Dermatol* 1995; 33:729–733.

88. Lobitz WC. Sweat retention syndrome. In: Rees RB, ed. *Dermatoses Due to Environmental and Physical Factors*. Springfield, IL: Charles C Thomas; 1962: 146–156.

89. Kirk JF, Wilson BB, Chun W, Cooper PH. Miliaria profunda. *J Am Acad Dermatol* 1996; 35:854–856.

90. Cage GW, Sato K, Schwachman H. Eccrine glands. The management and evaluation of the thermally injured patient. In: Fitzpatrick TB, Eisen AZ, Wolff K, et al., eds. *Dermatology in General Medicine*, 3rd ed. New York: McGraw-Hill; 1987: 691–704.

91. Zalar GL, Harber LC. Reactions to physical agents. In: Moschella SL, Hurley HJ, eds. *Dermatology*, 2nd ed. Philadelphia: WB Saunders, Co.; 1985: 1672–1690.

92. Kligman LH, Kligman AM. Reflections on heat. *Br J Dermatol* 1984; 110:369–375.

93. Dvoretzky I, Silverman NR. Reticular erythema of the lower back. *Arch Dermatol* 1991; 127:405–410.

94. Mok DWH, Blumgart LH. Erythema ab igne in chronic pancreatic pain: A diagnostic sign. *J R Soc Med* 1984; 77:299–301.

94a. Kligman LH. Intensification of UV induced dermal damage by IR radiation. *Arch Dermatol Res* 1982; 272:229.

95. Heller Page E, Shear NH. Disorders due to physical factors. In: Fitzpatrick TB, Eisen AZ, Wolff K, et al., eds. *Dermatology in General Medicine*, 4th ed. New York: McGraw-Hill; 1993: 1581–1592.

96. Drenth JPH, Michiels JJ. Erythromelalgia and erythermalgia: Diagnostic differentiation. *Int J Dermatol* 1994; 33:393–397.

97. Drenth JPH, Michiels JJ, Van Joost TH. Substance P is not involved in primary and secondary erythermalgia. *Acta Derm Venereol (Stockh)* 1997; 77:325–326.

98. Kaplan RP. Cancer complicating chronic ulcerative and scarifying mucocutaneous disorders. *Adv Dermatol* 1987; 2:19–46.

99. Laycock HT. The "Kangri cancer" of North-West China. *BMJ* 1948; 1:982.

100. Chowdri NA, Darzi MA. Postburn scar carcinomas in Kashmiris. *Burns* 1996; 22:477–482.

101. Cross F. On a turf (peat) fire cancer: Malignant change superimposed in erythema ab igne. *Proc R Soc Med* 1967; 60:1307.

102. Corson EF, Knoll GM, Luscombe HA, et al. Role of spectacle lenses in production of cutaneous changes, especially epithelioma. *Arch Derm Syphilol* 1949; 59:435–443.

103. Kulka JP. Cold injury of the skin. *Arch Environ Health* 1965; 38:484.

104. Knize DM, Weatherley-White LCA, Paton BC, et al. Prognostic factors in the management of frostbite. *J Trauma* 1969; 9:749–759.

105. Rossis CG, Yiacoumettis AM, Elemenoglou J. Squamous cell carcinoma of the heel developing at site of previous frostbite. *J R Soc Med* 1982; 75:715–718.

106. Daniels F. Physiologic factors in the skin's reactions to heat and cold. In: Fitzpatrick TB, Eisen AZ, Wolff K, et al., eds. *Dermatology in General Medicine*, 3rd ed. New York: McGraw-Hill; 1987: 1412–1424.

107. Miller BJ, Chasmar LR. Frostbite in Saskatoon: A review of 10 winters. *Can J Surg* 1980; 23:423–426.

108. Rietschel RL, Allen AM. Immersion foot: A method for studying the effects of protracted water exposure on human skin. *Military Med* 1976; 141:778–780.

109. Chow S, Westfried M, Lynfield Y. Immersion foot: An occupational disease. *Cutis* 1980; 25:662.

110. Francis TJR. Nonfreezing cold injury: A historical review. *J R Nav Med Serv* 1984; 70:134–139.

111. Dowd PM, Rustin MHA, Lanigan S. Nifedipine in the treatment of chilblains. *BMJ* 1986; 293:923–924.

112. Toback AC, Korson R, Krusinski PA. Pulling boat hands: A unique dermatosis from coastal New England. *J Am Acad Dermatol* 1985; 12:649–655.

113. Rycroft RJG, Smith WDL. Low humidity occupational dermatoses. *Contact Dermatitis* 1980; 6:488–492.

114. Rycroft RJG. Low humidity occupational dermatoses. *Dermatol Clin* 1984; 2:553–557.

115. Rycroft RJG. Low humidity and microtrauma. *Am J Ind Med* 1985; 8:371–373.

116. White IR, Rycroft RJG. Low humidity occupational dermatosis—An epidemic. *Contact Dermatitis* 1982; 8:287–290.

117. Blank IH: Factors which influence the water content of the stratum corneum. *J Invest Dermatol* 1952; 18:433–440.

118. Lidén C, Wahlberg JE. Does visual display terminal work provoke rosacea? *Contact Dermatitis* 1985; 13:235–241.

119. Berg M. Facial skin complaints and work at visual display units. Epidemiological, clinical and histopathological studies. *Acta Derm Venereol (Stockh)* 1989; 150 (suppl):1–40.

120. Bergqvist U, Wahlberg JE. Skin symptoms during work with visual display terminals. *Contact Dermatitis* 1994; 30:193–196.

121. Hamilton A. A vasomotor disturbance in the fingers of stonecutters. *Arch Gewerbepath Gewerbehyg* 1930; 1:348–358.

122. Agate JN, Druett HA, Tombleson JBL. Raynaud's phenomenon in grinders of small metal castings. *Br J Ind Med* 1946; 3:167–174.

123. Pyykkö I. Clinical aspects of the hand–arm vibration syndrome. *Scand J Work Environ Health* 1986; 12:439–447.

124. Taylor W. Vibration white-finger in the workplace. *J Soc Occup Med* 1982; 32:159–166.

125. Hellstrom B, Lange Andersen K. Vibration injuries in Norwegian forest workers. *Br J Ind Med* 1972; 29:255–263.

126. Gemne G, Ekenvall L, Hansson J-E, et al. Skadlig inverkan av hand-arm-vibrationer—en forsäkringsmedicinsk bedömningsmodell. Arbete Hälsa 1986;2.

127. American Conference of Governmental Industrial Hygienists (ACGIH). Background on vibration. In: *Documentation of the Threshold Limit Values for Physical Agents in the Workroom Environment*, 4th ed. Cincinnati: ACGIH; 1987:477–479.

128. Nielsen SL. Raynaud's phenomenon and finger systolic pressure during cooling. *Scand J Clin Lab* 1978; 38:765–770.

129. Dart EE. Effect of high speed vibrating tools on operators engaged in the airplane industry. *J Occup Med* 1946; 1:515–550.

130. Wener MH, Metzger WJ, Simon RA. Occupationally acquired vibratory angioedema with secondary carpal tunnel syndrome. *Ann Intern Med* 1983; 98:44–46.

131. Koskimies K, Pyykkö I, Starck J, Inaba R. Vibration syndrome among Finnish forest workers between 1972 and 1990. *Int Arch Occup Environ Health* 1992; 64:251–256.

132. Spittell JA. Raynaud's phenomenon and allied vasospastic disorders. In: Juergens JL, Spittell JA, Fairbarin JF II, eds. *Peripheral Vascular Diseases*, 5th ed. Philadelphia: WB Saunders, Co.; 1980:555–583.

133. Hashem CJ, Christina B, Sherertz EF. Is cryotherapy an occupational "contact" hazard for physicians with Raynaud's disease? *Am J Contact Dermatitis* 1997; 8:56–57.

134. Suciu I, Drejman I, Valaskai M. Contributions to the study of affections caused by vinyl chloride [in Romania]. *Med Intern* 1963; 15:967–978.

135. Mariqu HR. Vinyl chloride disease. In: Clark CM, Myers AR, eds. *Current Topics in Rheumatology*. New York: Grower Medical Publishing; 1985:105–113.

136. Cordier JH, Fieviez C, Lefévre MJ, Sevrin A. Acroosteolyse et lesions cutanées associées chez deux ouvriers affectés au nettoyage d'autoclaves. *Cah Med Travail* 1966; 4:3–39.

137. Dinman BD, Cook WA, Whitehouse WM, et al. Occupa-

tional acroosteolysis. I. An epidemiological study. *Arch Environ Health* 1971; 22:61–73.

138. Walker AE. Vinyl chloride disorder. *Br J Dermatol* 1981; 105(suppl 21):19.

139. Wilson RH, McCormick WE, Tatum CF, et al: Occupational acroosteolysis: Report of 3 cases. *JAMA* 1967; 201:557–580.

140. Walker AE. Clinical aspects of vinyl chloride disease. *Proc R Soc Med* 1976; 69:286.

141. Haustein UF, Ziegler V. Environmentally induced systemic sclerosis-like disorders. *Int J Dermatol* 1985; 24:747–757.

142. Zschunke E, Ziegler V, Haustein U-F. Occupationally induced connective tissue disorders. In: Adams RM, ed. *Occupational Skin Disease*, 2nd ed. Philadelphia: WB Saunders Co.; 1990:172–183.

143. Meyerson LB, Meyer GC. Cutaneous lesions in acroosteolysis. *Arch Dermatol* 1972; 106:224–227.

144. Conde-Salazar R, Guimaraens D, Romero LV. Occupational radiodermatitis from IR 192 exposure. *Contact Dermatitis* 1986; 15:202–204.

145. Yamada M, Kodama K, et al. Prevalence of skin neoplasms among the atomic bomb survivors. *Radiat Res* 1996; 146:223–226.

146. International Commission on Radiological Protection (ICRP). *Recommendations of the International Commission on Radiological Protection.* Annal ICRP 1991; 21:1–3.

147. Epstein J. Adverse cutaneous reactions to the sun. In: Malkinson FD, Pearson RW, eds. *Yearbook of Dermatology.* Chicago: Year Book Medical Publishers; 1971:7.

148. Rose RC III, Parker RL. Erythema and conjunctivitis outbreak caused by inadvertent exposure to ultraviolet light. *JAMA* 1979; 242:1155–1156.

149. Bruze M, et al. Dermatitis with an unusual explanation in a welder. *Acta Derm Venereol (Stockh)* 1994; 74:380–382.

150. Orentreich N, Harber LC, Tromovitch TA. Photosensitivity and photo-onycholysis due to demethylchlortetracycline. *Arch Dermatol* 1961; 83:730–737.

151. Appendix: Ultraviolet radiation. *IARC Monogr* 1986; 40:379–415.

152. Mackie RM, Elwood JM, Hawk JLM. Links between exposures to ultraviolet radiation and skin cancer. *Rep R Coll Phys* 1987; 21:1–6.

153. Elwood JM. Melanoma and sun exposure. *Semin Oncol* 1996; 23:650–666.

154. Schauder S, et al. Olaquindox induced airborne photoallergic contact dermatitis followed by transient or persistent light reactions in 15 pig breeders. *Contact Dermatitis* 1996; 35:344–354.

155. Willis I. Sunlight and skin. *JAMA* 1971; 217:1088–1093.

156. Klein LR, et al. Photo-exacerbation of cutaneous lupus erythematosus due to ultraviolet A emissions from a photocopier. *Arthritis Rheum* 1995; 38:1152–1156.

157. Ive FA, Magnus IA, Warin RP, et al. "Actinic reticuloid": A chronic dermatosis associated with severe photosensitivity and the histologic resemblance of lymphoma. *Br J Dermatol* 1969; 81:469–485.

158. Roelandts R, Huys I. Broad-band and persistent photosensitivity following accidental ultraviolet C overexposure. *Photodermatol Photoimmunol Photomed* 1993; 9:144–146.

159. Brown S, Lane PR, Magnus IA. Skin photosensitivity from fluorescent lighting. *Br J Dermatol* 1969; 81:420–428.

160. Harber LC. Dermatoses due to physical agents. In: Kopf AW, Andrade R, eds. *Yearbook of Dermatology.* Chicago: Year Book Medical Publishers; 1970:141.

161. IRPA/INIRC. *Guidelines, Fluorescent Lighting and Malignant Melanoma.* International Non-Ionizing Radiation Committee, International Radiation Protection Association. Health Phys 1990; 58:111–112.

162. Moss E, Murray W, Parr W, et al. Physical hazards. In: Key MM, ed. *Occupational Diseases: A Guide to Their Recognition.* Cincinnati: NIOSH; 1977:478.

163. Geeraets WJ, Berry ER. Ocular spectral characteristics as related to hazards from lasers and other light sources. *Am J Ophthalmol* 1968; 66:15–20.

164. Carmichael AJ, Roberts DL. Visual display units and facial rashes. *Contact Dermatitis* 1992; 26:63–64.

165. Bergqvist U, Wahlberg JE. Skin symptoms and disease during work with visual display terminals. *Contact Dermatitis* 1994; 30:197–204.

166. Stenberg B, et al. Facial skin symptoms in visual display terminal (VDT) workers. A case-reference study of personal, psychosocial, building and VDT-related risk indicators. *Int J Epidemiol* 1995; 24:796–803.

167. Wanderer AA. The spectrum of cold urticaria. *Immunol Allergy Clin North Am* 1995; 15:701–723.

Bibliography

Bäck O, Larsen A. Delayed cold urticaria. *Acta Derm Venereol (Stockh)* 1978; 58:369–371.

Bernhard J. Nonrashes. Atmoknesis. Pruritus provoked by contact with air. *Cutis* 1989; 44:143–144.

Bircher AJ. Water-induced itching. *Dermatologica* 1990; 181:83–87.

Black AK. Mechanical trauma and urticaria. *Am J Ind Med* 1985; 8:297–303.

Breathnach SM, Allen R, Milford-Ward A, et al. Symptomatic dermographism: Natural history, clinical features, laboratory investigations and response to therapy. *Clin Exp Dermatol* 1983; 8:463–476.

Chalamidas SL, Charles R. Aquagenic urticaria. *Arch Dermatol* 1971; 104:541–546.

Cho KH, Kim YG, Seo KI, Suh DH. Black heel with atypical melanocytic hyperplasia. *Clin Exp Dermatol* 1993; 18:437–440.

Cremer B, Henz BM. Heat contact urticaria. In: Henz BM, Zuberbier T, Grabbe J, Monroe E, eds. *Urticaria.* Berlin: Springer-Verlag; 1997.

Crow KD, Alexander E, Buch WHL. Photosensitivity due to pitch. *Br J Dermatol* 1961; 73:220–232.

Czarnetzki BM: *Urticaria.* Berlin: Springer-Verlag; 1986.

Czarnetzki BM, Meentken J, Rosenbach T, et al. Clinical, pharmacological and immunological aspects of delayed pressure urticaria. *Br J Dermatol* 1984; 111:315–323.

Henquet UF, Martens BPM, Van Vloten WA. Cold urticaria: A clinico-therapeutic study in 30 patients; with special emphasis on cold desensitization. *Eur J Dermatol* 1992; 2:75–77.

Henz BM, Jeep S, Ziegert FS, Niemann J, Kunkel G. Dermal and bronchial hyperreactivity in urticarial dermographism. *Allergy* 1996; 51:171–175.

Henz BM, Zuberbier T, Grabbe J, Monroe E. *Urticaria.* Berlin: Springer-Verlag; 1997.

Highet AS, Pye R, Felix RH. Vibratory urticaria. *Br J Dermatol* 1981; 105:40–41.

Hölzle E, Hadshiew IM. Mechanisms of solar urticaria. *Curr Opin Dermatol* 1996; 3:185–189.

Illig L, Kunick J. Klinik und diagnostik der physikalischen Urticaria I. *Hautarzt* 1969; 20:167–178.

Kirby JD, Matthews CNA, James J, et al. The incidence and other aspects of factitious whealing (dermographism). *Br J Dermatol* 1971; 85:331–335.

Kligman AM, Klemme JC, Susten AS. *The Chronic Effects of*

Repeated Mechanical Trauma to the Skin. New York: Alan R. Liss, Inc.; 1985.

Krüger-Krasagakes S, Henz BM. Delayed pressure urticaria. In: Henz BM, Zuberbier T, Grabbe J, Monroe E, eds. *Urticaria.* Berlin: Springer-Verlag; 1997.

Levine JI. *Medications that Increase Sensitivity to Light: A 1990 Listing.* HHS Publ. FDA 91-8280. Washington, DC. U.S. Department of Health and Human Services, Food and Drug Administration; December 1990.

Michaelsson G, Ros AM. Familial localized heat urticaria of delayed type. *Acta Derm Venereol (Stockh)* 1971; 51:279–283.

Möller A, Henning M, Zuberbier T, Czarnetzki BM. Epidemiologie und Klinik der Kälteurtikaria. *Hautarzt* 1997.

Möller A, Henz BM. Cold urticaria. In: Henz BM, Zuberbier T, Grabbe J, Monroe E, eds. *Urticaria.* Berlin: Springer-Verlag; 1997.

Neittaanmäki H. Cold urticaria. *J Am Acad Dermatol* 1985; 13:636–644.

Patterson R, Mellies CJ, Blankenship ML, et al. Vibratory angioedema: A hereditary type of physical allergy. *J Allergy Clin Immunol* 1972; 50:174–182.

Reinauer S, Lenutsphong V, Hölzle E. Fixed solar urticaria. *J Am Acad Dermatol* 1993; 29:161–165.

Rosenbach T, Henz BM. Solar urticaria. In: Henz BM, Zuberbier T, Grabbe J, Monroe E, eds. *Urticaria.* Berlin: Springer-Verlag; 1997.

Ryan TJ, Shim-Young N, Turk JL. Delayed pressure urticaria. *Br J Dermatol* 1968; 80:485–490.

Scott JR, Moris R, McPhaden AR, Knight SL, Webster MH. Malignant schwannoma in a burn scar. *Burns* 1996; 22:494–496.

Sheffer AL, Austen KF. Exercise-induced anaphylaxis. *J Allergy Clin Immunol* 1980; 66:106–111.

Sheffer AL, Soter NA, McFadden ER, et al. Exercise-induced anaphylaxis: A distinct form of physical allergy. *J Allergy Clin Immunol* 1983; 71:311–316.

Smith JA, Mansfield LE, Fokakis A, et al. Dermographia caused by IgE mediated penicillin allergy. *Ann Allergy* 1983; 51:30–32.

Songsiridej V, Busse WW. Exercise-induced anaphylaxis. *Clin Allergy* 1983; 13:317–321.

Soter NA. Urticaria and angioedema. In: Fitzpatrick TB, Eisen AZ, Wolff K, et al., eds. *Dermatology in General Medicine,* 4th ed. New York: McGraw-Hill; 1993: 1483–1493.

Soter NA, Joshi NP, Twarog FJ, et al. Delayed cold induced urticaria: A dominantly inherited disorder. *J Allergy Clin Immunol* 1977; 59:294–297.

Sussman GL, Harvey KP, Schoket AL. Delayed pressure urticaria. *J Allergy Clin Immunol* 1982; 70:337–342.

Villas-Martinez F, Contreras FJ, Lopez-Cazana JM, Lopez-Serrano MC, Martinez-Alzamora F. A comparison of new nonsedating and classical antihistamines in the treatment of primary acquired cold urticaria (AUC). *J Invest Allergol Clin Immunol* 1992; 2:258–262.

Warin RP. The role of trauma in the spreading wheals of hereditary angio-oedema. *Br J Dermatol* 1983; 108:189–194.

Wasserman D, ed. *Vibration White-Finger Disease in US Workers Using Pneumatic Chipping and Grinding Hand Tools. I. Epidemiology.* Publ. No. 82-118. Cincinnati: DHHS, NIOSH; 1982.

Willis I, Epstein JH. Solar vs heat-induced urticaria. *Arch Dermatol* 1974; 110:389–392.

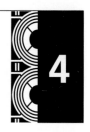

Systemic Toxicity from Percutaneous Absorption

KLAUS E. ANDERSEN, M.D., Ph.D.

Systemic toxicity caused by percutaneous absorption of toxic substances does occur, although systemic toxicity is more commonly caused by ingestion or inhalation. The amount of gases, volatile solvents, and aerosols taken into the lungs is often much more important than the amount of substance absorbed through the skin. However, more than one route is frequently involved in the exposure, and it may be difficult to determine the relative importance of each route. The relative importance of dermal exposure increases when airborne occupational exposure limits are reduced, unless steps to reduce skin exposure are undertaken.[1] Some substances do penetrate the skin, enter the circulation, and cause systemic toxicity in one or more target organs or elicit generalized hypersensitivity reactions. Evaluation of dermal exposure in the workplace is a very complicated task. The following variables are critical in the evaluation:

1. the form of the chemical,
2. the dose of the chemical,
3. the duration of dermal exposure,
4. the area exposed (size as well as location on the body),
5. the presence of other chemicals (mixture constituents, dispersant), and
6. workload and environmental factors (humidity and temperature).[2]

Previous reviews of disease and systemic toxicity following percutaneous absorption of chemicals include Wahlberg, Birmingham, Pascher, Grandjean, Freeman and Maibach, and de Groot et al.[3–8] This chapter does not attempt to list all references but surveys the current knowledge of systemic toxicity caused by percutaneous absorption based on experimental and clinical data. We are dependent not only on clinical observations but also on predictive test models in man, in animals, and in vitro for establishing the threshold limit values for exposure and for laying down the recommended precautions to be taken during work with the chemical.

Percutaneous Absorption

Over the past decades our knowledge about percutaneous absorption has increased.[9, 10] The principal barrier is the stratum corneum. The chemicals move across the barrier by passive diffusion and not by active transport. The toxicant must pass the epidermal cells and the cells of the sweat or sebaceous glands or enter through the hair follicles. The intercellular spaces between the corneocytes are filled with lamellar, nonpolar, lipid bilayers and constitute the major pathway of penetration for some substances.[11, 12] The stratum corneum also has a reservoir effect, as chemicals may penetrate the epidermis over a long period of time after exposure. It was suggested by Scheuplein[13] that absorption through ducts and follicles is predominant soon after application, whereas bulk diffusion through the intact stratum corneum is dominant in the steady-state stage. Once the corneal layer is penetrated, the chemical can pass relatively unimpeded into the systemic circulation of the body, but living epidermis also retains barrier properties to some extent. The skin thickness and resistance to penetration varies from individual to individual and with the body region (Table 4–1). The scrotal skin of a man is about 300 times more permeable by ^{14}C-hydrocortisone than is plantar skin[14]; and face, scalp, and axilla are about 3 to 6 times more penetrable than is forearm skin. Occupational physicians and toxicologists should be aware that highly absorbing skin areas such as face and scalp often are not covered with protective clothing. In general, the permeability increases severalfold if the stratum

TABLE 4–1 • **Comparative Relative Permeability of Human Skin to Topical ^{14}C Hydrocortisone, ^{14}C Parathion, and ^{14}C Malathion**[a]

Regional Variation	Hydrocortisone	Parathion	Malathion
Forearm	1.0	1.0	1.0
Palm	0.8	1.3	0.9
Foot, ball	—	1.6	1.0
Abdomen	—	2.1	1.4
Hand, dorsum	—	2.4	1.8
Scalp	3.5	3.7	—
Jaw angle	13.0	3.9	—
Forehead	6.0	4.2	3.4
Axilla	3.6	7.4	4.2
Scrotum	42.0	11.8	—

[a] Maibach HI, Feldmann RJ, Milby TH, Serat WF. Regional variation in percutaneous penetration in man: pesticides. *Arch Environ Health* 1971;23:208–211.

corneum is damaged or occluded.[15] Structural changes in the epidermis made by detergents or solvents may produce a similar effect. Changes in the water content—hydration or environmental chapping (dehydration)—may dramatically increase permeability. Even when the epidermis is intact, there may still be a thousandfold difference in penetration rate of different substances. The amount of a chemical absorbed depends on a number of factors: physicochemical properties, vehicle release, absorption kinetics, cellular distribution, substantivity, volatility, wash-and-rub resistance, and binding.[16] In general, lipid-soluble compounds are more easily absorbed than water-soluble compounds.

The penetration potential of a compound is best studied in human volunteers because one avoids the problems connected with extrapolation from one species to another. However, many compounds are too toxic to test in vivo in humans, so their percutaneous absorption must be investigated in animal models or in in vitro models. The animal models most predictive of percutaneous absorption in humans appear to be the pig and the monkey. The animal model of choice may be determined by the test compound. Smaller laboratory animals such as rats, guinea pigs, and rabbits may also be utilized, but correlations and predictions of results must be evaluated with utmost care.[17] Excised human skin is preferable for in vitro studies. The primary barrier to percutaneous absorption, the stratum corneum, is nonliving tissue and it retains its barrier properties after excision. Conduct of experiments in in vitro skin penetration requires attention to technical details in order to reduce intra- and interlaboratory variation.[18] The integrity of the skin samples should be checked by testing the permeability of a reference compound.[9]

Biotransformation

When a compound has penetrated the stratum corneum, it is subjected to a host of biological systems in the skin and internal organs that affect the concentration of the compound in the various parts of the body. Viable epidermis and dermis have significant metabolizing properties, and usually the chemical agent is deactivated or detoxified. However, the skin also contains several classes of metabolizing enzymes, such as arylhydrocarbon hydroxylase, epoxide hydratase, and gluthathione-S-epoxide transferase, which can be induced and which then convert nonactive substances into active pharmacological and toxicological agents.[19, 20] Cytochrome P-450 is a hemoprotein known from microsomal hepatic cell fractions. It functions as an oxidase of the metabolizing enzyme systems. It is present in the skin and can be induced by topical administration of agents such as polycyclic aromatic hydrocarbons (PAHs). These chemicals are metabolically activated in the skin and they induce skin carcinomas. The biotransformation systems in the skin further include oxidative, reductive, hydrolytic, and conjugative reactions. The significance of the biotransformation systems in the skin demands further study. There may be a difference in the cutaneous metabolic potential between normal and diseased skin.[21, 22]

Exposure and Reaction Patterns

Systemic toxicity from percutaneous absorption occurs in industry, in agriculture, in therapeutic medicine, and during leisure time. The clinical examples from the literature are usually case reports based on after-the-fact observations, and the route of exposure is often established by the nature of patients' histories. Many of the case reports

TABLE 4–2 • Important Elements of the Various Methods of Estimating Dermal Exposure[a]

Method/Technique	Validation Tests	Key Factors
Surrogate skin	Retention/absorption Breakthrough	Fabric weight (g/cm^2) Fabric yarn (yarns/cm)
Removal	Removal efficiency	Solubility in liquid Elapsed time Uptake through skin cohesion Forces
Tracer	Relative transfer Contaminant and tracer	
Biological monitoring	Pharmacokinetics Collection time	All routes of entry Internal exposure Irrelevant for local effects
Surface sampling	Removable residue Transferability	Fabric type Pressure/method Repeatability

[a] Van Hemmen UJ, Brouwer DH. Assessment of dermal exposure to chemicals. *Sci Tot Environ* 1995;168:131–141.

describe extreme and unintentional conditions of exposure, and this must be taken into consideration when evaluating the hazards involved in intentional use of a chemical. Several factors in the work environment can increase the risk of percutaneous toxicity: insufficient education of workers, simple negligence, failure to use protective gloves or clothing, and wearing soaked or defective protective clothing, gloves, or boots, which can lead to prolonged skin contact with a hazardous chemical. After accidental or unintended skin exposure to a hazardous substance, decontamination of the skin is warranted. Maibach and Feldmann[23] studied systemic absorption of pesticides and showed that washing with soap and water seemed to be the most practical and safest way to decontaminate skin.

Following contact with a chemical, the skin can react in several different ways, depending on the nature and dose of the chemical. The skin may:

1. act as an efficient barrier preventing penetration,
2. show mild to severe irritation that is confined to the skin,
3. be severely damaged by corrosive chemicals followed by systemic toxic effects (or the initial skin contact with a corrosive chemical may lead to the formation of a new barrier, resulting in reduced absorption during succeeding exposure to chemicals such as mercuric chloride),[24]
4. show an allergic contact dermatitis,
5. function as a reservoir for delayed release of the material, or
6. be permeable and allow absorption of the material to a degree that causes systemic effects.

Assessment of dermal exposure to a chemical or product in an occupational setting is very complicated and the methods vary in complexity. They include:

1. surrogate skin techniques in which a chemical collection medium is placed on the skin,
2. removal techniques such as washing and wiping of the skin,
3. fluorescent tracer techniques, in which a fluorescent compound is added to the product in question and contamination of exposed workers is quantified by measuring the fluorescence from the skin after work by using video imaging techniques, and
4. biological monitoring in which detailed pharmacokinetic analysis of the chemical involved in quantification has been performed.[1, 25]

The choice of method depends on the chemical in question as well as on practical and economic factors. All methods should be regarded as providing only estimates of dermal exposure until proper validation studies have been concluded. Table 4–2 shows some important details to be considered when dermal exposure is measured.

The following overview contains information about the systemic effects of percutaneous absorption of compounds in industry and agriculture and lists examples of systemic toxicity resulting from topical drugs and toiletries.

INDUSTRY

Carcinogens

More than 200 years ago the English physician Percival Pott described an association between exposure to soot and coal tars and cancer of the scrotum in chimney sweeps. For about 80 years it has been known that workers handling certain aromatic amines and chromium compounds have increased incidences of carcinoma of the urinary bladder and of the lung, respectively.[26] Organic solvents can also be hazardous. Components in gasoline are carcinogenic in experimental as well as in human epidemiological studies. This finding supports the implementation of preventive measures to reduce exposure of the human population to gasoline vapors.[27] There is evidence that benzene exposure carries a risk of producing leukemia.[28] The main route of absorption is through the respiratory and upper gastrointestinal tracts. However, the skin may be the port of entry for 4,4′-diaminodiphenyl (benzidine), which causes carcinoma of the bladder.

The industrial chemicals that cause other types of systemic effects through cutaneous penetration fall into the following groups: aromatic nitro and amino compounds, hydrocarbons, metals and their derivatives, and others.

Aromatic Nitro and Amino Compounds

Aniline dyes and aromatic amines are known to pass readily through intact skin. They can give rise to methemoglobinemia, dermatitis, and injury to the kidney, bladder, and liver. Methylenedianiline, 4,4′-diaminodiphenylmethane (MDA), is widely used as an epoxy hardener and as an antioxidant in the manufacture of rubber, urethane, and other elastomers. Toxic hepatitis developed in 12 male workers exposed to MDA during the manufacture of insulating material. They developed fever, chills, and right-upper-quadrant pain, with subsequent jaundice. All patients recovered within 7 weeks and reexamination years later showed no sign of chronic liver disease. There was circumstantial evidence that the route of entry was percutaneous. The workers kneaded a doughy mixture of curing epoxy resin and MDA by hand, which resulted in prolonged skin contact with MDA until the fully polymerized product became inert. They were often covered with dust, but air concentrations of MDA were low, so that the dust most probably did not contain noteworthy concentrations of MDA.[29]

Aromatic nitro compounds are used in the production of explosives and in medicine. Nitroglycerin transdermal devices have been developed for treatment of angina. Nitroglycerin (glyceryltrinitrate) is also used in dynamite. Workers engaged in the manufacture and use of dynamite may develop acute toxic reactions during the workday, including headache, weakness, tachycardia, and

hypotension. Nitroglycerin evaporates easily and contaminates the air and is also easily absorbed through the skin by direct contamination. Blood samples from exposed workers showed significantly higher concentrations in cubital vein blood than in femoral vein blood, indicating that absorption through the skin is of great importance.[30] Even sudden deaths have been reported. A certain degree of tolerance may develop; for some workers, symptoms are worse when starting at work after vacation when they have been free from exposure.

Solvents

The capability of hydrocarbon solvents to cause systemic effects varies. The poorly absorbed solvents cause more skin damage but low systemic toxicity in contrast to the solvents that penetrate easily and cause systemic toxicity without causing considerable skin damage. The saturated hydrocarbons are more irritating than the solvents from the aromatic series.[31] The health and safety aspects of solvent exposure were reviewed by Riihimäki and Ulfvarson.[32]

In most cases of solvent toxicity, it is not known how many of the systemic effects are caused by percutaneous absorption rather than by inhalation. Acute high-dose exposure can produce a transient narcotic effect on the central nervous system. Chronic exposure to organic solvents can produce an increased frequency of peripheral neuropathies and of toxic encephalopathies that lead to alterations in affect, to memory loss, and to impaired cognition—perhaps even to premature and persistent dementia in certain workers.[33, 34] Hansbrough and coworkers[35] reported four cases of contact injuries. One patient developed full-thickness skin loss following gasoline immersion, and another developed severe systemic complications after contact with a carburetor-cleaning solvent; it involved pulmonary, neurological, renal, and hepatic insufficiency. Gasolines containing lead may be more hazardous.

Although cutaneous absorption of gasoline and other hydrocarbons may cause systemic effects, the lungs are the primary site of systemic absorption in many cases. In severe contact injuries, surgical débridement should be considered if there is suspicion of continued absorption from the wound.

The percutaneous absorption of organic solvent vapors at the threshold limit level is insignificant compared to the inhalation route. It resulted in an absorption of 0.5 to 2.0% of the amount that would have been absorbed via the lungs during exposure to the same concentration during the same period. However, disease-affected skin may lead to increased absorption. A volunteer with atopic dermatitis absorbed 3 times more xylene vapor through the skin than did subjects with normal skin.[36]

Pure solvents in liquid form may be absorbed through the skin in significant amounts. Butanol absorption amounts to 8.8 μg/min/cm^2 which equals a total uptake of 195 mg if both hands are immersed in solvent for 30 minutes.[37] For xylene and methyl ethyl ketone, the corresponding calculated figures are 44 mg/30 min.[38, 39] Riihimäki and Pfäffli[36] found that a 15-minute immersion of a subject's hands in xylene produced blood levels comparable to those following an 8-hour inhalation exposure at 100 ppm (the threshold limit value).

The percutaneous toxicity of solvents may be evaluated in animal models. Wahlberg and Boman[40] used guinea pigs to compare 10 industrial solvents. A single application of 0.5 to 2 mL of the solvents was administered to a skin depot subsequently covered to prevent inhalation and licking. The animals were observed for 35 days for clinical symptoms and weight gain. Five solvents caused mortalities among the guinea pigs; in declining order, they were 2-chloroethanol, 1,1,2-trichloroethane, ethyleneglycolmonobutylether, carbon tetrachloride, and dimethylformamide. Four solvents affected weight gain significantly: benzene, toluene, 1,1,1-trichloroethane, and trichloroethylene. However, n-hexane produced no effect after percutaneous administration to guinea pigs. The clinical implication of these animal data is to be determined. Chlorinated hydrocarbons such as methyl chloride, methylene chloride, vinyl chloride, chloroform, and tetrachloroethylene probably do not cause systemic effects in humans through percutaneous absorption, even though many of them are well known to be toxins when inhaled. However, carbon tetrachloride can be absorbed by the skin in sufficient quantities to produce liver injury.

The same animal model was used to study the effect of two barrier creams and protective gloves on the skin absorption of solvents.[41] A combination of toluene and benzene was applied on skin treated with barrier cream and on skin covered with a glove membrane made of polyvinylchloride or rubber. The protective effect was temporary. After 2 to 3 hours, the blood concentrations were about the same as for unprotected skin.

Water solubility seems to be an essential factor in the regulation of percutaneous absorption of solvents. The absorption of n-butanol, a hydrophilic solvent, was increased by such skin injuries as stripping and contact dermatitis, whereas the

absorption of toluene and 1,1,1-trichloroethane, hydrophobic solvents, was reduced by the same factors.[42] The administration of solvents in mixtures that include detergents may reduce vapor pressure and the percutaneous absorption of solvents following skin contact. One cannot generalize; each combination of solvent and detergent should be evaluated in model systems to assure a reduced skin absorption. Hydrophobic solvents such as toluene and 1,1,1-trichlorethane were absorbed less through guinea pig skin in vivo when emulsified in water with the help of sodium dodecyl sulphate and Berol 065 (ethoxylated fatty alcohol), respectively, or when mixed with Triton 100 (octoxynol 9). In contrast, a hydrophilic solvent such as n-butanol was absorbed more readily when mixed with anionic detergent and water.[42]

Glycol ethers are used as industrial solvents for resins, lacquers, paints, dyes, and inks and as emulsifiers or detergents. Two workers in a textile printing plant developed clinical manifestations of encephalopathy, bone marrow injury, and pancytopenia after the use of ethylene glycol monomethyl ether (2-methoxyethanol) (EGMME) as a cleansing agent. Air samples obtained during the use of EGMME showed air concentrations well below the threshold limit value, indicating that poisoning was due primarily to cutaneous exposure.[43] Ethylene glycol monobutyl ether (2-butoxyethanol) (EGBE) was subjected to toxicokinetic studies in humans and animals.[44] The solvent was easily absorbed through the lungs and through the skin. The percutaneous absorption was higher from aqueous solutions containing 5 to 80% solvent than from neat EGBE. The metabolism of EGBE was inhibited by ethanol. However, it was distributed in a relatively low volume, and it cleared rapidly, suggesting that it would probably not be accumulated in the body.

A number of glycol ethers used in multicolor offset and ultraviolet curing printing processes are suspected of provoking bone marrow injuries after extensive exposure. The relative importance of inhalation and percutaneous absorption is not known.[45] Chlorinated biphenyls and naphthalenes can produce severe cutaneous and systemic effects. Dioxin (2,3,7,8-tetra-chlorodibenzo-p-dioxin) (TCDD) produces chloracne, which was the most prominent clinical sequela of the 1976 Seveso, Italy, accident. Among industrial populations exhibiting chloracne, a variety of ill-defined neurological abnormalities have been found together with porphyria cutanea tarda and hepatotoxicity.[46] The relative importance of percutaneous absorption compared to inhalation has not been determined. The serum level of polychlorinated biphenyls in workers at an electrical capacitor manufacturing plant was found to be a function of duration of employment and cumulative occupational exposure, indicating the importance of both exposure level and opportunity for contact, perhaps via percutaneous absorption.[47]

Occupationally Induced Scleroderma or Scleroderma-like Disease

It is suspected that systemic scleroderma or scleroderma-like disease may be provoked by solvents. Systemic scleroderma is a rare disease with unknown etiology. Genetic factors seem to play an important role, and women constitute 80 to 90% of the patients.[48] In male patients, environmental factors have been suspected to be the cause of the disease (Table 4–3). Haustein and Ziegler[49] found that 93 of 120 male patients with systemic sclerosis had been exposed to silica dust and 49 had silicosis. Similar findings have been reported among miners in South Africa.[50] Scleroderma-like disease may be caused by occupational exposure to vinyl chloride[51] and the chlorinated organic solvents trichloroethylene and perchloroethylene.[52] Similar clinical pictures have been seen in patients exposed to epoxy resins[53] and pesticides.[54] The mechanism by which these compounds provoke scleroderma-like disease and the relative importance of skin and pulmonary exposure is unknown. The anecdotal reports on the relationship between systemic scleroderma and scleroderma-like disease and occupational exposure to certain chemicals should be supplemented with larger epidemiological studies in several centers, including a sufficient number of controls, and should be designed in a way that allows for meta-analyses before an association between disease and exposure is convincing.

Metals and Their Derivatives

Skog and Wahlberg[55] performed a systematic study of the percutaneous absorption of aqueous solutions of isotope-labeled metal compounds in guinea pigs using a disappearance measurement technique. The relative mean absorption was less than 1% per 5 hours for cobalt chloride, zinc chloride, and silver nitrate. For mercuric chloride, potassium mercuric iodide, and methyl mercury dicyandiamide the absorption increased with increasing concentrations up to a certain level (3.2–4.5%/5 hours). A further increase in concentration resulted in reduced relative absorption. When the percutaneous toxicity of nine metal solutions was compared using the guinea pig model, it appeared that the mercury compounds showed the highest toxicity.[56] This is in accordance with the reported percutaneous toxicity of mercury in humans. Mercury is used in the electrical, pharmaceutical, and chemical industries. Vapor and dust are readily inhaled, and certain mercurials can penetrate skin to cause discoloration and systemic toxicity, which appears as mucosal changes, gingivitis, loose teeth, central nervous system changes, tremors, ataxia, mental confusion, and renal damage[57, 58] Bourgeois and coworkers[59] reported two cases of mercury poisoning caused by the use of an over-the-counter metallic mercury ointment. Of 70 psoriasis patients treated with an ointment containing ammoniated mercury, 33 showed signs and symptoms of mercury poisoning.[60] Topical silver nitrate may induce argyria which can closely mimic cyanosis and methemoglobulinemia. A woman used topical silver nitrate for bleeding gingiva secondary to poorly fitting dentures. After 2 years of heavy usage, diagnosis was made. She was deeply and confluently pigmented, most strikingly on sun-exposed skin. Gastroduodenoscopy and laparotomy showed extreme pigmentation of abdominal viscera.[61]

Lead is the most ubiquitous toxic metal. Alkyl lead compounds used as gasoline additives are readily absorbed through skin and may cause neurotoxicity.[4] Boranes are used as high-energy fuels, in nuclear reactors, in the hardening of steel, and as fire retardants. They may produce central nervous system toxicity.[62]

TABLE 4–3 • **Compounds Suspected to Be Causative Factors in the Induction or Elicitation of Systemic Scleroderma and Scleroderma-like Disease**[a]

Systemic Scleroderma	Scleroderma-like Disease
Silica	Vinyl chloride
	Aromatic solvents
	Aliphatic solvents
	Epoxy resins
	Bis(4-amino-3-methylhexyl)methane
	Bleomycin
	Pentazocine
	Penicillamine
	Paraffin
	Silicone
	Aniline

[a] Zschunke E, Ziegler V, Haustein U-F. Occupationally induced connective tissue disorders. In: Adams RM, ed. *Occupational Skin Disease,* 2nd ed. Philadelphia: W.B. Saunders; 1990:172–183.

Other Examples

Severe allergic reactions with systemic effects may occur after skin contact with certain industrial chemicals. Benzene sulfonyl chloride absorbed through the skin caused anaphylactic reactions and reversible liver damage in three workers.[63] Contact dermatitis complicated by gastrointestinal symptoms and finger paresthesia developed in a laboratory technician; it was related to a hydroxyethyl-methacrylate (2-HEMA) contact allergy. The gastrointestinal symptoms were reproduced by patch testing.[64] Another laboratory technician, who was working with the manufacture of disposable contact lenses, developed neurological and gastrointestinal symptoms after working with UV-curable acrylic monomers. After an accidental spill in which a major part of her skin surface was contaminated with 2-HEMA for a few hours, she experienced increased sensitivity to exposure to the acrylates. She had a recurrence of her systemic symptoms following patch tests with the acrylates. However, she showed no sign of contact allergy.[65] The only skin symptom was transient onycholysis of the finger nails. The systemic toxicity of acrylic monomers may affect multiple organs—those in the nervous, cardiovascular, cutaneous, gastrointestinal, and respiratory systems. The inhalation of vapor may be the most common route of exposure.[66]

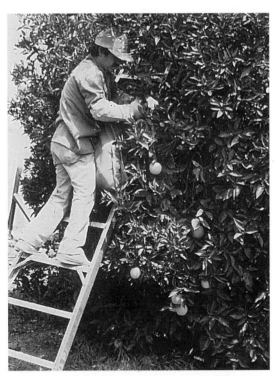

FIGURE 4–1 • A major concern for agricultural workers is the threat of systemic poisoning by pesticides. The organophosphates are highly likely to be absorbed through the skin if workers enter the field or orchard too soon after the pesticide's application.

AGRICULTURE

Pesticides

Workers exposed to a variety of pesticides in agriculture and gardening are at risk for development of toxic effects. This is an area that is attracting increasing attention from public health and environmental officials, from industry, and from consumers at large because pesticides can enter the food chain and contaminate drinking water, and reports of epidemics of poisoning by pesticides have been published in the scientific literature and by the mass media. During the period between 1960 and 1971, 5,500 farm workers in California had occupational illnesses attributed to pesticides, exclusive of eye and skin disorders.[4] In spite of preventive measures (Fig. 4–1) implemented to avoid pesticide toxicity, epidemics still occur.[67] Pesticides can be divided into five categories: insecticides, rodenticides, fungicides, herbicides, and fumigants. They can be further classified into phosphate esters, chlorinated hydrocarbons of various types, and a group of miscellaneous compounds of botanical, inorganic, or organic chemical origin.[68]

Potential dermal exposure to pesticides is generally much greater than potential respiratory exposure.[69, 70] The percutaneous absorption of pesticides varies considerably from compound to compound in experimental studies on normal skin of human volunteers.[71] With the same concentration applied to normal human forearm skin, the percentage of dose absorbed varied from 0.3% for paraquat to 73.9% for carbaryl (Table 4–4). The greatest toxicological potential for cutaneous pesticide absorption occurs when a high concentration of the compound is in contact with a large part of the body. The regional variation in pesticide absorption through the skin follows the general pattern: a high total absorption for scrotal skin, and for head and neck where environmental exposure is greater. Occlusion or skin damage increases absorption of pesticides by a factor of 2 to 9.[71] The amount of contact time is also important. Some pesticides seem to be absorbed very rapidly. In the case of a malathion dose, 9.6% was absorbed even after an immediate wash of the skin site with soap and water.[71]

Working conditions are of equal importance. Wolfe et al.[69, 70] examined 31 separate work activities involving 21 different pesticides. There were

TABLE 4–4 • In Vivo Percutaneous Absorption of Pesticides in Humans[a]

Pesticide	Percentage of Dose Absorbed
Paraquat	0.3
Diquat	0.4
Ethion	3.3
2,4-D	5.8
Malathion	6.8
Dieldrin	7.7
Aldrin	7.8
Parathion	8.6
Lindane	9.3
Azodrin	14.7
DDT	15.0
Guthion	15.9
Baygon	19.6
Carbaryl	73.9

[a] Wester RC, Maibach HI. In vivo percutaneous absorption and decontamination of pesticides in humans. *J Tox Environ Health* 1985;16:25–37.

wide ranges in exposure levels for a given pesticide, as they were determined by type of work activity, environmental conditions such as wind, and the technique of the operator. The loading operation was the most hazardous part of the cycle during spraying or dusting. During orchard spraying with air-blast application equipment, the highest total exposure to carbophenothion, an organophosphorous compound, was calculated to be about 1% of a toxic dose per hour, indicating that the hazard of systemic toxicity can be reduced by the use of the appropriate spraying equipment.

The potential exposure of agricultural workers during application of the herbicide 2,4-dichlorophenoxy acetic acid (Fernimine) was examined during the use of five types of application equipment. The dermal exposure was higher during mixing and loading than during spraying. Tractor-powered sprayers fitted with hydraulic nozzles produced lower exposure than did knapsack sprayers. The hands were the most highly exposed part of the body during mixing and loading operations for all sprayers as well as during spraying with tractor-powered sprayers. The lower legs of workers were exposed when knapsack sprayers were used. The potential respiratory exposure was negligible compared with the dermal exposure.[72]

There is no internationally agreed-upon approach to the evaluation of workers' exposure to pesticides. Harmonization is needed to satisfy scientific and regulatory requirements. However, exposure assessment is a complex issue.[73] Several techniques may be applied and they supplement each other. Whole-body sampling involving the use of clothing similar to that normally used during work is recommended as the first method of choice. A handwashing technique is also useful. For selected chemicals, biological monitoring may be conducted simultaneously. Urine is the preferred sampling matrix for analysis of excreted pesticides or metabolites as an index of absorption. Ideally, a suitable biological monitoring marker metabolite is one that represents a minimum of 30% of the administered dose.[73]

Phosphate Esters

A large number of well-known pesticides are phosphate esters: malathion, parathion, guthion, chlorothion, diazinon, and tetraethylpyrophosphate, for example. They vary in penetrability and in toxicity. Their toxicity is due to their capacity to inhibit cholinesterase, which controls the function of the neural transmitter acetylcholine. The clinical picture of poisoning with phosphate ester pesticides is characterized by overstimulation of the central nervous system and organs innervated by the parasympathetics. The patient suffers from nausea, vomiting, diarrhea, respiratory insufficiency, cyanosis, sweating, salivation, pupil contraction, convulsions, and eventually death from respiratory failure. The symptoms develop within minutes to a few hours after exposure.

The exposure to organophosphorous pesticides may be monitored by environmental air sampling at work sites and by the measurement of blood cholinesterase activity in workers both before and after exposure.[74] A Chinese field study of dipterex toxicity (trichlorifon) confirmed that percutaneous absorption was the major route of exposure and that poisoning was observed only in the warmer seasons, when several factors facilitated percutaneous absorption, such as larger areas of exposed skin, higher dermal temperatures, and increased sweating.[75] Similar climatic conditions may be in effect in greenhouses, thus increasing the risk of toxicity.[76] Further, under uncomfortable, hot conditions, workers may be more willing to risk poisoning than to use suitable protective gear.

Chlorinated Hydrocarbons

Chlorinated hydrocarbon insecticides are neurotoxins. They include such products as aldrin, chlordane, dieldrin, endrin, heptachlor, toxaphene, kepone, and lindane. They are fat-soluble and are often used in solvent vehicles which facilitates skin absorption. Clinical poisoning is characterized by anxiety, tremor, ataxia, convulsions, and so forth. Their use has been reduced in recent years because of their persistence in the environment.

Nicotine has been in use in commercial insecticides and has caused severe toxicity through percutaneous absorption.[77, 78] Benowitz and coworkers[79] described a woman who developed nausea, vomiting, lethargy, and abdominal cramps minutes to a few hours after soaking her skin with a diluted solution of 40% nicotine sulfate. Measurement of nicotine and metabolite levels in the blood showed prolonged absorption despite vigorous skin decontamination. In spite of the very high blood levels, the patient showed substantial clinical improvement, indicating a rapid development of tolerance.

Paraquat (1,1′dimethyl,4,4′bipyridylium dichloride) (Gramoxone) is a locally irritating bipyridyl compound used as an herbicide. It has a limited capability of skin penetration. However, serious and even fatal paraquat poisonings have been reported. A man used, by mistake, a paraquat solution to clean his perineum and subsequently developed severe local irritation and reversible renal, respiratory, and hepatic damage.[80] Five cases of fatal paraquat poisoning have been reported in adult Papua New Guinea men after skin absorption. Three cases followed occupational accidents, and two cases occurred in men who used paraquat for self-treatment of infestations.[81] They all had local blistering and excoriation and died of respiratory failure. Paraquat lung may develop rapidly after percutaneous poisoning and can lead to pulmonary fibrosis when it is not fatal.[82]

Pentachlorophenol is still used for wood preservation and as a fungicide, herbicide, and disinfectant. It is highly toxic because of its interference with oxidative phosphorylation, and poisoning may affect multiple organs. Chronic poisoning has been described in sawmill workers and in people living in log homes treated with pentachlorophenol-containing wood-protecting formulations.[83] Use of pentachlorophenol-based products as indoor wood preservatives poses an unacceptable risk to human health. Pentachlorophenol may also be absorbed extensively from contaminated soil, an important source of exposure.[84]

Ammonia is a colorless gas with a characteristic pungent odor. It is readily liquefied under pressure and combines easily with water to form ammonium hydroxide, which is corrosive. Liquid ammonia is manufactured in enormous quantities and is shipped by truck or railroad tank car to be used as a fertilizer, as a refrigerant, and in the chemical industry. Persons subjected to acute intoxication can be severely injured. Respiratory problems may be life-threatening, and skin injuries may be extensive and painful. A concentration of 10,000 ppm is sufficient to evoke skin damage. Ammonia in liquid form freezes the skin, but the chemical burn caused afterwards is much more significant. The alkali burn injury appears as a gray-yellow soft area and may extend to a liquefactive necrosis, fat saponification, and protein precipitation.[85, 86]

TOPICAL DRUGS AND TOILETRIES

The field of drugs and toiletries produces many case reports in which extreme exposure conditions explain the percutaneous toxicity. The use of high concentrations and the long-term treatment of babies and patients with burns or percutaneous absorption through dermatitis resulted in systemic toxicity. Most of the compounds have been continously in use and appear to be safe in low concentrations and under the supervision of a physician. Examples of compounds causing organ-related toxicity are shown in Tables 4–5 to 4–9.

Among topically used drugs that can induce systemic toxicity, *boric acid* is a classic example. It caused a number of fatalities in children when applied on damaged skin.[87, 88] The toxicity appeared as generalized erythema accompanied by signs of central nervous system irritation, such as exaggerated reflexes, convulsions, delirium, and coma and such gastrointestinal symptoms as nausea, vomiting, and diarrhea as well as renal injury. Only small amounts can penetrate normal skin. A water-emulsifying ointment containing a glycerol-boric acid/sodium borate buffer in an amount equivalent to 3% boric acid has been used for decades in caring for the skin of babies in Europe and it appears to be safe. It produced no rise in blood boron levels in 22 newborn infants following repeated application to the napkin area.[89]

Hexachlorophene has been widely used as a disinfectant in medicine, industry, and the manufacture of household products. Because of its toxicity, it has become obsolete in medicine. It induced encephalopathy, peripheral nerve damage, and renal disturbance in babies bathed daily with soaps containing this compound in high concentration. Four children treated by accident with a 6% hexachlorophene talc powder died.[90] It should not be used in patients with widespread areas of diseased skin or on small infants.[91] After 3 or more days of dermal applications at low concentration in humans, the skin became a reservoir, resulting in a constant blood level.

An epidemic of a hemorrhagic syndrome of sudden onset with signs of neuromeningeal involvement occurred in Vietnamese infants after accidental use of talc contaminated with a dicoumarin-type anticoagulant, probably because of accidental confusion with a rodenticide. Two months

TABLE 4–5 • Compounds Reported to Have Caused Blood Disorders Through Percutaneous Absorption

Methemoglobinemia	
Benzocaine	Haggerty, 1962[109]
Castellani's solution	Lundell and Nordman, 1973[118]
Mafenide acetate	Ohlgisser et al., 1978[101]
Resorcinol	Cunningham, 1956[123]
Phenol	
Silver nitrate	Geffner et al., 1981[135]
Trichlorocarbanilide?	Ponté et al., 1974[136]
Aromatic amines	
Marrow Depression	
Chloramphenicol	Abrams et al., 1980[96]
Podophyllin	Stoehr et al., 1978[97]
Povidone-iodine	Alvarez, 1979[98]
Sulfadiazine	Fraser and Beaulieu, 1979[99]
Ethylene glycol monomethyl ether	Ohi and Wegman, 1978[43]
Other glycol ethers?	Cullen et al., 1983[45]

after the beginning of the epidemic, 741 cases had been detected, with 177 deaths.[92]

A shampoo containing selenium sulfide provoked a systemic toxic reaction in a woman with a scalp eruption after 8 months of shampooing her hair 2 to 3 times a week. Within hours after the shampoo, she developed tremor, perspiration, metallic taste, and abdominal pain. She felt weak and anorectic for 3 days. Urinary selenium was 32 μg/mL and there were increased levels of uroporphyrin and coproporphyrin in the urine. She recovered completely in 5 days.[93] This is a rare case, considering the widespread use of selenium sulfide in shampoos.

Clindamycin-induced pseudomembranous colitis is a well-recognized side effect following systemic administration, but it has also been reported after topical use in an acne patient. She developed diarrhea 5 days after starting local treatment with a 1% solution of clindamycin hydrochloride. Examination of stool specimens revealed a significant titer of the clostridium difficile toxin; colonoscopy and mucosal biopsy showed changes consistent with pseudomembranous colitis.[94] Again, this is a

rare case considering the widespread topical use of the drug.

Chloramphenicol may cause aplastic anemia following systemic administration. Anemia may appear late during the course of therapy and is not related to dosage. It is estimated to occur in 1 out of every 18,000 to 50,000 patients treated.[95] One case described followed topical application of chloramphenicol in an eye ointment.[96] Marrow depression has also been reported following absorption of podophyllin,[97] povidone-iodine,[98] and sulfadiazine.[99] (See Table 4–5.)

Mafenide acetate (Sulfamylon) cream is a potent carbonic anhydrase inhibitor. In a patient with 50% full-thickness thermal burn and renal insufficiency, Sulfamylon cream caused a respiratory acidosis and increased carbon dioxide tension in arterial blood.[100] Two children with severe burns developed methemoglobulinemia after topical application of mafenide acetate.[101]

Gentamycin and neomycin are known ototoxins after systemic administration, and both have been connected with the development of moderate to severe hearing loss following topical administra-

 TABLE 4–6 • Compounds Reported to Have Caused Renal Toxicity Through Percutaneous Absorption

Boric acid	Skipworth et al., 1967[87]
Henna and paraphenylene diamine	D'Arcy, 1982[125]
Aromatic amines	
Gasoline	Hansbrough et al., 1985[35]
Carburetor cleaning solvent	
Mercury	Marzulli and Brown, 1972[58]
Paraquat	Tungsanga et al., 1983[80]

TABLE 4–7 • Compounds Reported to Have Caused Nervous System Toxicity Through Percutaneous Absorption

Gentamycin (ototoxicity)	Dayal et al., 1974[102]
Neomycin (ototoxicity)	Bamford and Jones, 1978[103]
Boric acid	Skipworth et al., 1967[87]
Hexachlorophene	Kimbrough, 1973[91]
Selenium sulfide?	Ransone et al., 1961[93]
Salicylic acid	Weiss and Lever, 1964[105]
Diphenylpyraline hydrochloride (psychosis)	Cammann et al., 1971[110]
N,N-diethyl-m-toluamide (DEET) (psychosis)	Snyder et al., 1986[112]
Lindane	Telch and Jarvis, 1982[115]
Podophyllin	Cassidy et al., 1982[116]
Phenol, resorcinol	DelPizzo and Tanski, 1980[120]
Ethyl and methyl alcohol	Giménez et al., 1968[126]
Acetyl ethyl tetramethyl tetralin (AETT)?	Spencer and Bischoff, 1983[137]
Musk ambrette?	Spencer and Bischoff, 1983[137]
Hydroxyethylmethacrylate	Mathias et al., 1979[64]
Gasoline	Hansbrough et al., 1985[35]
Carburetor cleaning solvent	
Ethylene glycol monomethyl ether	Ohi and Wegman, 1978[43]
n-Hexane	Spencer and Bischoff, 1983[137]
Methyl butyl ketone	
Acrylamide	
Other organic solvents	Baker et al., 1985[34]
Dioxin?	Poland et al., 1971[46]
Mercury	Stokinger, 1981[57]
Boranes	Roush, 1959[62]
Alkyl lead	Klaassen et al., 1986[138]
Organophosphorous compounds and other pesticides	Hayes, 1975[68]

 TABLE 4–8 • Compounds Reported to Have Caused Metabolic Disorders Through Percutaneous Absorption

Povidone-iodine (thyroid)	Block, 1980[117]
Resorcinol (thyroid)	Thomas and Gisburn, 1961[121]
Mafenide acetate (respiratory acidosis)	Liebman et al., 1982[100]
Neomycin (magnesuria)	Bamford and Jones, 1978[103]
Selenium sulfide? (porphyria)	Ransone et al., 1961[93]
Dioxin? (porphyria)	Poland et al., 1971[46]

 TABLE 4–9 • Compounds Reported to Have Caused Gastrointestinal Disorders Through Percutaneous Absorption

Boric acid	Skipworth et al., 1967[87]
Selenium sulfide?	Ransone et al., 1961[93]
Clindamycin (colitis)	Milstone et al., 1981[94]
Aromatic amines	
4,4'-diaminodiphenylmethane	McGill and Motto, 1974[29]
Gasoline (liver)	Hansbrough et al., 1985[35]
Carburetor cleaning solvent	
Carbon tetrachloride	
Dioxin? (liver)	Poland et al., 1971[46]
Benzene sulfonyl chloride (liver)	Stasik, 1975[63]
Hydroxyethylmethacrylate (2-HEMA)	Mathias et al., 1979[64]

tion in patients with extensive burns.[102] Bamford and Jones[103] described six children who developed deafness, and three of them showed a metabolic disorder suspected to be related to neomycin toxicity—magnesuria and consequent hypomagnesemia and hypocalcemia with hypocalcemic tetany. Antibiotic eardrops containing aminoglycosides may also provoke hearing loss. However, neomycin is a minimal penetrant through normal skin in accordance with the use of a 20% concentration for patch testing.[104]

Ointments containing *salicylic acid* 3 to 6% have caused nausea, dyspnea, hearing loss, confusion, and hallucinations in three patients with extensive psoriasis. They had two soap and water baths daily combined with UV therapy and six ointment applications. The symptoms developed in 4 days and the patients had significant salicylic acid levels in serum, which documented the absorption through psoriatic skin. The symptoms disappeared rapidly after discontinuation of the ointment applications.[105] Treatment with intravenous bicarbonate to prevent acidemia and induce urinary alkalinization, electrolyte replacement, and hemodialysis may be needed when serum concentration is above 0.1%.[106] Two fatal cases of percutaneous salicylate poisoning were described by Lindsey.[107] They were caused by the treatment of a fungal infection with an alcoholic solution containing 20% salicylic acid. In a recent case, salicylism developed in 2 days in a man with widespread psoriasis that covered 80% of his body surface after treatment with 10% topical salicylic acid on all involved areas of the skin.[108] Salicylic acid ointments are frequently prescribed by dermatologists and are safe when extreme exposure conditions (high concentrations over a large body area) are avoided. However, it is vital to be careful when treating children because intoxication has been reported predominantly in that age group.

Benzocaine has caused methemoglobinemia following topical use in small children with damaged skin. A 1-month-old infant with a weeping diaper rash developed methemoglobinemia about 3 hours after application of an ointment containing 3% benzocaine.[109] A number of other topical remedies may induce methemoglobinemia in rare cases, mainly in children and in patients with extensive wounds (see Table 4–5). Fatalities have been reported.

Diphenylpyraline hydrochloride, an antihistamine used topically for itching dermatoses, provoked a psychosis in 12 patients, mainly children. They showed restlessness, disorientation, and hallucinations. The symptoms disappeared in 4 days following withdrawal of the drug.[110]

The insect repellant *N,N′-diethyl-m-toluamide*

(DEET) is widely used and the general safety of DEET has been established during 30 years of human experience in applying it episodically to skin or bedclothes. However, local side effects may occur—contact urticaria and skin irritation—and excessive use in children and in adults too can induce a toxic encephalopathy. Four boys aged 3 to 7 years and one adult had generalized seizures temporally associated with use of DEET as an insect repellant.[111] A 30-year-old man applied DEET to his body daily for a few weeks to treat a rash. After each application he entered a homemade sauna for 60 to 90 minutes. He developed an acute manic psychosis and was admitted to a psychiatric ward. He improved completely in 6 days, which is atypical for classic endogenous mania. DEET and its metabolites were identified in his urine more than 2 weeks after the last drug application.[112]

Lindane is a potentially toxic agent. The hazards of industrial exposure and accidental ingestion are well documented. It may induce toxic reactions, including neurological, gastrointestinal, respiratory, cardiac, and hemopoietic disorders. Intoxication from topical application has been documented. Several authors have described scabies patients who developed seizures, anxiety, insomnia, dizziness, and amblyopia.[113–115] Percutaneous lindane absorption is considerable. When applied in acetone on intact human forearm skin, at least 9.3% of the substance was absorbed and subsequently excreted in the urine during the following 5 days.[71] Nearly all of the applied dose was absorbed when the skin was occluded. Treatment should follow certain recommendations: do not apply after a hot bath; do not use for more than 8 to 12 hours; do not use on pregnant or nursing women, on infants, or on people with extensive excoriations. However, permethrin, a synthetic pyrethroid, is now the scabicide of first choice because it has a lower mammalian toxicity and is poorly absorbed. It may reduce the occurrence of lindane intoxication.

Podophyllin is a natural product that contains numerous lignins and flavenols, including podophyllotoxin and alfa- and beta-peltatins. It is a skin irritant and is widely used in the local treatment of condylomata accuminata. Percutaneous absorption may induce severe marrow depression, neuropathy, confusional states, vomiting, coma, and death.[97, 116]

Povidone-iodine is used as antimicrobial agent. It may be absorbed through diseased skin and also through normal skin in children.[117] It caused TSH elevation in 4 of 7 family members using a povidone-iodine solution for treatment of recurrent skin infections, and it may also cause marrow depression.[98]

Castellani's solution contains *phenol* and *resorcinol*. It caused a severe methemoglobinemia in a 6-week-old infant whose head and eczematous skin folds had been painted with the solution.[118] Phenol is obsolete as an antiseptic, but in a dilution of 0.5 to 2%, it is sometimes prescribed as an antipruritic. Severe, even fatal phenol reactions following application to wounds have been reported.[119] Phenol exerts a markedly toxic action when topical applications are made over large areas of skin. Several cases of acute death have been reported after phenol face peels.[120] The systemic effects include CNS stimulation, dizziness, cardiovascular depression, abdominal pain, hemoglobinuria, cyanosis, and coma. Resorcinol is significantly less toxic than phenol but may elicit the same pattern of toxic reactions. Leg ulcer patients treated with continued applications of ointments containing resorcinol have developed myxedema.[121] Resorcinol 2% appears to be safe for topical use in adult humans. Volunteers treated with 2% resorcinol in a hydroalcoholic vehicle, 20 mL applied twice a day, 6 days a week, for 4 weeks had no resorcinol in their blood, nor were there any abnormalities in thyroid function or blood chemistry at week 2, 3, or 4.[122] However, fatal cases of severe hemolytic anemia and hemoglobinuria have been reported in small children after the topical application of 2 to 10% resorcinol.[123]

Peeling paste containing *naphthol* is a potential hazard in patients with widespread acne because 2-naphtol is readily absorbed through the skin. It should be used only on limited areas (150 cm²) and for a limited period of time.[124]

Henna is a reddish-brown dyestuff for coloring leather, hair, skin, and fingernails. It contains the dried leaves of *Lawsonia alba*, a shrub that grows in India, Sri Lanka, and North Africa. The dye is a hydroxynaphthoquinone. Henna has been used in Sudan in combination with paraphenylenediamine (PPD) in order to accelerate the dyeing process. This combination is highly toxic, and several cases of systemic toxicity following percutaneous absorption have been reported from Khartoum. The patients developed angioneurotic edema within hours of exposure, and the toxic reaction progressed, in some cases, to anuria and acute renal failure.[125] When PPD is used as a hair dye, it has been reported to produce vertigo and anemia in addition to the well-known cases of allergic contact dermatitis.

Compresses soaked in *ethyl* and *methyl alcohol* have been used in children with normal skin to relieve abdominal pain, but 48 children were intoxicated by percutaneously applied alcohol.[126] They developed CNS depression, alcoholic breath, abdominal erythema, and secondary hypoglycemia. Fatal cases were also described.

It is well known that *topical corticosteroids* may be absorbed and elicit laboratory and clinical evidence of iatrogenic hypercorticism when used on large surfaces of the body over an extended period of time. Corticosteroid absorption increases on dermatitic skin, and infants are more susceptible than adults.

Calcipotriol, a vitamin D derivative used topically for the treatment of psoriasis, may also be absorbed extensively through psoriatic skin. If weekly consumption exceeds 100 g, a patient may develop hypercalcemia.[127]

Systemic Contact Allergy Reactions These may be provoked in individuals previously sensitized by topical exposure. Most cases are elicited by a subsequent exposure by oral route or inhalation, as reviewed by Menné and Maibach.[128] There are several patterns of clinical reaction. The most common findings are vesicular hand dermatitis (pompholyx), flare of eczema, and flare of patch tests following test procedures or provocations in patients with strong nickel sensitivity. Generalized rash is a less common sign of systemic contact dermatitis reported after exposure to benzoin and propylene glycol. The rapid onset of the exanthema in some cases suggests that mechanisms other than the delayed type of hypersensitivity may be active.

The "baboon syndrome" is a catchword for a distribution pattern of systemic allergic contact dermatitis characterized by diffuse erythema of the buttocks, upper inner thighs, and axillae.[129] It has been provoked by nickel, mercury, and ampicillin. However, the systemic reaction may also develop following cutaneous and mucosal reexposure. Erythema multiforme-like eruptions have been caused by ophthalmic preparations.[130–132]

Contact dermatitis may be complicated by systemic symptoms presumably related to the cutaneous allergen exposure such as acute laryngeal obstruction due to thimerosal hypersensitivity.[133] Generalized immediate reactions of the anaphylactic type have been reported after cutaneous exposure to several topical drugs and cosmetic ingredients (Table 4–10).[8]

CONCLUSIONS

The bulk of the information on systemic toxicity resulting from percutaneous absorption comes from case reports which, although important to a

TABLE 4–10 • Chemicals Reported to Have Caused Generalized Immediate Reactions Following Skin Exposure[a]

Balsam of Peru	
Caraway seed oil	Heygi and Dolezalova, 1976[139]
Aminophenazone	Camarasa et al., 1978[140]
Ammonium persulfate	Fisher and Dooms-Goossens, 1976[141]
Ampicillin	Pietzker and Kuner, 1975[142]
Bacitracin	Katz and Fisher, 1987[143]
Chloramphenicol	Kozáková, 1976[144]
Triphenylmethane dyes	Michel et al., 1958[145]
Benzocaine	Kleinhans and Zwissler, 1980[146]
Mechlorethamine	Daughters et al., 1973[147]
Benzene sulfonyl chloride	Stasik, 1975[63]

[a] Lahti A. Immediate contact reactions. In: Rycroft RJ, Menné T, Frosch P, Benezra C, eds. *Textbook of Contact Dermatitis,* 2nd ed. Berlin: Springer-Verlag; 1995:62–74.

given patient, do not provide the most valuable way of looking at the subject. For topical drugs, controlled experiments have been performed to evaluate the extent of systemic absorption resulting from topical exposure. Epidemiological data from exposed populations are needed as is more information derived from human studies and from animal and in vitro models developed to study percutaneous toxicity. The continued development of methods of assessing occupational dermal exposure is seriously warranted.[1, 25]

Considering the current knowledge of the health risks that follow accidental skin exposure to toxic substances, emergency departments should implement treatment protocols that ensure that patients accidentally exposed to hazardous chemicals receive optimal decontamination. One protocol that has been reported to be effective prescribes external decontamination that is performed in a specially designed decontamination area; the treatment includes skin and hair decontamination and mucosal and ocular irrigation when necessary. The skin is washed three times with a detergent and cornmeal mixture and rinsed with water irrigation or shower for three minutes. This procedure was effective in a retrospective study comprising 72 patients.[134]

References

1. Fenske RA. Dermal exposure assessment techniques. *Ann Occup Hyg* 1993;37:687–706.
2. Fiserova-Bergerova V. Relevance of occupational skin exposure. *Ann Occup Hyg* 1993;37:673–685.
3. Wahlberg JE. Percutaneous absorption. *Curr Probl Dermatol* 1973;5:1–36.
4. Birmingham DJ. Cutaneous absorption and systemic toxicity. In: Drill VA, Lazar P, eds. *Cutaneous Toxicity.* New York: Academic Press; 1977:53–62.
5. Pascher F. Systemic reactions to topically applied drugs. *Int J Dermatol* 1978;17:768–775.
6. Grandjean P. *Skin Penetration: Hazardous Chemicals at Work.* London: Taylor & Francis; 1990.
7. Freeman S, Maibach HI. Systemic toxicity caused by absorption of drugs and chemicals through the skin. In: Marzulli FN, Maibach HI, eds. *Dermatotoxicology,* 4th ed. New York: Hemisphere Publishing; 1991:851–875.
8. De Groot AC, Weyland JW, Nater JP. *Unwanted effects of cosmetics and drugs used in dermatology,* 3rd ed. Amsterdam: Elsevier; 1994:228–285.
9. Bronaugh RL, Maibach HI. *Percutaneous Absorption,* 2nd ed. New York: Marcel Dekker; 1989.
10. Wester RC. Twenty absorbing years. In: C Surber, P Elsner, AJ Bircher, eds. *Exogenous Dermatology. Curr Prob Dermatol.* Basel: Karger; 1995:112–123.
11. Elias PM, Cooper ER, Kore A et al. Percutaneous transport in relation to stratum corneum structure and lipid composition *J Invest Dermatol* 1981;76:297–301.
12. Ghadially R, Halkier-Sørensen L, Elias P. Effects of petrolatum on stratum corneum structure and function. *J Am Acad Dermatol* 1992;26:387–396.
13. Scheuplein RJ. Mechanism of percutaneous absorption. *J Invest Dermatol* 1967;48:79–88.
14. Feldmann RJ, Maibach HI. Regional variation in percutaneous penetration of ^{14}C hydrocortisone in man. *J Invest Dermatol* 1967;48:181–183.
15. Feldmann RJ, Maibach HI. Penetration of ^{14}C hydrocortisone through normal skin. *Arch Dermatol* 1965;91:661–666.
16. Wester RC, Maibach HI. Cutaneous pharmacokinetics: 10 steps to percutaneous absorption. *Drug Metab Rev* 1983;14:169–205.
17. Wester RC, Maibach HI. Animal models for percutaneous absorption. In: Maibach HI, Lowe NJ, eds. *Models in Dermatology.* Basel: Karger; 1985b:159–169.
18. Skelly JP, Shah VP, Maibach HI et al. FDA and AAPS report of the workshop on principles and practices of in vitro percutaneous penetration studies: relevance to bioavailability and bioequivalence. *Pharm Res* 1987;4:265–267.
19. Bickers DR. The skin as a site of drug and chemical metabolism. In: Drill VA, Lazar P, eds. *Current Concepts in Cutaneous Toxicity.* New York: Academic Press; 1980:95–126.
20. Kao J, Carver MP. Skin metabolism. In: Marzulli FN, Maibach HI, eds. *Dermatotoxicology,* 4th ed. New York: Hemisphere Publishing; 1991:143–150.
21. Loomis TA. Skin as a portal of entry for systemic effects.

In: Drill VA, Lazar P, eds. *Current Concepts in Cutaneous Toxicity.* New York: Academic Press; 1980:153–169.

22. Noonan PK, Wester RC. Cutaneous biotransformations and some pharmacological and toxicological implications. In: Marzulli FN, Maibach HI eds. *Dermatotoxicology,* 2nd ed.: New York: Hemisphere Publishing; 1983:71–90.

23. Maibach HI, Feldmann RJ. Systemic absorption of pesticides through the skin of man, App. B: Occupational exposure to pesticides. Federal Working Group on Pest Management, Washington, D.C.: U.S. Government; 1974:120–127.

24. Wahlberg JE. Some attempts to influence the percutaneous absorption rate of sodium and mercuric chlorides in the guinea pig. *Acta Derm Venereol* 1965a;45:335–343.

25. Van Hemmen JJ, Brouwer DH. Assessment of dermal exposure to chemicals. *Sci Total Environ* 1995;168:131–141.

26. Ryser HJ-P. Chemical carcinogenesis. *N Engl J Med* 1971;285:721–734.

27. Mehlman MA. Dangerous and cancer-causing properties of products and chemicals in the oil refining and petrochemical industry. *Environ Res* 1992;59:238–249.

28. Grasso P. Cancer hazard from exposure to solvents. In: Riihimäki V, Ulfvarson U, eds. *Safety and Health Aspects of Organic Solvents.* New York: Alan Liss; 1986:187–202.

29. McGill DB, Motto JD. An outbreak of toxic hepatitis due to methylenediamine. *N Engl J Med* 1974;291:278–282.

30. Sivertsen E. Glyceryltrinitrate as a problem in industry. *Scand J Clin Lab Invest* 1984;173 [suppl]:81–84.

31. Schwartz L, Tulipan L, Birmingham DJ. *Occupational Diseases of the Skin,* 3rd ed. Philadelphia: Lea & Febiger; 1957.

32. Riihimäki V, Ulfvarson U, eds. *Safety and Health Aspects of Organic Solvents.* New York: Alan Liss; 1986.

33. Arlien-Søborg P, Bruhn P, Gyldenstedt C, Melgaard B. Chronic painter's syndrome. *Acta Neurol Scand* 1979;60:149–156.

34. Baker EL, Smith TJ, Landrigan PJ. The neurotoxicity of industrial solvents: a review of the literature. *Am J Industr Med* 1985;8:207–217.

35. Hansbrough JF, Zapata-Sirvent R, Dominic W, Sullivan J, Boswick J, Wang X-W. Hydrocarbon contact injuries. *J Trauma* 1985;25:250–252.

36. Riihimäki V, Pfäffli P. Percutaneous absorption of solvent vapors in man. *Scand J Work Environ Health* 1978;4:73–85.

37. DiVincenzo GD, Hamilton ML. Fate of n-butanol in rats after oral administration and its uptake by dogs after inhalation or skin application. *Tox Appl Pharmacol* 1979;48:317–325.

38. Riihimäki V. Percutaneous absorption of m-xylene from a mixture of m-xylene and isobutyl alcohol in man. *Scand J Work Environ Health* 1979;5:143–150.

39. Riihimäki V. Nordiska expertgruppen för gränsvärdedokumentation 43. *Metyl-etylketon. Arbeta och Hälsa* 1983;25:3–44.

40. Wahlberg JE, Boman A. Comparative percutaneous toxicity of ten industrial solvents. *Scand J Work Environ Health* 1979;5:345–351.

41. Boman A, Wahlberg JE, Johansson G. A method for the study of the effect of barrier creams and protective gloves on the percutaneous absorption of solvents. *Dermatologica* 1982;164:157–160.

42. Boman A, Wahlberg JE. Some factors influencing percutaneous absorption of organic solvents. In: Chambers PL, Gehring P, Sakai F, eds. *New Concepts and Developments in Toxicology.* Amsterdam: Elsevier; 1986:175–177.

43. Ohi G, Wegman DH. Transcutaneous ethylene glycol monomethyl ether poisoning in a work setting. *J Occup Med* 1978;20:675–676.

44. Johanson G. Toxicokinetics of 2-butoxyethanol. *Arbete och Hälsa* 1988;3:1–78.

45. Cullen MR, Rado T, Waldron JA, Sparer J, Welch LS. Bone marrow injury in lithographers exposed to glycol ethers and organic solvents in multicolor offset and ultraviolet curing printing processes. *Arch Environ Health* 1983;38:347–354.

46. Poland AP, Smith D, Metter G, Possick P. A health survey of workers in a 2,4-D and 2,4,5-T plant. *Arch Environ Health* 1971;22:316–327.

47. Acquavella JF, Hanis NM, Nicolich MJ, Phillips SC. Assessment of clinical, metabolic, dietary, and occupational correlations with serum polychlorinated biphenyl levels among employees at an electrical capacitor manufacturing plant. *J Occup Med* 1986;28:1177–1180.

48. Medsger TA, Masi AT. Epidemiology of systemic sclerosis (scleroderma). *Ann Intern Med* 1971;74:714–721.

49. Haustein U-F. Ziegler V. Environmentally induced systemic sclerosis-like disorders. *Int J Dermatol* 1985;24:147–151.

50. Erasmus L. Scleroderma in gold-miners on the Witwatersrand with particular reference to pulmonary manifestations. *S Afr Lab Clin Med* 1957;3:209–231.

51. Veitman C, Lange C, Juhe S, Stein G, Bachner V. Clinical manifestations and course of vinyl chloride disease. *Ann NY Acad Sci* 1975;246:6–17.

52. Silman A, Jones S. What is the contribution of occupational environmental factors to the occurrence of scleroderma in man? *Ann Rheum Dis* 1992;51:1322–1324.

53. Yamakage A, Ishikawa H, Saito Y, Hattori A. Occupational scleroderma-like disorder occurring in men engaged in the polymerisation of epoxy resins. *Dermatologica* 1980;161:33–44.

54. Dunnill MG, Black MM. Sclerodermatous syndrome after occupational exposure to herbicides—response to systemic steroids. *Clin Exp Dermatol* 1994;19:518–520.

55. Skog E, Wahlberg JE. A comparative investigation of the percutaneous absorption of metal compounds in the guinea pig by means of the radioactive isotopes ^{51}Cr, ^{58}Co, ^{65}Zn, ^{210}Ag, ^{115}Cd, ^{203}Hg. *J Invest Derm* 1964;43:187–192.

56. Wahlberg JE. Percutaneous toxicity of metal compounds: a comparative investigation in guinea pigs. *Arch Environ Health* 1965b;11:201–204.

57. Stokinger HA. Mercury. In: *Patty's Industrial Hygiene and Toxicology IIa,* 3rd ed. New York: Wiley Interscience; 1981:1769–1792.

58. Marzulli FN, Brown DWC. Potential systemic hazard of topically applied mercurials. *J Soc Cosmet Chem* 1972;23:875–886.

59. Bourgeois M, Dooms-Goossens A, Knockaert D, Van Boven M, Van Tittelboom T. Mercury intoxication after topical application of a metallic mercury ointment. *Dermatologica* 1986;172:48–51.

60. Young E. Ammoniated mercury poisoning. *Br J Dermatol* 1960;72:449–455.

61. Marshall JP, Schneider RP. Systemic argyria secondary to topical silver nitrate. *Arch Dermatol* 1977;113:1077–1079.

62. Roush G. The toxicology of the boranes. *J Occup Med* 1959;1:46–52.

63. Stasik MJ. Klinische Erfahrung mit Benzolsulfonsäurechlorid. *Arch Toxicol* 1975;33:123–127.

64. Mathias CGT, Caldwell TM, Maibach HI. Contact dermatitis and gastrointestinal symptoms from hydroxyethylmethacrylate. *Br J Dermatol* 1979;100:447–449.

65. Andersen KE. Systemic symptoms related to patch tests with UV curable acrylic monomers. Contact Dermatitis 1986;14:180.
66. Scolnick B, Collins J. Systemic reaction to methylmethacrylate in an operating room nurse. *J Occup Med* 1986;28:196–198.
67. Ferrer A, Cabral R. Recent epidemics of poisoning by pesticides. *Toxicol Lett* 1995;82/83:55–63.
68. Hayes WJ. *Toxicology of Pesticides*. Baltimore: Williams & Wilkins; 1975.
69. Wolfe HR, Durham WF, Armstrong JF, Wenatchee BS. Exposure of workers to pesticides. *Arch Environ Health* 1967;14:622–633.
70. Wolfe HR, Armstrong JF, Staiff DC, Comer SW. Exposure of spraymen to pesticides. *Arch Environ Health* 1972;25:29–31.
71. Wester RC, Maibach HI. In vivo percutaneous absorption and decontamination of pesticides in humans. *J Tox Environ Health* 1985a;16:25–37.
72. Abbott IM, Bonsall JL, Chester G, Hart TB, Turnbull GJ. Worker exposure to a herbicide applied with ground sprayers in the United Kingdom. *Am Ind Hyg Assoc J* 1987;48:167–175.
73. Chester G. Evaluation of agricultural worker exposure to, and absorption of, pesticides. *Ann Occup Hyg* 1993;37:509–523.
74. Lander F, Pike E, Hinke K, Brock A, Nielsen JB. Anticholinesterase agents uptake during cultivation of greenhouse flowers. *Arch Environ Contam Toxicol* 1992; 22:159–162.
75. Hu X, Lu Y, Xue S, Ling Y, Gu X. Toxicity of dipterex: a field study. *Br J Industr Med* 1986;43:414–419.
76. Adamis Z, Antal A, Füzesi I, Molnár J, Nagy L, Susán M. Occupational exposure to organophosphorous insecticides and synthetic pyrethroid. *Int Arch Occup Environ Health* 1985;56:299–305.
77. Wilson DJB. Nicotine poisoning by absorption through the skin. *Br Med J* 1930;ii:601–602.
78. Faulkner JM. Nicotine poisoning by absorption through the skin. *JAMA* 1933;100:1664–1665.
79. Benowitz NL, Lake T, Keller KH, Lee BL. Prolonged absorption with development of tolerance to toxic effects after cutaneous exposure to nicotine. *Clin Pharmacol Ther* 1987;42:119–120.
80. Tungsanga K, Chusilp S, Israsena S, Sitprija V. Paraquat poisoning: evidence of systemic toxicity after dermal exposure. *Postgrad Med J* 1983;59:338–339.
81. Wohlfahrt DJ. Fatal paraquat poisonings after skin absorption. *Med J Aust* 1982;1:512–513.
82. Papiris SA, Maniati MA, Kyriakidis V, Constantopoulos SH. Pulmonary damage due to paraquat poisoning through skin absorption. *Respiration* 1995;62:101–103.
83. Jorens PG, Schepens PJC. Human pentachlorophenol poisoning. *Hum Exp Toxicol* 1993;12:479–495.
84. Wester RC, Maibach HI, Sedik L, Melendres J, Wade M, DiZio S. Percutaneous absorption of pentachlorophenol from soil. *Fundam Appl Toxicol* 1993;20:68–71.
85. Helmers S, Top FH, Knapp LW. Ammonia injuries in agriculture. *J Iowa Med Soc* 1971;61:271–280.
86. Birken GA, Fabri PJ, Carey LC. Acute ammonia intoxication complicating multiple trauma. *J Trauma* 1981; 21:820–822.
87. Skipworth GB, Goldstein N, McBride WP. Boric acid intoxication from "medicated talcum powder." *Arch Dermatol* 1967;95:83–86.
88. Valdes-Dapena MA, Arey JB. Boric acid poisoning. *J Pediatrics* 1962;61:531–546.
89. Friis-Hansen B, Aggerbeck B, Aas Jansen J. Unaffected blood boron levels in newborn infants treated with boric acid ointment. *Food Chem Toxicol* 1982;20:451–454.
90. Goutieres F, Aicardi J. Accidental percutaneous hexachlorophene intoxication in children. *Br Med Bull* 1977;2:663–665.
91. Kimbrough RD. Review of the toxicity of hexachlorophene including its neurotoxicity. *J Clin Pharmacol* 1973;13:439–444.
92. Martin-Bouyer G, Linh PD, Tuan LC, et al. Epidemic of haemorragic disease in Vietnamese infants caused by warfarin-contaminated talcs. *Lancet* 1983;1:230–233.
93. Ransone JW, Scott NM, Knoblock CC. Selenium sulfide intoxication. *N Engl J Med* 1961;264:384–385.
94. Milstone EB, McDonald AJ, Scholhamer CF. Pseudomembranous colitis after topical application of clindamycin. *Arch Dermatol* 1981;117:154–155.
95. Wallerstein RO, Condit PK, Kasper CK, Brown JW, Morrison FR. Statewide study of chloramphenicol therapy and fatal aplastic anemia. *JAMA* 1969;208:2045–2050.
96. Abrams SM, Degnan TJ, Vinciguerra V. Marrow aplasia following topical application of chloramphenicol eye ointment. *Arch Intern Med* 1980;140:576–577.
97. Stoehr GP, Petersen AL, Taylor WJ. Systemic complications of local podophyllin therapy. *Ann Intern Med* 1978;89:362–363.
98. Alvarez E. Neutropenia in a burned patient being treated topically with povidone-iodine foam. *Plast Reconstr Surg* 1979;63:839–840.
99. Fraser GL, Beaulieu JT. Leukopenia secondary to sulfadiazine silver. *JAMA* 1979;241:1928.
100. Liebman PR, Kenelly MM, Hirsch EF. Hypercarbia and acidosis associated with carbonic anhydrase inhibition: a hazard of topical mafenide acetate use in renal failure. *Burns* 1982;8:395–398.
101. Ohlgisser M, Adler M, Ben-Dov B, Taitelman U, Birkhan HJ, Bursztein S. Methemoglobinemia induced by mafenide acetate in children: a report of two cases. *Br J Anaesth* 1978;50:299–301.
102. Dayal VS, Smith EL, McCain WG. Cochlear and vestibular gentamycin toxicity: a clinical study of systemic and topical usage. *Arch Otolaryng* 1974;100:338–340.
103. Bamford MFM, Jones LF. Deafness and biochemical imbalance after burns treatment with topical antibiotics in young children. *Arch Dis Child* 1978;53:326–329.
104. Panzer JD, Epstein WL. Percutaneous absorption following topical application of neomycin. *Arch Dermatol* 1970;102:536–539.
105. Weiss JF, Lever WF. Percutaneous salicylic acid intoxication in psoriasis. *Arch Dermatol* 1964;90:614–619.
106. Temple AR. Acute and chronic effects of aspirin toxicity and their treatment. *Arch Intern Med* 1981;141:364–369.
107. Lindsay CP. Two cases of fatal salicylate poisoning after topical application of an antifungal solution. *Med J Austr* 1968;1:353–354.
108. Jabarah A, Gilead LT, Zlotogorski A. Salicylate intoxication from topically applied salicylic acid. *J Eur Acad Dermatol Venereol* 1997;8:41–42.
109. Haggerty RJ. Blue baby due to methemeglobinemia. *N Eng J Med* 1962;267:1303.
110. Cammann R, Hennecke H, Beier R. Symptomatische Psychosen nach Kolton-Gelee-Applikation. *Psychiatr Neurol Med Psychol* 1971;23:426–431.
111. Oransky S, Roseman B, Fish D, et al. Seizures temporally associated with use of DEET insect repellent: New York and Connecticut. *MMWR* 1989;38:33–35.
112. Snyder JW, Poe RO, Stubbins JF, Garrettson LK. Acute manic psychosis following the dermal application of N,N-diethyl-m-toluamide (DEET) in an adult. *Clin Tox* 1986;24:429–439.
113. Lee B, Groth P. Scabies: transcutaneous poisoning during treatment. *Pediatrics* 1977;59:643.

114. Matsuoka LY. Convulsions following application of gamma benzene hexachloride. *J Am Acad Dermatol* 1981;5:98–99.

115. Telch J, Jarvis DA. Acute intoxication with lindane (gamma benzene hexachloride). *Can Med Assoc J* 1982;126:662–663.

116. Cassidy DE, Drewry J, Fanning JP. Podophyllum toxicity: a report of a fatal case and a review of the literature. *J Toxicol Clin Toxicol* 1982;19:35–44.

117. Block SH. Thyroid function abnormalities from the use of topical betadine solution on intact skin of children. *Cutis* 1980;26:88–89.

118. Lundell E, Nordman R. A case of infantile poisoning by topical application of Castellani's solution. *Ann Clin Res* 1973;5:404–406.

119. Baranowska-Dutkiewics B. Skin absorption of phenol from aqueous solutions in men. *Int Arch Occup Environ Health* 1981;49:99–104.

120. DelPizzo A, Tanski E. Chemical face peeling: malignant therapy for benign disease. *Plast Reconstr Surg* 1980; 66:121–123.

121. Thomas AE, Gisburn MA. Exogenous ochronosis and myxoedema from resorcinol. *Brit J Dermatol* 1961; 73:378–381.

122. Yeung D, Kantor S, Nacht S, Gans EH. Percutaneous absorption, blood levels, and urinary excretion of resorcinol applied topically in humans. *Int J Dermatol* 1983;22:321–324.

123. Cunningham AA. Resorcin poisoning. *Arch Dis Child* 1956;31:173–176.

124. Hemels HGWM. Percutaneous absorption and distribution of 2-naphtol in man. *Brit J Dermatol* 1972;87:614–622.

125. D'Arcy PF. Fatalities with the use of a henna dye. *Pharm Int* 1982;3:217–218.

126. Giménez ER, Vallejo NE, Roy E, et al. Percutaneous alcohol intoxication. *Clin Tox* 1968;1:39–48.

127. Bourke JF, Berth-Jones J, Hutchinson PE. Hypercalaemia with topical calcipotriol. *Br Med J* 1993;306:1344–1345.

128. Menné T, Maibach HI. Systemic contact-type dermatitis. In: Marzulli FN, Maibach HI, eds. *Dermatotoxicology*, 4th ed. New York: Hemisphere Publishing; 1991:453–472.

129. Andersen KE, Hjorth N, Menné T. The baboon syndrome: systemically induced allergic contact dermatitis. *Contact Dermatitis* 1984;10:97–100.

130. Gottshalk HR, Stone OJ. Stevens-Johnson syndrome from phthalmic sulfonamide. *Arch Dermatol* 1976; 112:513–514.

131. Rubin A. Ophthalmic sulfonamide induced Stevens-Johnson syndrome. *Arch Dermatol* 1977;113:235–236.

132. Guill MA, Goette DK, Knight CG, Peck CC, Lupton GP. Erythema multiforme and urticaria. *Arch Dermatol* 1979;115:742–743.

133. Maibach HI. Acute laryngeal obstruction presumed secondary to thiomersil (Merthiolate) delayed hypersensitivity. *Contact Dermatitis* 1975;1:221–222.

134. Lavoie FW, Coomes T, Cisek JE, Fulkerson L. Emergency department external decontamination for hazardous chemicals exposure. *Vet Hum Toxicol* 1992;34:61–64.

135. Geffner ME, Powars DR, Choctaw WT. Acquired methemoglobinemia. *West J Med* 1981;1347:7–10.

136. Ponté C, Richard J, Bonte C, Lequien P, Lacombe A. Méthémoglobinémies chez le nouveau-né: discussion du role étiologique du trichlorcarbanilide. *Ann Pediat* 1974;21:359–365.

137. Spencer PS, Bischoff MC. Skin as a route of entry for neurotoxic substances. In: Marzulli FN, Maibach HI, eds. *Dermatotoxicology*, 2nd ed. Washington: Hemisphere Publishing; 1983:611–626.

138. Klaassen CD, Amdur MO, Doull J. *Casarett and Doull's Toxicology*, 3rd ed. New York: Pergamon Press; 1986.

139. Heygi E, Dolezalova A. Urticarial reaction after patch tests of toothpaste with a subshock condition: hypersensitivity to caraway seed. *Cs Dermatologie* 1976;51:19–22.

140. Camarasa JMG, Alomar A, Perez M. Contact urticaria and anaphylaxis from aminophenazone. *Contact Dermatitis* 1978;4:243–244.

141. Fisher AA, Dooms-Goossens A. Persulfate hair bleach reactions: cutaneous and respiratory manifestations. *Arch Dermatol* 1976;112:1407–1409.

142. Pietzker F, Kuner V. Anaphylaxie nach epikutanem Ampicillin-Test. *Z Hautkr* 1975;50:437–438.

143. Katz BE, Fisher AA. Bacitracin: a unique topical antibiotic sensitizer. *J Am Acad Dermatol* 1987;17:1016–1024.

144. Kozáková M. Sub-shock brought on by epidermic test for chloramphenicol. *Cs Dermatol* 1976;51:82–84.

145. Michel PJ, Buyer R, Delorme M. Accidents généraux (cyanose, collapse cardiovasculaire) par sensibilisation à une solution aqueuse de violet de gentiane et vert de méthyle en applications locale. *Bull Soc Fr Dermatol Syphiligr* 1958;65:183.

146. Kleinhans D, Zwissler H. Anaphylaktischer Schock nach Anwendung einer Benzocain-haltigen Salbe. *Z Hautkr* 1980;55:945–947.

147. Daughters D, Zackheim HS, Maibach HI. Urticaria and anaphylactic reactions after topical application of mechlorethamine. *Arch Dermatol* 1973;107:429–430.

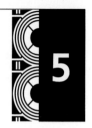

Biological Causes

ARMANDO ANCONA, M.D.

Almost any kind of infection can occur at work if the conditions are favorable. Many different occupations may be affected. Outdoor and agricultural workers, mainly in tropical and subtropical climates, may acquire certain fungal diseases. Bacterial infections affect individuals who are exposed to animals or their products. Viruses cause disease in workers who are in contact with infected animals, but viruses may also affect medical and laboratory personnel. Outdoor occupations provide many opportunities to be exposed to parasites and helminths; arthropod bites and stings affect entomologists, food handlers, and floriculture and forestry workers. Establishing a relationship between an occupation and a disease is not an easy matter. Isolating microorganisms from the environment and adding epidemiological data and a thorough job history can support the connection.

BACTERIAL INFECTIONS

Staphylococcal and Streptococcal Infections

The most common bacterial infections are secondary infections from minor lacerations, abrasions, burns, and puncture wounds. Folliculitis and boils caused by staphylococci and streptococci are especially common in construction workers as well as in farm workers.[1] A report on skin infections among meat packers[2] showed that pustular and inflamed lesions were present in 32 of 69 plant workers (Fig. 5–1). Acquisition of infection showed a clear association with job category. Occupations in which injuries and lacerations from bones and knives were present, such as boning and killing, provided the majority of the cases. Cultures from those lesions isolated group A β-hemolytic streptococcus, in 18 cases and *Staphylo-*

coccus aureus in 12 cases. In 20 instances, both germs were found. In this study, meat specimens contained the same streptococcal strain and may have acted as the vehicle of transmission. Barnham and Neilson[3] cultured group L β-hemolytic streptococci and *Staphylococcus aureus* from paronychia and infected wounds in 15 workers involved in the slaughter and processing of chickens and pigs. These same authors had previously published similar studies.[4–6]

The role of the carrier of *Staphylococcus aureus* among workers in a machine-building plant has been studied, and it showed that isolation of *S. aureus* from the nasal and pharyngeal mucosa as well as on the skin was more frequent in such workers than in a control group. Workers exposed to oils and microtrauma were prone to develop pyoderma in hands and fingers.[7]

Streptococcus suis, a commensal and pathogenic microorganism in pigs, has been reported to cause severe infections in pig farmers and abattoir workers; illnesses include meningitis, pneumonia, and endocarditis. Fresh cuts and abrasions of the hands was a common finding, suggesting that prompt disinfection of skin injuries constitutes a preventive measure.[8, 9]

Severe streptococcal axillary lymphadenitis, an unusual syndrome, may constitute a risk in health workers, as in the case reported by Boyce[10] in which an accidental prick by a contaminated needle produced a pustule at the site of the prick and, subsequently, a severe infection accompanied by marked swelling of the arm and forearm. A culture of the pustule on the patient's finger grew *Streptococcus pyogenes,* and the patient subsequently died from *S. pyogenes* bacteremia.

Recidivant ulcerative pyoderma caused by *Staphylococcus aureus* and *Streptococcus pyogenes* A in a butcher[11] and ecthyma in a fish seller[12] have also been reported. Skin infections

FIGURE 5–1 • Pustular lesion of
the palm caused by *Staphylococcus
aureus* in a meat handler.

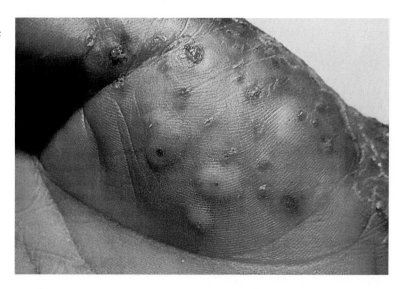

from streptococci and staphylococci in these trades seem to be underreported and thus constitute a risk. Other diseases acquired in these occupations include anthrax, erysipeloid, orf, and viral warts, which are particularly frequent in meat handlers.

Anthrax

Anthrax, a malignant pustule caused by *Bacillus anthracis,* a spore-forming bacterium, is chiefly an animal disease, but humans can be infected by contact with animals or their products. It is one of the oldest diseases known and the first infectious disease for which a bacterial vaccine was found effective (by Pasteur in 1881). Animals are infected by eating grass growing on soil contaminated with the vegetative form of the organism. The bacillus is a gram-positive, nonmotile, spore-forming rod that elaborates a highly toxic endotoxin that rapidly causes the death of infected animals. In the soil, the vegetative form is extremely resistant. The ability of these spores to remain viable for many years in animal products, soil, and the industrial environment is an important factor in the epidemiology of anthrax.[13]

Anthrax is found throughout the world; in developing countries, occupational anthrax morbidity is related to the incidence of the disease in animals. Occupation-oriented infection in industrialized countries is determined by the contamination of imported animal products. Infections in humans occur in agricultural workers, in stock farmers and breeders, and in those who work in abattoirs, in the butchery trade, and in bone and bone meal processing. In the United States, almost all anthrax infections are cutaneous and are limited to workers who handle imported goat hair, wool, and hides from regions where adequate disease-control programs are lacking, such as the Middle East, Africa, and South America, where the disease is endemic. Workers at greatest risk include longshoremen, freight handlers, warehouse workers, and employees of processing industries in which the products are treated for use. Sorters in tanneries are especially susceptible prior to disinfection of the hides. Other workers at risk include upholsterers, carpet makers, herders of goats and sheep, and slaughterers. Meneghini et al.[14] reported 18 cases of occupational cutaneous anthrax that occurred in a rural community. Most of the patients were farmworkers; meat and hide handlers were also infected. Human anthrax continues to be an occupational hazard, and erradication depends on the ability to control it in domestic animals. Strong clinical suspicion should be maintained about those who work in high-risk occupations.[15] Because of the lack of extensive data about human exposure, assesment of risk depends on information from animal tests. Such information must be interpreted in the light of strain-to-strain differences in virulence of *B. anthracis* and host susceptibility to infection.

Estimating the critical dose of *B. anthracis* spores in humans is only the first step in assessing the risk to workers. It is also necessary to quantify the virulence of the anthrax strain, as well as to list potential exposure sources.[16]

Infection almost always occurs on exposed parts of the body, such as the face, neck, hands, and arms and especially on areas of minor injury (Fig. 5–2). Direct inoculation can occur through a puncture wound or abrasion, and the inhalation of spores may induce a severe respiratory infection

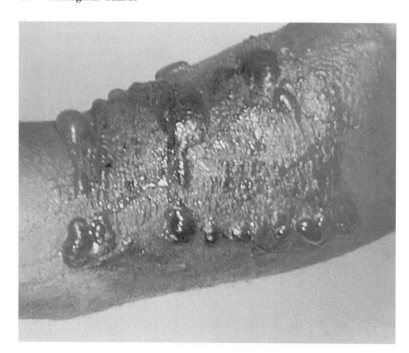

FIGURE 5–2 ● Anthrax. Hemorrhagic vesicles with satellite lesions. (Courtesy of Dr. C. Moreno.)

called wool-sorter's disease. Pulmonary anthrax from inhalation of spores[17] is usually fatal if untreated. A gastrointestinal form of the disease has also been described. The systemic form of the disease is commonly fatal; without treatment septicemia and death may occur in up to 20% of patients. The primary lesion is a small papule that rapidly enlarges to form a boggy, purplish-red, sharply marginated mass topped with a hemorrhagic vesicle or bulla. After a few days, the bulla becomes necrotic and satellite vesicles appear (Fig. 5–3). Because pain is nearly always absent, the lesion is often ignored for days or weeks. Regional lymph nodes become enlarged, but lymphangitis does not occur.

Systemic signs include fever, malaise, weakness, and tachycardia. Diagnosis is made on the basis of characteristic clinical indolent lesions, culture from the pustule, and occupational and epidemiological data. Anthrax responds to treatment with penicillin and tetracycline. Incision and drainage must be avoided to prevent systemic dissemination. Preventive measures include antianthrax vaccination in susceptible animals, elimination of soil pollution, and decontamination of hides. These methods have been quite successful in the United States since 1930. Reported cases today are therefore exceedingly rare.

Brucellosis

The skin is an important portal of entry for brucellosis (Malta fever, undulant fever), still a fairly common infection for veterinarians, slaughterhouse workers, meat packers and inspectors, and laboratory technicians. The disease is usually an acute illness characterized by chills, high fever, headache, and extreme weakness. A chronic form of the disease was common; it caused, splenic abscesses, renal disease, and bladder complications.[18]

Despite advances in the control of the disease in animals, brucellosis still has great economic impact in the United States. Cases in humans are underdiagnosed and underreported, which constitutes a major health hazard.[19] Three *Brucella* organisms are responsible, each a nonmotile gramnegative rod: *B. suis* from pigs, *B. abortus* from cattle, and *B. melitensis* from sheep and goats. Contact results from handling contaminated animals or ingesting milk or cheese that is contaminated and unpasteurized. The skin manifestations are nonspecific and range from a maculopapular eruption to petechiae, which occur in less than 5% of patients. A chronic ulcer may develop at the site of inoculation or injury and may occur in slaughterhouse workers and veterinarians from accidental self-injection while inoculating calves against the disease. Other cutaneous manifestations include a contact urticaria-like eruption and a subsequent vesicopustular reaction that is attributable to hypersensitivity to bacterial antigens by individuals occupationally exposed to contact with fluids from infected animals.[20]

An outbreak of brucellosis affecting 18 employees at a pork processing plant was reported in

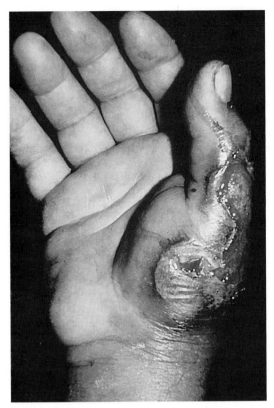

FIGURE 5–3 • Anthrax. Large bulla with necrosis. (Courtesy of Dr. Y. Ortíz.)

North Carolina in 1992. Risk for brucellosis was highest among workers in the kill department. The vast majority of the patients had histories of more frequent cuts and scratches at work, compared with healthy employees.

Occupational transmission of brucellosis occurs primarily among packing plant workers, veterinarians, livestock producers, and laboratory workers.[21] A laboratory research worker performing experiments on the products of conception from cattle and sheep to investigate possible infectious causes of abortion was infected by *B. melitensis*.[22] An epidemic of brucellosis caused by sniffing bacteriological cultures, a habit common in certain laboratories, has been reported recently.[23] Brucellosis continues to be an occupational hazard for medical laboratory personnel. Five cases of laboratory-acquired infection with *B. melitensis* were reported, which raises the importance of serological surveys and instruction to laboratory workers so that early recognition of cases is possible.[24]

Prevention should include animal prophylaxis by elimination of infected animals and vaccination of healthy ones; however, this goal may be difficult to achieve for economic reasons. Individual hygiene and the cleaning of the working area may

be difficult to maintain, particularly in rural areas. Vaccination by live vaccine (strain 19-BA) is effective in reducing human cases, but allergic reactions may be a contraindication to its use. Treatment with tetracycline, 500 mg four times a day for 3 weeks, is effective; however, chronic forms may be difficult to cure. Treatment may be combined with streptomycin, 1 g daily intramuscularly, the first 7 to 14 days.

Tularemia

Tularemia is a disease that occurs in many North American animals, including rabbits, deer, squirrels, skunks, muskrats, and numerous others, but 90% of human cases result from contact with cottontail rabbits. The disease was first discovered in 1911 in Tulare County, California, in ground squirrels—hence its name.[25] The first human infection was reported in 1914. The vectors of the causative bacterium, *Francisella tularensis,* are fleas, ticks, and deerflies.

The bacterium is a pleomorphic gram-negative coccal bacillus that produces an ulcer at the site of inoculation, followed by marked bubonic-plague–like enlargement of regional lymph nodes. The ulcer rapidly becomes necrotic and produces a characteristic black eschar. In many cases, severe constitutional symptoms may occur; they resemble the symptoms of typhoid: headache, chills, fever, and a generalized aching of muscles and joints. A maculopapular, hemorrhagic, generalized eruption may appear during the course of the febrile illness.

Recreational hunters are at the greatest risk, but the disease also affects veterinarians, farmers, butchers, foresters, and laboratory workers.[26]

Treatment with streptomycin, 1 to 2 g per day for 3 days, half the dose 3 more days in adults, is curative, but the organism rapidly develops resistance to this antibiotic. Other drugs that can be used are tretracycline or chloramphenicol.

Erysipeloid

Erysipeloid is an infectious disease that is commonly related to occupation. The causative organism is a slender gram-positive rod that infests the skin of freshwater and saltwater fish, crabs and other shellfish, and poultry, especially turkeys. The route of entry is through breaks in the skin caused by scratches, puncture wounds, and abrasions. Fishermen and butchers may develop erysipeloid, as may poultry dressers and retailers of fish and poultry. The disease is common in areas where fishing is the main industry. In 1954 Proctor and Richardson[27] reported 235 cases in Aberdeen, Scotland. Popuga et al.[28] reported an outbreak of erysipeloid in workers at a shoe factory. The infection spread through contact with infected raw materials. The causal microorganism was isolated from the water of the soaking baths. Bacteriological confirmation supported the occupational origin of the cases.

Seven workers at a quail processing plant developed localized inflammation of the fingers, which responded to antibiotic therapy for erysipeloid. *Erysipelothrix rhusiopathiae* was cultured from visceral organs of flocks of coturnix that had died from the disease.[29] Erysipeloid may coexist with other infections such as orf, as in the case of sheep farmers.[30]

Infection affects the hands more commonly than other sites. Between 3 and 7 days after inoculation a painful, raised, purplish papule appears and enlarges to form a characteristic sharply demarcated, painful, purplish-red lesion with associated lymphangitis and lymphadenitis. A low-grade fever and joint pains may be present. Endocarditis has been reported.[31] Septicemia may occur as a result of systemic spread of infection and manifests in the form of constitutional effects and a generalized purpuric, petechial rash. Cutaneous lesions regress slowly without suppuration and disappear spontaneously after 3 to 4 weeks.

Diagnosis is based on the characteristic clinical picture and the absence of suppuration and systemic symptoms as well as on the patient's occupational history. Erysipelas and cellulitis are most likely to be confused with erysipeloid.

Preventive measures should be directed toward elimination of decaying nitrogenous material, which is the main source of infection. Adequate hygiene of factory premises, as well as personal protective equipment and opportune treatment of cuts and abrasions may contribute to reducing its incidence.

Treatment with penicillin, 2 to 3 million units per day for 10 days is usually curative, but recurrences may develop.

Cutaneous Tuberculosis

Tuberculosis of the skin acquired through inoculation of *Mycobacterium tuberculosis hominis* or *bovis* is called tuberculosis verrucosa cutis, a warty granulomatous lesion usually seen in pathologists and morgue attendants (anatomic tubercle or necrogenic wart). Surgeons, veterinarians, farmers, and butchers also may acquire the infection. Needle-prick injuries might be important in cutaneous inoculation of tuberculosis in laboratory workers handling virulent tubercle bacilli, as in the case reported by Sharma et al.[32] Nosocomial spread of tuberculosis among hospital workers

should be considered possible from contact with cutaneous lesions of a tuberculous nature.[33] This was the case for hospital personnel caring for a patient with a skin ulcer in which subsequent noncaseating granulomas and acid-fast bacilli were demonstrated. Of the workers, 10 of 11 who were skin-test converters, two of whom did not received prophylaxis, developed pleural effusion that gradually resolved with antituberculous chemotherapy; all affected workers recalled being present during the dressing or débridement of the ulcer. Tuberculosis should be considered in the differential diagnosis of skin lesions of unknown cause, and appropriate protective measures should be used during wound care.[34]

Tuberculosis verrucosa cutis may be associated with *Mycobacterium bovis*. This was the case of a dairy farmer whose herd had been slaughtered because of tuberculosis; an open sore on the neck of an animal seemed to be the source of infection.[35]

The bacille Calmette-Guérin vaccine, used for tuberculosis prophylaxis as well as for the treatment of neoplastic diseases, represents a risk for health workers. Accidental prick with a contaminated syringe while treating urinary bladder cancer resulted in bacille Calmette-Guérinitis on the extensor surface of the fingers of a surgical resident.[36] Although a rare occupational risk,[37] it may still be diagnosed in countries where tuberculosis continues to be a problem.

With a predilection for the fingers and hands, the disease usually results from a minor injury that permits entry of the tubercle bacillus. Progress is slow, with regression eventually occurring after many months or years and leaving a delicate scar. In other instances it may progress slowly to form a warty hyperkeratotic plaque, which usually presents a chronic course (Fig. 5–4). Treatment consists of a course of INH (isoniazid) combined with streptomycin or other antituberculous drugs.

Atypical Mycobacterial Infections

The most common atypical mycobacterial infection is caused by *Mycobacterium marinum*. Most patients acquire the infection from exposure to infected fish, to aquariums, or to aquatic environments. Persons who clean fish tanks and fishermen in the Gulf of Mexico[38] are at greatest risk for developing this disease. In 1951 in Colorado, 290 cases occurred in persons swimming in a pool infected with this organism.[39]

The clinical picture consists of granulomatous papules and nodules that ulcerate and exude a clear thin serum. A pattern resembling sporotrichosis may develop,[40] with lesions occurring along

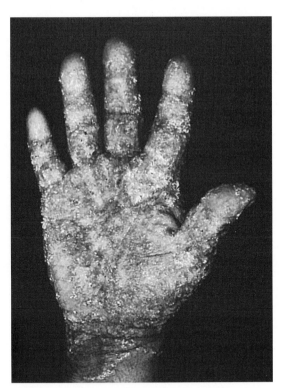

FIGURE 5–4 • Tuberculosis verrucosa cutis. Warty hyperkeratotic plaque caused by *Mycobacterium tuberculosis bovis* in a butcher.

the regional lymphatics. The organism enters through small breaks in the skin, usually involving fingers and hands (Fig. 5–5). An unusual form of occupational infection from *M. marinum*[41] was seen in a pump mechanic who acquired the infection while working with water pumps through inoculation in a cut by an impeller contaminated by the organism.

Mycobacterium ulcerans infections have also

been reported as possible occupational risks. Exner and Lemperle[42] studied a plastic surgeon who developed a necrotizing infection of the hand attributable to this atypical mycobacterium. This clinical picture, also called Buruli ulcer, responds poorly to chemotherapy; early and wide surgical excision proved to be the treatment of choice.

Atypical mycobacterial infections[43] seem to occur more frequently. Disturbances of the immune system, outdoor activities, and occupation influence their presentation. Precise mycobacterial identification requires specialized techniques, and response to treatment is variable. When the lesions are single and localized, surgical extirpation may be the treatment of choice. Otherwise, various antitubercular drugs as well as tetracycline[44] have been recommended.

Salmonella Infections

Salmonella dublin, an important bovine pathogen that causes dysentery, abortion, and septicemia, may produce a characteristic dermatitis in individuals occupationally exposed to fluids of infected animals. Williams,[21] after examining 105 veterinary surgeons in Wales, found five cases that presented certain common features. All the patients had carried out obstetric work requiring prolonged intrauterine manipulations without wearing gloves. Shortly afterwards, an erythematous rash appeared, followed by a papular pustular eruption with some painful red nodules. *S. dublin* was isolated from pus of those lesions. In most instances, *S. dublin* infection was confirmed in vaginal swabs from the cows. Veterinary surgeons may act as vectors of this disease, as pustules in salmonella dermatitis are a source of viable organisms. Similar cases have been reported in Australia.[45]

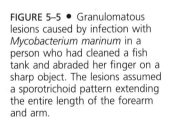

FIGURE 5–5 • Granulomatous lesions caused by infection with *Mycobacterium marinum* in a person who had cleaned a fish tank and abraded her finger on a sharp object. The lesions assumed a sporotrichoid pattern extending the entire length of the forearm and arm.

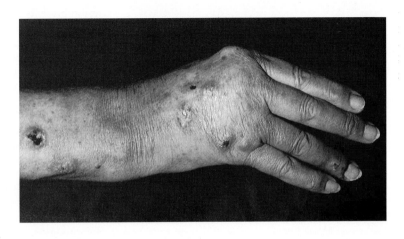

VIRAL INFECTIONS

Herpes Simplex

Herpes simplex infection of the hand, caused by virus type 1 or type 2, is a well-recognized occupational hazard of health professionals exposed to contact with secretions of the mouth and respiratory tract.[46–48] When localized to the fingers, primary or recurrent infection (herpetic whitlow) is characterized by edema and swelling that may resemble acute bacterial cellulitis accompanied by regional lymph node enlargement. In a second stage, coalescent vesicles appear, giving a more definite clinical picture (Fig. 5–6).

The recurrence of herpetic whitlow suggests that infection creates a reservoir for the virus that remains latent until reactivated.[49]

Several studies have shown that dental professionals are frequently exposed to the herpes simplex virus (HSV) and that they develop infections in the fingers more frequently than the general population. In a study at the Michigan School of Dentistry,[50] it was found that dentists are more likely to have a history of the disease and are at increased risk of contracting the virus than the general adult population. Rowe et al.[51] carried out a survey of dental practitioners and concluded that herpetic whitlow was more frequent in practicing dentists than in a control population. A similar study[52] also indicates that HSV infection constitutes an occupational risk among dentists.

On the other hand, health-care professionals with undiagnosed infections may pose a risk to their patients. This was shown by an outbreak of herpes simplex type 1 gingivostomatitis that occurred in a dental practice[53] and affected 20 out of 46 patients. Preventing the transmission of herpes simplex virus should be based on the following precautions: Work on the teeth of patients with active lesions should be deferred until healing has taken place, and dental personnel with negative complement-fixing and neutralizing antibodies to the HSV should take special care to avoid contamination, such as using disposable gloves and safety glasses.[54]

Nosocomial transmission of herpes virus type 1 infection may produce not only herpetic whitlow but also other infections such as keratoconjunctivitis; a cluster of cases occurred in an intensive care unit.[55]

Seroepidemiological studies for herpes virus type 1 infection in dental personnel showed no significant differences in the presence of antibodies between preclinical and clinical dental students or between qualified dental surgeons and a matched control group. That study design indicated no evidence of significant risk of occupational infection.[56]

Orf

Orf (ecthyma contagiosum) is endemic in sheep and goats and is readily transmitted to humans through direct contact. The infectious agent, a paravaccinia subgroup of poxviruses, enters the body through minor breaks in the skin, usually on the hands. A favorite site is the dorsal aspect of the right index finger (Fig. 5–7).

Johannessen et al.[57] observed more than 200 cases and described the following clinical stages. Between 3 and 6 days after a person has come into contact with infected sheep or goats, a macule appears. After a few days, it evolves into a papulous stage and begins to look like a target; the lesion presents a red center surrounded by a white ring and a red halo. A subsequent nodular stage shows a weeping surface and central umbilication resembling a keratoacanthoma. Finally, a granulomatous lesion is followed by ulceration and then healing occurs without scarring, about 7 weeks after infection.

Almost all lesions appear on the hands, and they may be multiple. Regional adenopathy is present along with a low-grade fever. Occasionally, a generalized vesiculopapular rash may be seen.[58] Bullous pemphigoid can complicate human orf and follow 2 to 3 weeks after infection; this has been considered significant rather than a coincidental association.[59] The disease resembles milkers' nodules, with which it may be confused.

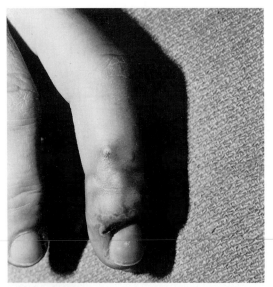

FIGURE 5–6 • Herpetic whitlow, an infection caused by the herpes simplex 1 virus.

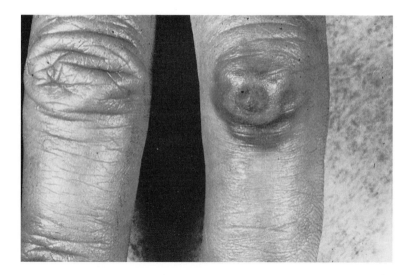

FIGURE 5–7 • Orf on the right index finger (the usual location), was contracted by bottle-feeding infected lambs.

Workers at greatest risk are shepherds, veterinarians, farmers, and sheep and goat shearers, especially workers who feed infected animals milk from a bottle. Infection occurs by animal lesions localized to nostrils, lips, or buccal mucosa. However, infection may also be acquired through indirect contact with contaminated objects.

Although seldom reported in North America, orf should be considered when diagnosing cutaneous lesions in patients who have exposure to animals associated with it.[60] A study of a farming community in Wales demonstrated that orf is recognized in both sheep and farmers in the vast majority of cases, suggesting that it is a common disease. As there is no effective treatment, preventive measures should be taken.[61]

Milkers' Nodules

The paravaccinia virus in infected cows causes this benign skin disease of milkers, dairy farmers, veterinarians and, especially, newly employed workers who have not yet developed immunity. Transmission to humans occurs by direct contact with infected teats and udders of cattle. Hand milking provides a particularly high-risk environment for exposure to the virus.

There are usually one to four 1-cm nodules on the hands or forearms; the nodules closely resemble those of orf (Fig. 5–8), and regional lymph nodes may be enlarged. The disease is self-limited and confers lasting immunity.[62] Prevention of milkers' nodules includes use of rubber gloves when handling affected animals, isolation of infected dairy cows, and hygienic milking procedures.

An epidemic of 15 cases in Denmark showed, besides classical lesions, an erythema-multiforme–like eruption. Microscopy and electron microscopy studies were consistent with parapox virus infection.[63] The symptoms are treated.

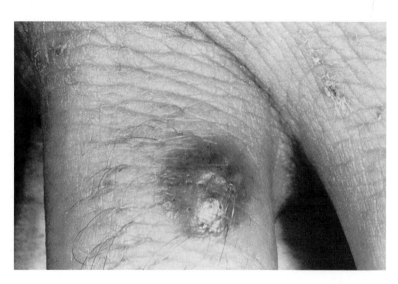

FIGURE 5–8 • Milkers' nodules are caused by the paravaccinia virus and are usually ignored by farm workers.

Other paravaccinia infections in humans were reported in eight persons from a veterinary school.[64] In those cases, cutaneous lesions were similar to those of orf and milkers' nodules and originated in cattle with bovine papular stomatitis. This disease occurs in cattle and is usually without observable lesions, which makes the source of transmission difficult to trace. Cowpox infections in humans are very rare. Marennikova et al.[65] reported two cases that occurred in Poland and note that wild rodents could have been the source of transmission in those cases.

Buffalopox has been reported in a dairy in India. Two workers exposed to affected buffaloes developed multiple bullous and dry-crusted lesions on the palmar aspects of the fingers. The diagnosis was confirmed by injecting cell culture harvests into embryonated chicken eggs on the chorioallantoic membrane; all virus isolates produced characteristic lesions.[66]

Cat-Scratch Disease

Small-animal veterinarians are most likely to develop this presumably viral disease, which is manifested by the development of a lichenoid, papular nodule at the site of a recent scratch by a cat. Enlargement of regional lymph nodes begins approximately 3 to 4 weeks after injury. The nodes are single or multiple and may become fluctuant and suppurative. Mild to moderate constitutional symptoms occur in many patients, including myalgia, headache, chills, and fever.[67] A rare complication is encephalopathy, which may be serious. Erythema nodosum, erythema multiforme, and thrombocytopenic purpura have also been observed.[68]

The causative organism has never been isolated, although an extensive search has been made.[69] That a virus is the cause is presumed, as Koch's postulates have never been fulfilled. The symptoms are treated.

Viral Wart

Several studies have shown an increased frequency of warts in meat handlers. Affected workers include butchers and those engaged in slaughtering of cattle, pigs, and poultry. Clinically, warts present the common appearance, affecting either the palms or the dorsa of the hands.

In a large epidemiological survey conducted in the meat-processing industry, De Peuter et al.[70] found an increased frequency of palmar and dorsal warts in comparison with a control group. Similar findings were reported by Taylor[71] in a poultry-processing and -packing station. In an epidemiological study of 1,141 meat and pork handlers, 687 of whom were constantly handling meat, Wall et al.[72] found an overall prevalence of hand warts in 46.4%. Personnel who handled meat most of the time were more seriously affected (54.1%) than workers who did so for less time (34.6%). Mergler et al.[73] found a 28.5% prevalence of hand warts in workers in a poultry slaughterhouse; the authors concluded that high humidity and abrasions of the skin facilitated cutaneous infections by the virus. In a study of the prevalence of warts in meat-industry workers in a large meat plant and in a control group, Funkel and Funkel[74] reported similar findings.

Poultry slaughterers were found to have an incidence of warts of 47.5%. Workers in certain specific jobs in which they were exposed to chicken claws, skin, and blood seemed to be the most seriously affected; wart distribution coincided with areas that were most commonly exposed during the process.[75] Retail butchers appear to be in a different situation. Bouchet and de la Brassinne[76] found no difference in the prevalence of viral warts on the hands of 113 workers in butchers' shops when compared with a control group of mechanics. The authors explain this difference on the basis of exposure; in large companies, direct contact among individuals and indirect contact through tools and working surfaces is higher, so virus propagation under such conditions would result in a larger number of cases.

Identification of papillomaviruses in butchers' warts was carried out by Orth et al.[77] Four known types of human papillomaviruses were identified, and a new papillomavirus (HPV-7) was found; the authors concluded that it may represent a new type of human papillomavirus. To date, there is no evidence that nonhuman papillomaviruses can cause infections in humans. Possible explanations for occupational infections may lie in environmental factors that might facilitate virus transmission among infected individuals. The possibility of human infection by nonhuman papillomaviruses requires further study.

FUNGAL INFECTIONS

Dermatophytic Infections

Occupational infections by dermatophytes occur (1) through contact with geophilic or zoophilic species by individuals exposed to soil products or animals or (2) through contact with anthropophilic fungi that may be transmitted among individuals if working conditions create a suitable environment, for example, humidity, occlusion, and microtrauma. In some instances, occupational origin may be easily presumed. For example, *Trichophyton verrucosum,* a zoophilic dermatophyte, infects farmers and cattle tenders. Anthropophilic dermatophytes such as *T. rubrum* and *T. mentagrophytes* cause tinea pedis in the general population. However, increased perspiration, as when wearing protective shoes in industry or crossinfections among individuals sharing shower facilities in factories, may result in greater frequency in a limited group of workers.

Many dermatophytes are associated with certain occupations. *Microsporum gypseum,* a geophilic fungus found in certain types of soil containing clay and sand, causes infections in agricultural workers. It has also been reported in metal-processing products and in association with other occupations involving the soil. Animals can transmit the disease to humans.

Zoophilic species, when they affect humans, produce inflammatory lesions that may resemble pyogenic infections. *Microsporum canis,* a fungus that frequently infects small animals, constitutes a source of transmission of dermatophytosis to workers in pet shops, to veterinarians, and to personnel in contact with laboratory animals. Occupational relationship is established by isolating the same dermatophyte from both the workers and the animals in their care.

Trichophyton verrucosum is associated mainly with infections of cattle, although other animals may also be affected. Humans are infected as a result of direct contact or secondary contact with contaminated barns, fences, straw, or soil. This fungus may remain viable in the environment for longer than a year. The lesions are inflammatory and resemble staphylococcal pyoderma. Farmers, milkers, cattle tenders, veterinarians, and tannery workers, especially hide sorters, are at risk (Fig. 5–9).

Another dermatophyte that can cause disease in animals and in humans is *Microsporum nanum.* Roller and Westblom[78] reported three cases of hog farmers who were infected with this fungus. The clinical features were those of common dermatophytic infections, which responded to griseofulvin. Although it was not possible to isolate *M. nanum* from the animals, lesions were characteristic, showing circinate, erythematous patches with indurated peripheries. This dermatophyte affects pigs predominantly but has also been isolated in cattle, dogs, and laboratory animals.

Trichophyton mentagrophytes is found in the soil as a saprophyte. Humans acquire infection from infected cattle, dogs, cats, and birds. It is one of the most common causes of tinea pedis, although it may produce infection in other areas, too, including onychomycosis. *T. mentagrophytes* infections have been described in a wide variety of occupations. Mycological studies of miners with tinea pedis reported that *T. mentagrophytes* was isolated from rubber boots and bathing premises. On the other hand, an epidemiological study in coal miners[79] demonstrated that dermatophytes accounted for only one-third of foot infections. Gram-negative bacilli were responsible for the remainder. The authors concluded that wetness of the feet predisposes to bacillary but not to dermatophytic infection. Grosshans et al.[80] studied the epidemiological and economic aspects of foot dermatophytoses in workers in a coking plant, a potash mine, and an automobile factory. Barn workers and cattle with dermatophytic infections were

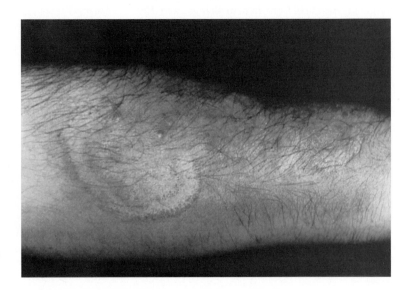

FIGURE 5–9 • Infection with the cattle fungus *Trichophyton verrucosum* is highly inflammatory, resembling a pyogenic infection. (Courtesy of Dr. A. Arévalo.)

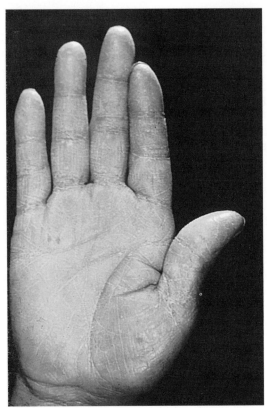

FIGURE 5–10 • Tinea manuum, dry scaling and nonpruritic, may accompany tinea pedis. Certain occupations that include humidity and mild trauma may favor this location.

studied by Kakepis et al.[81] *T. mentagrophytes* var. *granulare* was isolated in 35% of workers suspected of being infected and in 25% of apparently healthy animals.

Trichophyton rubrum, the dermatophyte most frequently isolated from human beings, and *Epidermophyton floccosum* are the main infectious agents in tinea pedis and other infections such as tinea manum, in which it produces a dry, scaling, mildly erythematous eruption, often unilateral and nonpruritic (Fig. 5–10). This localization often accompanies tinea pedis or onychomycosis. Certain workers are considered to be at risk, especially those engaged in mildly traumatic work in humid surroundings. In such cases, an occupational origin may be presumed, as the activity creates a local environment conducive to the establishment of the fungal infection. Such a conclusion is easy to refute, but today most compensation boards accept the relationship. Differential diagnosis includes psoriasis and chronic contact dermatitis. Cases treated previously with local steroids modify their clinical characteristics and are difficult to diagnose.[82]

Candida Infections

Infections with *Candida albicans* constitute the most common fungal disease of occupational origin. Infection appears on normal or previously irritated skin. The hands and fingernails are the main areas of involvement in occupationally acquired disease when environmental conditions favor proliferation of the fungus. Intertrigo of interdigital spaces presents as an erythematous exudative lesion with a fissure in the depth. Sometimes there is a desquamative collar at the periphery. Moisture and apposition of surfaces favor this condition (Fig. 5–11). Paronychia and onychia affect one or several fingers, producing painful inflammation of periungual tissue. There is a detachment of the cuticle and skin in the lateral nail folds. Infection of the nail plate is manifested as a yellow-green discoloration different from alterations produced by dermatophytes (Fig. 5–12). Differential diagnosis includes onychomycosis, psoriasis, and onychodystrophy secondary to eczema.

Candida species are ubiquitous saprophytes. Exposure of the skin to moisture, occlusion, emulsifying agents, and other irritants compromises local defenses and provides favorable environmental conditions for proliferation. It is generally admitted that activities that expose the skin to moisture, such as dishwashing, laundering, canning, and food handling, constitute significant risk for developing candidal infections. Exposure to cutting oils, because of their irritant and degreasing effects, seems to present an unusually high potential for yeast infections.[83]

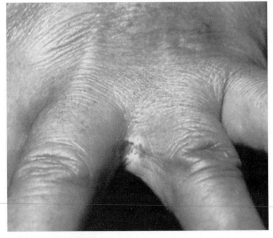

FIGURE 5–11 • Intertriginous candidosis presents as an erythematous, fissured, exudative lesion. Prolonged exposure to moisture favors this condition.

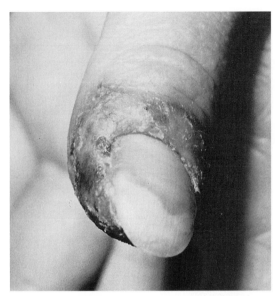

FIGURE 5–12 • Chronic paronychia due to *Candida albicans* is a common condition in persons who must keep their hands immersed in water during their work. In this case the nail plate is also involved, showing a yellow-green discoloration in the lateral nail fold.

Sporotrichosis

Sporotrichosis is a chronic disease of cutaneous and subcutaneous tissues that is characterized by the formation of subcutaneous nodules that ulcerate and drain; lymph nodes in the drainage pathway are involved. The etiological agent is a dimorphic fungus, *Sporothrix schenckii*, that has a widespread saprophytic distribution.

Cutaneous forms may be divided in two distinct clinical manifestations. The fixed type, which is restricted to the site of inoculation, may be nodular, ulcerative, or verrucous (Fig. 5–13). The lymphocutaneous type, the classic form of this disease, appears at the inoculation site of the microorganism and produces a painful papule that slowly enlarges and frequently ulcerates; secondary lesions develop along the lymphatics draining the initial lesion (Figs. 5–14 and 5–15).

This fungal disease is acquired by persons who work with soil—nursery, agricultural, and forestry workers—as well as by miners. The largest epidemic occurred in miners in South Africa, 3,000 of whom developed the disease from contact with timber on which the organism was growing. In none of the cases was dissemination found, however.[84]

Sporotrichosis may be inoculated by trauma with thorns, sticks, splinters, and sphagnum moss.[85] In three workers in a commercial nursery who presented with sporotrichosis, *Sporothrix schenckii* was cultivated from the clinical lesions and from sphagnum moss used for packing plant roots.[86] In 1988, the largest documented outbreak of cutaneous sporotrichosis to date in the United States occurred; 84 cases erupted in persons from 15 states who were exposed to Wisconsin-grown sphagnum moss used in packing evergreen tree seedings. The risk of infection increased as length of worktime exposure to the moss increased. Samples of moss from the Wisconsin supplier were negative, but *S. schenckii* was cultured from multiple samples of the sphagnum moss obtained from a nursery in Pennsylvania, the nursery that was

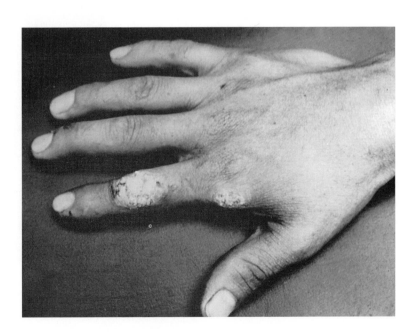

FIGURE 5–13 • Sporotrichosis may present as a fixed verrucous lesion restricted to the site of inoculation. (Courtesy of Drs. A. Saúl and A. Bonifaz.)

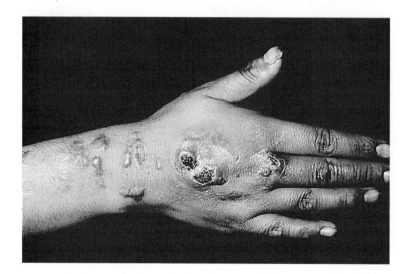

FIGURE 5–14 • Sporotrichosis caused by the fungi *Sporothrix schenckii* characteristically follows the distribution of the lymphatics. (Courtesy of Dr. Y. Ortiz.)

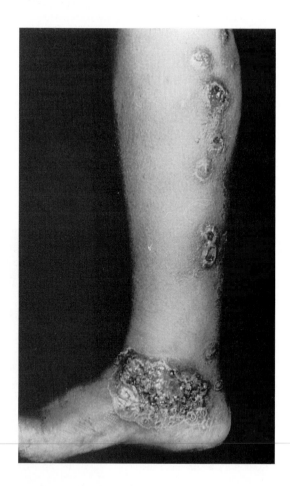

FIGURE 5–15 • Sporotrichosis may ulcerate. The development of secondary lesions along the lymphatics in a lower limb is frequent in agricultural workers. (Courtesy of Drs. A. Saúl and A. Bonifaz.)

identified as the location of 94% of the cases. Differences in tree-handling procedures and packing suggested possible explanations for the association.[87, 88]

Bonsai trees have been reported as a source of disseminated sporotrichosis.[89] Research activities involving *S. schenckii* and related to the 1988 epidemic in the United States spawned a case of laboratory-acquired sporotrichosis that occurred in the absence of any apparent trauma or other predisposing factors, which suggests the possibility that *S. schenckii* can invade healthy and intact skin.[90]

Zoonotic transmission of sporotrichosis is rare. Veterinarians and their assistants are at greatest risk when handling cats with cutaneous ulcers, even if they are without any penetrating skin injuries.[91]

Prevention of this disease should include environmental measures, such as monitoring and decontaminating sphagnum moss when it is used and maintaining the working area so as to reduce the possibility of injury by scratches, punctures, or lacerations. Personal measures should include informed workers, the wearing of protective clothing to prevent trauma to exposed skin areas, and opportune medical attention.

Treatment consists of 10 drops of saturated solution of potassium iodide, administered orally three times daily until the lesions clear. For more serious cases, amphotericin B or the new imidazoles are the drugs of choice.

Mycetoma

Mycetoma (Madura foot) is a localized swollen lesion, usually on a foot or hand, involving skin, subcutaneous tissue, fascia, and bone. The lesion contains granulomas and abscesses that suppurate and drain through sinus tracts. The pus contains granules that vary in size from microscopic to more than 2 mm in diameter.[92]

Mycetoma arises from both bacteria and fungi. Five species of actinomycetes (*Streptomyces madurae, S. pelletieri, S. somaliensis, Nocardia brasiliensis,* and *N. caviae*) and 13 species of true fungi have been implicated.[93]

The disease is acquired by traumatic implantation of the organism beneath the skin. Most persons acquire the disease while walking barefoot; agricultural workers are particularly at risk. Expanding areas of soft-tissue swelling and draining sinus tracts occur, accompanied by little pain or limitation of motion (Fig. 5–16). Osteomyelitis may also occur, but dissemination is rare. Other frequent sites are the side of the neck (Fig. 5–17) and the back (Fig. 5–18), where the infectious

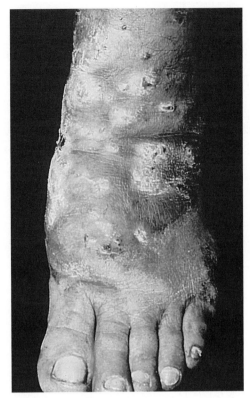

FIGURE 5–16 • Mycetoma is acquired by traumatic implantation of the organisms beneath the skin. The foot is a common location, mainly in agricultural workers who have walked barefoot. (Courtesy of Dr. F. Quintana.)

agent is introduced when contaminated materials are being carried. These two localizations are relatively frequent in workers living in rural areas where the agents are endemic. The microorganism can invade deeper tissues, producing pleuropulmonary involvement.

An atypical mycetoma localized to the anterior aspect of the neck and characterized by hard, nondraining nodules was present in a peasant living in the neighborhood of Acapulco. He was an iguana hunter and had suffered accidental bites from the animals. Clinical diagnosis of this nonsuppurative form, not suspected initially, was confirmed by a biopsy that demonstrated large granules corresponding to *Madurella mycetomatis.* Wild animals that are herbivorous may act as vectors, as in this case[94] (Fig. 5–19).

Treatment is difficult. Sulfones, streptomycin, and rifampicin may be helpful; imidazoles and amphotericin B are used in cases produced by fungi. Advanced disease, mainly in the limbs, requires amputation.[95]

As with other deep mycoses, relationship with occupation is not always easy to establish. Epidemiological evidence, existence of the fungus in the

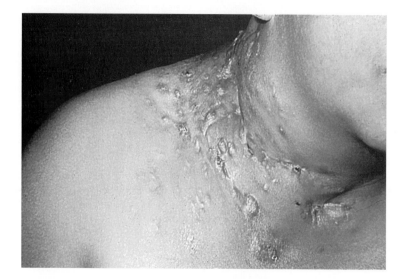

FIGURE 5–17 • Mycetoma in this location occurs frequently in rural areas where people carry infected vegetal materials. (Courtesy of Drs. A. Saúl and A. Bonifaz.)

FIGURE 5–18 • Mycetoma on the back commonly occurs in agricultural workers carrying burdens of infected materials, as in this sugarcane worker. (Courtesy of Drs. A. Saúl and A. Bonifaz.)

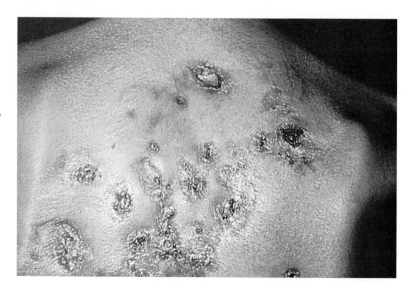

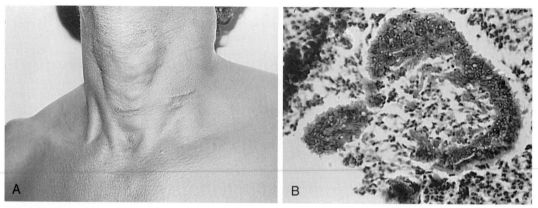

FIGURE 5–19 • *A,* Atypical mycetoma characterized by hard, nonsuppurative nodules caused by the bite of an iguana, a herbivorous animal that can serve as a vector, as in this case of a peasant. *B,* Biopsy of this lesion demonstrated large granules corresponding to *Madurella mycetomatis.* (Courtesy of Drs. G. Chávez and R. Estrada.)

workplace, and occupational factors that promote infection must be taken into account.

Chromomycosis

Chromomycosis, one of the deep mycoses, occurs by traumatic implantation of the fungus, which generally remains localized at the site of inoculation in the skin, mucous membrane, and underlying tissue. It may be caused by several species of dematiaceous or pigmented fungi that are saprophytes of soil, decaying vegetation, and rotting wood. The five main fungi that cause chromomycosis are *Phialophora verrucosa, Fonsecaea pedrosoi, F. compactum, F. dermatitidis,* and *Cladosporium carrionii.*[96]

The initial lesion is a scaly papule that enlarges to a warty tumor, spreading later to form a plaque (Fig. 5–20). Verrucous plaques may have central scarring (Fig. 5–21). Other lesions show induration with fistulas, recalling mycetoma. The legs are most often affected, and it may take years for the whole limb to be involved. There is no invasion of muscle or bone, and hematogenous spread is rare. Workers at risk are those in occupations that involve outdoor activities, mainly in tropical and subtropical climates requiring contact with contaminated soil, barks, grasses, and debris. The possibility of infection after trauma depends on the frequency of scratching and subsequent contamination by soil and the amount of the inoculum in the wound. Agricultural workers in areas where chromomycosis occurs more frequently are particularly at risk.

Differential diagnosis should be established primarily among sporotrichosis, blastomycosis, tuberculosis verrucosa cutis, leishmaniasis, and mycetoma. Preventive measures such as wearing protective cloth and following other practices to avoid accidental injuries are difficult to undertake in rural places where the weather is hot. Treatment is surgical removal of early, individual lesions. Chemotherapy with amphotericin B and 5 fluorocytosine is indicated in more advanced cases.[97]

Blastomycosis

Blastomycosis is caused by a dimorphic fungus, *Blastomyces dermatitidis,* that is found most commonly in the southeastern United States, although recent publications have reported cases in Africa, India, and Israel. The primary infection occurs in the lungs. Pulmonary infection is present in all patients, but it is clinically important in only about half.[98] Systemic disease may disseminate to other organs, with a predilection for skin, bone, and prostate. The skin is involved secondarily through dissemination from a primary focus in the lung. However, primary cutaneous forms have been observed in accidental inoculation in laboratory workers. The characteristic lesion is a slowly growing verrucose pustule with a serpiginous border that shows a tendency toward central healing. The face, arms, neck, and hands are most commonly involved.

Although the ecological niche of this organism is not known with certainty, organic debris and materials associated with soil and moisture appear to be sources of infection; workers involved with farming, forestry, construction, and heavy earthmoving equipment may be infected.[99] Amphotericin B is the treatment drug of choice.

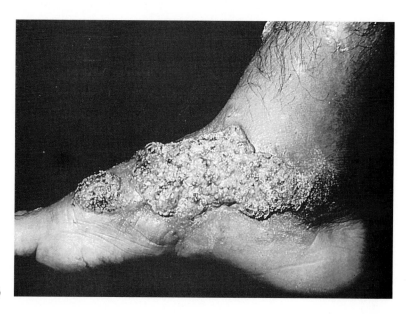

FIGURE 5–20 • Chromomycosis, verrucous plaque type, affects mainly the lower limbs. Unlike mycetoma, there is no invasion of muscle and bone. Workers in outdoor occupations in tropical climates are most commonly affected. (Courtesy of Dr. Y. Ortíz.)

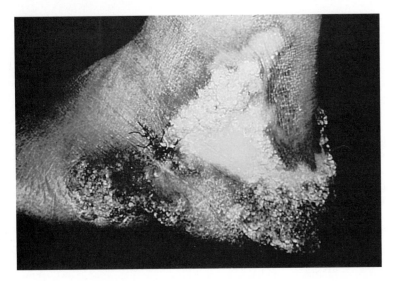

FIGURE 5–21 • Chromomycosis may present with scarring alternating with verrucous plaques. Workers who have contact with soil, barks, and contaminated grass are at higher risk. (Courtesy of Dr. F. Quintana.)

Coccidioidomycosis

Caused by inhalation of dust that contains spores of the fungus *Coccidioides immitis,* coccidioidomycosis is endemic to arid and semiarid regions of California, New Mexico, Arizona, northern Mexico, and Argentina.[100] The usual infection is a self-limited, often asymptomatic, influenza-like respiratory illness that resolves in 3 to 4 weeks. During this illness, hypersensitivity reactions may occur, the most common being erythema nodosum, erythema multiforme, and urticaria.[101] In a small percentage of persons, often blacks and Asians, dissemination occurs, producing multiple cutaneous abscesses (cold abscesses) (Fig. 5–22) and widespread abscess formation in the lungs and other body areas, including the brain. The death rate among Mexicans is 5 times greater than among whites; among blacks, 23.5 times greater; among Filipinos, 192 times greater.[102]

A rare inoculation type of local granulomatous lesion may occur.[103, 104] Coccidioidal infection may disseminate following corticosteroid therapy.[105]

Persons at greatest risk are migrant workers, farmers, construction workers, military personnel, bulldozer operators, laboratory workers, and others exposed to dust in areas where the fungus is endemic. The greatest number of cases occur during the summer months. Fatal disseminated coccidioidomycosis occurred in a cotton mill worker in Durham, North Carolina, who contracted it from cotton grown and baled in California's San Joaquin Valley. The bales contained spores of the fungus, which the worker inhaled while opening

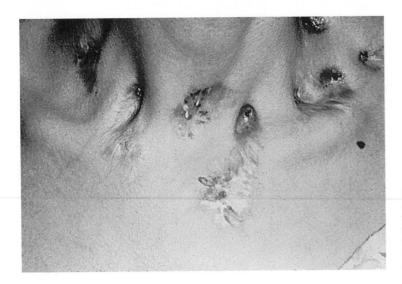

FIGURE 5–22 • "Cold abscesses" of disseminated coccidioidomycosis of the chest and neck in a young farm worker who contracted the disease while working in an area in which it is endemic. (Courtesy of Drs. A. Saúl and A. Bonifaz.)

the bales and feeding them into hoppers. This early processing of the cotton was the dustiest part of the operation.[106]

Coccidioidomycosis may also pose a risk for veterinarians. The disseminated form of the disease developed in a veterinarian who had autopsied a horse with disseminated disease, but in that case there were no draining lesions and no productive cough. Because the infectious form of *Coccidioides immitis* is not produced in humans and other mammalian hosts, it is postulated that in that case, transmission occurred through inhalation of tissue-phase endospores aerosolized in the course of dissection.[107]

Treatment of disseminated coccidioidomycosis demands intravenous amphotericin B. Prevention requires dust control and perhaps preselecting workers to be employed in certain high-risk jobs in areas where the fungus is endemic; discrimination must be avoided, however.

TREPONEMAL INFECTIONS

Syphilis

Occupational syphilis may be defined as syphilis contracted or transmitted in the course of a person's working. Nonvenereal occupational syphilis may be acquired among workers who share mouthpieces, for example, glassblowers. It has been reported, although rarely, to occur as a primary infection on the hands of health personnel and laboratory technicians. High-risk occupations include hostesses, entertainers, and people that facilitate sex for the public. The aggregation and industrialization of the population increase the risk of venereal syphilis. It may occur in large industrial complexes established in rural areas.[108]

RICKETTSIAE AND CHLAMYDIAE

Many of these infections are transmitted by blood-sucking insects and mites. The manifestations of Rocky Mountain spotted fever, Q fever, typhus, and trench fever are fairly characteristic, consisting of maculopapular eruptions that are often petechial or hemorrhagic. Workers at high risk for Rocky Mountain spotted fever are farmers, foresters, rangers, trappers, hunters, construction workers, surveyors, and guides. Workers with the potential for exposure to Q fever include dairy farmers, ranchers, abattoir personnel, tannery workers (especially hide sorters), and laboratory technicians.

PARASITES

Various parasites may cause skin disease; as with bacteria, any of them can cause occupational disease, given favorable conditions. The main groups include protozoa; helminth worms, which include platyhelminths and nemathelminths; and the phylum Arthropoda, which comprises the classes Arachnida and Insecta, among others.[109]

Protozoa

Many protozoa cause general health problems rather than occupational disease. Amebiasis, trypanosomiasis, and toxoplasmosis are examples. Cutaneous leishmaniasis (Oriental sore, bouton d'Orient), produced by *Leishmania tropica* which is transmitted by a minute fly, commonly *Phlebotomus papatasii,* is endemic to warm climates.

Clinically, it presents as an ulcerative form at the beginning, and can turn into a chronic scarring nodular form. Mucocutaneous and disseminated forms produced by *L. brasiliensis* constitute an endemic and rural disease in Central and South America.[110] Leishmaniasis becomes endemic in individuals working in tropical forests, as it occurs in southeastern Mexico (chiclero ulcer). The tropical forest in southeastern Mexico is an endemic area for leishmaniasis; individuals working on the extraction of sap from chicle trees are exposed. Görtz et al.[111] reviewed two cases of leishmaniasis and discussed its significance to occupational health as well as applicable preventive and therapeutic measures.

Helminths

Cercarial dermatitis (swimmer's itch, swamp itch, clam digger's itch), a highly pruritic eruption, is caused by penetration of the cercariae of a schistosome into the papillary dermis, causing an itchy papular eruption. Urticaria may occur, followed by widespread macules and papules.[112] Itching is intense. The disease lasts for 1 to 2 weeks, and secondary infection of the excoriated lesions is common. Persons who may develop this disease are skindivers, lifeguards, dock workers, and caretakers who maintain lakes and ponds.

The symptoms are treated. Immediately after leaving the water, the patient should vigorously rub the skin with a towel to try to remove most of the cercariae. Occasionally systemic steroids may be required. Secondary infections must be treated with appropriate antibiotics. Prevention may be accomplished by treating infected water with copper sulphate. Other platyhelminths produce general health problems rather than occupa-

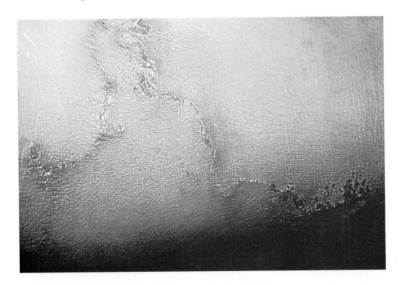

FIGURE 5–23 • Creeping eruption of larva migrans, showing the linear pattern. Chronic cases show desquamation. (Courtesy of Dr. A. Saúl.)

tional disease, as is the case in sparganosis and cysticercosis.

Larva migrans (creeping eruption, sandworm eruption) is caused by various nematode parasites. It is prevalent in subtropical and tropical regions where people work in and on moist soil infected with hookworm larvae. Sandy beaches are likely areas. The feces of dogs and cattle and occasionally humans carry the larvae, and humans are the final hosts. *Ancylostoma braziliense* is the parasite that most frequently causes this condition in the United States.

The disease has a characteristic appearance, showing a thin, red or flesh-colored, slightly raised line (Fig. 5–23), which is due to larval movement of between 1 and 2 mm and 1 cm a day. Scaling is seen in older lesions. The larvae of *Ancylostoma duodenale* and *Necator americanus* infect humans, penetrate the skin, and enter the circulation. They then travel to the lungs and from there enter the gastrointestinal tract and repeat the life cycle. Nonspecific gastrointestinal symptoms occur as well as intestinal bleeding that produces iron deficiency anemia. The larvae enter the skin between the toes and on the soles of the feet, where they produce a papulovesicular eruption that often ulcerates[113] (Fig. 5–24).

Agricultural workers, sewer workers, ditchdiggers, and lifeguards are at greatest risk.

Treatment consists of oral administration of thiobendazole, 25 to 60 mg/kg of body weight, for 2 to 4 days only. In the early stages, topical thiobendazole may be effective.

Other nematodes that cause skin diseases are unlikely to be occupational in origin, for example, trichinosis, dracunculosis, filariasis, loiasis, onchocerciasis, enterobiasis, strongyloidiasis, and toxocariasis.

Arthropods

The phylum Arthopoda comprises about nine classes, some of which are of dermatological interest and may cause occupationally related diseases.[114]

Arachnida, one of the most important classes, comprises mites, ticks, spiders, and scorpions. Insecta includes a large number of classes. Moths, bees, wasps, ants, flies, mosquitoes, fleas, and blister beetles, among others are the frequently reported causes of occupation-related bites and stings. Millipedes and centipedes, through bites or simple contact, may induce severe skin reactions. Crustacea may induce injury by biting with their claws. Sea lice, which frequent tropical seas, cause punctate hemorrhagic dermatitis with their powerful biting parts.[115]

Reactions caused by arthropods may be related to toxins or allergenic products that can reach the individual directly or through the air. Many of

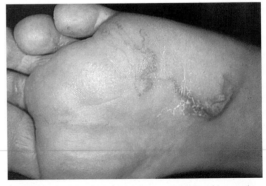

FIGURE 5–24 • Larva migrans may enter the skin on the soles of the feet, producing a papulovesicular linear eruption.

these reactions are often occupational in nature, affecting entomologists, food handlers, and outdoor workers.

Human skin lesions have been associated with only about 50 species of mites, which have various feeding habits—parasitic, predacious, saprophagous, graminivorous, herbivorous, and so forth. Skin lesions vary somewhat depending on the species of mite, the degree of host reaction, and the number of exposures to the mite. Lesions produced by biting are characterized by pruritic papular eruptions that may progress to urticaria. Papules are recognized by a central punctum or vesicle. Irritation and discomfort are the result of hypersensitivity to mite secretions during feeding.

Many occupations involve exposure to mites. Farming exposes workers to bird, chicken, and rodent mites. Mites associated with straw or hay may produce a disseminated varicelliform eruption accompanied in some cases by constitutional symptoms. Betz et al.[116] reported an outbreak of occupational dermatitis associated with *Pyemotes ventricosus* that had infested wheat. In an excellent monograph of dermatoses associated with mites and ticks, Krinsky[117] states that the straw itch mite actually corresponds to *P. tritici* and not to the frequently cited species *P. ventricosus*. The same article reviews publications related to occupational exposure to mites, which occurs in the following activities: grain processing, food processing, floriculture, and forestry, as well as among dock and restaurant workers. Factory workers may also be affected, as buildings harbor rodents and birds, which serve as sources of mites. Laboratory personnel may be at risk, as shown by the outbreak due to a tropical rat mite that occurred in research and animal technicians.[118] IgE-mediated contact urticaria, rhinitis, and conjunctivitis occurring in workers in a greenhouse and attributable to a spider mite, have been documented by Reunala et al.[119]

Mites can also be associated with human pathogens, for example, rickettsiae. Prevention requires localization and removal of the source of mites; this may include the fumigation and control of infested animals. Symptoms are treated.

Ticks ingest blood from a diversity of vertebrate hosts, including humans. Humans become infested by their association with domestic animals or contact with vegetation. Soft ticks produce small erythematous macules and papules that are mildly symptomatic. Extreme reactions that include pain, intense pruritus, necrosis, and ulceration may be due to previous exposure and sensitization to tick secretions. Bites of hard ticks become papular or nodular and may persist for months (Fig. 5–25). Occasionally, a febrile episode may ensue until the tick and its head are removed from the skin.[120] Erythema chronicum migrans may occur following a tick bite and is usually quite persistent, lasting for months.

Lyme disease, so called because it was first recognized in Lyme, Connecticut, is an inflammatory disease that may follow tick-induced erythema chronicum migrans weeks or months later. Intermittent attacks of mono- or oligoarticular arthritis occur, especially in the knees, and they are often associated with neurological abnormalities, myocardial conduction alterations, serum cryoprecipitates, elevated serum IgM levels, and an increased sedimentation rate. Erythema chronicum migrans is an important diagnostic marker of this disease.[121, 122] Epidemiological evidence suggests that Lyme disease is caused by an infectious agent transmitted by ticks of the genus *Ixodes*, such as *I. dammini* in the Northeast and Midwest and *I. pacificus* in the West. Attempts to isolate the causative organism from ticks have been unsuccessful, but recently a treponema-like spirochete was detected in and isolated from *I. dammini*. Serum of patients with Lyme disease was shown by indirect immunofluorescence to contain antibodies to this agent.[123] Tick paralysis is a serious disease associated with ticks; it is caused by a neurotoxin, chiefly seen from bites of *Dermacentor andersoni*, the tick responsible for Rocky Mountain spotted fever.

Tick bites are common in outdoor workers such as loggers, construction workers in wilderness areas, and ranchers. Prevention of tick bites depends on avoidance of tick-infested animals and environments as well as on the use of protective clothing and repellents. Treatment requires removal of the tick's mouth part in order to avoid the development of granulomatous lesions.

Although spider bites can be harmless, two well-defined clinical pictures are of interest and have clinical relevance to individuals at work. Arachnidism originated by the genus *Lactrodectus* (black widow spider) causes both local and systemic reactions. Most individuals recover in a few days, and fatalities are rare. Occupation-related problems caused by this arthropod have been reported in South African vineyard workers. Spiders of the genus *Loxosceles* (brown recluse spider) produce painful lesions that become necrotic (Fig. 5–26). Systemic intoxication may be followed by death in some cases.[124]

Allergic reaction to Hymenoptera venom produces a wide variety of clinical pictures, ranging from local reactions to anaphylaxis. Bee and wasp stings occur among beekeepers (Fig. 5–27). In a study population of 191 beekeepers, the occurrence of systemic and intense local reactions after

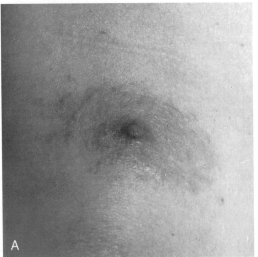

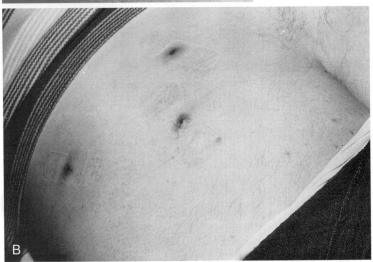

FIGURE 5–25 ● *A*, Inflammatory lesions from tick bites may persist for months. *B*, Infestation with bot fly in a surveyor who was planning road construction in Guatemala.

bee stings was high; a history of atopy was associated with systemic reactions and was more frequent in individuals who presented symptoms in the eyes and nose while working at hives and who had a history of beekeeping of fewer than 15 years.[125] In an attempt to correlate the clinical symptoms and the immunological reactivity to bee venom, 102 beekeepers were prick-tested with various concentrations of bee and wasp venom ranging from 10 to 300 μg/mL at the same time radioallergosorbent (RAST) tests were performed in order to screen for IgE antibodies. Prick-tests correlated significantly with the presence of specific IgE for both venoms, but no correlation was observed between venom allergy and atopy.[126]

In a clinical and immunological survey of sensitivity to Hymenoptera in Japanese forestry workers, it was concluded that the number of stings may contribute to the occurrence of systemic reactions to Hymenoptera stings, and that some mech-

anism other than IgE-mediated hypersensitivity may also be involved in these reactions.[127] Occupation-related allergy to bumblebee venom was reported on a farm that cultured this species for agriculture purposes. Because these insects do not sting deliberately, anaphylactic reactions to bumblebee venom occur only occasionally, but beekeepers, who commonly are sensitized to honey bee venom, are more at risk because of the cross-reactivity between the two venoms. Immunotherapy with honey bee venom proved to be successful in allowing beekeepers to continue in their jobs.[128]

The invasion of human tissue by the larvae of flies is termed myiasis; it develops in workers exposed to soil in which the flies lay their eggs, especially in warm, moist sand in tropical and subtropical regions. Surgical extirpation after local anesthesia with lidocaine is the treatment of choice. Antibiotics should be administered if secondary infection develops.

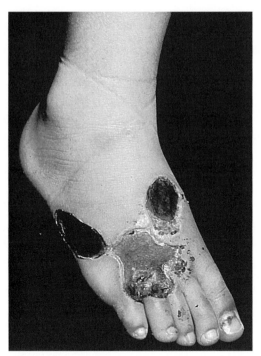

FIGURE 5–26 ● Necrotic lesions produced by the bite of a brown recluse spider (*Loxosceles reclusa*), which may also produce severe systemic reactions. (Courtesy of Dr. Y. Ortíz)

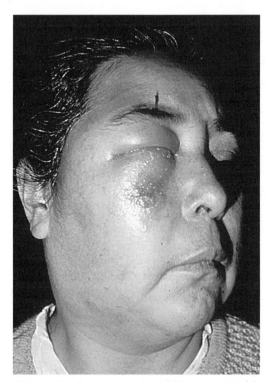

FIGURE 5–27 ● Hymenoptera (wasp) bites cause painful and edematous lesions. Symptoms are attributable to both toxic and antigenic substances. (Courtesy of Dr. M. Magaña-Lozano.)

Nonstinging arthropods may cause toxic or allergic reactions. This can occur either by direct contact or by airborne exposure. For example, cockroaches may cause not only allergic eruptions but also asthma.[129, 130] An occupational case was studied by Monk and Pembroke[131] in a medical-records clerk who developed urticated erythematous papules after inadvertent contact with insect debris. Prick-testing with cockroach extracts was positive; 20 healthy controls gave negative results. In some instances it may be difficult to determine whether clinical symptoms are due to hypersensitivity or to reaction to nonallergenic components of the arthropod. These reactions are more widespread than is generally recognized. Preventive measures should be directed to limit exposure to the causative agents; sanitation, use of protective equipment, and education could reduce the risk of these reactions.[132]

References

1. Peachey RDG. Skin hazards in farming. *Br J Dermatol* 1981; 105 [suppl 21]:45–50.
2. Fehrs LJ, Flanagan K, Kline S, et al. Group A beta-hemolytic streptococcal skin infections in a US meat-packing plant. *JAMA* 1987; 258:3131–3134.
3. Barnham M, Neilson DJ. Group L beta-haemolytic streptococcal infection in meat handlers: another streptococcal zoonosis. Epidemiol Infect 1987; 99:257–264.
4. Barnham M, Kerby J, Skillin J. An outbreak of streptococcal infection in a chicken factory. *J Hyg (Lond)* 1980; 84:71–75.
5. Barnham M, Kerby J. Skin sepsis in meat handlers: observations on the causes of injury with special reference to bone. *J Hyg (Lond)* 1981; 87:465–476.
6. Barnham M, Kerby J. A profile of skin sepsis in meat handlers. *J Infect* 1984; 9:43–50.
7. Malanchyn IM, Sytnyc OM. The *Staphylococcus aureus* carrier state among the workers of a machine-building plant. *Lik-Sprava* 1993; 7:97–100.
8. Baterlink AKM, van Kregten. *Streptococcus suis* as threat to pig-farmers and abattoir workers. *Lancet* 1995; 346:1707.
9. Clarke D, Almeyda J, Ramsay I, et al. Primary prevention of *Streptococcus suis* meningitis. *Lancet* 1991; 338:1147.
10. Boyce JM. Severe streptococcal axilliary lymphadenitis. *N Engl J Med* 1990; 323:655–658.
11. Kölmel KV, Proksch E. Rezivierende pyodermien als Berufskrankheit bei einem Schlachter. *Dermatosen* 1985; 33:223–224.
12. Gehrke U, Leyh F. Vogelaugenartige ekthymata bei einer Fischverkäuferin. *Dermatosen* 1983; 31:95–96.
13. Merchant IV. Anthrax. In: *Veterinary Bacteriology and Virology,* 4th ed. Ames, Ia: State College Press; 1953: 490–500.
14. Meneghini CL, Lospaluti M, Angelini G. Cutaneous anthrax: observation in 18 cases. *Berufs-Dermatosen* 1974; 22:233–237.
15. Jalaludin BB. Human cutaneous anthrax. *Med J Austral* 1991; 155:280.
16. Watson A, Keir D. Information on which to base assessments of risk from environments contaminated with anthrax spores. *Epidemiol Infect* 1994; 113:479–490.

17. Severn M. A fatal case of pulmonary anthrax. *Br Med J* 1976; 1:748.
18. McDevitt DG. Symptomatology of chronic brucellosis. *Br J Ind Med* 1973; 30:385–389.
19. Young EJ. Human brucellosis. *Rev Infect Dis* 1983; 5:821–842.
20. Trunnel TN, Waisman M, Trunnel TL. Contact dermatitis by brucella. *Cutis* 1985; 35:379–381.
21. Williams E. Veterinary surgeons as vectors of *Salmonella dublin. Br Med J* 1980; 280:815–818.
22. Taylor-Robinson SD. A case of laboratory acquired brucellosis. *Br Med J* 1996; 313:1130–1132.
23. Grammont-Cupillard M, Berthet-Badetti L, Dellamonica P. Brucellosis from sniffing bacteriological cultures. *Lancet* 1996; 348:1733–1734.
24. Gruner E, Bernasconi E, Galeazzi RL. Brucellosis: an occupational hazard for medical laboratory personnel: report of five cases. *Infection* 1994; 22:33–36.
25. McCoy GW, Chapin CW. Bacterium tularense, a plague-like disease in rodents. *Public Health Bull* No. 53 1912; 5:17–23.
26. Boyce JM. Recent trends in the epidemiology of tularemia in the United States. *J Infect Dis* 1975; 131:197–199.
27. Proctor DM, Richardson IM. A report on 235 cases of erysipeloid in Aberdeen. *Br J Ind Med* 1954; 11:175–179.
28. Popuga V, Podkin IA, Gurvich VB, et al. Erysipeloid as an occupational disease of workers in shoe enterprises. *Zh Mikrobiol Epidemiol Immunobiol* 1983; 10:46–49.
29. Mutalib A, Keirs R, Austin F. Erysipelas in quail and suspected erysipeloid in processing plant employees. *Avian Dis* 1995; 39:191–193.
30. Connor MP, Green AD. Erysipeloid infection in a sheep farmer with coexisting orf. *J Infect* 1995; 30:161–163.
31. Grieco MH, Sheldon C. *Erisipelothrix rhusiopathiae. Ann NY Acad Sci* 1970; 174:523–532.
32. Sharma V, Kumar B, Radotra BD, et al. Cutaneous inoculation tuberculosis in laboratory personnel. *Int J Dermatol* 1990; 29:293–294.
33. Hutton MR, Stead WW, Cauthen GM, et al. Nosocomial transmission of tuberculosis associated with a draining abscess. *J Infect Dis* 1990; 161:286–295.
34. Frampton MW. An outbreak of tuberculosis among hospital personnel caring for a patient with a skin ulcer. *Ann Intern Med* 1992; 117:312–313.
35. Healy, E, Rogers S. Tuberculosis verrucosa in association with bovine tuberculosis. *J Roy Soc Med* 1992; 85:704–705.
36. Atiyeh BS, Wazzan WC, Kaddoura IL, et al. Bacille Calmette-Guérin (BCG)-itis of the hand: a potential hazard for health workers. *Ann Plast Surg* 1996; 36:325–329.
37. Konetzke G, Beck B, Braunlich A, et al. Tuberculosis as an occupational disease. *Z Gesamte Hyg* 1982; 28:149–153.
38. Miller WC, Toon R. *Mycobacterium marinum* in Gulf fishermen. *Arch Environ Health* 1963; 27:8–10.
39. Philpott JA Jr, Wooburne AR, Philpott OS, et al. Swimming pool granuloma. *Arch Dermatol* 1963; 88:158–162.
40. Adams RM, Remington J, Steinberg J, et al. Tropical fish aquariums: a source of *Mycobacterium marinum* infection resembling sporotrichosis. *JAMA* 1970; 211:457–461.
41. Cole G. *Mycobacterium marinum* infection in a mechanic. *Contact Dematitis* 1987; 16:283.
42. Exner K, Lemperle G. Buruli ulcer: necrotizing infection of the hand of a plastic surgeon. *Handchir Mikrochir Plast Chir* 1987; 19:230–232.
43. Krüger M, Qadripur S, Ippen H. Erkrankungen durch atypische Mykobakterien. *Dermatosen* 1984; 32:195–205.
44. Wolinsky E, Gómez F, Zimpfer F. Sporotrichoid *Mycobacterium marinum* infection treated with rifampin and ethambutol. *Am Rev Respir Dis* 1972; 105:964–967.
45. Gillians JA, Palmer HW, Dyte OH. Follicular dermatitis caused by *Salmonella dublin. Med J Aust* 1982; 1:390–391.
46. Jones JG. Herpetic whitlow: an infectious occupational hazard. *J Occup Med* 1985; 10:725–728.
47. Gill MJ, Arlette J, Buchan K. Herpes simplex virus infection of the hand: a profile of 29 cases. *Am J Med* 1988; 84:89–93.
48. Watkinson AC. Primary herpes simplex in a dentist. *Br Dent J* 1982; 153:190–191.
49. Klotz RW. Herpetic whitlow: an occupational hazard. *AANA J* 1990; 58:8–13.
50. Brooks S. Rowe N, Drach J, et al. Prevalence of herpes simplex virus disease in a professional population. *JAM Dent Assoc* 1981; 102:31–34.
51. Rowe N. Heine C. Kowalsky C. Herpetic whitlow: an occupational disease of practicing dentists. *J Am Dent Assoc* 1981; 105:471–473.
52. Rames S, Folkmar T, Roed-Petersen B. Herpes simplex as a possible occupational disease in dentists of the county of Aarhus, Denmark. *Acta Derm Venereol* 1984; 64:163–165.
53. Manzella J, McConville J, Valenti W, et al. An outbreak of herpes simplex virus type 1 gingivostomatitis in a dental hygiene practice. *JAMA* 1984; 252:2019–2022.
54. Rowe N, Shipman C Drach J. Herpes simplex virus disease: implications for dental personnel. *J Am Dent Assoc* 1984; 108:381–382.
55. Perl TM, Haugen TH, Pfaller M, et al. Transmission of herpes simplex virus type 1 infection in an intensive care unit. *Ann Intern Med* 1992; 117:584–586.
56. Herbert AM, Bagg J Walker DM, et al. Seroepidemiology of herpes virus infections among dental personnel. *J Dent* 1995; 23:339–342.
57. Johannessen JV, Krogh HC, Kjeldsberg E. Orf. *Contact Dermatitis* 1980; 6:36–39.
58. Moore RM Jr. Human orf in the United States. *J Infect Dis* 1973; 127:731–732.
59. Murphy JK, Ralfs IG. Bullous pemphigoid complicating human orf. *Br J Dermatol* 1996; 134:929–930.
60. Gill MJ, Arlette J, Buchan K. Human Orf. *Arch Dermatol* 1990; 126:356–358.
61. Buchan J. Characteristics of orf in a farming community in mid-Wales. *Br Med J* 1996; 313:203–204.
62. Leavell UW Jr, Phillips IA. Milkers' nodules: pathogenesis, tissue culture, electron microscopy and calf inoculation. *Arch Dermatol* 1975; 111:1307–1311.
63. Hansen SK, Mertz H, Krogdahl A, et al. Milkers' nodules: a report of 15 cases in the county of North Jutland. *Acta Derm Venereol* 1996; 76:88.
64. Bowman KF, Barbery RT, Swango LJ, et al. Cutaneous form of bovine papular stomatitis in man. *JAMA* 1981; 246:2813–2818.
65. Marennikova SS, Wojnarowska Y, Bochanek W, et al. Cowpox in man. *Zh Mikrobiol Epidemiol Immunobiol* 1984; 8:64–69.
66. Ramanan C, Ghorpade A, Kalra SK, et al. Buffalopox. *Int J Dermatol* 1996; 35:128–129.
67. Spaulding WB, Hannessey JN. Cat-scratch disease (a study of 53 cases). *Am J Med* 1960; 28:504–509.
68. Carithers HA. Cat scratch disease (its natural history). *JAMA* 1969; 207: 312–316.
69. Emmons RW. Continuing search for the etiology of cat-scratch disease. *J Clin Microbiol* 1976; 4:112–114.
70. De Peuter M, de Clereq B, Minette A, et al. An epidemiological survey of virus warts of the hands among butchers. *Br J Dermatol* 1977; 96:427–431.

71. Taylor SW. A prevalence study of virus warts on the hands in a poultry processing and packing station. *J Soc Occup Med* 1980; 30:20–23.

72. Wall LM, Oakers D, Rycroft RJG. Virus warts in meat handlers. *Contact Dermatitis* 1981; 7:259–267.

73. Mergler D, Vezina N, Beauvais A. Warts among workers in poultry slaughterhouses. *Scand J Work Environ Health* 1982; 8 [suppl 1]: 180–184.

74. Funkel ML, Funkel DJ. Warts among meat handlers. *Arch Dermatol* 1984; 120:1314–1317.

75. Guillet G, Borredon J, Duboseq JM. Prevalence of warts on hands of poultry slaughterers, and poultry warts. *Arch Dermatol* 1987; 123:718–719.

76. Bouchet C, de la Brassinne M. Prevalence of viral warts on the hands of retail butchers. *Dermatosen* 1986; 34:108–109.

77. Orth G, Jablonska S, Favre M, et al. Identification of papillomaviruses in butchers' warts. *J Invest Dermatol* 1981; 76:97–102.

78. Roller JA, Westblom UT. *Microsporum nanum* infection in hog farmers. *J Am Acad Dermatol* 1986; 15:935–938.

79. Hope YM, Clayton YM, Hay RJ, et al. Foot infection in coal miners: a reassessment. *Br J Dermatol* 1985; 112:405–413.

80. Grosshans E, Schwaab E, Samsoen M, et al. Clinique, épidémiologie et incidences économiques des épidermomycoses des pieds en milieu industriel. *Ann Dermatol Venereol* 1986; 113:521–533.

81. Kakepis E. Marcelou-Kindi U, Stratigos J. Bovine ringworm: an outbreak caused by *Trichophyton mentagrophytes* var. *granulare* in Greece. *Int J Dermatol* 1986; 5:580–583.

82. Lachapelle JM. *Dermatologie Professionnelle.* Paris: Masson; 1984:95–97.

83. Cooper BH. Yeast infections. In: Di Salvo AF, ed. *Occupational Mycoses.* Philadelphia: Lea & Febiger; 1983: 183–200.

84. Helm MAF, Bermann C. Sporotrichosis infection in miners of the Witwatersrand: a symposium. In: *Proceedings of the Transvaal Mine Medical Officers Association.* Johannesburg, S. Afr.: Transvaal Chamber of Mines; 1947.

85. D'Allessio DJ, Leavens LJ, Strumpf GB, et al. An outbreak of sporotrichosis in Vermont associated with sphagnum moss as the source of infection. *N Engl J Med* 1965; 272:1054–1058.

86. Grotte M, Younger B. Sporotrichosis associated with sphagnum moss exposure. *Arch Pathol Lab Med* 1986; 105:50–57.

87. Coles FB, Schuchat A, Hibbs JR, et al. A multistate outbreak of sporotrichosis associated with sphagnum moss. *Am J Epidemiol* 1992; 136:475–487.

88. Dixon DM, Salkin IF, Duncan RA et al. Isolation and characterization of *Sporothrix schenkii* from clinical and environmental sources associated with the largest US epidemic of sporotrichosis. *J Clin Microbiol* 1991; 29:1106–1113.

89. Dong JA, Chren MM, Elewski BE. Bonsai tree: risk factor for disseminated sporotrichosis. *J Am Acad Dermatol* 1995; 33:839–840.

90. Cooper CR, Dixon DM, Salkin IF. Laboratory-acquired sporotrichosis. *J Med Vet Mycol* 1992; 30:169–171.

91. Reed KD, Moore FM, Geiger GE, et al. Zoonotic transmission of sporotrichosis case report and review. *Clin Infect Dis* 1993; 16:384–387.

92. Emmons CW, Binford CH, Utz JP. *Medical Mycology.* Philadelphia: Lea & Febiger; 1963:305–322.

93. Utz JP, Shadomy HJ. Deep fungous infections. In: Fitzpatrick TB, Arndt KA, Clark Wh, et al., eds. *Dermatology in General Medicine,* 2nd ed. New York: McGraw-Hill; 1979:1537.

94. Chávez G, Estrada R. Personal communication, 1997.

95. Zaias N, Taplin D, Rebell G. Mycetoma. *Arch Dermatol* 1969; 99:215–225.

96. Vollum ID. Chromomycosis: a review. *Br J Dermatol* 1977; 96:454–458.

97. Al-Doory Y. Chromomycosis. In: Di Salvo AF, ed. *Occupational Mycoses.* Philadelphia: Lea & Febiger; 1983:95–121.

98. Albernathy RS. Clinical manifestations of pulmonary blastomycosis. *Ann Intern Med* 1959; 51:707–727.

99. Di Salvo A. Blastomycosis. In: Di Salvo AF, ed. *Occupational Mycoses.* Philadelphia: Lea & Febiger; 1983:79–94.

100. Fiese MJ. *Coccidioidomycosis.* Springfield, Ill.: Charles Thomas; 1958.

101. Basler RSW, Lagomarsino SL. Coccidiodomycosis: clinical review and treatment update. *Int J Dermatol* 1979; 18:104–110.

102. Wilson JW. Factors which may increase severity of coccidioidomycosis. *Lab Invest* 1962; 11:1146–1150.

103. Levan EN, Huntington RW. Primary cutaneous coccidioidomycosis in agricultural workers. *Arch Dermatol* 1965; 92:215–220.

104. Wilson JW. Cutaneous (chancriform) syndrome in deep mycoses. *Arch Dermatol* 1963; 87:81–85.

105. Bayer AS, Yoshikawa TT, Galpin JE, et al. Unusual syndrome of coccidioidomycosis and diagnostic and therapeutic considerations. *Medicine* 1976; 55:131–149.

106. Gehlbach SH, Hamilton JD, Conant NF. Coccidioidomycosis. *Arch Intern Med* 1973; 131:254–255.

107. Kohn GJ, Linne SR, Smith CM, et al. Acquisition of coccidioidomycosis at necropsy by inhalation of coccidioidal endospores. *Diagn Microbiol Infect Dis* 1992; 15:527–630.

108. Wilcox RP. *Syphilis.* In: Parmeggiani L, ed. *Encyclopaedia of Occupational Health and Safety.* Vol. 2. Geneva International Labour Office; 1985: 131–133.

109. Ebling FJ. Introduction to cutaneous parasitology. In: Rook A, Wilkinson DS, Ebling FJ, eds. *Textbook of Dermatology.* Oxford: Blackwell Scientific; 1972: 806–808.

110. Harman RRM. Parasitic worms and protozoa. In: Rook A, Wilkinson DS, Ebling FJ, eds. *Textbook of Dermatology.* Oxford: Blackwell Scientific; 1972: 809–844.

111. Görtz H, Borneman H, Lang E, et al. Arbeitsmedizinische Aspekte der Kutanen Leshmaniose. *Dermatosen* 1986; 34:171–174.

112. Fisher AA. *Atlas of Aquatic Dermatology.* New York: Grune & Stratton; 1987: 62.

113. Schwartz L, Tulipan L, Birmingham DJ. *Occupational Diseases of the Skin.* Philadelphia: Lea & Febiger; 1957: 133.

114. Burns DA. Diseases caused by arthropods and other noxious animals. In: Champron RH, Burton JL, Elbing FJG, eds. *Textbook of Dermatology.* Oxford: Blackwell Scientific, 1992: 1265–1324.

115. Derbes VJ. Arthropod bites and stings. In: Fitzpatrick TB, Arndt KA, Clark WH, et al., eds. *Dermatology in General Medicine.* New York: McGraw-Hill; 1971: 1940–1954.

116. Betz TG, Davis BL, Fournier PV, et al. Occupational dermatitis associated with straw itch mites (*Pyemotes ventricosus*). *JAMA* 1982; 247:2821–2823.

117. Krinsky WL. Dermatoses associated with the bites of mites and ticks (Arthropoda: Acari). *Int J Dermatol* 1983; 22:75–91.

118. Fox JG. Outbreak of tropical rat mite dermatitis in laboratory personnel. *Arch Dermatol* 1982; 118:676–678.

119. Reunala T, Björkstén L, Forström L, et al. IgE-mediated occupational allergy to a spider mite. *Clin Allergy* 1983; 13:383–388.

120. Feder JA. Tick bite pyrexia. *JAMA* 1944; 126:293–294.
121. Steere AC, Hardin JA, Malawista SE. Erythema chronicum migrans and Lyme arthritis: cryoimmunoglobulins and clinical activity of skin and joints. *Science* 1977; 196:1121–1122.
122. Steere AC, Malawista SE, Hardin JA, et al. Erythema chronicum migrans and Lyme arthritis. *Ann Intern Med* 1977; 86:685–698.
123. Burgdorfer W, Barbour AG, Hayes SF, et al. Lyme disease: a tick-borne spirochetosis? *Science* 1982; 216: 1317–1318.
124. Rook A. Skin diseases caused by arthropods and other venomous or noxious animals. In: Rook A, Wilkinson DS, Ebling JF, eds. *Textbook of Dermatology.* Oxford: Blackwell Scientific; 1972: 845–884.
125. Annila IT Karjalainen ES, Annila PA, et al. Bee and wasp sting reactions in current beekeepers. *Ann Allergy Asthma Immunol* 1996; 77:423–427.
126. Annila IT, Karjalainen ES Morsky P, et al. Clinical symptoms and immunologic reactivity to bee and wasp stings in beekeepers. *Allergy* 1995; 50:568–574.
127. Shimizu T, Hori T, Tokuyama K, et al. Clinical and immunological surveys of Hymenoptera hypersensitivity in Japanese forestry workers. *Ann Allergy Asthma Immunol* 1995; 74:495–500.
128. Kochuyt AM, Van Hoeyveld, Stevens EAM. Occupational allergy to bumble bee venom. *Clin Exp Allergy* 1993; 23:190–95.
129. Zschunke E. Contact urticaria dermatitis and asthma from cockroaches. *Contact Dermatitis* 4:313–314, 1978 a.
130. Zschunke E: Contact urticaria, contact dermatitis and asthma from cockroaches. *Arch Dermatol* 1978; 114:1715–716.
131. Monk BE, Pembroke AC. Cockroach dermatitis: an occupational hazard. *Br Med J* 1987; 294:935.
132. Wirtz RA. Allergic and toxic reactions to non-stinging arthropods. *Annu Rev Entomol* 1984; 29:47–69.

Bibliography

Etkind PH, Odell TM, Canada AT. The gypsy moth caterpillar: a significant new occupational and public health problem. *J Occup Med* 1982; 24:659–662.

Goodman NL. Sporotrichosis. In: Di Salvo AF, ed. *Occupational Mycoses.* Philadelphia: Lea & Febiger; 1983: 65–78.

Groves RW, Wilson-Jones E, MacDonald DM. Human orf and milkers' nodules: clinicopathlogical study. *J Am Acad Dermatol* 1991; 25:706–711.

Jennings LC, Ross AD, Faoagali LJ. The prevalence of warts on the hands of workers in a New Zealand slaughterhouse. *NZ Med J* 1984; 97:473–476.

Kane J, Kradjen S. Dermatophytosis. In: Di Salvo AF, ed. *Occupational Mycoses.* Philadelphia: Lea & Febiger; 1983: 143–183.

Sampaio RN, de Lima LM, Vexenat A, et al. A laboratory infection with Leishmania brasiliensis. *Trans R Soc Med Hyg* 1983; 77:274.

Stevens WJ, Van den Abbeele J, Bridts CH. Anaphylactic reactions after bites by *Glossina morsitans* (tsetse fly) in a laboratory worker. *J Allergy Clin Immunol* 1996; 98:700–701.

Wilson JW, Plunkett OA. *The Fungous Diseases of Man.* Berkeley: University of California Press; 1985.

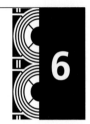

Contact Urticaria

JAMES S. TAYLOR, M.D.
YUNG-HIAN LEOW, M.D.
ALEXANDER A. FISHER, M.D.

It has been recognized that contact urticaria is an important skin disorder in the general population, and it is becoming increasingly so in occupational skin disease.[1–167] The contact urticaria syndrome was defined as a biological entity by Maibach and Johnson in 1975.[100] There are *four varieties of contact urticaria:*

1. nonimmunological reactions (NICU) (responses to primary urticariogenic agents);
2. immunological reactions (ICU) (allergic responses);
3. uncertain mechanisms—combined immunological and nonimmunological urticarial reactions; and
4. combined allergic eczematous and urticarial reactions.[1, 3]

Some contactants affect normal (intact) skin, whereas others require damaged (eczematized or fissured) skin to produce urticaria. In the nonimmunological variety, the reaction is produced without any previous sensitization in almost all exposed individuals. The immunological variety appears only on previously sensitized skin. The cause of the third variety of contact urticaria is uncertain but includes both immunological and nonimmunological mechanisms. Some contactants seem capable of being primarily urticariogenic in most individuals, but in certain sensitized patients they can also produce allergic reactions on immediate contact as well as delayed eczematous reactions.

The term "contact urticaria" typically refers to a wheal-and-flare reaction elicited within 20 to 30 minutes of exposure.[1] Delayed contact urticaria (up to 4 to 6 hours) has been described, as has delayed-onset and prolonged-contact urticaria.[4]

The spectrum of contact urticaria also includes wheals, erythema, and pruritus.[5] The concept of contact urticaria has been expanded to include all types of immediate contact reactions.[2, 7]

1. Immediate contact reaction: urticarial, eczematous, and other immediate reactions[2, 7];
2. Contact urticaria: allergic and nonallergic contact urticaria reactions[1, 2];
3. Protein contact dermatitis: allergic or nonallergic eczematous reactions (including vesicles) caused by proteins or proteinaceous material[5, 7–9];
4. Atopic contact dermatitis: immediate urticarial or eczematous IgE-mediated contact reaction,[2, 7, 9] and
5. Contact urticaria syndrome: both local and systemic immediate reactions precipitated by contact urticaria agents (ICU and NICU).[1, 2, 7] There are a number of instances in which immediate contact urticaria and delayed contact eczema have coexisted.[10–13]

Other than for latex, there is a very little statistical data on occupational contact urticaria. Data from Finland list farmers with the most cases (341 out of 815 cases) and show bakers as having the highest rate (140.4 per 100,000 workers). Cow dander was the number one cause (362 of 815 cases, or 44%), and natural rubber latex (NRL) was next (193 of 815 cases, or 24%). Cow dander was almost the most common cause of occupational rhinitis and asthma in Finland.[9] This is in contrast to other reports of respiratory and food allergies that have only occasionally been associated with contact urticaria. This association is assumed to be uncommon because it is thought that the responsible large protein molecules do not ordinarily penetrate intact skin but require in-

111

flamed skin.[14] The Finnish data have also identified several low-molecular-weight chemicals as a cause of contact urticaria: methyltetrahydrophthalic anhydrides, diglycidyl ether of bisphenol A epoxy resin, polyfunctional aziridines, nickel, and reactive dyes. Nonroutine laboratory methods are required to diagnose these cases.[9]

PRINCIPLES OF SKIN-TESTING FOR CONTACT URTICARIA

The following procedures may be followed when it is suspected that a contactant may be producing contact urticaria.[3]

1. Test the substance open (uncovered) on normal skin that has apparently never previously been the site of dermatitis. When testing foods, fresh raw items are generally preferred.

2. If negative, test open on previously affected skin even though the skin at present appears to be normal. Previously affected skin may remain in a state of increased responsiveness for a long time as compared to skin that has never been the site of dermatitis.

3. Testing open on eczematous skin may be worthwhile, provided that the tested area shows only light erythema, so that an urticarial reaction can be readily perceived on the eczematious skin.

4. If all these test procedures are negative, the suspected contactant can be occluded as a patch test on unaffected or previously affected skin.

5. If still negative, perform prick-testing. Scratch and scratch-chamber tests are more likely to produce false-positive responses. Intradermal tests are more likely to be associated with anaphylaxis and have been rarely reported to document contact urticaria.

6. It should be noted that, as a rule, certain substances produce nonimmunological contact urticaria on normal skin that has never been the site of dermatitis.

7. The use of controls is much more significant in immunological contact urticaria than in the nonimmunological variety. Thus, such nonimmunological contact urticants as sorbic acid or benzoic acid may react in only about one-half of the population.

8. The upper back, the antecubital space, and the volar aspect of the forearm are suitable sites for testing. Some nonimmunological contact urticants, however, such as sorbic and benzoic acid, may react only on the face and not elsewhere.

9. Reading of test sites for immediate urticarial reactions should be done in intervals of 10 minutes to 45 minutes. Delayed readings should be done in atypical cases.[4]

10. Precautions: Because anaphylactic reactions may occur from skin testing in highly allergic patients, epinephrine and resuscitation equipment should be available.

Kanerva et al.[15] and Hannuksela[16] have described skin-testing for immediate hypersensitivity in more detail, including the rub, scratch chamber, other challenge tests, and in vitro tests. At present, the "proof" of allergic contact urticaria is established mostly by direct in vivo testing of the patient's skin with the suspected contactant. It is hoped that in the future in vitro testing may help to identify specific agents in food and other contactants that are the actual causes of allergic contact urticaria.[3]

NONIMMUNOLOGICAL CONTACT URTICARIA

Nonimmunological contact urticaria (NICU), occurring without previous sensitization in nearly all individuals exposed, is the most common type. A direct influence on dermal vessel walls or a nonantibody-mediated release of vasoactive substances such as histamine, prostaglandins, leukotrienes, substance P, or other inflammatory mediators, is the probable cause.[6, 7]

Certain agents commonly used as preservatives or flavoring agents in foods, soft drinks, ice cream, chewing gum, soaps, shampoos, perfumes, and mouthwashes and in pharmaceutical products such as creams and ointments are primarily urticariogenic in many normal people. These agents include the widely used benzoic acid, sodium benzoate, sorbic acid, cinnamic acid, cinnamic aldehyde, balsam of Peru, acetic acid, butyric acid, and ethyl, butyl, isopropyl, and cetyl alcohol.[3, 6, 7]

The strongest and best-studied NICU agents are benzoic acid, sorbic acid, cinnamic acid, cinnamic aldehyde, and nicotinic acid esters. A majority of individuals react with a localized urticarial response 45 minutes after application of relatively high concentrations to intact skin, such as 5% in petrolatum. Lower concentrations considerably lessen the urticarial reactions, although many still react with some degree of erythema. Atopic persons were no more liable to get NICU from these substances than nonatopic individuals, and scratching or stripping the skin did not seem to alter the urticarial response.[3, 6, 7]

NICU caused by several of these substances is not inhibited by the antihistamines hydroxyzine or terfenadine or by pretreatment with capsaicin. However, NICU does seem to be inhibited by oral acetylsalicylic acid and indomethacin, by the topical NSAIDs diclofenac and naproxen gels, and by ultraviolet B (UVB) and ultraviolet A (UVA). Guinea pig earlobe swelling may be an animal model for study of some NICU agents. Human skin responds similarly, including tachyphylaxis to certain NICU agents.[7]

Table 6–1 lists agents that can produce NICU. They include foods, fragrances and flavors, animals, plants, preservatives, miscellaneous substances and medicaments, and therapeutic agents.

Therapeutic Agents that Can Cause NICU

Dimethyl Sulfoxide

Dimethyl sulfoxide (DMSO) is also known as sulfinyl-bis (methane). In the United States, DMSO, which is sold as Rimso-50, is FDA-approved for treatment of interstitial cystitis.[17] Unlabeled, non-FDA-approved therapies using DMSO have included its use as a local analgesic and anti-inflammatory agent in scleroderma, arthritis, tendinitis, and other musculoskeletal disorders and as a promoter for percutaneous penetration of certain chemicals.[17] However, in some cases, ordinarily safe topical chemicals such as camphor and menthol may produce systemic toxicity when dissolved in DMSO. Erythema or whealing can be caused by DMSO on contact.[18] Industrial and veterinary grades of DMSO may not be safe for humans.

Kellum identified no cases of allergic contact sensitization to DMSO.[18] With repeated and continuous daily skin applications of 90% DMSO under occlusion, hardening (acquired tolerance to irritating compounds) was achieved by the skin of most individuals within approximately 1 month.[18]

Sorbic Acid

Sorbic acid is a widely used antimicrobial agent that is a natural preservative occurring in berries of the mountain ash (*Sorbus*). It is active against molds and yeasts and to a lesser degree against bacteria. Creams and ointments containing sorbic acid caused erythema and slight itching and sometimes slight edema on the face in about half of the 20 persons tested.[19, 20] Rietschel saw a female patient who had contact urticaria and respiratory symptoms from a shampoo containing sorbic acid.[21] The contact urticaria could be elicited on intact skin of the face only by open testing. Fisher also reported a case in which sorbic acid produced nonimmunological contact urticaria only on the face.[22] In addition to each of the types of contact urticaria, sorbic acid may also produce an allergic eczematous reaction.

Benzoic Acid

Benzoic acid occurs in balsam of Peru and balsam of Tolu, in many of the essential oils of flowers and spices, and in berries (cranberries and others). It has antibacterial and antifungal properties and is commonly used as a preservative in acidic food products. Whitfield's ointment contains benzoic acid 6% as an antifungal agent and salicylic acid 3%. Severe and immediate systemic allergic reactions have been reported after occupational handling of materials containing benzoic acid, which shows that some of the compounds that are capa-

TABLE 6–1 • Agents that Cause Nonimmunological Contact Urticaria

Foods	Capsaicin	Caterpillars	**Miscellaneous**
Fish	Choloroform	Corals	Acetic acid
Mustard	Dimethyl sulfoxide	Jellyfish	Ammonium persulfate
Cayenne pepper (capsicum)	Friar's balsam	Moths	Benzophenone
Thyme	Iodine	Sea anemones	Butyric acid
	Methyl salicylate	Stinging insects	Cobalt chloride
Fragrances and Flavorings	Methylene green		Diethyl fumarate
Balsam of Peru	Mustard (black)	**Plants**	Histamine
Benzaldehyde	Myrrh	Nettles	Naphtha 21/99
Cassia (cinnamon) oil	Nicotinic acid esters	Seaweed	Pine oil
Cinnamic acid	Resorcinol		Pyridine carboxaldehyde
Menthol	Tar extracts	**Preservatives and Germicidals**	Sulfur
Vanilla	Tincture of benzoin	Benzoic acid	Turpentine
	Thyme oil	Chlorocresol	
Medicaments	Witch hazel	Formaldehyde	
Alcohols		Sodium benzoate	
Benzocaine	**Animals**	Sorbic acid	
Camphor	Arthropods		
Cantharides			

Adapted and updated from Burdick and Mathias[189] and Lahti, et al.[190]

ble of evoking NICU may, exceptionally, also be true sensitizers under proper conditions.[23]

Balsam of Peru

Hjorth studied balsam of Peru, which contains many aromatic substances and can produce both NICU and delayed allergic eczema.[24] Among the components of balsam of Peru, cinnamic aldehyde, cinnamic acid, benzoic acid, and benzaldehyde elicited the same reactions. The reactions could not be passively transferred and were abolished by antihistamine given before testing and by pretreatment with compound 40/80. Seite-Belleza et al.[25] reported a 19-year-old confectioner with contact urticaria to various pastry components. He reacted immediately to balsam of Peru, cinnamic aldehyde 1% in petrolatum and benzaldehyde 5% in petrolatum on open patch-testing. Avoidance of direct skin contact with pastry prevented recurrence of lesions.

Cinnamic Acid

Cinnamic acid has been found among the constituents of the essential oils of basil, Chinese cinnamon, styrax, oil of cinnamon, coca leaves, and balsam of Peru. It is used as a flavoring ingredient in pharmaceutical preparations and also in food products and perfumery. Cinnamic acid has antibacterial and antifungal properties similar to those of benzoic acid. Contact urticaria from cinnamic acid 5% in petrolatum occurs in most normal individuals.[26] Cinnamic acid may be present in sunscreens that contain cinnamates. The stinging, burning sensation that occurs with the application of such sunscreens may be due to the primary urticariogenic properties of the esters of the cinnamic acid such as methyl and benzyl cinnamates. In addition, the coniferyl alcohol ethers of cinnamic acid may be present not only in balsam of Peru, but also in balsam of Tolu and benzoin (gum benzoin).

Cinnamic Aldehyde

Cinnamic aldehyde is a constituent of cinnamon and is one of the substances responsible its typical odor and flavor. It is used as a flavoring agent in soft drinks, chewing gum, ice cream, baked goods, dentifrices, mouthwashes, and soaps. Cinnamic aldehyde at concentrations as low as 0.01% may evoke an erythematous response associated with a burning and tingling feeling of the skin.[27] Higher concentrations produce lip swelling or contact urticaria in normal skin.[7]

Chlorocresol

Chlorocresol was identified as a contact urticant in a 28-year-old woman who developed red, swollen eyelids each time she washed chicken incubators[86] An open test with the cleaning solution Prophyl (20% water) was positive, and eyelid swelling occurred. Prick-testing to p-chloro-m-cresol (one of two active constituents of Prophyl) was strongly positive at a 10% concentration and questionably positive at 1%, with associated superficial necrosis at the test site and on the eyelids. Chlorocresol tested in 10 controls produced slight erythema without edema or necrosis. Prick-testing with chickens was not performed. Unusual features are the high concentration of chlorocresol required to induce urticaria, as well as the superficial necrosis. Harvell et al. previously classified chlorocresol contact urticaria as nonimmunological.[28]

Naptha 21/99

Naphtha 21/99 is an aromatic hydrocarbon solvent containing propylbenzene mesitylene (1,3,5-trimethyl-benzene), xylene, and toluene. Several cigarette-packing workers developed urticaria after the introduction of a new ink that caused the clogging of the printing machines and an associated increase in the use of cleaning solvent.[29] Thirty-minute closed patch tests with the solvent were positive in 4 of 8 employees, and the same 4 tested positive to Naphtha 21/99, one of six ingredients in the solvent. Of 20 controls, 7 developed erythema and edema to Naphtha 21/99, and 6 developed mild erythema. Because of the positive controls, the authors considered the mechanism to be nonimmunological.

Grevillea juniperina may cause nonimmunological contact urticaria, and it is discussed under "Plants that can cause ICU."

IMMUNOLOGICAL CONTACT URTICARIA

Contactants that produce allergic contact urticaria are playing an ever-increasing role in occupational dermatitis, particularly in hand dermatitis.

The usual criteria for regarding a reaction as allergic are (1) a history of previous exposure without symptoms; (2) the degree of specific sensitization, which tends to increase with further exposure; and (3), as a rule, the small proportion of exposed subjects who are usually affected.[3] More and more chemicals are being reported as being responsible for immunological contact urticaria (ICU) (Table 6–2). Selected materials that cause contact urticaria in industry are listed in Table 6–3.[1–6, 30–169]

The most common immediate immunological mechanism is probably the one mediated by IgE.

TABLE 6–2 • Agents that Cause Immunological Contact Urticaria

Food	Vegetables	Antineoplastics	Cotoneaster	Chlorothalonil
Dairy	Beans	Cisplatin	Elm tree	Citraconic anhydride
Cheese	Cabbage	Mechlorethamine	*Eruca sativa*	Denatonium benzoate
Eggs	Carrots	Topical immunotherapy	Eucalyptus	Diethyltoluamide
Milk	Castor bean	Diphenylcyclopro-	*Ficus benjamina*	Dicyanidiamide
Seafood	Celery	penone	*Grevillea juniperina*	Epoxy resin
Cod	Chives	Ionotophoresis	*Hakea suerveoleus*	Ethylenediamine
Crab	Cucumbers	Mexiletine hydro-	Larch	Hypochlorite
Fish	Cucumber pickles	chloride	Lichens	Lanolin alcohol
Oysters	Endive	Phenothiazines	Lilies	Methylethylketone
Prawns	Garlic	Chlorpromazine	Limba	Methylhexaphydropthal-
Shellfish	Lettuce	Levomepromazine	Mahagony	icanhydrides
Shrimp	Maize[32]	Promethazine	Mulberry	Methyltetrahydropthali-
Fruits	Onions	Pyrazolones	Obeche	canhydrides
Apples	Parsley	Aminophenzone	*Phaseolus multiflorus*	Naphthylacetic acid
Apricots	Potatoes	Methimazole	*Semecarpus anacar-*	Nylon
Apricot stones	Rutabagas (swede)	Prophylphenazone	*dium*	Oleylamide
Bananas	Soybeans		Teak	Papain
Kiwis[30]	Tomatoes	**Metals**	Tulips	Patent blue dye
Litchis[31]	Winged beans	Iridium		Perlon (synthetic fiber)
Limes		Mercuric fluorescein	**Preservatives and**	Phosphorus susquisul-
Mangos[32]	**Fragrances and**	compound	**Germicidals**	fide
Oranges	**Flavorings**	Nickel	Ammonia	Plastic
Peaches	Balsam of Peru	Platinum	Benzyl alcohol	Polyethelyne glycol
Plums	Benzoic acid	Rhodium	Butylated hydroxytolu-	Potassium ferricyanide
Strawberries	Cinnamic aldehyde		ene	Silk
Watermelons[33]	Menthol	**Organisms, Tissue**	Chloramine	Sodium silicate
Grains		**Fluids, and**	Chlorhexidine	Sodium sulfide
Buckwheat flour	**Hair-Care Products**	**Secretions**	Formaldehyde	Sulfur dioxide
Flour	Basic blue 99	*Argus reflexus*	o-Phenylphenate	Tinofix S (chemical tex-
Maize	Henna	Blood	Parabens	tile finish)
Malt (beer)	Hydrolyzed animal pro-	Chironomids	Phenylmercuric acetate	Terpinyl acetate
Rice[32]	teins	Cockroaches	Phenylmercuric propio-	1,1,1-Trichloroethane
Wheat bran	Paraphenylenediamine	Dander	nate	Tobacco
Honey		Gut	Polysorbate	Vinyl pyridine
Nuts	**Medicaments**	Hair	Sodium hypochlorite	Xylene
Peanuts[32]	Antibiotics	Jellyfish	Sorbitan monolaurate	
Peanut butter	Ampicillin	Liver	Sorbitan sesquioleate	**Rubber**
Sesame seeds	Bacitracin	Placenta, amniotic fluid		Natural rubber latex
Sunflower seeds	Benzoyl peroxide	Saliva	**Miscellaneous**	proteins
Meats	Cephalosporins	Seminal fluid	Acrylic acid	Zinc diethyldithiocarba-
Beef	Chloramphenicol	Silk	Alcohols	mate
Chicken	Gentamicin	Spider mite	Amyl	Zinc pentamethylene-
Lamb	Iodochlorhydroxy-	Worm (*Nereis diversi-*	Butyl	dithiocarbamate
Liver	quin	*color*)	Ethyl	Zinc dibutyldithiocar-
Pork	Mezlocillin		Isopropyl	bamate
Sausage	Neomycin	**Plant Substances**	p-Aminodiphenylamine	Zinc dimethyldithiocar-
Turkey	Penicillin	Algae	Ammonthioazole	bamate
Mustard	Rifamycin	Birch	Ammonium chloride	Morpholinylmercapto-
Salami casing mold	Streptomycin	*Bougainvillea*	Aliphatic polyamide	benzothiazole
Spices	Antiparasitics	Chrysanthemum	Benzophenone	Black rubber mix
	Lindane	Cinchona	Carbonless copy paper	Rubber glove powder

Adapted and updated from Burdick and Mathias[189] and Lahti, et al.[190]

Nonspecific elevation of IgE has been reported frequently in association with ICU, and elevation of IgE specific for particular offending antigens has been found in some cases. Although the prevalence of NICU is the same in atopic and nonatopic individuals, it is likely that ICU is more common among atopic patients. Urticaria, however, may also be caused by allergic mechanisms not requiring IgE; specific IgG and perhaps also IgM might be responsible for activation of the complement flow through the classical pathway.

Foods that Can Cause ICU

Occupational allergic contact dermatitis of the hands of food handlers is a common cause of chronic hand dermatitis. According to Lahti, foodstuffs are the most common causes of ICU.[7] It

TABLE 6–3 • Materials that Cause Contact Urticaria in Industry

Material	Industry
Aliphatic polyamines	Epoxy resin workers
Aminothiazole	Pharmaceutical workers
Ammonia	Ammonia workers
Castor bean pomace	Castor oil extractors, fertilizers workers, and farmers
Complex platinum salts	Platinum refiners
Formaldehyde	Phenolic and amino resin workers, fumigators, and laboratory workers
Latex (natural rubber)	Health-care and rubber workers
Lindane	Insecticide workers and cotton dusters
Penicillin	Pharmaceutical workers and nurses
Sodium sulfide	Photographers and workers with dyes, tanning, and hides
Sorbic acid	Chemical workers
Spices	Spice workers, bakers, and sausage makers
Sulfur dioxide	Paper mill workers
Vinyl pyrrolidine	Chemistry research workers
Xylene	Chemistry research workers

Adapted and updated from Key.[76]

should be stressed that in cases of immediate urticarial contact dermatitis resulting from food, the classic delayed 48-hour patch tests are negative—unless both immediate and delayed responses coexist in the patient.[3]

At present, it appears that patients with ICU due to food-handling can eat such foods without experiencing a flare of the dermatitis. It is likely that either the cooking of the food or the action of digestion renders the food hypoallergenic for these patients. At present, however, it is not clear whether the food "antigens" that allergists use in testing for allergic rhinitis, asthma, and gastrointestinal allergy are also the antigens that are responsible for the immediate ICU of hands that results from handling certain foods.[3] Very often, when the food handler is examined, the hands are so eczematized that contact urticaria is not suspected as the cause of the eczema.

Potatoes

Sensitivity to potatoes can be so severe that merely rubbing the intact skin with a raw potato may cause a wheal to form.[34, 35] More often, a strongly positive scratch-test reaction to potato is obtained in sensitized individuals; it consists of a large wheal that forms within 20 minutes. Intracutaneous prick or scratch tests with cooked potatoes usually give negative results. Potato sensitivity can cause "housewife's hand eczema" and can be classified as an occupational allergy in cooks. Most patients who have allergic contact sensitivity can eat cooked potatoes without any reaction.

Fish

Hjorth and Roed-Petersen reported the first cases of protein contact dermatitis. Several homemakers with atopic dermatitis noted an aggravation of their eczema after contact with fish, particularly white haddock and herring, which caused an itching erythema within 30 minutes after contact with the allergen.[36] An open epicutaneous test with fish on the site of preceding eczema produced a blister (dyshidrotic blister formation) in the sensitized patient. On normal skin (on which there was no preceding eczema), an open epicutaneous test with fish (mostly haddock) resulted in an urticarial reaction at the contact site. Those patients noted that their eczema worsened with contact with fish, and they also showed a higher IgE serum level with contact with fish.

Mitchell reported a homemaker with chronic hand eczema that was attributed to handling fresh shrimp.[37] Scratch tests were carried out on the forearm flexure to the flesh (the edible portion) of the shrimp (Pandalus). The raw and the boiled shrimp flesh were applied to the scratch site without covering; a drop of sea water (Millipore-filtered) was applied to a scratch test site as a control. Five physicians served as concomitant controls.

Maibach reported a 24-year-old atopic caterer who requested testing because of marked, recurrent facial burning after handling seafood. She provided fresh samples of crab, lobster, prawns, and shrimp which, when applied to the intact skin of her forearm and the slightly abnormal skin of her dorsal hands, failed to reproduce her symptoms. However, application to the forehead (intact skin) produced a large (highly pruritic) wheal and flare only with the shrimp. Ten controls (forehead and intact skin) were negative. A passive transfer study and a radioallergosorbent test (RAST) were not performed.[38]

In retrospect, we suspect that the facial burning was, in fact, a flare due to hand transfer and not to hematogenous spread. Thus, human skin is not homogeneous but is, in fact, a mosaic, and in this case, the face was more permeable than the arm; other differences undoubtedly exist. Until better methodology becomes available, it may be necessary to apply contact urticariogens to unusual test sites suggested mainly by the patient's history.

Patch-testing might have provided an alternative method; obtaining appropriate controls using raw seafood is more complex, as is clinical interpretation.[3]

According to Melino et al., contact urticaria in response to foods is more frequent in atopic persons and in food handlers. Their patient, with a history of atopy, was admitted because of a suspicion of contact urticaria in reaction to fish. She observed that every time she handled fresh or frozen uncooked fish, she developed erythema, edema, itching, and burning on the backs of her hands; in the same way, she developed angioedema of the lips and tongue combined with nausea whenever she ate fish.[39] These symptoms started within 10 minutes of contact with fish and slowly settled, over the course of the day. Total IgE was high (3,900 U/mL). The RAST was positive to cod, the only fish available as a specific allergen. Prick tests with the most common foods showed a strong localized wheal reaction to fish. Histamine was used as a positive control and physiological saline as a negative control. The test was regarded as positive if a localized wheal reaction equivalent to the positive histamine control developed. Twenty-minute closed patch tests with the five different fresh fish (anchovy, cod, mullet, pilchard, and tuna) suspected to be responsible for contact urticaria were carried out on normal and affected skin on the volar side of the forearms. The fresh fish were cleaned of slime, and the skin was removed from them. Results of the patch tests with raw fish were positive; results with cooked fish were negative.

In a survey done by Kavli and Moseng on workers at a fish-stick factory in northern Norway,[40] eight had contact urticaria to fish and three had immediate reactions to mustard, which was added as flavoring. Eight of these workers were atopics.

Seafood

A 34-year-old atopic Japanese man experienced eczematous lesions on his hands, forearms, and face immediately after occupational contact with pearl oysters.[41] He also had recurrent episodes of acute urticaria with nausea after ingestion of oysters, clams, and other shellfish. Scratch and patch tests to pearl-oyster meat and extract in saline were positive, with the development of immediate whealing and delayed (2-day) eczema, respectively. Four controls were negative. IgE-RAST was positive for mussels and crab. This is the first report of coexistent contact urticaria and contact dermatitis from pearl oysters.

Meat

The following meats have been reported as causing allergic contact urticaria, particularly in individuals with chronic hand dermatitis: chicken, lamb, turkey, calves' liver, beef, and sausage.[42–46]

Fisher and Stengel reported a 50-year-old butcher who had chronic hand dermatitis for 6 years.[44] His dermatitis became worse when he handled raw calves' liver which, when placed at the site of a scratch on his forearm, produced a large wheal and flare in 15 minutes. Six control subjects were negative. A scratch test with chicken liver on the opposite forearm was negative.

Fisher reported a 60-year-old homemaker whose chronic hand dermatitis was worsened by wearing rubber gloves.[45] Routine patch-testing revealed positive reactions to nickel and mercapto-benzothiazole. The patient stated emphatically that whenever she prepared beef hamburgers, the hand dermatitis flared severely. In addition, when she ate a medium-rare beef hamburger, she developed angioedema of her lips with perlèche; when she ate a well-done hamburger, no symptoms occurred. The patient was tested on normal skin and had no reaction to beef, pork, or chicken. The three meats were then applied to normal skin of the back, on which a small scratch and been made. Each meat was gently rubbed in with a Q-tip, and within 15 minutes, an urticarial wheal without any flare appeared at the site at which the beef had been applied. No reaction was obtained with the pork or chicken, and scratch tests with raw beef were negative in six controls. Subsequently, she did not react to a scratch test with cooked beef. A biopsy at the site of the wheal reaction to raw beef was consistent with urticaria.

Moseng reported that a butcher's assistant, who was feeding a machine daily with pig's gut (Taiwanese import) as part of sausage production, developed urticarial, crusted, erosive lesions, mainly on the extremities. He developed urticaria when eating hot dogs.[46]

Jovanovic et al. reported a 21-year-old baker who experienced aggravation of his hand eczema after handling beef mince and raw beef. His hands immediately began to itch, and whealing occurred on his neck. Prick-testing to the above were positive but were negative to cooked beef.[47]

A 34-year-old nonatopic woman experienced urticaria on previously healthy skin after contact with fresh pork. Open and prick tests were positive to pork in less than 10 minutes, and three controls were negative. Total serum IgE was 84 U/mL, and RAST was positive (class 4) for pork.[48]

Fruits

Andersen and Lowenstein reported the possibility of contact urticaria from handling apples. They stated that most of the patients with reactions to raw potatoes and apples were atopic.[49] Patients without any evidence of atopy, however, may also develop immediate-type reactivity to protein-like materials.

A 50-year-old cook developed face and hand dermatitis associated with burning and stinging after handling pickles for 15 years.[50] Open immediate skin tests on normal skin of the arm were strongly positive for cucumber pickle and strawberry. Five controls were negative to cucumber pickle. The hand eczema was considered multifactorial, with contact urticaria from pickles and strawberries and irritation from grease, detergents, and bleaches. The authors postulated an immunological mechanism for this contact urticaria because most individuals handle pickles and strawberries without wheal and flare reactions.

Apricot stones were identified as an allergen in a 19-year-old nonatopic woman who, after 6 weeks of working at a marzipan factory, developed urticaria following contact with mixtures of sweet almond, apricot stone, and spices.[51] Patch tests were positive at 30 minutes with peeled apricot stone only. Fifteen controls were negative.

Litchis are a type of fruit with a close botanical affinity to mangos, an established cause of ICU. A 34-year-old woman with a history of atopy developed generalized urticaria, edema, and bronchospasm after eating litchi fruits.[52] Patch tests were positive to whole litchi epicarp and litchi epicarp extract and negative in five controls. Also, prick and scratch tests were positive to mango mesocarp extract, indicating possible crossreactivity.

Temesvari and Becker reported a 45-year-old woman with seasonal rhinitis and conjunctivitis who experienced urticaria and swelling of her lips after eating watermelon; on repeated exposures, the response advanced to generalized urticaria, angioedema, dyspnea, and hypotension.[53] She had a total IgE level of 81 kU/L and specific IgE levels to perennial rye grass (0.8 PRU/mL) and ragweed (4.5 PRU/mL). Patch tests with fresh watermelon and with watermelon previously soaked for 1 hour in acetone, water, and 70% alcohol were positive at 40 and 60 minutes but were negative in three controls. The authors comment that only a few cases of fruit allergy have been identified by specific IgE, with the diagnosis usually established by positive prick tests with fresh fruits. Two other cases of allergies to fruits and vegetables associated with pollen sensitivity have been reported, with pollen allergy occurring first.

Green Vegetables

Krook reported four patients with occupational contact dermatitis in response to lettuce (*Lactuca sativa*), who had cross-sensitivity to *Circhorium endiva*.[54] One of the patients also had contact urticaria to *Lactuca* and *Circhorium,* and another reacted positively to scratch tests with these plants with signs of immediate allergy. In two cases such immediate allergy was considered the cause of a vesicular, intense itching eruption within a few minutes of contact with fresh leaves of *Lactuca* on previously eczematous skin. The severe chronic dermatitis of the hands of these patients is ascribed to combined delayed and immediate allergy.

Carrots

Munoz et al. presented a case of urticaria and rhinoconjunctivitis, IgE-mediated, from contact with carrot.[55] Scratch tests were positive. Carrots are considered the vegetable that is most frequently sensitizing.

Beans

Lovell and Rycroft reported that a food chemist who operated a machine that extracted bean oil from various seeds developed edema of the face and eyes within 3 hours of working at the machine.[56] The skin lesions cleared within 6 hours of his leaving his place of work. The beans in question are related to soybeans. Patch tests were negative to the standard series, the face series, and the foodstuffs that he handled. Intradermal tests of response to winged-bean meal were strongly positive, and there was a weak positive reaction to soybean meal. Prick tests to other seeds that he handled, namely, mustard seed, rape seed, and cottonseed meals, were negative. Since avoiding contact with winged bean and soya bean, he has had no further skin lesions.

Castor-bean allergy was found by Kanerva et al. in a 50-year-old male stockroom worker in a coffee-roasting plant who, after 22 years of employment, developed rhinitis, facial dermatitis, and periodic dermatitis on the backs of his hands on work days.[57] Scratch and nasal provocation tests (diluted to 1:10,000 in saline) were positive with crushed castor bean. Patch-testing with crushed beans showed an urticarial reaction at 5 hours, 24 hours, and 48 hours, which had disappeared at the 3-day reading; at 4 days, a strong vesicular response was observed. Twenty controls were negative on scratch-testing for both urticarial and delayed reactions. The concomitant type I and type IV reactions in this patient were postulated to involve three components: an immediate IgE-mediated reaction followed by an IgE-mediated late reaction and a delayed IgE hypersensitivity reaction.

Similarly, another patient was identified with both immediate and delayed hypersensitivity to soybean and garlic.[58] A 31-year-old atopic man developed urticaria, rhinitis, conjunctivitis, and dyspnea as well as eczema on the hands and face when at work. Specifically, his reactions occurred when he entered the department of the factory where garlic and soybean powders were used. Patch tests, prick tests, and RASTs were positive to both garlic and soybean; 15 controls were negative. Inhalation challenge tests with soybean powder induced an asthmatic crisis.

Sorbic Acid and Potassium Sorbate

Fisher reported that bakers can acquire NICU from the presence of sorbic acid or potassium sorbate in the preservatives in blueberry filling, German chocolate cream, and lemon filling.[59, 60]

Miscellaneous Food Items

Maibach reported a 35-year-old supervisor in a salami manufacturing plant with episodic erythematous "burned" lesions on his hands and face and with associated sneezing.[61] He had a strong wheal-and-flare reaction to the mold on the salami casing and had positive prick tests to *Aspergillus* and *Hormodendrum* molds that were added to age the salami. Tosti and Guerra reported positive open 20-minute patch test reactions to tomatoes, dairy products, and meat derivatives in eight professional food handlers.[62] They were a barman, a cook, a pizza maker, a dairyman, two pastry cooks, and two food sellers.

Grains

Buckwheat flour was found to be an allergen in a 29-year-old atopic woman who, after working for 4 years in a creperie, experienced work-related sneezing, rhinitis, nasal itching, dyspnea, and contact urticaria.[63] She also developed urticaria after eating buckwheat pancakes. Prick-testing with heated and unheated buckwheat flour extract was positive at 15 minutes and negative in five controls. Rub-testing was also positive. Specific IgE against buckwheat was demonstrated by histamine-release testing and by reverse enzyme immunoassay (REIA). There was no demonstrable crossreactivity between buckwheat and other cereal flours or related pollen and seeds.

Di Lernia et al. reported the first case of contact urticaria from rice.[64] A 17-year-old woman developed erythema of the hands, edema of the eyelids, dyspnea, and cough after throwing raw rice during a wedding, although she ate and continued to eat cooked rice without problems. Prick tests with rice, maize, peanuts, and beans caused immediate urticarial reactions. A few weeks later, open, scratch, and handling tests with raw rice were positive. IgE was normal, and RASTs were positive for rice and peanuts.

Antibiotics that Can Cause ICU

Table 6–2 lists the antibiotics from which medical personnel and chemists may acquire contact urticaria by administering these drugs to patients or otherwise handling them.

Rudzki et al. describe a nurse working in a tuberculosis sanitorium who developed contact dermatitis from streptomycin.[65] Two minutes after several drops of streptomycin prepared for injection were placed on her forearm, a large wheal appeared; a few minutes later, rhinitis and lacrimation developed and required hydrocortisone administration.

Tuft studied an instance of contact urticaria in a chemist that resulted from an acquired sensitization to cephalosporin compounds.[66] Patch tests elicited an immediate urticarial response. Similar control tests with other antibiotics produced negative results. Although the patient's primary complaint was urticaria, prolonged or excessive contact with the cephalosporin also caused coryza and syncope. There was, however, no recurrence of symptoms after the patient transferred to another laboratory where he worked with other chemicals.

Occupational mezlocillin allergy occurred in a 32-year-old nurse who, after 5 years of work, experienced urticaria and dyspnea following local contact with injectable mezlocillin (Baypen).[13] She also had hand and flexural eczema. Open patch-testing with mezlocillin 1% produced urticaria at 10 minutes and eczema at 2 and 3 days. Total IgE was 84 kU/L, and specific IgE of penicillins G and V were found. No RASTs or control tests were performed, but the patient's urticaria and eczema cleared following a job change.

A 51-year-old nonatopic man developed contact urticaria followed in 40 minutes by generalized urticaria and anaphylactic shock after application of Rifocin-soaked gauze to a leg ulcer.[67] Open tests, 20-minute patch tests, and scratch tests were positive to Rifocin solution and Rifamycin SV, but were negative to all other constituents of Rifocin solution. Scratch tests with Rifocin solution were negative in 11 controls. Prausnitz-Kustner passive transfer tests on the patient's mother and father were positive.

Miyahara et al. reported two Japanese nurses with contact urticaria and anaphylactoid reactions to cefotiam hydrochloride, a parenteral cephalosporin that was one of the most commonly used antibiotics in Japan.[68]

Miscellaneous Medications that Can Cause ICU

Benzocaine

Contact urticaria may occur in dentists who apply this topical anesthetic to their patients prior to injection of a local anesthetic.[69]

Nitrogen Mustard

Dermatologists and nursing personnel who apply nitrogen mustard to patients with mycosis fungoides may acquire contact urticaria even if they wear rubber gloves, which are not impervious to nitrogen mustard.[70, 71]

Levomepromazine

Johansson reported a 41-year-old nurse working in a mental hospital who had episodic itchy swelling of her face and eyelids and urticaria.[72] She noticed that symptoms occurred with opening and drawing levomepromazine from injection ampoules. Open immediate patch-testing to levomepromazine hydrochloride, a phenothiazine derivative, was positive.

Cisplatin

Schena et al. reported a 35-year-old nurse who developed generalized urticaria after preparing cisplatin infusion solutions.[73] Immediate open testing to ammonium tetrachloroplatinate 0.25% aq. and ammonium hexachloroplatinate 0.10% aq. were positive. Cisplatin is an intravenous alkylating agent used in the treatment of certain solid tumors.

Metals that Can Cause ICU

Nickel

Occupational exposure to nickel can produce immediate and allergic contact urticaria and delayed eczematous contact urticaria.[74]

Rhodium

Nakayama and Imai reported that 17 out of 50 workers at a major precious metals factory had been suffering from contact urticaria, contact dermatitis, and asthma for the preceding 9 years.[75] Scratch-patch tests for 1 hour using Finn chambers revealed immediate hypersensitivity reactions to platinum in 9 out of 12 patients and to rhodium in 7 out of 12 patients. A 48-hour closed patch test revealed that the patients had delayed-type hypersensitivy to rhodium, platinum, and mercury.

Platinum

Osmundsen,[74] Key,[76] and Levene[77] investigated allergic contact urticaria in reaction to industrial exposures to platinum salts.

Iridium

Contact urticaria and anaphylaxis occurred in a 26-year-old nonatopic male process operator who worked in an electrochemical factory manufacturing titanium anodes.[78] The reactions developed when he sprayed the anodes with a coating solution containing various metal salts. A prick test to iridium chloride was positive, and a scratch test produced an anaphylactoid reaction. Prick tests in 14 factory coworkers were negative. Iridium is one of the platinum-group metals in the periodic table, but prick-testing with hexachloroplatinate solution was negative. No RASTs were performed.

Chemicals in Industry that Can Cause ICU

A wide variety of chemicals have been implicated in causing an immunological type of contact urticaria. Table 6–3 lists various chemicals that can produce industrial contact urticaria. Chemists experimenting with new chemicals are particularly prone to developing ICU.

Epoxy Resin Hardener

Jolanki et al. reported a worker in an electrical factory who had to fill condensers with a slightly warmed, uncured mixture of an epoxy resin, a hardener, an accelerator, and a colorant. Within 2 months she developed urticarial eruptions on her face, neck, breast, and arms. Two weeks after she changed jobs, the skin eruptions disappeared.[79] Open tests with the filling mixture and the hardener, tested separately, were positive, but tests with all the other components, both mixed and separately applied, were negative. Prick tests were negative, too. Tests with the undiluted hardener in 12 control patients were all negative.

Tarvainen et al. reported two patients who developed occupational airborne contact urticaria and respiratory symptoms from methylhexahydrophthalic anhydride (MHHPA) and methyltetrahydrophthalic anhydride (MTHPA).[80] They are both dicarboxylic anhydrides used as hardeners for epoxy resins. Both workers were exposed to the anhydride fumes in the course of their work as an assembler of ski poles and winder of electrical machines, respectively.

Additives to Plastics (Butylhydroxytoluene and Oleylamide)

Osmundsen stated that plastics had not previously been reported as a cause of contact urticaria.[74] In one case, plastic folders and polyvinyl chloride (PVC) provoked strong urticarial reactions on unbroken skin after 20 minutes. These reactions correlated with the clinical history. The plastic materials that provoked the contact urticaria contained butylhydroxytoluene (BHT) or oleylamide. BHT is used as an antioxidant in plastics, and oleylamide is used as a shipping agent for plastics.

Xylene

Altman described an acute urticarial reaction to xylene in a patient who was allergic to this solvent in her work.[81] Palmer and Rycroft reported a cytology technician with occupational airborne contact urticaria to xylene.[82] She processed a large number of slides and began experiencing attacks of generalized urticaria after her extractor fan malfunctioned. Most occurred in the evening, but the worst episodes were witnessed at work. Fifteen-minute closed patch-testing on her forearm with xylene produced severe erythema with whealing that spread beyond the test area and persisted for 1 hour. Although four controls demonstrated slight transient erythema, the authors concluded an immunological mechanism was operative. Goodfield and Saihan described three factory workers with urticaria from Naphtha 21/99, an aromatic hydrocarbon solvent that contains xylene[83] (see the discussion under "Naphtha").

Methyl Ethyl Ketone

Varigos and Nurse described a 48-year-old man who experienced hand, forearm, and facial dermatitis 18 months after he started spray-painting with an epoxy-polyamide paint;[84] eye irritation and itching after exposure to an epoxy glue; and severe hand, arm, and face irritation after touching methyl ethyl ketone (MEK).[76] MEK is a solvent widely used in industry, especially in plastics manufacture. Open tests on two occasions with MEK produced bright erythema in 10 minutes that maximized at 15 minutes. MEK from the same container was negative on five controls. The authors felt that this represented contact urticaria, possibly immunological, given the negative controls, despite the known mild irritation usually produced by MEK. He was also patch-test positive to epoxy resin.

Trichloroethane

Fowler reported a woman working as an eyeglass manufacturer who developed occupational airborne contact urticaria from trichloroethane (TCE).[85] It was used as an organic solvent for cleaning glass lenses.

Acrylic Acid

A 39-year-old male chemist developed recurrent urticaria followed several weeks later by recurrent facial dermatitis after he moved from factory production to a laboratory where he had more intense chemical exposure. Open testing with 2% acrylic acid in olive oil showed wheal-and-flare reactions at 2 minutes and 30 minutes and an eczematous response at 48 hours. No other chemical produced immediate or delayed hypersensitivity reactions, and six controls were negative.[87] A 24-year-old Lebanese woman who was undergoing patch-testing to evaluate her chronic eczema developed contact urticaria from the acrylic acid present in the tape used in the test. At day 1, she had urticaria that was strictly confined to the area under the Fixomull tape; in 24 hours it had progressed to generalized urticaria accompanied by edema of the face and uvula, which required intravenous corticosteroids. Subsequent patch-testing with the individual components of the tape showed multiple urticarial lesions at the site of acrylic acid 2% petrolatum within 20 minutes. No RASTs or controls were performed.[88]

Chlorothalonil

Dannaker et al. reported a 49-year-old tree nursery worker with contact urticaria and respiratory symptoms that resulted from handling seedlings that were treated with the fungicide chlorothalonil. She developed an anaphylactic reaction during skin-testing with the allergen.[89]

Chloramine

Dooms-Goossens reported a nurse who developed contact urticaria and respiratory symptoms from chloramine powder that was being used as a disinfectant for bedpans.[90]

Henna

Leonie Majoie and Bruynzeel reported a hairdresser who developed urticaria, rhinitis, and bronchial asthma from henna which she used as a hair colorant on her own hair and on that of her clients. Prick-testing was positive for henna, but negative for the dye 2-hydroxy-1,4-naphthoquinone, which had been reported previously as an allergen. They suspected that the putative allergen may be an undetermined ingredient of the henna powder.[91]

Other Hair-care Chemicals

Nonoccupational contact urticaria has been reported to be caused by basic blue 99 in a hair-setting lotion, hydrolyzed animal protein present in hair conditioners, and paraphenylenediamine.[92–95]

Colophony

Rivers and Rycroft reported a 34-year-old female inspector of printed circuit boards who developed contact urticaria from the colophony in solder flux fumes.[96]

Phenylmercuric Acetate

Torresani et al. reported a 54-year-old farmer's wife who developed contact urticaria and respiratory symptoms in response to the mercurial compound phenylmercuric acetate, which was present in pesticides and herbicides used on farm crops. Open tests on her back with phenylmercuric acetate (0.01%) produced erythema at 30 minutes and urticaria at 60 minutes, followed by facial edema and bronchospasm. Three controls were negative. Other mercurial compounds applied to the patient's back did not produce a reaction.[97]

Pyridine Carboxaldehyde

Archer and Cronin reported a 23-year-old postgraduate student of chemistry who developed airborne contact urticaria in response to pyridine carboxaldehyde. Indomethacin 25 mg was unable to suppress the wheal-flare response.[98]

Phenylmercuric Propionate

Mathews studied a physician who had asthma and urticaria that was traced to hospital-laundered bed linens and uniforms. Scratch tests with phenylmercuric propionate, an antibacterial fabric softener used in the hospital laundry, produced a wheal-and-flare response. Provocative inhalation tests produced asthma within 5 minutes.[99]

Diethyltoluamide

Maibach and Johnson showed that diethyltoluamide (DEET), a popular insect repellent, can cause an allergic contact urticaria syndrome.[100] This was the first report of the contact urticaria syndrome.

Carbonless Copy Paper

LaMarte et al. have proved that an alkylpheonl novolac resin present in carbonless copy paper can produce contact urticaria, laryngeal edema, and potentially life-threatening reactions in susceptible workers.[167] Marks had also previously described such reactions but without identifying the chemical culprit; plasma thromboxane B2 and prostaglandin PGF$_2$ levels increased during the provocation test.[168] Hannuksela and Bjorksten described immediate type dermatitis, contact urticaria, and rhinitis in four office workers who handled carbonless copy paper for several hours a day. Contact urticaria was produced with the back side of the top sheet in all four and with the front side of the bottom sheet in two. RAST results were inconclusive.[169] Marks also reported allergic contact dermatitis from carbonless copy paper[170] and airborne irritant dermatitis has also been observed.[171] Murray has reviewed associated controversial subjective systemic symptoms.[172]

Plants that Can Cause ICU

Wood

Hausen stated that some species of wood may produce nonimmunological types of reactions, although immediate reactions based on immunological mechanisms are more characteristic.[101] Species that have induced such immunological reactions include obeche, larch, limba, and occasionally teak. A state of allergic sensitivity is proved by rubbing the skin of the patient's forearm moistened slightly with water, 20 to 30 times, with a piece of the suspected wood species. An urticarial reaction is produced within several minutes. Reaction to a species results in a large wheal and flare, whereas the nonoffending species produce no reaction. No reactions to the offending wood occur in the control group.

Exotic Woods

Garces Sotillos et al. reported a 31-year-old female who had occupational asthma and contact urticaria that was caused by the dust of maukali wood, an exotic tree from the Sapotaceae family.[102] Goransson reported a 33-year-old worker in a caravan-building plant who had contact urticaria and rhinoconjunctivitis from launau (Philippine red mahogany) sawdust.[103]

Apted reported a 63-year-old amateur gardener who developed contact urticaria from the prickly leaves of *Grevillea juniperina* and *Hakea Snaveolens*. Within 15 minutes of brushing prickly *Grevillea juniperina* leaves along his forearm, localized urticaria developed at the site and persisted for 60 minutes. Two of three controls were positive, suggesting that the reaction may have been nonimmunologic.[104, 105]

Dooms-Goossens et al. reported a 31-year-old warehouseman who developed airborne contact urticaria from unloading bags of dried bark of cinchona (family Rubiaceae). Immediate tests with cinchona produced urticaria in 15 minutes. Water, ethanol, and acetone extracts of cinchona were negative, whereas ether and ethanol cinchona extract residues were strongly positive at 15 minutes. This indicated that the urticariogenic substance is a polar, water-soluble though labile substance. Control tests were not performed, but none of the patient's coworkers reported reactions.[106]

Contact urticaria to obeche wood was detailed by Hinojosa et al. in a study involving eight woodworkers who developed rhinitis at work. That was followed several weeks later by nonproductive cough and whealing as well as itching and erythema, especially on the palms.[14] Later the symptoms progressed from contact urticaria on exposed body surfaces to occasional generalized urticaria. All patients had positive prick tests with obeche wood extracts. Skin-provocation rubbing tests with obeche sawdust on the eight patients were positive after 20 minutes but were negative in 20 controls. Allergen-specific IgE antibodies to obeche were confirmed by a REIA technique in all eight patients. Obeche is a West African tree of the Sterculiaceae family, and it is the African wood most frequently exported commercially.

An Indian man showed a localized urticarial reaction on his thigh that corresponded to a mark on his pants made by his launderer, or dhobi, with a marking nut.[107] Testing was done with 1-cm square pieces of fabric soaked in water and juice from the marking nut, *Semecarpus anacardium,* and dried onto filter paper. Response was positive after 6 minutes of occlusion. Ten controls were negative after up to 45 minutes of occlusion. The Indian marking nut belongs to the Anacardiaceae family, which includes poison ivy. It is a well-known cause of allergic contact dermatitis, but this apparently was an unusual cause of contact urticaria. Urticaria did not recur after the patient discarded the indelibly marked pants.

Tulips and Lilies

Lahti described an atopic florist who, after 8 years of work, developed contact urticaria and respiratory symptoms that were caused by lilies and tulips.[108] Contact with the bulb or stem of either plant produced erythema, edema, and itching of the fingers, dorsal hands, and face, along with rhinitis, hoarseness, and dyspnea within 20 minutes. Patch tests with fresh Monte Carlo tulip bulb, stem, and petal were negative, but a rub test with the same tulip stem was positive on the hands and fingers within 30 minutes. Scratch chamber tests were positive to fresh bulbs and stems of all five varieties of tulip and to lily; 40 controls were negative. Prick and scratch tests with extracts of tulip and lily bulbs were positive, whereas alcohol and acetone extracts (often positive in delayed tulip allergy) were negative. The allergen was present in all varieties of tulips tested and in all parts of the plant, suggesting that it was a protein.

Tobacco

Tosti et al. reported a 38-year-old cigarette factory worker with generalized urticaria, bronchial asthma, and rhinoconjunctivitis resulting from exposure to tobacco leaves and dust.[109] Open patch tests were positive to several tobacco blends at 30 minutes. Prick tests with tobacco dust were positive. No RASTs were performed, but open patch tests on 20 controls were negative, indicating a probable immunological mechanism.[80]

Gaseous Compounds

Ammonia fumes and simple gaseous compounds, such as sulfur dioxide, have also been associated with urticaria.[110–112]

Textiles and Fabrics that Can Cause ICU

Silk, wool, nylon, and rubber may produce allergic contact urticaria. Three divergent views are held as to the source of the silk allergen: (1) the silk fiber itself, (2) the gum, or glue, (sericin) contained in raw silk or (3) the silkworm. The silkworm pupa contains 10 times more allergen than does the cocoon. Because there is undoubted sensitization to silk cloth that contains no pupa and relatively little sericin, some of the allergen must persist in finished silk.

Silk allergy may manifest as inhalant symptoms, urticaria, or atopic dermatitis.[113]

Nylon

Dooms-Goossens and coworkers reported that a nurse who was required to wear nylon stockings during nurses' training acquired contact urticaria. A patch test with colorless nylon pants caused a wheal-and-flare response after 90 minutes.[114]

Formaldehyde in Clothing

Andersen and Maibach described an unusual type of contact urticaria in response to formalin, based on 4 patients and experiments in 14 volunteers.[115] The contact urticaria appeared on healthy skin only following repeated open applications, or after a single application on slightly diseased skin. This phenomenon is possibly relevant for patients claiming textile intolerance.

Formaldehyde in Leather

Helander described a patient who developed contact urticaria after she handled foreign leather that was found qualitatively to contain minimal amounts of formaldehyde.[116] The patient worked as a carver and model setter in a factory that made leather dresses. She had urticaria almost daily, most severely on the hands, and occasionally, edema of the lip. During weekends and vacations, when the patient had no contact with leather, she remained clear of hives. The patient was transferred to another department where she handled only domestic leather that did not contain formaldehyde.

Chemical Textile Finish

DeGroot and Gerkens reported a 55-year-old man who developed contact urticaria and anaphylaxis to Tinofix S, which was the chemical textile finish found in the inner lining of his trousers.[117] It is a cationic condensation product of dicyandiamide, formaldehyde, ammonium chloride, and ethylenediamine. The patient did not react to the individual ingredients, only to Tinofix S.

Rubber

Natural Rubber Latex. Natural rubber latex (NRL) is one of the most important causes of immunologically mediated contact urticaria. The number of reported cases has increased more dramatically during the past decade than have reported cases for any other agent. As a result, NRL allergy is a major medical, occupational health, medicolegal, and regulatory problem (Fig. 6–1).[118–142]

Although NRL gloves have been used in medicine since the 1890s, it was not until 1979 that Nutter described NRL glove allergy that was manifested by contact urticaria.[143] Contact urticaria is probably more common than allergic contact dermatitis in response to rubber gloves.[124]

Individuals at highest risk are patients with spina bifida, health-care workers, and other workers with significant NRL exposure. Most reported series of occupational cases involve health-care workers, affecting 5 to 11% of those studied. Stud-

ies of populations of nonhealth-care workers are infrequent and include kitchen workers, cleaners, manufacturers of rubber bands, surgical gloves, latex dolls, and miscellaneous other occupations.[124] Predisposing risk factors are hand eczema, allergic rhinitis, allergic conjunctivitis, or asthma in individuals who frequently wear NRL gloves; mucosal exposure to NRL; and multiple surgical procedures. The spectrum of clinical signs ranges from contact urticaria, generalized urticaria, allergic rhinitis, allergic conjunctivitis, angioedema, and asthma to anaphylaxis. More than 600 serious reactions to latex, including 16 fatal anaphylactic reactions, have been reported to the U.S. Food and Drug Administration. The majority of cases involve reactions to NRL gloves—that is, donning NRL gloves or being examined by individuals wearing NRL gloves.

Reactions to other NRL devices, both medical and nonmedical, have occurred; they include balloons, rubber bands, condoms, vibrators, dental dams, anesthesia equipment, and toys for animals and children. The route to exposure to NRL proteins is important; it includes direct contact with intact or inflamed skin and mucosal exposure, such as inhalation of powder from NRL gloves, especially in medical facilities and in operating rooms.[118–125]

NRL allergy is sometimes associated with allergic reactions to fruit, especially bananas, kiwis, chestnuts, and avocados.[129–131] This results from crossreactivity between proteins in NRL and those found in the fruits. Symptoms range from oral itching and angioedema to asthma, gastrointestinal upset, and anaphylaxis. The list of foods with crossreactivity to NRL continues to increase with the addition of kiwis, hazel nuts, peanuts, celery, melons, potatoes, papayas, figs, passion fruit, tomatoes, grapes, pineapples, cherries, and peaches. Other stone-fruit allergens include apricots, nectarines, and plums. As many as 50% of latex-allergic patients have reported symptoms after eating bananas. NRL-allergic patients with severe fruit allergy should probably be counseled to avoid all fruits to which they are skin-test positive; they should also be skin-tested with fresh food material prior to eating any new fresh fruits or vegetables that carry a risk of NRL crossreactivity.[129–131]

Preexisting hand eczema is often mentioned as a significant risk factor for NRL allergy, but patch-test results are infrequently reported. Several articles discuss concomitant delayed hypersensitivity to latex gloves. Turjanmaa alone and with coworkers summarized data on 124 patients with latex allergy, of whom 83 were patch-tested.[125, 128, 144] Of these, 11 of 83 (13%) had positive patch tests in response to rubber chemicals or mixes, 7 of 11

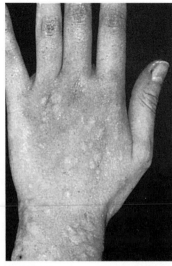

FIGURE 6–1 • Contact urticaria caused by latex. (Courtesy of Drs. Kristina Turjanmaa and Arto Lahti.)

(64%) to thiurams only, and 2 of 11 (18%) to both thiurams and carbamates. We recently reported 44 patients with latex allergy, 38 of whose cases were occupationally related, all but two of them in health-care professions. Hand eczema was present in 36, and 26 had relevant positive patch tests that included glutaraldehyde, latex and vinyl gloves, rubber chemicals, and preservatives in lotions and creams used by the patients. Preexisting hand eczema with or without allergic contact dermatitis may easily mask signs of contact urticaria. Latex allergy should be suspected in the presence of directly elicited symptoms of pruritus or burning and stinging on donning gloves or after exposure to other latex devices.[124]

Diagnosis of NRL allergy is strongly suggested if the patient has a history of angioedema of the lips when inflating balloons or itching, burning, urticaria, or anaphylaxis when donning rubber gloves or undergoing surgical, medical, or dental procedures or following exposure to condoms or other NRL items. Diagnosis is confirmed by a positive wear-or-use test with NRL gloves, a valid positive intracutaneous prick test to NRL, or a positive RAST to NRL. Severe allergic reactions have occurred as a result of prick-and-wear tests; epinephrine and resuscitation equipment free of NRL should be available during these procedures.[124]

NRL allergy is an IgE-mediated, immediate type I reaction to one or more of 240 proteins present in NRL or cured rubber latex.[124, 125, 140] High-pressure liquid chromatography has shown allergenic protein fractions with peaks at molecular weights between 2 and 30 kd in natural rubber as well as in latex surgical and examination gloves.[119, 125] Immunoblotting techniques have revealed that IgE4 binds to 12 rubber proteins in the range of 14 to 53 kd and that IgE antibodies bind to 9 antigens. The major antigen from both antibodies was a 21-kd rubber protein.[119, 140]

Immunoblot assays from a study of eight different glove brands identified a total of 14 protein bands, ranging from 11 to 200 kd.[145] Allergenic peptides and neoantigens of lower molecular mass (<10 kd) may also be present. Turjanmaa et al. summarized the major NRL allergens. Prohevein (20 kd) and hevein (4.72 kd) are the major allergens in health-care workers. In contrast, rubber elongation factor (REF) (14.6 kd) and a 27-kd NRL protein are the major allergens in multioperated children. Other molecularly characterized NRL allergens include hevein C domain (14 kd), hevamine (29.6 kd), a 36-kd endogluconase, and a 46-kd protein.[146]

Hyposensitization to NRL is not yet possible, so avoidance of and substitution for NRL are imperative. Because many patients with NRL allergy are atopic and have hand eczema, immediate allergic symptoms, or both, the most important issues for physicians are accurate diagnosis, appropriate treatment, and counseling. Dermatological evaluation to exclude other causes of hand eruptions and allergy or pulmonary evaluation of associated rhinitis, conjunctivitis, asthma, angioedema, or anaphylaxis is important. Prevention and control of NRL allergy includes latex avoidance in health-care settings for affected workers and patients. Substitute synthetic non-NRL gloves should be available; and in many cases, low-allergen NRL gloves should be worn by coworkers to accommodate those with NRL allergy, in order to minimize symptoms and to decrease induction of NRL allergy. Synthetic, non-NRL gloves include those made of polyvinyl chloride (vinyl), tactylon, elastyren, neoprene, and nitrile.[124] Allergen content of gloves should be requested from manufacturers and suppliers; lists of glove allergen content have also been published.[147, 148] Patients with NRL allergy should obtain Medic-Alert bracelets and inform health-care providers of their diagnosis and be given lists of substitute gloves, other non-NRL devices, potentially allergenic fruits, and occult sources of NRL exposure such as dog and child toys and dental prophylaxis cups.

Some of this information is available in published sources and from latex allergy support groups. Two of those groups are Education for Latex Allergy Support Team and Information Coalition (ELASTIC), which provides Latex Allergy News at 860/482-6869, and Allergy to Latex Education and Support Service (ALERT) at 414/677-9707. The National Institute for Occupational Safety and Health (NIOSH) has recently issued a review on preventing allergic reactions to NRL in the workplace.[149] Other information on latex allergy is available on the Internet. The FDA has issued a proposed rule requiring labeling of NRL devices and proposing substitute language to replace the "hypoallergenic" label.[150] As currently labeled, hypoallergenic gloves are still made of NRL and should not be worn by people with an NRL allergy.

Multidisciplinary task forces on latex allergy have been established in many medical centers. The same approach is also needed in physicians' offices. Continued cooperation among government, industry, and health-care professionals is necessary to control latex allergy.[151]

Turjanmaa et al. have suggested that future challenges in NRL allergy include (1) diagnosis of asymptomatic NRL-allergic patients, (2) understanding of the mechanisms of NRL sensitization, (3) elucidation of the significance of NRL exposure (especially airborne NRL) in health-care workers, (4) assessment of the consequences of coexistent food and NRL allergy, (5) further identification and characterization at a molecular level of NRL allergens for more specific in vivo and in vitro diagnostic tests and whether food allergy predisposes to NRL allergy, (6) production of purified NRL allergens for possible immunotherapy, and (7) prevention of NRL allergy, including a lowering of the NRL allergen levels in gloves and other NRL devices.[152]

Rubber Chemicals. Contact urticaria or immediate-type hypersensitivity to accelerators have also been reported. Wrangsjo et al. found a patient with positive scratch tests to rubber latex, zinc pentamethylene dithiocarbamate, and zinc dibutyldithiocarbamate.[132] Helander and Makela evaluated a glove-allergic kitchen worker with relapsing eyelid edema, and he was found to be sensitized to zinc diethyldithiocarbamate.[133] Heese et al. also found a latex-allergic patient with a strong wheal-flare reaction to zinc dimethyldithiocarbamate.[134] Belsito investigated seven cases of contact urticaria caused by rubber and found three patients who were scratch-test positive to black rubber mix, carba mix, and mercaptobenzothiazole, respectively.[135] Brehler reported a case of an allergic dental assistant who redeveloped contact urticaria 1 year after switching to NRL–free nitrile gloves that contained morpholinyl mercaptobenzothiazole.[136]

It is, however, not clear whether development of contact urticaria in response to these chemicals is of pseudoallergic origin or is mediated through specific IgE.

Cornstarch in Rubber Gloves. Van der Meeren and van Erp[137] and Fisher[138] have reported contact urticaria in medical personnel that results from the presence of cornstarch in rubber gloves.

Assalve et al.[139] reported a 29-year-old obstetrician who developed urticaria, rhinitis, and asthma after wearing latex gloves. She was patch-test negative to cornstarch powder and to both washed and unwashed latex gloves, but an urticarial reaction was observed with cornstarch powder and unwashed gloves at 48- and 72-hours. Use tests with both washed and unwashed gloves and an inhalation test with powdered gloves were both positive. It is now generally believed that powder is the depository and vehicle for the latex protein. Inhalation-triggered reaction in a sensitized individual working in an environment where fellow employees don powdered gloves is significant, as is touch transfer of the powder.[140–142]

Animals and Animal Secretions that Can Cause ICU

Allergic contact urticaria can occur because of animal hair, dander, saliva, serum, placenta, and even human seminal fluid. This type of urticaria is not uncommon among investigators performing animal research.

Rat Saliva

Burrows noted that in facilities in which large numbers of experimental rats are used, asthma, hay fever, and urticaria are common among research workers.[153] The animal attendants were less likely to be affected. This finding suggests that the allergen is contained in internal secretions such as saliva rather than in hair or skin. This problem was so great in some laboratories that a staffing problem occurred.

Bovine Blood and Amniotic Fluid

Degreef reported protein contact dermatitis with positive RASTs in response to fresh bovine blood with amniotic fluid in a veterinary surgeon with a 2-year history of itching skin lesions on his arms and face that were aggravated when he performed a cesarean section on a cow.[154] Roger et al. reported a similar clinical presentation in a veterinarian who had positive intradermal and patch tests in response to bovine amniotic fluid.[155]

Placenta of Cow

Schmidt observed immunological contact urticaria in a veterinary surgeon who, after 2 years of work, noticed itching localized to his arms. Symptoms occurred only when he loosened the placenta from a cow, a procedure that normally occurs between 12 and 24 hours after delivery. He had no symptoms when working with horses, pigs, or other domestic animals. His total serum IgE was 91 mg/mL, and RAST was positive to cow but negative to cat and horse. With a prick test, a + + + reaction to cow was produced. The patient showed a 3-mm reaction to amniotic fluid and a large 25-mm reaction to chorion-allantoic fluid and to the placenta from a cow. As his reaction became worse, he had to leave his job as a veterinary surgeon for one in which he had no direct contact with domestic animals.[156]

Von den Driesch reported an unusual case of immediate hypersensitivity to calf placenta extract that was used by a cosmetician during her work. Prick and scratch-chamber tests with the extract were positive.[157]

Cockroaches

Zschunke observed dermatitis, urticaria, rhinitis, bronchitis, and asthma in four agricultural insecticide research assistants whose job was breeding cockroaches. They had patch tests with a cockroach extract on the volar aspect of the forearm. Dilutions of 1:1000 produced 5- to 10-mm wheals within 15 minutes that lasted about 30 minutes. Zschunke concluded that dermatitis due to cockroaches should be classified as allergic contact urticaria.[158]

Rat Tails

Rudzki et al. showed that a psychologist who experimented with rats developed urticaria, rhinitis, and conjunctivitis. He developed contact urticaria 5 minutes after his forearm touched a rat's tail.[159]

Guinea Pigs

Rudzki et al. described a nurse who developed contact urticaria because of handling guinea pigs.[159]

Mouse Hair

Karches and Fuchs reported on a 29-year-old animal research laboratory assistant who developed contact urticaria from rat and mouse hair. Her job required her to feed bullfrogs and toads with live mice.[160]

Spider Mite

Reunala et al. reported on two greenhouse workers who developed allergic rhinoconjuctivitis and contact urticaria from two spotted spider mites (*Tetranychus urticae*, Koch). There was no crossreactivity between spider mite and house dust mite allergen.[161]

Locusts

Monk described a case of allergic contact urticaria provoked by locusts in a laboratory research worker. One of her colleagues also had locust-induced contact urticaria and another had asthma provoked by locust exposure. Contact urticaria to locusts is an occupational hazard apparently well known to professional entomologists, but one that has not previously been described in the dermatological literature. Prick-testing showed positive reactions to grass, pollens, house dust mite, cockroach antigen, and extemporaneously prepared locust antigen. Her total blood IgE level was mildly elevated at 302 IU/L. A direct provocation test with live locust produced an immediate whealing reaction at the sites of contact, developing within 1 minute. No reaction was seen in a control subject.[162]

Amphibian Serum

Contact with amphibian serum by research investigators may produce an immediate hypersensitivity reaction that results in hand dermatitis.[163]

Larvae in Fish Food

A 35-year-old atopic chemist who kept fish as a hobby developed contact urticaria following exposure to fish food containing red midge larvae (*Chironomus*). He had a 6-year history of contact urticaria that developed 15 minutes after handling both fresh and frozen fish food. Specific IgE for *Chironomus thummi* was strongly positive at 56.1 kU/L (Class 5 RAST); total IgE was normal. Frozen and dried *Chironomus* extracts were strongly positive on prick-testing, and a rub test with the fish food produced local urticaria in 15 minutes. Prick tests in 10 controls were negative.[164]

Fishing Worms

Nereis diversicolor, or north worm, is a popular fishing worm produced in large numbers in Korea and exported worldwide. A 46-year-old atopic fisherman developed acute facial angioedema, conjunctivitis, and dyspnea when handling north worms. Open testing with the worm's celomic fluid showed mild erythema at 40 minutes, and closed patch tests showed mild erythema and edema at 2 and 4 days. Closed patch-testing with a small piece of whole worm was negative at 2 and 4 days. The authors suggested that the mechanism was probably immunological contact urticaria caused by an active agent released when hooking the worm, although no controls or RASTs were performed.[165]

Red Spider Mite

Fifty-six Italian farmworkers with exposure to the macroscopic mite *Tetranychus urticae* were described with one or more findings: contact urticaria, protein contact dermatitis, allergic contact dermatitis, urticaria, rhinitis, and asthma. Diagnoses were confirmed by open tests for urticaria and eczema, patch tests, RAST, and skin prick tests. One worker had positive patch tests to mite extract without dermatitis. Cutaneous findings were termed the "overlapping contact cutaneous syndrome."[166]

Physical Causes of Contact Urticaria

Approximately 20 types of physical urticaria have been reported. The most common types are dermographism, cholinergic urticaria, cold urticaria, and delayed pressure urticaria. The various urticarias due to cold, heat, sun, and water may be immunological or nonimmunological in nature. Certain occupations may make it impossible for some individuals to avoid being exposed to these agents. Most physical urticarias are chronic, lasting for a number of years.[173]

Dermographism

Dermographism is caused by a rubbing, stroking, or writing on the skin by exerting pressure with a hard object. Red dermographism occurs after 15 to 20 seconds and can fade, or a second-reaction reflex erythema can occur. Urticarial dermographism occurs in some patients 3 to 5 minutes after a pressure stimulus; rarely, it develops after 3 to 6 hours and can persist for up to 24 hours.[177] The palms, soles, genitalia, and scalp are less commonly involved.[173]

Cholinergic Urticaria

In cases of cholinergic urticaria, highly pruritic follicular wheals appear after physical exertion or emotional stimuli. Lesions may be disseminated and accompanied by systemic symptoms such as headache, palpitation, abdominal cramps and, rarely, exercise-induced anaphylaxis. Reactions usually last up to 1 hour.[173, 177]

Delayed Pressure Urticaria

A delayed response to pressure can occur alone but often occurs in conjunction with chronic urticaria. Whealing occurs 4 to 6 hours after a stimulus, which could be wearing a tight belt, standing on a ladder rung, or working with a screwdriver. Lesions can last up to 48 hours and may be accompanied by systemic symptoms.[173]

Cold Urticaria

Cold urticaria is heterogeneous disorder that is classified according to the nature of response to a cold-provocation test.[173] Essential acquired contact cold urticaria is the most common type and is regarded as immunological in nature. Lesions appear usually within minutes of contact with, for example, an ice cube. The now outdated passive transfer test was positive in about 50% of reported cases. The transferable agent has been suggested to be IgE or IgM.[174] Although immunoglobulins may be involved pathogenically, causing mast cell degranulation, the biochemical sequences initiating this type of humoral response remain obscure.

Secondary cold urticaria may be caused by infectious diseases, cryoglobulinemia, drugs, and other systemic diseases, all of which should be excluded before diagnosing essential cold urticaria. Systemic atypical cold urticaria patients do not react to cold-contact testing.[173] Fitzgerald et al. reported a 45-year-old pottery worker who developed cold urticaria in the course of her work as a lithographer. She had to manually immerse transfers in a cold solution and apply them to pieces of finished pottery. The patient also had primary antiphospholipid syndrome.[175]

Swimming in cold water or exposure to cold wind may produce a shock-like syndrome, with a risk of drowning. Presumably, this reaction is due to histamine release.[176]

Heat Urticaria

Heat urticaria is extremely rare and is considered to be nonimmunological in nature. Immediate hives may be produced by applying a test tube filled with water (38–44°C) to the forearm. There is a hereditary delayed type of the condition.[177] In spite of numerous investigations, the pathophysiology of this syndrome has not been delineated. Moragas et al. implicated the kininogen-kinin system and possibly histamine,[178] whereas Daman et al. suggested the activation of the alternative complement pathway in the genesis of increased vascular permeability as the cause of this rare type of contact urticaria.[179]

Solar Urticaria

Solar urticaria is also uncommon. It is characterized by the rapid development of an urticarial reaction on areas of skin exposed to nonionizing electromagnetic radiation.[173, 180] There are at least four groups, and the wavelengths usually responsible for solar urticaria fall between 290 and 700 nm.[173] Mast cell degranulation is associated with the development of solar urticaria and elevated levels of histamine; eosinophil and neutrophil chemotactic factors have been found in the venous blood draining the site of reaction. Over 50% of patients are reported to be symptomatic after 10 years.[173]

Aquagenic Urticaria

In aquagenic urticaria, perifollicular hives similar in appearance to those of cholinergic urticaria appear on skin exposed to tap water, distilled water, salinated water, or the patient's own sweat or sebum after 2 to 30 minutes.[177, 181] It has been proposed that a toxic histamine-releasing substance is formed through the combination of water and sebum.[181]

CONTACT URTICARIA OF UNCERTAIN MECHANISM

Ammonium Persulfate

Beauty parlor operators and their patrons who are exposed to ammonium persulfate may suffer severe urticarial reactions, including anaphylactoid reactions. Ammonium persulfate is used widely to boost peroxide hair bleaches in order to obtain a platinum blond shade. The persulfates can produce a variety of cutaneous and respiratory responses, including allergic eczematous contact dermatitis, irritant dermatitis, localized edema, generalized urticaria, rhinitis, asthma, and syncope. Some of these reactions appear to be truly allergic, whereas others appear to be due to the release of histamine on a nonimmunological basis.[182, 183]

Patch tests may be performed with a 2 to 5% aqueous solution of ammonium persulfate. Scratch tests may result in asthma and syncope. In some patients, merely rubbing a saturated solution of ammonium persulfate into the skin will evoke a large urticarial wheal. Hairdressers should be made aware that these ammonium persulfate hair bleach preparations may provoke severe reactions. They should seek medical attention if the client complains of severe itching. tingling, a burning sensation, hives, dizziness, or weakness. The variety of reaction patterns, which include toxic dermatitis, localized or generalized urticaria, rhinitis, asthma, and even vascular collapse, is puzzling.

CONCLUSION

Although NICU is said to be more common than ICU, most cases studied appear to be immunological. Contact urticaria occurs as a result of direct contact with skin (most examples) or mucosa (e.g., latex and chlorhexidine; the latter may be associated with systemic toxicity),[70, 184, 185] or through airborne contact (e.g., chincona, mulberry, xylene).[82, 106, 186] Exposure may be accidental or due to equipment failure (e.g., xylene).[82] Ingredients (e.g., Tinofix S) or trace contaminants or impurities (e.g., an anhydride present in sorbitan sesquioleate) may be responsible.[117, 187] Contact urticaria may be associated with other urticaria (e.g., delayed pressure urticaria).[188]

Further delineation of distinctions between immunological and nonimmunological causes should include RASTs and control-patient testing whenever possible. Passive transfer tests risk the transfer of blood-borne viral infections such as HIV.

The list of agents that cause contact urticaria is large and dynamic. The purpose of accumulating such a list is to create a source that will help to provide insight into a patient's history and indicate the choice of testing methods. Thus, it remains important to continue to report all agents that cause contact urticaria. Finally, contact urticaria should be thought of in the broadest context to include immediate contact eczema as well as accelerated type I reactions with urticaria, angioedema, and anaphylaxis.

References

1. Von Krogh G, Maibach HI. The contact urticaria syndrome. *Semin Dermatol* 1982; 1:56.

2. Tanglertsampan C, Maibach HI. Contact urticaria. In: Hogan DJ, ed. *Occupational Skin Disorders*. New York: Igaku-Shoin, 1994; 81–88.

3. Fisher AA. Contact urticaria due to occupational exposures. In: Adams RM, ed. *Occupational Skin Disease,* 2nd ed. Philadelphia: W.B. Saunders; 1990.

4. Czarnecki D, Nixon R, Beckhor P, et al. Delayed prolonged contact urticaria from the elm tree. *Contact Dermatitis* 1993; 28:196–197.

5. Kligman AM. The spectrum of contact urticaria. *Dermatol Clin* 1990; 8:57–60.

6. Lahti A. Nonimmunologic contact urticaria. *Acta Derm Venereol* 1980; 60 [suppl 91]:1.

7. Lahti A. Immediate contact reactions. In: Rycroft RJG, Menne T, Frosch PJ, eds. *Textbook of Contact Dermatitis.* Berlin: Springer-Verlag; 1995: 62–74.

8. Tosti A, Guerra L, Bardazzi F. Contact urticaria during topical immunotherapy. *Contact Dermatitis* 1989; 21:196–197.

9. Kanerva L, Toikkanen J, Jolanki R, et al. Statistical data on occupational contact urticaria. *Contact Dermatitis* 1996; 35:229–233.

10. Kanerva L, Estlander T, Jolanki R. Long-lasting contact urticaria: type I and type IV allergy from castor bean and a hypothesis of systemic IgE-mediated allergic dermatitis. *Dermatol Clin* 1990; 8:181–188.

11. Goncalo M, Chieira L, Goncalo S. Immediate and delayed hypersensitivity to garlic and soybean. *Am J Contact Dermatitis* 1992; 3:102–104.

12. Majoie ML, Bruynzell DP. Occupational immediate-type hypersensitivity to henna in a hairdresser. *Am J Contact Dermatitis* 1992; 7:38–40.

13. Keller K, Schwanitz HJ. Combined immediate and delayed hypersensitivity to mezlocillin. *Contact Dermatitis* 1992; 27:348–349.

14. Hinojosa M, Subiza J, Moneo I, et al. Contact urticaria caused by obeche wood (*Triplochiton scleroxylon*): report of eight patients. *Ann Allergy* 1990; 64:476–479.

15. Kanerva L, Estlander T, Jolanki R Skin testing for immediate hypersensitivity in occupational allergology. In: Menne T, Maibach HI, eds. *Exogenous Dermatoses: Environmental Dermatitis.* Boca Raton, Fla.: CRC Press; 1991.

16. Hannuksela M. Skin tests for immediate hypersensitivity. In: Rycroft RJG, Menne T, Frosch PJ, eds. *Textbook of Contact Dermatitis.* Berlin: Springer-Verlag; 1995.

17. *Drug Facts and Comparisons.* Facts and Comparisons, St. Louis: 1991; 731b,c.

18. Kellum RE, ed. Selected reviews of the literature. *Arch Dermatol* 1966; 93:135.

19. Fryklof L-E. A note on the irritant properties of sorbic acid in ointments and creams. *J Pharm Pharmacol* 1968; 10:719.

20. Fisher AA. Erythema limited to the face from sorbic acid. *Cutis* 1987; 40:303.

21. Rietschel RL. Contact urticaria from synthetic cassia oil and sorbic acid limited to the face. *Contact Dermatitis* 1978; 4:347.

22. Fisher AA. Erythema limited to the face from sorbic acid. *Cutis* 1987; 40:303.

23. Pevny I, von Rauscher E, Lechner W, Metz D. Excessive Allergie gegen Benzoesaure mit anaphylktischem Schock nach Expositionstet. *Dermatosen* 1981; 29:123.

24. Hjorth N. Eczematous allergy to balsams, allied perfumes and flavoring agents. Acta Derm Venereol Suppl (Stockh) 1981; 41:216.

25. Seite-Bellezza D, El Sayed F, Bazex J. Contact urticaria from cinnamic aldehyde and benzaldehyde in a confectioner. *Contact Dermatitis* 1994; 31:272.

26. Lahti A. Skin reactions to antimicrobial agents. *Contact Dermatitis* 1978; 4:302.
27. Mathias CGT, Chappler RR, Maibach HI. Contact urticaria from cinnamic aldehyde. *Arch Dermatol* 1980; 116:74.
28. Harvell J, Bason M, Maibach HI. Contact urticaria (immediate reaction syndrome). *Clin Rev Allergy* 1992; 10:303–323.
29. Goodfield MJD, Saihan EM. Contact urticaria to naphtha present in a solvent. *Contact Dermatitis* 1988; 18:187.
30. Veraldi S, Schianchi-Veraldi. Contact urticaria from kiwi fruit. *Contact Dermatitis* 1990; 22:244.
31. Giannattasio M, Serafini M, Guarrera P, Cannistraci C, Cristando A, Santucci B. Contact urticaria from litchi fruit (litchi Chinese Sonn.). *Contact Dermatitis* 1995; 33:67.
32. Lernier VD, Albertinis G, Bisighini G. Immunologic contact urticaria syndrome from raw rice. *Contact Dermatitis* 1992; 27:196.
33. Temesvari E, Becker K. Contact urticaria from watermelon in a patient with pollen allergy. *Contact Dermatitis* 28:185.
34. Nater JP, Swartz JA. Atopic allergic reaction due to raw potato. *J Allergy* 1967; 40:202.
35. Pearson RSB. Potato sensitivity: an occupational allergen in housewives. *Acta Allergol* 21:507, 1966.
36. Hjorth N, Roed-Petersen J. Bernfsekzeme durch proteine. *Z Hautkr* 1975; 50:851.
37. Mitchell JC. Contact urticaria from a shrimp *(Pandalus)*. *Contact Dermatitis Newsletter* 1974; 16:486.
38. Maibach HI. Regional variation in elicitation of contact urticaria syndrome: shrimp. *Contact Dermatitis* 1986; 15:100.
39. Melino M, Toni F, Rignzzi G. Immunologic contact urticaria to fish. *Contact Dermatitis* 1987; 17:182.
40. Kavli G, Moseng D. Contact urticaria from mustard in fish-stick production. *Contact Dermatitis* 1987; 17:153.
41. Nakamori M, Matsus I, Ohkido M. Coexistence of contact urticaria and contact dermatitis due to pearl oysters in an atopic dermatitis patient. *Contact Dermatitis* 1996; 34:438.
42. Hjorth N, Roed-Petersen J. Occupational protein contact dermatitis in food handlers. *Contact Dermatitis* 1976; 2:23.
43. Maibach HI. Immediate hypersensitivity in hand dermatitis: role of food-contact dermatitis. *Arch Dermatol* 1976; 112:1289.
44. Fisher AA, Stengel F. Allergic occupational hand dermatitis due to calves' liver: an urticarial "immediate" type hypersensitivity. *Cutis* 1977; 19:561.
45. Fisher AA. Allergic contact urticaria to raw beef-histopathology of the specific wheal reaction at the scratch test site. *Contact Dermatitis* 1982; 8:425.
46. Moseng D. Urticaria from pig's gut. *Contact Dermatitis* 1982; 8:135.
47. Jovanovic M, Oliwiecki, Beck, MH. Occupational contact urticaria from beef associated with hand eczema. *Contact Dermatitis* 1992; 27:188.
48. Valsecchi R, DiLandro A, Pansera B, et al. Contact urticaria from pork. *Contact Dermatitis* 1994; 30:121.
49. Andersen KE, Lowenstein H. An investigation of the possible immunological relationship between allergen extracts from birch, pollen, hazelnut, potato and apple. *Contact Dermatitis* 1978; 4:73.
50. Weltfriend S, Kwangsukstith C, Maibach HI. Contact urticaria from cucumber, pickle and strawberry. *Contact Dermatitis* 1995; 32:173.
51. Goransson K. Contact urticaria to apricot stone. *Contact Dermatitis* 1981; 7:282.
52. Giannattasio M, Serafini M, Guarrera P, et al. Contact urticaria from litchi fruit. *Contact Dermatitis* 1995; 33:67.
53. Temesvari E, Becker K. Contact urticaria from watermelon in a patient with pollen allergy. *Contact Dermatitis* 1993; 28:185–186.
54. Krook G. Occupational dermatitis from *Lactuca sativa* (lettuce) and *Cichorium* (endive). *Contact Dermatitis* 1977; 3:27.
55. Munoz D, Leanizbarrutia I, Lobera T, Fernandezde Corres L. Anaphylaxis from contact with carrot. *Contact Dermatitis* 1985; 13:345.
56. Lovell CR, Rycroft RJG. Contact urticaria from winged bean (*Psophocarpus tetragonolobus*). *Contact Dermatitis* 1984; 10:315.
57. Kanerva L, Estlander T, Jolanki R. Long-lasting contact urticaria: type I and type IV allergy from castor bean and a hypothesis of systemic IgE-mediated allergic dermatitis. *Dermatol Clin* 1990; 8:181.
58. Goncalo M, Chieira L, Goncalo S. Immediate and delayed hypersensitivity to garlic and soybean. *Am J Contact Dermatitis* 1992; 3:102.
59. Fisher AA. The contact dermatitis syndrome (contact urticaria). *Cutis* 1983; 31:28.
60. Fisher AA. Hand dermatitis: a baker's dozen. *Cutis* 1982; 29:214.
61. Maibach HI. Contact urticaria syndrome from mold on salami casing. *Contact Dermatitis* 1995; 32:120.
62. Tosti A, Guerra L. Protein contact dermatitis in food handlers. *Contact Dermatitis* 1988; 19:149.
63. Valdivieso R, Moneo I, Pola J, et al. Occupational asthma and contact urticaria caused by buckwheat flour. *Ann Allergy* 1989; 63:149.
64. Di Lernia V, Albertini G, Bisighini G. Immunologic contact urticaria syndrome from raw rice. *Contact Dermatitis* 1992; 27:196.
65. Rudzki E, Rebandel P, Rogozinski T. Contact urticaria from rat tail, guinea pig, streptomycin and vinyl pyridine. *Contact Dermatitis* 1981; 7:186.
66. Tuft L. Contact urticaria from cephalosporins. *Arch Dermatol* 1975; 111:1609.
67. Mancuso G, Masara N. Contact urticaria and severe anaphylaxis from rifamycin SV. *Contact Dermatitis* 1992; 27:124–125.
68. Miyahara H, Koga T, Imayamer S, Honi Y. Occupational contact urticaria syndrome from defotian hydrochloanole. *Contact Dermatitis* 1993; 29:210.
69. Ryan ME, Davis BM, Marks JG Jr. Contact urticaria and allergic contact dermatitis to benzocaine gel. *J Am Acad Dermatol* 1980; 2:221.
70. Grunnet E. Contact urticaria and anaphylactoid reaction induced by topical application of nitrogen. *Br J Dermatol* 1976; 94:101.
71. Daughters D, Zackheim H, Maibach H. Urticaria and anaphylactoid reactions after topical application of mechlorethamine. *Arch Dermatol* 1976; 94:101.
72. Johansson G. Contact urticaria from levomepromazine. *Contact Dermatitis* 1988; 19:304.
73. Schena D, Barba A, Costa G. Occupational contact urticaria due to cisplatin. *Contact Dermatitis* 1996; 34:220.
74. Osmundsen PE. Contact urticaria from nickel and plastic additives (butylhydroxytoluene, oleylamide). *Contact Dermatitis* 1980; 6:452.
75. Nakayama H, Imai T. Occupational contact urticaria, contact dermatitis and asthma caused by rhodium hypersensitivity. Sixth International Symposium on Contact Dermatitis and Joint Meeting between ICRG and JCDRG. Tokyo: May 21, 1982.
76. Key MM. Some unusual allergic reactions in industry. *Arch Dermatol* 1961; 83:3.

77. Levene GM. Platinum sensitivity. *Br J Dermatol* 1971; 85:5.

78. Bergman A, Svedberg U, Nilsson E. Contact urticaria with anaphylactic reactions caused by occupational exposure to indium salt. *Contact Dermatitis* 1995; 32:14.

79. Jolanki R, Estlander T, Kanerva L. Occupational contact dermatitis and contact urticaria caused by epoxy resins. Acta Derm Venereal Suppl (Stockh) 1987; 134:90.

80. Tarvainen K, Jolanki R, Estlander T, Tupasela O, Pfaffli P, Kanerva L. Immunologic contact urticaria due to airborne methylhexahydrophthalic and methyltetrahydrophthalic anhydrides. *Contact Dermatitis* 1995; 32:204.

81. Altman AT. Facial dermatitis (xylene) *Arch Dermatol* 1977; 113:1460 [letter].

82. Palmer KT, Rycroft RJG. Occupational airborne contact urticaria due to xylene. *Contact Dermatitis* 1993; 28:44.

83. Goodfield MJD, Saihan EM. Contact urticaria from naphtha present in a solvent. *Contact Dermatitis* 1988; 18:187.

84. Varigos GA, Nurse DS. Contact urticaria from methyl ethyl ketone. *Contact Dermatitis* 1986; 15:259.

85. Fowler JF. Contact urticaria to 1,1,1-trichloroethane. *Am J Contact Dermatitis* 1991; 2:239.

86. Freitas JP, Brandao FM. Contact urticaria to chlorocresol. *Contact Dermatitis* 1986; 15:252.

87. Fowler JF Jr. Immediate contact hypersensitivity to acrylic acid. *Dermatol Clin* 1990; 8:193.

88. Daecke C, Schaller S, Schaller J, et al. Contact urticaria from acrylic acid in Fixomull tape. *Contact Dermatitis* 1993; 29:216–217.

89. Dannaker CJ, Maibach HI, Malley MO. Contact urticaria and anaphylaxis to the fungicide chlorothalomil. *Cutis* 1993; 52:312.

90. Dooms-Goossens A, Gevers D, Mertens A, Vanderheyden D. Allergic contact urticaria due to chloramine. *Contact Dermatitis* 1983; 9:319.

91. Leonie Majoie IM, Bruynzeel DP. Occupational immediate-type hypersensitivity to henna in a hairdresser. *Am J Contact Dermatitis* 1996; 7:38.

92. Jagtman BA. Urticaria and contact urticaria due to basic blue 99 in a hair dye. *Contact Dermatitis* 1996; 35:52.

93. Freeman S, Lee MS. Contact urticaria to hair conditioner. *Contact Dermatitis* 1996; 35:195–196.

94. Pasche-Koo F, Claeys M, Hauser C. Contact urticaria with systemic symptoms caused by bovine collagen in a hair conditioner. *Am J Contact Dermatitis* 1984; 57–58.

95. Temesvari E. Contact urticaria from paraphenylenediamine. *Contact Dermatitis* 1984; 11:125.

96. Rivers JK, Rycroft RJG. Occupational allergic contact urticaria from colophony. *Contact Dermatitis* 1987; 17:181.

97. Torresani C, Caprari E, Manaka QC. Contact urticaria syndrome due to phenylmercuric acetate. *Contact Dermatitis* 1993; 29:282.

98. Archer CB, Cronin E. Contact urticaria induced by pyindine carboxyaldehyde. *Contact Dermatitis* 1986; 15:308.

99. Mathews KP. Immediate-type hypersensitivity to phenylmercuric compounds. *Am J Med* 1968; 44:310.

100. Maibach HI, Johnson HL. Contact urticaria syndrome: contact urticaria to diethyltoluamide (immediate-type hypersensitivity). *Arch Dermatol* 1975; 111:726.

101. Hausen B. Woods injurious to human health—a manual. Berlin: Walter de Gruyter; 1981:7.

102. Garces Sotillos MM, Blanco Carmona JG, Juste Picon S, Rodriguez Gaston P, Perez Gimenez R, Alonso Gil L. Occupational asthma and contact urticaria caused by maukali wood dust *(Aningeria robusta). J Allergy Clin Immunol* 1995; 5:113.

103. Goransson K. Contact urticaria and rhinoconjunctivitis from tropical wood (lanan, Philippine red mahogany). *Contact Dermatitis* 1980; 6:223.

104. Apted J. Acute contact urticaria from *Grevillea juniperina. Contact Dermatitis* 1988; 18:126 [letter].

105. Apted J. Acute contact urticaria from *Hakea snaveolens. Contact Dermatitis* 1988; 18:126 [letter].

106. Dooms-Goossens A, Deveylder H, Dunon C, Dooms M, Degreef H. Airborne contact urticaria due to cinchona. *Contact Dermatitis* 1986; 15:258.

107. Krupa Schankar DS. Contact urticaria induced by *Semecarpus anacardium. Contact Dermatitis* 1992; 26:200.

108. Lahti A. Contact urticaria and respiratory symptoms from tulips and lilies. *Contact Dermatitis* 1986; 14:317–319.

109. Tosti A, Melino M, Veronesi S. Contact urticaria to tobacco. *Contact Dermatitis* 1987; 16:225.

110. Combes FC, Morris GE. Contact sensitivity to inappreciable exposures. *Indiana Med* 1956; 25:289.

111. Morris GE. Urticaria following exposure to ammonia fumes. *AMA Arch Health* 1956; 13:480.

112. Zschunke E. Occupational urticaria due to sulfur dioxide. *Berufsdermatosen* 1967; 15:23.

113. Rudzki E. Contact urticaria from silk. *Contact Dermatitis* 1997; 3:53.

114. Dooms-Goossens A, Dunon C, Loncke J, Degreet H. Contact urticaria due to nylon. *Contact Dermatitis* 1986; 14:63.

115. Andersen KE, Maibach HI. Multiple application delayed-onset contact urticaria: possible relation to certain unusual formalin and textile reactions? *Contact Dermatitis* 1984; 10:227.

116. Helander I. Contact urticaria from leather containing formaldehyde. *Arch Dermatol* 1977; 113:1443.

117. DeGroot AC, Gerkens F. Contact urticaria from a chemical textile finish. *Contact Dermatitis* 1989; 20:63.

118. Estlander T, Jolanki R, Kanerva L. Dermatitis and urticaria from rubber and plastic gloves. *Contact Dermatitis* 1986; 14:20.

119. Slater JE. Latex allergy. *J Allergy Clin Immunol* 1994; 94:139.

120. Tarlo MS, Wong L, Roos J, Booth N. Occupational asthma caused by latex in a surgical glove manufacturing plant. *J Allergy Clin Immunol* 1990; 85:626.

121. Taylor JS, Cassetari J, Wagner W, Helm T. Contact urticaria and anaphylaxis to latex. *J Am Acad Dermatol* 1989; 21:874.

122. Matthew SN, Melton AL, Wagner WO. Latex hypersensitivity: a case study. *Ann Allergy* 1993; 70:483.

123. Taylor J, Evey P, Helm T. Contact urticaria and anaphylaxis from latex. *Contact Dermatitis* 1990; 23:277.

124. Taylor JS, Praditsuwan P. Latex allergy: review of 44 cases including outcome and frequent association with allergic hand eczema. *Arch Dermatol* 1996; 132:265.

125. Turjanmaa K, Makinen-Kiljunen S, Reunala T, Alenins H, Palosuo T. Natural rubber latex allergy: the European experience. *Immunol Allergy Clin North Am* 1995; 15:71.

126. Van der Walle HB, Brunsveld VM. Latex allergy among hairdressers. *Contact Dermatitis* 1995; 32:177.

127. Heese A, Peters K-P, Hornsein OP. Anaphylactic reaction to unexpected latex in a polychlorphene glove. *Contact Dermatitis* 1992; 27:336.

128. Turjanmaa K. Update on occupational natural rubber latex. *Dermatol Clin* 1994; 12:561.

129. Crisi G, Belsito DV. Contact urticaria from latex in a patient with immediate hypersensitivity to banana, avocado and peach. *Contact Dermatitis* 1993; 28:247.

130. Blanco C, Carillo T, Costillo R, Quiralte J, Cuerae M. Latex allergy: clinical feature and cross-reactivity with fruits. *Ann Allergy* 1994; 73:309.

131. Taylor JS. Latex allergy update: four vignettes. *Am J Contact Dermatitis* 1998; 9:45–48.

132. Wrangsjo K, Mellstrom G, Axelsson T. Discomfort from

rubber gloves indicating contact urticaria. *Contact Dermatitis* 1986; 15:79.

133. Helander I, Makela A. Contact urticaria to zinc diethyldithiocarbamate (ZDC). *Contact Dermatitis* 1983; 9:326.

134. Heese A, van Hinzenstern J, Peters K-P, Koch HU, Hornstein OP. Allergic and irritant reactions to rubber gloves in medical health services. *J Am Acad Dermatol* 1993; 25:831.

135. Belsito DV. Contact urticaria caused by rubber. *Dermatol Clin* 1990; 8:61.

136. Brehler R. Contact urticaria caused by latex-free nitrile glove. *Contact Dermatitis* 1996; 34:296.

137. Van der Meeren HLM, Van Erp PEJ. Life-threatening contact urticaria from glove powder. *Contact Dermatitis* 1986; 14:190.

138. Fisher AA. Contact urticaria due to cornstarch surgical glove powder. *Cutis* 1986; 38:307.

139. Assalve D, Cicioni C, Perouo P, Lisi P. Contact urticaria and anaphylactoid reaction from cornstarch surgical glove powder. *Contact Dermatitis* 1988; 19:61.

140. Slater JE, Chabra SK. Latex antigens. *J Allergy Clin Immunol* 1992; 89:673.

141. Bauer X, Jager D. Airborne antigens from latex gloves. *Lancet* 1990; 335:912.

142. Truscott W. The industry perspective on latex. *Immunol Allergy Clin North Am* 1995; 15:89.

143. Nutter AF. Contact urticaria to rubber. *Br J Dermatol* 1979; 101:597–598.

144. Turjanmaa K. Contact urticaria from latex gloves. In: Maibach HI, Mellstrom G, Walberg JE, eds. *Protective Gloves for Occupational Use.* Boca Raton, Fla.: CRC Press; 1994:241–254.

145. Alenius H, Makinen-Kihjunen S, Turjanmaa K, et al. Allergen and protein content of latex gloves. *Ann Allergy* 1994; 73:315–320.

146. Turjanmaa K, Alenius H, Makinen-Kiljunen S, et al. Natural rubber latex allergy. *Allergy* 1996; 51:593–602.

147. Yuninger J, Jones R, Fransway A, et al. Extractable latex allergens and proteins in disposable medical gloves and other rubber products. *J Allergy Clin Immunol* 1994; 93:836.

148. Palosuo T, Turjanmaa K, Reunala T, Makinen-Kiljunen S, Alenius H. Allergen content of latex gloves used in 1994–1996 in health care in Finland: results of renewed market survey in 1995. Helsinki: National Agency for Medicines, Medical Devices Center; 1996.

149. NIOSH alert: preventing allergic reactions to natural rubber latex in the workplace. DHHS (NIOSH) Publication No. 97–135. Cincinnati: National Institute for Occupational Safety and Health; 1997.

150. Latex-containing devices; user labeling; proposed rule. *Federal Register* June 24, 1996; VII, 61:32618–32621.

151. Hunt LW, Boone-Orke JL, Fransway AF, et al. A medical-center-wide, multidisciplinary approach to the problem of natural rubber latex allergy. *J Occup Envir Med* 1996; 38:765–770.

152. Turjanmaa K, Alenius H, Makinen-Kiljunen S, Reunala T, Palosuo T. Natural rubber latex allergy. *Allergy* 1996; 51:593–602.

153. Burrows D. Urticaria from rats. *Contact Dermatitis* 1979; 5:122.

154. Degreef H. Protein contact dermatitis with positive RAST tests to fresh bovine blood and amniotic fluid in a veterinary surgeon. Sixth International Symposium on Contact Dermatitis and Joint Meeting between ICRG and JCDRG. Tokyo: May 21, 1982.

155. Roger A, Giuspi R, Garcia-Patos V, et al. Occupational protein contact dermatitis in a veterinary surgeon. *Contact Dermatitis* 1995; 32:248.

156. Schmidt H. Contact urticaria. *Contact Dermatitis* 1978; 4:239.

157. Von den Driesch P, Fartasch M, Diepgen TL, Peters KP. Protein contact dermatitis from calf placenta extracts. *Contact Dermatitis* 1993; 28:46.

158. Zschunke E. Contact urticaria, dermatitis and asthma from cockroaches. *Contact Dermatitis* 1978; 4:313.

159. Rudzki E, Rebandel P, Rogozinski T. Contact urticaria from rat tail, guinea pig, streptomycin and vinyl pyridine. *Contact Dermatitis* 1981; 7:186.

160. Karches F, Fuchs T. A strange manifestation of occupational contact urticaria due to mouse hair. *Contact Dermatitis* 1993; 28:200.

161. Reunala T, Bjorksten F, Forstrom L, Kanerva L. IgE-mediated occupational allergy to a spider mite. *Clin Allergy* 1983; 13:383.

162. Monk BE. Contact urticaria to locusts. *Br J Dermatol* 1988; 118:707.

163. Thomsen RJ, Honsinger RW Jr. Immediate hypersensitivity reactions amphibian serum manifesting as hand eczema. *Arch Dermatol* 1987; 123:1426.

164. Galindo PA, Melero R, Garcia R, et al. Contact urticaria from chironomids. *Contact Dermatitis* 1996; 34:297.

165. Camarasa JG, Serra-Baldrich E. Contact urticaria from worm *(Nereis diversicolor). Contact Dermatitis* 1993; 28:248.

166. Astarita C, Di Martino P, Scala G, Franzese A, Sproviero S. Contact allergy: another occupational risk to *Tetranychus urticae. J Allergy Clin Immunol* 1996; 98:732–738.

167. LaMarte FP, Merchant JA, Casale TB Acute systemic reactions to carbonless copy paper associated with histamine release. *JAMA* 1988; 260:242–243.

168. Marks JG Jr, Trautlein JJ, Zwillich CW, DeMers LM. Contact urticaria and airway obstruction from carbonless copy paper. *JAMA* 1984; 252:1038–1040.

169. Hannuksela M, Bjorksten F. Immediate-type dermatitis, contact urticaria, and rhinitis from carbonless copy paper: report of four cases. In: Frosch PJ, RJG, Scheper RJ, eds. *Current Topics in Contact Dermatitis.* Berlin: Springer-Verlag, Berlin; 1989:453–456.

170. Marks JG Jr. Allergic contact dermatitis from carbonless copy paper. *JAMA* 1986; 245.

171. Frosch PJ. Cutaneous irritation, In: Rycroft RJG, Menne T, Frosch PJ, Benezra C, eds. *Textbook of Contact Dermatitis.* Berlin: Springer-Verlag; 1992:28–61.

172. Murray R. Health aspects of carbonless copy paper. *Contact Dermatitis* 1991; 24:321–333.

173. Mahmood T. Physical urticarias. *Am Fam Physician* 1994; 49:1411–144.

174. Kaplan AP, Gray L, Shaff RE et al. *In vivo* studies of mediator release in cold urticaria and cholinergic urticaria. *J Allergy Clin Immunol* 1975; 55:394.

175. Fitzgerald DA, Heagenty AHM, English JSC. Cold urticaria as an occupational dermatosis. *Contact Dermatitis* 1995; 32:238.

176. Highet AS, Tittenington A. Treatment of cold urticaria. *Br J Dermatol* 1979; 51:101.

177. Braun-Falco O, Plewig G, Wolff HH, Winkelmann RK, eds. Urticaria. In *Dermatology.* Berlin: Springer-Verlag; 1991: 292–315.

178. Moragas JM, Gimenez-Camarasa JM, Noguera J. Localized heat urticaria. *Arch Dermatol* 1973; 108:684.

179. Daman L, Lieberman P, Ganier M, Hashimoto K. Localized heat urticaria. *Allerg Clin Immunol* 1978; 61:273.

180. Parrish JA, Jaenicke KF, Morison WL, et al. Solar urticaria: treatment with PUVA and mediator inhibitors. *Br J Dermatol* 1982; 106:575.

181. Tkach JR. Aquagenic urticaria. *Cutis* 1981; 28:454.

182. Calnan CD, Shuster S. Reactions to ammonium persulfate. *Arch Dermatol* 1968; 88:812.

183. Fisher AA, Dooms-Goossens A. Persulfate hair bleach reactions. *Arch Dermatol* 1976; 112:1407.

184. Bergqist-Karlsson A. Delayed and immediate-type hypersensitivity to chlorhexidine. *Contact Dermatitis* 1988; 18:84–88.

185. Wong WK, Goh CL, Chan KW. Contact urticaria from chlorhexidine. *Contact Dermatitis* 1990; 22:52.

186. Munoz FJ, Delgado J, Palma JL et al. Airborne contact urticaria due to mulberry pollen. *Contact Dermatitis* 1995; 32:61.

187. Hardy MP, Maibach HI. Contact urticaria syndrome from sorbitan sesquioleate in a corticosteroid ointment. *Contact Dermatitis* 1993; 29:282–283.

188. El Sayed F, Manzur F, Bayle P, et al. Contact urticaria from abietic acid. *Contact Dermatitis* 1995; 32:361–362.

189. Burdick AE, Mathias CG. The contact urticaria syndrome. *Dermatol Clin* 1985; 3:71–84.

190. Lahti A, vonKrogh G, Maibach HI. Contact urticaria syndrome. An expanding phenomenon. In: Stone JF, ed. *Dermatologic Immunology and Allergy*. St. Louis, Mosby, 1985:379–390.

Acne, Folliculitis, and Chloracne

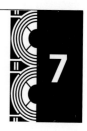

JOSEPH F. FOWLER, JR., M.D.

ACNE AND FOLLICULITIS

Various occupational and environmental factors can cause or exacerbate acne and folliculitis, including mechanical effects such as occlusion and friction and chemical effects such as certain chlorinated hydrocarbons. Chronic workplace exposure to oils and greases can lead to the onset of acne and folliculitis on exposed skin surfaces.[1] At sites of contact, especially when there is occlusion by clothing, comedones, follicular papules and pustules, and furuncles may appear. Common locations are areas in contact with oil-soaked clothing, such as the anterior thighs and the lateral aspects of the arms. Machinists and other metalworkers are especially at risk for development of acne and oil folliculitis (Fig. 7–1), the usual cause being contact with oil-based cutting oils or with oils used to coat metals for corrosion resistance. Water-based cutting fluids are less likely to cause

folliculitis but are more frequently responsible for contact dermatitis. Oil acne and oil folliculitis may also develop in auto and truck mechanics, roofers, rubber workers, asphalt paving workers and workers in the oil industry and in coal-tar plants. Actually, any worker exposed to oils, grease, coal tar, pitch, or creosote may be affected with occupational acne and folliculitis. Even those employed in fast-food restaurants where fried foods are prepared may develop acne and folliculitis, a condition that has been termed "McDonald's acne"[2] (Table 7–1).

Acne that occurs in areas chronically exposed to friction and heat, termed acne mechanica,[3] may be present on the thighs and buttocks. It is caused by the friction and pressure of tight-fitting clothing such as bluejeans. Heat and perspiration exacerbate the condition. Professional truck and taxi drivers sometimes develop acne mechanica on their backs (Fig. 7–2) and legs because of friction with a vehicle's seat. Horseback riders such as mounted police may develop this condition on their buttocks and inner thighs. Acne mechanica is also common in athletes, especially in areas where protective clothing rubs against the skin. Persons with keratosis pilaris may develop frank acne in the areas involved as a result of the same factors that induce acne mechanica. Actors, dancers, and other entertainment professionals often develop acne because of their use of greasy cosmetics.[4]

Treatment

Successful treatment of acne mechanica, oil acne, and folliculitis requires the elimination or reduction of exposure to the agent causing the friction or occlusion. Topical application of comedolytic agents such as tretinoin or adapalene can be help-

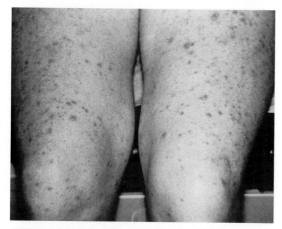

FIGURE 7–1 • Folliculitis on the anterior thighs is common among machinists who fail to protect their skin from the heavy machine oils, usually the insoluble types.

135

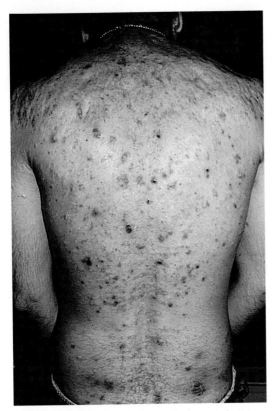

FIGURE 7–2 • This 22-year-old man had acne prior to beginning his job as a long-distance truck driver. The many hours behind the wheel of a large truck caused severe aggravation of his condition.

Type	Occupations
Cosmetic acne	Actors, actresses, models, cosmetologists
Acne mechanica	Truck drivers, professional and amateur athletes, telephone users
Oil acne	Auto mechanics, machinists working with oil-based cutting fluids, roofers, petroleum refiners, rubber workers, road pavers, workers subject to McDonald's acne
Chloracne	Those involved in the manufacture of pesticides, wood preservatives, etc.

TABLE 7–1 • Examples of Environmental Acne in the Workplace

most important distinctions are lesion morphology and distribution and the timing of occurence.[7–10]

Individual lesions of chloracne consist primarily of comedones (blackheads and whiteheads) and cysts[8] (Fig. 7–3). Although these lesions also occur in acne vulgaris, the chief difference is the presence of inflammation in ordinary acne, especially the inflammatory papules and pustules in acne vulgaris.[11] Frank inflammation almost never

ful, as can topical and systemic antibiotics, which are prescribed as for regular acne.

CHLORACNE

Chloracne is the term used to describe a well-defined symptom complex consisting of acneiform lesions caused by exposure to various halogenated hydrocarbons. The condition was first described nearly a century ago by von Bettman[5] and was given its name and further detailed by Herxheimer.[6] Since then, numerous reports of chloracne have been published; causes lie in industrial and agricultural sources and also result from accidental environmental contamination and even from ingestion of contaminated food and food products.

Clinical Findings

Chloracne shares some features of ordinary acne vulgaris, but significant differences exist, and they permit separation of the two (Table 7–2). The

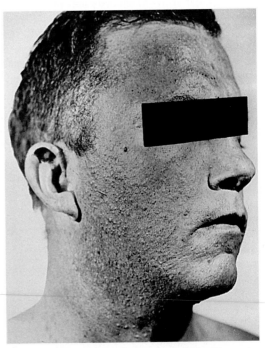

FIGURE 7–3 • Chloracne showing cysts, folliculitis, and hyperpigmentation in a transformer mechanic.

TABLE 7–2 • Features of Acne Vulgaris and Chloracne

Feature	Acne Vulgaris	Chloracne
Exposure to chloracnegens	Absent	Present
Aggravation of acne within 2 to 8 weeks of exposure	Absent	Present
Inflammatory lesions	Present	Absent until late in course
Distribution	Central face, back, and chest	Malar crescent of face (crow's foot area), behind ears, axillae, scrotum; absence around nose
Age	Younger patients but rarely younger than 8 years old	Any age
Meibomian gland involvement	Absent	Present
Sebaceous glands	Present and active	Absent with "dry" features
Comedones	Smaller in size and number	Large straw-colored cysts, sheets of open and closed comedones

occurs in chloracne until very late in the course of the disease. In acne vulgaris, the cysts are usually red and tender; in chloracne, the cysts are predominantly straw-colored and noninflamed. Numerous tiny milial cysts are often found in chloracne, and some investigators have considered their presence a hallmark of the disease.

An additional difference between acne vulgaris and chloracne is the location of the lesions. Chloracne commonly involves the malar crescent, the "crow's feet" areas beside the eyes, and the retroauricular areas.[7] The nose is almost never involved in chloracne but is a common site in acne vulgaris.[12, 13] Chloracne occurs chiefly on exposed skin surfaces, but following intensified external or systemic exposure, lesions may appear in other regions, especially the genital area, groin, and axillae.[12, 13] In contrast, acne vulgaris is almost always limited to the face, neck, back, chest, and shoulders.

Chloracne usually begins several weeks or months after exposure, and new lesions may continue to appear even after exposure has ceased.[8, 14, 15] Any age group may be affected. Although chloracne may persist indefinitely, in cases with limited exposure, regression usually takes place within 4 to 6 months.[8, 14, 16] The classic pattern of the disease is the occurrence of noninflammatory comedones on the malar crescent and behind the ears and the appearance of numerous straw-colored cysts. With sparing of the nose, and the absence of inflamed papules and cysts, the diagnosis of chloracne is more likely. In severe cases, sheets of comedones may involve virtually every follicle, giving the skin a peculiar grayish cast.[13]

Hyperpigmentation is common, especially on the face, and in severe cases it may become generalized.[17] In persons affected by Yusho poisoning in Japan in 1968, pigmentation of the nails, lips,

and even mucous membranes was seen.[18] The pathogenesis of pigmentation is uncertain, but because chloracnegens are also irritants and may also cause irritant contact dermatitis, it has been thought that the cause is simply postinflammatory hyperpigmentation.

Porphyria cutanea tarda may follow exposure to tetrachlorodiabenzodioxin (TCDD),[19, 20] in which case the full spectrum of cutaneous manifestations is seen, including hyperpigmentation, hypertrichosis, milia, and vesicular, scarring lesions on the hands.[21]

Other cutaneous findings that often accompany chloracne include xerosis, follicular hyperkeratosis, conjunctivitis, and meibomian cysts.[8, 12, 13, 22, 23] Cutaneous erythema may also occur, most likely as a result of irritation. Photosensitivity has been suggested but not verified.[13]

Histopathology

The chief finding on biopsy is the plugging of hair follicles with keratotic debris. The absence of inflammation seen clinically is also found histologically. The sebaceous glands are absent or greatly reduced in size, and many are replaced with keratinous cysts.[24] Dilatation of the follicular infundibulum is a prominent histological finding.[25]

Chloracne as a Marker of Chemical Exposure

Chloracne has been called the most sensitive indicator of toxicity resulting from exposure to halogenated hydrocarbons.[26, 27] Its presence should prompt physicians to search for systemic toxicity, and it is important to remember that the external dose required to induce chloracne is much lower than that required to cause systemic poisoning,[28] which emphasizes the fact that chloracne may occur in the absence of systemic toxicity. Conversely, absence of chloracne suggests that systemic toxicity is highly unlikely.[12, 28]

Noncutaneous Effects of Halogenated Hydrocarbons

Liver damage with or without porphyria may occur as a result of exposure to halogenated hydrocarbons.[29, 30] It is important to remember that other causes of liver damage may account for hepatic findings in exposed individuals; for example, Tamburro[31] found that alcoholism and viral hepatitis, not exposure to chemicals, were the major causes of liver disease in a group of Vietnam war veterans, even though they had been exposed to Agent Orange (2,4-D and 2,4,5-T).

Peripheral neuropathy has been reported, especially in those persons with severe systemic exposure. Other nonspecific complaints, such as headaches, fatigue, irritability, and insomnia are difficult to confirm as having a relationship to exposure.[13, 15, 19, 32] Other reported noncutaneous findings include elevated levels of serum triglycerides and pulmonary changes such as bronchitis.

A major area of controversy is whether these agents are also carcinogenic. Tetrachlorodibenzodioxin (TCDD) has been demonstrated to be a carcinogen in rats and mice, but only at chronic, high-dose levels.[33, 34] Aylward[35] has declared that humans are far less sensitive than rats to the carcinogenic effects of TCDD. Collins et al.[36] reported increased mortality rates from soft-tissue sarcomas and bladder and respiratory cancers in workers exposed to 4-aminobiphenyl, but they were unable to rule out confounding factors. In that study, no worker who was exposed only to TCDD showed any increased cancer risk. Following the 1976 explosion of a large chemical plant in Seveso, Italy, the surrounding population was exposed to TCDD.[37, 38] In a 10-year follow-up study, there appeared to be a slight increase in death from leukemia (relative risk, 2.2), but not from any other cancer.[39] Following accidental exposure of 1,583 workers to TCDD in a German chemical plant, a small increase in total cancer mortality was found (relative risk, 1.24), with a slightly higher risk in those workers with the longest exposure.[40] However, other long-term studies have shown no increase in cancer risk.[41–43]

The conclusion today is that dioxins appear to pose little, if any, risk of human carcinogenicity. Nevertheless, for a definitive answer on this issue, more extensive and longer-lasting studies should be done.

Chemicals Reported to Cause Chloracne

The various halogenated hydrocarbons reported to cause chloracne are shown in Table 7–3. Although the term "chloracne" has been well-established for nearly a century, it is now known that both chlorine- and bromine-containing compounds produce similar effects.

Contaminants in Polychlorophenol Compounds

Polychlorophenol compounds are the so-called dioxins, such as TCDD. Large amounts of these chlorinated phenolic compounds are produced worldwide and are used as insecticides, fungicides, herbicides, antiseptics, mold-inhibitors, dyes, and pigments.[13] At one time, exposure of workers was common, but today engineering controls and enclosed processes have greatly limited contact. Now most exposure is the result of industrial accidents and explosions, which affect not

 TABLE 7–3 • Chloracne-Producing Chemicals*

Polyhalogenated Naphthalenes*
  Polychloronaphthalenes
  Polycromonaphthalenes†

Polyhalogenated Biphenyls*
  Polychlorinated biphenyls (PCBs)
  Polybrominated biphenyls (PBBs)

Polyhalogenated Dibenzofurans*
  Polychlorodibenzofurans, especially tri-, tetra-, penta-, and hemachlorodibenzofurans
  Polybromodibenzofuran, especially tetrabromodibenzofuran

Contaminants of Polychlorophenol Compounds, Especially Herbicides
  (2,4,5-T and pentachlorophenol) and herbicide intermediates
  (2,4,5-troichlorophenol)
  2,3,7,8-Tetrachlorodibenzo-p-dioxin (TCDD)
  Hexachlorodibenzo-p-dioxin
  Tetrachlorodibenzofuran

Contaminants of 3,4-Dichloroaniline and Related Herbicides (Propanil, Methazole, etc.)
  3,4,3′,4′-Tetrachloroazoxybenzene
  e,r,e′,4′-Tetrachloroazobenzene

Others
  1,2,3,4-Tetrachlorobenzene (experimental)
  Dichlobenil (Casoron), a herbicide (clinical only)
  DDT (crude trichlorobenzene)†

*Polychlorodibenzofurans and hexachloronaphthalenes may occur as contaminants in some PCBs.
†Not confirmed as chloroacnegens.
From Taylor JS: Environmental acne update and review: Ann NY Acad Sci 320:295–307, 1979, with permission.

only workers but also individuals living in the vicinity of the factories. In Nitro, West Virginia, in 1949, and in Seveso, Italy, in 1976, major contaminations of the surrounding environment occurred[37, 44, 45]; the effects of those accidents have been summarized by Tindall.[13]

Dioxin exposure may also occur during the spraying of pesticides such as 2,4-D (2,3-dichlorophenoxyacetic acid) and 2,4,5-T (2,4,5-trichlorophenoxacetic acid), chemicals that were combined to make the herbicide Agent Orange during the Vietnam war. Agent Orange (and Agents Pink, Purple, and Green) contained from 0.02 to 15 parts per million of TCDD as a contaminant; thus, large numbers of American and other soldiers and the civilian population were exposed to these agents.[46]

A dioxin-containing oil was sprayed on roadways at Times Beach, Missouri, to control dust. As a result, the entire area had to be evacuated and long-lasting lawsuits were filed.[47] The contaminated land was finally purchased by the U.S. government.

Pentachlorophenol (PCP) is also reported to be a chloracnegen. A widely used fungicide, bactericide, herbicide, and wood preservative, it can be contaminated with various dioxins, but because it is very irritating to mucous membranes, chronic exposure is not likely.

The toxicity of dioxins increases with the increasing halogenation of the molecule. The half-life of TCDD is very long, approximately 7.5 years.[35] Routes of entry include inhalation, ingestion, and percutaneous penetration, but because dioxins are not especially volatile, inhalation is unlikely except in situations where there is direct exposure such as working in confined spaces or spraying the chemical.[12, 13] Sources of dioxin exposure are shown in Table 7–4.

TABLE 7–4 • Sources of Dioxin Exposure

Activity	Chemical
Spraying herbicides	2,4,5-T
Manufacturing herbicides	Various chlorinated phenolins
	Hexachlorophene
	Wood preservatives
Transformer accidents	Polychlorinated biphenyls
	Pentachlorophenol
Ship-building	Chlorinated naphthalenes
Eating fish from contaminated waters	

Polyhalogenated Biphenyls

Polyhalogenated biphenyls (PCBs, PBBs) are a complex group of chemicals that includes various hexachloronaphthalenes and polychlorodibenzofurans.[48, 49] Widely used since the late 1920s, they are usually found at low levels in the environment and mostly in closed systems such as electrical transformers.[13]

Two major incidents of poisoning with PCBs have occurred, both in Asia: the Yusho incident in 1968 in Japan and the Yu-Cheng incident in 1979 in Taiwan. In both, cooking oil was contaminated with PCBs.[18, 50] The dermatological manifestations were prominent early in the course of the outbreaks—chloracne and hyperpigmentation of face, mucous membranes, and nails.[51] Although the mucocutaneous manifestations improved over time in most patients, their systemic complaints increased.[13] In the Yu-Cheng incident, one-third of the children who were exposed transplacentally or through breast milk were found to have nail abnormalities, which became the most persistent cutaneous finding even 11 years after the event.[52]

In 1973 in Michigan, cattle feed was found to be contaminated with PBBs from a flame-retardant called Firemaster BP-6.[53] Many of the animals died or had to be destroyed, and contamination of humans occurred as a result of handling the feed or consuming dairy products. Chloracne was found in 13% of workers in plants that manufactured Firemaster BP-6 and in 3% of the exposed farm workers, as well.[9]

A 1981 building fire in Binghamton, New York, exposed firefighters and clean-up workers to PCBs as well as to combustion products that contained dioxins and dibenzofurans.[54] Exposure levels were low, and chloracne was not found in the workers.

Chloracne has been reported as a result of various other occupational PCB exposures, particularly among those who work with chemicals, such as the makers of electrical capacitors.[55]

Polychlorinated Dibenzofurans

Chlorinated phenols may be contamined with polychlorinated dibenzofurans (PCDFs), chemicals that were present in the cooking oil in the Yusho incident. Tindall[13] reported that these chemicals were no longer manufactured because of their extreme toxicity, but in 1994 Coenraads et al.[56] found high levels of PCDFs in the blood of workers in a Chinese factory where PCP was made. These workers also showed high levels of polychlorodibenzodioxins.

Halogenated Naphthalenes

Sold under the trade name Halowax, halogenated naphthalenes have been used for years as insulation waxes in the electronics industry, in lubricants, wood preservatives, metal coatings, and wire coverings and as sealing compounds such as for boat hulls.[9, 57] In 1970 Crow found these chemicals to be more acnegenic as fumes than as solids.[7] The most acnegenic were the pentachloronaphthalenes and hexachloronaphthalenes; those with more or less chlorine were not acnegenic.[24, 58] Kleinfeld et al. studied workers exposed to these chemicals at an electric plant. Of 59 workers, 56 had skin lesions that were thought to be chloracne caused by exposure to chlorinated naphthalenes. Other complaints included eye irritation, pruritus, headache, and fatigue.[57]

Other Chemicals

In 1977, Taylor reported chloracne caused by exposure to tetrachloroazooxybenzene (TCAB), a chemical intermediary used in the manufacture of an herbicide.[16] Of workers, 41 of 47 developed chloracne, as did 4 of their family members who had never been in the plant, most likely from exposure to the workers' clothing. Poland et al.[59] found that TCAB is similar to TCDD in its ability to induce chloracne.

After accidental exposure to dichloraniline derivatives, 17 workers developed chloracne 6 to 12 weeks after exposure. Xerosis and folliculitis were common complaints among these workers.[22]

Chloracne has been reported to have erupted in a research chemist during work with dihydrotrifluoromethylphenol benzothiopyranopyrazolone, which was being developed as an antirheumatic agent.[15] In addition to treatment-resistant chloracne, the chemist developed a severe sensory neuropathy, bursitis, and abnormal liver enzymes.

Treatment of Chloracne

Chloracne is markedly resistant to treatment.[9, 13, 15, 60] The usual treatments for acne vulgaris, such as oral and topical antibiotics and peeling agents, are of little value in treating chloracne, which is to be expected because the pathogeneses of the two conditions are so different. Berkers et al.[61] have shown in vitro that retinoids effectively block the ability of TCDD to induce the terminal differentiation of keratinocyte, suggesting that topical and systemic retinoids such as tretinoin, isotretinoin, and others could be of value in treating this condition.

Using EMLA cream (Astra Corp., Westborough, MA) a eutectic mixture of lignocaine and prilocaine, followed by light cautery, Yip et al. reported successful management of six patients with chloracne, even after only one or two treatments.[62] No evidence of scarring was seen after 24 months.

References

1. Plewig G, Braun-Falco O. Treatment of comedones in Favré-Rachouchot disease and acne venenata with vitamin A acid. *Hautartz* 1971;22:341–345.
2. Litt JZ. McDonald's acne. *Arch Dermatol* 1974;110:956.
3. Mills OH Jr, Kligman AM. Acne mechanica. *Arch Dermatol* 1975;111:481–483.
4. Kligman AM, Mills ON Jr. Acne cosmetica. *Arch Dermatol* 1972;106:843–853.
5. Von Bettman S. Chlorakne ein besondere Form Von professioneller Hauterkrankung. *Disch Med Wochenschr* 1901;27:437.
6. Herxheimer K. Weitere Mitteilungen über Chlorakne. VII Dermat. kougr. Breslau, Germany: 1901:152.
7. Crow KD. Chloracne: a critical review including a comparison of two series of acne from chloronaphthalene and pitch fumes. *Trans St. Johns Hosp Derm Soc* 1970;56:79–99.
8. Crow KD. Chloracne and its potential clinical implications. *Clin Exp Dermatol* 1981;6:243–257.
9. Taylor JS. Environmental chloracne: update and overview. *Ann NY Acad Sci* 1979;320:296–307.
10. Veterans Administration Chloracne Task Force. *Guidelines for the Diagnosis of Chloracne.* 1984.
11. Webster GF. Inflammation in acne vulgaris. *J Am Acad Dermatol* 1995;33:247–253.
12. Zugerman C. Chloracne: clinical manifestations and etiology. *Dermatol Clin* 1990;8:209–213.
13. Tindall JP. Chloracne + chloracnegens. *J Am Acad Dermatol* 1985;13:539–558.
14. May G. Chloracne from the accidental production of tetrachlorodibenzo-dioxin. *Br J Ind Med* 1973;30:276–283.
15. Scerri L, Zaki I, Millard LG. Severe halogen acne due to a trifluoromethylpyrazole derivative and its resistance to isotretinoin. *Br J Dermatol* 1995;132:144–148.
16. Taylor JS, Wuthrich RC, Lloyd KM, et al. Chloracne from the manufacture of a new herbicide. *Arch Dermatol* 1977;113:616–619.
17. Moore JA. Toxicity of 2,3,7,8-TCCD. *Ecol Bll* (Stockh) 1978;27:134–144.
18. Kurasune M, Yoshimura J, Matsuzaka J, et al. Epidemiologic study on Yusho, a poisoning caused by ingestion of a rice oil contaminated with a commercial branch of polychlorinated biphenyls. *Environ Health Perspect* 1972;1:119–128.
19. Jirasek L, Kalensky K, Kubec J, et al. Acne chlorina, porphyria cutanea tarda and other manifestations of general intoxication during the manufacture of herbicides. II. *Cestra Dermatol* 1974;49:145–157.
20. Bleiberg J. Industrially acquired porphyria. *Arch Dermatol* 1964;89:793–799.
21. Jund G, Konietzko J, Reill-Konietzko G, et al. Porphyrin studies in TCDD-exposed workers. *Arch Tox* 1994;68:595–598.
22. McDonaghi AJ, Gawkrodger DJ, Walker AE. Chloracne study of an outbreak with new clinical observations. *Clin Exp Dermatol* 1993;18:523–525.
23. Rosas Vasquez E, Campos Macias P, Ochoa Tirado J, et al. Chloracne in the 1900's. *Int J Dermatol* 1996;35:643–645.
24. Hambrick GW. The effects of substituted naphthalenes on the pilosebaceous apparatus of rabbit and man. *J Invest Dermatol* 1957;28:89–103.
25. Moses M, Prioleu PG. Cutaneous histologic findings in chemical workers with and without past exposure to

2,3,4,7,8 tetrachlorodibenzo-*p*-dioxin. *J Am Acad Dermatol* 1985;12:497–506.

26. Crow KD. Significance of cutaneous lesions in the symptomatology of exposure to dioxins and other chloracnegens. In: Tucker RE et al., eds. *Human and Environmental Risks of Chlorinated Dioxins and Related Compounds.* New York: Plenum Publishing; 1983:605–612.

27. Suskind RR. The "hallmark" of dioxin intoxication. *Scand J Work Environ Health* 1985;11:165–168.

28. Crow KD. Chloracne: an up-to-date assessment. *Ann Occup Hyg* 1978;21:297–298.

29. Kimbrough RD. The toxicity of polychlorinated polycyclic compounds and related chemicals. *Crit Rev Toxicol* 1974;2:445–498.

30. Goldman PJ. Severe acute chloracne. A mass intoxication by 2,3,6,7-tetrachlorobenzodioxin. *Hautarzt* 1973;24:149–152.

31. Tamburro CH. Chronic liver injury in phenoxy herbicide exposed Viet Nam veterans. *Environ Res* 1992;59:175–188.

32. Poland AP, Smith D, Metter G, Possick P. A health survey of workers in a 2,4D and 2m,4,5-T plant. *Arch Environ Health* 1971;22:316–327.

33. Kociba RJ, Keyes DG, Beyer JE, et al. Results of a two-year chronic toxicity and oncogenecity study of 2,3,7,8-tetrachlorodibenzo-*p*-dioxin in rats. *Toxicol Appl Pharmacol* 1978;46:279–303.

34. Poland A, Palen D, Glover E. Tumor promotion by TCDD in skin of ITRS/hairless mice. *Nature* 1982;300:271–273.

35. Aylward LL, Hays SM, Karch NJ, Paustenbach DJ. Relative susceptibility of animals and humans to the cancer hazard posed by 2,3,7,8-tetrachlorodibenzo-*p*-dioxin using internal measures of dose. *Environ Sci Tech* 1996;30:3534–3543.

36. Collins JJ, Strauss ME, Levinskas GJ, Conner PR. The mortality experience of workers exposed to 2,3.7.8-tetrachlorodibenzo-*p*-dioxin in a trichlorophenol process accident. *Epidemiology* 1993;4:7–13.

37. Hay A. Toxic cloud over Seveso. *Nature* 1976;262:636–638.

38. Reggiani G. Medical problems raised by the TCDD contamination in Seveso, Italy. *Arch Toxicol* 1978;40:161–188.

39. Bertrazzi PA, Zocchetti C, Pesatori C, et al. Mortality of a young population after accidental exposure to 2,3,7,8-tetrachlorodibenzodioxin. *Int J Epidemiol* 1992;21:118–123.

40. Manz A, Berger J, Dwyer JH, et al. Cancer mortality among workers in a chemical plant contaminated with dioxin. *Lancet* 1991;338:959–964.

41. Zack A, Suskind RR. The mortality experience of workers exposed to tetrachlorodibenzodioxin in a trichlorophenol-process accident. *J Occup Med* 1980;22:11–14.

42. Thiess AM, Frentzel-Beyme R, Link R. Mortality study of persons exposed to dioxin in a trichlorophenol-process accident that occurred in the BASF AG on November 17, 1953. *Am J Ind Med* 1982;3:179–183.

43. Dalderup LM, Zellenrath D. Dioxin exposure: 20-year follow-up. *Lancet* 1982;2:1134–1135.

44. Ashe W, Suskind RR. Chloracne cases of the Monsanto Chemical Company, Nitro, West Virginia. In: *Reports of the Kettering Laboratory.* Cincinnati: University of Cincinnati, October 1949, April 1950, July 1953.

45. Pocchiari F, Silano V, Zampieri A. Human health effects from accidental release of tetrachlorodiabenzo-*p*-dioxin

(TCDD) at Seveso, Italy. *Ann NY Acad Sci* 1979;320:311–320.

46. Council on Scientific Affairs. The health effects of "Agent Orange" and polychlorinated dioxin contaminants: technical report. American Medical Association; October 1981:1–2.

47. Sun M. Missouri's costly dioxin lesson. *Science* 1983;219:367–369.

48. Kimbrough RD. Toxicity of chlorinated hydrocarbons and related compounds. *Arch Environ Health* 1972;25:125–131.

49. Vos JG. Toxicology of PCBs for mammals and birds. *Environ Health Perspect* 1972;1:105–118.

50. Wong CR, Chen CJ, Cheng PC, Chen PH. Mucocutaneous manifestations of polychlorinated biphenyls (PCBs) poisoning: a study of 122 cases in Taiwan. *Br J Dermatol* 1982;107:327–333.

51. Urabe H, Koda H, Asahi M. Present state of Yusho patients. *Ann NY Acad Sci* 1979;320:273–276.

52. Hsu MM, Mak CP, Hsu CC. Follow-up of skin manifestations of Yo-Cheng children. *Br J Dermatol* 1995;132:427–432.

53. Carter LJ. Michigan PBB incident: chemical mix-up leads to disaster. *Science* 1976;192:240–243.

54. Schecter A. Contamination of an office building in Binghamton, New York, by PCB's, dioxins, furans, and diphenylenes after an electrical panel and electrical transformer incident. *Chemosphere* 1983;12:669–680.

55. Fischbein A, Wolff MS, Lilis R, et al. Clinical findings among PCB-exposed capacitor manufacturing workers. *Ann NY Acad Sci* 1979;320:703–715.

56. Coenraads PJ, Broower A, Olie K, Tano NJ. Chloracne, some recent issues. *Dermatol Clin* 1994;12:569–576.

57. Kleinfeld M, Messite J, Swencicki R. Clinical effects of chlorinated naphthalene exposure. *J Occup Med* 1972;14:377–379.

58. Shelley WB, Kligman AM. Experimental production of acne by penta- and hexachloronaphthalenes. *Arch Dermatol* 1972;75:689–695.

59. Poland A, Glover E, Kende AS, et al. 3,4,3′4′-Tetrachloroazoxybenzene and azobenzene: potent inducers of aryl hydrocarbon hydroxylase. *Science* 1977;194:627–630.

60. Taylor JS. Chloracne: a continuing problem. *Cutis* 1974;13:585–589.

61. Berkers JA, Hassing I, Spenkelink B, et al. Interactive effective of 2,3,7,8-tetrachlorodibenzo-*p*-dioxin and retinoids on proliferation and differentiation in cultured human keratinocytes: quantification of cross-linked envelope formation. *Arch Toxicol* 1995;69:368–378.

62. Yip J, Peppall L, Gawkrodger D, Cunliffe W. Light cautery and EMLA in the treatment of chloracne lesions. *Br J Dermatol* 1993;128:313–316.

Bibliography

Baader EW, Bauer HJ: Industrial intoxication due to pentachlorophenol. *Ind Med Surg* 1951;20:286–290.

Council on Scientific Affairs. The health effects of "Agent Orange" and dioxin contaminants. *JAMA* 1982;248:1985–1987.

Hirayama C. Clinical aspects of PCB poisoning. In: Higuchi K, ed. *PCB Poisoning and Pollution.* New York: Academic Press; 1976:97–99.

May G. Tetrachlorodibenzodioxin: a survey of subjects ten years after exposure. *Br J Med* 1982;39:128–135.

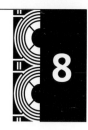

Occupational Skin Cancer

JOHN H. EPSTEIN, M.D.
ALICE ORMSBY, M.D.
ROBERT M. ADAMS, M.D.

Nonmelanoma skin cancers (NMSCs), basal cell carcinomas (BCCs), and squamous cell carcinomas (SCC) are by far the most common cancers that occur in the United States each year.[1] The American Cancer Society estimated that there would be 800,000 new NMSCs in the United States in 1996. Four-fifths of these would be BCCs and one-fifth would be SCCs.[2] However, these statistics appear to be low. Miller and Weinstock[3] estimated that there were between 900,000 and 1.2 million new NMSCs in the United States in 1994. This equaled the total number of cancers reported in all other organs in the body. In addition, these cancers have been increasing in incidence at a rapid rate in the past several decades in many parts of the world.[4-8] For example, Gallagher and coworkers[9] compared the incidence in the years 1971 to 1973 with the years 1985 to 1987. They noted an increased incidence in BCC of 60.6% in men and 48.4% in women and in SCC of 59.2% in men and 67.4% in women. The vast majority of these cancers occurred on the head and neck, supporting the importance of sun exposure as the causative stimulus, even in British Columbia, which receives much less sun than more southern latitudes. Indeed, we are in what has been considered a quiet 20th-century epidemic.[10]

The causative role of the sun in the induction of these growths was suggested by a number of astute clinical observations around the turn of the 20th century.[11-14] Since that time a large body of circumstantial evidence has been accumulated to support this concept. However, studies directly confirming this relationship as well as determination of the action spectrum, dose responses, energy requirements, relationships to chemical stimuli,

immune responsiveness, oncogene expression, and suppressor gene inactivity have been confined to experimental animal investigations, not only because of the impropriety of such experimentation in humans, but also because of impracticality.[15] Such tumor induction most likely would require 10 to 20 years or more of frequently repeated, closely monitored exposures.

Evidence for the relationship of skin cancer in humans to sunlight is derived primarily from epidemiological studies, which have become more exact in recent years.[16-18]

EXPERIMENTAL AND EPIDEMIOLOGICAL EVIDENCE

Action Spectrum

Although action spectrum studies are most difficult, even in experimental systems, the bulk of the data indicates that the primary carcinogenic action spectrum falls in the UVB range (290–320 nm)[15, 19] (Table 8–1). UVC (100–280 nm) can induce cutaneous cancers in experimental animals[20, 21] and also can transform mammalian cells in culture.[22-24] Because these rays do not reach the Earth from the sun, they have little relationship to human skin cancer. It should be noted, however,

TABLE 8–1 • Ultraviolet Spectra	
Wave	**Nanometer Range**
UVA	320 (315) − 400 nm
UVB	280 (290) − 320 nm (315 nm)
UVC	100 − 280 nm

that exposure to such rays does occur in certain industrial settings, including exposure to germicidal lamps[25] and welding arcs.[26] Such exposures could add to the carcinogenic influences of the sun. There is also evidence that UVA rays (320–400 nm) can augment UVB carcinogenesis and in large amounts may induce cancer formation by themselves.[27–29]

Physical Influences

Heat, wind, and humidity have been shown to accelerate photocarcinogenesis in experimental animals.[30–33] The tumor-promoting effects of physical stimuli, including freezing, scalding, and wounding, have been reported in chemically induced carcinogenesis.[15] The studies of Argyris[34] suggest that epidermal hyperplasia induced by cutaneous injury is responsible for these promoting effects in experimental chemical carcinogenesis.

There is evidence that chronic heat exposure induces precancerous and cancerous cutaneous changes in humans.[35–41] Dermal deposition of abnormal elastic fibers is a striking effect of chronic sun exposure. In areas of high insolation, infrared (as well as UV radiation) is increased in amount. Kligman[42] demonstrated that repeated infrared exposures alone will induce the formation of many fine feathery elastic fibers in mice. With UV radiation alone, numerous thick, twisted elastic fibers are seen in the dermis. The combination of UV and infrared radiation resulted in dense mat-like elastic fiber deposition that was much more notable than were changes produced by either form of radiation alone. Thus, it seems likely that these changes in human skin are due to injury by chronic infrared as well as UV radiation. Under certain circumstances it is impossible to separate the effects of thermal and mechanical or chemical stimuli in human skin.[43] The skin cancers on the legs of railway stokers were due to heat and mechanical trauma, and those on the abdomens of older women carrying earthenware pots of heated charcoal—called a kangri in Kashmir, a kang in China, and a kairo in Japan—next to their abdominal skin for warmth were caused by heat and chemical influences.

As noted, mechanical trauma can accelerate experimental chemical carcinogenesis.[34] The role it plays in human cutaneous carcinogenesis is not clear.[44]

Chemical Carcinogenesis

Although UV is the primary cause of human skin cancers, chemical agents appear to be responsible for at least some of these malignancies.[45] Studies of cutaneous chemical carcinogenesis in animal models have supplied important concepts for cancer pathogenesis in general. The monoclonal origin of most benign and malignant chemically induced skin tumors was noted.[46] Experimental skin carcinogenesis has been divided into three stages. The first phase, initiation, consists of an irreversible, heritable event that is most likely mutational in nature. This can be accomplished by a variety of stimuli, including several polycyclic hydrocarbons, alkylating agents, nitrosamines, and ultraviolet radiation.[45, 47] These stimuli are generally complete carcinogens and if applied in large enough amounts or repeatedly will supply the next two stages and result in cancer formation. The mechanism of initiation is interaction of the chemicals (and UV) or their metabolites with DNA.[48–53] Recent studies indicate that the initiating events are the result of or are associated with the activation of certain transforming proto-oncogenes.[49] It should be noted that physical carcinogens also activate similar proto-oncogenes.[28, 54, 55]

The second stage promotion can be accomplished by the application of a number of noncarcinogenic agents. These stimuli induce benign tumor formation in skin that has been treated with an initiator. All of these stimuli induce inflammation and hyperplasia. However, other agents that produce inflammation and hyperplasia are not tumor promoters. Thus, specific events must be induced by promoting stimuli. In the case of the phorbol ester 12-0-tetradecanoylphorbol (TPA) binding to and activation of membrane-associated protein kinase C is the essential step.[56, 57] Similarly, aplysiatoxin also promotes through protein kinase C activation. Other promoters such as anthralin and the peroxides function through other, as yet undetermined mechanisms.[58]

The third stage is the conversion of benign tumors into carcinomas. This is a spontaneous step that can be accelerated by the application, topically or systemically, of chemical mutagens that may be initiating agents.[59, 60] This may involve a genetic change in the benign tumor's cells.

Chemical Influences on Photocarcinogenesis

Chemicals can effect photocarcinogenesis in a number of ways. They can act as photosensitizers, as additive carcinogens, or as promoters. Again, knowledge of these processes derives primarily from animal experimentation.

The UVB rays (290–320 nm) bear primary responsibility for the acute and chronic effects (including skin cancers) of the sun on the skin. Photosensitizing chemicals with suitable action spectra can induce acute phototoxic reactions and, with repeated exposures, skin cancers with UVA radiation (320–400 nm) in amounts that normally do not produce such responses.[61–66] Clinical correlations with this carcinogenic effect have been demonstrated with 8-methoxypsoralen and UVA (PUVA) therapy of psoriasis.[67, 68]

The additive effects of a complete chemical carcinogen and UV-induced carcinogenesis were first demonstrated by showing initiation by means of a single application of dimethylbenzanthracene (DMBA) followed by repeated exposures to UVB radiation.[69, 70] Similar responses were noted when UVB was used as the initiator and was followed by DMBA.[71] Subsequently, an additive effect has been noted in the cases of a number of carcinogens, including nitrogen mustard[72, 73] and certain nitrosoureas.[74, 75]

Chemical promotion of UV-initiated carcinogenesis has also been demonstrated. In 1968[76] and 1970[77] croton oil was shown to promote UV-initiated carcinogenesis, and the effect was later confirmed.[78] In addition, TPA, the primary promoting molecule in croton oil, has been shown to promote PUVA-induced cancer formation[79] and all transretinoic acid has been shown to both promote and inhibit photocarcinogenesis.[80] Chemicals can also inhibit carcinogenesis. Sunscreens have been shown to inhibit photocarcinogenesis in experimental animals[42, 81] and precancerous actinic keratoses in people.[82, 83] Low dietary fat has also been shown to inhibit precancerous lesions and NMSC in human skin.[84, 85] Antioxidants have been shown to inhibit and accelerate both chemical- and UV-induced carcinogenesis in experimental animals.[86–95] Their effect, if any, on human cancer formation is also unclear. Interferons have been shown to have antitumor effects in experimental UV-induced tumors[96] as have a number of other naturally occurring and synthetic chemicals.[97] In addition to sunscreens and reduced dietary fat, retinoids, especially 13*cis*-retinoic acid[98–100] and indomethacin,[101] have demonstrated cancer prevention effects in humans.

Epidemiology

The epidemiological evidence that ultraviolet radiation from the sun is the primary cause of nonmelanoma skin cancers derives from several observations.[4, 17, 18, 102, 103]

1. Skin cancer occurs most commonly on the head, neck, arms, and hands.
2. Pigmented races who sunburn much less readily than do people with white skin have a much lower incidence of skin cancer, and, when

it does occur, it is not found predominantly on sun-exposed skin.
3. Skin cancers occur in people with white skin who spend more time out of doors than in those who work indoors.
4. Skin cancers are more common in white-skinned people who live in areas of high insolation.

Mechanisms of UV or Sun-induced Human Skin Cancers

How UV radiation induces skin cancers poses a most interesting question. Immune suppression such as occurs in kidney transplant patients leads to a high incidence of skin cancers, mostly SCC, in sun-exposed skin.[104, 105] Subcarcinogenic exposures to UVB rays prevent rejection of highly antigenic UVB-induced transplanted cancers due to the activation of specific suppressor T cells in experimental animals.[106, 107] In addition, an acute exposure to UVB radiation will induce tolerance to a subsequently topically applied antigen, again due to activation of specific suppressor T cells. As yet, no similar system has been described in humans. However, Yoshikawa et al.[108] reported on a group of people in whom previous UVB irradiation inhibited sensitization to DNCB, a very potent contact allergen. When compared with another similar group in whom previous UVB radiation did not prevent DNCB sensitization, they noted that 92% of those with skin cancers were in the former UVB-inhibited group. Thus, people with skin cancers may not have the immunological ability to reject their sun-induced skin cancers.

UV-induced DNA damage and repair are important issues when considering the role of the sun in skin cancer formation.[109, 110] Most of what is known of the functioning of this system in human skin derives from studies on the rare genetic disease xeroderma pigmentosum (XP).[111–113] Patients with this disorder have a defective DNA-repair enzyme system. In addition, they have an inordinate susceptibility to the carcinogenic effects of UV rays. Thus, it would seem reasonable to assume that the defects in DNA repair are responsible for this susceptibility. In addition, enhancing DNA repair does reduce the incidence of skin cancer in animal models.[114] However, definitive proof of this relationship in XP remains to be established. Also, there is no specific evidence that defects in DNA repair are responsible for sun-induced cancers in the general human population.

One of the most intriguing areas of interest concerns the relationship of oncogene activation and suppressor gene inactivation to human carcinogenesis.[54, 115–117] These genes are part of the normal genetic wiring that directs the growth and development of normal cells. However, they are susceptible to carcinogenic stimuli such as UV radiation, ionizing radiation, chemicals, and age. Such exposures can activate oncogenes to produce more of their normal gene products or to produce aberrant gene products or they may inactivate normal suppressor gene function. In addition, there is evidence that specific carcinogenic stimuli dictate the oncogene activation or the suppressor gene inactivation or both.[54, 115, 118] Along this line, Brash et al.[119] reported specific UV-induced mutations in the P53 suppressor gene in over 50% of the invasive SCC they studied. Campbell et al.[120] reported similar findings in Bowen's lesions, Nagano et al.[121] in actinic keratoses, and Nakazawa et al.[122] even in chronically sun-damaged skin without histological neoplasia. The SCCs studied indicate that these specifically UV-induced mutations are early events in sun-induced skin cancers.

MELANOMA

The third most common skin cancer is the malignant melanoma. This cancer makes up about 5% of all skin cancers but accounts for three-quarters of the deaths due to skin cancer. Melanomas account for 3% of all reportable cancers from all sites of the body in the United States and were estimated to be responsible for 2% of cancer deaths in men and 1% in women in 1996.[2] The American Cancer Society estimated that there would be 38,300 new melanomas in the United States in 1996, 21,800 in men and 16,500 in women.[2] This cancer was also estimated to cause 7,300 deaths in 1996, 4,600 in men and 2,700 in women. It is the seventh most common reportable cancer and is increasing in incidence more rapidly than any other reportable cancer in the United States. Indeed, its worldwide incidence is increasing faster than that of any other cancer.[123] The lifetime risk of developing a melanoma in the United States was 1 in 1,500 in 1930; in 1996, it was 1 in 87. And if it continues to rise at this 6% per year rate, it will reach 1 in 75 by the year 2000. The death rate also continues to rise at 2% per year. However, survival rates for stage I melanomas have increased from 50% in the 1950s to 90% at present. To put this into some perspective, the number of melanomas diagnosed in the United States in 1980 was 14,000; in 1989 it was 27,000, an increase of 94%. The population increased only 11% in that time period.[124]

As noted, the UV rays, primarily UVB rays, from the sun are the primary cause of nonmelanoma skin cancers. This is most notable for SCC, which has an almost one-to-one relationship to cumulative sun exposure.[125] Although the sun's rays do appear to have an important influence on melanoma formation, this association is much less clear than it is for nonmelanoma skin cancers.[1, 126, 127] However, Scotto and Fears[16] reported a statistically significant correlation between geographic UVB exposure and melanoma incidence. Epidemiological studies have suggested various possible patterns of relationship to the sun, ranging from excessive total sun exposure to intense intermittent exposures.[128, 129]

Experimentally, melanomas have been induced by nonionizing radiation or chemical carcinogens and promoters in a variety of animals, including rodents, marsupials, and fish.[1] Unfortunately none of these models has been satisfactory for determining the action spectrum, time-dose relationship, or mechanisms by which sunlight causes these cancers in human skin. It has been assumed that the more energetic UVB rays are primarily responsible for this response. However, recent epidemiological studies have noted a relationship to the use of artificial sun-tanning equipment and increased melanoma risk, which suggests that UVA may contribute as well.[130, 131]

In summary, a melanoma epidemic has been going on for several decades. Although sun exposure appears to play an important role, the reason for the increasing incidence is not completely understood. It appears likely that at least some of these tumors are industrial in origin.[132]

OCCUPATIONAL CANCER

Occupational cancer is a malignancy that results from exposure to carcinogenic forces in an occupational environment.

The first notation of an occupational cancer was written by Percival Pott in 1775 when he described scrotal cancers in English chimney sweeps. They were caused by the friction and soot that the sweepers were exposed to in the course of their work. Interestingly, as late as 1955, such cancers were reported in chimney sweeps.[133]

Incidence

As noted, approximately 900,000 to 1.2 million new cases of nonmelanoma skin cancer from all causes occur in the United States each year.[3] This makes up about 50% of cancers in all sites that occurred in a given year, and they are continuing to increase in incidence rapidly. Approximately 3% of all cancers that occur each year are melanomas, excluding nonmelanoma skin cancer and carcinoma in situ.[2] It has been estimated that 70 to 90% of human cancers are likely to be caused by environmental factors.[134] However, the importance of occupational exposures is probably far less significant than are other factors, such as smoking, for certain cancers.[135]

Data concerning the incidence of occupational skin cancer are more readily obtained in countries where there is greater efficiency in reporting all occupational injuries and illnesses. Unfortunately, good data for the United States are wanting. In the United Kingdom, where incidence data are reported and tabulated with reasonable accuracy each year, occupational skin cancer accounts for less than 1% of all skin cancers.[136]

Nevertheless, certain cancers can easily be related to occupational exposure. Angiosarcoma of the liver, which occurs in workers exposed to the monomer of polyvinyl chloride, has been directly related to a specific occupation: the cleaning of the vats in which the monomer is manufactured.[137] Scrotal cancers have long been considered almost entirely occupational.[138] Workers in the manufacturing of dyestuffs such as benzidine and derivatives have been known for decades to have an increased incidence of bladder cancer.[139] Among men 20 to 74 years old, approximately 20% of bladder cancer is caused by an occupational exposure.[140] Selikoff et al.[141] clearly showed a relationship between asbestos exposure and lung carcinoma, which they found to be greatly enhanced by cigarette smoking.

More often, however, a predominant risk factor cannot be identified, probably because several factors operate at approximately the same level of influence. An example may be mycosis fungoides, for which Cohen et al.[142, 143] showed data that suggest that it occurs more commonly among persons who work in manufacturing and construction. Genetic factors may also be important, as demonstrated by the prevalence of skin cancer in fair-skinned persons, particularly those of Celtic descent. Deeply pigmented individuals, especially African-Americans, rarely develop actinic skin cancer, regardless of the amount and duration of sunlight exposure. As already noted, a striking example of the influence of heredity is XP in which defective enzymes cause incomplete DNA repair following ultraviolet exposure, which leads ultimately to multiple skin cancers of a particularly aggressive nature.[109–113, 144, 145]

Immunological factors are also important. Immunological control has become a popular concept in cancer research in recent years, and alterations in immunological characteristics have provided methods of cancer identification.

Experimentally, antilymphocyte serum has been shown to accelerate UVR-induced tumor formation.[146] Clinically, immunosuppression that has been induced for organ transplantation has also been associated with sunlight-induced squamous cell carcinomas.[104, 147–149] This is usually noted after 5 years of immune suppression. In contrast, Ferrandiz and coworkers[150] reported a high incidence of cutaneous malignancy, mainly BCCs, in the early posttransplant period. Occupational sun exposure was an important risk factor in the development of these lesions. We were unable to detect any acceleration of UV carcinogenesis when methotrexate or hydroxyurea was administered in low doses over long periods of time, as they might be in the treatment of benign diseases such as psoriasis, and this has also been noted under clinical conditions.[151, 152]

Perhaps the most exciting of the immunological relationships to cutaneous carcinogenesis is the experimental demonstration that chronic subcarcinogenic doses of UVR result in the susceptibility of mice to transplanted, highly antigenic UVR-induced cancers.[106] This effect appears to result from the production of suppressor T cells with antigen specificities directed toward specific UV-induced tumor antigens. This may be one of the mechanisms that allows sun-induced tumors to occur and grow in human skin.

Etiology of Occupational Skin Cancer

Polycyclic hydrocarbons derived from oil, gasoline, kerosene, lubricating oils, cutting oils, paraffin waxes, pitch, and tars have been considered the primary industrial carcinogens. A minority of reported work-related cancers have been associated with inorganic metals and chemicals, physical burns and trauma, and ionizing and nonionizing radiation. However, it seems most likely that the primary cause of occupational skin cancer is the primary cause of skin cancer in general—that is, nonionizing radiation from the sun. Also, combinations of carcinogenic stimuli are probably of the utmost importance (Fig. 8–1).

Skin cancer occurs significantly more frequently in outdoor than in indoor workers,[153–157] especially those with light skin, light eye color, and light hair color who sunburn easily and tan poorly. Persons of Celtic descent appear to be particularly vulnerable, possibly even in the absence of these phenotypic characteristics.[17, 102, 158] It is more common in men than women because of occupation categories and also because of the use of protective cosmetics by women. Thus, agricultural workers, sailors, ski instructors, tennis professionals, and the like are at greater risk for developing nonmelanoma skin cancers than are

FIGURE 8–1 • Chronic severe actinic skin changes in a 63-year-old man who worked for many years in Southern California oil fields. The combination of oil and sunlight accelerated his disease.

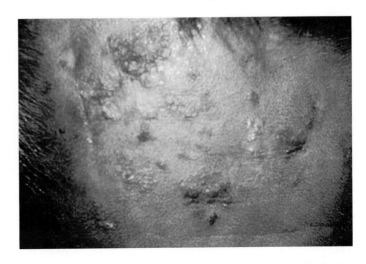

office or other indoor workers. However, there are indoor sources of occupational exposure to UV radiation.[159] Table 8–2 lists many of the workers at risk for UV-induced cancers. Some of these sources of UV, such as arc welding, plasma torches, and germicidal ultraviolet lamps, emit significant amounts of UVC energy as well as some UVB energy.[25, 26, 159, 160] This energy has been shown to be carcinogenic in experiments, but its exact role in occupationally induced skin cancers is not clear.[148] Emmett et al.[161] detected no rela-

tionship between arc welding and precancerous or cancerous skin lesions.

Clinical Features

Nonmelanoma skin cancers, the common malignancies induced by sun exposure, are primarily epidermal in origin, that is, they are either basal cell carcinomas or squamous cell carcinomas. They represent distinct malignancies that differ not only in their microscopic anatomy but also in

TABLE 8–2 • Workers Potentially Exposed to Ultraviolet Radiation

Natural Sunlight	**Arc Welding Ultraviolet**
Agricultural workers	Welders
Brick masons	Pipeline workers
Ranchers	Pipecutters
Construction workers	Maintenance workers
Farmers	
Fishermen	**Plasma Torch Ultraviolet**
Gardeners	Plasma torch operators
Greenskeepers	
Horticultural workers	**Germicidal Ultraviolet**
Landscapers	Physicians
Lifeguards	Nurses
Lumberjacks	Laboratory technicians
Military personnel	Bacteriology laboratory personnel
Oilfield workers	Barbers
Open-pit miners	Cosmetologists
Outdoor maintenance workers	Kitchen workers
Pipeline workers	
Police officers	**Laser Ultraviolet**
Postal carriers	Laboratory workers
Railroad track workers	
Road workers	**Drying and Curing Processes**
Sailors	Printers
Ski instructors	Lithographers
Sports players	Painters
Surveyors	Wood curers
	Plastics workers
	Food irradiation workers

their biological growth patterns, ability to metasta-size, and association with sun exposure. Sun-in-duced prenonmelanoma skin cancers include ac-tinic keratoses and, at times, keratoacanthomas.

Actinic keratoses have been characterized as grade ½ squamous cell carcinomas with irregular proliferation, individual cell keratinization, loss of cellular polarity, increased density of the nuclear chromatin pattern, irregular loss of basement membrane staining, and increased mitoses.[162] These keratoses are caused by sun exposure and so are found exclusively in sun-exposed skin. If untreated, a small number will progress to squa-mous cell carcinomas.[163, 164] These generally are not aggressive cancers, and metastases occur in less than 0.5%.[165, 166] The incidence of squamous cell carcinomas of the lower lip is higher in out-door workers at least in part because of UV radia-tion, though other factors may play a role.[167] This is a much more aggressive tumor and 10 to 16% metastasize.[10, 164]

Squamous cell carcinomas are invasive cancers that can usually be differentiated from basal cell carcinomas histologically by a more eosinophilic staining tint with hematoxylin and eosin stain (H&E) due to partial or complete keratinization. More advanced SCCs may not keratinize, so the cells will be stained darker, but they will have more atypicality and mitotic figures than BCCs, which are characterized by darkly stained cells that commonly separate in masses from the sur-rounding stroma. This separation is an artifact of fixation, but it is characteristic of this tumor. With very few exceptions, these tumors do not metasta-size.

Basal cell carcinomas are much more common than squamous cell carcinomas; about 80% of nonmelanoma skin cancers are BCCs.[4] SCCs ac-count for only 20% of such tumors, but they are responsible for three-quarters of the deaths due to nonmelanoma skin cancer.[168] These two cancers differ in their relationship to sun exposure, as well. SCC occurs most commonly on the face, head, and neck, especially in males, followed by involvement of the upper extremities and the legs of women. Generally, BCC is four times more common than SCC in men and six times more common in women. The incidence of cancers of both cell types increases with decreasing latitude and, presumably, greater UVB exposure. How-ever, SCCs increase in incidence to a much greater degree,[4, 125] which supports the distinct relationship of SCC to sun exposure (Fig. 8–2).

Scotto et al.[4] reported that in 81.2% of men and 84.1% of women, BCCs occur on the head and neck, and in 12% of men and 8.9% of women, they occur on the trunk. It has been estimated that

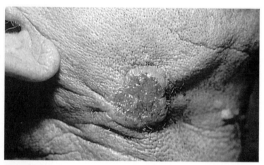

FIGURE 8–2 • Squamous cell carcinoma on the neck, induced by chronic sun exposure.

about one third of BCCs on the face, head, and neck occur in customarily shaded areas, whereas SCCs occur in the most heavily exposed areas.[169] Thus, some other factors in addition to the sun must play a role.

The relationship of sun exposure and malignant melanoma is not so clear. Hutchinson's precancer-ous melanosis occurs on the face primarily, is associated with chronic actinic damage, and is undoubtably caused by the sun's rays. Therefore, the slow-growing melanomas that occur in these lesions are caused by the sun. The melanomas that occur in patients with XP are also caused by the sun. In addition, melanomas have been induced in experimental animals by UV radiation.[88, 170] Thus, it is reasonable to consider that UV rays stimulate melanoma formation and progression. However, it seems unlikely that the sun is the single cause of the increasing incidence of melanoma, even though it may be one of a number of factors involved.[78]

Beral and Robinson[153] reported that outdoor work was associated with melanomas of the head, face, and neck as were squamous cell carcinomas and basal cell carcinomas. In contrast, indoor of-fice work was associated with melanomas of the trunk and limbs.[171, 172] This suggests that prolonged occupational exposure to sunlight is an important cause of melanomas of the head, face, and neck as well as of nonmelanoma skin cancer. It is of interest that the high rate of melanomas of the trunks and limbs in office workers contrasts not only with the rate found in outdoor workers but also with the rate in other indoor workers, who generally have a low rate of all forms of skin can-cer.

The data concerning indoor and outdoor work-ers suggest that sunlight does not play a role in melanomas other than those of the head, face, and neck. However, Austin and Reynolds[132] reported that other factors, such as the exposure to unusual chemicals of petrochemical workers and chemists and the exposure to PCBs or ionizing radiation, may be in play, although the data is somewhat fragmented as yet. Pion and coworkers[173] found no difference in melanoma incidence in indoor and outdoor workers, but they did note that white-collar workers and workers with upper-pay-scale jobs had an increased incidence of melanomas. Among specific occupational exposures, only x-rays significantly raised the melanoma risk. Carpenter et al.[174] also reported an increased risk of melanomas and NMSC associated with ionizing radiation in three U.K. nuclear workforces. Hardell and associates[175] reported an increased risk of developing melanomas associated with occupational exposure to low-frequency electromagnetic fields.

Similar to the findings of Pion et al.,[173] Streetly and Markowe[176] reported that the mortality rates were higher in men with nonmanual occupations than in those with manual occupations, at least into the early 1980s. This appears to reflect social class rather than occupation. A report from Scotland noted that the incidence of melanoma was much higher in wealthy than in poor men and women;[177] however, the mortality rate was the opposite.

The relationship of melanoma to occupational sun exposure is not clear. Pion et al.[173] found no difference in incidence between indoor and outdoor workers, but Nelemans et al.[178] reported that sun-sensitive indoor workers had a higher relative risk of developing a melanoma than did outdoor workers as a whole. This study supported the theory of intermittent sun exposure. Wiklund and Dich[179] found no increased incidence in either NMSC or melanomas in 140,208 Swedish farmers, and farmers in Alberta, Canada, were found to have a considerably lower risk for developing melanomas than were nonfarmers.[180]

In contrast, other investigators noted an increased incidence of melanomas as well as of cancers of the lip among farmers.[181, 182] Delzell and Grufferman[155] noted an increase in melanoma-induced mortality in nonwhite as well as in white farmers in North Carolina. They did not note the distribution of the lesions. Miller and Beaumont[183] reported that mortality from melanomas was higher in male veterinarians than in the general population. In summary, the relationship of melanoma formation to occupational exposures remains unclear.

The keratoacanthoma is usually a benign, self-limited tumor of the epidermis that is characterized by rapid growth and downward regular extension of epithelial squamous cells.[184] The tumor evolves with a central keratinization process that appears to destroy the growth. There are three clinical forms—the solitary growth, which is the most common; the multiple form (Ferguson-Smith), which is quite uncommon; and the eruptive form, which is rare. The solitary keratoacanthoma may have an occupational origin. It usually begins after 45 years of age, and men are more commonly affected than women. A number of environmental factors appear to play causative roles. Exposure to sun and tar and oil products, mechanical trauma, burns, and the like are among the potential occupation-environment factors. These lesions commonly occur on sun-exposed skin of the head, neck, and upper extremities, which are sites exposed to other carcinogenic stimuli. Though most are benign in behavior, a small number of lesions follow a progressive course and occasionally metastasize.

Evaluation and Prevention

In evaluating workers with actinic skin damage, including carcinoma, that is suspected to be of occupational origin, the physician must determine how much time the patient actually spends exposed to ultraviolet light while at work in relation to that spent during nonoccupational activities, especially recreational pursuits. A thorough occupational history must be obtained, including the first job after leaving school as well as the activities engaged in as a child and teenager. Nonoccupational pursuits, particularly sports and hobbies, can be significant. After this information is obtained, it may be possible to arrive at a decision regarding the significance of work-related exposure to ultraviolet radiation. Physicians are often asked to make such a determination and to consider actinic damage as "cumulative trauma" which, of course, it is.

Prevention of skin cancer due to UV radiation depends primarily on protection. Special attention to protection should be paid by those at high risk—phenotypically light-complexioned people and genotypically vulnerable people, including those of Scottish, Irish, or Welsh descent and, of course, individuals with XP, albinism, or extensive vitiligo, who should avoid outdoor occupations altogether and indoor jobs in which they are exposed to UV radiation.

Protection consists of wearing tightly woven clothing and wide-brimmed hats and avoiding the midday sun whenever possible. Sunblocks that contain particulate materials, such as zinc oxide and titanium dioxide, reflect the sun's rays. These can be quite effective if used in high enough concentrations, but that is generally cosmetically unacceptable. In contrast, sunscreens absorb the UV rays and can be used in lotions or creams that are essentially invisible.[185] These preparations contain *para*-aminobenzoic acid (PABA), PABA esters, benzophenones, cinnamates, salycylates, and anthralates in alcohol gels or solutions, moisturizing lotions, or creams. These agents in various combinations can be formulated to provide sun protective factors ranging from 2 to 50 or more. The sun protective factor (SPF) is defined as the amount of UVB energy required to induce a minimal erythema (MED) with the sunscreen in place divided by the MED without the sunscreen protection. Thus, if a person requires 20 minutes of noonday sun to induce a minimal erythema, a sunscreen with an SPF of 15 would allow the individual to remain out of doors for 5 hours before developing this degree of reaction. Since the UVB rays are generally minimal before 10 a.m. and after 3 p.m., such a sunscreen would be quite effective for most people. However, for those who are more sensitive, the more potent sunscreens might be of value. Using a sunscreen with an SPF of less than 15 has no place in the concept of photoprotection. Potent PABA-free sunscreens can be used if the person is allergic to PABA. Experimental evidence has established that the use of sunscreens does inhibit photocarcinogenesis and photodamage to dermal connective tissue in animal models.[42, 81]

Studies have shown that the consistent use of a good sunscreen reduces the formation of precancerous solar keratoses.[82, 83] Because UVA can augment UVB carcinogenesis and can even be photocarcinogenic in itself, the incorporation of UVA absorbers is of value. Higher concentrations of benzophenones reduce UVA penetration of sunscreens, and a group of molecules, the dibenzoyl methanes, have significant UVA absorption characteristics.[186, 187] It should be noted that sunscreen preparations have varying substantivity properties. Some remain intact despite significant exposure to water such as swimming. These are said to be waterproof. Others are moderately resistant to washing off and are called water resistant, whereas others do not resist water well at all. It is probably a good idea to reapply sunscreens after swimming or sweating or at 1- to 2-hour intervals at midday, because mechanical removal is common.

Career counselors should be aware of the possible presence of genetic diseases that predispose an individual to the development of actinic skin cancer, such as albinism, XP, Celtic genes, and others. Gallagher and coworkers[188] reported that subjects with pale skin and red hair have an elevated risk of developing SCCs. Subjects whose mothers are of southern European ancestry have a reduced risk of developing SCCs. From an occupational point of view, there was a strong trend for increasing risk with increased chronic occupational sun exposure in the 10 years prior to the diagnosis of the first SCC. Table 8–2 lists many of the occupations in which workers are exposed to large amounts of sunlight.

POLYCYCLIC AROMATIC HYDROCARBONS

When Percival Pott observed the high frequency of scrotal cancers in London chimney sweeps, the cancers were considered to be caused by exposure to soot, lack of protective clothing, and poor personal hygiene. In the next century it was recognized that a number of coal tar products and certain forms of mineral oil used in industry could cause cutaneous cancers.[189]

Schwartz and his coauthors believed that coal tar and its derivatives were the most frequent causes of occupational cancer, with 35% caused by tar, 54% by pitch, and 5% by heavy tar oil. Gas works contributed 70% of the cases and coke ovens about 5%.[43]

Although it seems clear that radiation from the sun is the primary cause of occupationally induced skin cancers, coal tar and petroleum products play an important role in work-related carcinogenesis. These products include tar, pitch, carbon black (soot), creosote, crude paraffin, asphalt, and mineral oil from coal, petroleum, and shale. The complex mixtures contain polycyclic aromatic hydrocarbons, which can act as initiators and promoters of carcinogenesis,[36, 190–193] and noncarcinogenic accelerators, such as n-dodecane and certain phenols and catechols that can promote cancer formation. Studies have established that exposure of mammalian skin to tar solutions induces aryl hydrocarbon hydroxylase (AHH) activities.[41] AHH is one of the cytochrome P450-dependent mono-oxygenases present in the skin, and it is capable of converting polycyclic aromatic hydrocarbons into reactive metabolic species such as diolepoxides that may initiate tumor formation.

Shale oil products appear to be particularly carcinogenic.[194] A recent comparison between U.S. shale oil workers and coal miners revealed skin cancers in each group but more actinic keratoses in the shale oil group.[195] Also, coal tar pitch is more carcinogenic than are petroleum-derived tars.[196, 197] One report noted that roofers and road pavers who are exposed to bitumen and coal tar fumes suffer more internal cancers as well as skin cancers.[198] In the roofers, an increased risk was suggested for lung cancers, stomach cancers, NMSC, and leukemia. The relative risk in road pavers was consistently lower than in the roofers for cancers of the lung and leukemias. The risk of skin cancer was significantly increased, according to one study.

Creosote, a tar product, has also been found to be carcinogenic. Karlehagen et al.[199] evaluated 922 creosote-exposed wood impregnators employed between 1950 and 1975. They noted an increased risk for skin and lip cancer, which may have in part been a result of sun exposure as well as of contact with creosote. An increased risk of malignant melanoma mortality was noted in oil industry workers in Canada due to petroleum contact and perhaps to sun exposure as well.[200] No increase in NMSC was noted in this study as opposed to previous findings in oil refinery workers. Locomotive drivers in the steam engine era who were exposed to coal and diesel combustion products had a 1.5-fold increase in incidence of NMSC.[201]

Oils used by machine operators may be carcinogenic. Cruickshank and Squire[202] noted an association between scrotal cancers and the use of cutting oils that is perhaps related to their incorporation of shale oil. Axelson et al.[203] noted that trichloroethylene (TRI) is present in some degreasing oils. There is limited evidence for mutagenicity and carcinogenicity of TRI in experimental test systems. In a cohort of 1,670 persons, these authors noted a doubled incidence of NMSC. However, they concluded that there was no evidence that TRI is a human carcinogen.

Polycyclic aromatic hydrocarbons can act additively to produce cutaneous cancers in experiments. It appears likely that such effects can occur in human skin as well, suggesting that outdoor workers who contact polycyclic aromatic hydrocarbons would be at a greater risk of developing skin cancer than would those exposed to one or the other. UVB has an additive effect on the catalytic activity essential for cancer initiation that is induced by crude coal tar. This suggests a possible mechanism for the enhancement of carcinogenesis by the combination of these two stimuli.[204]

Clinical Features

The first observable sign following exposure to fumes of tar and asphalt is diffuse erythema of the exposed skin, accompanied by a burning sensation. Later, edema, thickening of the skin, and a yellow-brown hyperpigmentation develop. Areas of folliculitis with numerous comedones are seen, accompanied by pruritus (tar itch). Large black comedones and keratotic follicles occur, even on the trunk and thighs, where oil-soaked clothing rubs against the skin. Conjunctivitis is common.[205]

Photosensitization has been shown to be a contributing factor to the evolution of the chronic skin changes caused by tar and pitch exposure. This was demonstrated experimentally by Epstein and coworkers,[170] who found that administration of subtumorigenic doses of ultraviolet light after a single application of 7,12-dimethyl benzanthracene (DMBA) produced an increased number of malignant tumors in mice. These studies confirmed what had been known for years from clinical observations. Emmett et al.[196] found that roofers working with coal tar pitch develop a phototoxic keratoconjunctivitis that is markedly enhanced by ultraviolet exposure. Photosensitizing chemicals known to be present in tar include anthracene, acridine, methylanthracene, pyrene, fluoranthene, and 3,4-benzopyrene.[195]

As exposure to tar continues, the skin shows poikilodermatous changes that are manifested by irregular areas of atrophy, loss of pigment with patchy areas of hyperpigmentation, and diffuse telangiectasis. These changes are particularly noticeable on the sides of the neck and the cheeks. The scrotum, because of the thinness of the skin and the difficulty of removing tar residues from the rugae, commonly becomes atrophic and hyperpigmented.

Keratotic papillomas (tar warts) also begin to appear on the poikilodermatous skin. Most workers recognize these as harmless and usually scrape them off with their fingernails. Areas of predilection are the face, forearms, and hands and also the dorsum of the feet and ankles, as well as the scrotum.[195] These verrucous growths may develop into squamous cell carcinomas, but probably only a small number ever do. Basal cell carcinomas and keratoacanthomas also occur. Older skin appears to be much more susceptible to these changes.

Exposure time for the development of the skin changes ranges from 1 year to more than 20 years, but the majority of cases occur between the 6th and 20th years of work.[195] Henry, in an excellent study, found the maximum number of malignancies in pitch and tar workers to occur between 20 and 24 years after beginning to work. By contrast, shale oil and mineral oil workers appear to develop malignancy much later, after 50 to 54 years, suggesting that pitch and tar have a greater potential for inducing skin cancer than does mineral oil.[207] As noted previously, this may be because of a difference in the types and quantities of promoters present.

Experimental and clinical data support the concept that cutaneous cancers and precancerous lesions due to polycyclic hydrocarbons are primarily epithelial in nature. However, Savitz and Moure[208] reported melanomas associated with oil refinery exposures and pointed out that skin cancer incidence by cell type had not been examined.

Methods of Prevention

Substitution of a noncarcinogenic oil, although not always possible, can markedly reduce the chance of developing skin carcinoma. Emmett[159] described how such substitution in the British cotton industry in 1953 reduced the incidence of mule spinner's cancer from an average of 54 cases yearly between 1920 and 1943 to only 7 in 1965.

Unprocessed petroleum-derived lubricating oils have varying degrees of carcinogenicity. Refining processes have been shown to reduce or eliminate such activity.[209] Solvent refining removes polycyclic aromatic hydrocarbons as well as some other materials and appears to abolish experimental carcinogenicity.[210] A combination of hydroprocessing and moderate solvent refining was effective in removing the cancer stimuli. Thus, it is possible to develop petroleum oil distillates that are virtually free of cancer-inducing activities.

Engineering Controls

Engineering controls must be instituted so that skin contact is minimized or prevented altogether, if possible. This entails using closed systems and controlling dust and oil mists. Protective clothing,

adequate and convenient facilities for cleaning the skin, including showers, and good housekeeping of the work place are also essential. Clothing must be changed frequently and kept free of encrusted oil and tars. Shielding the skin from sunlight during work is also important. Protective creams are not very helpful, with the exception of sunscreening lotions and creams.

Employee education in the nature of the hazards, the consequences of prolonged contact with the carcinogenic materials, and the importance of using protective measures, even those found cumbersome, are valuable and necessary measures.

Good personal hygiene has been recognized for more than a century as being extremely important in preventing the harmful effects of these substances.[211]

Periodic physical examination of workers and monitoring of the types of oils, tars, etc. in the work place are also vital. Emmett[175] describes a simple method for determining the presence or absence of carcinogens in a given soil or tar.

Workers at Risk

Table 8–3 lists many of the occupations in which a worker can come into contact with polycyclic hydrocarbons. The total numbers are not well established, but at least 100,000 U.S. workers are employed in oil refineries,[212] so the overall num-

---

TABLE 8–3 • Workers Potentially Exposed to Polycyclic Aromatic Hydrocarbons

Soot or Carbon Black	**Creosote Oil**
Chimney sweeps	Timber proofers
Soot manufacturing workers	Brick & pottery workers
Coal Tar, Pitch, Tarry Products	**Anthracene**
Tar distillers	Chemical workers
Coal tar manufacturers	
Cable layers	**Oil Fractionation and Distillation Products**
Road workers	Refining workers
Fabric proofers	Cotton mule spinners
Net fixers	Shale oil workers
Wharfmen	Mineral cutting oil users
Electrical equipment workers	Machine tool setters
Brake and clutch lining makers	Machine tool operators
Caulking material makers	Paraffin workers in
Insulation makers	Match factories
Linoleum makers	Munitions
Protective coatings workers	Naphthalene
Roofers	Paper industry
Rope makers	
Rubber workers	
Ship stokers	
Shoemakers	
Briquette manufacturers (from pitch)	

bers exposed to these carcinogens must be quite large.

ARSENIC

Experimental Evidence

Of all known human carcinogens, arsenic remains unusual in that experimental proof of carcinogenicity is lacking. Epidemiological data, however, strongly links exposure to inorganic arsenic to both skin and lung cancer.

Tumorigenesis in laboratory animals following administration of arsenic has never been conclusively demonstrated. Rats and mice fed drinking water tainted with arsenic trioxide did not show an increased rate of carcinogenesis.[213] The topical application of arsenic compounds, likewise, has not provided evidence of carcinogenicity. Furthermore, neither tumor promotion nor tumor initiation has ever been clearly demonstrated for arsenicals.[214, 215] The explanation most commonly offered for the inability to induce arsenical cancers in experimental animals is that animals do not survive the long latent period characteristic of arsenic malignancy.

The mechanism of arsenic tumorigenesis is not yet known, but DNA repair mechanisms may be involved. Inorganic trivalent arsenic functions as an enzyme inhibitor by blocking enzyme protein linkage to sulfhydryl groups.[216] One theory suggests that arsenic inhibits the dark repair enzymes that repair the DNA damage caused by ultraviolet irradiation. Sodium arsenate has been shown to decrease the incorporation of nucleotides in both dermal cells and lymphocytes.[217] Other evidence suggests that arsenic replaces phosphorus in the DNA chain.[217] Sodium arsenite decreases the survival of both the wild type and the excision-repair-deficient strains of *Escherichia coli* when they are exposed to increasing doses of ultraviolet irradiation.[218] Further work using the same bacterial strains showed that sodium arsenite can inhibit both single-strand DNA break formation and post-replication repair, possibly mediated through diminished cellular ATP levels.[219]

More convincing is the in vitro production of chromosomal aberrations by inorganic arsenic, perhaps by blocking oxidative phosphorylation.[220] Chromosomal aberrations were five times more frequent in cultured human leukocytes exposed to trivalent arsenic than in those exposed to pentavalent arsenic. Similar results were found in human skin fibroblasts.[221] Epidemiological studies have shown an increased frequency of chromosomal aberrations in workers exposed to arsenic compounds and in individuals exposed to arsenic-containing medicinals.[217, 222]

Epidemiology and Historical Background

In 1823, J. A. Paris was the first to implicate arsenic as a carcinogen. He described how cattle grazing in the vicinity of a copper smelter were losing their hoofs and developing "cancers" on their rumps from arsenic in the air. The occurrence was probably due to selenium rather than arsenic toxicity.[223] Jonathan Hutchinson, in 1887, reported six cases of plantar keratosis and carcinoma from Fowler's solution (1% sodium arsenite) given for the treatment of psoriasis. Skin and lung malignancies as well as keratoses and pigmentary changes in sheep-dip workers were first reported in 1902 by Legge.[224] Further reports in the 1930s[225] verified the presence of arsenic intoxication in sheep-dip workers.

The first acceptable epidemiological study of the arsenic problem was done in 1948 by Hill and Faning,[226] who compared the incidence of cancer of the skin and lungs in a group of factory workers exposed to large amounts of inorganic arsenic with the incidence found in a similar population of nonfactory workers. The workers exposed to arsenic also showed pigmentation, hyperkeratinization of exposed skin, and wart formation, with increased levels of arsenic in their hair and urine. The greatest incidence of carcinoma was in those who actually worked in areas where the levels of inorganic arsenic were high, such as chemical workers; workers in the same plant who were not exposed had the lowest incidence. Although the actual number of cases was small, the study added considerably to the evidence, albeit associative, for the carcinogenic properties of arsenic.

The most convincing evidence appeared in 1969, when Lee and Fraumeni[227] found that smelter workers exposed to arsenic for over 15 years had a three to eight times greater risk of respiratory cancer than did the U.S. white male population in general. In pesticide manufacturing, workers showed an excess respiratory and lymphatic cancer rate that was two to seven times the expected rate among adult white males.[228] Among workers retired from pesticide manufacturing, Baetjer et al.[229] found an excess mortality rate for respiratory cancer of 6.7 and for lymphatic cancer of 3.0.

Further persuasive evidence comes from a study of an area in Taiwan where the water supply from artesian wells was contaminated with arsenic. A complete and detailed study of the population of 37 villages demonstrated a marked incidence of skin carcinoma that increased with age, so that by the age of 50, 100% of the exposed people were affected. The youngest patient with melanosis was 3, with keratosis 4, and with skin cancer 24. A large control population showed none of these changes.[230]

Clinical Features

Arsenic keratoses are characteristic of chronic arsenicalism. They are multiple yellow, punctate keratoses distributed symmetrically on the palms and soles. Mild erythema and hyperhidrosis can precede their development. The usual size is 1 to 2 mm in diameter, but they may grow to 5 to 6 mm. Flat, white keratoses may also be seen on the dorsum of the hands, shins, and ankles. Rarely, squamous cell carcinoma can develop from an arsenical keratosis, occasionally preceded by erythema or thickening.[184]

Squamous cell carcinoma can also develop from apparently normal skin, most often after a very long latent period. Bowen's disease, or intraepidermal squamous cell carcinoma, is most commonly seen after arsenic exposure. These erythematous, slightly hyperpigmented, scaling round plaques are asymmetrically distributed over the trunk and limbs and can reach 3 to 5 cm in diameter. Aggressive squamous cell carcinoma develops in lesions of Bowen's disease only rarely and only after a many-year latent period. A recent Japanese study of a restricted neighborhood with a history of possible arsenic exposure demonstrated that Bowen's disease appeared within 10 years, invasive skin cancers after 20 years, and pulmonary cancers 30 years after arsenic exposure.[231]

Most controversial is the association of Bowen's disease and internal malignancy. Graham and Helwig[232] were the first to show an 80% increased incidence of visceral carcinoma in patients with Bowen's disease. In a follow-up study, arsenic was listed as one possible causative factor.[233] Several subsequent studies reported an increased incidence of 15 to 30%.[234–237]

In a retrospective study of 207 patients with Bowen's disease diagnosed at the Finsen Institute, Denmark, no significant differences were found between observed and expected numbers for internal malignancies.[238] An extended study of 581 patients with Bowen's disease diagnosed at the same institution during the 40-year period between January 1, 1943, and December 31, 1982, confirmed their original findings.[239]

Thus, the relationship of Bowen's disease to internal cancer remains unclear. Callen[240] points out that patients with Bowen's disease have approximately a 10% risk of developing an internal malignancy, which is close to the risk in the general population matched for age. He advises regular physical examinations appropriate to their age and symptoms for these patients but does not recommend an extensive search for internal malignancy.

Basal cell carcinomas are also seen after arsenic exposure. They are usually multifocal and superficial and are frequently pigmented (Fig. 8–3).

Workers at Risk

In 1975, the National Institute of Occupational Safety and Health (NIOSH) estimated that 1,500,000 workers are potentially exposed to arsenic, mostly as arsenic trioxides[241] (Table 8–4). Its major uses are in insecticides and herbicides, copper and lead smelting, glass and drug production, and animal feed stock. Arsenic is also the primary carcinogen used in appreciable amounts in the semiconductor and electronics industry.[242] Gallium arsenide, used as an alternative to silicon as the base material in device fabrication, accounts for only 5% of semiconductor manufacturing, but its future role will probably be significant. One industrial hygiene concern is its dissolution into gallium and arsenic.[243]

Pharmacy technicians come into contact with a number of pharmaceuticals and chemicals, many of which are carcinogens. In one study there was a 1.5-fold elevated risk of developing an NMSC in this population.[244] No specific relationship to a particular chemical was noted.

Female hairdressers in Finland had a relative risk of 2 for developing NMSC.[245] Here, too, the reason was not clear. In contrast, the premalignant and malignant skin lesions in 133 of 242 paraquat workers appeared to be the result of a synergistic effect of bipyridines and solar exposure.[246]

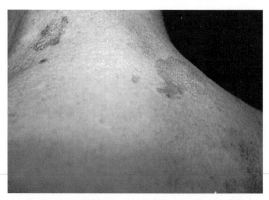

FIGURE 8–3 • Multiple superficial basal cell carcinomas on the trunk in a woman who had received arsenic treatment (Fowler's solution) many years previously for acne vulgaris.

TABLE 8–4 • **Workers Potentially Exposed to Arsenic**

Alloy makers	Fireworks makers	Printing ink workers
Aniline color makers	Gold refiners	Rodenticide makers
Arsenic workers	Herbicide makers	Semiconductor component
Babbitt metal workers	Hide preservers	makers
Brass makers	Insecticide makers	Silver refiners
Bronze makers	Lead shot makers	Taxidermists
Ceramic enamel makers	Lead smelters	Textile printers
Ceramic makers	Leather workers	Tree sprayers
Copper smelters	Painters	Type metal workers
Drug makers	Paint makers	Water weed controllers
Dye makers	Petroleum refinery workers	Weed sprayers
Enamelers	Pigment makers	

CUTANEOUS T-CELL LYMPHOMA

Clinical Features

Cutaneous T-cell lymphoma (CTCL), encompassing both mycosis fungoides (MF) and the Sézary syndrome, is an uncommon malignant lymphoma of helper T cells. Initially limited to the skin, involvement of lymph nodes, visceral organs, and peripheral blood can occur and lead to subsequent death. Fewer than 100 deaths per year due to CTCL have been reported in the United States.

Three cutaneous forms exist, usually in sequential order: an often pruritic eczematous or erythematous macular eruption, an infiltrated plaque form, and a tumor stage. Diagnosis at the initial stage may be difficult, and there may be an interval of 6.1 years between onset of skin disease and diagnosis.[247] Many patients are reported to have a preceding chronic dermatitis, such as chronic contact dermatitis, atopic dermatitis, nummular eczema, psoriasis, or neurodermatitis, lasting 10 to 20 years. Such eruptions are often steroid-responsive and can involute spontaneously.[248]

Considerable information regarding the clinical and histologic picture of CTCL exists, but causal factors have yet to be clearly identified. It has been proposed that an alteration in cellular immune responsiveness mediated by Langerhans' cells is the primary event.[249] Under this scheme, T lymphocytes are transformed into reactive cells after initial antigen processing by the Langerhans' cells. These transformed cells, seen by light microscopy as the "mycosis fungoides cell" in the epidermis and upper dermis, may induce an inflammatory reaction and clinical dermatitis. Chronic antigenic stimulation could conceivably produce a malignant clone of antigen-responsive T cells, resulting in CTCL. With this perspective in mind, several retrospective and case-controlled studies have attempted to correlate occupational exposure with the development of CTCL.

Epidemiological Evidence

Fischmann et al.[250] reported a group of 44 patients with MF, or Sézary syndrome, who had entered into an approved human experimentation protocol at the National Cancer Institute-Veterans Administration Medical Oncology Branch between July 1976 and November 1978. Detailed histories were obtained regarding exposure to chemicals, drugs, radiation, and allergens at the time of onset of skin disease. All but 1 of the 44 patients had multiple exposures, with prolonged exposure ranging from 13 years for chemicals to 18 years for drugs. Chemical exposures included air pollutants (39%), pesticides (36%), solvents and vapors (30%), and detergents and disinfectants (14%). Tobacco (86%) was the most frequent drug, followed by analgesics (20%), tranquilizers (18%), and thiazides (14%). Exposure to physical agents included radiation (18%), and burns (2%); allergen exposure included bacteria (9%), mold (5%), pollen (5%), and house dust (2%). The authors concluded that individuals with a prolonged exposure to various combinations of chemicals, drugs, physical agents, and biological agents may be at increased risk for developing the Sézary syndrome. Unfortunately, the lack of a comparison group and the small size of the test population limit any conclusions that can be drawn from these results.

In a similar uncontrolled study, Greene et al.[251] evaluated data collected by the Mycosis Fungoides Cooperative Study Group and the county-by-county survey of cancer mortality conducted by the National Cancer Institute for 1950–1975. A life-time occupational history was requested on the intake questionnaire of 211 patients designated as having MF. These patients had a high frequency of allergic conditions, fungal and viral skin infection, family history of malignancy (especially leukemia and lymphoma), sun sensitivity, and employment in a manufacturing occupation (especially the petrochemical, textile, metal, and machinery industries). The U.S. cancer mortality data showed excessive rates due to MF in counties where petroleum, rubber, metal, machinery, and printing industries are located.

Using a matched case-control design, Cohen et al.[143] examined occupational exposure history in 59 patients with a clinical diagnosis of MF seen at the Yale-New Haven Hospital or the West Haven Hospital during the years 1965 through 1976. Patients and controls were matched on the basis of age, sex, and race. The relative risk of encountering a history of employment in manufacturing or construction industries among the patients with MF was 4.3 times that for controls. Occupations such as machinist, machine operator, construction work foundry operatives, hatters, and industrial electricians were found in apparent excess compared to controls. Furthermore, shortened survival was seen in the patients with an industrial occupation versus a nonindustrial occupation, suggesting more severe disease.

Subsequent work by Tuyp et al.[252] did not confirm an association between occupational exposure and the development of MF[53]; patients with histologically proven MF were matched by age and sex to a hospital-based control population, and occupation; recreation; exposure to petrochemicals, pesticides, insecticides, and potential carcinogens; tanning and sun exposure history; smoking and drug ingestion history; other skin disease; and personal and family history of other malignancies were evaluated. No statistically significant difference regarding occupational history or exposure to potential carcinogens, noxious chemicals, or radiation was seen.

Thus, the issue of an industrial origin of cutaneous T-cell lymphoma has not been clearly established. Further studies are needed to clarify this issue.

Trauma

Although Virchow proposed, in 1863, a theory of carcinogenesis arising from repeated trauma, the possibility that skin cancer can be caused by a single trauma has been a controversial subject for many years. Most of the early reports were anecdotal and poorly documented. Patients, however, often tell physicians that a skin cancer was preceded by some type of single trauma.

Litigation based on the claim that malignant tumors were caused by a single injury has been increasing since the 1950s.[253] More of these cases are appearing from within the workplace. Because the cause of cancer is still essentially unknown, the courts will accept a relationship between trauma and cancer if evidence is produced show-

ing a greater than 50% probability that a given cancer was caused by trauma.[254]

Ewing's criteria have traditionally been used to establish the relationship between a single trauma and an ensuing malignancy. Ewing first published his ideas regarding this relationship in 1926 and enlarged them in 1935.[255, 256] In 1979, Stoll and Crissey[257] combined Ewing's criteria with those of others[258–260] and formulated a useful list of criteria for diagnosis:

- The skin must previously have been normal.
- Adequate and authenticated trauma must have occurred, preferably confirmed by medical personnel.
- A positive diagnosis of a nonmetastatic carcinoma must be made, and the tumor must be histologically consistent with the tissues of that site.
- The carcinoma must originate from the exact point of injury.
- A reasonable time interval between the trauma and the first appearance of the carcinoma must be present.
- There must be continuity of physical signs from the traumatic event to the appearance of the carcinoma.

Because single trauma is an uncommon cause of skin cancer, the criteria used to establish causation are inexact. In 1960, Dix reviewed 25 patients with 27 skin cancers recorded at the Wisconsin State Industrial Accident Commission between 1942 and 1960.[261] Most of the patients were welders or machinists, and the precipitating event was usually a burn from a welding spark or a hot metal chip from a lathe. All the patients fulfilled Ewing's criteria. The initial wound in each case was relatively insignificant, but the site failed to heal, and later a low-grade cancer appeared. All were basal cell carcinomas; two were basosquamous. Most appeared within 1 to 5 months; one occurred as late as 2 years after the trauma.

Malignancy occurring in scars, especially burn scars, has been known since at least 1828 when the French surgeon Jean Marjolin described a tumor arising from a traumatic scar. The term Marjolin's ulcer, originally applied to a neoplasm occurring in a burn scar, is now loosely applied to a carcinoma originating in any type of scar tissue. The ratio of squamous cell carcinomas to basal cell carcinomas is approximately 3:1. The growth arises from the edge of the scar and is usually single. Metastases are uncommon.[262] The latent period ranges from a few months to 35 years or more,[263] which may present considerable difficulties for occupational physicians, insurance companies, and compensation boards.

Long-recognized examples of burn scar neoplasms are kangri and kairo cancers. The kangri type occurs in India in persons who carry bowls of hot charcoal against the body for warmth.[264] Similarly, the kairo cancer occurs in Japan in those who carry a box, also containing hot coals, against the abdomen for warmth. In these cases, erythema ab igne precedes the development of cancer by many years, and the majority of tumors are squamous cell. The development of cancer is probably enhanced by the coal tar products present in the charcoal. A case of neuroendocrine carcinoma mixed with squamous cell carcinoma arising in an area of erythema ab igne was reported. The patient, an elderly black woman, had sat in front of wood- and coal-burning fires for many winters.[39] The extensive use of electric space heaters in recent years may lead to an increased incidence of erythema ab igne and possibly associated skin cancer.

IONIZING RADIATION

Ionizing radiation is a well-established carcinogenic stimulus. Cancer of the skin from x-rays was reported only a few years after Roentgen's discovery in 1895. A technician who had demonstrated x-ray tubes for over 4 years by holding his hand under them developed a squamous cell carcinoma and later died of metastases.[265] By 1914, 104 cases had been collected from the world's literature. Of these, 95% were occupationally induced. Until the 1930s, most of the radiation cancers were occupationally induced and occurred in physicians, dentists, nurses, orderlies, and laboratory technicians, when exposure was not controlled because the machines were uncalibrated. These lesions occurred on the hands and feet, with only a few appearing on the face, and were most commonly squamous cell carcinoma rather than basal cell carcinoma (Fig. 8–4).

By the early 1930s, adequate protective measures had been developed, and occupational radiation dermatitis and cancers gradually disappeared. However, recent years have seen an increase in the number of basal cell epitheliomas induced by fractionated radiotherapy, which is used for dermatological disease such as acne, dermatitis, and hirsutism. These lesions occur almost exclusively on the face, usually in an area of chronic radiation dermatitis, and are primarily basal cell carcinomas.

Two types of chronic radiation injury may occur. The first is the result of relatively high doses delivered over a short period of time, such as those

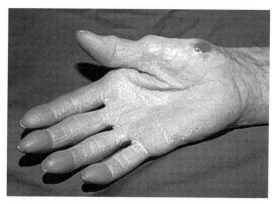

FIGURE 8–4 • A squamous cell carcinoma developing in an area of old radiodermatitis in an x-ray technician who previously restrained children by hand, without protection, during x-ray examinations.

used for skin cancers. This results in ulceration, followed by atrophy, telangiectasia, hyper- and hypopigmentation, and a smooth, pliable scar.

In contrast, low doses delivered over a long period of time and leading to a relatively high total dose are the type of injury that usually leads to carcinoma production. In this case, the chronic injury leads to a dryness of the skin, atrophy of the sebaceous and sweat glands, loss of hair, thickening of the skin, warty keratotic growths, brittleness and cracking of the nails, persistent ulceration, and various premalignant and malignant neoplasms.[266]

The histological types include squamous cell carcinomas, basal cell carcinomas and, rarely, melanomas and sebaceous and sweat gland tumors.[266] Squamous cell carcinomas of x-ray origin tend to be more invasive than are those of actinic origin, with metastases occurring in 20 to 26% of cases as opposed to 3% for actinically induced cancers.[267] Tumors are usually multiple. The latent period ranges from 7 weeks to 56 years, with an average of 25 to 30 years. The duration varies inversely with the dose.[268] The dose equivalent to produce skin carcinoma appears to be 3,000 rem. Emmett has urged reduction in this "permissible" dose in the United States.[159] In 1981, the EPA recommended a new federal radiation guideline for occupational exposure to ionizing radiation.

Radiation carcinomas constitute less than 1% of all occupational skin cancers. The occupational sources of ionizing radiation include curing plastics, painting radium compounds on watch dials, manufacturing electronic tubes, working in nuclear power plants, performing medical diagnoses and treatments, mining uranium, and sterilizing materials (Table 8–5).

TABLE 8–5 • Workers Potentially Exposed to X-Irradiation

Aircraft workers	Nurses
Atomic energy plant workers	Oil well loggers
Biologists	Ore assayers
Cathode ray tube makers	Petroleum refinery workers
Chemists	Physicians
Dental assistants	Pipeline oil-flow testers
Dentists	Pipeline weld radiographers
Dermatologists	Plasma torch operators
Drug makers	Plastics technicians
Drug sterilizers	Prospectors
Electron microscope makers	Radar tube makers
Electron microscopists	Radiologists
Electrostatic eliminators	Radium laboratory workers
Embalmers	Radium refinery workers
Fire alarm makers	Research workers
Food preservers	Television tube makers
Food sterilizers	Thickness gauge operators
Gas mantle makers	Thorium-aluminum alloy workers
H-V television repairman	Thorium-magnesium alloy workers
H-V vacuum tube makers	Thorium ore producers
H-V vacuum tube users	Tile glazers
Industrial fluoroscope operators	Uranium dye workers
Industrial radiographers	Uranium miners
Klystron tube operators	Veterinarians
Liquid level gauge operators	X-ray aides
Luminous dial painters	X-ray diffraction machine operators
Machinists for fabricated metal products	X-ray technicians
Military personnel	X-ray tube makers

References

1. Epstein JH. Experimental models for primary melanoma. *Photodermatol Photoimmunol Photomed* 1992; 9:91–98.
2. Parker SL, Tong T, Bolden S, et al. Cancer statistics. *CA Cancer J Clin* 1996; 46:7–29.
3. Miller DL, Weinstock MA. Nonmelanoma skin cancer in the United States: incidence. *J Am Acad Dermatol* 1994; 30:774–780.
4. Scotto J, Fears TR, Fraumeni JF Jr. *Incidence of Nonmelanoma Skin Cancer in the United States.* Washington, D.C.: U.S. Department of Health, Education and Welfare (NIH), Publication No. 82-2433; 1981.
5. Marks R, Staples M, Giles GG. Trends in nonmelanoma skin cancer treated in Australia: the second national survey. *Intl J Cancer* 1993; 53:585–590.
6. Glass AG, Hoover RN. The emerging epidemic of melanoma and squamous cell carcinoma. *JAMA* 1989; 262:2097–2100.
7. Lloyd-Roberts D. Incidence of nonmelanoma skin cancer in West Glamorgan, South Wales. *Br J Dermatol* 1990; 122:399–403.
8. Magnus K. The Nordic profile of skin cancer incidence: a comparative epidemiologic study of the three main types of skin cancer. *Intl J Cancer* 1991; 47:12–19.
9. Gallagher RP et al. Trends in basal cell carcinoma, squamous cell carcinoma and melanoma of the skin from 1973 through 1987. *J Am Acad Dermatol* 1990; 23:413–421.
10. Marks R. Nonmelanotic skin cancer and solar keratoses: the quiet 20th century epidemic. *Intl J Dermatol* 1987; 26:201–205.
11. Dubreuilh W. Des hyperkeratoses circonscriptes. *Ann Dermatol Syphiligr (Paris)* 1896; 7;3:1158–1204.
12. Hyde J. On the influence of light in the production of cancer of the skin. *Am J Med Sci* 1906; 31:1–22.
13. Shield AM. A remarkable case of multiple growths of the skin caused by exposure to the sun. (1899). *Lancet* 1980; 1:22–23.
14. Unna P. *Histopathologie der Hautkrankheiten.* Berlin: August Hirschwald; 1894.
15. Epstein JH. Photocarcinogenesis, skin cancer and aging. In: Balin AK, Kligman AM, eds. *Aging and the Skin.* New York: Raven Press; 1989:307–329.
16. Scotto J, Fears TR. The association of solar ultraviolet and skin melanoma incidence among Caucasians in the United States. *Cancer Inv* 1987; 5:275–283.
17. Urbach F, Epstein JH, Forbes PD. Ultraviolet carcinogenesis: experimental, global and genetic aspects. In: Fitzpatrick TB, et al., eds. *Sunlight and Man.* Tokyo: University of Tokyo Press; 1974:259–283.
18. Urbach F. Photocarcinogenesis. In: Regan JD, Parrish JA, eds. *The Science of Photomedicine.* New York, London: Plenum Press; 1982:261–292.
19. van der Leun JC. UV carcinogenesis. *Photochem Photobiol* 1984; 39:861–868.
20. Blum HF. *Carcinogenesis by Ultraviolet Light.* Princeton, N.J.: Princeton University Press; 1959.
21. Lill PH. Latent period and antigenicity of murine tumors induced in C3H mice by short-wavelength ultraviolet radiation. *J Invest Dermatol* 1983; 81:342–346.
22. Chan GL, Little JB. Induction of transformation in vitro by ultraviolet light. *Nature* 1976; 264:422–444.
23. Dipaolo JA, Donovan PJ. Transformation frequency of

Syrian golden hamster cells and its modulation by ultraviolet irradiation. *Natl Cancer Inst Monogr* 1978; 50:75–80.

24. Withrow TJ, Lugo MH, Dempsey MJ. Transformation of BALB 3T3 cells exposed to a germicidal UV lamp and a sunlamp. *Photochem Photobiol* 1980; 31:135–141.

25. Rose RC III, Parker RL. Erythema and conjunctivitis outbreak caused by inadvertent exposure to ultraviolet light. *JAMA* 1979; 242:1155–1156.

26. Zenz C, Knight AL. Ultraviolet microwave, laser and infrared radiation in occupational medicine. In: Zenz C, ed. *Occupational Medicine*. Chicago: Year Book Medical Publishers; 1975:564.

27. Staberg B et al. Carcinogenic effect of sequential artificial sunlight and UVA radiation in hairless mice. *Arch Dermatol* 1983; 119:641–643.

28. Strickland PT. Photocarcinogenesis by near-ultraviolet (UVA) radiation in Sencar mice. *J Invest Dermatol* 1986; 87:272–275.

29. Willis I, Menter JM, Shyte HJ. The rapid induction of cancers in the hairless mouse utilizing the principle of photoaugmentation. *J Invest Dermatol* 1981; 76:404–408.

30. Bain JA, Rusch HP, Kline BE. Carcinogenesis with ultraviolet radiation of wavelength 2,800–3,400 A. *Cancer Res* 1943; 3:610–612.

31. Owens DW et al. Influence of wind on ultraviolet injury. *Arch Dermatol* 1974; 109:200–201.

32. Owens DW et al. Influence of humidity on ultraviolet injury. *J Invest Dermatol* 1975; 64:250–252.

33. Owens DW, Knox JM. Influence of heat, wind and humidity on ultraviolet radiation injury. *Natl Cancer Inst Monogr* 1978; 50:161–167.

34. Argyris TS. Tumor promotion by abrasion-induced epidermal hyperplasia in the skin of mice. *J Invest Dermatol* 1980; 75:360–362.

35. Arrington JH III, Lockman DS. Thermal keratoses and squamous cell carcinoma in situ associated with erythema ab igne. *Arch Dermatol* 1979; 115:1226–1228.

36. Cross F. On a turf (peat) fire cancer: malignant change superimposed on erythema ab igne. *Proc R Soc Med* 1967; 60:1307–1308.

37. Funlayson GR, Sams WM, Smith JG Jr. Erythema ab igne: a histopathological study. *J Invest Dermatol* 1966; 46:104–108.

38. Johnson WC, Butterworth T. Erythema ab igne elastosis. *Arch Dermatol* 1971; 104:128–131.

39. Jones CS, Tyring SK, Lee PC, Fine JD. Development of neuroendocrine (Merkel cell) carcinoma mixed with squamous cell carcinoma in erythema ab igne. *Arch Dermatol* 1988; 124:110–113.

40. Peterkin GAG. Malignant change in erythema ab igne. *Br Med J* 1955; 2:1599–1602.

41. Shahrad P, Marks P. The wages of warmth: changes in erythema ab igne. *Br J Dermatol* 1977; 97:178–186.

42. Kligman LH. Intensification of ultraviolet-induced dermal damage by infrared radiation. *Arch Dermatol Res* 1982; 272:229–238.

43. Schwartz L, Tulipan L, Birmingham DJ. Occupational Diseases of the Skin. Philadelphia: Lea & Febiger; 1957:726–737.

44. Gellin GA. Occupational Dermatoses. Chicago: American Medical Association; 1972.

45. Yuspa SH. Cutaneous carcinogenesis: natural and experimental. In: Goldsmith L, ed. *Biochemistry and Physiology of the Skin*. Oxford: Oxford University Press; 1983:1115–1138.

46. Iannaccone PM, Gardner RL, Harris H. The cellular origin of chemically induced tumors. *J Cell Sci* 1978; 29:249–269.

47. Epstein JH. Photocarcinogenesis, skin cancer, and aging. *J Am Acad Dermatol* 1983; 9:487–502.

48. Allen-Hoffman BL, Rheinwald JG. Polycyclic aromatic hydrocarbon mutagenesis of human epidermal keratinocytes in culture. *Proc Natl Acad Sci USA* 1984; 81:7802–7806.

49. Androphy EJ, Lowy DR. Tumor viruses, oncogenes and human cancer. *J Am Acad Dermatol* 1984; 10:125–141.

50. Bickers DR. Drug, carcinogen and steroid hormone metabolism in skin. In: Goldsmith L, ed. *Biochemistry and Physiology of the Skin*. Oxford: Oxford University Press; 1983: 1169–1186.

51. Brookes P, Lawley PD. Evidence for the binding of polynuclear aromatic hydrocarbons to the nucleic acids of mouse skin: relation between carcinogenic hydrocarbons and their binding to deoxyribonucleic acid. *Nature* 1964; 202:781–784.

52. Mukhtar H et al. Chlortrimazole, an inhibitor of epidermal benz(a)pyrene metabolism and DNA binding and carcinogenicity of the hydrocarbon. *Cancer Res* 1984; 44:4233–4240.

53. Nakayama J, Yuspa SH, Poirier MC. Benzo(a)pyrene-DNA adduct formation and removal in mouse epidermis in vivo and in vitro: relationship of DNA binding to initiation of skin carcinogenesis. *Cancer Res* 1984; 44:4087–4095.

54. Ananthaswamy HN, Kanjilal S. Oncogenes and tumor suppressor genes in photocarcinogenesis. *Photochem Photobiol* 1996; 63:428–432.

55. Suarez HG, Nardeux PC, Andeol Y, Sarasin A. Multiple activated oncogenes in human tumors. *Oncogene Res* 1987; 1:201–207.

56. Berridge MJ. Inositol triphosphate and diacylglycerol as second messengers. *Biochem J* 1984; 220:345–360.

57. Blumberg PM et al. Mechanism of action of the phorbol ester tumor promoters: specific receptors for lipophilic ligands. *Biochem Pharmacol* 1984; 33:933–940.

58. Klein-Szanto AJP, Slaga TJ. Effects of peroxides on rodent skin: epidermal hyperplasia and tumor promotion. *J Invest Dermatol* 1982; 79:30–34.

59. Hennings H et al. Malignant conversion of mouse skin tumours is increased by tumour initiators and is unaffected by tumour promoters. *Nature* 1983; 304:67–69.

60. Hennings H, Yuspa SH. Two-stage tumor promotion in mouse skin: an alternative interpretation. *J Natl Cancer Inst* 1985; 74:735–740.

61. Bungeler W. Ober den einfluss photosensibilisierender Substanzen auf die enstehung von Hautgeschwulsten. *Z Krebsforsch* 1937; 46:130–167.

62. Epstein JH. Adverse cutaneous reactions to the sun. In: Malkinson FD, Pearson RW *Year Book of Dermatology*. Chicago: Year Book Medical Publishers; 1971:5–43.

63. Epstein JH. Photosensitivity, 1: mechanisms. In: Fellner MJ, Zeide DA, eds. *Clinics in Dermatology*. Philadelphia: J.B. Lippincott; 1986:81–87.

64. Forbes PD, Davies RE, Urbach F. Phototoxicity and photocarcinogenesis: comparative effects of anthracene and 8-methoxypsoralen in the skin of mice. *Food Cosmet Toxicol* 1976; 14:303–306.

65. Grube DD, Ley RD, Fry RJ. Photosensitizing effects of 8-methoxypsoralen on the skin of hairless mice. II. strain and spectral differences for tumorigenesis. *Photochem Photobiol* 1977; 25:269–276.

66. Urbach F. Modification of ultraviolet carcinogenesis by photoactive agents. *J Invest Dermatol* 1959; 32:373–378.

67. Stern RB et al. Cutaneous squamous cell carcinoma in patients treated with PUVA. *N Engl J Med* 1984; 310:1156–1161.

68. Stern RB, Laird N, Melskin J, et al. Cutaneous squamous

cell carcinoma in patients treated with PUVA. *N Engl J Med* 1984; 310:1156–1161.

69. Epstein JH, Epstein WI. Cocarcinogenesis effects of ultraviolet light on DMBA tumor initiation in albino mice. *J Invest Dermatol* 1962; 39:455–460.

70. Epstein JH. Comparison of the carcinogenic and cocarcinogenic effects of ultraviolet light on hairless mice. *J Natl Cancer Inst* 1965; 34:741–745.

71. Stenbäck F. Studies on modifying effect of ultraviolet radiation on chemical skin carcinogenesis. *J Invest Dermatol* 1975; 64:253–257.

72. Epstein JH. Nitrogen mustard (mechlorethamine) and UVB photocarcinogenesis: a dose response. *J Invest Dermatol* 1984; 83:320–322.

73. Epstein JH. How important is the role of radiation from the sun in the rising incidence of melanomas. In: Epstein E, ed. *Controversies in Dermatology.* Philadelphia: W.B. Saunders; 1984:10–12.

74. Epstein JH. Stimulation of ultraviolet-induced carcinogenesis by 1,3,-Bis(2chlorethyl)-1-nitrosourea. *Cancer Res* 1979; 39:408–410.

75. Epstein JH. Effects of mechlorethamine (HN$_2$, nitrogen mustard) on UV-induced carcinogenesis in hairless mouse skin. *J Natl Cancer Inst* 1984; 72:383–385.

76. Epstein JH, Roth HL. Experimental ultraviolet light carcinogenesis. *J Invest Dermatol* 1968; 50:387–389.

77. Pound AW. Induced cell proliferation and the initiation of skin tumor formation in mice by ultraviolet light. *Pathology* 1970; 2:269–275.

78. Epstein JH. Photocarcinogenesis promotion studies with benzoyl peroxide (BPO) and croton oil. *J Invest Dermatol* 1988; 91:114–116.

79. Fry RJM, Ley RD, Grube DD. Photosensitized reactions and carcinogenesis. *Natl Cancer Inst Monogr* 1978; 50:39–43.

80. Epstein JH. All-trans retinoic acid and cutaneous cancers. *J Am Acad Dermatol* 1986; 15:772–778.

81. Pathak MA. Sunscreens: principles of photoprotection. In: Mukhtar H, ed. *Pharmacology of the Skin.* Boca Raton, Fla.: CRC Press; 1991:229–248.

82. Naylor MF et al. High sun protection factor sunscreens in the suppression of actinic neoplasia. *Arch Dermatol* 1995; 131:170–175.

83. Thompson SC, Jolley D, Marks R. Reduction of solar keratoses by regular sunscreen use. *N Engl J Med* 1992; 329:1147–1151.

84. Black HS et al. Effect of low-fat diet on the incidence of actinic keratosis. *N Engl J Med* 1994; 330:1272–1275.

85. Black HS et al. Evidence that a low-fat diet reduces the occurrence of nonmelanoma skin cancer. *Int J Cancer* 1995; 62:165–169.

86. Black HS, Chan JT. Suppression of ultraviolet-induced tumor formation by dietary antioxidants. *J Invest Dermatol* 1975; 65:412–414.

87. Black HS, Chan JT, Brown GE. Effects of dietary constituents on ultraviolet light-mediated carcinogenesis. *Cancer Res* 1978; 38:1384–1387.

88. Epstein JH. Examination of the effect of topical tocopherol on photocarcinogenesis. *Photochem Photobiol* 1994; 59:59S.

89. Gensler HL, Magdalino M. Topical vitamin E inhibition, immunosuppression and tumorigenesis induced by ultraviolet irradiation. *Nutr Cancer* 1991; 15:97–106.

90. McIntosh GH. The influence of dietary vitamin E and calcium status on intestinal tumors in rats. *Nutr Cancer* 1992; 17:47–55.

91. Mitchel REJ, McCann R. Vitamin E is a complete tumor promoter in mouse skin. *Carcinogenesis* 1993; 14:659–662.

92. Odukoya O, Hawach F, Shklar G. Retardation of experimental oral cancer by topical vitamin E. *Nutr Cancer* 1984; 6:98–104.

93. Perchellet J-P et al. Inhibitory effects of glutathione level-raising agents and d-alpha-tocopherol on ornithine decarboxylase induction and mouse skin tumor promotion by 12-O-tetradecanoylphorbol-13-acetate. *Carcinogenesis* 1985; 6:567–573.

94. Shklar G, Schwartz JL, Tuckler DL, Reed S. Prevention of experimental cancer and immunostimulation by vitamin E. *J Oral Pathol Med* 1990; 19:60–64.

95. Slaga TJ, Bracken WM. The effects of antioxidants on skin tumor initiation and aryl hydrocarbon hydroxylase. *Cancer Res* 1977; 37:1631–1635.

96. Brysk MM et al. The activity of interferon on ultraviolet light-induced squamous cell carcinomas in mice. *J Am Acad Dermatol* 1981; 5:61–63.

97. Agarwal R, Mukhtar H. Chemoprevention of photocarcinogenesis. *Photochem Photobiol* 1996; 63:440–444.

98. Chen L-C, De Luca LM. Retinoid effects of skin cancer. In: Mukhtar H, ed. *Skin Cancer: Mechanism and Human Relevance.* Boca Raton, Fla.: CRC Press; 1995: 401–424.

99. Lippman SM, Kessler JF, Meyskens FL Jr. Retinoid as preventive and therapeutic anticancer agents, II. *Cancer Treat Rep* 1987; 71:493–515.

100. Lippman SM, Meyskens FL Jr. Results of the use of vitamin A and retinoid in cutaneous malignancies. *Pharmacol Ther* 1989; 40:107–122.

101. Al-Saleem T, Ali ZS, Gassab M. Skin cancer in xeroderma pigmentosum: response to indomethacin and steroids. *Lancet* 1980; 1:264–265.

102. Gellin GA, Kopf AW, Garfinkel L. Basal cell epithelioma: a controlled study of assorted factors. *Arch Dermatol* 1965; 91:38–45.

103. Vitaliano PP, Urbach F. The relative importance of risk factors in nonmelanoma skin carcinoma. *Arch Dermatol* 1980; 116:454–456.

104. Boyle J et al. Cancer, warts and sunshine in renal transplant patients. *Lancet* 1984; 1:702–705.

105. Smith SE et al. Absence of human papilloma virus in squamous cell carcinomas of nongenital skin from immunocompromised renal transplant patients. *Arch Dermatol* 1993; 129:1585–1588.

106. Kripke ML. Immunology and photocarcinogenesis: a new light on an old problem. *J Am Acad Dermatol* 1986; 14:149–155.

107. Kripke ML. Immunosuppressive action of UV radiation. In: de Gruijl FR, ed. *The Dark Side of Sunlight.* Utrecht, Neth.: Utrecht University; 1993:77–85.

108. Yoshikawa T et al. Susceptibility to effects of UVB radiation on induction of contact sensitivity as a risk factor for skin cancer in humans. *J Invest Dermatol* 1990; 95:530–536.

109. Cleaver JE. DNA damage and repair in light-sensitive human skin diseases. *J Invest Dermatol* 1970; 54:181–195.

110. Cleaver JE. Repair processes for photochemical damage in mammalian cells. *Adv Radiat Biol* 1974; 4:1–75.

111. Cleaver JE, Epstein JH. Xeroderma pigmentosum. In: Arndt K, Robinson J, LeBoit P, Wintroub B, eds. *Cutaneous Medicine and Surgery,* Vol. 2, *An Integrated Program in Dermatology.* Philadelphia: W.B. Saunders; 1996: 1747–1752.

112. Kraemer KH, Lee MM, Scotto J. Xeroderma pigmentosum: cutaneous, ocular and neurologic abnormalities in 830 published cases. *Arch Dermatol* 1987; 123:241–250.

113. Kraemer KH. Twenty years of research on xeroderma pigmentosum at the National Institutes of Health. In: Riklis E, ed. *Photobiology.* New York: Plenum Press; 1991:211–221.

114. Yarosh D et al. Enzyme therapy of xeroderma pigmentosum: safety and efficacy testing of T4N5 liposome lotion containing a prokaryotic DNA repair enzyme. *Photodermatol Photoimmunol Photomed* 1996; 12:122–130.

115. Ananthaswamy HN, Piercell WE. Molecular mechanisms of ultraviolet radiation carcinogenesis: yearly review. *Photochem Photobiol* 1990; 52:1119–1136.

116. Bishop MJ. The molecular genetics of cancer. *Science* 1987; 235:305–311.

117. Nataraj AJ, Trent JC II, Ananthaswamy HN. p53 gene mutations and photocarcinogenesis. *Photochem Photobiol* 1995; 62:218–230.

118. Elder JT. C-Ha-ras and UV photocarcinogenesis. *Arch Dermatol* 1990; 126:379–382.

119. Brash DE et al. A role for sunlight in skin cancer: UV-induced p53 mutations in squamous cell carcinoma. *Proc Natl Acad Sci USA* 1991; 88:10124–10128.

120. Campbell C et al. p53 mutations are common and early events that precede tumor invasion in squamous cell neoplasia of the skin. *J Invest Dermatol* 1993; 100:746–748.

121. Nagano T, Ueda M, Ichihashi M. Expression of p53 protein is an early event in ultraviolet-induced cutaneous squamous cell carcinogenesis. *Arch Dermatol* 1993; 129:1157–1161.

122. Nakazawa H et al. UV and skin cancer: specific p53 gene mutation in normal skin as a biologically relevant exposure measurement. *Proc Natl Acad Sci USA* 1994; 91:360–364.

123. Rigel DS. Malignant melanoma: perspectives on incidence and its effects on awareness, diagnosis, and treatment. *CA Cancer J Clin* 1996; 46:195–198.

124. Rigel DS, Kopf AW, Friedman RJ. Incidence and mortality of malignant melanoma in the U.S. *Melanoma Letters* 1989; 7:1–2.

125. Johnson TM, Rowe DE, Nelson BR, Swanson NA. Squamous cell carcinoma of the skin (excluding lip and oral mucosa). *J Am Acad Dermatol* 1992; 26:467–484.

126. Koh HK, Kligler BE, Leu RA. Sunlight and cutaneous melanoma: evidence for and against causation—yearly review. *Photochem Photobiol* 1990; 51:765–779.

127. Koh HK, Leu RA. Sunscreens and melanoma: implications for prevention. *J Natl Cancer Inst* 1994; 86:78–79 [editorial].

128. Katsambas A, Nicolaidov E. Cutaneous malignant melanoma and sun exposure: recent developments in epidemiology. *Arch Dermatol* 1996; 132:444–450.

129. Marks R. Prevention and control of melanoma: the public health approach. *CA Cancer J Clin* 1996; 46:199–216.

130. Walter SD et al. The association of cutaneous malignant melanoma with the use of sunbeds and sunlamps. *Am J Epidemiol* 1990; 131:232–243.

131. Westerdahl J et al. Use of sunbeds or sunlamps and malignant melanoma in southern Sweden. *Am J Epidemiol* 1994; 140:691–698.

132. Austin DF, Reynolds P. Occupation and malignant melanoma of the skin. In: Gallagher RP, ed. *Epidemiology of Malignant Melanoma: Recent Results in Cancer Research.* Berlin: Springer-Verlag; 1986:98–107.

133. Goldblatt MW. Occupational carcinogenesis. *Br Med Bull* 1958; 14:136–141.

134. Schottenfeld P, Haas F. Carcinogens in the workplace. *CA Cancer J Clin* 1979; 29:144–168.

135. Doll R. Relevance of epidemiology to policies for the prevention of cancer. *J Occup Med* 1981; 23:601–609.

136. Kipling MD. Oil and the skin. In: *Annual Report of HM Chief Inspector of Factories, 1967.* London: HM Stationery Office; 1968:105–119.

137. Lloyd JW. Angiosarcoma of the liver in vinyl chloride/ polyvinyl chloride workers. *J Occup Med* 1975; 17:33–334.

138. Hotchkiss RS. Cancer of the skin of the male genitalia. In: Andrade R et al., eds. *Cancer of the Skin,* Vol. 2. Philadelphia: W.B. Saunders; 1976:1432.

139. Beard RR, Noe JT. Aromatic nitro and amino compounds. In: Clayton GD, Clayton F, eds. *Patty's Industrial Hygiene and Toxicology,* Vol. 2A. New York: John Wiley & Sons; 1981:2422–2425.

140. Cole P. A population study of bladder cancer. In: Doll R, Vodopija I, eds. *Host Environment Interaction in the Etiology of Cancer in Man.* IARC Sci Publ, 1973:83–87.

141. Selikoff IJ, Mannond EC, Churg J. Asbestos exposure, smoking and neoplasia. *JAMA* 1968; 204:106–112.

142. Cohen SR et al. Mycosis fungoides: a retrospective study with observations on occupation as a new prognostic factor. *J Invest Dermatol* 1978; 70:221.

143. Cohen SR et al. Mycosis fungoides: clinicopathologic relationships, survival, and therapy in 59 patients, with observation on occupation as a new prognostic factor. *Cancer* 1980; 46:2654–2666.

144. Epstein JH, Fukuyama K, Reed WB, Epstein WL. Defect in DNA synthesis in xeroderma pigmentosum. *Science* 1970; 168:1477–1478.

145. Setlow RV et al. Evidence that xeroderma pigmentosum cells do not perform the first step in repair of UV damage to their DNA. *Proc Natl Acad Sci USA* 1969; 64:1035–1041.

146. Nathanson RB, Forbes PD, Urbach F. Modification by antilymphocytic serum of 6-mercaptopurine. *Proc Am Assoc Cancer Res* 1973; 14:46.

147. Blohme I, Larko O. Premalignant and malignant skin lesions in renal transplant patients. *Transplantation* 1984; 37:165–167.

148. Kelley GE, Sheil AGR, Taylor R. Nonspecific immunological studies in kidney transplant patients with and without skin cancer. *Transplantation* 1984; 37:368–372.

149. Koranda FC et al. Cutaneous complications in immunosuppressed renal homograft recipients. *JAMA* 1974; 229:419–424.

150. Ferrandiz C et al. Epidermal dysplasia and neoplasia in kidney transplant recipients. *J Am Acad Dermatol* 1995; 33:590–596.

151. Epstein JH. Photocarcinogenesis: a review. *Natl Cancer Inst Monogr* 1978; 50:13–25.

152. Nyfors A, Jensen H. Frequency of malignant neoplasms in 248 long-term methotrexate-treated psoriatics: a preliminary study. *Dermatologica* 1983; 167:260–261.

153. Beral V, Robinson N. The relationship of malignant melanoma, basal cell and squamous skin cancers to indoor and outdoor work. *Br J Cancer* 1981; 44:886–891.

154. Blair A, Hayes HM Jr. Mortality patterns among US veterinarians 1947–1977: an expanded study. *Int J Epidemiol* 1982; 11:391–397.

155. Delzell E, Grufferman S. Mortality among white and nonwhite farmers in North Carolina, 1976–1978. *Am J Epidemiol* 1985; 121:391–402.

156. Hogan DJ, Lane P. Dermatologic disorders in agriculture. *Occup Med* 1986; 1:285–300.

157. Stellman SD, Garfinkel L. Cancer mortality among woodworkers. *Am J Ind Med* 1984; 5:343–357.

158. Hall AF. Relationship of sunlight, complexion, and heredity to skin carcinogenesis. *Arch Dermatol Syphilol* 1950; 61:589–610.

159. Emmett EA. Occupational skin cancer: a review. *J Occup Med* 1975; 17:44–49.

160. Birmingham DJ. Occupational dermatoses. *Prog Dermatol* 1968; 3:1–8.

161. Emmett EA et al. Skin and eye diseases among arc

welders and those exposed to welding operations. *J Occup Med* 1981; 23:85–90.

162. Epstein JH. Ultraviolet light carcinogenesis. In: Montagna W, Dobson RL, eds. *Advances in Biology of Skin,* Vol. 7. *Carcinogenesis.* Oxford: Pergamon Press; 1966: 215–236.

163. Marks R, Rennie G. Malignant transformation of solar keratoses to squamous cell carcinoma. *Lancet* 1988; 1:795–797.

164. Moller R, Reymann F, Hou-Jensen K. Metastasis in dermatological patients with squamous cell carcinoma. *Arch Dermatol* 1979; 115:703–705.

165. Bendl BJ, Graham JH. New concepts on the origin of squamous cell carcinomas of the skin: solar (senile) keratosis with squamous cell carcinoma—a clinico-pathogenic and histochemical study. In: *Proceedings of the Sixth National Cancer Conference, 1968, Denver, Colo.* Philadelphia: J.B. Lippincott; 1970:471–488.

166. Lund HZ. How often does squamous cell carcinoma of the skin metastasize? *Arch Dermatol* 1965; 92:635–637.

167. Lindquest C, Tepps L. Epidemiologic evaluation of sunlight as a risk factor of lip cancer. *Br J Cancer* 1978; 37:983–989.

168. Dunn JE et al. Skin cancer as a cause of death. *Calif Med* 1965; 102:361–363.

169. Emmett EA. Occupational skin cancers. *Occup Med* 1987; 2:165–177.

170. Epstein JH, Epstein WL, Nakai T. Production of melanomas from DMBA-induced "blue nevi" in hairless mice with ultraviolet light. *J Natl Cancer Inst* 1967; 38:19–30.

171. Lee JAH, Strickland D. Malignant melanoma: social status and outdoor work. *Br J Cancer* 1980; 41:757–763.

172. Teppo L et al. Way of life and cancer incidence in Finland. *Scand J Soc Med* 1980; 19[suppl].

173. Pion IA et al. Occupation and the risk of malignant melanoma. *Cancer* 1995; 75:637–644.

174. Carpenter L et al. Combined analysis of mortality in three United Kingdom nuclear industry workforces, 1946–1988. *Radiat Res* 1994; 138:224–238.

175. Hardell L, Holmberg B, Malker H, Paulsson LE. Exposure to extremely low frequency electromagnetic fields and the risk of malignant disease: an evaluation of epidemiological and experimental findings. *Eur J Cancer Prev* 1995; 1:3–107.

176. Streetly A, Markowe H. Changing trends in the epidemiology of malignant melanoma: gender differences and their implications for public health. *Intl J Epidemiol* 1995; 24:897–907.

177. Mackie RM, Hole DJ. Incidence and thickness of primary tumours and survival of patients with cutaneous melanoma in relation to socioeconomic status. *Br Med J* 1996; 312:1125–1128.

178. Nelemans PJ et al. Effect of intermittent exposure to sunlight on melanoma risk among indoor workers and sun-sensitive individuals. *Environ Health Perspect* 1993; 101:252–255.

179. Wiklund K, Dich J. Cancer risks among male farmers in Sweden. *Eur J Cancer Prev* 1995; 4:81–90.

180. Fincham SM, Hanson J, Berkel J. Patterns and risks of cancer in farmers in Alberta. *Cancer* 1992; 69:1276–1285.

181. Blair A et al. Clues to cancer etiology from studies of farmers. *Scand J Work Environ Health* 1992; 18:209–215.

182. Davis DL, Blair A, Hoel DG. Agricultural exposures and cancer trends in developed countries. *Environ Health Perspect* 1993; 100:39–44.

183. Miller JM, Beaumont JJ. Suicide, cancer, and other causes of death among California veterinarians, 1960–1992. *Am J Indust Med* 1995; 27:37–49.

184. Schwartz RA, Stoll HL. Epithelial precancerous lesions. In: Fitzpatrick TB et al., eds. *Dermatology in General Medicine,* 3rd ed. New York: McGraw Hill; 1987.

185. Pathak MA. Sunscreens: topical and systemic approaches for protection of human skin against harmful effects of solar radiation. *J Am Acad Dermatol* 1982; 7:285–312.

186. Lowe NJ et al. Indoor and outdoor efficacy testing of a broad spectrum sunscreen against ultraviolet A radiation in psoralen-sensitized subjects. *J Am Acad Dermatol* 1987; 17:224–230.

187. Lowe NJ. Ultraviolet A claims and testing procedures for OTC sunscreens: a summary and review. In: Lowe NJ, Sheath NM, Pathak MA, eds. *Sunscreens, Development, Evaluation and Regulatory Aspects,* 2nd ed. New York: Marcel Dekker; 1996:527–535.

188. Gallagher RP et al. Sunlight exposure, pigmentation factors, and risk of nonmelanocytic skin cancer. II. Squamous cell carcinoma. *Arch Dermatol* 1995; 131:164–169.

189. Decoufle P. Occupation. In: Schottenfeld P, Fraumeni JF Jr, eds. *Cancer Epidemiology and Prevention.* Philadelphia: W.B. Saunders; 1982:318–335.

190. Bourguet CC, Checkoway H, Hulka BS. A case control study of skin cancer in the tire and rubber manufacturing industry. *Am J Indust Med* 1987; 11:461–473.

191. Kaden DA, Hites RA, Thilly WG. Mutagenicity of soot and associated polycyclic aromatic hydrocarbons to Salmonella typhi-murium. *Cancer Res* 1977; 39:4152–4159.

192. NIOSH. Criteria for a recommended standard: occupational exposure to coal tar products. US Department of Health, Education and Welfare; 1977.

193. Saperstein MD, Wheeler LA. Mutagenicity of coal tar preparations used in psoriasis. *Tox Lett* 1979; 3:325–329.

194. International Agency for Research on Cancer. Polynuclear aromatic compounds. 4. Bitumen, coal-tar and derived products, shale-oils, and soots, Vol. 35. Lyon, France: WHO, IARC; 1985.

195. Ron WN et al. Morbidity survey of US oil shale workers employed during 1948–1969. *Arch Environ Health* 1985; 40:58–62.

196. Emmett EA, Bingham EM, Barkley W. A carcinogenic bioassay of certain roofing materials. *Am J Ind Med* 1981; 2:59–64.

197. Emmett EA. Cutaneous and ocular hazards of roofers. *Occup Med* 1986; 1:307–322.

198. Partanen T, Boffetta P. Cancer risk in asphalt workers and roofers: review and meta-analysis of epidemiologic studies. *Am J Indust Med* 1994; 26:721–740.

199. Karlehagen S, Andersen A, Ohlson CG. Cancer incidence among creosote-exposed workers. *Scand J Work Environ Health* 1992; 18:26–29.

200. Schnatter AR et al. A retrospective mortality study within operating segments of a petroleum company. *Am J Indust Med* 1992; 22:209–229.

201. Nokso-Koivisto P, Pukkala E. Past exposure to asbestos and combustion products and incidence of cancer among Finnish locomotive drivers. *Occup Environ Med* 1994; 51:330–334.

202. Cruickshank CN, Squire JR. Skin cancer in the engineering industry from the use of mineral oil, 1949. *Br J Indust Med* 1993; 50:289–300.

203. Axelson O et al. Updated and expanded Swedish cohort study on trichlorethylene and cancer risk. *J Occup Med* 1994; 36:556–562.

204. Mukhtar H et al. Additive effects of ultraviolet B and crude coal tar on cutaneous carcinogen metabolism: possible relevance to the tumorigenicity of the Goeckerman regimen. *J Invest Dermatol* 1986; 87:348–353.

205. Goetz H: Tar keratoses. In: Andrade R et al., eds. *Cancer of the Skin.* Philadelphia: W.B. Saunders; 1976:495.

206. Emmett EA, Stetzer L, Taphorn B. Phototoxic keratoconjunctivitis from coal-tar pitch volatiles. *Science* 1977; 198:841–842.

207. Henry SA. Occupational cutaneous cancer attributable to certain chemicals in industry. *Br Med Bull* 1947; 4:389–401.

208. Savitz DA, Moure R. Cancer risk among oil refinery workers: a review of epidemiologic studies. *J Occup Med* 1984; 26:622–670.

209. Bingham E, Thrust RP, Warshawsky D. Carcinogenic potential of petroleum hydrocarbons: a critical review of the literature. *J Environ Pathol Toxicol* 1979; 3:483–563.

210. Halder CA et al. Carcinogenicity of petroleum lubricating oil distillates: effects of solvent refining, hydroprocessing, and blending. *Am J Indust Med* 1984; 5:265–274.

211. Butlin HT. Three lectures on cancer of the scrotum in chimney-sweeps and others. Lecture II. Why foreign sweeps do not suffer from scrotal cancer. *Br Med J* 1892; 1:1–6.

212. Cantrell A. Annual refining survey. *Oil Gas J* 1980; 78:130–160.

213. Hueper WC, Payne WW. Experimental studies in metal carcinogenesis: chromium, nickel, iron, arsenic. *Arch Environ Health* 1962; 5:445–462.

214. Baroni C, Van Esch GJ, Saffiotti U. Carcinogenesis tests of two inorganic arsenicals. *Arch Environ Health* 1963; 7:668–674.

215. Sanderson KC. Arsenic and skin cancer. In: Andrade R et al., eds. *Cancer of the Skin.* Philadelphia: W.B. Saunders; 1976:478.

216. Thompson RHS. The effect of arsenical vesicants on the respiration of skin. *Biochem J* 1946; 40:525–529.

217. Petres J et al. Effects of arsenic cell metabolism and cell proliferation: cytogenic and biochemical studies. *Environ Health Perspect* 1977; 19:223–227.

218. Rossman T, Meyn MS, Troll W. Effects of sodium arsenite on the survival of UV-irradiated *Escherichia coli*: inhibition of a recA-dependent function. *Mutat Res* 1975; 30:157–161.

219. Fong K, Lee F, Bockrath R. Effects of sodium arsenite on single-strand DNA break formation and post-replication repair in *E. coli* following UV irradiation. *Mutat Res* 1980; 70:151–156.

220. Oppenheim JJ, Fishbein WN. Induction of chromosome breaks in cultured normal human leucocytes by potassium arsenite, hydroxyurea and related compounds. *Cancer Res* 1965; 25:980.

221. Nakamuro K, Sayato Y. Comparative studies of chromosomal aberration induced by trivalent and pentavalent arsenic. *Mutat Res* 1981; 88:73–80.

222. Nordenson I, Beckman G, Beckman L, Nordstrom S. Occupational and environmental risks in and around a smelter in northern Sweden. II. Chromosomal aberrations in workers exposed to arsenic. *Hereditas* 1978; 88:47–50.

223. Frost DV. Arsenicals in biology: retrospect and prospect. *Fed Proc* 1967; 26:194–208.

224. Legge TM. Annual report of HM Chief Inspector of Factories. London: HM Stationery Office; 1902:262.

225. Henry SA. Industrial arsenical poisoning. In: Legge TH, ed. *Industrial Maladies.* London: Oxford University Press/Hogarth Milford; 1934:83–84.

226. Hill AB, Faning EL. Studies on the incidence of cancer in a factory handling inorganic compounds of arsenic. I. Mortality experience of the factory. *Br J Ind Med* 1948; 5:1–6.

227. Lee AM, Fraumeni JF Jr. Arsenic and respiratory cancer in man: an occupational study. *J Natl Cancer Inst* 1969; 42:1045–1052.

228. Ott MG, Holder BB, Gordon HL. Respiratory cancer and occupational exposure to arsenicals. *Arch Environ Health* 1974; 29:250–255.

229. Baetjer AM, Levin ML, Lilienfeld A. *Analysis of Mortality Experience of Allied Chemical Plant.* Unpublished report submitted to Allied Chemical Corp. July 1974.

230. Tseng WP, Chu HM, How SW. Prevalence of skin cancer in an endemic area of chronic arsenicism in Taiwan. *J Natl Cancer Inst* 1968; 40:453–463.

231. Miki Y et al. Cutaneous and pulmonary cancers associated with Bowen's disease. *J Am Acad Dermatol* 1982; 6:26–31.

232. Graham JH, Helwig EB. Bowen's disease and its relationship to systemic cancer. *Arch Dermatol* 1959; 80:133–159.

233. Graham JH, Helwig EB. Bowen's disease and its relationship to systemic cancer. *Arch Dermatol* 1961; 83:738–758.

234. Epstein E. Association of Bowen's disease with visceral cancer. *Arch Dermatol* 1960; 82:349–351.

235. Peterka ES, Lynch FW, Goltz RW. An association between Bowen's disease and internal cancer. *Arch Dermatol* 1961; 84:623–629.

236. Hugo NE, Conway H. Bowen's disease: its malignant potential and relationship to systemic cancer. *Plast Reconstr Surg* 1967; 39:190–194.

237. Callen J, Headington J. Bowen's and non-Bowen's squamous intraepidermal neoplasia of the skin. *Arch Dermatol* 1980; 116:422–426.

238. Andersen SLC et al. Relationship between Bowen's disease and internal malignant tumors. *Arch Dermatol* 1973; 108:367–370.

239. Raymann F et al. Bowen's disease and internal malignant diseases. *Arch Dermatol* 1988; 124:677–679.

240. Callen JP. Bowen's disease and internal malignant disease. *Arch Dermatol* 1988; 124:675.

241. NIOSH. *Criteria for a Recommended Standard: Occupational Exposure to Inorganic Arsenic.* Cincinnati: U.S. Department of Health, Education and Welfare, Public Health Service; 1975.

242. Sheehy JW, Jones JH. Assessment of arsenic exposures and controls in gallium arsenide production. *Am Indust Hyg Assn J* 1993; 54:61–69.

243. Wald PH, Jones J. Semiconductor manufacturing: an introduction to processes and hazards. *Am J Ind Med* 1987; 11:203–221.

244. Hansen J, Olsen JH. Cancer morbidity among Danish female pharmacy technicians. *Scand J Work Environ Health* 1994; 20:22–26.

245. Pukkala E, Norso-Koivisto P, Roponen P. Changing cancer risk pattern among Finnish hairdressers. *Intl Arch Occup Environ Health* 1992; 64:39–42.

246. Jee SH et al. Photodamage and skin cancer among paraquat workers. *Intl J Dermatol* 1995; 34:466–469.

247. Epstein EH Jr. Mycosis fungoides: survival, prognostic features, response to therapy and autopsy findings. *Med* 1972; 51:61–72.

248. Patterson JAK, Edelson RL. Cutaneous T-cell lymphoma and other leukemic and lymphomatous infiltrates of the skin. In: Fitzpatrick TB et al., eds. *Dermatology in General Medicine,* 3rd ed. New York: McGraw-Hill; 1987.

249. Rowden G, Lewis MG. Langerhans cells: involvement in the pathogenesis of mycosis fungoides. *Br J Dermatol* 1976; 95:665–672.

250. Fischmann AB et al. Exposure to chemicals, physical agents, and biologic agents in mycosis fungoides and the Sézary syndrome. *Cancer Treat Rep* 1979; 63:591–596.

251. Greene MH et al. Mycosis fungoides: epidemiologic observations. *Cancer Treat Rep* 1979; 63:597–606.

252. Tuyp E, Burgoyne A, Aitchinson T, Mackie R. A case-

control study of possible causative factors in mycosis fungoides. *Arch Dermatol* 1987; 23:196–200.

253. Auster LS. The role of trauma in oncogenesis: a juridical consideration. *JAMA* 1961; 175:946–950.

254. Vickers CFH. Industrial carcinogenesis. *Br J Dermatol* 1981; 105:57–61.

255. Ewing J. Relation of trauma to malignant tumors. *Am J Surg* 1926; 40:30–36.

256. Ewing J. Modern attitudes toward traumatic cancer. *Arch Pathol* 1935; 19:690–728.

257. Stoll HL Jr, Crissey JT. Epithelioma from single trauma. In: Helm F, ed. *Cancer Dermatology*. Philadelphia: Lea & Febiger; 1979:25–30.

258. Jordan A. Uber die Ehtstehungnvon Tumoren, Tuberkulose, und anderen Organerkrankheiten noch Einwirkung, stumpfer Gewalt (unter Ausschuluss von Frakturen, Luxationen, Hernien und traumatischen Neurosen). *Munch Med Wchnschr* 1901; 48:1741–1746.

259. Lowenstein S. Zur Frage der "Posttraumatischen Krebse." *Beitrage Kin Chir* 1911; 74:715–743.

260. Mock HE, Ellis JD. Trauma and malignancy. *JAMA* 1926; 86:257–261.

261. Dix CR. Occupational trauma and skin cancer. *Plastic Reconstr Surg* 1960; 26:546–554.

262. Coburn RJ. Malignant cancer ulcers following trauma. In: Andrade R, et al., eds. *Cancer of the Skin*. Philadelphia: W.B. Saunders; 1976:941.

263. Arons MS et al. Scar tissue carcinoma. I. A clinical study with special reference to burn scar carcinoma. *Ann Surg* 1965; 161:170–188.

264. Neve EF. Kangri-burn cancer. *Br Med J* 1923; 2:1255.

265. Frieben E. Demonstration eines Cancroids des rechten Handruckens, dass sich nach langdauernder Einwirkung von Roentgenstrahlen entwickelt hatte. *Fortschr Roentgenstr* 1902; 6:106.

266. Goldschmidt H, Sherwin WK. Reactions to ionizing radiation. *J Am Acad Dermatol* 1980; 3:551–579.

267. Stoll HL Jr. Squamous cell carcinoma. In: Fitzpatrick TB et al., eds. *Dermatology in General Medicine,* 3rd ed. New York: McGraw-Hill; 1987:746–758.

268. Mole RH. Radiation-induced tumors: human experience. *Br J Radiol* 1972; 45:613.

Bibliography

Adams RM. *Occupational Skin Disease.* New York: Grune and Stratton; 1983:83.

Hutchinson J. Arsenic cancer: reports of societies. *Br Med J* 1887; 2:1280–1281.

Joust J, Oppenheim JJ, Fishbein WN. Induction of chromosome breaks in cultured normal human leukocytes by potassium arsenite, hydroxyurea and related compounds. *Cancer Res* 1965; 25:980–985.

Kopf AW, Rigel DS, Friedman RJ. The rising incidence and mortality rate of malignant melanoma. *J Dermatol Surg Oncol* 1982; 8:760–761.

Paris JA. *Pharmacologia, Comprehending the Art of Prescribing upon Fixed and Scientific Principles Together with the History of Medicinal Substances.* New York: F&R Lockwood; 1823:61–66.

Pott P. *Cancer Scroti.* In: *Chirurgical Observations.* London: Hawes, Clarke, and Collins; 1775:63–68.

Rigel DS, Friedman RJ. The rate of malignant melanoma in the United States: are we making an impact? *J Am Acad Dermatol* 1987; 17:1050–1053.

Silverberg E, Lubera JA. Cancer statistics, 1987. *CA Cancer J Clin.* 1987; 37:2–19.

Silverberg E, Lubera JA. Cancer statistics, 1988. *CA Cancer J Clin.* 1988; 38:5–27.

Yuspa SH. Cutaneous chemical carcinogenesis. *J Am Acad Dermatol* 1986; 15:1031–1044.

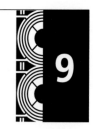

Occupational Nail Disorders

MARTHA J. MASO, M.D., M.P.H.
RICHARD K. SCHER, M.D.

Since time immemorial, the skin and integument have provided physicians with clues to an individual's occupation or position in life. It was not until 1700, however, when Ramazzini[1] wrote the first formal treatise on occupational medicine, that recognition was given to the area of occupational medicine in general and to occupational dermatology in particular.

Perhaps because medical schools, medical residency training programs, and even occupational medicine residency programs offer limited training in dermatology, diagnosis of occupational skin diseases continues to challenge even the most talented physicians in occupational medicine, despite the fact that as much as 50% of occupational disease involves skin.[2] Taking the intricacies of subspecialization and modern medicine a step farther, nail disease and especially occupational nail disease continue to test the skills of—if not confound—the most astute of dermatologists. With this in mind, we have attempted, in the following pages, to summarize the salient issues in the identification of occupational nail disease.

CATEGORIES OF DIAGNOSIS

Mechanical Factors

Mechanical trauma, chemical exposures, and physical or biological factors are the major categories of occupational nail disease.[3] In turn, manifestations of nail disease usually fall into one of a few distinct clinical reaction patterns, the most common of which include trauma to the nail plate, nail matrix injuries, discoloration of the nail, onycholysis, onychorrhexis, onychia, koilonychia, clubbing, and paronychia-induced nail plate changes.[3–5]

The effects of mechanical trauma on nails have been well described by Adams[4] and may be associated acutely with one significant injury or chronically with repeated minor injury. The most common result of trauma to the nail unit is probably subungual hematoma, which the clinician must be able to differentiate from malignant melanoma or other pigment-associated phenomena.[5] Hematomas have been well described in the large toes of tennis players (Fig. 9–1) and squash and raquetball players, in the second and third toes of soccer and football players, and in the fourth and fifth toes of runners and joggers[6] (Fig. 9–2). Obviously, any

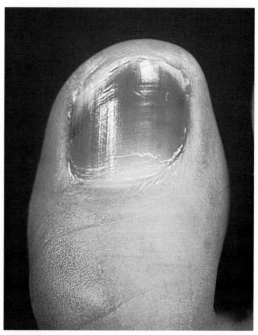

FIGURE 9–1 • Subungual hematoma of the hallux of a tennis player—"tennis toe."

165

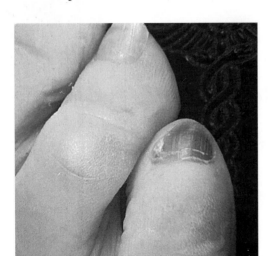

FIGURE 9–2 • Subungual hematoma of the fifth toe of a jogger—"jogger's toe."

athlete can injure any toe, so biopsy, if indicated, is the gold standard for diagnosis, particularly because up to 25% of acral lentiginous melanomas are seen in the context of preceding nail trauma.[5] Splinter hemorrhages, leukonychiae striae, onychauxis, onycholysis, pincer nails, splits and ridges, hook nails, and ectopic nails are other well-described nail injuries in athletes.[7] Additionally, worn-down fingernails have been seen in bowlers.[8]

Repeated trauma in association with increased pressure on the nail plate may result in nail hypertrophy, onychogryphosis[4] and onycholysis.[9] The recently described entity of frictional longitudinal melanonychia[10] also has been attributed to increased pressure on the nail plate, causing pigmentation of the toenails in individuals wearing tightly fitting shoes, and melanonychia striata of the fingernails in association with Hutchinson's sign in a boxer of 40 years.[11] Repetitive trauma, as seen in association with keypunching, has been linked to leukonychia striae.[12] Hand-arm vibration syndrome, synonymous with Raynaud's phenomenon of occupational origin or vibration white finger syndrome has been reported in workers using vibrating hand tools such as chain saws.[13] In these individuals, a reduction in the number of nail-fold capillaries has been noted, although this may not translate to nail plate changes. Spooning of the nails, or koilonychia, is a reaction usually seen with minor repetitive trauma in conjunction with exposure to organic solvents, oils, and acids. Groups at risk include cabinetmakers, mechanics, housespouses, glassworkers, mushroom growers,[14] and hairdressers.[15]

Penetrating injury to the nail is another frequent occupational hazard. A worker involved in the production of small appliances sustained a penetrating injury to the dorsal fingertip and nail and 4½ months later, proved to have a foreign-body reaction from two of her own retained fingernail fragments.[16] Another interesting example of a foreign-body reaction secondary to a penetrating injury was reported in a Mediterranean diver and a sea urchin fisherman who developed sea urchin granulomas of the nails due to the embedding of the spines in the skin.[17] The affected nails exhibited periungual nodules, partial detachment from the nail bed and splitting of the nail plates distally. Traumatic pterygia resulting from hammer injuries to the nail matrix are not uncommon among carpenters and construction workers.[5] A more subtle manifestation of penetrating injury was described recently in a hairdresser who developed a subungual trichogranuloma due to subungual penetration by sharp hair clippings.[18] Onycholysis due to embedded hair has been reported previously in beauticians.[19]

Chemical Exposures

Chemical exposures also produce recognizable clinical reactions in nails. Just as contact dermatitis is one of the most frequently encountered problems in occupational dermatology, so too is it one of the major players in occupational nail disease, and it can lead to onycholysis, onychorrhexis, subungual hyperkeratosis, paronychia, crumbling of the nail plate, and Beau's lines.[5] In a 1995 study of occupational hand dermatitis in a dermatology clinic in Taipei,[20] authors identified 164 affected patients. Of these, 58.5% and 41.5%, respectively, demonstrated irritant vs. allergic contact dermatitis. Patients with nail-fold involvement were at greater risk for allergic contact dermatitis, with the most important allergens being dichromate, nickel, cobalt, fragrance mix, epoxy resin, thiram mix, and paraphenylenediamine (Fig. 9–3).[20]

Reactions to nail cosmetics are seen widely in both manicurists and their clients. Reaction patterns include transient or permanent nail dystrophy, paronychia, onycholysis and, in severe cases, permanent nail loss (Fig. 9–4).[21, 22] Exposure to methyl methacrylate, methacrylate ester monomers, dimethacrylates, and trimethacrylates are most frequently implicated.[21, 23] Most likely, the methacrylate monomers, more widely used today, crossreact with methyl methacrylate, which was more commonly used in the past. Additionally, cyanoacrylate nail preparations have been reported to cause nail dystrophy and paronychia.[23] Before

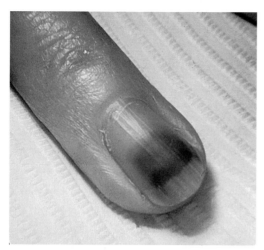

FIGURE 9–3 • Nail plate staining by paraphenyl-enediamine in a hairdresser.

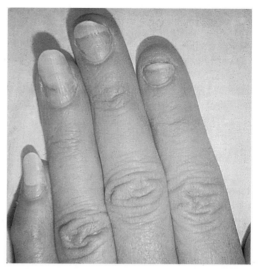

FIGURE 9–5 • Onycholysis caused by nail hardener.

formaldehyde was removed from nail hardeners (Fig. 9–5) in the United States, the use of these products had been linked to subungual hemorrhage, inflammatory and noninflammatory onycholysis, paronychia, chromonychia, onychomadesis, pterygium inversum unguis, subungual hyperkeratosis, and lip hemorrhages in onychotillomania.[25] These days, products containing formaldehyde-releasing agents rather than formaldehyde itself may be problematic. Sulfonamide resins in nail polish may cause contact dermatitis, and the dyes in nail polish may lead to photosensitization, possibly leading to concomitant reactions in nails as described above.[5]

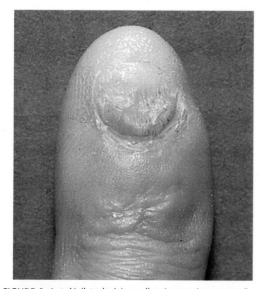

FIGURE 9–4 • Nail technician; allergic reaction to acrylic, with partial nail plate loss.

Workers employed in the production of paraquat, weed killers, and insecticides can exhibit localized white transverse bands at low levels of exposure, whereas with severe exposure, transverse ridging and furrowing, onycholysis, and onychia may ensue.[26] Onychia also has been known to result from exposure to hair products that restore split ends, as well as to depilatories and thioglycolates in permanent-wave preparations.[25] Tulip workers who separate bulbs may develop contact dermatitis in association with onycholysis.[27] Exposure to vinyl chloride has been associated with acro-osteolysis and the widening and shortening of the nail plate.[5] Sensitivity to quaternium 15 in the context of trauma may produce onycholysis without nail-fold changes.[28]

Chromonychia is a reaction that nails exhibit to occupational damage from a number of sources (Fig. 9–6), and chemically induced chromonychia, in particular, has myriad origins (Table 9–1). To distinguish chromonychias of environmental as opposed to endogenous origin, Zaias[29] suggests that the latter follows the shape of the lunula in contrast to exogenous chromonychias which follow the proximal nail fold. When examining the nail, certain steps should be taken.[3, 30] First, fingers should be relaxed, with no pressure on the tips. Next, the nail bed should be blanched by depressing the nail plate. The underside of the nail's free edge should then be illuminated. Pigment limited to the nail plate will persist after both tests, whereas illumination probably will cause pigment in the nail bed to disappear. Additionally, topical staining should be ruled out by scraping, cleansing, or applying solvent such as acetone to the nail bed.

Some interesting examples of chemically induced occupational chromonychia follow, and other examples are listed in Table 9–1. Chestnut-brown pigmentation of the nail plate has been described with the use of hydroquinone depigmenting cream.[31] Pigmentation deepened during periods of sun exposure and resolved when nails were protected or removed from the hydroquinone. Yellow staining has been noted on fingernails of molded-plastics workers exposed to 4,4'- methylenedianiline (MDA). This finding may assist in diagnosing exposure to MDA,[32] a hepatotoxin known to cause cholestasis. Harris and Rosen[33] describe orange-brown discoloration of the nails that arose in a nonsmoking individual who had constructed a mahogany bannister and used no stains, varnishes, or paints. Occupational or exogenous factors reported to cause nail staining in the yellow-to-brown spectrum include nail treatments,[5] contact with rural well water high in elemental iron,[34] and exposure to tobacco, pecans, walnuts, coffee, burnt sugar, varnishes, formaldehyde, dyes, weed killers, and insecticides.[30, 35] Purple-blue discoloration of the nails has been reported in workers exposed to aromatic amines or aromatic compounds, leading to methemoglobinemia. Those at risk are employed in the manufacturing of pigments, dyes, explosives, rubber, textiles, and paper.[36] Blue-gray discoloration of the nails is also associated with generalized argyria seen in silver refinery workers.[37]

Physical Agents

Physical factors contributing to occupational nail disease are varied and diverse. Occupational expo-

TABLE 9–1 • Sources of Occupational and Environmental Chromonychia[25, 31-33]

Yellow Nails	Orange-Brown Nails
Amphotericin	Anthralin
Dinitroorthocresol	Arning's tincture
Fluorescein	Burnt sugar
Hatter's chemicals	Chromium salts
Hydrofluoric acid	Chrysarobin
4,4'-methylenedianiline	Coffee
Nail treatments	Dinitrotoluene
	Dithranol
Green Nails	Dyes
Chlorophyll	Formaldehyde
Copper salts	Glutaraldehyde
Pseudomonas	Henna
(Figure 9–6)	Hydroquinone
	Iodohydroxyquinolone
Gray-Blue Nails	Iron
Ammoniated mercury	Mahogany
Mercuric chloride	Mepacrine
Silver	Nicotine
	Paraquat
Dark Blue Nails	Pecans
Oxalic acid	Picric acid
Silver cyanide	Potassium
	permanganate
Lilac-Blue Nails	Pyrogallol
Aromatic amines	Resorcin combined with
	nail lacquer
Purple Nails	Rivanol
Gentian violet	Thermal injury
	Varnishes
Red Nails	Vioform
Carbolfuchsin	Walnuts
Black Nails	
Phenol sulfate	
hydroquinone	
Red wine	
Silver nitrite	

sure to x-rays (Fig. 9–7) has been implicated in the genesis of Bowen's disease (Fig. 9–8) of the nail matrix, which has presented as a rapidly growing pigmented nail streak with nail deformity in a Japanese physician.[38] Clearly, the differential diagnosis of subungual melanoma would have to be ruled out in cases such as these. Interestingly, inadvertent exposure to microwave radiation has been implicated in the development of Beau's lines in two snackbar employees.[39]

Exposure to the cold, wet mud used to repair walls and irrigation canals has been related to seasonal, reversible koilonychia.[40] The anomaly has been reported to occur primarily in spring and summer and to resolve during the winter. Wet work in general has been reported to increase brittleness of nails, a factor more common among women, possibly because of weaker bridges in nail plate corneocytes in females than in males.[41]

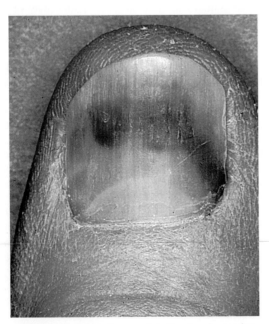

FIGURE 9–6 • *Pseudomonas* infection in a bartender.

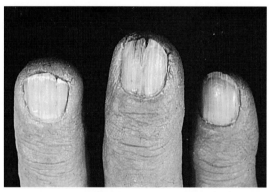

FIGURE 9–7 • Brittle nails caused by years of fluoroscopy in a radiologist.

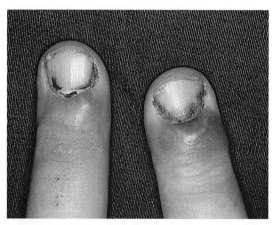

FIGURE 9–9 • Milkers' nodules, the paravaccinia virus, in farmworker.

Biological Agents

Infectious causes of occupational nail disease commonly involve *Candida albicans* and *Candida parapsilosis* in association with paronychia,[3] although the latter also can be seen with tuberculosis.[42] *Pseudomonas aeruginosa* frequently colonizes the onycholytic nail, imparting a green-black color to the nail bed (see Fig. 9–6).[5] *Scytalidium dimidiatum* and *Scytalidium hyalinum* toenail and fingernail infections are less common in the United States but have been well described in West African, West Indian, and Pacific Island immigrants to the United Kingdom.[43] Onychomycosis has been estimated to account for some 50% of nail problems and can lead to psychological disorders, occupational limitations, cosmetic disfigurement, and reduced quality of life.[44] *Trichophyton rubrum* and *Trichophyton mentagrophytes* cause onychomycosis most frequently, although zoophilic dermatophytoses may occur more commonly in veterinarians, farmers, butchers, abattoir workers, and zookeepers.[3] Herpes simplex virus infection of the nail plate or herpetic whitlow has been well described in health-care workers, and milkers' nodules have been observed in farmworkers (Fig. 9–9).[5]

TREATMENT AND PREVENTION

Treatment of occupational nail disease is accomplished most obviously by prevention, although clearly most infectious causes can be treated medically. Preventive strategies parallel general principles of prevention in occupational medicine, such as substitution of a nontoxic material for a toxic one, engineering controls (enclosure, isolation, ventilation), controls on human behavior (e.g., administrative personnel issues and changes, work practices), and the use of personal protective equipment.[45]

NAIL CHANGES RESULTING FROM PREGNANCY AND FROM TRANSPLACENTAL EXPOSURE TO TOXINS

Physiological skin changes during pregnancy have been reviewed by Wong and Ellis.[46] Nail changes, in particular, have been reported as early as the sixth week of gestation and include transverse grooving, increased brittleness (Fig. 9–10), softening, distal onycholysis, and subungual hyperkeratosis.[46] Although the causes of these findings are unknown, it may be hypothesized that capillary blood flow velocity, which significantly increases

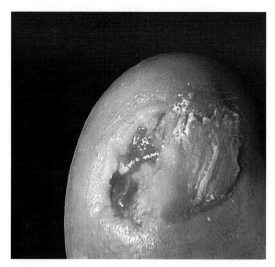

FIGURE 9–8 • Bowen's disease in an elderly dentist resulting from x-ray exposure many years earlier.

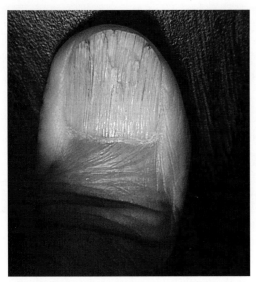

FIGURE 9–10 • Brittle nails developed during pregnancy.

in the first trimester, may play a contributory role.[47] Exposures that may exacerbate nail changes should be avoided—wet work, nail treatments, and infections.

Transplacental exposure to chemicals or toxins during pregnancy has been linked to nail changes in both nonhuman and human offspring. Rhesus macaque monkeys fed diets containing polychlorinated biphenyl (PCB) mixtures, dioxin (TCDD or 2,3,7,8 tetrachlorodibenzo-*p*-dioxin), and 2,3,7,8 tetrachlorodibenzofuran (TCDF) exhibited nailbed metaplasia such that the nail-bed epidermis became keratinizing.[48] This led to the lifting away and breaking of the nail plate due to the keratin accumulating under it. In children exposed in utero to PCBs and dibenzofurans through consumption of contaminated rice and bran cooking oil, a higher rate of dystrophic fingernails and pigmented or dystrophic toenails was noted than in nonexposed children.[49] A follow-up study of these individuals 11 years later[50] suggested that (1) transplacental exposure to PCBs may lead to developmental retardation of the fetal nail matrix, (2) maternal storage of PCBs could affect nail growth in children even several years after the initial intoxication, and (3) nail deformities in children were the most persistent abnormality associated with transplacental exposure to PCBs. Particular deformities included transverse grooves, irregular depressions, koilonychia, and nail flattening. Hypoplastic nails also have resulted from in utero exposure to phenytoin, either alone or in combination with other anticonvulsant agents.[51]

More devastating from a societal standpoint in terms of frequency of occurrence and potential for

prevention is exposure to ethanol in utero, which can lead to fetal alcohol syndrome (FAS).[52] FAS may occur in 1 to 2:1,000 births and may be partially expressed in as many as 1:200 births. Of note is that nail dysplasia has been identified in more than 20% of people with FAS,[53] making this finding a potential early clue for detection, diagnosis, and intervention.

METAL LEVELS IN NAILS AS AN INDICATOR OF OCCUPATIONAL EXPOSURE

Although controversial, there is some evidence to suggest that monitoring the nail concentrations of certain metals may identify individuals at occupational risk for exposure. Agahian et al.[54] reported a formula to estimate air arsenic exposure levels by testing the arsenic content of fingernails. Similarly, Peters et al.[55] concluded that the higher the levels of nickel in the fingernails, the greater the likelihood of pinpointing individuals exposed to nickel in the workplace.

CONCLUSIONS

As technology and computer algorithms come to be used increasingly in the diagnosis and treatment of disease, and as external variables exist to direct patients to seek care from general practitioners, it is critical that we not lose sight of the importance of clinical diagnosis, particularly in so uniquely a visual a specialty as dermatology. Training in the recognition and diagnosis of occupational skin and nail disorders should be emphasized in dermatology residency programs, and dermatologists should be the experts and consultants from whom patients seek direct treatment for occupationally related skin and nail conditions.

References

1. Ramazzini B. De mortis artificium diatriba. 1700.
2. Mathias CGT. The cost of occupational skin disease. *Arch Dermatol* 1985;121:332–334.
3. Kern DG. Occupational disease. In: Scher RK, Daniel III CR. *Nails: Therapy, Diagnosis and Management.* Philadelphia: W.B. Saunders; 1997. [In press.]
4. Adams RM. Effects of mechanical trauma on nails. *Am J Ind Med* 1985;8:273–280.
5. Scher RK. Occupational nail disorders. *Dermatol Clin* 1988;6:27–33.
6. Scher RK. Jogger's toe. *Int J Dermatol* 1978;17:719.
7. Mortimer PS, Dawber RD. Trauma to the nail unit including occupational sports injuries. *Dermatol Clin* 1985;3: 415–420.
8. Ronchese F. Occupational marks. New York: Grune and Stratton; 1948.

9. Menne T, Roed-Petersen J, Hjorth N. Pressure onycholysis in slaughterhouse workers. *Acta Derm Venereol Suppl* 1985;120:88–89.

10. Baran R. Frictional longitudinal melanonychia: a new entity. *Dermatologica* 1987;174:280–284.

11. Bayerl C, Moll I. Striped nail pigmentation with Huchinson sign in a boxer. *Hautarzt* 1993;7:476–479.

12. Honda M, Hattori S, Koyama L, et al. Leukonychia striae. *Arch Dermatol* 1976;112:1147.

13. Vayssairat M, Patri B, Mathieu JF, et al. Raynaud's phenomenon in chain saw users: hot and cold finger systolic pressures and nailfold capillary findings. *Eur Heart J* 1987;8:417–422.

14. Ancona-Alayon A. Occupational koilonychia from organic solvents. *Contact Dermatitis* 1975;1:367–369.

15. Alanko K, Kanerva L, Estlander T, et al. Hairdresser's koilonychia. *Australas J Dermatol* 1997 [suppl 2];38:90 [abstract].

16. Brown CK, Wooter SL, Fair LK. Retained foreign body: a fingernail fragment? *J Emerg Med* 1993;11:259–264.

17. Haneke E, Tosti A, Piraccini B. Sea urchin granuloma of the nail apparatus: report of two cases. *Dermatology* 1996;192:140–142.

18. Hogan DJ. Subungual trichogranuloma in a hairdresser. *Cutis* 1988;42:105–106.

19. Stubbart FJ. Onycholysis of fingernails of beauticians due to imbedded hair. *Arch Dermatol* 1956;74:430.

20. Sun C, Guo Y, Lin R. Occupational hand dermatitis in a tertiary referral dermatology clinic in Taipei. *Contact Dermatitis* 1995;33:414–418.

21. Freeman S, Lee M, Gedmundsen K. Adverse contact reactions to sculptured acrylic nails. *Contact Dermatitis* 1995;33:381–385.

22. Norton LA. Common and uncommon reactions to formaldehyde-containing nail hardeners. *Semin Dermatol* 1991;10:29–33.

23. Kanerva L, Lauerma A, Estlander T, et al. Occupational allergic contact dermatitis caused by photobonded sculptured acrylics and a review of (meth)acrylates in nail cosmetics. *Am J Contact Dermatitis* 1996;7:109–115.

24. Shelley ED, Shelley WB. Nail dystrophy and periungual dermatitis due to cyanoacrylate glue sensitivity. *J Am Acad Dermatol* 1988;19:574–576.

25. Rietschel RL, Fowler JF. *Contact Dermatitis*, 4th ed. Philadelphia: Williams & Wilkins; 1995:82–87.

26. Baran RL. Nail damage caused by weed killers and insecticides. *Arch Dermatol* 1974;110:467.

27. Baran RL. Occupational nail disorders. In: Adams RM, ed. *Occupational Skin Disease*. New York: Grune and Stratton; 1983.

28. Marren P, deBerker D, Dawber RPR, et al. Occupational contact dermatitis to quaternium 15 presenting as nail dystrophy. *Contact Dermatitis* 1991;25:253.

29. Zaias N. *The Nail in Health and Disease*. Norwalk, Conn.: Appleton & Lange; 1990.

30. Daniel CR, Osment LS. Nail pigmentation abnormalities. *Cutis* 1980;25:595.

31. Coulson IH. Fade-out photochromonychia. *Clin Exp Dermatol* 1993;18:87–88.

32. Cohen SR. Yellow staining caused by 4,4'-methylenedianiline exposure. *Arch Dermatol* 1985;121:1022–1027.

33. Harris A, Rosen T. Nail discoloration due to mahogany. *Cutis* 1989;43:55–56.

34. Olsen T, Jatlow P. Contact exposure to iron causing chromonychia. *Arch Dermatol* 1984;120:102.

35. Jeanmougin M, Civatte J. Nail dyschromia. *Int J Dermatol* 1983;22:279.

36. Beard RR, Noe JT. Aromatic nitro and amino compounds. In: Clayton GD, Clayton FE, eds. *Patty's Industrial Hygiene and Toxicology*. New York: John Wiley & Sons; 1981.

37. Bleeker SS, Gould DJ, Harrington CI, et al. Occupational argyria; light and electron microscopic studies and x-ray microanalysis. *Br J Dermatol* 1981;104:19.

38. Saijo S, Kato T, Tagami H. Pigmented nail streak associated with Bowen's disease of the nail matrix. *Dermatologia* 1990;181:156–158.

39. Brodkin RH, Bleiberg J. Cutaneous microwave injury. *Acta Derm Venereol* 1973;53:50.

40. Dolma T, Norboo T, Yayha M, et al. Seasonal koilonychia in Ladakh. *Contact Dermatitis* 1990;22:78–80.

41. Lubach D, Beckers P. Wet working conditions increase brittleness of nails, but do not cause it. *Dermatology* 1992;185:120–122.

42. O'Donnell TF, Jurgenson PF, Weyerich NF. An occupational hazard—tuberculosis paronychia. *Arch Surg* 1971;103:757.

43. Gugnanni HC, Oyeka CA. Foot infections due to *Hendersonula toruloidea* and *Scytalidium hyalinum* in coal miners. *J Med Vet Mycology* 1989;27:169–179.

44. Scher RK. Onychomycosis is more than a cosmetic problem. *Br J Dermatol* 1994;130 [suppl 43]:15

45. Fowler DP. Industrial hygiene. In: LaDou J, ed. *Occupational Medicine*. East Norwalk, Conn.: Appleton & Lange; 1990:499–513.

46. Wong RC, Ellis CN. Physiologic skin changes in pregnancy. *J Am Acad Dermatol* 1984;10:929–940.

47. Linder HR, Reinhart WH, Hanggi W, et al. Peripheral capillaroscopic findings and blood rheology during normal pregnancy. *Eur J Obstet Gynecol Reprod Biol* 1995;58:141–145.

48. McNulty WP. Toxicity and fetotoxicity of TCDD, TCDF and PCB isomers in rhesus macaques (*Macaca mulatta*). *Environ Health Perspect* 1985;60:77–88.

49. Gladen BC, Taylor JS, Wu YC, et al. Dermatological findings in children exposed transplacentally to heat-degraded polychlorinated biphenyls in Taiwan. *Br J Dermatol* 1990;122:799–808.

50. Hsu MM-L, Mak C-P, Hsu C-C. Follow-up of skin manifestations in Yu-Cheng children. *Br J Dermatol* 1995;132:427–432.

51. D'Souza SW, Robertson IG, Donnai D, et al. Fetal phenytoin exposure, hypoplastic nails and jitteriness. *Arch Dis Child* 1991;66:320–324.

52. Clarren SK, Smith DW. The fetal alcohol syndrome. *N Engl J Med* 1978;298:1063–1067.

53. Crain LS, Fitzmaurice NE, Mondry C. Nail dysplasia and fetal alcohol syndrome. *Am J Dis Child* 1983;137:1069–1072.

54. Agahian B, Lee J, Nelson J, et al. Arsenic levels in fingernails as a biological indicator of exposure to arsenic. *Am Ind Hyg Assoc* 1990;51:646–651.

55. Peters K, Gammelgaard B, Menne T. Nickel concentrations in fingernails as a measure of occupational exposure to nickel. *Contact Dermatitis* 1991;25:237–241.

Phototoxicity and Photosensitivity Reactions

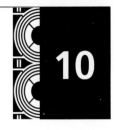

EDWARD A. EMMETT, M.D.

The term "photodermatosis" is applied to any of a number of abnormal reactions of the skin caused by light. The responsible wavelengths are usually in the ultraviolet range.

The classification of these photosensitivity disorders is rather complex. Two kinds of occupational factors are particularly significant in the production of photodermatoses. First, industrial chemicals may induce photosensitivity. Second, occupational exposure to sunlight or to artificial sources of ultraviolet radiation may provoke a preexisting photodermatosis. Photosensitivity induced by industrial chemicals is particularly important and is discussed in this chapter. The effects of occupational exposure to ultraviolet radiation are considered in chapter 8.

CHEMICAL PHOTOSENSITIZATION

Industrial chemicals may induce photosensitization reactions of two major types: phototoxic reactions and photoallergic reactions.

There are some other ways in which industrial chemicals may, less commonly, contribute to photosensitivity. Thus, agents that cause depigmentation, such as p-tertiary-butylphenol[1, 2] lower the protection of the skin against ultraviolet radiation, and exogenous chemicals may induce a systemic disease of which photosensitivity is one manifestation. The induction of porphyria cutanea tarda by hexachlorobenzene[3] illustrates the latter phenomenon, although examples of occupational significance are rare.

PHOTOTOXICITY

In phototoxicity, the dermatitis occurs as a result of chemically induced reactivity to ultraviolet or visible radiation on a nonimmunological basis, the feature that distinguishes it from photoallergy. Phototoxic responses, as far as is known, are governed by a direct dose-response relationship between the intensity of the reaction and both the concentration of the inciting chemical in the target tissue and the amount of radiation of the appropriate wavelength to which that target is exposed.[4]

In phototoxic reactions, the responsible chemical is a light-absorbing molecule, a chromophore, which absorbs radiation. The precise wavelengths of radiation that a molecule is capable of absorbing are defined by the absorption spectrum of that molecule. After absorbing the energy of the incoming radiation, the molecule is in an excited state; it is a highly energetic species. This species of molecule exists for a fraction of a second before the energy dissipates. This very short time may, however, be sufficient for one or more photochemical reactions to occur, such as the formation of a specific chemical product, a photoproduct, that may induce a toxic reaction. Such photoproducts can include new compounds formed by combining with surrounding molecules, for example, the photo adducts formed by psoralens and DNA. The biochemical processes initiated by these photoproducts may lead to subsequent cell proliferation, mutagenesis, and other consequences. The action spectrum for phototoxic agents is specific for the responsible agent, as it depends on the absorption spectrum, and may include the UVC, UVB, UVA, and visible wavebands.

Although an enhanced sunburn reaction is characteristic of most phototoxic reactions in industry, a variety of clinical types of reactions are seen, depending on the specific photosensitizing agent. The morphology of phototoxic responses depends on the particular phototoxic agent responsible and the circumstances of contact, but in general, features include fairly immediate burning sensations, erythema, and urticarial swelling. The burning sensation is more pronounced than in ordinary sunburn and may be described as "smarting" or "like a lighted cigarette being pressed into the skin." This sensation usually resolves rapidly when the affected skin is shaded. Delayed erythema and edema may occur after a few hours or even after 1 to 2 days following exposure. Blistering may occur in severe reactions. Localized hyperpigmentation may be noted after the reaction and, in some instances, may be the only manifestation.

Other morphological reactions may be seen when phototoxic agents are administered systemically. They may include damage to the fingernails, including elevation of the nail plate above the bed, termed photo-onycholysis[5, 6]; papular reactions[7]; changes indistinguishable from those seen in porphyria cutanea tarda[8]; and severe localized edema with massive soft tissue swelling of the hands and periorbital region.[9] Phototoxic changes in skin may also be accompanied by phototoxic eye damage.[4]

Phototoxic lesions are confined to areas of the skin exposed to light, typically one or more areas of the face, the pinnae of the ears, the V and the nuchal area of the neck, the extensor surfaces of the forearms, and the dorsa of the hands. Other areas may be involved, depending on work practices and clothing. Where short trousers are worn, a dermatitis confined to the dorsa of the hands and anterior aspects of the legs can suggest a phototoxic reaction. Hairy areas of the body are usually protected. The magnitude of phototoxic reactions is also influenced by the degree of natural pigmentation, being greatest in light-skinned individuals and least in those who are heavily pigmented.[10, 11]

It has been shown experimentally that the vehicle in which a phototoxic agent is applied affects the extent of subsequent phototoxic reactions through its influence on percutaneous absorption.[12] Increased temperature and humidity also enhance phototoxic reactions.[13] Other variations in the circumstances of application influence subsequent phototoxic reactions; for example, amyl-dimethylamino-benzoic acid, a demonstratedly effective sunscreen ingredient, may be phototoxic in human skin if the site of application is occluded for 6 to 24 hours prior to irradiation.[4, 14] In this case, the difference between a phototoxic and a screening effect appears to be a function of the distribution of the absorbing molecules within the skin. If they are predominantly on the surface or in the stratum corneum, there is screening; if they are predomi-

nantly in the living layers of the epidermis, however, there is a phototoxic reaction on irradiation.[4]

Causes of Phototoxic Reactions

Table 10–1 lists some of the more important phototoxic agents. Phototoxic agents are found not just in industry but also in consumer products, medications, and various plants.

Coal tar and pitch cause phototoxic dermatitis, particularly in lightly pigmented individuals.[10, 11] The dermatitis varies in severity from a burning sensation on exposure to the sun (termed "pitch smarts") to erythema or extensive formation of bullae on exposed areas. The burning sensation begins within 15 to 60 minutes of sun exposure and continues to worsen as long as sun exposure continues. Window glass does not protect against this effect. Scaling may occur subsequently in the absence of erythema. Little appreciable tan is left in those affected, although some gradual darkening may occur. The action spectrum is from 340 to 430 nm.[10] Experimental studies have shown the reaction to be biphasic.[15] Roofers exposed to coal tar fumes also develop photophobia and painful phototoxic keratoconjunctivitis, which may progress to corneal ulceration from subsequent exposure to sunlight.[16] Skin pigmentation, though protective against phototoxic dermatitis, does not protect against the ocular phototoxicity. Photosensitizers in coal tar include acridine, anthracene, pyrene, B-methylanthracene, phenanthrene, ben-

---

 TABLE 10–1 • Selected Phototoxic Drugs and Chemicals

Coal Tars and Related Products
Acridine
Anthracene
Coal tar
Creosote

Furocoumarins
Psoralen
8-Methoxypsoralen
4,5,8-Trimethylpsoralen

Aminobenzoic Acid Derivative
Amyl-ortho-dimethylaminobenzoic acid

Dyes
Disperse blue 35

Drugs and Pharmaceuticals
Sulfonamides
Phenothiazides
Sulfonylureas
Tetracyclines
Thiazides

zo(a)pyrene, and fluoranthene.[17] Petroleum-derived tars and vegetable tars do not usually exhibit this phototoxic effect.

Products derived from coal tar, notably creosote, may be phototoxic. Jonas[18] described 450 subjects with creosote "burns" caused by fine sawdust produced by sawing wood saturated with creosote or by skin contact with creosoted roof paper. Most had mild erythema in exposed areas; more severely affected individuals had intense burning and itching followed by desquamation and hyperpigmentation. Photosensitization was most pronounced in fair-skinned workers. Heyl and Mellett[19] described irritant dermatitis and photodermatitis caused by contact with ammunition boxes impregnated with creosote.

Davies[20] described the development of cutaneous and ocular photosensitivity in at least 28 dockyard workers exposed to fine dust containing bitumen. A bitumen-containing black paint on a drydock gate had been removed by shotblasting. No problems occurred during shotblasting, as the workers wore full protective equipment; the symptoms occurred during a subsequent cleanup operation.

Repeated exposure to coal tars and related substances containing polycyclic aromatic hydrocarbons leads to chronic skin changes, as described in chapter 8. It is likely that ultraviolet radiation contributes to these effects, and certainly ultraviolet radiation and tar interact in the development of skin cancer in experiments.

Amyl-ortho-dimethylaminobenzoic acid was found to cause phototoxicity in workers formulating UV-cured inks.[21] The workers complained of sharp burning sensations on exposed areas of the body while in sunlight, followed by erythema and swelling within less than 1 hour. The reaction was biphasic; the initial erythema and swelling disappeared 1 or 2 hours later, only to recur within a few more hours and remain for 2 to 5 days. Sunscreens that were effective against both UVA and UVB, but not those effective against UVB alone, would block the reaction. Employees at other plants where most of the same ingredients, except for amyl-ortho-dimethylaminobenzoic acid, were used in formulating similar inks did not suffer from photosensitivity.[22]

Workers manufacturing the dye disperse blue 35 (a mixture of intermediates rather than a single product) noted transient erythema and burning of the skin after leaving the factory on sunny days. Sunlight exposure through window glass produced similar symptoms. Irradiation in the 400 to 700 nm waveband was shown to reproduce the dermatitis.[23]

The term "phytophotodermatitis"[24] is applied to phototoxic reactions caused by contact with plants and subsequent exposure to sunlight. The responsible chemicals are usually psoralens (furocoumarins), for which the most active wavelengths of light are from 300 to 340 nm.[25] However, other phototoxic substances are present in some plants, including alpha-terthienyl in plants of the Compositae (chrysanthemum) family.[26] No doubt there are many others also.

Several plant species can produce phytophotodermatitis,[27] including Rutaceae (e.g., lime, lemon, bergamot, bitter orange, gas plant, burning bush); Umbelliferae (carrots, cow parsley, wild chervil, celery, parsnip, fennel, dill); Compositae (yarrow, stinking mayweed); Moraceae (fig); Cruciferae (mustard); and Ranunculaceae (buttercup). Exposures of workers to psoralen-rich fluid from crushed plants of these types lead to photosensitivity. Moist skin, friction, sweating, and heat enhance development of the reaction. Heavily pigmented workers are less affected by dermatitis but may suffer more pronounced hyperpigmentation.[28] Vegetable harvesters, dairy workers, cannery pickers, gardeners, florists, and bartenders exposed to limes are among those at risk. The phytophotodermatitis usually develops 18 to 24 hours after exposure. Irregularly shaped bullae characteristically occur and may become very large and numerous. These heal rapidly but characteristically leave residual hyperpigmentation. Phototoxicity in celery harvesters in Israel is associated with a kind of celery grown in southern Israel that has a particularly high psoralen content; fair skin, lack of protective clothing, and harvesting a postmature crop contribute to the phototoxicity.[29]

Phytophotodermatitis was described in women working in a celery-packing cannery who were stationed next to large windows so that they had sufficient light to see insects deep in the celery heart.[24] Celery pickers develop phytophotodermatitis almost exclusively in the presence of pink-rot disease, a fungal parasite of celery.[28]

Cashiers, baggers, and produce clerks at supermarkets in the United States have developed papular, well-circumscribed dermatitis confined to the upper extremities, with residual blistering or hyperpigmentation. The rates of this dermatitis are highest in those who bag food and have frequent contact with unpackaged celery and exposure to sunlight during the work shift. An interaction between produce exposure and use of tanning salons was also seen. Although contact with celery seems the most likely cause, contact with other fruits and flowers could also play a role.[30]

Carrots[31] and lime oil[32] are also common causes of occupational phytophotodermatitis. Phytophotodermatitis has occurred on the hands of workers milking cows who grazed on fields containing cow parsnip.

Repeated exposure to both 8-methoxypsoralen and UV is carcinogenic in experimental animals.[33, 34] There is also evidence that this combination may be carcinogenic in patients treated with oral photochemotherapy with psoralens and UVA (PUVA).[35, 36] To date, however, there is no indication that a carcinogenic effect has been observed in those who have had occasional phyto-photodermatitis such as that which occurs in occupational situations.

Occupational factors can result in exposure to phototoxic medications. For example, photosensitivity reactions from doxycycline, which is used for malaria prophylaxis, were seen in the U.S. troops stationed in Somalia.[37]

Bilateral maculopathy attributable to photochemical injury has been described in an arc welder who was being treated with the antidepressant drug fluphenazine.[38]

Prevention of Phototoxicity

Prevention of phototoxicity requires the identification of phototoxic agents, the provision of appropriate information to alert users or potential users of this effect, the minimization of exposure to phototoxic chemicals, and, when necessary, the minimization of exposure to the inciting wavelengths of light.

Phototoxic agents may be identified in a variety of systems,[4] including in vitro systems, so that screening of industrial chemicals is possible. Candidates should be those compounds that absorb visible wavelengths and ultraviolet wavelengths that range above about 260 nm. Such screening should also detect most potential photoallergens, although additional testing is necessary to establish the specific potential to cause photoallergy. Once a phototoxic agent is identified, if occupational exposure is likely, the hazard should be brought to the attention of management and workers through appropriate notification, labeling, and education programs. Such education should include both protective and preventive measures and recognition of symptoms. Contact with the agent should be minimized by means appropriate to its specific use, including administrative and engineering controls, personal protective clothing, and personal hygiene. Substitution of suitable agents free of phototoxic potential should be considered.

Minimization of ultraviolet radiation or sunlight exposure is less desirable and much more difficult in practice, but may be necessary. This can be accomplished by avoiding outdoor and indoor UV sources, by wearing broad-brimmed hats and tightly woven clothing, by and covering exposed skin, and by using sunblocks that incorporate agents such as titanium dioxide or zinc oxide, which are effective against all wavelengths. Less effective are broad-spectrum sunscreens that are effective against both UVA and UVB. Narrow-spectrum sunscreens effective only against UVB are of little or no use. In extreme situations, work may be rescheduled so that it is performed at night.

PHOTOALLERGY

General Features

Photoallergic reactions differ from phototoxic reactions in the immunological nature of the response. This type of response is elicited only in those individuals who have been previously sensitized by simultaneous exposure to the photosensitizing substance and the appropriate radiation. Photoallergy is distinctly less common than phototoxicity.

Photoallergy appears to involve biological processes similar to those of allergic contact dermatitis, except for the role of ultraviolet radiation or light in the conversion of the hapten to the complete allergen. This may occur through the conversion of a compound into an oxidation product that is a more potent allergy sensitizer than is the parent compound, as occurs in sulfanilamide photoallergy[39] or through the binding of light-excited molecules with cutaneous proteins to form a complete allergen.[40] The responsible radiation generally lies in the UVA range, although it may extend into or, rarely, be primarily in the UVB range.[41, 42]

Photoallergic reactions are usually characterized by sun-induced pruritic eczematous eruptions or lichenoid papules.[43] The eruption often has a sudden onset and consists of an acute eczematous dermatitis, lichenoid papules, or a thickened lichenified dermatitis similar to that seen in chronic atopic dermatitis. Lesions may extend beyond exposed areas, and flares of distant, previously involved sites may occur with recrudescences of the eruption. Widespread milder dermatitis may be seen. As the dermatitis subsides, pigmentary changes and thickening of the involved skin may be quite prominent. Exacerbations are characteristically delayed for 1 to 2 days after sun exposure. Some patients, however, react to extraordinarily small amounts of light energy, and both this relationship and a clear distribution on exposed areas may be obscured. In those who are highly photosensitive, exposure to sunlight through clothing, especially loosely woven clothing or exposure to long-wavelength ultraviolet radiation from fluorescent lighting may be sufficient to provoke dermatitis. Photoallergic reactions are seen predominantly in males in the fifth to eighth decades, for reasons that are not fully explained. Members of races with dark pigmentation can develop severe photoallergic reactions.

The diagnosis is often suggested by the distribution and character of the eruption. Confirmation requires careful interrogation and photopatch-testing. Histological changes are not diagnostic but are similar to those in allergic contact dermatitis. There is a characteristic dense, perivascular, round-cell dermal infiltrate. Epidermal changes vary from spongiosis and vesicle formation to acanthosis. In addition to phototoxic reactions and other photosensitive states, differentiation of photoallergy from airborne contact dermatitis and contact allergy to plants demands particular attention.

A serious complication of photoallergy is the development of a persistent reaction to light. This disease is characterized by extreme photosensitivity that persists despite apparent removal of all contact with the photoallergen. Additionally, there is a broadening of the action spectrum so that even brief small exposure to UVB elicits the photosensitivity.[6] Persistent light reaction has been described following photoallergic reactions to halogenated salicylanilides, promethazine, chlorpromazine, and musk ambrette.

Causes of Photoallergic Reactions

A list of agents that have been reported to cause photoallergy following topical contact appears in Table 10–2. Some patients treated with systemic medications may also develop photosensitivity, often described as photoallergy. However, many of the described reactions caused by systemic medications may actually be phototoxicity, although in the cases of sulfanilamide and chlorpromazine, true photoallergy may occur.[44]

The agents that have been reported to cause photoallergy are commonly found in consumer products, such as drugs, cosmetics, soaps, shampoos, sunscreens, and fragrances, but in a significant number of instances the disease appears in an occupational setting. A major epidemic of photoallergic contact dermatitis occurred in Great Britain in 1960 following the use of two new soaps in which tetrachlorosalicylanilide (TCSA) was incorporated as an antibacterial agent.[45, 46] In a single factory, 29 out of 106 workers exposed to these soaps developed photodermatitis. An estimated 10,000 cases of photoallergy occurred throughout Britain before TCSA was withdrawn in 1962, but

 TABLE 10–2 • Selected Causes of Photoallergic Reactions

Halogenated salicylanilides and related compounds
  Tetrachlorosalicylanilide
  3,4',5-tribromosalicylanilide
  4',5-dibromosalicylanilide
  Bithional
  Hexachlorophene
  Dichlorophene
  Fentichlor
  Jadit (Buclosamide)
  Bromochlorosalicylanilide

Sulfanilamide

Phenothiazines
  Chlorpromazine
  Promethazine

4,6-Dichlorophenylphenol

Diphenhydramine

Quinoxaline 1,4-di-N-oxide

Olaquindox

Fragrances
  Musk ambrette
  6-Methylcouramin

Optical brighteners (stilbenes)

Sunscreens
  PABA esters
  Digalloyl trioleate

Plants of the Compositae family

Photosensitivity component in allergic reactions
  Chromium
  Lichens

the most dramatic experience occurred in industry. Subsequently, additional cases of photoallergy occurred as a result of contact with structurally related materials, particularly tribromosalicylanilide and dibromosalicylanilide, that had been incorporated into germicides in many areas of the world. Although most of these agents have been withdrawn from most products, a recent analysis of product compositions using the Material Safety Data Sheet database of the Canadian Centre for Occupational Health and Safety revealed that a number of products containing tribromosalicylanilide were still in industrial use in North America.[47]

Photoallergic reactions due to occupational contact with chlorpromazine have been seen in nurses, pharmacists, and other health-care personnel.

Photoallergic dermatitis from quindoxin, a growth-promoting factor, occurred in British workers handling animal foodstuffs.[48, 49] Quindoxin was subsequently withdrawn from the market.

More recently, photoallergic dermatitis caused by airborne exposure to a related substance, olaquindox, has been reported in 15 pig breeders. Of the 15, 10 developed persistent light reactions.[50]

Photoallergic dermatitis caused by the Compositae species of plants occurs in outdoor workers in various parts of the world; for example, ragweed causes it in the United States,[51] and in Australia, a variety of Compositae causes a condition described as "Australian bush dermatitis."[52]

With increasing frequency, outdoor workers are being encouraged to use sun-protective agents to prevent the acute and chronic effects of sun. Although the incidence of photoallergic reactions is rare, considering the very widespread use of these agents, sunscreens are currently among the common causes of photoallergic reactions.[53] Allergic contact dermatitis caused by sunscreen agents appears on exposed areas. Photoallergy and plain contact allergy to sunscreens can be differentiated by photopatch-testing.

Chrome dermatitis may be associated with apparent photosensitivity.[54] Tronnier[55] suggested that this relationship may be due to the change of hexavalent to trivalent chrome in the skin by UV. Wahlberg and Wennersten[56] reported more intense patch-test reactions in subjects allergic to chromium when the patch was irradiated with UV.

Photosensitivity may coexist with allergic contact dermatitis in forestry or horticultural workers exposed to lichens.[57]

Photopatch-testing

The standard diagnostic technique used to confirm photoallergic dermatitis and determine its cause is photopatch-testing. A recommended technique for photopatch-testing[58] is described in Table 10–3. Most, if not all, photoallergens are also phototoxic under appropriate circumstances, so photopatch-testing relies on the use of dilutions of potential allergens to a level at which phototoxic reactions are not seen.

Over the past several decades, there has been considerable variation in the photopatch-test techniques used by different investigators. Comparative studies of the significance of these technical variations have been few, so that it is difficult to identify all the essential elements of testing. Selection of vehicle, occlusion, duration of application, and concentration of allergen have been shown to significantly alter the results of photopatch-testing. Modern techniques of patch-testing owe much to the seminal work of Stephan Epstein. The test procedure recommended here is based in large measure on the Scandinavian standard photopatch-test procedure described by Jansen et al.[59] A more detailed and referenced discussion of the evaluation of a photosensitive patient, including photopatch-testing, can be found in the work of Emmett.[58]

The composition of a recommended photopatch-test series for North America is shown in Table 10–4. The choice of the chemicals to be used in photopatch-testing should reflect photoallergens to which the patient is likely to have been exposed. Thus, a standard series of photopatch-test allergens may vary considerably from one region of the world to another. It is often important to include certain stronger photoallergens such as the halogenated salicylanilides to which current exposure is not necessarily anticipated. The reasons for this can include the following: (1) the substance, though no longer used, was the initial cause of a persistent light reaction; (2) the substance is still used in some areas of the world, and travelers and others might therefore be exposed— for example, bithional was used until quite recently in Scandinavia, and fentichlor has been used in Canada; (3) the substance is still present in an old product no longer on the market but to which the patient might have been exposed; (4) the substance is still used despite some applications' being discontinued or even prohibited.

Experience indicates that the last possibility is more common than might be thought. Tetrachlorosalicylanilide should not, however, be included in photopatch-testing because of its extraordinarily strong capacity to photosensitize.

In addition to the standard series, patients should be photopatch-tested with sunscreens they are currently using. Because of the difficulty in distinguishing between photoallergic dermatitis and simple contact dermatitis, plain patch-testing with plants and plant oleoresins appropriate to the area is strongly recommended in patients with suspected photoallergic contact dermatitis.

A positive photopatch test establishes that the patient has a photoallergy to that substance but does not establish that the substance is the cause of the patient's dermatitis. In a transient light eruption, clinical relevance should be established—that is, there should be a history of contact with the photoallergen and with light in a relationship that could reasonably be expected to exacerbate the dermatitis. In a persistent light eruption, recent exposure to the photoallergen is not a requirement for diagnosis. Furthermore, a negative photopatch test in the presence of strong clinical evidence of a photoallergic contact dermatitis in response to the agent in question may raise the need to repeat the tests under altered conditions.

TABLE 10–3 • Photopatch-Test Procedure

Outline of Recommended Photopatch-Test Procedure
The procedure described here is designed to require three visits, the first two on consecutive days and the final visit on the fourth or fifth day.
Day 1
    (i) Application of duplicate sets of test substances, one on either side of the back and preferably in the lumbosacral area, using either Finn chambers or the Al test delivery system with hypoallergenic adhesive such as Scanpor tape.
    (ii) Determination of threshold of sensitivity to the UVA source, if not previously known, with 1, 5, and 10 J/cm² total exposure on normal back skin. The tested area of skin should be clearly identified using a skin-marking pen or small pieces of hypoallergenic adhesive tape (e.g., Scanpor or Blenderm).
    (iii) Determination of threshold of sensitivity to UVB, using an appropriate source, may also be performed at this time.
Day 2 (24 hours after application)
    (i) Read results of determination of sensitivity to UVA source.
    (ii) Remove patches in dim light. Inspect and record reactions.
    (iii) Recover one set of patches (the dark control patches) with opaque paper fixed in place using hypoallergenic adhesive tape such as Scanpor. This step will avoid the occurrence of so-called masked photopatch-test reactions on the control site precipitated by diffuse room light through clothing. Make sure that patch-testing sites are clearly marked for later identification.
    (iv) Irradiate the second set of patches, together with a small area of adjacent skin, with 5J/cm² from the UVA source or if the UVA threshold was less than 10J/cm², with one-half the minimal UVA erythema threshold dose. Mark area clearly for later identification.
    (v) If UVB sensitivity was determined, read results.
Day 4 or 5 (72 or 96 hours after application)
Inspect irradiated and control sets of patches and record both sets of reactions.

Acceptable Light Sources
Acceptable light sources should contain, at most, only small proportions of UVB, certainly insufficient to produce erythemal reactions at UVA doses of 5J/cm². Acceptable sources include:
    Hot quartz (high pressure mercury arc) lamps with window-glass filter
    Bank of fluorescent blacklights
    Waldman PUVA-500
    Airam PUVA-4
    Xenon arc lamp with Schott and IR filters
    UVATEC (median pressure mercury arc lamp with window-glass filter)
Application of patches and patient instructions follow generally similar guidelines to those for standard testing. Excess substance is removed from the skin prior to irradiation. Subjects must also be instructed to avoid sun exposure of the tested areas prior to the final reading. Because delayed photopatch-test reactions occur more frequently than delayed patch-test reactions, patients should be instructed to have their skin inspected subsequent to the final reading and to report any reactions.
    Although most photoallergies will be detected using the procedure outlined above, in the case of 6-methylcoumarin, the application should be made within 6 hours of the light exposure, conveniently 30 to 60 minutes beforehand.

Recording and Interpretation
Photopatch test results are recorded with the prefix "Ph." Accepted designations by the International Contact Dermatitis group are:
    Ph −   Negative reaction
    Ph? +   Doubtful reaction; faint or macular erythema only
    Ph +   Weak positive reaction; erythema and infiltration, possibly papules
    Ph + +   Strong positive reaction; edematous or vesicular
    Ph + + + Extreme bullous or ulcerative reaction
    PhT   Phototoxic reaction
    PhNT   Not photopatch tested
A negative reaction on the dark control site serves to exclude a plain allergic contact reaction. Identical reactions on both control and irradiated sites are seen in contact allergy without photoallergy. Contact photoallergy and contact allergy may coexist; in this case, a more severe reaction is seen on the irradiated site.

TABLE 10–4 • Suggested Photoallergen Tray for Photopatch-Testing in North America

Chlorpromazine hydrochloride 0.1% pet
Musk ambrette 1% pet
Para-aminobenzoic acid 5% alcohol
Amyl dimethyl PABA 5% in alcohol
Parsol 1789 5% pet
Octyl dimethyl PABA 5% in alcohol
Tribromosalicylanilide 1% pet
Benzophenone-2 1% pet
Promethazine 1% pet
Oak moss (synthetic) 1% pet
Bithionol 1% pet
Fentichlor 1% pet
Atranorin 0.5% pet
6-Methylcoumarin 1% alcohol[a]
Petrolatum control

[a]In the case of 6-methylcoumarin, the allergen should be applied to the skin 30 to 60 minutes prior to irradiation.

Treatment

The treatment regimen should be designed to minimize exposure both to light and to the photoallergen.[4, 60]

Exposure to ultraviolet radiation, particularly UVA, in sunlight and, in extreme cases, fluorescent light sources, should be minimized. Work outdoors should be arranged to minimize exposure. Protective, closely woven, dark clothing as well as gloves and wide-brimmed hats should be worn. Topical sunscreens that block out UVA, particularly those containing opaque titanium dioxide or zinc oxide, or selective UVA absorbers such as benzophenone, should be used. Symptomatic topical treatment or, in severe cases, short courses of oral steroids may be required. The photoallergen must be identified, and this must be followed by rigorous measures to avoid further contact. Potential cross-sensitizers must also be identified and the patient carefully instructed to avoid contact with them.

Prevention

Photoallergy can be induced experimentally in guinea pigs[61] and mice,[62] so predictive testing is possible, although strict attention to detail is required for successful results.[63] Predictive testing for photoallergy can be performed in humans, but the potential for induction of persistent light eruption limits its desirability. Photoallergens generally have a resonating structure, have a molecular weight of less than 500, and absorb ultraviolet radiation. Most, if not all, photoallergens are pho-

totoxic in appropriate experimental systems, which may help to identify them using in vitro tests.

The prevention of photoallergy depends on the identification of photoallergens, appropriate warnings about their use, and reduction of their contact with skin. In some cases, such as with tetrachlorosalicylanilide, potent photoallergens have been effectively removed from commerce.

References

1. Kahn G. Depigmentation caused by phenolic detergent germicides. *Arch Dermatol* 1970; 102:177–187.
2. Gellin GA, Possick PA, Perone VD. Depigmentation for 4-tertiary butyl catechol—an experimental study. *J Invest Dermatol* 1970; 55:190–197.
3. Schmid R. Cutaneous porphyria in Turkey. *N Engl J Med* 1960; 263:397–398.
4. Emmett EA. Phototoxicity from endogenous agents. *Photochem Photobiol* 1979; 30:429–436.
5. Frank SB, Cohen HJ, Minkin W. Photo-onycholysis due to tetracycline hydrochloride and doxycycline. *Arch Dermatol* 1971; 103:520–521.
6. Harber LC, Bickers DR. *Photosensitivity Diseases: Principles of Diagnosis and Treatment.* Philadelphia: W.B. Saunders; 1981.
7. Frost P, Weinstein GD, Gomez EC. Methacycline and demeclocycline in relation to sunlight. *JAMA* 1971; 216:326–329.
8. Epstein JH et al. Porphyria-like cutaneous changes induced by tetracycline hydrochloride photosensitization. *Arch Dermatol* 1976; 112:661.
9. Zalar GL, Poh-Fitzpatrick M, Krohn DL, Jacobs R, Harber LC. Induction of drug photosensitization in man after parenteral exposure to hematoporphyrin. *Arch Dermatol* 1977; 113:1392–1397.
10. Crow KD, Alexander E, Buck WHL, Johnson BE, Magnus IA, Porter AD. Photosensitivity due to pitch. *Br J Dermatol* 1961; 73:220–232.
11. Emmett EA. Cutaneous and ocular hazards of roofers. *Occup Med* 1986; 1:307–322.
12. Kaidbey KH, Kligman AM. Topical photosensitizers: influence of vehicle on penetration. *Arch Dermatol* 1974; 110:868–870.
13. Levine GM, Harber LC. The effect of humidity on the phototoxic response to 8-methoxypsoralen in guinea pigs. *Acta Derm Venereol* 1969; 49:82.
14. Kaidbey KH, Kligman AM. Phototoxicity to a sunscreen ingredient. *Arch Dermatol* 1978; 114:547–549.
15. Kaidbey KH, Kligman AM. Clinical and histological study of coal tar phototoxicity in humans. *Arch Dermatol* 1977; 113:592.
16. Emmett EA, Stetzer W, Taphorn B. Phototoxic keratoconjunctivitis from coal-tar pitch volatiles. *Science* 1977; 198:841–842.
17. Kochevar IE, Armstrong RB, Einbinder J, Walther RR, Harber LC. Coal tar phototoxicity: active compounds and action spectra. *Photochem Photobiol* 1982; 38:65–69.
18. Jonas AD. Creosote burns. *J Ind Hyg Toxicol* 1943; 25:418–420.
19. Heyl T, Mellett WA. Creosote dermatitis in an ammunition depot. *S Afr Med J* 1982; 62:66–67.
20. Davies MG. A large outbreak of bitumen-induced phototoxicity in a dockyard. *Contact Dermatitis* 1996; 35:188–189.
21. Emmett EA, Taphorn BR, Kominsky JR. Phototoxicity

occurring during the manufacture of ultraviolet-cured ink. *Arch Dermatol* 1977; 113:770–775.

22. Emmett EA. Contact dermatitis from polyfunctional acrylic monomers. *Contact Dermatitis* 1977; 3:245–248.

23. Gardiner JS, Dickson A, Macleod TM, Frain-Bell W. The investigation of photocontact dermatitis in a dye manufacturing process. *Br J Dermatol* 1972; 86:264.

24. Klaber R. Phytophotodermatitis. *Br J Dermatol* 1942; 54:193–211.

25. Moller H. Phototoxicity of *Dictamus alba*. *Contact Dermatitis* 1978; 4:264–269.

26. Chan GFQ, Prihoda M, Towers GNH, Mitchell JC. Phototoxicity evoked by alpha-terthienyl. *Contact Dermatitis* 1977; 3:215–218.

27. Pathak MA, Daniels F Jr, Fitzpatrick TB. The presently known distribution of furocoumarins (psoralens) in plants. *J Invest Dermatol* 1962; 39:225–239.

28. Birmingham DJ, Key MM, Tubich GE, Perone VB. Phototoxic bullae among celery harvesters. *Arch Dermatol* 1961; 83:73–87.

29. Finkelstein E, Ajek U, Gross E, Aharoni N, Rosenberg L, Halevy S. An outbreak of phytophotodermatitis due to celery. *Int J Dermatol* 1994; 33:116–118.

30. MMWR. Phytophotodermatitis among grocery workers. *JAMA* 1985; 253:753.

31. Peck SN, Spolyar LW, Mason HS. Dermatitis from carrots. *Arch Dermatol Syphilol* 1944; 49:266–269.

32. Sams WM. Photodynamic action of lime oil (citrus aurantifola). *Arch Dermatol Syphilol* 1941; 44:571–587.

33. Griffin AC, Hakim RE, Knox I. The wavelength effect upon erythemal and carcinogenic response in psoralen-treated mice. *J Invest Dermatol* 1958; 31:289–295.

34. Urbach F. Modification of ultraviolet carcinogenesis by photoactive agents. *J Invest Dermatol* 1959; 32:372–378.

35. Stern RS, Thibodeau LA, Kleinerman RA, Parrish JA, Fitzpatrick TB. Risk of cutaneous carcinoma in patients treated with oral methoxsalen photochemotherapy for psoriasis. *N Engl J Med* 1979; 300:809–813.

36. Stern RS, Lange BFA. Non-melanoma skin cancer occurring in patients treated with PUVA five to ten years after first treatment. *J Invest Dermatol* 1988; 91:120–124.

37. Sanchez JL, DeFraites RF, Sharp TW, Hanson RK: Mefloquine or doxycycline prophylaxis in US troops in Somalia. Lancet 341:1021–1022, 1993.

38. Power WJ, Travers SP, Mooney DJ. Welding arc maculopathy and fluphenazine. *Br J Ophthalmol* 1991; 75:433–435.

39. Schwarz K, Speck M. Experimentelle untersuchungen zur frage der photoallergie der sulphonamide. *Dermatologica* 1957; 114:232–243.

40. Kochevar IE, Harber LC. Photoreactions of 3,3′,4′,5-tetrachlorosalicylanilide with proteins. *J Invest Dermatol* 1977; 68:151–156.

41. Freeman RG, Knox JM. The action spectrum of photocontact dermatitis. *Arch Dermatol* 1968; 97:130–136.

42. Emmett EA. Diphenhydramine photoallergy. *Arch Dermatol* 1974; 110:249–252.

43. Emmett EA. Drug photoallergy. *Int J Dermatol* 1978; 17:370–378.

44. Guidici P, Maguire HC Jr. Experimental systemic photoallergy. *J Invest Dermatol* 1985; 84:355.

45. Wilkinson DS. Photodermatitis due to tetrachlorosalicylanilide. *Br J Dermatol* 1961; 73:213–219.

46. Calnan CD, Harman RRM, Wells GC. Photodermatitis from soaps. *Br Med J* 1961; 2:1266.

47. Storrs F. Personal communication, University of Oregon Health Science, 1988.

48. Scott KW, Dawson TAJ. Photocontact dermatitis arising from the presence of quindoxin in annual feeding stuffs. *Br J Dermatol* 1974; 90:543–546.

49. Frain-Bell W, Gardiner J. Photocontact dermatitis due to quindoxin. *Contact Dermatitis* 1976; 1:256–257.

50. Schauder S, Schroder W, Geier J. Olaquindox-induced airborne photoallergic contact dermatitis followed by transient or persistent light reactions in 15 pig breeders. *Contact Dermatitis* 1996; 35:344–354.

51. Epstein S. Role of dermal sensitivity in ragweed contact dermatitis. *Arch Dermatol* 1960; 82:48–55.

52. Burry JM, Kuchel R, Reid JG, Kirk J. Australian bush dermatitis: Compositae dermatitis in South Australia. *Med J Aust* 1973; 1:110–116.

53. Thune P. Contact and photocontact allergy to sunscreens. *Photodermatology* 1984; 1:5–9.

54. Feuerman EJ. Chromates as the cause of contact dermatitis in housewives. *Dermatologica* 1971; 143:292–297.

55. Tronnier H. Zur lichtempfindlichkeit von ekzematikern (unter besonderer berucksichtigung des chromat-ek-zems). *Arch Klin Exp Derm* 1970; 237:494–506.

56. Wahlberg JE, Wennersten G. Light sensitivity and chromium dermatitis. *Br J Dermatol* 1977; 97:411–416.

57. Thune PO, Solberg YJ. Photosensitivity and allergy to aromatic lichen acids, Compositae oleoresins and other plant substances. *Contact Dermatitis* 1980; 6:81–87.

58. Emmett EA. Evaluation of the photosensitive patient. *Dermatol Clin* 1986; 4:195–202.

59. Jansen CT, Wennersten F, Rystedt I, Thune P, Brodthagen H. The Scandinavian standard photopatch test procedure. *Contact Dermatitis* 1982; 8:155–158.

60. Elmets CA. Drug-induced photoallergy. *Dermatol Clin* 1986; 4:231–241.

61. Kochevar IE, Zalar GL, Einbinder J, Harber LC. Assay of contact photosensitivity to musk ambrette in guinea pigs. *J Invest Dermatol* 1979; 73:144–146.

62. Maguire HC Jr, Kaidbey K. Experimental photoallergic contact dermatitis: a mouse model. *J Invest Dermatol* 1982; 79:147–152.

63. Harber LC. Current status of mammalian and human models for predicting drug photosensitivity. *J Invest Dermatol* 1981; 77:65–70.

Occupational and Environmental Connective Tissue Disorders

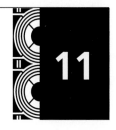

11

LINDA MORSE, M.D.

Dermatological manifestations of occupationally and environmentally induced connective tissue disorders are rare. They are also difficult to differentiate from the idiopathic versions or those due to other causes. With few exceptions, occupational and environmental agents rarely provoke rheumatological disorders in those exposed. Conversely, identification of one of these disorders as industrial or environmental in origin may be regarded as a "sentinel health event"—a sign that others are probably also being exposed to the same hazards, a situation that requires intervention and protection of those exposed.[1]

New causes and syndromes continue to be identified, and more can be expected as humans develop new chemicals and industrial processes and venture off the planet. Most chemicals used in modern industrial operations did not exist 100 years ago. Human immune systems have no evolutionary experience with chlorinated hydrocarbons or epoxy resins, for example. Regulations in the United States and western Europe have dramatically reduced exposures in large industrial operations, but hazardous exposures still exist in smaller industries and in countries moving rapidly into the industrial age. Alert clinicians will consider and explore the possibility of an occupational or environmental cause of a patient's presentation even though a clear relationship may be difficult to prove. Identification of an industrial or environmental cause not only allows intervention for the protection of other exposed individuals, it also creates an opportunity for superb directed research, which can add to our general understanding of the pathogenesis of these disorders.

The most commonly reported and widely studied of the occupational environmentally caused connective tissue diseases is scleroderma, which has many proven and suspected chemical causes. Raynaud's phenomenon is commonly found in those exposed to hand-arm vibration (discussed in Chapter 3). It is also found in those exposed to chemicals, notably to vinyl chloride but usually associated also with scleroderma. Other conditions reported much less frequently include eosinophilic fasciitis, which is often confused with scleroderma.

This chapter first reviews specific disorders, subdivided by the exposure type. The medicolegal issue of causation and treatment options is discussed.

SCLERODERMA

Scleroderma ("hardening of the skin") is a rare disease of the connective tissue of the skin and often of other specific organs; it has a prevalence rate of two to eight cases per million. It affects females more frequently than males (between three and eight cases to one) and is found in a wide variety of countries and races. Evidence reveals an association with histocompatibility antigens (HLA), but this is controversial.[2] Silman, in his comprehensive review of the epidemiology of sclerosis, found the association weak and the relative risks low.[3] Some favor the hypothesis that a genetic predisposition exists in many, if not most, cases whereas others postulate two forms of the disease: a genetically susceptible, idiopathic version and a version resulting from toxic exposure, which is not linked to genetic factors. The disease is classified into systemic and localized forms.[4, 5] Alteration of capillaries and arterioles has been identified as the marker of the disease process, and it includes devascularization, alteration of endothelial cells, duplication of the basement membrane, and perivascular fibrosis of superficial dermal capillaries.[6] Cell damage causes the release of mediators of inflammation, with resultant cellular infiltration of lymphocytes, macrophages, and plasma cells. Skin ischemia and capillary reduction are demonstrated by nail capillaroscopy.

The pathophysiology of scleroderma has not been elucidated yet, and even less is known about the occupational and environmental versions. A number of immunological markers and abnormalities have been associated with progressive systemic sclerosis, pointing toward an immunological basis for the disorder.[6,7] Examples include studies associating the disease with different HLA allele, presence of antinuclear antibodies or other antibodies in 60 to 90% of patients with the progressive systemic form of sclerosis (PSS), and increased circulating immune complexes in up to 50% of these same patients.

Perivascular infiltrates in scleroderma are composed primarily of T cells, with corresponding normal B-cell but decreased T-cell populations in peripheral blood. Further evidence for T-cell activation is the association of scleroderma-like findings with graft vs. host disease in which T-cell activation plays a part in pathogenesis. Local mast cell infiltration has been associated with other processes in which inflammation results in fibrosis, such as keloid formation, and is also implicated in the pathophysiology of fibrotic lung disorders such as asbestosis and silicosis.[7] Moreover, mast cell populations are increased in the involved areas of the skin of those with early active disease compared with controls.

Hawkins et al. evaluated biopsies from involved and noninvolved sites in 12 patients with PSS and 21 controls, all age- and sex-matched, and the former divided into three disease stages.[7] They found an increased mast cell density in the early indicative form of PSS. They noted that mast cells are involved with fibrosis development and postulated that a stimulus led to lymphocyte activation which resulted in the hallmarks of PSS: vascular endothelial cell proliferation, cytotoxicity, and fibroblast collagen synthesis. Slow degranulation of mast cells, they noted, promotes collagen production. Finally, they noted that mast cell populations decreased in the later stages of PSS, when the skin softens, and noted that mast cells are naturally present in large numbers in the skin, lungs, and GI tract, all of which are affected in PSS, and are not found, for example, in the nervous system, which is not affected in PSS.

Occupational and environmental causes have been reported since the early 1900s. Predominant occurrence in the female gender disappears when occupational causes are studied, which may result only from the far greater numbers of males in risk occupations or which may be further evidence favoring two forms of the disease. Links between scleroderma and silica, vinyl chloride, some other halogenated and nonhalogenated hydrocarbons in solvent form, and certain medications are now well established, although the pathophysiological mechanisms are not understood. Reports of case-control studies, individual case reports, and a few large studies implicate diverse chemical compounds with little structural or other similarities. Silica, a simple SiO_2 molecule is a nonorganic, very common natural substance found all over the world, whereas the halogenated chlorinated hydrocarbons, including vinyl chloride, trichloroethylene, and perchloroethylene have existed on the planet only for the past 60 to 75 years.

Silicon

Silicon (Si) is the most abundant element on the Earth's surface except for oxygen. It is not found naturally in its free form but is always bound to oxygen in crystalline or amorphous silica (SiO_2) which is present in over 90% of the rock on this planet.[8] It has many industrial applications, and the United States produces approximately 200,000 tons annually. A major use of it during the past 2 decades has been in the electronics industry, which requires increasing quantities of high-purity silicon for the manufacture of microelectronic chips. New uses for this abundant cheap material are being identified continually.

Bramwell is said to have reported, in 1914, nine cases of diffuse scleroderma, five of whom worked as stonemasons.[9] Scleroderma was reported by Rodnan et al. in 1966 in 60 males, 73% of whom had worked as miners or in other job categories that involved heavy exposure to silica dust; many of them presented with Raynaud's phenomenon and had associated systemic findings, including esophageal motility abnormalities.[10] An evaluation of the frequency of PSS from 1958 to 1962 in 10 hospitals of the Miners Memorial Hospital Association in the Appalachian region near Pittsburgh, Pennsylvania, revealed a prevalence of 17 per 100,000 hospital discharges among coal miners compared with 6 per 100,000 in male nonminers and 9 out of 100,000 in females.[11]

In Germany, 72 cases of systemic sclerosis in uranium miners were evaluated by Baur et al. in 1996.[12,13] The prevalence rate was 11 out of 100,000. Most of them were exposed to very high concentrations of dust and radiation in the 1940s and 1950s. The authors noted significant increases in alleles DR3 and DQ2, especially in anti-Scl-70 positive miners, among other abnormalities.

Scleroderma in black South African coal miners has also been reported, with an annual incidence rate calculated at 81.8 per million black men aged

33–57, compared with the expected 3.4 per million black men of similar age in the general population.[14] A cohort of white South African gold miners has also been described.[14a]

Evidence associating scleroderma with silica dust exposure includes not only the above studies but also a decrease in the number of cases in recent years, possibly associated with a significant decrease in dust exposure in mining industries.

The pathophysiology of silica in the cause of fibrotic diseases has been best studied in silicosis.[15] Silica dust does not penetrate the skin, but it is able to enter the respiratory system. Large particles are trapped in the upper airways, those that are 5 to 10μ lodge in the bronchi and those that are smaller than 5μ can be inhaled into the alveoli. After ingestion by pulmonary alveolar macrophages, particulate silica is incorporated into a membrane-bound vesicle called a phagosome, which then is merged with an enzyme containing lysosome. Normal macrophage action includes both destruction of many kinds of particles via lysosomal action and migration toward large bronchi, with eventual expectoration via the mucociliary escalator. Silica particles damage the macrophage cell membranes instead, resulting in release of the particle into the cell cytoplasm along with release of the lysosomal enzymes and lysis of the macrophage itself, which releases the silica. This process repeats itself many times while damaged macrophages accumulate in the alveoli and bronchioles, fibroblasts are attracted, and a thin network of reticulin fibers form around the macrophages, which results in the lesions of simple silicosis. A large percentage of silica-exposed workers with scleroderma also have silicosis.

Activation of the immune system can occur as part of this process, including generation of autoantibodies, delayed hypersensitivity reactions, and alterations in resistance to infection. The development of the skin lesions of scleroderma resulting from inhaled silica dust requires the systemic circulation of factors that act locally. Activation of T cells or mast cells by a circulating humoral factor produced by the repeated macrophage lysis has been postulated. Alternatively, destruction of the macrophages has been proposed to cause sensitization to altered intracellular components. Activation of lymphocytes might occur due to PAM destruction, leading to release of lymphokines which promote fibroblast growth and collagen production.

Vinyl Chloride

Vinyl chloride (CH_2CHCl) monomer is a gas that has been used in the production of polyvinyl chloride (PVC) plastic since the 1930s. The monomer is pumped into large reactor vessels, catalysts and emulsifiers are added, and the vessel is put under high pressure. The monomer gas is transformed by this process into powdered vinyl chloride and polyvinyl chloride, which is later used for the production of PVC items. The reaction leaves residue on the container walls, which require periodic cleaning; this used to be performed by workers who entered the vessel and cleaned the walls using putty knives or chisels.

In 1967 Wilson et al. reported 31 cases of acroosteolysis among 3,000 personnel (3% prevalence) in vinyl chloride production operations.[16] Scleroderma-like skin changes and Raynaud's phenomenon were also observed in this group, which was limited to cleaners of reactor vessels. By 1971, Dinman et al. had published results of a large epidemiological and industrial hygiene study of 32 plants in the PVC industry in the United States.[17, 18] Both confirmed that the reactor vessel cleaning operations were the problem area, with industrial hygiene measurements revealing exposures of 50 to 1,000 ppm during hand scraping of the residue. The authors noted that vinyl chloride disease was a systemic disorder that was probably initiated only in susceptible individuals, as it affected approximately 41 out of 1,047 at risk.

Reports from a number of other studies confirm this low rate. Scleroderma-like skin changes affected 10% of Wilson's cohort of 31.[19] Black et al. studied a group of 44 PVC production workers with scleroderma as part of their disease processes, and compared the presence or absence of certain immunological markers in that group, a group of 50 patients with classic scleroderma, and 148 controls.[20] The patients who worked with PVC had far less severe clinical problems than did the idiopathic scleroderma patients, with the exception of Raynaud's phenomenon, arthralgias, and abnormal lung function. Scleroderma was present in only approximately 10% of this group, and no anticentromere or antiscleroderma antibodies were found in these patients. Increased frequencies of HLA antigen B8, DR3, and DR5 were found. Veltman reported an 11.4% prevalence of scleroderma-like changes among 70 workers and later a 10% prevalence in a group of 98 workers reported on in another year (although it is unclear if there is overlap in the populations, as the first paper is in German, and a translation is not available to this author).[21, 22] Lilis reported edematous thickened skin with decreased elasticity in 6.4% of 354 exposed workers.[23] Ward reported evaluation of 58 vinyl chloride–exposed workers (28 with vinyl chloride–related disease), finding scleroderma-like changes in 6 of the group (approximately 10%).[24]

Histological evaluation of the skin of affected workers was performed by Veltman,[22] and he noted endothelial swelling, lymphocytic infiltrate, thickening of collagen, and rarefaction, fissuration, and fragmentation of the elastic fibers of the skin. The changes in the elastic fibers were not found in similar biopsies of patients with PSS.[21]

Suciu et al. examined 168 PVC production workers in an extensive clinical evaluation which included skin symptoms and signs.[25] Of the workers, 80% complained of transient dermatitis at some point, with pruritus in 4.8% of those with no skin changes. Scleroderma-like changes were found in only 3.6% of the cases. Three cases of papulomucinosis were found as was a 7.4% rate of contact dermatitis.

Epoxy Resin

Yamakage reported the cases of two workers who developed skin edema, hair loss, and subsequent sclerodermatous changes within 2 months of assignment to work in an epoxy resin polymerization process.[26] Both had systemic symptoms including fatigue and weight loss and were found to have indurated sclerotic skin and erythema, muscle atrophy, weakness, and slightly decreased vital capacity on pulmonary function testing. Histological evaluation showed thickening of the lower dermis and hyalinized collagen. Treatment was begun with prednisone and removal from exposure. Both were followed-up every 2 to 3 years for 2 decades, and Ishikawa reported that laboratory tests remained negative, and lung, liver, and esophagus function normal. Hair loss was reversed by 1977, the sclerosis disappeared by 1980, and the sclerodactyly was gone by 1993. Skin biopsy of one patient in 1993 revealed atrophy but normal collagen.

Yamakage, through elegant animal research, identified bis(4-amino-3-methyl-cyclohexal) methane as the toxin responsible. The lack of other reported cases is presumed to be due to Yamakage's work in bringing this "sentinel health event" to corporate, medical, and public attention, resulting in decreased exposure for others. These cases are excellent examples of the preventive nature of occupational medicine and of the key role of alert clinicians in public health.

Organic Solvents

Aliphatic and aromatic solvents are being reported with increasing frequency as a cause of skin sclerosis. Most solvents vaporize rapidly and can easily penetrate into systemic circulation through the lungs. Many can also pass through the skin, too—the chemical term "solvent" implies fat solubility.[27]

Most reports that describe an association between sclerosis and solvents are case descriptions. They are especially likely to involve chlorinated hydrocarbons such as trichloroethylene (TCE), trichloroethane, and perchloroethylene.[28–30] The first two are common industrial solvents (under much more controlled use now because of extensive water table contamination) and "perc" is the fluid used in dry cleaning. Significantly, these commonly associated solvents are all very similar in chemical structure to vinyl chloride.

Czirjak et al. reviewed data from 21 patients with PSS and found exposure to chemicals, including TCE, polyethylene, and other organic chemicals, in 8 of them.[31] They postulated dysfunction of the immune system for the pathogenesis.

Bovenzi et al. evaluated 21 cases of scleroderma in a group of patients admitted to their local hospitals from 1990 through 1991, matching them by age and gender to two controls each.[32] They found a significant association between exposure to organic solvents and scleroderma.

While some suggest a specific criterion of duration of exposure such as 6 months as a minimal dose to cause sclerosis, Lockey at al. reported a compelling case of a woman exposed to TCE in a degreaser tank.[33] A 2½-hour exposure produced fatigue, swelling of hands and forearms, and a pruritic macular rash over the exposed areas. Over the next months the patient developed scleroderma and related pulmonary, esophageal, cardiac, and renal signs and symptoms, which resulted in death in the 10th month. Her immediate dermal reaction to the exposure of her hands and arms to TCE was a key point in linking her rapidly fatal PSS to the exposure.

Herbicides

Dunnill and Black reported, in 1994, a patient presenting with a 1-year history of progressive thickening of the skin, that began with the symptoms of burning fingertips and skin tightening. The problem progressed to involve his face and parts of his chest, abdomen, and thighs.[34] He was reported to have spent 3 months spraying weed killer along railroad tracks 6 months prior to symptom onset. His skin was exposed mainly when he dipped his bare hands into the weed killer to unblock the mechanism and when wind blew the liquid back onto his face, trunk, and thighs. The patient had an elevated erythrocyte sedimentation rate (ESR) and liver function test and antinuclear antibodies (ANA) of 1:10 (Scl 70 and Jo-I were negative). Muscle biopsy was abnormal for focal areas of perivascular inflammatory cells and skin histology showed hylanization and bands of new connective tissue.

The authors noted that the active ingredients in the weed killer were aminotriazole, bromouracil, and diuron; a review of the literature revealed no other cases of these chemicals' causing similar problems. Unfortunately, although discussing solvents and other chemical causes of scleroderma, they did not discuss the chemical composition of the liquid vehicle of the weed killer. Commonly, pesticides and herbicides make up a tiny percentage of the solution sprayed, with the "inert" ingredients usually composed of a hydrocarbon solvent or mixture of solvents. The toxic effect may possibly have been due to the solvent carrier rather than the herbicides themselves.

Welding

Fessel noted scleroderma in two clinic patients who were welders, and he proceeded to study all cases of scleroderma in his clinic, comparing the 14 scleroderma cases with 54 controls taken from an industrial population.[35] Of the group with scleroderma, five were welders or had close exposure to welding, which was a statistically significant number. He noted that only one patient with scleroderma had had exposure to silica and none to vinyl chloride, and postulated a multifactorial pathogenesis for the disease.

Hypothenar Hammer Syndrome

Hypothenar hammer syndrome is a rare vascular disorder of the ulnar artery of the hand due to repeated trauma which causes degeneration and thrombosis. It is caused by work involving repeated striking of the palms and is often misdiagnosed as Raynaud's phenomenon. Bhatha et al. reported a case of hypothenar hammer syndrome in a 45-year-old male who developed pain and cyanosis in both hands on exposure to cold.[36] He worked in a sawmill, pushing logs onto a conveyor belt, which was postulated to be the cause of the cumulative microtrauma to his ulnar arteries. Angiography was abnormal and he underwent surgical repair of his dilated, thrombosed ulnar arteries. Within 6 months he complained of shortness of breath and skin symptoms and was found on reexamination to have evidence of systemic sclerosis. The authors discussed other cases and postulated that mechanical damage to the arteries of the hand may trigger regional or even, through other mechanisms, systemic disease.

Drugs

Ethosuximide was postulated as a cause after systemic lupus erythematosus (SLE) and scleroderma developed in a 16-year-old with epilepsy.[37] The disorder developed after treatment with the drug was begun, resolved when it was withdrawn, reappeared when ethosuximide was readministered after 6 months, and remitted again when it was withdrawn. Skin biopsy confirmed the diagnosis of scleroderma. The authors note that lupus has been associated with other anticonvulsants, too. Scleroderma-like disorders have also been reported with other drugs, including bleomycin,[38] an antibiotic used in cancer chemotherapy. In two patients, remission was reported after cessation of the drug.

Appetite suppressants were identified as the cause in 2 other cases, and the authors identified 4 more who had also been exposed among 32 patients with systemic sclerosis.[39] They postulated a serotonin-mediated mechanism.

Human Adjuvant Disease

Progressive systemic sclerosis and localized morphea as well as rheumatoid arthritis, mixed connective tissue disease, and other rheumatological disorders have been reported to be associated with petroleum jelly or silicon breast implants and with paraffin or petroleum insertion for cosmetic purposes.[40, 41] The literature is controversial, although silicon could be postulated to have immunological properties similar to the silica from which it is made.

EOSINOPHILIC FASCIITIS AND OTHER SYNDROMES

Eosinophilic faciitis, with eosinophilia inflammation and sclerosis of the deep fascia, is rare and is often confused with scleroderma. The disease presents as tender swelling in the arms and legs which changes into brawny induration. However, Raynaud's phenomenon is rare in patients with fasciitis, as are systemic symptoms, and nailfold capillaries are normal.

The cause is unknown and cases are rare and sporadic. L-tryptophan consumption caused an epidemic of eosinophilia-myalgia syndrome, and one-third of those affected developed extremity pitting edema, peau d'orange dimpling, and induration.[42] Treatment with 25 hydroxytryptophan (L5HTP) also caused a scleroderma-like illness in one patient,[43] and Stachow et al. postulated impaired transformation of serotonin, with an excess of tryptamine as the mechanism.[44]

Trichlorethylene, reported numerous times to cause scleroderma, has also been reported to cause fasciitis in two cases, one occupational and one environmental, through exposure to TCE-contaminated water.[45]

Environmental exposure through ingestion of contaminated rapeseed oil caused an epidemic of eosinophilic fasciitis scleroderma, myalgias, muscle atrophy, and neuropathy in 1981 in thousands of patients.[46]

Diagnosis is made by deep biopsy that includes the deep fascia and skeletal muscle. Spontaneous resolution occurs within 5 years in most cases, and although prednisone may bring eosinophilia and the ESR back to normal, the disease process may progress.

CAUSALITY

Cause is a most difficult issue to deal with, far more so with dermatological manifestations of connective tissue disorders than with most industrial skin problems. Occupational and environmental specialists and dermatologists who focus on causes of skin disorders are being asked more and more often to comment, as treating physicians or expert witnesses, on environmental and product liability cases.

An approach to the problem is manageable if cause is carefully pursued in a logical fashion. First, a specific diagnosis must be identified. This may seem self-evident but there can be a number of possible causes of similar complaints or presentations. Making a specific diagnosis involves a complete medical history, including a history of the present illness, past medical history, family history, current medications, and a review of systems, habits, allergies, and social behavior. A fully detailed occupational and environmental history is also critical, including hobbies and secondary jobs. If chemical exposures are suspected, it is important to identify exactly which chemicals are present in the environment and the conditions of exposure. Material-safety data sheets (MSDS) obtained from the employer are most helpful. However, the presence of a toxin in the workplace does not mean that exposure has occurred or that the disease identified has been caused by that exposure. The toxin must be in a form in which it can get into the body and conditions must exist to allow that to happen at a sufficient dose and duration of exposure to possibly cause disease. For

example, TCE use in milliliter quantities by a trained employee wearing appropriate gloves and working under a laminator flow hood that is checked and calibrated routinely poses no hazard. On the contrary, low levels of the same contaminant in ground waters have been found to cause high levels of exposure to those showering in the contaminated water because the TCE was both heated and aerosolized, greatly increasing skin and respiratory tract absorption.

Obtaining current information about exposure in the workplace is comparatively easy now, with right-to-know laws and MSDS present in most large workplaces, but the clinician and patient will both be challenged when attempting to obtain information about exposures in years past or specifics about the content of a toxic waste dump or multitoxin contamination such as a hazardous-material spill. It can be helpful to identify coworkers still living or working at the facility and safety personnel who may have records going back years and to locate purchasing department information and inspection records of local, state, or federal environmental agencies, health departments, or other government organizations such as the Occupational Safety and Health Administration (OSHA). For environmental exposures that occur through water, air, earth, or food, the patient is commonly forced to pay for very expensive private toxicological testing or to organize with others affected to pressure appropriate public agencies (often underfunded and understaffed) to do the testing.

Once the relevant history, physical examination and biopsy, and toxicological or other tests have been done, the issue of causation is faced. A careful computerized search of the medical literature for case reports, epidemiological studies, and experimental research citations must be performed, and these articles should be reviewed critically. Causation is a complicated subject in workers' compensation and environmental and product liability cases. Use of the term "probably associated" which means "a 51% or greater likelihood" or "more likely than not" is required to initiate a case in most states. For example, the author was referred an unusual case of scleroderma by a local rheumatologist in the mid-1980s, with a question about whether the patient's disease was of industrial origin. She had had significant unprotected occupational exposure to TCE and trichloroethane and epoxy resins, and her case was unusual because of a history of swelling and blanching of the skin of her arms after working with TCE and trichlorethane and because of the absence of rheumatological markers and the presence of bilateral, peripheral ulnar and median nerve neuropathy. When she was first evaluated, the conclusion was that the case was "possibly" caused by her work environment. Five years later, more information had been published, including Lockey's description of a patient (who also had the same swelling and blanching as this patient) with rapidly progressive PSS after a 2½-hour exposure to TCE[33] and also including Yamakage's description of epoxy resin as a cause of scleroderma.[26] The patient was called back to the clinic and completely reevaluated; an industrial claim was filed and, after the workers' compensation appeals process, the case was affirmed as being industrial in origin. The first time, the diagnosis was "scleroderma, unusual variant, possibly industrial," but it was changed to "probably" 5 years later.

The causation issue is complicated by the fact that patients and many health workers believe that medical practitioners can test blood or urine and identify which toxins are present. Patients will often present, insisting that the medical problem is associated with an exposure and requesting a "chemistry panel," or they will bring in a bottle of liquid for identification. Actually, of the over 100,000 chemicals used daily in U.S. industrial processes, there are biological monitoring tests for only approximately 100. Testing for unknowns is complicated by the various test processes for different chemical groups and by the fact that many, if not most, chemicals are rapidly metabolized into many other forms by enzymes in the liver, blood, lungs, and other organs.

Two other "tests of proof" must be met before ascribing a patient's disease process to a particular exposure. First, other causes of the problem must be ruled out, if possible. This is difficult for connective tissue disorders as we are still unclear about the causes and pathogenic processes. However, absence of ingestion of drugs known to cause scleroderma or Raynaud's phenomenon must be ascertained and there must be a search for, and exclusion of, other diseases associated with those findings. The clinician must be able to say that probably "but for this exposure" the disease would likely not have occurred. Finally, the connection between the exposure and the disease process must be "biologically plausible," another difficult issue in cases of dermatological connective tissue disorders, as the pathogenesis is not well understood. However, unusual sensitization reactions to the chemical, presence of other disease processes such as peripheral neuropathy associated with exposure to the chemical but not with the suspected disease, and sufficient dose and duration of exposure are helpful findings. Because of recently reported cases, significant short duration is plausible if it is documented as having been heavy and unprotected, but other symptoms of heavy exposure such as solvent narcosis, blanching of the skin, and so forth, must also be elucidated.

TREATMENT

Treatment involves immediate removal from exposure to the suspected toxin. In vinyl chloride disease and the epoxy resin cases identified by Yamakage, removal from exposure led to reversal of the skin changes.[26] Similarly, Raynaud's phenomenon and most of the acro-osteolysis in vinyl-chloride-exposed workers resolved on removal from exposure.

Given the systemic nature of most of the disease presentations and the suspected activation of the immune system as a common mechanism of pathogenesis, removal from exposure should be permanent. The scleroderma or Raynaud's phenomenon will not result in mortality, but pulmonary fibrosis, liver disease, thrombocytopenia, and other organ system problems associated with the skin manifestations can lead to death.

A number of authors have advocated corticosteroids as part of the treatment protocol. These agents have been effective to varying degrees in different studies, and their effectiveness makes sense, given what we know of the pathophysiology. Provision of a warm workplace and use of gloves is advocated for those with Raynaud's phenomenon, and calcium-channel-blockers may also be helpful.

Long-term follow-up by both a dermatologist and an internist/rheumatologist is appropriate. Provision under workers' compensation for future medical care should be reserved for life, as significant advances in the treatment of diseases are being developed yearly.

References

1. Spieler, E. Legal issues in occupational medicine. In: Herington TN, Morse LH, eds. *Occupational Injuries, Evaluation Management and Prevention*. St. Louis: Mosby; 1997:89.
2. Briggs D, Welsh KI. Major histocompatibility complex II: genes and systemic sclerosis. *Ann Rheum Dis* 1983;119:957–961.
3. Silman AJ. Epidemiology of scleroderma. *Ann Rheum Dis* 1991;50:846–853.
4. Rodnan, GP. When is scleroderma not scleroderma? The differential diagnosis of progressive systemic sclerosis. *Bull Rheum Dis* 1981;31:7–10.
5. Silver RM. Clinical aspects of systemic sclerosis (scleroderma). *Ann Rheum Dis* 1991;50:854–861.
6. Haustein UF, Herrmann K, Bohme HJ. Pathogenesis of systemic sclerosis. *Int J Derm* 1986;25:286–293.
7. Hawkins RA, Claman HN, Clark AF, et al. Increased mast

cell populations in progressive systemic sclerosis: a link to chronic fibrosis? *Ann Int Med* 1985;102:182–186.

8. Stokinger HF. The halogens and the non-metals boron and silicon. In: *Patty's Industrial Hygiene and Toxicology*, 3rd ed. Vol. 2B, 3005–3019, John Wiley and Sons, New York, 1981.

9. Straniero NR, Furst DE. Environmentally-induced systemic sclerosis-like illness. *Clinical Rheumatology* 1989;3:63–88.

10. Rodnan GP, Benedek TG, Medsger TA, et al. The association of progressive systemic sclerosis (scleroderma) with coal miner's pneumoconiosis and other forms of silicosis. *Ann Int Med* 1967;66:323–334.

11. Benedek TG, et al. Serum immunoglobulins, rheumatic factor and pneumoconiosis in coal miners. *Arthritis Rheum* 1976;19:731–738.

12. Baur X, Rihs HP, Altmeyer P, et al. Systemic sclerosis in German uranium miners under special consideration of auto-antibody subsets and HLA class II alleles. *Respiration* 1996;63:368–375.

13. Rihs HP, Conrad K, Mehlhorn J, et al. Molecular analysis of HLA-DPB$_1$ alleles in idiopathic systemic sclerosis patients and uranium miners with systemic sclerosis. *Int Arch Allergy Immunol* 1996;109:216–222.

14. Cowie RL. Silica dust exposed mine workers with scleroderma (systemic sclerosis). *Chest* 1981;92:260–262.

14a. Erasmus LD. Scleroderma in gold miners on the Witwatersrand with particular reference to pulmonary manifestations. *S Afr J Lab Clin Med* 1957;3:209–231.

15. Uber CL, Reynolds RA. Immunotoxicology of silica. *Crit Rev Toxicol* 1982;10:303–319.

16. Wilson RH, McCormick WE, Tatum CF, et al. Occupational acro-osteolysis. *JAMA* 1967;201:83–87.

17. Dinman BD, Cook WA, Whitehouse WM, et al. Occupational acro-osteolysis, an epidemiological study. *Arch Environ Health* 1971;22:61–73.

18. Cook WA, Gieves PM, Dinman BD, et al. Occupational acro-osteolysis, an industrial hygiene study. *Arch Environ Health* 1971;22:74–82.

19. Wilson RI, McCormic WE, Tatum CF. Occupational acro-osteolysis, *JAMA* 1967;201:83–87.

20. Black CM, Welsh KI, Walker AE, et al. Genetic susceptibility to scleroderma-like syndrome induced by vinyl chloride. *Lancet* 1983;1:53–55.

21. Veltman G, Lange CE, Jiihe S, et al. Clinical manifestations and course of vinyl chloride disease. *Ann NY Acad Sci* 1975;246:6–17.

22. Veltman VG. Clinical manifestations and aspects of occupational medicine in vinyl chloride disease (Eng. summary). *Dermatol Monatsschr* 1980;166:705–712.

23. Lilis R, Anderson H, Nicholson WJ, et al. Prevalence of disease among vinyl chloride and polyvinyl chloride workers. *Ann NY Acad Sci* 1974;22–41.

24. Ward AM, Udnoon S, Watkins J, et al. Immunological mechanisms in the pathogenesis of vinyl chloride disease. *Br Med J* 1976;1:936–938.

25. Suciu L, Prodan EA, Paduranu A, et al. Clinical manifestations in vinyl chloride poisoning. *Ann NY Acad Sci* 1975;246:53–69.

26. Yamakage A, Ishikawa H, Saito Y, et al. Occupational scleroderma-like disorder occurring in men engaged in the polymerization of epoxy resins. *Dermatologica* 1980;161:33–44.

27. Bauer M, Rabens SF. Trichlorethylene toxicity. *Int J Dermatol* 1977;16:113–116.

28. Walder BK. Do solvents cause scleroderma? *Int J Dermatol* 1983;22:157–158.

29. Flindt-Hansen H, Isager H. Scleroderma after occupational exposure to trichloroethylene and trichloroethane. *Acta Derm Venereol (Stockh)* 1987;67:263–264.

30. Sparrow GP. A connective tissue disorder similar to vinyl chloride disease in a patient exposed to perchlorethylene. *Clin Exp Derm* 1977;2:17–22.

31. Czirjak L, Danko K, Schlammadinger J, et al. Progressive systemic sclerosis occurring in patients exposed to chemicals. *Int J Dermatol* 1987;26:374–378.

32. Bovenzi M, Barbone F, Betta A, et al. Scleroderma and occupational exposure. *Scand J Work Environ Health* 1995;21:289–292.

33. Lockey JE et al. Progressive systemic sclerosis associated with exposure to trichloroethylene. *J Occup Med* 1987;29:493–496.

34. Dunnill MGS, Black MM. Sclerodermatous syndrome after occupational exposure to herbicides: response to systemic steroids. *Clin Exp Dermatol* 1994;19:518–520.

35. Fessel WJ. Scleroderma and welding [letters to the editor]. *N Engl J Med* 1977;269:1537.

36. Bhatha A, Bulatao IS, Walker SE. Accelerated progressive systemic sclerosis in a patient with hypothenar hammer syndrome. *J Rheumatol* 1996;23:388–392.

37. Teoh PC, Chan HL. Lupus-scleroderma syndrome induced by ethosuximide. *Arch Dis Child* 1975;50:658–661.

38. Finch WR, Rodnan GP, Buehingham RB, et al. Bleomycin-induced scleroderma. *J Rheumatol* 1986;7:651–658.

39. Tomlinson IW, Jayson MI. Systemic sclerosis after therapy with appetite suppressors. *J Rheumatol* 1984;11:254.

40. Kumagai Y, Chiyuki A, Shiokawa Y. Scleroderma after cosmetic surgery. *Arthritis Rheum* 1979;22:532–537.

41. Nabunaga M, Oribe K, Oshishi S. A case of scleroderma with Sjogren's syndrome developed after mammoplasty. *Clin Rheum* 1984;3:375–397.

42. Silver RM, Heyes MP, Maize JC, et al. Scleroderma, fasciitis and eosinophilia associated with the ingestion of tryptophan. *N Engl J Med* 1990;322:874–881.

43. Sternberg EM, van Woert MH, Young SN, et al. Development of a scleroderma-like illness during therapy with 1-5 hydroxytryptophan and carbidopa. *N Engl J Med* 1990;303:782–787.

44. Stachow A, Jablonska S, Skiendzielewsha A. 5-hydroxytryptamine and tryptamine pathways in scleroderma. *Br J Derm* 1977;97:147–153.

45. Walker PA, Clauw D, Cupps T, et al. Fasciitis (not scleroderma) following prolonged exposure to an organic solvent (trichloroethylene). *J Rheumatol* 1994;21:1567–1570.

46. Mateo IM, Izgurerdo M, Fernandez-Dapica MP, et al. Toxic epidemic syndrome. *J Rheumatol* 1984;11:333–338.

Diagnosis and Differential Diagnosis

SUSANNE FREEMAN, M.D.

A patient who believes that his or her skin disease is work-related and who may be seeking workers' compensation is more time-consuming for a physician than is the average patient with nonoccupational skin disease. Hence, many dermatologists shrink from trying to establish a diagnosis for such an individual and often refer him or her to others who have a special interest in this field. In fact, this need not be the case if certain guidelines are followed.

The diagnosis and management of possibly work-related dermatoses can be very satisfying, although it requires a certain discipline. First and foremost, these cases cannot be dealt with as part of a list of general dermatology cases. The average workers' compensation patient needs about twice as much time for the first consultation. Time spent initially on taking a careful, detailed history and examining the patient fully undressed is well repaid later, when a report must be sent to an attorney or insurer. In addition, the patient is commonly strongly influenced by the first diagnosis, and it is often very difficult to change his or her mind later. There is a natural tendency on the part of a physician to want to help the patient. This often produces a bias in favor of a diagnosis of work-related disease, and this is often what the patient wants to hear.

A patient who develops a dermatitis for the first time in adult life naturally wants to find a cause for it. It seems that the work must be responsible, especially if it involves "chemicals" or "dirt." The concept of an endogenous or constitutional eczema or dermatitis is very difficult for the worker to accept. Yet it is not uncommon for atopic eczema to begin for the first time in adult life with no obvious precipitating cause.

A physician must resist a hasty diagnosis of work-related disease. This can have a detrimental effect and militate against the patient's speedy recovery. Often, further investigations, including patch tests, fungal and bacterial cultures, biopsies, and plant visits, are necessary before a diagnosis of occupational skin disease can be made. Perhaps the most important aid to diagnosis in difficult cases is observation of the course of the dermatosis when the patient is away from work for a suitable period of time, followed by observation of the course on return to work.

HISTORY-TAKING

It is extremely helpful to have a special form for recording the history and physical examination. Vital questions are easily omitted if a checklist is not adhered to. A suggested form for recording the history and physical examination is shown in Table 12–1. Every history of a current illness should begin with the following questions:

1. Where did the rash first begin? (That is, exactly which anatomical site was affected first?) Most occupational skin disease is contact dermatitis, which must begin at the site of contact with the offending agent. Later, spread to other sites can occur, especially in cases of allergic contact dermatitis. Very often a worker with dermatitis on the hand will admit, in response to questioning, that the foot or some other area of the skin not exposed during work was affected first, thus suggesting an endogenous dermatitis. If the dermatitis began on the hand, it is important to ask exactly which part was first involved. If the eruption is unilateral, note whether the patient is right- or lefthanded.

2. When did the dermatitis begin? If the job is the principal cause, the dermatitis must have commenced during the course of employment. An endogenous dermatitis, present before the current

Table 12–1. SUGGESTED FORM FOR RECORDING MEDICAL HISTORY AND PHYSICAL EXAMINATION OF PATIENTS WITH SKIN DISEASE SUSPECTED TO BE OF OCCUPATIONAL ORIGIN

Name _____ Date _____

Address _____ Age _____ Sex _____

Home phone _____ Soc.sec.no. _____ Referred by _____

Current employer (name and address) _____

_____ Job title at present _____

Employer at onset of injury (name and address) _____

_____

Date employed _____ Date terminated _____

Job title at onset of injury _____ Date _____

Insurance carrier (name and address) _____

_____

Present Illness

Date of onset _____ Dates of disability _____

Location at onset _____

Patient's description _____

_____

_____

_____

Time off work (incl. vacations)? _____

Effect of return to work? _____

Workers' Compensation claim? _____

Previous job(s)? _____ How long? _____

Previous Treatment

1. Plant dispensary _____

2. Other physician _____

_____

3. Self-treatment _____

_____

Description of Work

_____

_____

_____

_____

Materials contacted _____

_____

Other workers affected? Yes _____ No _____ No. affected _____

How many workers on this job? _____

Methods of cleaning skin at work (and frequency) _____

_____

Protective creams (names) _____

_____

Protective clothing (incl. gloves) _____

Past History

Previous compensation claims? Yes _____ No _____ Explain _____

_____

Previous skin diseases _____

Relation to occupation? Yes _____ No _____ Place of birth _____

Past health _____

Allergic history: Hay fever _____ Asthma _____ Eczema _____ Allergic to cosmetics, medications, creams, ointments, jewelry, drugs, perfumes? (circle which)

Describe _____

Family history of atopy or psoriasis? Yes _____ No _____ Second job _____

Hobbies

Contacts at Home

Housework _____ Full-time _____ Part-time _____

Married _____ Single _____ Widow _____ Divorced _____

Children _____ Yes _____ Number _____ Ages _____

Emotional factors _____

Table 12–1. (*Continued*)

Physical Examination

General appearance _____

Description of disease _____

Other skin diseases _____

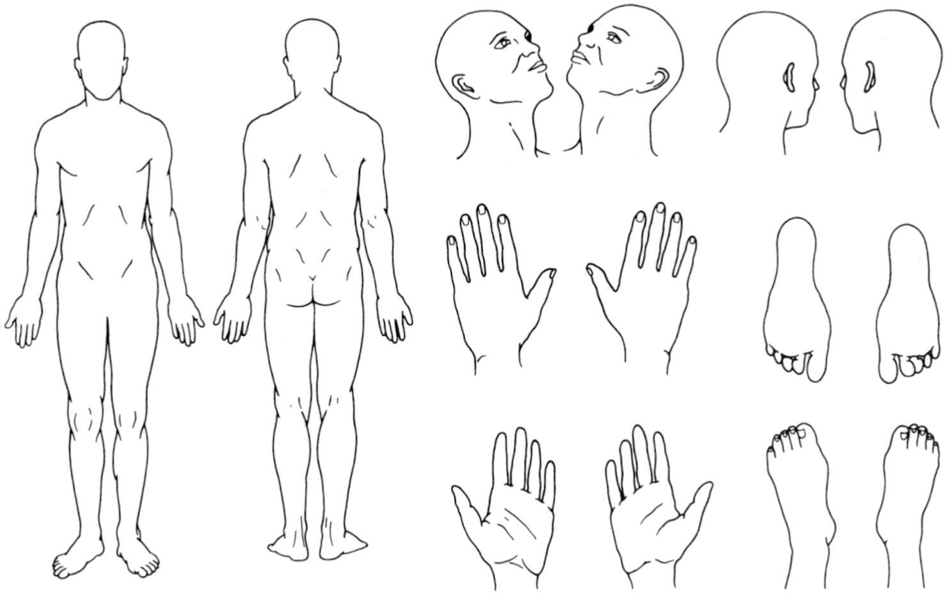

Diagnosis

Eczema	Yes _____	No _____	Different _____
Contact dermatitis	Entirely _____	Partially _____	No _____
Endogenous dermatitis	Atopic _____	Discoid _____	Seborrheic _____
	Hand _____	Foot _____	Asteatotic _____
	Face _____	Stasis _____	Unclassified _____

Pre–Patch Test Diagnosis

Sensitizers		Relevance	
Irritants		Relevance	
Occupational	Yes _____	No _____	Don't know _____

Special Tests

KOH _____ Fungal culture _____ Bacterial culture _____

Biopsy _____

Patch testing (results)   Sensitizers _____

Relevance _____

Occupational   Yes _____   No _____   Clinical photographs?   Yes _____   No _____

Treatment _____

Disability   Yes _____   No _____   Occupational   Yes _____   No _____

Remarks and Recommendations _____

Post–Patch Test Diagnosis

Sensitizers _____	Relevance _____	
Irritants _____	Relevance _____	
Occupational _____	Yes _____	No _____

job, can, of course, be aggravated by factors present at the job.

3. Does the rash itch? Eczema, or dermatitis (the two terms are virtually interchangeable), is characteristically pruritic, whereas psoriatic hand dermatitis is usually not. A nonitching hand "dermatitis" is usually not caused primarily by situations at work and is often psoriatic.

4. Does the dermatitis improve when the worker is away from work for a reasonable period of time? Does the dermatitis worsen on return to work? The answers to these questions are probably the most important of all the pieces of evidence that can be used to decide whether or not a case is work-related. The careful observation and documentation of the severity of the dermatitis before and after, say, 2 weeks off work, is the most telling evidence in a workers' compensation case. Of course, it is important to know what the worker was doing while away from work. Sometimes, a hobby such as gardening, home cementing, or car maintenance can prevent improvement of a job-related dermatitis despite absence from the workplace.

5. What treatments have been used? The answer may suggest a medicament as the cause or enhancer of the contact dermatitis, especially if a particular treatment seemed to worsen the condition or failed to produce the expected improvement. A history of clearing with systemic corticosteroids followed by a rebound flare, despite absence from work, is suggestive of an endogenous eczema. An allergic contact dermatitis treated with systemic corticosteroids in adequate dosage, with gradual tapering of the dose, will usually not rebound, provided that there is no further contact with the offending allergen.

Occupational History

1. What job does the patient do? The job title can be important but is often misleading. What the worker actually does and the work contactants present during a typical working day are the details that must be determined. Job titles such as "operator" and "technician" convey very little. When asked to explain, the worker often uses trade jargon that may be meaningless to the physician, who must be prepared to admit ignorance. The worker should be pressed for a full explanation of the relevant technical details of the work. In certain cases a real understanding can be achieved only by a visit to the site. Without detailed questioning, assumptions regarding contact factors may be erroneous. For example, a cleaner may be assumed to be susceptible to hand derma-

titis, yet many do no wet work at all and may only vacuum floors, sweep, and dust.

2. How long has the worker been in the present job? The answer to this question can be of vital importance. An apprentice hairdresser, chef, or auto mechanic who develops a hand dermatitis within the first year of the apprenticeship usually has an irritant contact dermatitis and commonly will not be able to complete the training, whereas a worker developing a hand dermatitis after many years in the trade is more likely to have an allergic contact dermatitis due to sensitization. In these cases, identification of the allergen and making a substitution for it can enable resumption of the job. There are many exceptions, however. Allergic contact dermatitis can sometimes develop early, especially with strong allergens such as epoxies. Irritant contact dermatitis, on the other hand, may develop after many years if the work process changes, the work load increases, or home and hobby irritants add to the cumulative insults.

3. What was the previous job? Did it involve handling irritants or potential allergens? Did the skin react at that time? If the answer is yes, it may be useful to compare the present skin reaction with that of the past. Previous occupations may also be relevant to a positive patch test.

4. What protective clothing is worn? Are gloves worn, and if so, what type? Protective clothing can be effective, but it is often inadequate. Gloves tear, allow liquids to enter at the top, are often permeable to chemicals, and become contaminated on the inside when taken off and placed on the workbench. Worst of all, they are hot, uncomfortable, and clumsy for jobs requiring manual dexterity. Allergy may develop to antioxidants and accelerators in rubber gloves, which can often be the whole or partial cause of the hand dermatitis.

5. Does the worker like the job and want to continue in it? An honest answer to this question can be a helpful pointer to prognosis.

6. What does the worker believe to be the cause? The answer can illuminate both valid possibilities and misconceptions. In any case, it is helpful to ask the question and to record the answer.

7. Are other workers affected? If there is a convincingly high incidence of contact dermatitis in other workers, an allergenic or irritant work material may well be responsible. A site visit may be needed to investigate such a problem.

Hobbies or Part-time Jobs

A 40-hour work week occupies only about a third of a week's waking hours. This leaves ample opportunity for other factors to present themselves in hobbies, part-time jobs, or housework. In any case of possible occupational skin disease, these nonoccupational activities must not be overlooked.

The hobbyist who works with cement or epoxy, the gardener exposed to plant allergens, the housekeeper exposed to cleaning solutions—all are handling materials that may be partially or wholly contributing to the dermatitis. The marital status and number and ages of children should always be noted. A hand dermatitis may be related to or wholly caused by wet housework, especially when the care of young children is involved. This is now true of both men and women.

Past History

A past history of any contact allergies may be relevant, as the same allergen or a related one may again be causing irritation. A patient with a past history or a family history in a first-degree relative of eczema, asthma, or hayfever is considered an atopic individual for most practical purposes. An atopic history may weight the diagnosis in favor of an endogenous rather than a work-related dermatitis. However, patients with atopic eczema are thought to be more susceptible to irritant contact dermatitis. It is a common misconception that the diagnosis must be either endogenous (atopic) dermatitis or exogenous (contact) dermatitis. It is not uncommon for both to play a part.

Family History

A family history of atopic disease is significant, as is a family history of psoriasis when a differential diagnosis of psoriasis and eczema is being considered. If the whole family or many of the workmates are feeling itchy, scabies must always be considered.

General Health

Questions about general health may be revealing. The existence of diabetes, arteriosclerosis, stasis dermatitis, fungal infection, or a psychiatric disorder may be relevant.

Drug Intake

Cutaneous reactions to medicaments can take many forms and can at times resemble an occupational dermatosis (see the section on differential diagnosis). The response or lack of response to systemic corticosteroids, antibiotics, and sedatives can be important in aiding diagnosis.

PHYSICAL EXAMINATION

It is important that the patient undress completely. Otherwise, patches of clearly endogenous eczema (flexural, lichenified, or discoid), plaques of psoriasis on elbows, knees, scalp, and feet (Fig. 12–1), psoriatic nail pits, tinea pedis, or tinea cruris might be missed. Although these conditions can coexist with an occupational dermatosis, their presence can influence the diagnosis in doubtful cases.

Which Patterns Are Suggestive of an Occupational Contact Dermatitis?

Most occupational contact dermatitis affects the hands. If the worker's hands are normal and no

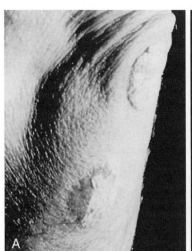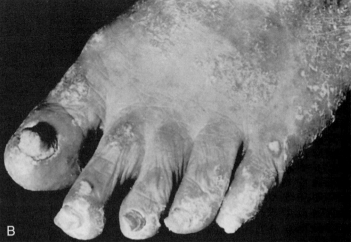

FIGURE 12–1 • A and B, typical plaques of psoriasis such as these can be missed if the patient has not undressed completely during the physical examination.

gloves are worn, a contact dermatitis is very un-likely. If gloves are worn, the arms above the gloves may be affected. Airborne contact factors (dusts, fumes, vapors) affect the face and neck.

Allergic contact dermatitis may later become generalized, as it is mediated by circulating T cells. Alternatively, allergens such as epoxies can be transferred from gloved hand to face.

It is often said that contact dermatitis first af-fects the thinner epidermis of the dorsal surfaces of the hands and the finger webs, whereas endoge-nous hand dermatitis affects the palms and sides of the fingers. The latter, especially in the vesicu-lar form, has been called dyshidrotic eczema or pompholyx. Both these terms are of doubtful value and are best replaced by the term "endogenous hand dermatitis." Although the pattern of hand dermatitis may at times be helpful in differentiat-ing an endogenous from a contact dermatitis, it is not reliable. Chronic nickel and chromate allergy, for example, may produce an "endogenous" pat-tern, and contact dermatitis can certainly affect palmar surfaces. In any case, contact factors often operate together with an atopic diathesis, so a mixed picture would be expected.

Cronin's study[10] of patterns of hand eczema in 263 women is extremely interesting. She has shown that, at least in women, allergens, irritants, and endogenous factors can all produce similar and indistinguishable patterns of hand eczema. She states that elucidation of the cause rests more on a detailed history and the results of patch-testing than on the clinical distribution of the hand eczema. Low-grade, repeated, frictional skin irritation can produce an irritant contact derma-titis. The distribution of the dermatitis corresponds exactly to the cutaneous sites exposed to friction. For example, a carpenter developed a dermatitis involving thumb and index finger at the sites that came into contact with screws and nails.[19]

Which Patterns Are Suggestive of Endogenous Dermatitis?

Cronin recognizes only two clinical patterns of hand eczema that are associated with cause, and both are endogenous.[10] The first is a localized eczema of the central palm that spreads proximally toward the base or heel of the hand; it is probably always endogenous (Fig. 12–2). The second is a palmar eczema in an "apron pattern," and it is also endogenous. This is eczema that extends from the proximal fingers to the contiguous distal part of the palms to form a half circle or apron pattern. However, it is often complicated by an irritant, allergic, or endogenous spread of eczema to other parts of the hands.

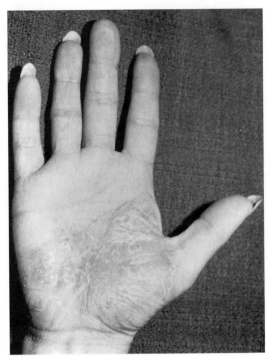

FIGURE 12–2 • Eczema localized to the central palm is almost always endogenous.

Eczema affecting other parts of the body pro-duces patterns well known to be endogenous. Involvement of antecubital and popliteal fossae is nearly always endogenous (atopic) eczema. An-other endogenous pattern consists of excoriated papules surrounded by normal skin. When these affect the back, only that part accessible to the fingers is involved (Fig. 12–3).

In other words, with the exception of the fore-going patterns, which are typically endogenous, contact dermatitis cannot be confidently diagnosed or ruled out by pattern alone.

INVESTIGATIONS

Patch Testing

The only certain way to diagnose allergic contact dermatitis caused in the workplace is through di-agnostic patch testing. However, the results must be carefully interpreted in the light of the history, and the relevance of a positive patch test must be determined. Great care must be taken before test-ing with unknown industrial chemicals, for they can product toxic reactions. Irritant contact derma-titis cannot be diagnosed by patch testing.

Details of patch-testing techniques are dealt with in chapter 14.

FIGURE 12–3 • Excoriated papules surrounded by normal skin is a pattern of endogenous eczema. Note that only the part of the back accessible to the scratching fingers is involved.

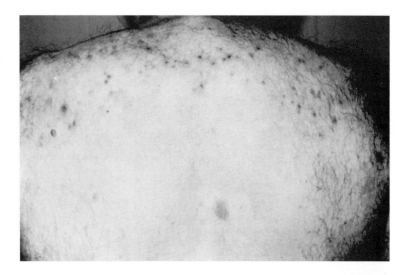

Prick-Testing

Food handlers such as chefs (Fig. 12–4), butchers, and caterers can develop a hand dermatitis that is caused by an immediate, or type I, hypersensitivity to foods, particularly seafood and meats. Although this is actually contact urticaria, it usually manifests itself not as urticaria but as dermatitis. Diagnosis can be made by prick-testing with the foods responsible (Figs. 12–5 and 12–6); positive tests produce a wheal-and-flare reaction. In cases such as these, 48- to 72-hour patch testing with the foods is negative.

This subject is dealt with in detail in chapter 6. In the past 10 years there has been increasing awareness of immediate, type I hypersensitivity to natural rubber latex (NRL) gloves. Prick-testing is the most sensitive diagnostic test for this and is very important as this allergy is a potential source of anaphylaxis.[35]

Other occupation-based allergens that can be detected by prick-testing include flour and grains

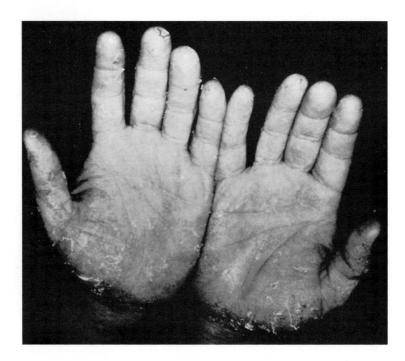

FIGURE 12–4 • Hand dermatitis in a chef who presented initially with contact urticaria to seafood.

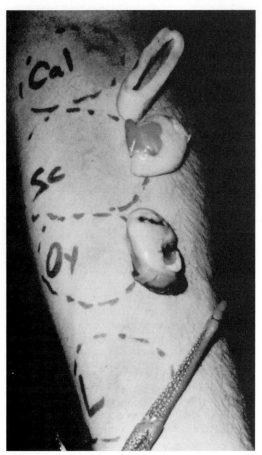

FIGURE 12–5 • Positive prick tests to samples of seafood (calamari, scallops, oysters, and lobster).

(bakers), cow dander (farmers), and industrial enzymes added to cleaning and soap products (factory workers).[26]

Biopsy

Biopsy can help differentiate occupational skin disease from that of nonoccupational origin, such as psoriasis, lichen planus, and tumors. Often neglected by nondermatologists, the biopsy is simple to perform and often reveals vital information that cannot be otherwise obtained. Psoriasis of hands and feet can be difficult to distinguish clinically from dermatitis. Unfortunately, these cases are often indistinguishable histologically too.

Fungal Examination

Tinea of the hands and feet can often mimic a contact dermatitis. It can be excluded by examining skin scrapings for fungi, using a potassium hydroxide mount and culturing fungi on Sabouraud's glucose agar.

Special Chemical Tests

Dimethylglyoxime Spot Test for Detecting Nickel

Nickel-sensitive workers can react to contact with materials containing nickel. This spot test can be used to determine nickel content. The kit consists of 1% dimethylglyoxime in alcohol and a 10% ammonium hydroxide solution. The addition of a few drops of each solution to the metallic object produces a reddish color if the test is positive. This pink precipitate occurs in the presence of available nickel in sufficient concentration (at least 1:10,000) to produce dermatitis in nickel-sensitive persons (see also chapter 24).

Test for Chromates

Chromates are commonly used in industry, and in a chromate-sensitive worker it is important to detect chromate in work materials. The object is placed in hot water to extract any chromium present. The solution is acidified with diluted hydrochloric acid. Then a 1% alcoholic solution of diphenyl carbazide is added. The development of

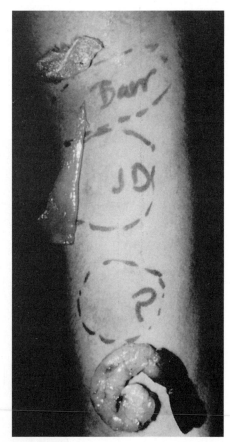

FIGURE 12–6 • Positive prick tests to barramundi fish, John Dory fish, and prawns.

a persistent red color is specific for hexavalent chromium salts. The test is sensitive to 10 parts per million.

Test for Detection of Formaldehyde

Formaldehyde is an allergen that is used in many industrial processes. The chromotropic acid method can be used for qualitative formaldehyde determination.[11] The principle is that if formaldehyde is present, a violet color appears with the addition of chromotropic acid in concentrated sulfuric acid. However, this method sometimes produces a masking discoloration. A complementary method using acetylacetone as the reagent has been described by the same authors.[17] It can be used for both qualitative and quantitative determination of the presence of formaldehyde.

OCCUPATIONAL SITE SURVEY

Industrial Plant Visits

Material Safety Data Sheets, when properly used, are indispensable for learning about the chemical hazards of a given workplace, but additional information can be obtained by making a visit to the plant; doing so can be profitable in many ways. Familiarity with work materials, job processes, the plant's environment, and the attitudes of workers and management can facilitate diagnosis and treatment of occupational skin disease arising from working conditions in the plant. It also puts the physician in a better position to recommend preventive measures and to assist in the placement of workers.

A visit must not be made unannounced and can be arranged with the manager of a small industrial plant, or the safety or personnel departments of larger industrial plants. If the industrial plant has a part-time or full-time physician, arrangements can usually be made readily. Another method is to obtain an appointment through an industrial engineer of the local or state health department. Visits should be made early in the day, at the beginning of the day shift (at 7 a.m.) and can usually be completed within an hour or so. It must be emphasized that there is no substitute for personally viewing the patient's work and work environment (see chapter 17).

DIFFERENTIAL DIAGNOSIS OF OCCUPATIONAL DERMATITIS

The following nonoccupationally caused conditions are frequently encountered and may be confused with occupational disease; in certain instances, the condition may be aggravated by the occupation.

Contact Dermatitis from Nonoccupational Sources: Home, Hobbies, Cosmetics, Clothing, Jewelry, Medicaments, and Plants

Only 35 to 40 of a possible 168 hours are spent at work during an average week, and the substances encountered off the job rival those found at work for variety and potential toxicity. Indeed, the number of hazardous substances present in the average home makes many work environments seem harmless by comparison.[14] Among the most common are dermatitis-producing plants, especially poison ivy and oak. Other substances include soaps and detergents, furniture polishes, medications, and many other materials (Tables 12–2 and 12–3).

Cosmetics

Cosmetics must be considered in the differential diagnosis of occupational dermatitis. Most severe

 TABLE 12–2 • The Most Common Irritants Found in the Home

Soaps and detergents, including shampoos
Oven cleaners
Scouring pads and powders
Toilet bowl and drain cleaners
Window cleaners
Rug shampoos
Pet shampoos
Copper and metal brighteners
Bleaches
Pesticides
Fertilizers
Furniture polishes and waxes
Vegetables, fruits, and meats (contact urticaria)

 TABLE 12–3 • The Most Common Allergens Found in the Home

Rubber: gloves, elastic, rubber bands, adhesive tape
Nickel: jewelry, zippers, buttons, hand tools, coins, keys
Cosmetics: fragrances, germicidal agents, lanolin
Medications, including those for pets
Plants, especially *Rhus*
Plastics: epoxy resin in adhesive
Dichromate: leather gloves, belts, leashes; cement; paint; matches; anticorrosion compounds for automobiles

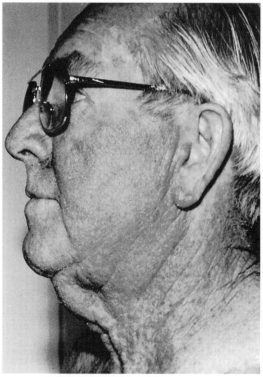

FIGURE 12–7 ● Allergic contact dermatitis due to cosmetics. This patient suspected his work as the cause of his dermatitis, but patch-testing showed him to be allergic to the fragrance in his shaving cream.

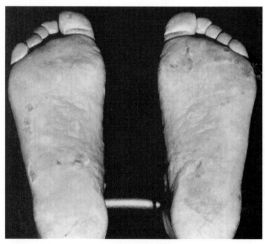

FIGURE 12–9 ● Allergic contact dermatitis due to tetramethylthiuram disulfide in the inner soles of shoes.

cosmetic reactions are allergic in nature (Fig. 12–7). The most common causes are fragrances and preservatives, such as quaternium-15, formaldehyde, imidazolidinyl urea, and parabens.[1] Chapter 22 deals with cosmetics in detail.

Clothing, Including Gloves and Shoes

Dermatitis caused by formaldehyde-based textile finishes[24] or dyes[21] is a possibility to consider. Rubber sensitivity, particularly to rubber gloves

(Fig. 12–8) or footwear (Fig. 12–9), is a frequent cause of dermatitis (see chapter 29).

Shoes are an important source of allergic contact dermatitis of the feet.[34] If an allergy can be traced to work boots or shoes, an occupational cause is implicated. Constituents of rubber, adhesives, and leather are the most common causes of this type of allergic contact dermatitis. Because there are many unknown chemicals in shoes, patch testing with samples cut from every part of the shoe is the best form of diagnosis. Samples must be thin and wide (7 to 10 mm) and should be soaked in water for 15 min before testing. Samples should be left on the skin for 4 to 5 days instead of the usual 2 days.

Medicaments

Medicaments applied at home or at work are common causes of contact dermatitis. Neomycin, benzocaine, wool alcohols, and preservatives used in creams are all well-known potential contact

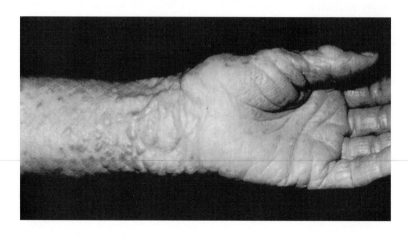

FIGURE 12–8 ● Allergic contact dermatitis due to mercapto-benzothiazole in rubber gloves.

allergens. In recent years many publications have shown that even topical corticosteroids are potential contact allergens.[18]

Nickel

Nickel sensitivity had a very high incidence in women in Prystowsky's study; it was found in 9% of women and in only 0.9% of men (Fig. 12–10). Nickel sensitivity is more often acquired from ear piercing than from industry.[30] Women with nickel allergy can develop chronic hand dermatitis despite minimal contact with nickel. This may be caused by nickel that has been ingested (see also chapter 24).

Photocontact Dermatitis

Persistent dermatitis on exposed areas may be photocontact dermatitis. The most common causes of photocontact dermatitis at this time are sunscreen agents—PABA and octyl dimethyl PABA, cinnamates, benzophenones, and dibenzoylmethanes.[4] Pig farmers may develop photocontact allergy to olaquindox, a growth promoter in feed additives for pigs.[32]

Plants

Allergic contact dermatitis that is caused by plants can mimic an occupational dermatitis. House plants, especially chrysanthemums, philodendrons, and *Primula obconica* (Fig. 12–11), as well as outdoor plants such as *Rhus, Grevillea,* and *Compositae* species must be considered. For further

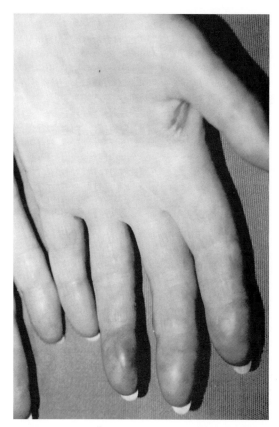

FIGURE 12–11 • Allergic contact dermatitis due to *Primula obconica*. This woman tended the plants in the museum where she was employed.

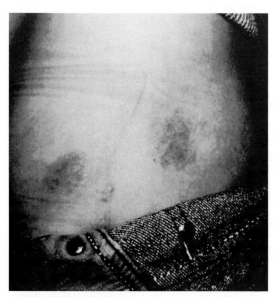

FIGURE 12–10 • Nickel allergy can manifest as "jeanodermatosis." Nickel sensitivity in women usually originates from ear piercing, often done many years previously.

details about contact dermatitis caused by plants, see chapter 31.

Atopic Eczema

Atopic eczema is dealt with in detail in chapter 13. For practical purposes, an individual with a personal or family history of eczema, asthma, and hayfever is considered atopic. Atopic eczema usually commences in infancy but can appear for the first time in adulthood and can be limited to the hands or the face. It is this type that causes the greatest difficulty when it comes to determining possible work-related causation. Many times, these cases are partially due to contact dermatitis (more often irritant rather than allergic in nature) that has been superimposed on an atopic diathesis.

Nummular Eczema

Nummular eczema is an entity by virtue of its morphology, that is, its characteristic coinlike lesions of erythema with vesicles, in acute cases, or erythema with scaling, in subacute cases (Fig.

12–12). The precise cause is not known. Predisposing factors include atopy, bacterial organisms, xerosis, and primary irritation.[9, 23] Nummular eczema is not specifically related to occupation, but widespread allergic contact dermatitis in certain patients may assume this pattern.

Dyshidrotic Eczema, or Pompholyx

Itching vesicles on the palms, soles, and sides of the fingers has been called dyshidrotic eczema, or pompholyx (Fig. 12–13). Although hyperhidrosis may be present and appears to be a complicating factor, a disorder of sweating has not been proved to be the cause. Hence, this condition is now often termed simply "endogenous hand and/or foot dermatitis." However, as discussed earlier, Cronin[10] has shown that it is very difficult to make a diagnosis of endogenous hand dermatitis based on morphology alone. The clinical appearance of endogenous hand dermatitis (dyshidrotic eczema, or pompholyx) may be indistinguishable from that of contact dermatitis. In addition, many cases are altered by the effects of medication, work contactants, and secondary infection. Occupational contactants may aggravate and prolong the condition. Some patients have an atopic background.

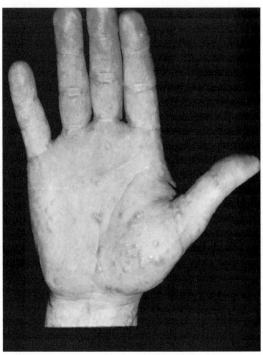

FIGURE 12–13 • This endogenous hand dermatitis, sometimes termed dyshidrotic eczema or pompholyx, is at times difficult to differentiate from contact dermatitis.

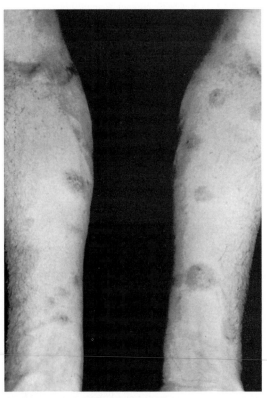

FIGURE 12–12 • "Discoid" or nummular eczema, a condition that is only rarely work-related.

Acrodermatitis Perstans (Continua)

Also called pustular acrodermatitis or dermatitis repens, acrodermatitis perstans, or acrodermatitis continua, is characterized by a persistent eruption of sterile pustules particularly on the skin of the distal phalanx of fingers or toes. Burning and itching are often present. The blisters burst and peel off, leaving a bright red area. It is considered to be related to psoriasis, which can occur in its typical or pustular form at any time in these patients.

Trauma and chemical irritation may provoke an episode, but the condition is not an occupational disease. The cause is basically unknown, and occupation can be only an aggravating factor. Yet because the condition is chronic, recurrent, and commonly disabling, it is important to establish the exact role played by occupation early in the course of the disease. Home contactants and emotional stress can also play significant roles.

Lichen Simplex Chronicus

Also called localized neurodermatitis, lichen simplex chronicus is a response of predisposed skin to repeated rubbing (Fig. 12–14). The typical lesion is a thickened, scaling plaque in which the skin markings are greatly exaggerated. Paroxys-

FIGURE 12–14 • Lichen simplex chronicus is caused by persistent rubbing of the skin and is rarely related to the occupation.

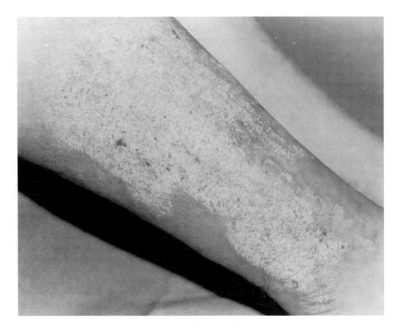

mal itching is a prominent feature. Lichenification is characteristic of the atopic state, although this is not an invariable accompaniment. The condition is more common in women and in patients of Asian descent. Common sites are the back of the neck, the lateral aspect of the lower leg, and the vulva or scrotum. However, any site can be affected, including the dorsum of the hand. The condition is rarely of occupational origin.

Psoriasis

When psoriasis presents in its classic form, diagnosis can be made easily, and a work relationship immediately determined. Sometimes the work is responsible for initiating psoriasis in predisposed persons. The diagnosis can be difficult, however, when the lesions are few and limited to the palms (Fig. 12–15). Thickened, erythematous, scaling, nonpruritic plaques are characteristic. Differentiation from dermatitis is necessary and may be made easier by the usual absence of itching in psoriasis. Patients complain of painful cracks and fissures in psoriatic hand dermatitis, but rarely complain of itching.

Psoriasis, like atopic eczema, can be limited to the hands and can appear for the first time at any age. Although, like atopy, it is an endogenous, genetically determined condition, it can be precipitated by occupational trauma, even of mild form.

Pressure and friction from occupational procedures may produce psoriasis of the hands, particularly the palms and volar surface of the fingers. This Koebner phenomenon was seen in a pharma-

cist (caused by the pressure of opening and closing containers with child-resistant caps), a surgeon, a dentist (caused by the pressure of various instruments), a bus driver (caused by the pressure of the steering wheel), and an office worker (caused by pounding a stapler).[15]

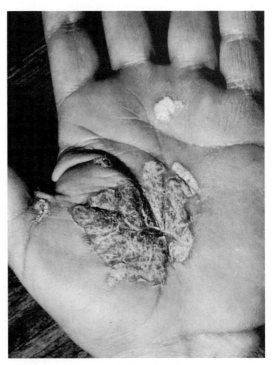

FIGURE 12–15 • These thickened, scaling, sharply marginated, nonpruritic lesions are examples of psoriasis.

Also, fresh lesions of psoriasis that appear following trauma resulting from scratching, abrasions, lacerations, folliculitis, and acne have led many workers to press for compensation in the belief that the disease was caused or activated by their occupations. If a "Koebnerized" lesion is followed quickly by a severe flare of the disease, the idea of occupational causation seems even more likely to the worker. Trauma may undoubtedly incite the development of new lesions of psoriasis, but this occurs only in persons who already have the disease, if only in latent form. Thus, the Koebner phenomenon is medicolegally important when it follows industrial injuries.

Lichen Planus

Lichen planus has some features similar to those of psoriasis: Both commonly show the Koebner phenomenon, good patient health, and sometimes widespread involvement. Lichen planus is an inflammatory, pruritic dermatosis of unknown origin in which the lesions are discrete, occasionally grouped, polygonal, flat-topped, violaceous, papular, and commonly located on the wrists (Fig. 12–16A), ankles, and genitalia. The oral and vaginal mucous membranes usually show white papules in a lacelike pattern. When palms or soles are involved, a worker may be markedly disabled. Lesions on the soles of the feet may become painful ulcerations, necessitating skin grafts. Lichen planus is more common in men than in women.

The cause of lichen planus, like that of psoriasis, is unknown, and there is rarely a direct relationship to the occupation. Occasionally the onset is blamed on an emotional experience at work, although this is usually very difficult to prove. Because new lesions occur following scratches and abrasions, work injury is often claimed, but aggravation of the disease by occupation is difficult to establish at times. Hellgren[22] has found a greater incidence of lichen planus in so-called dirty occupations such as agriculture, forestry, engineering, construction, and metalworking.

The so-called lichenoid eruptions, which closely resemble lichen planus, have occurred in persons working with color film developers, which are derivatives of *p*-phenylenediamine (Fig. 12–16B).[5, 27, 29] However, since the advent of automation in this industry, such cases are rare. Similar contact-type lichenoid eruptions have been reported to result from fur dyeing, gasoline manufacture, and rubber compounding.[5] Differentiation from true lichen planus can be difficult, but the history and the examination of histological sections may be helpful.

Mite Infestation

Infestation of the skin with sarcoptic mites, animal or human, produces a dermatitis resembling contact dermatitis, especially fibrous glass dermatitis. The eruption caused by animal scabies is usually less severe and more self-limited than that caused by human scabies, but both produce a widespread eruption consisting of small papules with linear streaks ("burrows"), vesicles, and pustules (Fig. 12–17). Excoriations and secondary eczematization are always present. Differentiation from fibrous glass dermatitis may be made on the basis of localization: The groin and genitalia, the webs of the fingers, and the wrists are most commonly involved in scabies.

Mites readily invade stored food such as grains, cheese, figs, and copra. Although ordinarily nonpathogenic, they may occasionally cause dermatitis.[2] Workers who risk mite infestation include

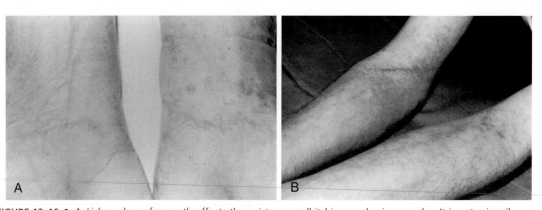

FIGURE 12–16 ● *A*, Lichen planus frequently affects the wrists as small itching, coalescing papules. It is not primarily work-related but lesions may appear in areas of trauma (Koebner phenomenon). *B*, When due to contact with color developers during work, the condition is clearly work-related and may resemble lichen planus.

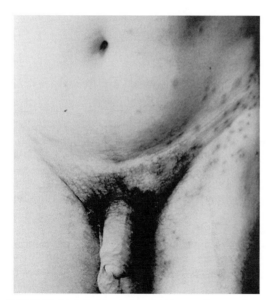

FIGURE 12–17 • Scabies involves widespread areas of skin, typically in the groin area.

dock workers exposed to grain and copra and those in the food industry who handle stored produce, such as bakers, mill hands, and storage hands.

Photosensitivity Eruptions

Polymorphous light eruptions and discoid lupus erythematosus may resemble eczematous dermatitis, especially early in their development. When these conditions occur in workers heavily exposed to sunlight or artificial ultraviolet light, as in welding, the occupation may clearly aggravate the condition. Solar urticaria may also be triggered by sunlight exposure and becomes eczematized by rubbing and scratching.

This subject is dealt with in detail in chapter 10.

Acne Vulgaris

Acneiform lesions that closely resemble acne vulgaris are common in workers exposed to greases and oils. Acne cosmetica, caused by contact with lanolin, petrolatum, certain vegetable oils, butyl stearate, lauryl alcohol, and oleic acid[28] may be seen in persons demonstrating and selling cosmetics.

Occupational acne, including chloracne, is dealt with in detail in chapter 7.

Perioral Dermatitis

Perioral dermatitis is a common clinical problem that affects the face. As the name implies, it af-

fects principally the area around the mouth (Fig. 12–18). It is usually seen in women.[8] The condition consists of tiny erythematous papules on an erythematous background with some scaling. The cause is obscure, and the condition is primarily cosmetic. It disappears without leaving a trace. When several women workers are simultaneously affected, as is sometimes the case, an occupational cause may be suspected. But the condition is not occupational, and there are no known occupational aggravating factors except perhaps the use of greasy makeup, as required of actors, actresses, and cosmetic salespersons. The only known environmental factors that have been incriminated are fluorinated topical corticosteroids,[36] sunlight, and heat.[6]

Fungal Infections

Tinea manuum can mimic hand dermatitis, especially after erroneous treatment with topical corticosteroids. However, an arcuate advancing edge is a sign of tinea (Fig. 12–19). If there is doubt, fungal scrapings should be made and the feet and groin examined for tinea.

Because fungal infections of the feet are so common, the finding of a fungus on a potassium

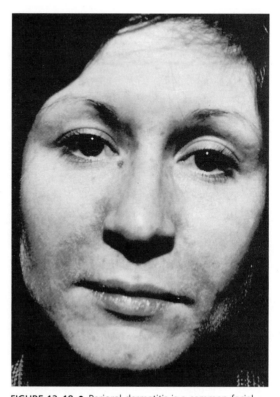

FIGURE 12–18 • Perioral dermatitis is a common facial eruption that is not of occupational origin.

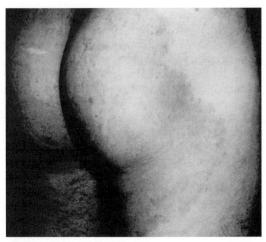

FIGURE 12–19 • A worker with a widespread tinea infection, showing the typical slightly raised, serpiginous border. This case was not work-related.

hydroxide mount or fungal culture does not necessarily prove that the disease in question is related to the fungus. Study of the patient's history as well as the appearance of the lesions are necessary to prove such a relationship. Specific occupational fungal infections are described in chapter 5.

Herpes Simplex Infections

Herpes simplex infections may superficially resemble contact dermatitis when located on fingers and hands (Fig. 12–20). These infections are especially common in medical and dental personnel and are seen also in masseurs, wrestlers, barbers, and hairdressers. The incubation period ranges from 3 to 7 days, and the condition lasts for

approximately 2 weeks.[20] Gloves protect the skin from the virus.[31]

Malingering

The experienced physician can usually recognize self-induced skin lesions at a glance. They often show bizarre geometric patterns, such as crosses, triangles, arcs, and circles and are frequently unilateral, erosive, and ulcerative. When liquids are used, streaking is produced. The patient may show strange or exaggerated behavior or exhibit a curious indifference to the lesions. Lesions may be induced by lye, strong acids, phenol, scissors, knives, manicure tools, a surgical scalpel or hemostat, or sandpaper and other abrasive materials. Figure 12–21 shows a patient with a self-induced eruption caused by burning the dorsum of the hand with cigarettes. At onset, the condition was thought to be porphyria cutanea tarda.

The malingerer often has much to gain and commonly plans the activity with great secrecy and care. Sometimes self-destructive acts follow a bona fide injury. These individuals may be psychotic or prepsychotic and should be handled with the utmost caution. Direct confrontation is ineffective and frequently inadvisable. If possible, psychiatric assistance should be sought.

According to Combes,[7] other types of malingerers include those who (1) conceal information regarding a previous dermatitis or allergic sensitivity at preplacement interviews and examinations, (2) deliberately expose themselves to harm-

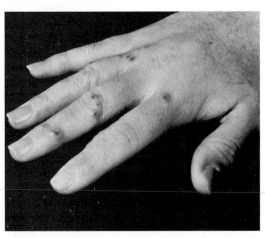

FIGURE 12–20 • Herpes simplex on the hands may superficially resemble contact dermatitis.

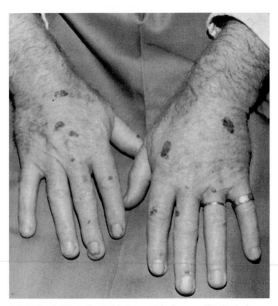

FIGURE 12–21 • Factitial dermatitis from self-inflicted cigarette burns.

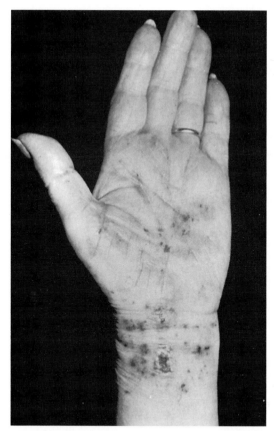

FIGURE 12–22 • This patient had delusions of parasite infection. The "dermatitis" was caused by continual excoriations with the intention to dig out the parasite.

ful chemicals, and (3) flagrantly refuse to facilitate treatment.

Malingerers must not be confused with persons suffering from delusions of parasite infestation. The latter are usually obsessed with the belief that there is "something," usually an insect, residing under the skin, which must be extracted even if painful, unsightly lesions are produced (Fig. 12–22). They may spend hours every day attempting to dig these invisible beasts from their skin, then present the physician with a paper bag or envelope containing minute bits of skin offered as "proof" of the existence of the offending creature. Such patients are extremely refractory to any treatment.

Dermatitis Medicamentosa

Cutaneous reactions to oral and systemic medications assume a wide variety of forms, at times closely resembling other diseases. Dermatitis medicamentosa has been termed today's "great imitator," supplanting syphilis in this regard. Drug eruptions have become much more common and

must be considered in the differential diagnosis of a great many skin diseases.

A fixed drug eruption, particularly if it occurs at a site where contact dermatitis is common, may be confused with occupational dermatitis. This lesion is peculiar in that it occurs repeatedly at the same site following ingestion of the offending drug. Often, multiple lesions are present. It appears soon after administration as a sharply marginated, round or oval edematous plaque of red-violet hue, ranging from 2 to 20 cm in diameter. Itching and burning usually occur, and occasionally the eruption is bullous or hemorrhagic. The lesion disappears in 2 or 3 weeks, usually leaving residual hyperpigmentation. Medications associated with fixed drug eruptions include salicylates, tetracyclines, phenylbutazone, sulfonamides, chloral hydrate, phenolphthalein, reserpine, quinine, phenacetin, barbiturates, and others.[12]

A unique type of dermatitis medicamentosa may be produced by the systemic administration of a drug that has previously caused allergic contact dermatitis (Fig. 12–23). Jadassohn[25] first reported this phenomenon in a young man previously sensitive to a mercury-containing salve

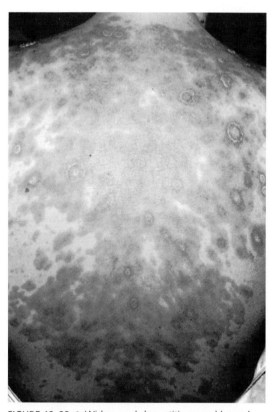

FIGURE 12–23 • Widespread dermatitis caused by oral administration of promethazine (Phenergan), to which the patient had previously been sensitized topically (Phenergan cream).

TABLE 12–4 • "External" Contact Sensitizers and Immunochemically Related Medicaments That Can Produce a Systemic Contact-Type Dermatitis

"External" Contactant	Immunochemically Related Medicaments
Alcohol	Alcoholic beverages
Aminophylline suppositories	Ethylenediamine antihistamines
Ammoniated mercury	Organic and inorganic mercurials, mercury amalgam
Antihistamine eye drops, nosedrops	Ethylenediamine antihistamines
Arnica, tincture of	Elixir terpene hydrate
Balsam of Peru	Tr. benzoin inhalation
Benadryl cream	Benadryl, Dramamine
Benzocaine	*See* para-amino compounds
Bismark brown	*See* para-amino compounds
Disphenol A (epoxy resin component)	Diethylstilbestrol
Caladryl cream, lotion	Benadryl, Dramamine
Chlorobutanol (preservative and local anesthetic)	Chloral hydrate
Chloroquin	Atabrine
Cobalt chloride	Vitamin B_{12}
Epoxy amine hardener, amine type	Ethylenediamine antihistamines, aminophylline
Ethylenediamine hydrochloride	Ethylenediamine antihistamines
Formaldehyde	Urotropin, Mandelamine, Urised, Methenamine
Glyceryl PABA sunscreens	*See* para-amino compounds
Halogenated hydroxyquinolines	Vioform, Dioquin
Hydralazine hydrochloride (industrial exposure)	Isoniazid, Apresoline, Nardil
Iodine	Iodides, iodinated organic compounds
Mercurochrome	Same as mercury
Mercury, metallic, bichloride	Mercurial diuretics, calomel, mercury amalgam fillings
Methylene blue	Phenothiazines
Neomycin sulphate	Streptomycin, kanamycin, framycetin, paromomycin
Orange peel, oil of	Elixir terpene hydrate
Para-amino compounds	Para-aminobenzoic acid (PABA), azo dyes in foods and drugs. Dymelor, Orinase, Diabinese, sulfonamides, Diuril, HydroDIURIL, Saluron, Renese, para-aminosalicylic acid (PAS)
Phenothiazine (insecticide)	Phenergan
Quinilor compound ointment	Vioform
Resorcin	Hexylresorcinol (Crystoids)
Thiram and disulfiram (rubber and insecticide compounds)	Antabuse
Triethylenetetramine (epoxy hardener)	Ethylenediamine antihistamines, aminophylline
Turpentine, cardamon flavor	Elixir terpene hydrate

From Fisher AA. Systemic dermatitis. In: Fisher AA, ed. *Contact Dermatitis*. Philadelphia: Lea & Febiger; 1986:128. Used with permission.

who erupted in a widespread dermatitis following ingestion of calomel. Jadassohn's observations in this case led to his discovery of the diagnostic patch test. Fisher[15] reemphasized the importance of this reaction and listed a number of sensitizers and related drugs that may produce systemic eczematous contact-type dermatitis medicamentosa (Table 12–4).

Dermatitis medicamentosa is not related to an occupation as such but may be induced by administration of drugs provided by the plant dispensary.

Fluorinated topical steroids induce adverse reactions in many persons. Effects include atrophy, striae, purpura, steroid rosacea, perioral dermatitis,

and steroid-induced acne; they also mask the appearance of fungal infections.

References

1. Adams RM, Maibach HI. A five-year study of cosmetic reactions. *J Am Acad Dermatol* 1985; 13:1062–1069.
2. Alexander JOD. Skin eruptions caused by mites from stored food. In: *Arthropods and Human Skin*. Berlin: Springer-Verlag; 1984:345–352.
3. Bandmann HJ, Calnan CD, Cronin E, et al. Dermatitis from applied medicaments. *Arch Dermatol* 1972; 106:335–337.
4. British Photodermatology Group. Workshop report: photopatch testing—methods and indications. *Br J Dermatol* 1997; 136:371–376.

5. Buckley WR. Lichenoid eruptions following contact dermatitis. *Arch Dermatol* 1958; 78:454–457.

6. Cochran REI, Thomson J. Perioral dermatitis: reappraisal. *Clin Exp Dermatol* 1979; 4:75–80.

7. Combes FC. Dermatology problems in establishment of workmen's compensation claims. *Community Med* 1952; 1:5–10.

8. Cotterill JA. Perioral dermatitis. *Br J Dermatol* 1979; 101:259–262.

9. Cowan MA. Nummular eczema: review, follow-up, and analysis of a series of 325 cases. *Acta Derm Venereol (Stockh)* 1961; 41:453–460.

10. Cronin E. Clinical patterns of hand eczema in women. *Contact Dermatitis* 1985; 13:153–161.

11. Dahlquist I, Fregert S, Gruvberger B. Reliability of the chromotropic acid method for qualitative formaldehyde determination. *Contact Dermatitis* 1980; 6:357–358.

12. Derbes VJ. The fixed eruption. *JAMA* 1964; 190:765–766.

13. English JSC, White IR, Cronin E. Sensitivity to sunscreens. *Contact Dermatitis* 1987; 17:159–162.

14. Epstein S. Newer contact sensitizers in the home. In: Rees RB, ed. *Dermatoses Due to Environmental and Physical Factors*. Springfield, Ill.: Charles C Thomas; 1962.

15. Fisher AA. Systemic contact dermatitis. In: Fisher AA, ed. *Contact Dermatitis*. Philadelphia: Lea & Febiger; 1986:119–128.

16. Fisher AA, Adams RM. Occupational dermatitis. In: Fisher AA, ed. *Contact Dermatitis*. Philadelphia: Lea & Febiger; 1986:480–514.

17. Fregert S, Dahlquist I, Gruvberger B. A simple method for the detection of formaldehyde. *Contact Dermatitis* 1984; 10:132–134.

18. Freeman S. Corticosteroid allergy. *Contact Dermatitis* 1995; 33:240–242.

19. Freeman S, Rosen R. Friction as a cause of irritant contact dermatitis. *Am J Contact Dermatitis* 1990; 1:165–170.

20. Hambrick GW Jr, Cox RP, Senior JR. Primary herpes simplex infection of fingers of medical personnel. *Arch Dermatol* 1962; 85:583–589.

21. Hatch KL, Maibach HI. Textile dye dermatitis. *J Am Acad Dermatol* 1985; 12:1079–1092.

22. Hellgren L. Lichen ruber planus in occupational groups in total population. *Berufsdermatosen* 1976; 24:71–78.

23. Hellgren L, Mobacken H. Nummular eczema—clinical and statistical data. *Acta Derm Venereol (Stockh)* 1969; 49:189–196.

24. Hording G. The formaldehyde in textiles. *Acta Derm Venereol (Stockh)* 1959; 39:357.

25. Jadassohn J. Zur Kenntnis der medikamentosen Dermatosen. Graz, Austria: Fifth Congress of the German Academy of Dermatology; 1896.

26. Kanerva L, Susitaival P. Cow dander: the most common cause of occupational contact urticaria in Finland. *Contact Dermatitis* 1996; 35:309.

27. Kersey P, Stevenson CJ. Lichenoid eruption due to colour developer: a new occupational hazard of automatic self-photographing machines. *Contact Dermatitis* 1980; 6:503–504.

28. Kligman AM, Mills OH. Acne cosmetica. *Arch Dermatol* 1972; 106:843–850.

29. Mandel EH. Lichen planus-like eruptions caused by a color film developer. *Arch Dermatol* 1960; 81:516–519.

30. Prystowsky SD, Allen AM, Smith RW, et al. Allergic contact hypersensitivity to nickel, neomycin, ethylenediamine and benzocaine. *Arch Dermatol* 1979; 115:959–962.

31. Rosato FE, Rosato EF, Plotkin SA. Herpetic paronychia: an occupational hazard of medical personnel. *N Engl J Med* 1970; 283:804–805.

32. Schauder S, Schroder W, Geier J. Olaquindox-induced airborne photoallergic contact dermatitis followed by transient or persistent light reactions in 15 pig breeders. *Contact Dermatitis* 1996; 35:344–354.

33. Schwartz L, Tulipan L, Birmingham DJ. *Occupational Diseases of the Skin*. Philadelphia: Lea & Febiger, 1957; 677.

34. Storrs FJ. Dermatitis from clothing and shoes. In: Fisher AA, ed. *Contact Dermatitis*. Philadelphia: Lea & Febiger; 1986:283–337.

35. Turjanmaa K, Reunala T, Rasanen L. Comparison of diagnostic methods in latex surgical glove contact urticaria. *Contact Dermatitis* 1988; 19:241–247.

36. Wilkinson DS, Kirton V, Wilkinson JD. Perioral dermatitis: a 12-year review. *Br J Dermatol* 1979; 101:245–257.

37. Wojnarowska F, Calnan CD. Contact and photocontact allergy to musk ambrette. *Br J Dermatol* 1986; 114:667–675.

Atopy and Atopic Dermatitis

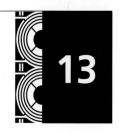

JON M. HANIFIN, M.D.

DEFINING ATOPIC CONDITIONS

Diagnostic Criteria for Atopic Dermatitis

The influence of atopic dermatitis on occupational skin disease is evident from many perspectives, most prominently in the overlap with irritant dermatitis and with atopic hand dermatitis (Fig. 13–1). Most dermatologists make the diagnosis of atopic dermatitis intuitively, with little need for a formalized approach. Diagnostic criteria are used

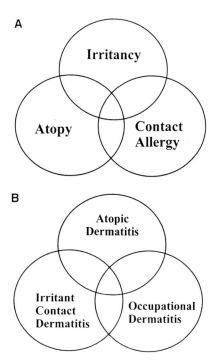

FIGURE 13–1 • These Venn diagrams illustrate the overlap between atopic dermatitis, irritant dermatitis, and occupational eczema.

primarily for research protocols but they can be helpful in distinguishing nummular eczema, mycosis fungoides, allergic contact dermatitis, scabies, seborrheic dermatitis, and even psoriasis, all of which are occasionally misdiagnosed as atopic dermatitis. Such criteria depend upon recognition of a constellation of features, a comprehensive list of which was originally developed to improve communication between disciplines,[1] then expanded during an international symposium,[2] subsequently adapted for children[3] and for practical clinical settings (Table 13–1),[4] and recently shortened and validated for a questionnaire used in epidemiological studies.[5]

The practitioner can usually clarify the diagnosis quite simply by using the major criteria, especially ascertaining current or past flexural involvement and onset in childhood. In the clinic, the most frequently asked ascertainment questions for adults are, "Did you ever have itchy rashes here or here (indicating scratching in the antecubitals and popliteals)?" and "Did you have eczema or food allergies as a child?" The latter is not to imply that food allergies are intrinsic to atopic dermatitis but to recognize its early onset and the practical reality that most pediatricians, allergists, and family practitioners tell children that their eczema is caused by foods. Other questions relate to personal and family history of atopy and are essential to an occupational assessment. Atopy is not required for the diagnosis of atopic dermatitis because at least 20% of patients with typical flexural eczema have neither history of atopy nor evidence of IgE reactivity (increased serum IgE, positive skin tests, or elevated RAST levels).[6] This entity has been called "pure atopic dermatitis," "nonatopic atopic dermatitis," or "intrinsic atopic dermatitis,"[7–9] all less than ideal terms. Tests for IgE reactivity are occasionally helpful in diagnosing atopic dermatitis when the history and signs

TABLE 13–1 • Abbreviated List of Characteristics for Diagnosis of Atopic Dermatitis

Major Features—Four Must Be Present
Pruritus
Early age of onset
Typical morphology and distribution:
  Flexural lichenification and linearity in adults
  Facial and extensor involvement during infancy
    and childhood
Chronic or chronically relapsing dermatitis
Personal or family history of atopy (asthma,
  allergic rhinoconjunctivitis, atopic dermatitis)

Minor or Less Specific Features
Xerosis
Ichthyosis/palmar hyperlinearity/keratosis pilaris
Immediate, type I skin-test response
Hand/foot dermatitis
Cheilitis
Nipple eczema
Susceptibility to cutaneous infection (especially
  S. aureus and herpes simplex)
Perifollicular accentuation

are equivocal, but these tests are very nonspecific and can be considered supportive only. They are quite sensitive, however, as indicators of generic atopy.

Meaning of Atopy

Many allergists consider that a singly positive prick test is a reasonable indicator of atopy.[10] It seems probable that increased irritancy, for example, reactivity to low concentrations of sodium lauryl sulfate (SLS), may become established as a more basic and comprehensive indicator of atopy.[11] Criteria for use of the term *"atopy"* have never been clear. As with atopic dermatitis, the base cause for the imprecise definition is the lack of an objective marker for atopy. The result is widely disparate usage and definition in almost every study mentioning atopy, which leads to meanings that might be *clinical atopy* (e.g., atopic dermatitis, allergic rhinitis, asthma), *subclinical atopy* (e.g., one or more positive immediate skin tests), or even atopic dermatitis itself (all too often dermatologists call atopic dermatitis "atopy").

For many years, the assumption has been that atopy relates only to IgE-mediated mechanisms. A weakness in that assumption has been the fact that many patients with atopic dermatitis, and probably asthma too, have normal serum IgE levels and no evidence of IgE-mediated reactivity. One study suggests that the presence of clinical

atopy reflects a state of cellular hyperreactivity that, in turn, represents irritancy and increased susceptibility to develop occupational dermatitis.[11] Whether subclinical atopy also confers this susceptibility remains to be determined, but we might speculate that it would. Obviously, a comprehensive biochemical or genetic marker for atopy would greatly aid research in this field but is not feasible at present.

Until there is a reliable marker for atopy, reports should include clear definitions. For this review of atopy and occupational skin disease, we will use the following definitions.

Atopy: a genetically predisposed tendency to react to certain environmental stimuli (e.g., irritants, allergens, pharmacological agents) with exaggerated responses such as bronchial constriction, IgE production, inflammation, vasodilatation, and pruritus. Note that although some authors have considered atopy synonymous with "allergy,"[12] the latter is a very imprecise term and should not be used unless referring to a specific clinical expression of an allergic response.[10] Many authors accept allergen skin-test reactivity as a definition of atopy,[13–15] but it is preferable to consider positive skin tests as one of several manifestations of subclinical atopy.

Subclinical atopy: one or more positive immediate skin tests, often in the setting of a family history of atopy, dry or "sensitive" skin, and airways reactivity, but no overt clinical disease.

Clinical atopy: current or previous well-documented atopic dermatitis, allergic rhinitis, or asthma.

Atopy and Occupational Fitness

It is crucial to understand that the interactions of individuals with their occupational environments are subject to all the variables that result from complex biological systems. No physician or researcher, no matter how astute, can accurately predict which atopic person will be susceptible to occupational injury. This would hold true even if we had precise genetic or biochemical markers for atopy. Efforts to stigmatize workers because of atopic sensitivity violate their personal rights, and physicians can do great harm to life and health by applying theoretical predictions to fitness assessments that might ban people from certain jobs. We can only advise patients in general terms; job choices should be made by well-informed patients who best know their personal limitations and abilities.

PREVALENCE

What is known of the prevalence of atopy? Because atopy is even less well-defined than atopic dermatitis, any attempt at estimating prevalence is hopelessly imprecise and varies greatly with the age group studied. Detection of atopy (except for atopic dermatitis) is always lowest in children. In this discussion of occupational effects, adults are the relevant group. For example, Carr and colleagues, in 1964, estimated a "true incidence of atopy" of 20%,[12] although they included recurrent urticaria, a condition that appears to affect atopics and nonatopics indiscriminately. In 1981, Taylor and colleagues found a prevalence of 33% symptomatic atopy among New Zealand medical students.[16] This seems to be a reasonable estimate, and it is accepted by allergists and epidemiologists.[17] There is also wide acceptance that atopy prevalence is increasing, as is atopic dermatitis specifically.[13, 17, 18]

Regarding atopic dermatitis specifically, Schultz-Larsen and coworkers demonstrated a cumulative incidence of 10% in children in Denmark.[19] He also suggested a rising incidence, and others have confirmed this trend in countries around the world.[13, 20–22] The implications of increasing atopy for the field of occupational medicine are potentially great, although only theoretical at present. Whether the incidence of dermatitis in workers will ascend in parallel with atopy is at present only speculative. This is an important area in need of well-designed prospective studies and efforts in prevention. Occupational choices for patients with atopic dermatitis (and, perhaps, atopy) appear to be major determinants in the natural course of their disease.

Prognosis of Atopic Dermatitis

Attempts at prognostication for atopic dermatitis require an understanding of the usual course of that disease. Atopic dermatitis is occasionally present at birth but generally does not appear until 6 to 8 weeks of age when coordinated motor activity begins. This indicates the important role that scratching, rubbing, and irritation play in the disease, although it is wrong to assume that the inflammation appears only when the skin is traumatized. It is useful to understand that atopic inflammatory cells are hyperreactive and that any physical or chemical insult from the environment causes exaggerated release of a whole range of inflammatory mediators.[23] The biochemical defect that causes this hyperreactivity is present in cord blood mononuclear leukocytes of atopic infants,[24] and this abnormality appears to persist through life. Typically, young infants are affected primarily on areas that can be rubbed against bedding and carpets, especially the face and the extensors of the extremities. Rajka showed that the onset of

atopic dermatitis occurred within the first year in 57% of 1,200 persons with atopic dermatitis, and by age 5, 87% had developed the disease.[6] Fewer than 2% had onset after age 20, an important diagnostic point, as late onset should alert physicians to the possibility of other conditions such as contact dermatitis or cutaneous lymphoma.

Longstanding uncertainty has surrounded the question of whether "infantile eczema" is the same entity seen in older children and adults. Longitudinal observations clearly demonstrate that the disease is the same and that the early extensor involvement gives way to the diagnostically important flexural lichenification and linearity that is the hallmark of atopic dermatitis at some point in its course. During the adult years, the stigmata of atopic dermatitis may be very subtle, with only mild dermatitis present in one or two localized areas, most commonly the hands and fingertips but also involving the nipples, face, eyelids, nuchal scalp, and ankles. At times, only dry skin is evident and many of these signs are indistinct except to the trained observer or during the winter months when low indoor humidity accentuates the typical tendency toward symptomatic dry skin.

Most studies of long-term prognosis have depended on retrospective recall surveys, using letters sent to patients previously seen during childhood in the dermatology department; replies were never in high proportion to the questionnaires sent. The data are difficult to interpret, but Purdy concluded that 68% of patients with infantile eczema had developed asthma, hay fever, or atopic dermatitis, alone or in combination, and that only 21% of those retained skin sequelae.[25] A home-visit study in England suggested that eczema was still present in 55% of patients by age 13, whereas the skin had cleared by age 3 in 27% of patients.[26] Meenan in 1959 reported a postal survey of 42 children previously hospitalized for severe infantile eczema, and results show that roughly 30% of the cases had residual eczema.[27]

Roth and Kierland reviewed case records of 492 consecutive patients seen for atopic dermatitis at the Mayo Clinic between 1940 and 1942.[28] Cases were grouped into mild and severe categories; the median age for clearing in both groups was 21 years. Approximately 60% of the mild group and 70% of the severe group retained some stigmata of atopic dermatitis. As with other surveys, however, only 45% of the 492 patients responded to the survey, raising some concern about whether patients no longer affected were less inclined to reply. However, a survey by Musgrove and Morgan in England[29] as well as other studies in Belgium[30] and Germany[31] have shown persistence of eczema features in 50 to 60% of cases, so the weight of evidence suggests that these estimates are roughly reliable.

Occupational Impact of Atopic Dermatitis

Perhaps the greatest social effect of atopic dermatitis is its role in predisposing to occupational dermatitis and, conversely, occupational injury is a major determinant of persistence of atopic dermatitis. For many years, atopic dermatitis has been a disqualifying condition for individuals entering military service in the United States. A number of studies have shown the frequent background of atopy among populations with atopic dermatitis. All are in close agreement that a large proportion of patients or compensable work-related cases have a relationship to atopy. Glickman and Silvers[32] in 1967 were perhaps the first to report this association. They questioned 50 housewives with hand eczema for the presence of atopy, as compared to a matched control group without dermatitis. Their data showed evidence of atopy in 85% of the patients with hand eczema. Again, definitions were imprecise and this figure may have been somewhat inflated by the inclusion of urticaria as an atopic condition, but the presence of atopy in 28% of the normal control group fits with the prevalence in the normal population.[12]

MECHANISMS OF ATOPIC PREDISPOSITION TO OCCUPATIONAL INJURY

Many biological factors contribute to occupational injury in atopy and atopic dermatitis (Table 13–2). Most of the factors listed in the table have considerable overlap and the sum of those influences establishes the biological milieu that represents atopic susceptibility. Atopy appears to be a genetically conferred condition in which the hyperreactivity of inflammatory and immune cells causes exaggerated responses to a panoply of stimuli.[23]

 TABLE 13–2 • Biological Determinants Predisposing to Occupational Injury in Atopic Dermatitis

Inflammatory cell hyperreactivity
Keratinocyte cytokines
Cutaneous irritancy
IgE-mediated reactions
Defective stratum corneum barrier

Irritants, bacteria, allergens, heat, and ultraviolet light can initiate the inflammation that leads to pruritus and to the epidermal hyperproliferation that causes the defective stratum corneum barrier that characterizes atopic dermatitis. This combination of defects helps to explain the well-demonstrated increase in transepidermal water loss and irritancy in atopic dermatitis.[33] Interestingly, irritant responses appear to be increased also in patients with allergic respiratory disease, even when there is no history of dermatitis.[11] This supports the concept that hyperirritability is not primary in epidermal cells because even in respiratory atopy, the circulating leukocytes are abnormally active.

Leukocyte hyperreactivity appears linked to inadequate control of cyclic AMP, a defect caused by overly active cyclic AMP phosphodiesterase enzymes, that results in hyperfunctional responses.[23] These include increased release of cytokines,[34, 35] prostaglandins,[36] histamine,[37, 38] and IgE.[39] The hyperreactivity of cells infiltrating atopic skin lowers the threshold to all manner of physical and chemical insults encountered in the workplace. The concept of leukocyte abnormalities underlying the features of atopy is supported by multiple reports of transferral of atopic dermatitis, and even antigenically specific allergies, by bone marrow transplantation.[40]

The basic defects in immune responses and inflammatory control manifest as a number of clinical features predisposing to occupational illness. The xerotic, defective stratum corneum barrier allows penetration of chemicals, ranging from small haptens to large proteins. This, combined with the exaggerated production of allergen-specific IgE antibodies, accounts for the high proportion of individuals with atopic dermatitis who develop contact urticaria to animals, foods, and latex. The impaired barrier may also explain the surprisingly frequent occurrence of allergic contact dermatitis in atopic dermatitis.[41] Whether the defective immunological control mechanisms associated with atopy enhance contact allergy, including aeroallergen contact hypersensitivity, is unknown at the present time.[42] Some investigators believe that atopic dermatitis is an antigen-induced reaction pattern composed of an early Th2 response, followed by a chronic Th1-mediated second phase.[43] At present, the relevance of these putative reactions to occupational dermatitis is unclear.

In addition to inflammatory cell hyperreactivity, one report has demonstrated overproduction of granulocyte macrophage colony stimulating factor (GM-CSF) by keratinocytes from nonlesional skin of patients with atopic dermatitis.[44] This cytokine appears to have an important role in regulating the function of epidermal dendritic cells, in recruiting and activating eosinophils, monocytes, and basophils, and in enhancing the proliferation of keratinocytes. Thus, the impaired epidermal permeability barrier in atopic dermatitis may be causally linked to increased keratinocyte cytokine production induced by acute epidermal injury.[33, 45–47]

These studies point up the need for expanded basic studies of irritancy in atopic dermatitis, a disease in which disproportionate attention has focused on immunological studies. Whether the abnormality is primary in atopic keratinocytes or the result of in situ influences of defective, infiltrating, marrow-derived cells, including Langerhans cells, remains to be established. It is difficult to dismiss the demonstrations of atopy transmission from marrow transplants[40] unless the marrow-derived cells required a coexisting defect in recipient epithelial cells, a situation that seems unlikely. Regardless of primacy, newer studies agree in concept that the skin and respiratory tissues of atopic individuals are primed to overreact to any of the multitude of stimuli encountered in the workplace.

ENVIRONMENTAL FACTORS

Irritants and Nonspecific Aggravants

Trigger factors for atopic dermatitis are well recognized, and avoidance of these exacerbants is a mainstay of standard dermatological management and prevention. In the workplace, the list of such factors is lengthy (Table 13–3). Heat can cause increased itching, both by initiating sweating and, in 10% of patients, by stimulating cholinergic urticaria. Humidity adds to the sweating and is cited by many patients as an aggravating condition, though for some, high humidity allows reparation of dry, brittle stratum corneum and remission of atopic dermatitis. This is likely to account for the fact that many patients clear completely when they travel to tropical regions.[21, 48] Conversely, working in low-humidity conditions in winter and at high altitudes can trigger relapses of atopic dermatitis or even initiate it in people who grew up in humid regions. This situation probably accounts for the atypical, and often diagnostically challenging, late-onset atopic dermatitis.

Irritants are the most obvious and the most common category of occupational aggravants for atopic individuals. The list of direct chemical irritants is essentially endless and needs little explanation. Most of the irritant effects are on hands, and a particularly notorious category is that of wet-work occupations, which will be discussed further in the section on hand eczema. Hands are the most prominent target, but certainly airborne chemicals (e.g., detergents, disinfectant sprays, and acid washes) can occasionally affect other exposed and unexposed skin regions, especially if protective clothing is inadequate. Physical irritants can also affect widespread body areas, especially fiberglass insulation, coarse woolen fabrics, and stiff or occlusive garments.

Dusty, dirty, and unhygienic working conditions are frequently cited by patients as contributory to the worsening of atopic dermatitis. These are highly individualized situations and must be evaluated on merit, but they can lead to both localized and widespread dermatitis and such conditions are best avoided, if possible, by the at-risk person. Plant irritants are an uncommon cause of problems in atopic patients. Emotional stress is one of the few triggers that has been demonstrated under controlled, experimental conditions,[49] and those reports are supported by clinical observations. Patients with atopic dermatitis have pruritus and scratching when confronted with emotionally uncomfortable situations. Onset is rapid, for example, during a stressful interview, and may regress just as rapidly, but it may initiate more chronic involvement as well. Most patients experience this emotional triggering phenomenon but its relevance to harmful occupational outcomes is probably uncommon.

Contact Urticaria

Contact urticaria encompasses both immunological (allergic, IgE-mediated) and nonimmunological (pharmacological) forms.[50] Both merge in the triggering of mast cell histamine release as the final effector pathway. Nonimmunological contact urticaria (NICU) is probably not highly germane to a discussion of occupational disease in atopics, so this section focuses primarily upon allergic problems encountered most commonly among food handlers, animal workers, and people work-

---

TABLE 13–3 • Occupational Factors that Aggravate Atopic Dermatitis

Heat	Animals
High humidity	Food handling
Low humidity	Latex exposure
Wet-work	Phytoirritants
Chemical irritants	Contact allergens
Physical irritants (e.g., wool and fiberglass)	Emotional stress
	Sunlight
Dirty conditions	Molds
Dust	

ing with latex products, especially in the health professions.[50–52] The atopic diathesis is a major factor in the development of hypersensitivity to all three categories of these contact allergens. This occurs because of the porous epidermal barrier that easily allows ingress of large-molecular-weight protein antigens and because of the propensity of atopic individuals to overproduce protein-specific IgE antibodies.

When latex or other protein allergens cross the clinical threshold (Table 13–4), patients usually present with concerns about worsening hand dermatitis. Prior to this clinical presentation, the dermatitis may be very subtle, with barely perceptible itch, erythema, and papulation or mild eczematous scaling.[50] After repeated exposure, symptoms become more troublesome and begin to require therapy. This progression may be so slow that the gloves or other allergens are not recognized as the cause of the dermatitis, and the source may be recognized only when the sensitivity progresses to the pont of immediacy, with itching, wheals, and edema. Other common presentations include eyelid dermatitis, edema, and eczematous changes over the face. When symptoms and signs are subtle and fleeting, the physician is apt to dismiss the occupational association. Realization that the patient is atopic and in contact with protein antigens can prevent serious progression from contact urticaria to anaphylactic responses.

Allergic Contact Dermatitis

Allergic contact dermatitis, especially when covert and masquerading as atopic dermatitis, is a very damaging condition. Recognition of it can have profound benefits, and misdiagnosis can be disastrous. A case illustrative of this trap was provided by a 47-year-old photographer with life-long atopic dermatitis. The eczema progressively worsened during adulthood, eventually requiring systemic corticosteroids to prevent disability. Alternate-day corticosteroid tablets were continued

TABLE 13–4 • Clinical Presentations of Occupational Contact Urticaria
Hand eczema
Facial dermatitis
Eyelid dermatitis
Genital itching/dermatitis
Erythematous papulation
Immediate urtication
Mucosal edema
Angioedema
Anaphylaxis

TABLE 13–5 • Combined Allergic Contact and Atopic Dermatitis
Coexistence is common.
The frequency of hybrids may be increasing.
Adult worsening of atopic dermatitis suggests possible allergic contact dermatitis.
Recalcitrant or steroid-dependent atopic dermatitis may be allergic contact dermatitis.
Patch-testing is difficult but often advisable.

for 15 years, until the patient was diagnosed with steroid-induced premature cataracts and osteopenia. He was referred for management suggestions, and patch testing revealed contact allergy to the highly relevant workplace chemicals, color developer #3 and chromate. When the photographer avoided the darkroom, the dermatitis subsided completely, revealing that there was no residual atopic dermatitis.

Several points about combined atopic and allergic contact dermatitis should be continually reemphasized (Table 13–5): (1) They do coexist, and the frequency of coexistence appears to be increasing.[41, 50, 53–56] (2) We should always consider allergic contact dermatitis when adults present with worsening atopic dermatitis. (3) Patch testing should be done more often in patients with atopic dermatitis, especially those with recalcitrant manifestations and particularly when systemic corticosteroid therapy is contemplated. (4) We should recognize that patch testing is difficult (see Prevention and Management). (5) Finally, the dermatologist must keep in perspective the oft-quoted studies showing altered cell-mediated immunity in atopic dermatitis.[1]

Reduced Cellular Immunity: a Paradox

Several studies have shown reduced contact allergy responses in subjects with atopic dermatitis.[1, 57–59] Early clinical observations led to in vitro studies that demonstrated T-cell abnormalities and formed the basis for many subsequent immunological investigations.[60–62] Later, one report suggested that reduced dinitrochlorobenzene (DNCB) sensitization may be significant only in severe, active atopic dermatitis,[63] but Rees et al.[59] demonstrated, using more sensitive methods, that reduced responsiveness was a general characteristic of atopic dermatitis. This is paradoxical because although the rate of experimentally induced contact allergy is diminished in subjects with atopic dermatitis,[57–59] multiple studies have shown that atopic individuals often have allergic contact dermatitis, presumably due to chronic, repeated induction.[41, 56]

There are other facets in the paradox. In long-term studies of atopic dermatitis, we have been impressed with the difficulty in finding control subjects with widespread allergic contact dermatitis who are clearly not atopic. Very few such people can be identified. Additionally, a significant proportion of patients referred to patch-test clinics for suspected contact dermatitis have the atopic diathesis. We carried out a study of the relationship between allergic contact dermatitis and atopy in that population and confirmed our impressions that a majority of patients with atopy had patch-test–proven allergic contact dermatitis, and over half of patients with allergic contact dermatitis were clinically atopic.[54] Also, atopic subjects averaged significantly more positive patch tests than did nonatopics.[54] We conclude that although cutaneous cellular immune responsiveness is diminished in atopic dermatitis, most patients can become sensitized with repeated, prolonged exposure to antigens.

HAND ECZEMA

Hand eczema is a very frequent accompaniment of atopic dermatitis. Agrup's studies showed that 70% of patients had hand involvement at some point.[64] Experience tells us that the clinical features and natural course of hand eczema in atopic dermatitis reflect all the characteristics of the generalized condition. Hand eczema is common in children, usually affecting dorsal surfaces, yet seemingly not irritant-induced in this young population. This may be a reflection of the constitutional or endogenous nature of the basic disease prior to the advent of exogenous aggravating factors.

A very helpful sign, at all ages, is volar wrist involvement, which is typical.[64] Vesiculation, particularly along the sides of the fingers, is common and, at times, along with the consequent fissuring, may involve finger pads and palms. Hand eczema may persist throughout life, although more usually it is remittent, reappearing sometimes after many years of quiescence. Most patients are well aware of their susceptibility to irritant insults and live on the margin of clinical dermatitis with winter chapping, paronychial scaling, and other daily reminders of the need for moisturizers.

The previous description roughly represents the natural course of atopic hand problems, but there can be no precise signs that distinguish this eczema from pompholyx/dyshidrosis, dermatophytids, or even allergic contact dermatitis. The volar wrist involvement, present or past, is helpful, as is early onset, past flexural eczema, atopic background, and irritant susceptibility during remissions (Table 13–6).

The most important clinical distinction for the physician is to suspect atopic diathesis in patients who otherwise might simply be relegated to the diagnostic scrap heap of "irritant dermatitis" because the presentation is predominantly dorsal, dry, and lichenified. Suspecting atopy gives a much clearer perspective, not only for recognizing irritant problems but also for considering possible contact urticaria as a causative factor. Occupational hand eczema in atopics results from endogenous predisposing influences that create a lower threshold for chemical and physical aggravators. The endogenous factors include hyperreactive cells producing inflammatory mediators, immune cells overproducing IgE, and hyperproliferative epidermal cells producing an inadequate stratum corneum barrier. All of these factors combine to promote development of occupational dermatitis, and multiple clinical and epidemiological studies have documented this propensity.

Investigations of Hand Eczema in Atopic Individuals

Prior to 1980, relatively little attention was paid to the association of atopy and occupational hand eczema. In 1967, Glickman and Silvers[32] reported that approximately 80% of housewives with hand eczema were atopic and it is interesting that this estimate coincided with subsequent studies.[65–67] Since 1980, many other studies have considered the contribution of atopy to work-related hand eczema,[65–69] including Scandinavian thesis dissertations that provided in-depth research into the problems associated with atopy.[65, 70, 71] These studies agree that hand eczema is significantly more prevalent in patients with atopy and atopic dermatitis than it is in nonatopics. The degree of these

 TABLE 13–6 • Features Suggestive of Atopic Dermatitis in Patients with Hand Eczema

Predominantly dorsal hand involvement
Past or present volar wrist involvement
Early age of onset
Chronically recurring
History of flexural eczema
Atopic background
History of contact urticaria
Chronic dryness
Irritant susceptibility

differences varies greatly, from one study to the next (estimates range from twofold to tenfold), in great part because of the varied definitions, methods of data collection, and levels of atopic severity.[68-70, 72]

Rystedt's studies have been particularly informative.[65, 68, 72, 73] She followed 955 patients who had been treated for atopic dermatitis during childhood, either as inpatients or as outpatients. Those with the more persistent and severe atopic dermatitis, and especially those with childhood hand eczema, were most prone to have problems as adults. Compared with nonatopics, those with childhood atopic dermatitis had more severe and more frequent recurrences of hand eczema. These patients tended to have more physician visits and work absences as well.[65, 72] Associated respiratory allergy also increased the frequency of hand eczema.

Occupational Factors

There is good concordance among studies indicating that certain types of work cause higher frequencies of hand eczema in persons with atopic dermatitis.[65-70] Almost all have identified the common factor of wet-work exposure such as in hospital employees, especially nurses, and in kitchen assistants, cleaners, domestics, hairdressers, and food handlers.[68-71, 74] The latter may reflect the tendency of atopic individuals to develop IgE-mediated contact urticaria to protein allergens.[51] It should be noted that the above exposures tend to parallel those of women in the home and that home exposures probably add to the occupational insults in many cases. Rystedt noted a correlation between household irritant exposure and hand eczema that was independent of occupational risk,[68] and studies have shown that the incidence of hand eczema in mothers increases with greater numbers of children and with younger children.[68, 69]

The presence of atopy in general appears to strongly influence development of occupational illness.[32, 66, 67] A striking proportion of work-related conditions, predominantly hand eczema, occurs in atopic persons. However, atopic dermatitis does not invariably confer occupational illness on workers, and one-fourth of those atopic individuals never experience problems, even in situations of high irritant exposure.[68, 69]

PREVENTION AND MANAGEMENT OF OCCUPATIONAL SKIN DISEASE IN ATOPIC INDIVIDUALS

Avoidance

Obviously, protection from environmental exacerbants is the key management goal for any patient with occupational dermatitis. The presence of atopy and especially of atopic dermatitis alters the threshold of tolerability and adds extra layers of complexity because both irritancy and contact urticaria reactivity are increased in such individuals. The workplace is designed for people with normal levels of sensitivity so the atopic person may need to take extra measures to protect against one or more factors that might trigger dermatitis. Even materials meant to help can be an unexpected liability, for example, skin cleansers that are too harsh and occlusive or stiff protective clothing.

Skin Protection

Whether problems relate to irritants, contact allergens, or contact urticants, the first line of defense is an intact stratum corneum barrier. Use of moisturizers to protect from evaporative damage is the single most important preventive and therapeutic measure we can advise. Moisturizers must be readily available to the worker in all areas of the workplace. They must be effective and, for people with atopic dermatitis, that means no lotions. Petrolatum or cream bases are essential, and frequent application must be constantly encouraged. Preparations promoted as "barriers" have not been demonstrated to provide any advantage; in fact, they may instill a false sense of security and undermine proper moisturizing. Gloves can be both good and bad. Latex is never a first choice because of the high rate of sensitization among atopics. Any occlusive glove causes wetting, thus moisturizing is required immediately when gloves are removed.

Problems with Patch-testing the Atopic

A crucial aspect of avoiding contact allergens is identifying those that are causing problems, and patch-testing is often required for that diagnosis. Patch-testing in patients with atopic dermatitis is difficult; the tape sticks poorly, adhesives irritate the skin, "angry back" phenomenon often occurs, allergic responses can be slow-arising, and true contact allergy is difficult to distinguish from the frequent irritant reactions. We must constantly remind other physicians, as well as insurers, that effective and optimal patch-testing of these patients may require hospitalization, a maneuver that is clearly justified in many cases to prevent corticosteroid toxicity.

Diagnostic patch-testing on patients with atopic dermatitis is beset by many obstacles, especially in the outpatient setting (Table 13–7). It may be

TABLE 13–7 • Problems Encountered in Patch-Testing Patients with Atopic Dermatitis

Finding an uninflamed, adequate area on the back for testing

Deciding which antigens to test

Keeping patch tests in place for sufficient time to allow early (two-day) readings

Keeping test sites marked for 2- to 5-day readings

Hyperirritability ("angry back" syndrome)

Ambiguous reactions including:

Irritant
- Rapid onset, usually within 24 hours
- Well demarcated
- Confined to exact test site
- Smooth, glazed, or cracked surface with slight erythema
- Develops in most subjects

Allergen
- Delayed onset, 48 to 96 hours
- Indistinct margins
- Reaction that spreads beyond test site
- Induration, papulation, and vesiculation
- Affects only a few, sensitized subjects

---

impossible to find an adequate area on the back for patch-testing because uninflamed skin is required. Sometimes application of topical steroids may reduce the inflammation enough to make patch-testing feasible; however, because immunosuppression is undesirable, the test site is best kept free of topical steroid medications for at least 48 hours prior to patch application. Ideally, systemic corticosteroids should be discontinued at least 1 week prior to patch-test readings. Patch tests are difficult to keep in place because tape almost never sticks well, as atopic dermatitis patients have very scaly skin, and their skin is often saturated with lipid moisturizers. The back should be bathed with lavish use of mild soap or detergent and then tested 1 hour later. Patch-test application can be reinforced by preparing the skin with tincture of benzoin or Mastisol. Patients should be warned that they will have itching associated with the patches but that the patches should be kept in place or the whole process must be repeated. Sedating antihistamines can be used for itching and sleep.

Exposing patients with atopic dermatitis to a wide range of antigens is another problem. Sometimes one or a few highly suspect antigens may be tested but usually a large array should be screened because there may not be an easy second chance. Materials used at work present a special problem when patch-testing atopics because of irritancy

characteristics. Occupational materials, although more likely to be irritants to the patient with atopic dermatitis, may be contact allergens, as may rubber, especially in gloves and shoes. It may be as important to the worker's well-being to identify products used at home as to rule out job-related products. An important group would include skin-care products used by the patient or the patient's partner, as well as topical medications, including corticosteroids. We use the North American Contact Dermatitis Group tray,[75] supplemented with other preservatives and materials commonly present in skin-care products. The TRUE Test is not recommended because its reliability in testing patients with atopic dermatitis has not been established.

Intrinsic to atopic dermatitis is the concern about skin hyperirritability,[76] which requires that the general level of dermatitis be stable and well-controlled throughout the patch-test process. For that reason, it is best to hospitalize these patients for the two-day patch applications. Even in the best-controlled situations, some patients flare completely or partially over the patch test area, making it necessary to reapply the patches at a later date.

Ambiguous reactions are often noted, especially on the skin of atopic dermatitis patients, even by examiners with extensive experience. We use as guidelines the characteristics of irritant responses and allergic responses listed in Table 13–7. A given test or group of tests should be repeated if allergic positivity or relevancy is questionable. If multiple irritant reactions are noted, the test must be repeated at a later date. When a patch-test site has all the characteristics of allergic contact dermatitis and they persist at least 72 to 96 hours, allergy to that material is indicated, if clinically relevant. Relevancy is not considered conclusive unless avoidance of the material leads to clearing and reexposure reproduces the clinical disease.

A diagnosis of relevant allergic contact dermatitis can provide a cure for the disease if the patient discontinues exposure to that allergen. Patients must be informed and encouraged always to read the chemical constituents of products they use, both in the workplace and at home if they develop allergies to ingredients in skin-care products. The simplest, least chemically adorned preparations are always preferable. This is especially true of workplace cleansers and other products that may contain allergens and irritants.

Immediate Contact Testing

Testing for contact urticaria is generally much easier than testing for allergic contact dermatitis because onset of reactions is rapid, and relevancy testing is much more precise. Diagnosis is confirmed by demonstrating reactions ranging from erythema to faint papulation to frank urtication when the allergen is rubbed on the skin or applied under nonocclusive adhesive for 5 to 30 minutes. This direct test is preferred because it readily reproduces the lesion, although false negatives are common. Skin-prick tests of the material can also be helpful but may be overly sensitive, causing false positives. Positive RAST, as with prick-testing, is diagnostic only if accompanied by a relevant history of reproducible lesions or itching with exposure to a substance.[54] It is important to realize that a combination of allergic contact dermatitis and contact urticaria in response to latex gloves is not uncommon, so 48-hour patch-testing should be done in parallel with contact urticaria testing.[77] Caution should be used in epicutaneous testing of patients who have a history of anaphylactoid reactions to latex; in such cases, RAST confirmation is sufficient to make a diagnosis.

Job Change

A change of job may be warranted in any situation in which relevant irritancy or allergy is temporally associated with occupational exposure. This is especially true when a trial of avoidance causes improvement and reintroduction consistently worsens the dermatitis. Rystedt's studies indicate that people with atopic dermatitis often make changes, especially to avoid wet-work.[78] She notes, however, that the healing rate after job change is lower among atopics, probably because the constitutional factors remain; so it is not appropriate to make any guarantees to such patients, and aggressive skin care is also essential. Although the rate of complete *healing* may be only 20%, *improvement* is expected and can convert a disabling situation into a productive vocational experience.

Job Counseling

Every child with atopic dermatitis should be made aware of risk factors associated with certain vocational choices. Rystedt has suggested that high- and low-risk individuals can be distinguished, in many cases, by identifying key characteristics: (1) presence of childhood hand eczema, (2) persistent atopic dermatitis in adulthood, and (3) chronic dry, itchy skin. The presence of all three would indicate high risk. In a group of such high-risk atopics, 90% had at some point developed hand eczema as adults when performing wet-work jobs, compared to only 13% for those without any risk factors.[65] Occupations considered especially risky

for susceptible atopics include ladies' hairdressing, food handling and other kitchen work, nursing, domestic work, and industrial work involving solvents and oils.

Vocational guidance should be provided not only for adolescents planning career choices but also for adults considering career or job changes. People with atopic dermatitis should be given a list to review, such as the one shown in Table 13–3. Those with eczema persisting past childhood should avoid hot, humid working conditions. Restrictions would be less stringent for people who have had remissions of atopic dermatitis, but high-risk jobs are still best avoided. For those with atopy but no eczematous history, job avoidance is not indicated unless symptoms are developing from exposure to latex, food, or animals. Continued exposure to such antigenic proteins carries the danger of progressive sensitization, with the risk of not only contact urticaria but also asthma and anaphylaxis; in an extreme case, this may occur even when the person enters a room containing airborne allergens.

References

1. Hanifin JM, Lobitz WC. Newer concepts of atopic dermatitis. *Arch Dermatol* 1977;113:663–670.
2. Hanifin JM, Rajka G. Diagnostic features of atopic dermatitis. *Acta Derm Venereol Suppl (Stockh)* 1980;92:44–47.
3. Hanifin JM. Atopic dermatitis in infants and children: pediatric dermatology. *Pediatr Clin North Am* 1991; 38:763–789.
4. Hanifin JM. Atopic dermatitis. In: Moschella SL, Hurley HJ, eds. *Dermatology*, 3rd ed. Philadelphia: W.B. Saunders; 1992:441–464.
5. Williams HC. Atopic dermatitis: new information from epidemiological studies. *Br J Hosp Med* 1994;52:409–412.
6. Rajka G. *Atopic Dermatitis*. London: W.B. Saunders; 1975.
7. Ohman S, Johansson SGO. Immunoglobulins in atopic dermatitis. *Acta Derm Venereol Suppl (Stockh)* 1974; 54:193.
8. Jones HE, Inouye JC, McGerity JL, et al. Atopic disease and serum immunoglobulin-E. *Br J Dermatol* 1975;92:17–25.
9. Wüthrich B. Atopic dermatitis flare provoked by inhalant allergens. *Dermatologica* 1989;178:51–53.
10. Nelson HS. The atopic diseases. *Ann Allergy* 1985;55:441–447.
11. Nassif A, Chan SC, Storrs FJ, Hanifin JM. Abnormal skin irritancy in atopic dermatitis and in atopy without dermatitis. *Arch Dermatol* 1994;130:1402–1407.
12. Carr DR, Berke M, Becker SW. Incidence of atopy in the general population. *Arch Dermatol* 1964;89:87–92.
13. Williams HC. Is the prevalence of atopic dermatitis increasing? *Clin Exp Dermatol* 1992;17:385–391.
14. Barbee R, Kaltenborn W, Lebowitz MD, Burrows B. Longitudinal changes in allergen skin test reactivity in a community population sample. *J Allergy Clin Immunol* 1987;79:16–24.
15. Sibbald B. Genetic basis of asthma. *Semin Respir Med* 1986;7:307–315.

16. Taylor B, Broom BC. Atopy in medical students. *Ann Allergy* 1981;47:197–199.

17. Shirakawa T, Enomoto T, Shimazu S-I, Hopkin JM. The inverse association between tuberculin responses and atopic disorder. *Science* 1997;275:77–79.

18. Strachan DP. Hay fever, hygiene, and household size. *Br Med J* 1989;299:1259–1260.

19. Schultz-Larsen F, Diepgen T, Svensson A. The occurrence of atopic dermatitis in north Europe: an international questionnaire study. *J Am Acad Dermatol* 1996;34:760–764.

20. Taylor B, Wadsworth M, Wadsworth J, Peckham C. Changes in the reported prevalence of childhood eczema since the 1939–45 war. *Lancet* 1984;ii:1255–1258.

21. Hanifin JM. Epidemiology of atopic dermatitis. In: Schlumberger H, ed. *Monographs in Allergy/Epidemiology of Allergic Diseases.* Basel: S. Karger; 1987:116–131.

22. Diepgen TL, Blettner M. Analysis of familial aggregation of atopic eczema and other atopic diseases by odds ratio regression models. J Invest Dermatol 1996;106:977–981.

23. Hanifin JM, Chan SC: Monocyte phosphodiesterase abnormalities and dysregulation of lymphocyte function in atopic dermatitis. *J Invest Dermatol* 1995;105:84S–88S.

24. Heskel NS, Chan SC, Thiel ML, Stevens SR, Casperson LS, Hanifin JM. Elevated umbilical cord blood leukocyte cyclic adenosine monophosphate-phosphodiesterase activity in children with atopic parents. *J Am Acad Dermatol* 1984;11:422–426.

25. Purdy MJ. The long-term prognosis in infantile eczema. *Br Med J* 1953;1:1366.

26. Vowles M, Warin RP, Apley J. Infantile eczema: observations on natural history and prognosis. *Br J Dermat* 1955;67:53–59.

27. Meenan FOC. Prognosis in infantile eczema. *Irish J Med Sci* 1959;28:79–83.

28. Roth HL, Kierland RR. The natural history of atopic dermatitis. *Arch Dermatol* 1964;89:209–214.

29. Musgrove K, Morgan JK. Infantile eczema *Br J Dermatol* 1976;95:365–372.

30. Van Hecke E, Leys G. Evolution of atopic dermatitis. *Dermatologica* 1981;163:370–375.

31. Wüthrich B, Schudel P. Atopic dermatitis after the childhood phase. *A Hautkr* 1982;58:1012–1023.

32. Glickman FS, Silvers SH. Hand eczema and atopy in housewives. *Arch Dermatol* 1967;95:487–489.

33. Agner T, Serup J. Sodium lauryl sulfate for irritant patch testing: a dose response study using bioengineering methods for determination of skin irritation. *J Invest Dermatol* 1990;95:543–547.

34. Ohmen JD, Hanifin JM, Nickoloff BJ, et al. Overexpression of IL-10 in atopic dermatitis: contrasting cytokine patterns with delayed-type hypersensitivity reactions. *J Immunol* 1995;154:1956–1963.

35. Chan SC, Li S-H, Hanifin JM. Increased interleukin 4 production by atopic mononuclear leukocytes correlates with increased cyclic AMP-PDE activity and is reversible by PDE inhibition. *J Invest Dermatol* 1993;100:681–684.

36. Chan SC, Henderson WR Jr, Li S-H, Hanifin JM. Prostaglandin E$_2$ control of T cell cytokine production is functionally related to the reduced lymphocyte proliferation in atopic dermatitis. *J Allergy Clin Immunol* 1996;97:85–94.

37. Butler JM, Chan SC, Stevens SR, Hanifin JM. Increased leukocyte histamine release with elevated cyclic AMP-phosphodiesterase activity in atopic dermatitis. *J Allergy Clin Immunol* 1983;71:490–497.

38. Sampson HA, Broadbent KR, Bernhisel-Broadbent J. Spontaneous release of histamine from basophils and histamine-releasing factor in patients with atopic dermatitis and food hypersensitivity. *N Engl J Med* 1989;321:228–232.

39. Cooper KD, Kang K, Chan SC, Hanifin JM. Phosphodies-terase inhibition by Ro 20-1724 reduces hyper-IgE synthesis by atopic dermatitis cells *in vitro. J Invest Dermatol* 1985;84:477–482.

40. Agosti JM, Sprenger JD, Lum LG, et al. Transfer of allergen-specific IgE-mediated hypersensitivity with allogeneic bone marrow transplantation. *N Engl J Med* 1988; 319:1623–1628.

41. Cronin E, McFadden JP. Patients with atopic eczema do become sensitized to contact allergens. *Contact Dermatitis* 1993;28:225–228.

42. Ring J, Darsow U, Abeck D. The atopy patch test as a method of studying aeroallergens as triggering factors of atopic eczema. *Dermatol Ther* 1996;1:51–60.

43. Grewe M, Walther S, Gyufko K, Czech W, Schöpf E, Krutmann J. The two-phase model for the pathogenesis of atopic dermatitis: further evidence. *J Invest Dermatol* 1996;426:103.

44. Pastore S, Fanales-Belasio E, Albanesi C, Chinni LM, Giannetti A, Girolomoni G. Granulocyte macrophage colony-stimulating factor is overproduced by keratinocytes in atopic dermatitis: implications for sustained dendritic cell activation in the skin. *J Clin Invest* 1997;99:3009–3017.

45. Wood LC, Elias PM, Calhoun C, Tsai JC, Grunfeld C, Feingold KR. Barrier disruption stimulates interleukin-1α expression and release from a pre-formed pool in murine epidermis. *J Invest Dermatol* 1996;106:397–403.

46. Wood LC, Jackson SM, Elias PM, Grunfeld C, Feingold KR. Cutaneous barrier perturbation stimulates cytokine production in the epidermis of mice. *J Clin Invest* 1992;90:482–487.

47. Nickoloff BJ, Naidu Y. Perturbation of epidermal barrier function correlates with initiation of cytokine cascade in human skin. *J Am Acad Dermatol* 1994;30:535–546.

48. Davis RH, Sarkany I. Atopic eczema in European and Negro West Indian infants in London. *Br J Dermatol* 1961;73:410–414.

49. Graham DT, Wolf S. The relation of eczema to attitude and to vascular reactions of the human skin. *J Lab Clin Med* 1953;42:238–254.

50. Hanifin JM, Klas PA. The spectrum of cutaneous patch test reactions in patients with atopic dermatitis: immunological aspects of dermatological disease. *Clin Rev Allergy Immunol* 1996;14:225–240.

51. Hjorth N, Roed-Peterson J. Occupational protein contact dermatitis in food handlers. *Contact Dermatitis* 1976;2:24–42.

52. Von Krogh G, Maibach HI. The contact urticaria syndrome—an updated review. *J Am Acad Dermatol* 1981; 5:328–342.

53. Cronin E, Bandmann HJ, Calnan CD, et al. Contact dermatitis in the atopic. *Acta Derm Venereol* 1970;50:183.

54. Klas PA, Corey G, Storrs FJ, Chan SC, Hanifin JM. Allergic and irritant patch test reactions and atopic disease. *Contact Dermatitis* 1996;34:121–124.

55. Lever R, Forsyth A. Allergic contact dermatitis in atopic dermatitis. *Acta Derm Venereol Suppl* 1992;176:95–98.

56. Whitmore SE. Should atopic individuals be patch tested? *Dermatol Clin* 1994;12:491–499.

57. Rostenberg A Jr, Sulzberger MB. Some results of patch tests. *Arch Dermatol* 1937;35:433–454.

58. Palacios J, Fuller EW, Baylock WK. Immunological capabilities of patients with atopic dermatitis. *J Invest Dermatol* 1966;47:484.

59. Rees J, Friedmann PS, Matthews JNS. Contact sensitivity to dinitrochlorobenzene is impaired in atopic subjects: controversy revisited. *Arch Dermatol* 1990;126:1173–1175.

60. Byrom NA, Timlin DM. Immune status in atopic eczema: a survey. *Br J Dermatol* 1979;100:491–498.

61. Elliott ST, Hanifin JM. Delayed cutaneous hypersensitivity and lymphocyte transformation: dissociation in atopic dermatitis. *Arch Dermatol* 1979;115:36–39.

62. McGeady SJ, Buckley RH. Depression of cell-mediated immunity in atopic eczema. *J Allergy Clin Immunol* 1975;56:393.

63. Uehara M, Sawai T. A longitudinal study of contact sensitivity in patients with atopic dermatitis. *Arch Dermatol* 1989;125:366–368.

64. Agrup G. Hand eczema and other hand dermatoses in south Sweden. *Acta Derm Venereol Suppl* 1969;49:1–91.

65. Rystedt I. Hand eczema and long-term prognosis in atopic dermatitis. *Acta Derm Venereol Suppl* 1985;117:1–59.

66. Schmunes E, Keil JE. The role of atopy in occupational dermatoses. *Contact Dermatitis* 1984;11:174–178.

67. Schmunes E, Keil JE. Occupational dermatoses in South Carolina: a descriptive analysis of cost variables. *J Am Acad Dermatol* 1983;9:861–866.

68. Rystedt I. Work-related hand eczema in atopics. *Contact Dermatitis* 1985;12:164–171.

69. Nilsson E, Mikaelsson B, Andersson S. Atopy, occupation and domestic work as risk factors for hand eczema in hospital workers. *Contact Dermatitis* 1985;13:216–223.

70. Lammintausta K. Risk factors for hand dermatitis in wet work: atopy and contact sensitivity in hospital workers. Sweden: 1982 [thesis].

71. Nilsson E. Individual and environmental risk factors for hand eczema in hospital workers. Sweden: Uned University; 1986 [thesis].

72. Rystedt I. Hand eczema in patients with history of atopic manifestations in childhood. *Acta Derm Venereol Suppl* 1985;65:305–312.

73. Rystedt I. Atopic background in patients with occupational hand eczema. *Contact Dermatitis* 1985;12:247–254.

74. Lammintausta K. Hand dermatitis in different hospital workers who perform wet work. *Dermatosen* 1983;31:14–19.

75. Marks JG Jr, Belsito DV, DeLeo VA, et al. North American Contact Dermatitis Group standard tray patch test results (1992 to 1994). *Am J Contact Dermatitis* 1995;6:160–165.

76. Roper S, Jones H. A new look at conditioned hyperirritability. *J Am Acad Dermatol* 1982;7:643–650.

77. Rich P, Belozer M, Norris P, Storrs F. Allergic contact dermatitis to two antioxidants in latex gloves: 4,4′-thiobis (6-tert-butyl-meta-cresol) (Lowinox 44S36) and butyl-hydroxyanisole. *J Am Acad Dermatol* 1991;24:37–43.

78. Rystedt I. The role of atopy in occupational skin diseases. In: Adams RM, ed. *Occupational Skin Diseases*, 2nd ed. Philadelphia: W.B. Saunders; 1990:215–222.

Diagnostic Patch-Testing

14

TORKEL FISCHER, M.D.
ROBERT M. ADAMS, M.D.

Idiosyncratic reactions to various substances were recognized during the early 19th century (by Bateman in 1814[1] and by Staedler in 1847[2]), but Josef Jadassohn, in 1895 (Fig. 14–1),[3] was the first to devise a method for demonstrating these reactions in the skin, which he recognized as being different from ordinary irritant skin responses. His observations of a young man in whom sensitivity to a mercury-containing ointment had developed led to the first use of the patch test[3] more than a decade before the term "allergy" was defined by von Pirquet in 1906. Although the test occupied the interest of investigators in dermatology such as Bruno Bloch and others in the early part of the 20th century, it remained almost entirely a research tool until 1931, when Marion Sulzberger and Fred Wise of New York University wrote a major paper on the subject, "The Contact or Patch Test: Its Uses, Advantages, and Limitations."[4] Nevertheless, for the next 30 years, the test saw only limited use by clinicians. In the early 1960s, European dermatologists began to use the test with increasing frequency in their studies of patients with contact dermatitis, and they and a growing number of dermatologists, especially in the United States, Canada, and Japan, reported their observations in the international literature. Since then, the test has become an integral part of the work-up of patients with dermatitis in most parts of the world.

Although the patch test is not a perfect bioassay, it nevertheless possesses unique and valuable features. The opportunity to select the site of application and the ability to use only a minute concentration of test substance and confine it to a small area of skin are its most important advantages. The test is thus a model of the disease being investigated and is safer than using raw, undiluted (and unknown) substances as test materials. Because the organ tested is the same one affected with the disease, and because the same mechanism for production of the disease is used, the patch test is one of the most direct of all methods of medical testing. When used intelligently, the patch test is of inestimable value in managing dermatological patients, and at the same time, it solves many difficult clinical problems. Properly inter-

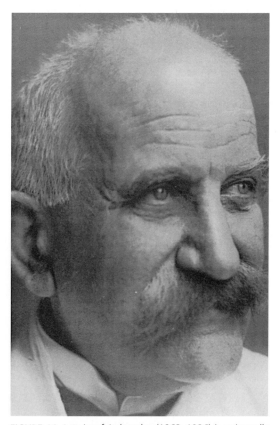

FIGURE 14–1 • Josef Jadassohn (1863–1936) is universally recognized as the "father" of patch-testing.

preted, patch-test reactions are acceptable as "scientific proof" of the cause of dermatitis and therefore are of medicolegal importance.

Standardized procedures are very important when patch-testing is used. The comparison of results is impossible if different concentrations, materials, or methods have been used. Most important are the concentration of the allergen and the type and characteristics of the vehicle. A change in concentration—from 0.1 to 1.0%, for example—may elicit irritant reactions with many allergens, and a reduction in concentration—as in the case of nickel sulfate from 5 to 2.5%—may result in false-negative reactions in a small but significant number of nickel-sensitive patients.[5] A petrolatum vehicle is suitable for most allergens, but for a few, water may be better. Formaldehyde is one example, and some investigators also prefer to use nickel in an aqueous vehicle.[6] In recent years there has been a worldwide movement toward the standardization of patch-testing. The methods of testing, allergen concentrations, and vehicles recommended in this chapter are those advocated by most dermatologists in patch-testing centers throughout the world. This information is also available in several important texts.[5–16] Although it is not always possible to avoid adverse, particularly irritant, reactions when patch-testing, by adhering to standard procedures as described in this text and the previously mentioned works such reactions can be greatly reduced.

SELECTION OF PATIENTS

The ideal patient for patch-testing is one with a recurring eczematous, pruritic dermatitis who, from the history, is found to be coming into contact with a substance that contains a recognized contact allergen. Less than one-half of the patients with contact dermatitis seen in daily practice fit this model, and if only these individuals are tested, large numbers of patients will remain undiagnosed and will continue to experience episodes of dermatitis. Itching is an important and usually indispensable symptom for diagnosis, but treatment with corticosteroids can markedly diminish this response. Furthermore, contact sensitization may become superimposed upon and aggravate other dermatoses, especially pustular psoriasis, nummular eczema, and others (see chapter 12). Patch-testing also may become part of a thorough work-up of a patient's puzzling diagnostic problem.

THE TAPE

Two tape methods are currently in use. The A1 test was a standard method for several years. It consists of a filter paper disk of cellulose attached to a strip of plastic-coated aluminum foil and is available in rolls. A more recent and more widely used method is the Finn chamber, which employs an aluminum or polypropylene cup, 8 mm in diameter, fixed to a strip of Scanpor tape (Fig. 14–2A and B), which is a finely meshed paper tape with a polyacrylate adhesive. Although it permits excellent adherence, Scanpor tape rarely induces miliaria because of the large number of perforations in the fabric per cm.[2] The Finn chamber occupies a smaller test area than does the A1 test, and thus many more allergens can be applied to the back.

An entirely new method, called the TRUE test (thin layer, rapid-use epicutaneous test) (Fig. 14–3), developed by Pharmacia in Sweden, is a ready-to-use test strip of tape in which a measured amount of allergen is placed in a thin hydrophilic gel film printed on a polyester patch that is 9 × 9 mm. These patches, containing different aller-

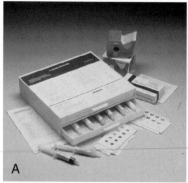
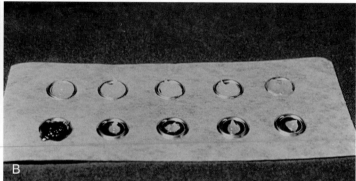

FIGURE 14–2 • *A* and *B,* Finn chambers on Scanpor tape consist of aluminum cups with an inner diameter of 8 mm and a chamber volume of 24 μK. The test material should be slightly more than one-half the volume of the chamber.

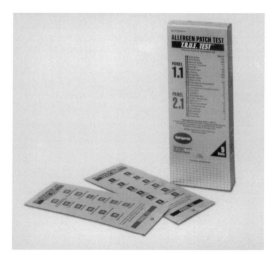

FIGURE 14–3 • The TRUE test consists of allergens placed on an impermeable backing of plastic and mounted on a strip of tape. The patches are covered with a protective sheet of plastic and packed in airtight and light-impermeable envelopes. This method eliminates the possibility of errors that exists with manual application. (Courtesy GlaxoWellcome Pharmaceuticals.)

tization was done with intradermal allergen extracts containing aluminum.[23]

THE VEHICLE

Most commercial allergens for use in the Finn chamber or A1 test are incorporated in a petrolatum vehicle; a few are incorporated in water. Other vehicles that have been recommended for specific allergens are ethanol, acetone, methyl ethyl ketone, ethyl ether, ethyl alcohol, olive oil, lanolin, and others. Petrolatum is almost universally used, but it has certain disadvantages, especially the slow release of hydrophobic allergens from the lipophilic petrolatum.[24, 25] This seems most likely to occur with metal allergens,[26] and slightly more reliable results occur when these allergens are used in distilled water. Petrolatum, however, has the advantages of a greater sealing capacity, less risk of decomposition, and ease of application, especially when nonocclusive tapes are used.[24]

In the TRUE test, the vehicle contains hydrophilic gel-forming substances such as hydroxypropylcellulose and polyvinylpyrolidone (PVP).[19]

gens, are mounted on strips of nonwoven cellulose tape with acrylic adhesive protected by sheets of plastic and are packaged in airtight envelopes. The thin sheet of plastic is removed, and the strips are placed on the skin. On contact with the skin and its moisture, the dry film dissolves into the gel and the allergen is released onto the skin.[17]

The TRUE test was evaluated on 2,678 consecutive patients tested on suspicion of contact dermatitis and compared with the Finn chamber method. Using 24 different patches including 47 different allergens, the concordance for positive reactions between the two methods was 69% where the TRUE test demonstrated 83% and the reference method 86% positive reactions. The advantages of TRUE test are a constant amount of allergen per patch, uniformity in materials and procedure, and considerable savings in time of performance of testing.[18–21]

All test methods should maintain firm occlusion of the test material within a small, well-defined area. When the Finn chamber or A1 test is used, the same measured amount of test substance should be applied; however, because application is done by hand, irregular amounts can easily be added, sometimes by spilling the test material beyond the confines of the patch, even onto an adjacent test site.

Allergic sensitization to the patch materials is a possibility, but this rarely occurs. Reactions to the aluminum patches have been described,[22] but nearly always in individuals in whom past desensi-

THE TEST SITES

The upper half of the back is the recommended test site[27, 28] (Fig. 14–4). The upper, outer arm can be used if necessary. Fisher recommends this area when a strong reaction is anticipated, as with nickel, to avoid the "angry back" reaction.[6]

The skin must be normal and hairless. If the patches are applied directly over a heavy coat of hair, lack of occlusion will result in false-negative reactions. Except for shaving, which should be done with an electric razor or a pair of scissors to avoid soap and shaving creams, no preparation of the skin is necessary.

THE ANTIGENS

Contact allergens are simple chemical substances, with molecular weights rarely higher than 1,000 daltons and almost always lower than 500 daltons. On entering the skin, the allergen is taken up by the Langerhans cells and is transformed into a complete antigen. In a complex process, this antigen is presented to T lymphocytes, which are stimulated to divide and develop clones of cells with specific sensitivity to the antigen. On repeated contact, such cells evoke the inflammatory response characteristic of contact dermatitis.[29] Most allergens used in patch-testing today are

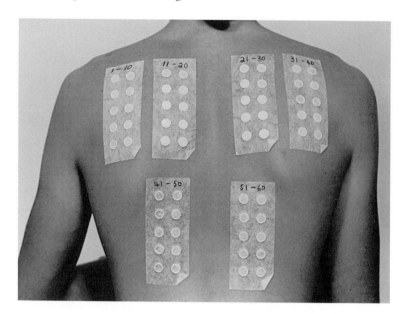

FIGURE 14–4 • The upper back is the site of application most likely to produce accurate results. As many as 50 to 60 tests can be applied.

well-defined chemical compounds, but for several test materials, such as natural resins, fragrances, and lanolin, detailed chemical information concerning their allergens is lacking. It is possible that they may contain several allergens. Among the 2 to 3 million chemicals known today, approximately 3,700 have been identified as sensitizers.[13] About 100 or so are common sensitizers, and of these the most frequently encountered have been selected by the various international patch-testing groups for inclusion in standard batteries of 20 to 30 different test materials. Some of them are mixes containing two to eight substances. There are several companies today that provide test substances arranged in groups for testing persons in various occupational settings, such as hairdressers, machinists, dental technicians, printers, and so forth.

When the history given by the patient fails to reveal a possible allergen, it is sometimes advisable to postpone testing to allow the patient to consider the questions raised by the physician and perhaps recall information that may shed some light on the cause, thus facilitating the choice of test materials. If no clues are forthcoming, the use of one or more standard series of screening allergens is helpful (Tables 14–1 and 14–2). When a positive result is found, it can then be included in the framework of information already obtained from the history and physical examination. Often a positive result does not represent the primary cause but instead uncovers a crossreacting chemical. This may lead to further investigation to determine previous contact with immunologically related chemicals and will possibly result in

identification of the causative agent, which might not have been discovered without using the standard battery. For example, a positive reaction to the mixture of "-caine" anesthetics may not be caused by the anesthetics themselves but may instead reflect sensitivity to *p*-phenylenediamine or its derivatives, to *p*-aminobenzoic acid (PABA) and certain sunscreens, or to other chemicals with the amino group in the para position. A crossreacting chemical may produce a weak reaction, which can then alert the dermatologist to look for the culprit in one of its relations.

MIXES

Testing with single allergens provides the most exact information, but the use of mixes of closely related allergens saves time and space. The area of skin on the average back permits application of no more than 50 to 55 test allergens at one time. By using mixes containing four to five related chemicals, this number can be considerably increased. Bonnevie first employed mixes in 1939[30] using wood tars, chrysarobin, and anthrarobin. In 1963, Hjorth used mixes of paraben esters, -caine anesthetics, and antibiotics.[31] Ernst Epstein and others[32, 33] advocated mixes of -caine anesthetics, antibiotics, rubber chemicals, and antibacterial agents. At present, the North American Contact Dermatitis Group recommends mixes of four sets of rubber chemicals.

Nevertheless, the use of mixes involves problems of concentration, interference, stability, and formulation. Because of a high total concentration

TABLE 14–1 • **Standard Allergens**

North American Contact Dermatitis Group	European Contact Dermatitis Group
1. Benzocaine, 5% pet	1. Potassium dichromate 0.5% pet
2. Mercaptobenzothiazole, 1% pet	2. Paraphenylenediamine base, 1% pet
3. Colophony, 20% pet	3. Thiuram mix, 1% pet
4. Paraphenylenediamine base, 1% pet	4. Neomycin sulfate, 20% pet
5. Imidazolidinyl urea, 2% aq	5. Cobalt chloride, 1% pet
6. Cinnamic aldehyde, 1% pet	6. Benzocaine, 5% pet
7. Lanolin alcohol, 30% pet	7. Nickel sulfate, 5% pet
8. Carbamix, 3% pet	8. Clioquinol, 5% pet
9. Neomycin sulfate, 20% pet	9. Colophony, 20% pet
10. Thiuram mix, 1% pet	10. Paraben mix, 8% pet
11. Formaldehyde, 1% aq	11. N-isopropyl-N-phenylparaphenylenediamine, 0.1% pet
12. Ethylenediamine dihydrochloride, 1% pet	12. Wool alcohols, 30% pet
13. Epoxy resin, 1% pet	13. Mercaptomix, 2% pet
14. Quaternium 15, 2% pet	14. Epoxy resin, 1% pet
15. p-tert-Butylphenol formaldehyde resin, 1% pet	15. Balsam of Peru, 25% pet
16. Mercaptomix, 1% pet	16. p-tert-Butylphenol formaldehyde resin, 1% pet
17. Black rubber mix, 0.6% pet	17. Mercaptobenzothiazole, 2% pet
18. Potassium dichromate, 0.25% pet	18. Formaldehyde, 1% pet
19. Balsam of Peru, 25% pet	19. Fragrance mix, 8% pet
20. Nickel sulfate, 2.5% pet	20. Sesquiterpene lactone mix
	21. Quaternium 15, 1% pet
	22. Primin, 0.01% pet
	23. Cl + Me-isothiazolinone, 0.01% aq

aq, aqueous; pet, petrolatum

of allergen, mixes may show irritant reactions. For example, all the present mixes in the standard series may occasionally induce irritation. To avoid this, the allergens are incorporated in suboptimal amounts, sometimes resulting in weak or negative reactions, which is the case with mercaptomix, which often results in false-negative reactions. Conversely, when there is a reaction to a mix that is suspected of being irritant, it may be advisable to repeat the test after a couple of weeks using the separate ingredients.[34]

Balsam of Peru, lanolin, and colophony are examples of natural mixes. Balsam of Peru contains several sensitizing ingredients that are also present in many fragrances. Thus, when a positive test result is found with balsam of Peru, it is possible that fragrance allergy exists in approximately 50% of those reacting. Conversely, when the fragrance mix produces positive results, fragrance allergy may be indicated in 70 to 80% of sensitive patients. However, as is the case with all mixes, one must beware of false-positive reactions.

It is possible that certain mixes are unnecessary in the standard tray. A positive reaction to carbamix, for example, provides little extra information than can be obtained from other tests, especially thiuram mix, and it has therefore been excluded from the European Standard series.[35] Carbamix also produces irritant reactions. In a large study, Logan and White[36] showed that the carbamix is actually redundant in a standard tray, because thiuram mix, paraphenylenediamine dihydrochloride (PPD) mix, and mercaptomix (MBT) almost always detect the presence of rubber sensitivity.

THE PACKING

The stability of contact allergens varies considerably, and there has been too little research on the stability of patch-test allergens. Metal salts appear to be quite stable, as is the case with formaldehyde in aqueous solution.[37] Paraphenylenediamine degrades rapidly, as evidenced by its change from colorless to blue-black after several months, but its allergenic properties apparently are not altered. As fragrances age, their antigenicity diminishes significantly.[38] Sunlight may also change the reactivity of allergens, especially those chemicals used for photopatch testing, which rapidly lose activity with exposure to sunlight, even through window glass.[39] The packing should mechanically protect

TABLE 14–2 • Standard Allergens (TRUE Test)

1. Nickel sulfate 0.2 mg/cm^2
2. Wool alcohols 1.00 mg/cm^2
3. Neomycin sulfate 0.23 mg/cm^2
4. Potassium dichromate 0.023 mg/cm^2
5. Caine mix 0.63 mg/cm^2
6. Fragrance mix 0.43 mg/cm^2
7. Colophony 0.85 mg/cm^2
8. Epoxy resin 0.05 mg/cm^2
9. Quinoline mix 0.19 mix/cm^2
10. Balsam of Peru 0.80 mg/cm^2
11. Ethylenediamine dihydrochloride 0.05 mg/cm^2
12. Cobalt dichloride 0.02 mg/cm^2
13. p-tert-Butylphenol formaldehyde resin 0.04 mg/cm^2
14. Paraben mix 1 m/cm^2
15. Carba mix 0.25 mg/cm^2
16. Black rubber mix 0.075 mg/cm^2
17. Cl + Me-Isothiazolinone 0.0040 mg/cm^2 (Kathon CG)
18. Quaternium 15 0.1 mg/cm^2
19. Mercaptobenzothiazole 0.075 mg/cm^2
20. Paraphenylenediamine (PPD), 0.090 mg/cm^2
21. Formaldehyde 0.18 mg/cm^2
22. Mercapto mix 0.075 mg/cm^2
23. Thimerosal 0.0080 mg/cm^2
24. Thiuram mix 0.025 mg/cm^2

against air, humidity, ultraviolet radiation, and loss of stability, and it should not interact with or contaminate either the allergen or the vehicle. The polypropylene used for syringes containing commercial petrolatum-based allergens is inert and also provides protection against air and humidity. The impermeable plastic-coated aluminum envelopes used for the TRUE test also afford stability and minimal interaction with the allergens.[19]

TEST TECHNIQUE

For a satisfactory test result, the amount of test material applied is critical. Although it must cover the test area completely, it should not spread beyond the area's limits, which would cause loss of occlusion. Using Finn chambers, which have a volume of 25 μl, 12 to 15 μl of test material, or slightly more than one-half of the chamber, should be applied.[40] With solutions, application of one drop to the filter paper disk is usually sufficient, and it must be applied immediately before the test is performed to avoid evaporation of vehicle and reduction of skin contact. When Finn chambers are used, 50 to 55 test allergens can be applied to the back at one time.

The tape strips should be applied from below with firm pressure to remove air bubbles and provide uniform adhesion (Fig. 14–5). Each test site should then be pressed lightly to ensure contact with the skin. Sometimes the ends of the strips require additional tape, but only as much as is necessary to hold the ends secure should be applied. The most frequent cause of tape-loosening is the application of too much tape. If the skin is very oily, washing with ethyl alcohol may improve adhesion; however, the back must be permitted to dry completely before the patches are applied. As previously mentioned, if shaving is necessary, it should be done with an electric razor, not with soap or a shaving foam or cream.

MARKING THE AREA

The most satisfactory marking material is one that will remain on the skin for at least 72 hours and at the same time will not discolor clothing or sensitize the patient. Various methods have been recommended, including gentian violet (which stains clothing and is messy), silver nitrate solution (which is irritating and expensive), a concentrated solution of dihydroxyacetone (which does not last), pyrogallol and ferric chloride,[7] and others. Additional locating with 8-mm-round stickers over the marking ink protects the clothing and

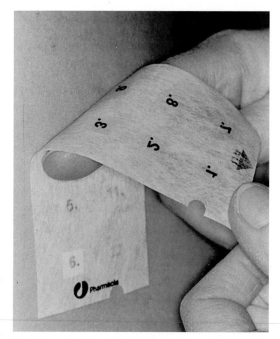

FIGURE 14–5 • To avoid air bubbles, the patches should be applied with a small amount of pressure from below upward.

FIGURE 14–6 • A handheld flashlight with a black lightbulb will outline the sites that have previously been circled with a felt pen containing a fluorescent ink. The fluorescence remains visible on the skin for 3 to 4 days.

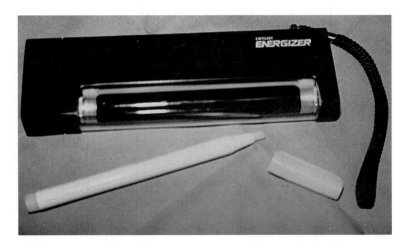

stays on the skin longer. A satisfactory identification material is an inexpensive marking pen containing ultraviolet fluorescent ink, which is available in most stationery stores (Fig. 14–6). When properly applied and not removed by bathing, the marking will last for 72 to 96 hours after application. Reapplication should be done at each return visit. To see the fluorescent ink, a conveniently sized flashlight with a blacklight bulb (Eveready) can be used (Fig. 14–6), which illuminates the ink surrounding the test sites as a bright yellow-green when the room is darkened.

The normal application time of 48 hours is a compromise. Shorter application times may be used for some allergens; for others, the yield of positive reactions would increase with application for 72 to 96 hours and with a decreased allergen dose.[41]

INSTRUCTIONS TO THE PATIENT

The patient should be instructed to keep the patches dry and undisturbed during the 2 days of application. If excessive burning or itching occurs under any patch, it may be carefully removed, making certain to leave the other patches undisturbed. It is important that the patient not shower or bathe or engage in strenuous activity during the 48 hours the patches are in place. Even nonstrenuous work activity that causes considerable sweating should be avoided. If the tape becomes loose, the patient can reaffix it with a small additional amount of tape. Scratching and rubbing should be cautioned against. Written instructions are very helpful, including a reminder of future appointments for readings.

INTERPRETATION OF THE RESULTS

Readings should be done at 72 hours, 96 hours, and 1 week. A single reading at 48 hours will lose approximately 30% of the positive reactions and at the same time will often show irritant reactions.[42] At the time of removal, the effects of occlusion and the tape reactions are most pronounced; thus, preliminary inspection should wait until these effects have subsided. Certain test substances, such as neomycin and organic dyes,[7] may show reactions only 4 to 6 days after removal. When a positive reaction appears after 2 to 3 weeks, active sensitization by the substance used for patch-testing has occurred. Fisher[6] states that this must be suspected even when positive reactions appear after only 7 to 10 days. Termed spontaneous flares, these reactions, fortunately, are rare.

The interpretation recommended by the International Contact Dermatitis Group (ICDG) and the North American Contact Dermatitis Group (NACDG) is shown in Table 14–3. The "?" and

 TABLE 14–3 • Patch Test Interpretation Codes

1 =	Weak (nonvesicular) reaction: erythema, infiltration, papules (+)
2 =	Strong (edematous or vesicular) reaction (+ +)
3 =	Extreme (spreading, bullous, ulcerative) reaction (+ + +)
4 =	Doubtful reaction, macular erythema only (?)
5 =	Irritant reaction (IR)
6 =	Negative reaction (−)
7 =	Excited skin
8 =	Not tested

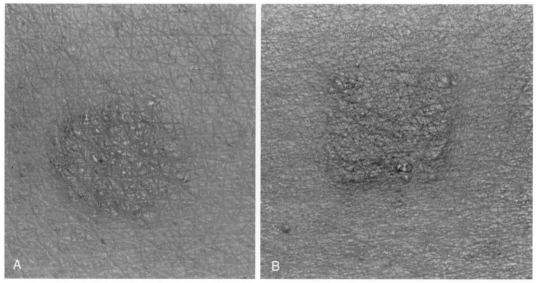

FIGURE 14–7 ● *A* and *B,* Reactions of 2 +, showing erythema, infiltration, and small, closely set vesicles. *A,* From testing with the Finn chamber. *B,* From testing with the TRUE test. *(See Color Plates.)*

"+" reactions are the most difficult to interpret. Erythema alone has an intensity parameter that does not discriminate between allergic and irritant reactions. If an increase in intensity develops by 96 hours and is accompanied by pruritus, a readily palpable infiltration, and small close-set vesicles, the result indicates an allergic reaction (Fig. 14–7A and B). *(See Color Plates.)* It is important to be critical of reactions showing only erythema with questionable infiltration (Fig. 14–8) *(See Color Plates)* and to avoid the assumption that they represent true, but weak, responses. Substances that commonly cause these reactions are formalin, potassium dichromate, wool wax alcohols, fragrance and paraben mixes, and propylene glycol. Other substances that occasionally cause marginal irritant reactions are balsam of Peru, nickel sulfate, carbamix, and thimerosal. Repeat testing may be necessary to clarify such weak reactions.

Irritant reactions exhibit varied patterns: fine wrinkling, erythematous follicular papules, petechiae, pustules, bullae, and necrosis (Figs. 14–9 to 14–11). *(See Color Plates.)* Petechiae, in addition to other signs of allergic reaction, may occasionally be present, especially from testing with black rubber chemicals[43] and cobalt.[44] Fortunately, + + + bullous reactions are rare (Fig. 14–12) *(See Color Plates)* and almost always represent irritation, usually from testing with substances of unknown composition brought to the office by the patient, such as coolants (tested in full concentration), soaps, detergents, solvents, or highly alkaline and corrosive materials. Hyperpigmentation and scarring may result, and in persons with a high degree of pigmentation, depigmentation of the test site may occur.

The classic positive patch-test reaction and the only reaction that can safely be interpreted as

FIGURE 14–8 ● A 1 + reaction, showing erythema and barely palpable infiltration. By the following day, this reaction will either disappear (if an irritant response) or will increase to a clearly positive allergic reaction. *(See Color Plates.)*

FIGURE 14-9 • A papular reaction for potassium dichromate is difficult to interpret. It is most likely due to irritation rather than to allergic sensitivity. *(See Color Plates.)*

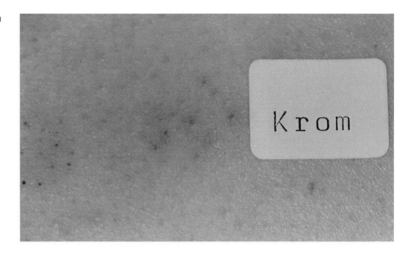

allergic contact sensitivity consists of erythema, edema, and small, closely set vesicles (Fig. 14–7A and B). Any reaction that is greater or less than this, or of different morphology, must be suspected as a possible false-positive reaction. By limiting observations to this result alone in interpretating patch tests, most of the pitfalls and problems associated with the procedure would be avoided. Physicians lose credibility when patients are told they are sensitive to a substance that they later learn from experience they are not.

CAUSES OF FALSE-POSITIVE REACTIONS

Use of Irritant Substances

Because it is often impossible to differentiate between allergic and irritant reactions on morpholog-

ical grounds alone, irritation is undoubtedly the common cause of reports of unexplained "positive" reactions. They can occur even from the use of substances in concentrations generally considered nonirritating, especially in persons with atopic and actinically damaged skins. In addition, the test materials themselves may be irritating, especially when occluded under the test patch, as is the case with many substances that patients bring to the office from the workplace, such as solvents, coolants, soaps, and detergents. It should be repeated that testing with substances of unknown composition and concentration should not

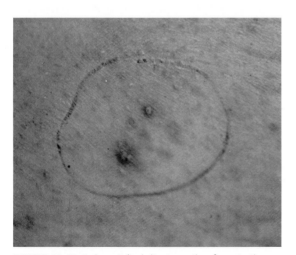

FIGURE 14-10 • A pustular irritant reaction from testing with nickel in a patient with atopic dermatitis. *(See Color Plates.)*

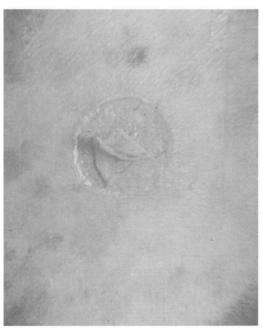

FIGURE 14-11 • A bullous reaction confined to the site of application. This reaction is clearly an irritant response. *(See Color Plates.)*

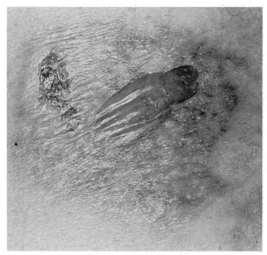

FIGURE 14-12 • A bullous reaction due to testing with an unknown substance that obviously contained a potent irritant. This reaction, which may leave an unsightly scar, can be avoided if substances of unknown composition are never used in testing. *(See Color Plates.)*

be attempted unless there are obvious reasons to believe the material is not irritating, even when occluded.

The active ingredient itself may be nonirritating, but the vehicle may be irritating or the test substance may be contaminated by an irritant.[7] Sometimes, especially with patch-test materials formulated by individuals unfamiliar with the test (such as druggists), the test material may be unevenly dispersed throughout the mixture, resulting in a false-positive irritant or false-negative reactions when tested, or the person compounding the test material may add a dispersant or surfactant to make the mixing easier, which then may act as an irritant or enhance the irritant properties of the test chemical.

An additional source of false-positive reactions is reading only at 48 hours. Studies of the NACDG have shown that reading solely at 48 hours may show reactions that disappear within 24 hours (and are presumed to be mostly irritant reactions) as often as 18% of the time, whereas second readings on the third through seventh days will detect an additional 34% positive reactivity.[42] The importance of reading beyond 48 hours must be emphasized.

Edge Effect

The edge effect is almost always an irritant reaction, consisting of a greater reaction at the periphery of the patch-test site but little or no reaction at its center (Fig. 14-13). *(See Color Plates.)* It

appears to be caused by an increased concentration of an irritating liquid at the margins of the patch.[8, 45] Following removal of the patch, the reaction disappears rapidly. Not all ring-shaped reactions are irritant in nature, however. Lachapelle and coworkers[46] described ring-shaped positive allergic patch-test reactions to formaldehyde, Kathon CG, hydrocortisone, and hexamidine diisothionate in liquid media. Allergic corticosteroid reactions are often of the "edge" type.[46a]

Pustular Patch-Test Reactions

Atopic individuals are especially likely to show pustular reactions from application of salts of nickel, mercury, copper, arsenic, and tungstate.[47, 48] Pruritus is usually minimal or absent. Pustular reactions may occasionally persist for several days.[49]

Pressure Reactions

Sometimes testing with a solid substance produces an edematous area with greater intensity at the margins and occasionally covering the entire test area. Individuals with dermographism are more likely to have pressure reactions, which are aggravated, of course, by rubbing and scratching.

Dermatitis Near the Test Sites

Patch-testing should be postponed until dermatitis on the back—or adjacent to the back, or an active widespread dermatitis anywhere—has subsided.

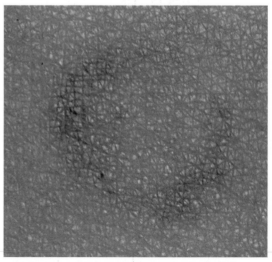

FIGURE 14-13 • A reaction showing the "edge effect," with greater reaction at the margins. This almost always denotes irritation rather than allergy. *(See Color Plates.)*

The Angry Back Reaction

The "angry back" reaction ("excited skin") is a regional phenomenon caused by the presence of either a single strong positive reaction or several strong reactions, which induce a state of skin hyperreactivity in which other patch-test sites become marginally reactive, especially at the sites of formalin or metal salt testing. The phenomenon was first described by Bruno Bloch early in the 20th century and more recently was studied by Mitchell,[50] who emphasizes the importance of dismissing these concomitant "positive" reactions. He first tested 35 patients who showed 90 positive reactions to 28 substances at 48 hours. He retested them on the seventh day. On reading them on the ninth day, 42% of the reactions were negative, suggesting that the original reactions were falsely positive. Mitchell emphasizes that the true index of sensitivity can be falsely exaggerated by over-interpreting these reactions. To confirm or deny the significance of "angry back" reactions, Mitchell recommends later sequential testing with each substance alone.

CAUSES OF FALSE-NEGATIVE REACTIONS

Concentration of Test Substance Too Low

The concentration is critical and should not be altered arbitrarily, because the threshold of reactivity often exists within a narrow margin; at even slightly higher concentrations many substances become irritating. Conversely, certain substances require an artificially high concentration in order to penetrate the skin's barrier layer. Neomycin, tested at an inflated concentration of 20% is an example. In the usual therapeutic concentration, it penetrates intact, normal skin with difficulty, but it easily enters skin altered by dermatitis, even at the lower concentration. To pass the skin's barrier at the healthy, normal test site, an increase in concentration to 20% is required; irritant reactions with this concentration are rare. Another example is lanolin, because the allergen, which probably is present in the wool wax alcohol fraction, exists in a very low concentration. The wool wax alcohol mixture is therefore a better test material because it has a higher concentration of allergen.

Insufficient Reproduction of the Conditions of the Original Dermatitis

The inability of the patch test to duplicate the conditions present during the dermatitis, such as sweating and friction, is an occasional cause of negative results when testing with clothing, especially sections of shoes. If the allergen fails to leach out of the material, it will not penetrate the stratum corneum to reach the effector cells and challenge the immune system.[13]

Failure to Read After 48 Hours

Perhaps the most common cause of false-negative readings today is reading only at 48 hours.[42] If a later reaction develops, the patient may be unaware of its presence, and a significant finding is lost forever.

Inappropriate Vehicle

The vehicle is very important; if the substance is insoluble in the vehicle, or if the vehicle itself evaporates before application of the test, the result may be negative.

Too Brief Duration of Contact

The optimal duration of occlusion for most allergens in closed patch tests is probably 48 hours. Earlier removal, especially as a result of traumatic loosening of the patches, sweating, or deliberate manipulation, may result in false-negative reactions.

Failure to Perform Photopatch Testing

Testing with substances that require ultraviolet light to become complete allergens may result in negative reactions.

Corticosteroid Treatment

Potent topical steroids applied to the test site for several days prior to testing may diminish or even obliterate positive results. Conversely, systemic steroids, in daily dosages of 20 mg or less, probably do not inhibit strong reactions.[51, 52]

Ultraviolet Radiation

Ultraviolet radiation has been shown by Morison and colleagues[53] to influence the induction and elicitation of allergic contact dermatitis in guinea pigs. Bruze,[54] testing a large number of patients in Sweden, demonstrated more positive routine test reactions during winter than during summer. Statistical comparison of the difference using X-analysis was significant. More recently, however,

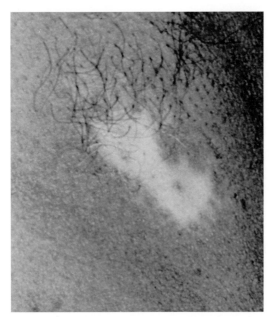

FIGURE 14–14 • Depigmentation resulting from testing, fortunately in the axilla, with monobenzyl ether of hydroquinone. *(See Color Plates.)*

Dooms-Goossens and colleagues[55] in Belgium found no seasonal influence of sunlight on patch-test reactions in humans over a 9-year period in a retrospective study of nearly 8,000 patients. Whether or not a recent sunburn alters patch-test reactions has not been clarified.

ADVERSE REACTIONS

Alterations in Pigmentation

Sunlight exposure immediately following removal of patches in which coal tar or fragrance materials have been employed may result in hyperpigmentation. Severe reactions, especially those caused by testing with irritants, may result in depigmentation. Irritant reactions may induce hyperpigmentation in certain patients from inflammation alone, independent of the chemical applied.[56, 57] Testing with chemicals that are known to cause depigmentation, such as monobenzyl ether of hydroquinone, may induce depigmentation at the test site (Fig. 14–14). *(See Color Plates.)*

Persistence of Reaction

Testing with gold compounds may result in persistent reactions that last for weeks or even months.[58]

Temporary Flare of Dermatitis Elsewhere

A mild flare of the existing dermatitis elsewhere on the skin may occur at the apex of a positive patch-test reaction, and this "focal flare" often, but not always, suggests relevance. Sometimes dyshidrotic eruptions and id-like dissemination occur and may be so severe that treatment with a short course of prednisone is required.[47]

Active Sensitization

Active sensitization is an extremely infrequent complication of patch-testing. It may occur from plant oleoresins or, rarely, from paraphenylenediamine and other potent allergens. If only the smallest concentration of a test substance is used, active sensitization is much less likely to occur. This emphasizes the hazard of testing with unknown materials provided by the patient or employer. Meneghini and Angelini believe that when proper techniques are used (and also standard, commercially prepared allergens), patch-testing rarely causes new sensitizations.[59]

Psoriasis

In susceptible persons, psoriasis may appear at the test sites 2 or 3 weeks later, either from irritant or from allergic test reactions (the Koebner phenomenon) (Fig. 14–15). *(See Color Plates.)*

Scarring

Testing with substances of unknown composition or concentration, or both, is usually responsible

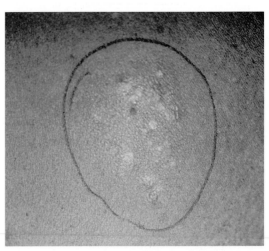

FIGURE 14–15 • Psoriasis developing 6 weeks after a positive patch test reaction to *p*-phenylenediamine in a patient sensitive to hair dye who has a history of having had psoriasis years previously. *(See Color Plates.)*

for intense reactions that result in scarring. When standard test concentrations are used, this reaction almost never occurs, even in the strongest allergic reactions.

Anaphylactoid Reactions

The serious, life-threatening reaction known as an anaphylactoid reaction can occur when potent urticaria-producing substances are used in testing, such as ammonium persulfate, which is a booster in the bleaching of hair,[60] and other substances.[61] Symptoms may develop within minutes following application. Fortunately, this reaction is extremely rare.

DETERMINATION OF RELEVANCE

When one or more allergic reactions are found, the relevance of each must then be determined. The most important question is whether the reaction is a manifestation of the dermatitis under study or whether it is an expression of allergic sensitization that developed years previously. The patient's history may reveal the source. For example, positive patch-test results to mercury are commonly found on investigation to be due to contact with mercury-containing antiseptics years previously, usually in childhood. When the clinical and historic facts are consistent with the patch-test results, one can be reasonably certain of the validity. Often, however, one must reverse the process and attempt to find a chemical in the patient's environment that unexpectedly appears reactive on patch-testing and then determine whether the clinical situation at the onset of the dermatitis could have been responsible.

Often, the patch-test result represents an aggravating factor and not the primary cause of the dermatitis. This is especially true for reactions to medications or rubber chemicals in gloves used to protect an irritant dermatitis.

A reaction may appear to have no relevance whatever. Judgments of unknown relevance, however, often reflect not only one's own ignorance of the chemical environment but also the patterns of cross-sensitivity rather than true irrelevancy.[62] Studies to define the relevance of positive nonirritant patch-test responses have been undertaken by NACDG each year for several years. The multiple studies show recovery of present or past relevance of 58% and relevance to the dermatitis under study of approximately 25%. In 1970, Wilkinson and others tested a large number of patients with hand eczema and found 40% with one or more contact allergies, of which two-thirds were deemed rele-

vant.[63] Such impressive results prompted Hjorth to emphasize that a more extensive use of patch-testing by physicians is indicated.[47]

PREVENTION OF RECURRENCE

After completing the work-up and finding a responsible allergen, the patient should be provided with sufficient information to avoid recurrence. In the case of allergens widely distributed in the environment, such as nickel, formaldehyde and many cosmetic preservatives, occasional recurrences may be impossible to avoid. If the patient has enough knowledge of which substances to avoid, however, recurrences can be reduced to an acceptable level and sometimes eliminated entirely. The exact name of the allergen, with its synonyms, should be given to the patient. Material Safety Data Sheets, required to be available at the workplace, may also provide information for the patient (the physician may have to obtain the specific chemical information, however). The labeling of cosmetics, required in the United States since 1977, has been indispensable for patients with cosmetic contact allergy.

Providing the patient with lengthy lists of substances that may (or may not) currently contain the allergen may be confusing and should not be routinely provided to every patient. An obsessive-compulsive individual may become an "iatrogenic" invalid by misinterpreting and overreacting to this information. The legal consequences can sometimes assume major proportions, especially in worker compensation cases. Helping the patient to avoid further contact by suggesting use of allergen alternatives when possible is a better approach.[64–66] Company personnel may be willing to make substitution of an offending chemical used in the workplace, but sometimes a simple measure (such as covering nickel-plated objects with plastic) will suffice.

CONCLUSION

Despite the considerable knowledge accumulated over the years through use of the patch test, many dermatologists and dermatology departments do not teach or use the test. They believe that it is too time-consuming, that the results are sometimes confusing, and that sufficient information can be obtained from a "use test" or by trial and error. Those who regularly use the patch test realize that the discovery of a specific chemical responsible for dermatitis is fundamental to the prevention of recurrence of a frequently disabling condition. It has been repeatedly demonstrated over the years that this knowledge can be obtained only through intelligent and careful patch-testing. Thus, training in the techniques of patch-testing is as essential to dermatologists as is that of surgical procedures and should become an integral part of the curriculum for all training institutions in dermatology.

For suggested allergens in specific occupations, see the Appendix.

References

1. Bateman T. Eczema. *A Practical Synopsis of Cutaneous Diseases.* London: 1814:250.
2. Staedler. Über die eigentümlichen Bestandteile der Anacardium Früchte. *Ann Chemie Pharmacie* 1847; 63:117–119.
3. Jadassohn J. *Zur Kenntnis der Medikamentösen Dermatosen.* Graz, Austria: Fifth Congress of the German Academy of Dermatology; 1895.
4. Sulzberger MB, Wise F. The contact or patch test: its uses, advantages, and limitation. *Arch Dermatol* 1931; 23:519–531.
5. Cronin E. *Contact Dermatitis.* Edinburgh: Churchill Livingstone; 1980.
6. Fisher AA. *Contact Dermatitis.* Philadelphia: Lea & Febiger; 1986.
7. Fregert S. *Manual of Contact Dermatitis.* Copenhagen: Munksgaard; 1981.
8. Lachapelle J-M. *Dermatologie Professionnelle.* Paris: Masson; 1984.
9. Foussereau J. *Les Eczemas Allergiques, Cosmétologiques: Thérapeutiques et Vestimentaires.* Paris: Masson; 1987.
10. Garcia-Perez A, Conde-Salazar L, et al. *Tratado de Dermatosis Profesionales.* Madrid: Eudema; 1987.
11. Grimalt F, Romaguera C. *Dermatitis de Contacto.* Barcelona: Syntex Latino; 1987.
12. Larsen WG, Adams RA, et al. *Color Text of Contact Dermatitis.* Philadelphia: W.B. Saunders; 1992.
13. de Groot AC. *Patch Testing: Test Concentrations and Vehicles for 3700 Chemicals.* Amsterdam: Elsevier; 1994.
14. Guin JD. *Practical Contact Dermatitis: Handbook for the Practitioner.* New York: McGraw-Hill; 1995.
15. Rietschel RL, JFJ Fowler. *Fisher's Contact Dermatitis.* Baltimore: Williams & Wilkins; 1995.
16. Rycroft RJG, Menné T, et al. *Textbook of Contact Dermatitis.* Berlin: Springer-Verlag; 1995.
17. Fischer T Maibach HI. The thin layer rapid use epicutaneous test (TRUE test), a new patch test method with high accuracy. *Br J Dermatol* 1985; 112:63–68.
18. Lachapelle JM, Bruynzeel DP, et al. European multicenter study of the TRUE Test. *Contact Dermatitis* 1988; 19:91–7.
19. Fischer T, Maibach HI. Easier patch testing with TRUE test. *J Amer Acad Dermatol* 1989; 20:447–453.
20. TRUE Test Study Group. Comparative multicenter studies with TRUE test and Finn chamber in eight Swedish hospitals. *J Am Acad Dermatol* 1989; 21:486–489.
21. Wilkinson JD, Bruynzeel DD, et al. European multicenter study of TRUE Test, Panel 2. *Contact Dermatitis* 1990; 22:218–225.
22. Fischer T, Rystedt I. A case of contact sensitivity to aluminium. *Contact Dermatitis* 1982; 8:343.
23. Clemmensen O, Knudsen HE. Contact sensitivity to aluminium in a patient hyposensitized with aluminium precipitated grass pollen. *Contact Dermatitis* 1980; 6:305–308.
24. Wahlberg JE. Petrolatum: a reliable vehicle for metal allergens? *Contact Dermatitis* 1980; 6:134–135 [letter].
25. Mendelow AY, Forsyth A, et al. Patch testing for nickel allergy: the influence of the vehicle on the response rate to topical nickel sulphate. *Contact Dermatitis* 1985; 13:29–33.
26. van Ketel WG. Petrolatum again: an adequate vehicle in cases of metal allergy? *Contact Dermatitis* 1979; 5:192–193.
27. Magnusson B, Hersle K. Patch test methods. II. Regional variations of patch test responses. *Acta Derm Venereol* 1966; 45:257–261.
28. Fischer T, Maibach HI. Patch testing in allergic contact dermatitis, an update. *Occupational and Industrial Dermatology.* Chicago: Year Book Medical Publishers; 1987:190–210.
29. Belsito D. The mechanism of allergic contact dermatitis. In: Larsen GW, Adams RM, Maibach H, eds. *Color Text of Contact Dermatitis.* Philadelphia: W.B. Saunders: 1–4.
30. Bonnevie P. *Etiology and Pathogenesis of the Eczemas.* Copenhagen: Busck, A. Nyk Nordisk, Copenhagen; 1939.
31. Hjorth N. Routine patch tests. *Trans St Johns Hosp Derm Soc* 1963; 49:99–107.
32. Epstein E. Simplified patch test screening with mixtures. *Arch Dermatol* 1967; 95:269–274.
33. Epstein E, Rees ST, et al. Recent experience with routine patch test screening. *Arch Dermatol* 1968; 98:18–22.
34. Lammintausta K, Kalimo K. Sensitivity to rubber: study with rubber mixes and individual rubber chemicals. *Dermatosen* 1985; 33:204–208.
35. Bruynzeel DP, Andersen KE, et al. The European standard series: European Environmental and Contact Dermatitis Research Group (EECDRG). *Contact Dermatitis* 1995; 33:145–148.
36. Logan RA, White IR. Carbamix is redundant in the patch test series. *Contact Dermatitis* 1988; 18:303–304.
37. Wahlberg JE, Kartus E. Stability of formalin test solutions. *Contact Dermatitis* 1981; 7:43–44.
38. Fisher AA, Dooms-Goossens A. The effect of perfume "ageing" on the allergenicity of individual perfume ingredients. *Contact Dermatitis* 1976; 2:155–159.
39. Bruze M, Fregert S. Studies on purity and stability of photopatch test substances. *Contact Dermatitis* 1983; 9:33–39.
40. Fischer T, Maibach H. Finn chamber patch test technique. *Contact Dermatitis* 1984; 11:137.
41. Bjarnason B, Fischer T. Objective assessment of nickel sulphate patch test reactions with laser Doppler perfusion imaging. *Contact Dermatitis* 1998; 39:112–118.
42. Rietschel RL, Adams RM, et al. The case for patch test readings beyond day 2: notes. *J Am Acad Dermatol* 1988; 18:42–45.
43. Roed-Petersen J, Clemmensen OJ, et al. Purpuric contact dermatitis from black rubber chemicals. *Contact Dermatitis* 1988; 18:166–168.
44. Schmidt H, Larsen FS, et al. Petechial reaction following patch testing with cobalt. *Contact Dermatitis* 1980; 6:91–94.
45. Sulzberger MB. Discussion of paper by Anderson WA, Shatin H, Canizaras O: influence of varying physical factors on patch test responses. *J Invest Dermatol* 1958; 30:77.
46. Lachapelle JM, Tennstedt D, et al. Ring-shaped positive allergic patch test reactions to allergens in liquid vehicles. *Contact Dermatitis* 1988; 18:234–236.
46a. Bjarnason B, Fischer T. Patch test edges may indicate a corticosteroid test response. Margins of budesonide patch tests. (In manuscript.)
47. Hjorth N. Diagnostic patch tests. In: Marzulli F, Maibach HI, eds. *Dermatotoxicology and Pharmacology.* New York: John Wiley & Sons; 1977; 344–349.

48. Fischer T, Rystedt I. Cobalt allergy in hard-metal workers. *Contact Dermatitis* 1983; 9:115–121.
49. Wahlberg J, Maibach HI. Sterile cutaneous pustules: a manifestation of primary irritancy? *J Invest Dermatol* 1981; 76:381–383.
50. Mitchell JC. The angry back syndrome: eczema creates eczema. *Contact Dermatitis* 1975; 1:193–194.
51. Condie MW, Adams RM. Influence of oral prednisone on patch test reactions to rhus antigen. *Arch Dermatol* 1973; 107:540–543.
52. Sukanto H, Nater JP, et al. Influence of topically applied corticosteroids on patch test reactions. *Contact Dermatitis* 1981; 7:180–185.
53. Morison WL, Parish TA, et al. Influence of PUVA and UVB radiation on delayed hypersensitivity in the guinea pig. *J Invest Dermatol* 1981; 76:484–488.
54. Bruze M. Seasonal influence on routine patch test results. *Contact Dermatitis* 1986; 14:184.
55. Dooms-Goossens A, Lesaffre E, et al. UV sunlight and patch test reactions in humans. *Contact Dermatitis* 1988; 19:36–42.
56. Shelley WB. The patch test. *JAMA* 1967; 200:874–878.
57. Rudzki E, Grzywa Z. Hyperpigmentation from irritant patch tests. *Contact Dermatitis* 1977; 3:53.
58. Bruze M, Björkner B, et al. Skin testing with gold sodium thiomalate and gold sodium thiosulfate. *Contact Dermatitis* 1995; 32:5–8.
59. Meneghini CL, Angelini G. Behaviour of contact allergy and new sensitivities on subsequent patch tests. *Contact Dermatitis* 1977; 3:138–142.
60. Fisher A. Urticarial and systemic reactions to contactants varying from hair bleach to seminal fluid. *Cutis* 1977; 19:715.
61. Maibach HI, Johnson HL. Contact urticaria syndrome. *Arch Dermatol* 1975; 111:726–730.
62. Jordan WPJ. *The Role of Patch Testing in Allergic Contact Dermatitis.* N.J.: Johnson & Johnson; 1980.
63. Wilkinson DE, Fregert S, et al. Terminology of contact dermatitis. *Acta Derm Venereol* 1970; 50:287–292.
64. Adams RM. Allergen replacement in industry. *Cutis* 1977; 20:511–516.
65. Fisher AA. Allergen replacement in allergic dermatitis. *Int J Dermatol* 1977; 16:319–328.
66. Adams RM, Fisher AA. Contact allergen alternatives. *J Am Acad Dermatol* 1986; 14:951–969.

Bibliography

Fregert S. Contact allergy to phenoplastics. *Contact Dermatitis* 1981; 7:170.
Lachapelle JM. Occupational allergic contact dermatitis to povidone-iodine. *Contact Dermatitis* 1984; 11:189–190.

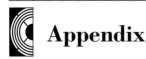

Appendix

Contact Allergens: Their Sources and Uses

Numerical Code for Uses of Allergens

1 = Cosmetics, hair, and manicure materials
2 = Dental materials
3 = Food additives, flavors, bakery materials
4 = Fragrances, perfumes, balsams
5 = Medications, local anesthetics, antibiotics
6 = Metals and metal compounds
7 = Oils, coolants, machining oils
8 = Organic dyes, textile colors, and finishes
9 = Paints, varnishes, lacquers
10 = Pesticides
11 = Photoallergens
12 = Photographic chemicals
13 = Plants, woods
14 = Plastics, adhesives
15 = Preservatives, antimicrobials
16 = Rubber chemicals
17 = Shoe chemicals
18 = Soldering chemicals
19 = Sunscreens
20 = Various sources
21 = Vehicles, emulsifiers

Columns

A = Inclusion in standard series:
    N = Included in NACDG standard series
    E = Included in EECDRG standard series
    J = Included in JCDS standard series
B = Marketed by:
    C = Chemotechnique
    H = Trolab/Hermal
C = Sources according to numerical code
D = Name of allergen/substance and common synonyms
E = Recommended test concentration and vehicle

A	B	C	D	E
	C, T	7, 14, 21	Abietic acid	5–10% pet
			Abitol (see Hydroabietyl alcohol)	
	C		*Achillea millefolium* (Yarrow)	1% pet
	C		Acid black 2 (see Nigrosin B)	
	C	8, 17	Acid yellow 36	1% pet
	C		Agerite resin D (see 2,2,4-Trimethyl-1,2-dihydroquinolone)	
	C		Agfa (see 4-Amino-*N,N*-diethylaniline sulfate)	
	C, T	13	Alantolactone (Helenin, in sesquiterpene lactone mix)	0.1% pet
	C	5	Aclometasone-1,7,21-dipropionate	1% pet
	C		Allocaine (see Procaine hydrochloride)	
		14	Allyl glycidyl ether	0.25% acetone
	C	6	Aluminum	as is
	C	1, 5	Aluminum chloride hexahydrate	2% pet
	T	5	Amcinonide	0.1% pet
	C, T	21	Amerchol L 101 (Wool alcohols and Mineral oil)	50% pet
			Amethocaine hydrochloride (see Tetracaine hydrochloride)	
	C	8, 17	4-Aminoazobenzene	0.25% pet
	C, T	11, 19	4-Aminobenzoic acid (PABA)	2–5% pet
		8, 12	4-Aminodiethylaniline	1% pet
	C	12	4-Amino-*N,N*-diethylaniline sulfate (TSS, AGFA)	1% pet
	T	8, 12	4-Aminodiphenylamine hydrochloride	0.25% pet
		18, 20	Aminoethylethanolamine	1% pet
		1, 8	2-Aminophenol	10% pet
	C, T	1, 8, 12	3-Aminophenol	1% pet
	C, T	1, 7, 8, 12	4-Aminophenol	1% pet
			Ammoniated mercury chloride (see Mercury chloride, ammoniated)	
	C	6	Ammonium hexachloroplatinate	0.1% aq
	C, T	1, 12	Ammonium persulfate	2.5% pet
	C, T	2, 6, 12	Ammonium tetrachloroplatinate	0.25% pet
	C, T	1	Ammonium thioglycolate	2.5% pet
	C, T	3, 4	α-Amyl cinnamaldehyde (in fragrance mix)	1% pet
	C	5	Amylocaine hydrochloride (Stovaine, 1-dimethylamino-2-methyl-2-butanolbenzoate hydrochloride, in some caine mixes)	1% pet
	C	3, 4	Anethole	5% pet
		4	Anisyl alcohol	5% pet
		4	Anisyl acetone	2% pet
			Antabuse (see Tetraethylthiuram disulfide)	
	C	13	*Anthemis cotula*	1% pet
			Anthemis nobilis (see Chamomilla Romana)	
		5, 8	Anthraquinone	2% pet
		6, 9	Antimony chloride	1% aq
	C		Arlacel 83 (see Sorbitan sesquioleate)	
	C, T	5	*Arnica montana* (Mountain tobacco)	0.5% pet
			Arnica tincture	20% pet
	C		Atosil (see Promethazine hydrochloride)	
	C, T	4, 11, 13	Atranorin (in lichen acid mix)	0.1–0.5% pet
			Aureomycin (see Chlortetracycline)	
	C		1-Aza-3,7-dioxa-5-ethyl-bicyclo(3,3,0)-octane (Bioban CS 1246)	1.0% pet
	C	14	Azodiisobutyrodinitrile	1% pet
	C, T	5	Bacitracin	5–20% pet
N, E, J	C, T	3, 4, 5, 9, 11	Balsam of Peru	25% pet
		4, 13	Balsam of pine	20% pet
		4	Balsam of spruce	20% pet
	C, T	4, 5	Balsam of Tolu	20% pet
		6, 9, 17	Basic chromium sulfate (Trivalent chromium)	5–10% pet

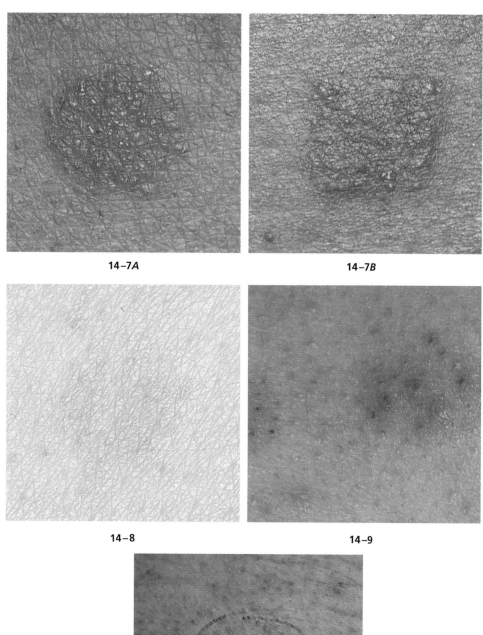

14–7A   14–7B

14–8   14–9

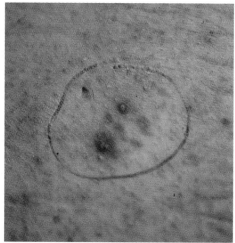

14–10

COLOR PLATE I

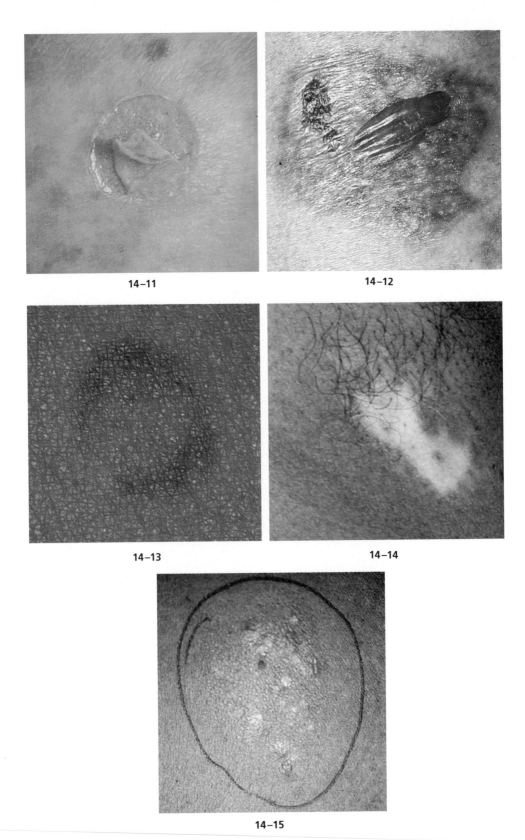

14–11

14–12

14–13

14–14

14–15

COLOR PLATE II

A	B	C	D	E
	C	8	Basic red 46	1% pet
		13	Beech (in wood mix)	5% pet
	C	5, 13	Beech tar (in wood tar mix)	3% pet
		9, 17, 21	Beeswax	30% pet
			Benlate (see Benomyl)	
	T	10	Benomyl (Benlate, (1-butylcarbamoyl)-2-benzimidazole-carbamic acid methylester)	0.1% pet
	T	3, 4, 15	Benzaldehyde	5% pet
	C, T	5, 15	Benzalkonium chloride	0.1% aq
		20	Benzidine	2% MEK
	C, T	1, 5, 9	1,2-Benz-isothiazolin-3-one (BIT, Proxel)	0.05–0.1% pet
N, E	C, T	2, 5	Benzocaine	5% pet
	C, T	15	Benzoic acid	5% pet
		4, 5	Benzoin tincture	10% alc
		19	Benzophenone-1 (2,4-Dihydroxybenzophenone)	1% pet
		19	Benzophenone-2 (2,2′,4,4′-Tetrahydroxybenzophenone)	1% pet
	C, T	19	Benzophenone-3 (2-Hydroxy-4-methoxybenzophenone, Eusolex 4360, Escalol 567, Oxybenzone)	2% pet
	C, T	19	Benzophenone-4 (2-Hydroxy-4-methoxybenzophenone-sulfonic acid, Sulisobenzone, Uvinyl MS-40)	5% pet
		19	Benzophenone-8 (2,2′-Dihydroxy-4-methoxybenzophenone; Dioxybenzone)	2% pet
	C	19	Benzophenone-10 (2-Hydroxy-4-methoxy-4′-methylbenzophenone, Mexenone)	2% pet
	C, T	7, 12, 14, 21	1H-Benzotriazole (Tinuvin P, 2(2′-Hydroxy-5′-methyl-phenyl) benzotriazole)	1% pet
	C, T	3, 5, 14	Benzoyl peroxide	1% pet
	C, T	3, 4, 5	Benzyl alcohol	1% pet
		4, 15	Benzyl benzoate	5% pet
	T	3, 4	Benzyl cinnamate	5% pet
	C	15	Benzyl-4-hydroxybenzoate (Benzyl paraben)	3% pet
		4	Benzylideneaceton	0.5% pet
	C, T	4, 19, 21	Benzyl salicylate	2% pet
		4	Bergamot oil	2% pet
		6	Beryllium chloride	0.5% aq
	C, T	5	Betamethasone-17-valerate	0.1–1% pet
		3, 14, 21	BHA (Butyl hydroxyanisole, 2-tert-Butyl-4-methoxyphenol)	2% pet
		3, 14	BHT (Butyl hydroxytoluene, 2,6-di-tert-Butyl-4-cresol)	2% pet
	C	7, 9, 15	Bioban CS 1135 (see also 4,4-Dimethyloxazolidine and 3,4,4-Trimethyloxazolidine)	1% pet
	C	7, 9, 15	Bioban CS 1246 (see 1-Aza-3,7-dioxa-5-ethylbicyclo(3,3,0)-octane)	1% pet
	C	7, 15	Bioban P 1487 (see also 4-(2-nitrobutyl)morpholine and 4,4-(2-ethyl-2-nitrotrimethylene)dimorpholine)	1% pet
	C	5, 13	Birch tar	3% pet
		13	Birch wood	3% pet
			Bis(dibutyl-dithiocarbamate)zinc (see Zinc dibutyl-dithiocarbamate)	
			Bis(diethyl-dithiocarbamate)zinc (see Zinc diethyldithiocarbamate)	
			BIS-EMA (see 2,2-bis(4-[2-Methacryloxyethoxy]phenyl)propane)	
			BIS-GMA (see 2,2,bis(4-[2-hydroxy-3-methacryloxypropoxy]phenyl) propane)	
			BIS-MA (see 2,2-bis(4-methacryloxyphenyl)propane)	
		11, 14	Bismark brown	1% pet
	C, T	11, 14	Bisphenol A	1% pet
		14	Bisphenol A dimethacrylate	2% pet
			BIT (see 1,2-Benzisothiazolin-3-one)	
	C, T	11, 15	Bithionol (2,2′-Thiobis[4,6-dichlorophenol])	1% pet

A	B	C	D	E
N, J	C, T	16	Black rubber mix (PPD-mix; N-Cyclohexyl-N-phenyl-4-phenyl-enediamin N,N-Diphenyl-4-phenylenediamine and N-Isopropyl-N-phenyl-4-phenylenediamin)	0.6% pet
			2-Bromo-2-nitropropane-1,3-diol (see Bronopol)	
	C, T	1, 15	Bronopol (2-Bromo-2-nitropropane-1,3-diol)	0.25–0.5% pet
			BUDA (see 1,4-Butanediol diacrylate)	
	C, T	5	Budesonide	0.1% pet
	C	2, 14, 20	1,4-Butanediol diacrylate (BUDA)	0.1% pet
			BUDMA (see Butanediol dimethacrylate)	0.1% pet
	T		Bufexamac	5% pet
	C	2, 14, 20	1,4-Butanediol dimethacrylate (BUDMA)	2% pet
			2-Butoxy-N-(2-[diethylamino]ethyl)-4-quinolinecarboxy-amide hydrochloride (see Dibucaine hydrochloride)	
	C	8, 9, 14	n-Butyl acrylate	0.1% pet
			4-(Butylamino)benzoic acid 2-(dimethylamino)ethyl-ester hydrochloride (see Tetracaine hydrochloride)	
	C	7	4-tert-Butylbenzoic acid	3% pet
	C, T	7, 9, 14	4-tert-Butylcatechol, 1-Butylcarbamoyl-2-benzimidazole-carbamic acid methyl ester (see Benomyl)	1% pet
			2,6,-di-tert-Butyl-4-cresol (see BHT)	
		14	N-Butyl glycidyl ether	0.25% acetone
	C, T	21	4-N-Butyl hydroquinone	1% pet
			Butylhydroxyanisole (see BHA)	
	C, T	3, 15	Butyl-4-hydroxybenzoate (Butyl paraben, in paraben mix)	3% pet
			Butylhydroxytoluene (see BHT)	
	C	2, 14	N-Butylmethacrylate	2% pet
		4	4-N-Butyl-α-methyl hydrocinnamic aldehyde (Lilial)	20% pet
	C, T	11, 19	N-Butyl-4-methoxy-4-dibenzoylmethan (Parasol 1789)	2–10% pet
			2-N-Butyl-4-methoxyphenol (see BHA)	
			Butyl paraben (see Butyl-4-hydroxybenzoate)	
	C, T	7, 9, 14	4-N-Butylphenol	2% pet
N, E, J	C, T	14, 17	4-N-Butylphenol formaldehyde resin (PTBF)	1% pet
	C	6, 9, 11, 12	Cadmium chloride	1% aq
J	C	5	Caine mixes (various compositions of Amylocaine hydrochloride, Benzocaine, Dibucaine hydrochloride, Lidocaine, Prilocaine, Procaine hydrochloride, Tetracaine hydrochloride)	3.5–10% pet
		5, 14, 15	Camphor	10% pet
	C	4	Canaga oil	2% pet
	T	10	Captafol (N-(1,1,2,2-Tetrachloroethylthio)-4-cyclohexene-1,2-dicarboximide, Dilolatan)	0.1% pet
	C, T	10, 15	Captan (N-(Trichloromethylthio)-4-cyclohexene-1,2-dicarboximide)	0.1% pet
N	C, T	15, 16	Carbamix (1,3-Diphenylquanidine, Zinc diethyldithiocarbamate, Zinc dibutyldithiocarbamate)	3% pet
			CBS (see N-Cyclohexyl-2-benzothiazylsulfenamide)	
	T	4, 11	Cedarwood oil	10% pet
	C	21	Cetyl alcohol	5% pet
	T	21	Cetyl/stearyl alcohol	20% pet
	C		Chamomilla Romana (Anthemis nobilis)	1% pet
			Chinoform (see Clioquinol)	
	T	15	Chloramine T	0.5% aq
	C, T	5	Chloramphenicol	5% pet
	C	11, 15	Chlorhexidine diacetate	0.5% aq
	C, T	11, 15	Chlorhexidine digluconate	0.5% aq
	C, T	7, 14, 15	2-Chloroacetamide	0.2% pet
N, E	C, T	5, 15	1-(3-Chloroallyl)-3 5,7-triaza-1-azoniaadamantane chloride (Quaternium 15, Dowicil 200)	1%
	C, T	1, 7, 15	4-Chloro-3-cresol (PCMC)	1% pet
		15	2-Chloro-N-hydroxy methylacetamide	0.2% pet
			5-Chloro-7-iodo-8-quinolinol (see Clioquinol)	

A	B	C	D	E
E, J	C, T	7, 15	5-Chloro-2-methyl-4-isothiazolin-3-one and 2-Methyl-4-isothiazolin-3-one 3:1 (Kathon CC)	0.01% aq
		15	Chlorothymol	2% pet
	C, T	1, 7, 15	4-Chloro-3-xylenol (PCMX)	1% pet
	C, T	5, 11	Chlorpromazine hydrochloride	0.1% pet
	C, T	5	Chlorquinaldol (5,7-dichloro-2-methyl-8-quinolinol, Sterosan, in quinoline mix)	5% pet
		5, 11	Chlortetracycline (Aureomycin)	3% pet
	C, T	10, 13	*Chrysanthemum cinerariaefolium* (Pyrethrum)	1–2% pet
	T	13	*Chrysanthemum parthenium* (Feverfew)	1% pet
			Cincaine hydrochloride (see Dibucaine hydrochloride)	
			Cinchocaine hydrochloride (see Dibucaine hydrochloride)	
	C, T	3, 4	Cinnamic alcohol (in fragrance mix)	1–2% pet
N	C, T	3, 4	Cinnamic aldehyde (in fragrance mix)	1% pet
		4	Citral	2% pet
		4	Citronella oil	2% pet
			Clioquinol (5-Chloro-7-iodo-8 quinolin, Chinoforum, Viotorm, Iodochlor-hydroxyquinoline, inquinoline mix)	
	C, T	5	Clobetasol-1,7-propionate	0.25–1% pet
	T	5	Clotrimazol	5% pet
	T	4	Clove oil (Madagascar)	2% pet
		5, 13	Coal tar	5% pet
E	C, T	6, 9	Cobalt (II) chloride hexahydrate	0.5 to 1% pet
		6, 9	Cobalt sulfate	2% aq
		6, 9, 12, 16	Cobalt naphthenate	2% pet
			Cocamide-DEA (see Coconut diethanolamide)	
	C, T	1, 7, 21	Cocamidopropyl betaine (Tegobetaine L7)	1% aq
	C, T	7, 21	Coconut diethanolamide	0.5% pet
N, E, J	C, T	2, 7, 9, 17, 21	Colophony (rosin)	20% pet
		12	CD-1 (Color Developer-1; 4-*N*,*N*-Diethyl-1,4-phenylenediamine sulfate monohydrate)	1% pet
	C, T	12	CD-2 (Color Developer-2; *N*,*N*-Diethyl-2-methyl-1,4-phenylenediamine hydrochloride)	1% pet
	C, T	12	CD-3 (Color Developer-3; 4-*N*-Ethyl-*N*-(2-methane sulfonamidoethyl)-2-methyl-1,4-phenylenediamine sesquisulfate hydrate)	1% pet
	C, T	12	CD-4 (Color Developer-4; (4-(*N*-Ethyl-*N*-2-hydroxyethyl)-2-methylparaphenylenediamine sulfate mono-hydrate)	1% pet
		12	CD-6 (Color Developer-6; (4-(*N*-Ethyl-*N*-2-methoxyethyl)-2-methylphenylenediamine ditoluene sulfonate)	1% pet
		8	Congo red	2% pet
		4	Coniferyl benzoate	2% pet
	C	6	Copper oxide	5% pet
	C	2, 6, 9, 10	Copper sulfate	1% aq
	C		Costunolide (in sesquiterpene lactone mix)	
		4, 13	Costus root oil	0.1% pet
		4, 11	Coumarin	5% pet
		4	Coumarin aldehyde	5% pet
			CPPD (see *N*-Cyclohexyl-*N*-phenyl-phenylenediamine)	
	T	14	Cresyl glycidyl ether	0.25% pet
		4	Cumin aldehyde	15% pet
		4	Cyclamen aldehyde	3% pet
	T	14	Cyclohexyl thiophthalimide	1% pet
	C, T	16	*N*-Cyclohexylbenzothiazyl sulphenamide (CBS, in mercapto mix)	1% pet
	C	16	*N*-Cyclohexyl-*N'*-phenyl paraphenylenediamine (in black rubber mix)	
			Dandelion (see *Taraxacum officinale*)	
			DDT (see Dichlorodiphenyltrichloroethane)	

A	B	C	D	E
			Dehydrocostus lactone (see Sesquiterpene lactone mix)	0.25% pet
			Derris root (see Rotenone)	
			DETA (see Diethylenetriamine)	
	C, T	5	Dexamethasone-21-phosphate disodium salt	1% pet
	C	13	Diallyl disulfide	1% pet
	C, T	14, 16	4,4′-Diaminodiphenylmethane (Methylenedianilin)	0.5% pet
	C, T	1, 14	2,5-Diaminotoluene sulfate (Toluene-2,5-diamine sulphate)	1% pet
	C, T	15	Diazolidinyl urea (Germall II)	2% pet
	C, T	16	Dibenzothiazyl disulfide (MBTS, in mercapto mix)	1% pet
	C, T	7, 9, 15	1,2-Dibromo-2,4-dicyanobutane (Tekamer 38, in Euxyl K400)	0.1% pet
		11, 15	Dibromosalicylanilide	1% pet
	C, T	5	Dibucaine dihydrochloride (2-butoxy-N-(2-[diethylamino]-ethyl]-4-quinolinecarboxamide monohydrochloride); Cincaine; Cinchocain; Nupercaine; Percaine, in some caine mixes)	5% pet
			2,6-Di-tert-butyl-4-cresol (see BHT)	
	C, T	3, 14, 21	Di-N-butyl phthalate	5% pet
	C, T	16, 17	Dibutylthiourea	1% pet
		15	Dichlorodiphenyltrichloroethane (DDT)	1% pet
			5,7-Dichloro-2-methyl-8-quinolinol (see Chlorquinaldol)	5% pet
	C, T	7, 15	Dichlorophene	0.5–1% pet
		5	Dienestrol (diethylstilbestrol)	1% pet
		5, 15	Diethylenediamine (Piperazine)	1% pet
	C	14	Diethylene glycol diacrylate (GEGDA)	0.1% pet
	C, T	14	Diethylenetriamine (DETA)	0.5% pet
			Diethylhexylphthalate (see Dioctyl phthalate)	
		4	Diethyl maleate	0.1% pet
	T	14	Diethyl phthalate	5% pet
			N,N-Diethyl-2-methyl-1,4-phenylenediamine hydrochloride (see CD-2, Color Developer 2)	
			4-N,N-Diethyl-1,4-phenylenediamine sulfate monohydrate (see CD-1, Color Developer 1)	
	C	16	Diethyl thiourea	1% pet
			2,4-Dihydroxybenzophenone (see Benzophenone 1)	
		4	Dihydroxycoumarin	5% pet
		16	4,4′-Dihydroxydiphenyl (DOD)	0.1% pet
			2,2′-Dihydroxy-4-methoxybenzophenone (see Benzophenone 8)	
		14	Diisodecylphthalate	5% pet
			Dilolatan (see Captafol)	
			1-Dimethylamino-2-methyl-2-butanolbenzoate hydrochloride (see Amylocaine hydrochloride)	
		4	Dimethylcitraconate	12% pet
			3,4-Dimethyloxazolidine (Bioban CS 1135)	1% pet
		14	Dimethyl phthalate	5% pet
	C	2, 14	N,N-Dimethylaminoethyl methacrylate	0.2% pet
	C	8	Dimethylol dihydroxy ethylene urea (Fixapret CPN)	4.5% aq
		8	Dimethylol methoxy propylene urea (Fixapret PCL)	5% aq
	C	8	Dimethylol propylene urea (Fixapret PH)	5% aq
			4,4-Dimethyloxazolidine (see Bioban CS 1135)	
		14	Dimethylphthalate	5% pet
	C, T	2, 14	N,N′-Dimethyl-4-toluide	2–5% pet
	C	16	N,N-Di-β-naphthyl-4-phenylenediamine (DBNPD, DNP, in naphthyl mix)	1% pet
	C	14	Dioctyl phthalate (Diethylhexylphthalate)	2–5% pet
		9	Dioxane	1% pet
			Dioxybenzone (see Benzophenone 8)	
	C, T	16, 17	Dipentamethylene thiuram disulfide (PTD, in Thiuram mix)	0.25–1% pet
	C, T	3, 4, 7, 9	Dipentene (D,L-limonene)	1–2% pet
	C	5, 11	Diphenhydramine hydrochloride	1% pet
	C, T	16	1,3-Diphenylguanidine (DPG, in carba mix)	1% pet
	C, T	9, 14, 16	Diphenylmethane-4,4-diisocyanate	0.1–2% pet
	C, T	16	N,N′-Diphenyl-4-phenylenediamine (DPPD, in black rubber mix)	0.25–1% pet

A	B	C	D	E
	C, T	14, 16, 17	Diphenylthiourea (Thiocarbanilide, DPTU)	1% pet
	T		Disperse blue 1	1% pet
	C, T	8	Disperse blue 3	1% pet
	C	8	Disperse blue 35	1% pet
	C	8	Disperse blue 85	1% pet
	C	8	Disperse blue 106	1% pet
	C	8	Disperse blue 124	1% pet
	C	8	Disperse blue 153	1% pet
	C	8	Disperse brown 1	1% pet
	C	8	Disperse orange 1	1% pet
	C, T	8	Disperse orange 3	1% pet
	C	8	Disperse orange 13	1% pet
	C, T	8	Disperse red 1	1% pet
	T		Disperse red 3	1% pet
	C, T	8	Disperse red 17	1% pet
	C, T	8	Disperse yellow 3	1% pet
	C, T	8	Disperse yellow 9	1% pet
			Disulfiram (see Tetraethylthiuram disulfide)	
J			Dithiocarbamate mix	2% pet
		16	4,4'-Dithiodimorpholine	1% pet
	T	14	Diurethane dimethacrylate	2% pet
	C, T	1, 21	DMDM hydantoin (Dimethylol dimethyl hydantoin)	1% pet
			DNP (see N,N-DI-β-naphtyl-4-phenylenediamine)	
			DOD (see 4,4'-Dihydroxydiphenyl)	
	C, T	3, 7, 21	Dodecyl gallate (Lauryl gallate)	0.25% pet
	C	14, 16, 17	Dodecyl mercaptan	0.1% pet
			Dog fennel (see Anthemis cotula)	
			DOP (see Di-N-butylphthalate)	
			Dowicil 200 (see 1-(3-Chloroallyl)-3 5,7-triaza-1-azonia-adamantane chloride)	
			Dowicide 1 (see 6-Phenylphenol)	
			DPG (see 1,3-Diphenylguanidine)	
			DPPD (see N,N-Diphenyl-4-phenylenediamine)	
			DPTU (see N,N-Diphenylthiourea)	
			Ebecryl 220 (see Urethane diacrylate, aromatic)	
			Ebecryl 270 (see Urethane diacrylate, aliphatic)	
	C		Econazole nitrate	1% alc
			EDTA (see Ethylenediaminetetraacetic acid disodium dihydrate)	
			EGDMA (see Ethylene glycol dimethacrylate)	
			EHA (see 2-Ethylhexyl acrylate)	
			EMA (see Ethyl methacrylate)	
		5, 8, 21	Eosin	50% pet
		14	Epichlorhydrin	0.1% pet
	C	9, 14	Epoxy acrylate	0.5% pet
N, E, J	C, T	14	Epoxy resin (Bisphenol A-epichlorhydrin)	1% pet
	C		Epoxy resin, cycloaliphatic	0.5% pet
	T	5	Erythromycin	1% pet
			Escalol 106 (see Glyceryl mono-4-aminobenzoic acid)	
			Escalol 507 (see 2-Ethylhexyl-4-dimethylaminobenzoate)	
			Escalol 557 (see 2-Ethylhexyl-4-methoxy cinnamate)	
			Escalol 567 (see Benzophenone 3)	
			6-Ethoxy-1,2-dihydroxy-2,2,4-trimethylquinoline (see Ethoxyquin)	
		19	Ethoxyethyl-4-methoxycinnamate	1% pet
	C	11, 16	Ethoxyquin (6-Ethoxy-1,2-dihydroxy-2,2,4-trimethylquinoline)	0.5% pet
	C	14	Ethyl acrylate	0.1% pet
		16, 17	Ethylbutyl thiourea	1% pet
N, J	C, T	5, 12, 14, 16, 21	Ethylenediamine dihydrochloride	1% pet
	C, T	5, 21	Ethylenediaminetetraacetic acid disodium dihydrate (EDTA)	1% pet
		9, 20	Ethylene glycol	5% alc
	C, T	2, 14	Ethylene glycol dimethacrylate	2% pet

A	B	C	D	E
	C	8, 16	Ethylene thiourea	1% pet
	C	8, 9, 10	Ethylene urea (in Fixapret AC)	10% pet
	C	14	2-Ethylhexyl acrylate (EHA)	0.5% pet
	C, T	19	2-Ethylhexyl-4-dimethylaminobenzoate (Eusolex 6007, Escalol 507, Octyldimethyl-PABA)	2–10% pet
	C, T		2-Ethylhexyl-4-methoxy cinnamate (Octyl methoxycinnamate, Parsol MCX, Escalol 557)	2–10% pet
	C, T	15	Ethyl-4-hydroxybenzoate (Ethyl paraben, in paraben mix)	3% pet
			4-(N-Ethyl-N-2-hydroxyethyl)-2-methyl-1,4-phenylene-diamine sulfate monohydrate (see CD-4, Color Developer 4)	
	C	14	Ethyl methacrylate	2% pet
			4-N-Ethyl-N-(2-methane-sulfonamidoethyl)2-methyl-1,4-phenylenediamine sesquisulfate hydrate (see CD-3, Color Developer 3)	
			4-(N-Ethyl-N-methoxyethyl)-2-methyl-phenylenediamine ditoluene sulfonate, (see CD-6, Color Developer 6)	
			4,4-(2-Ethyl-2-nitrotrimethylene) dimorpholine (see Bioban P1487)	
			Ethyl paraben (see Ethyl-4-hydroxy benzoate)	
	C	2, 14	N-Ethyl-4-toluenesulfonamide	0.1% alc
	T	2, 4	Eucalyptus oil	2% pet
		21	Eucerin	as is
	C, T	1, 2, 3, 4	Eugenol (in Fragrance mix)	1–2% pet
			Eusolex 232 (see Phenylbenzimidazol-5-sulphonic acid)	
			Eusolex 4360 (see Benzophenone 3)	
			Eusolex 6007 (see 2-Ethylhexyl-4-dimethylaminobenzoate)	
			Eusolex 6300 (see 3-(4′-Methylbenzylidene) camphor)	
			Eusolex 8020 (see 4-Isopropyl dibenzoyl methane)	
			Eusolex 8021 (see 3-(4′-Methylbenzylidene) camphor and 4-isopropyl dibenzoyl methane)	
	C, T	1	Euxyl K 400 (1,2-Dibromo-2,4-dicyanobutane and 2-Phenoxy-ethanol)	0.5% pet
	C	11, 13	Evernic acid (in lichen acid mix)	0.1% pet
		4	Farnesol	4% pet
			Fenazil (see Promethazine hydrochloride)	
	C	10, 11	Fenticlor	1% pet
			Feverfew (see *Chrysanthemum parthenium*)	
			Fixapret AC (see Ethylene urea and Melamine formaldehyde)	
			Fixapret CPN (see Dimethylol dihydroxyethyleneurea)	
			Fixapret PCL (see Dimethylol methoxypropylene urea)	
			Fixapret PH (see Dimethylol propylene urea)	
			Fixapret 140 (see Tetramethylol acetylene diurea)	
			Flectol H (see 2,2,4-Trimethyl-1,2-dihydroxyquinoline)	
		8	Fluorescein sodium (D and C yellow no. 8)	1% pet
	T	9, 10	Folpet (Phaltan, N-(Trichloromethylthio) phthalimide)	0.1% pet
N, E, J	C, T	7, 8, 9, 14, 15	Formaldehyde	1% aq
E. J J	C, T	4	Fragrance mix	8% pet
			Fradiomycin sulphate (see Neomycin sulphate)	
		5, 8	Fuchsin	1% pet
			2,5-Furandione (see Maleic anhydride)	
	T	5	Fusnic acid disodium salt	2% pet
			Galaxolide (see 1,3,4,6,7,8-Hexahydro-4,6,6,7,8,8-hexa-methyl cyclopenta-γ-2-benzopyran)	
			GEDA (see Diethylene glycol diacrylate)	
	C, T	5	Gentamycin sulfate	20% pet
		5, 8	Gentian violet	1% aq
	C, T	4	Geraniol (in fragrance mix)	1–2% pet
	C	4	Geranium oil of Bourbon	2% pet
			Germall II (see Diazolidinyl urea)	
			Germall 115 (see Imidazolidinyl urea)	
	C, T	12, 14, 15, 17	Glutaraldehyde	0.2–0.3% pet

A	B	C	D	E
		19	Glyceryl mono-4-aminobenzoic acid (Escalol 106)	5% pet
	C, T	1	Glyceryl monothioglycolate	1% pet
		14	Glycol dimethacrylate	2% pet
		2, 6, 12	Gold chloride	0.1% aq
		6	Gold leaf	as is
	C, T	2, 5, 6	Gold sodium thiosulfate (Sodiumthiosulfatoaurate)	0.25–0.5% pet
			Grotan BK (see Hexahydro-1,3-5-tris-(2-hydroxy-ethyl)triazine)	
			Grotan HD (see N-Methylolchloroacetamide)	0.1% pet
			Grotan K (see 5-Chloro-2-methyl-4-isothiazolin-3-one, and 2-Methyl-4-isothiazolin-3-one 3:1)	
		10	Haloprogin	1% pet
		5	Halquinol	1% pet
			HDDA (see 1,6-Hexanediol diacrylate)	
			HEA (see 2-Hydroxyethyl acrylate)	
			Helenin (see Alantolactone)	
			HEMA (see 2-Hydroxyethyl methacrylate)	
	C, T	11, 15	Hexachlorophene	1% pet
		4	1,3,4,6,7,8-Hexahydro-4,6,6,7,8,8-hexamethyl-cyclopenta-γ-2-benzopyran (Galaxolide)	25% pet
		14	Hexahydrophthalic anhydride	1% pet
	C	7, 15	Hexahydro-1,3,5-tris-(2-hydroxy-ethyl)triazine (Grotan BK)	1% pet
	C, T	7, 8, 14, 15	Hexamethylenetetramine (Methenamine, Hexamine)	1–2% pet
			Hexamine (see Hexamethylenetetramine)	
	C	14	1,6-Hexanedioldiacrylate (HDDA)	0.1% pet
		4	N-Hexyl cinnamic aldehyde	10% pet
		5, 15	Hexylresorcinol	1% pet
			HPMA (see 2-Hydroxypropyl methacrylate)	
		14	Hydrazine monobromide	1% pet
	C	7, 12, 15	Hydrazine sulfate	1% pet
		7, 14, 17, 21	Hydroabietic acid	10% pet
	C, T	4, 7, 9, 14, 21	Hydroabietyl alcohol (Abitol)	5–10% pet
		5	Hydrocortisone	25% pet
	C, T	5	Hydrocortisone-17-butyrate	0.1–1% alc
	C	1	Hydrogen peroxide	3% aq
	C, T	12, 14, 16	Hydroquinone	1% pet
	C	9, 16, 21	Hydroquinone monobenzylether (Monobenzone)	1% pet
			2,4-Hydroxybenzophenone (see Benzophenone 1)	
	C, T	4	Hydroxycitronellal (in Fragrance mix)	1–2% pet
	C	14	2-Hydroxyethyl acrylate (HEA)	0.1% pet
	C, T	14	2-Hydroxyethyl methacrylate (HEMA)	1–2% pet
			2-Hydroxy-4-methoxybenzophenone (see Benzophenone 3)	
	C	2, 14	2,2-bis(4-[Hydroxy-3-methacryloxypropoxy]-phenyl)propane (BIS-GMA)	2% pet
			2-Hydroxy-4-methoxy-4′-methyl benzophenone, (see Benzophenone 10)	
			Hydroxy-4-methoxy-5-sulfonic acid, 2-(see Benzophenone 4)	
	C	8, 12	Hydroxylammonium sulfate	0.1% aq
	C, T	7, 14, 15	2-Hydroxymethyl-2-nitro-1,3-propanediol (Tris-Nitro)	1% pet
			2(2′-Hydroxy-5′-methyl-phenyl) benzotriazole (see 1H-Benzotriazole)	
	C	14	Hydroxypropyl acrylate	0.1% pet
	C	14	2-Hydroxypropyl methacrylate (HPMA)	2% pet
		5, 15	8-Hydroxyquinoline	5% pet
		5	Idoxuridine	0.5% pet
N	C, T	15	Imidazolidinyl urea (Germall 115)	2% pet
E	C, T	5	Iodochlorhydroxyquin, (see Clioquinol)	
			Iodochlorhydroxyquinoline (see Clioquinol)	
			IPPD (see N-Isopropyl-N-phenyl-4-phenylenediamine)	

A	B	C	D	E
			IPDI (see Isophorone diisocyanate)	5% pet
			Irgasan BS 200 (see Tetrachlorsalicylanilide)	
			Irgasan OP 300 (see Trichlorsalicylanilide)	
	C, T	3, 4	Isoeugenol (in fragrance mix)	1–2% pet
	C, T	14	Isophorone diamine	0.1–0.5% pet
	C	14	Isophorone diisocyanate (IPDI)	1% pet
	C, T	11, 19	4-Isopropyl-dibenzoyl-methane (1-(4-Isopropylphenyl)-3-phenyl-1,3-propanedione, Eusolex 8020, in Eusolex 8021)	2–10% pet
	C, T	21	Isopropyl myristate	10–20% pet
			1-(4-Isopropylphenyl)-3-phenyl-1,3-propanedione (see 4-Isopropyl-dibenzoyl methane)	
E	C, T	16, 17	N-Isopropyl-N-phenyl-4-phenylene diamine (IPPD, in black rubber mix)	0.1% pet
			Cl-Me-Isothiazolinone (see 5-Chloro-2-methyl-4-iso-thiazolin-3-one and 2-Methyl-4-isothiazolin-3-one 3:1)	
	C	4	Jasmine absolute, Egyptian	10% pet
	C	4	Jasmine synthetic	10% pet
	C	4, 5, 13	Juniper tar (in wood tar mix)	3% pet
	C, T	5	Kanamycin sulfate	10–20% pet
E, J	C, T	7, 15	Kathon CG (see also 5-Chloro-2-methyl-4-isothiazolin-3-one and 2-Methyl-4-isothiazolin-3-one); in European standard: Cl + Me-Isothiazolinone	0.01% aq
			Kathon 893 (see 2-n-Octyl-4-isothiazolin-3-one)	
			Kaurit M 70 (see Melamine formaldehyde resin)	
			Kaurit S (see Urea formaldehyde resin)	
			Lanolin alcohols (see Wool alcohols)	
		21	Lanolin (anhydrous)	as is
			Lanolin wax (see Wool alcohols)	
			Lapis (see Silver nitrate)	
	T	4	Laurel oil	2% pet
			Lauryl gallate (see Dodecyl gallate)	
	C	3, 4, 11	Lavender, absolute	2% pet
	T	4	Lemon grass oil	2% pet
	T	3, 4	Lemon oil	2% pet
			Lergigan (see Promethazine hydrochloride)	
	C, T	2, 5	Lidocaine hydrochloride (Lignocaine, Xylocaine, in some caine mixes)	5–15% pet
			Lilial (see p-tert-Butyl-o-methyl-hydrocinnamic aldehyde)	
			D,L-Limonene (see Dipentene)	
		5, 10	Lindane (Kwell)	1% pet
		10	Malathion	0.5% pet
		7, 14	Maleic anhydride (2,5-Furandione)	1% alc
	T	10	Maneb (Manganese ethylenebis(dithiocarbamate))	1% pet
			Manganese ethylenebis(dithiocarbamate) (see Maneb)	
			MBT (see 2-Mercaptobenzothiazole)	
			MBTS (see Dibenzothiazyl disulfide)	
			MDI (see Diphenylmethane-4-4-diisocyanate)	
	C	8, 14	Melamine formaldehyde resin (Kaurit M-70, in Fixapret AC)	7% pet
			MEK peroxide (see Methyl ethyl ketone peroxide)	
	C	3, 4, 5	Menthol	2% pet
		5, 15	Merbromin (Mercurochrome)	0.1% aq
		16	Mercaptobenzimidazole	1% pet
N, E	C, T	7, 10, 15, 16, 17	2-Mercaptobenzothiazole (MBT, in Mercapto mix)	1–2% pet
N, E, J	C, T	16	Mercapto mix (Mercaptobenzothiazole, Dibenzothiazyl disulfide, Morpholinylmercaptobenzothiazole and N-Cyclohexyl-benzothiazyl sulfenamide)	1–2% pet
	C	5, 12, 15	Mercuric chloride	0.1% pet
			Mercurochrome (see Merbromin)	
	C	2, 6	Mercury	0.5% pet
			Mercury amide chloride (see Mercury chloride, ammoniated)	
			Mercury ammonium chloride (see Mercury chloride, ammoniated)	

A	B	C	D	E
J	C, T	5	Mercury chloride, ammoniated (Ammoniated mercury chloride, Mercury amide chloride, Mercury ammonium chloride)	1% pet
			Merthiolate (see Thimerosal)	
	C	2, 14	2,2-bis(4-(2-Methacryloxyethoxy)-phenyl propane (BIS-EMA)	1% pet
	C	2, 14	2,2-bis(4-(Methacryloxy)-phenyl propane (BIS-MA)	2% pet
			Methenamine (see Hexamethylenetetramine)	
E, J	C, T	13	6-Methoxy-2-N-pentyl-4-benzoquinone (Primin)	0.01% pet
		14	Methyl acrylate	0.1% pet
	C, T	1, 12	4-Methylaminophenol sulfate (Metol)	1% pet
		4	Methyl anisate	4% pet
	C, T	19	3-(4′-Methylbenzylidene)camphor (Eusolex 6300 in Eusolex 8021)	2–10% pet
	C	1	6-Methyl coumarin	1% pet
		2	Methyl dichlorbenzene sulfonate (catalyst in Impregum)	0.1% pet (alc)
		14	Methyl diisocyanate (MDI)	1% pet
	C	14	N,N-Methylene-bis-acrylamide	1% pet
	C	13	α-Methylene-γ-butyrolactone (Tulipaline A)	0.01% pet
			Methylenedianilin (see 4,4′-Diaminodiphenylmethane)	
	T	7	Methylene-bis (Methyloxazolidine)	1% pet
		14	Methyl ethyl ketone peroxide (MEK peroxide)	1% pet
		4	Methylheptide carbonate	0.5% pet
	C	2, 14	Methylhydroquinone	1% pet
	C, T	15	Methyl-4-hydroxybenzoate (Methyl paraben, in paraben mix)	3% pet
			2-Methyl-4-isothiazoline-3-one (see 5-Chloro-2-methyl-4-iso-thiazolin-3-one and 2-Methyl-4-isothiazolin-3-one 3:1)	
	C, T	2, 14	Methyl methacrylate (MMA)	2% pet
		9, 14	N-Methylol acrylamide	0.1% pet
	C	7, 15, 23	N-Methylol chloroacetamide (Grotan HD, Parmetol K 50)	0.1% pet
			Methyl paraben (see Methyl-4-hydroxybenzoate)	
		1, 2, 4, 5, 19	Methyl salicylate (Oil of wintergreen)	2% pet
			Metol (see 4-methylaminophenol sulfate)	
			Mexenone (see Benzophenone 10)	
	C	5	Miconazole	1% alc
			MMA (see Methyl methacrylate)	
			Monobenzone (see Hydroquinone monobenzylether)	
	C	5, 9, 15	2-Monomethylol phenol (Saligenin)	1% pet
	C, T	16, 17	2-(4-Morpholinyl-mercapto)benzothiazole (MOR, in mercapto mix)	0.5 to 1.0% pet
		4, 11	Muscone	5% pet
	T	4, 11	Musk ambrette	5% pet
	C	4	Musk ketone (in musk mix)	5% pet
	C		Musk mix (Musk ketone, Musk moskene, Musk tibetine and Musk xylene)	
	C	4	Musk moskene (in musk mix)	5% pet
	C	4	Musk tibetine (in musk mix)	5% pet
	C	4	Musk xylene (in musk mix)	5% pet
	T	8	Naphthol AS	1% pet
	C	16	Naphtyl mix (N,N-Di-β-naphthyl-4-phenylenediamine and N-phenyl-2-naphthylamine)	1% pet
			Neocaine (see Procaine hydrochloride)	
N, E	C, T	5	Neomycin sulfate (Fradiomycin sulfate)	20% pet
	T	4	Neroli oil (Orange flower oil)	2% pet
N, E, J	C, T	2, 6, 9	Nickel sulfate hexahydrate	2.5–5% pet
	C	8	Nigrosine B (Acid black 2)	1% pet
			Nipagin (see Methyl-4-hydroxybenzoate)	
	C	7	4-(2-Nitrobutyl)morpholine (see also Bioban P 1487)	1% pet
	C	5	Nitrofurazone	1% pet
		5	Nitroglycerin	0.02% aq
	C	1	2-Nitro-4-phenylenediamine	1% pet
			Novantisol (see Phenylbenzimidazol-4-sulfonic acid)	
			Novolac (see Phenol formaldehyde resin acid catalyzed)	

A	B	C	D	E
			Nupercaine (see Dibucaine)	
	T	5	Nystatin	2%
	C, T	4, 13	Oak moss absolute (in fragrance mix)	1–2% pet
			Octyl-dimethyl-4-aminobenzate (see 2-Ethylhexyl-4-dimethyl-aminobenzoate)	
	C, T	3, 21	Octyl gallate	0.25% pet
	C, T	7, 9, 15	2-N-Octyl-4-isothiazolin-3-one (Skane M-8; Kathon 893)	0.025–0.1% pet
			Octyl methoxycinnamate (see 2-Ethylhexyl-4-methoxycinnamate)	
	C, T	5	Olaquindox	1%
		1, 7, 8	Oleyl alcohol	10% pet
	C	9, 14	Oligotriacrylate 480 (OTA 480)	0.1% pet
	C	3, 5	Olive oil	as is
		10	Omite (see Propargite)	1% pet
			Orange flower oil (see Neroli oil)	
	T	4	Orange oil	2% pet
			OTA 480 (see Oligotriacrylate 480)	
	T	5	Oxytetracycline	3% pet
			Oxybenzone (see Benzophenone 3)	
			PABA (see 4-Aminobenzoic acid)	
	C, T	2, 6	Palladium chloride	1–2% pet
E, J	C, T	1, 5, 15	Paraben mix (Butyl-4-hydroxybenzoate, Ethyl-4-hydroxybenzoate, Methyl-4-hydroxybenzoate, Propyl-4-hydroxybenzoate)	16% pet
			Paraphenylenediamine (see 4-Phenylenediamine-base)	
			Parasol 1789 (see tert-Butylmethoxydibenzoylmethane)	
			Paratertiary butylcatechol (see 4-tert-Butylcatechol)	
			Paratertiary butylphenol (see 4-tert-Butylphenol)	
			Paratertiary butylphenol formaldehyde resin (see 4-tert-Butyl-phenol formaldehyde resin)	
			Parmetol K (see N-Methylol chloracetamide)	
			Parsol MCX (see 2-Ethylhexyl-4-methoxy cinnamate)	
	C	13	Partenolid	0.1% pet
			PCM (see 4-Chloro-3-xylenol)	
			PCMC (see 4-Chloro-3-cresol)	
			PCMX (see 4-Chloro-3-xylenol)	
			PCNB (see Pentachloronitrobenzene)	
			PEG 300/1500 (see Polyethylene glycol)	
		10	Pentachloronitrobenzene (PCNB, Terrachlor)	0.5% pet
		10	Pentachlorophenol	1% aq
			Pentadecylcatechols (see Urushiol of poison ivy/oak)	
	C	9, 14	Pentaerythritol triacrylate (PETA)	0.1% pet
	T	3, 4	Peppermint oil	2% pet
			Percaine (see Dibucaine dihydrochloride)	
			PETA (see Pentaerythritol triacrylate)	
J	C, T	21	Petrolatum	as is
			P-F-R-2 (see Phenol formaldehyde resin)	
			Phaltan (see Folpet)	
			Phenergan (see Promethazine hydrochloride)	
			Phenidone (see 1-Phenyl-3-pyrazolidinone)	
	C	8, 9, 14, 17	Phenol formaldehyde resin (P-F-R-2)	1% pet
	T	9, 14	Phenolformaldehyde resin, acid catalyzed (Novolac)	5% pet
	T	9, 14	Phenolformaldehyde resin, alkali catalyzed (Resol)	5% pet
	C, T	1, 5, 9	Phenoxyethanol (in Euxyl K 400)	1% pet
		4	Phenyl acetaldehyde	2% pet
	C, T	19	Phenylbenzimidazol-5-sulfonic acid (Eusolex 232, Novantisol)	2% pet
		8, 16	N-Phenyl-N'-cyclohexyl-4-phenylenediamine	1% pet
		8	2-Phenylenediamine	2% pet
		8, 12, 14, 16	3-Phenylenediamine	2% pet
N, E, J	C, T	1, 8, 12, 14, 16, 17	4-Phenylenediamine, base (PPD, Paraphenylenediamine)	1% pet

A	B	C	D	E
	C	1, 8, 12, 14, 16, 17	4-Phenylenediamine dihydrochloride	0.5% pet
	C	14	2-Phenylglycidyl ether	0.25% pet
	C	14	2-Phenylindole	2% pet
		14	Phenylisocyanate	0.1% pet
	CT	1, 10, 15	Phenylmercuric acetate	0.01–0.05% aq
		10, 15	Phenylmercuric nitrate	0.01% aq
	CT	16	N-Phenyl-2-naphthylamine (in naphthyl mix)	0.5 to 1% pet
	C	7, 10, 15, 16	2-Phenylphenol (Dowicide 1)	1% pet
	T	12	1-Phenyl-3-pyrazolidinone (Phenidone)	1% pet
	C, T	5, 19	Phenyl salicylate (Salol)	1% pet
	T	7, 20	Phosphorus sesquisulfide	1% pet
		14	Phthalic anhydride	1% pet
		14, 20	Pimaric acid	10% pet
		4, 13	α/δ-Pinene	15% pet
	C	5, 13	Pine tar (in wood tar mix)	3% pet
	C	13	Pine wood (in wood mix)	3% pet
			Piperazine (see Diethylenediamine)	
		2, 6	Platinum chloride	1% aq
			Poison ivy/oak (see Pentadecyl catechol)	
		14	Polyester resin monomer	10% pet
		21	Polyethylene glycol (PEG 300/1500)	as is
	C	3, 21	Polyoxyethylene sorbitan monooleate (Tween 80)	2% pet
E, N, J	C, H	6, 9, 12, 17	Potassium dichromate	0.25, 0.5% pet
	C, T	2, 6	Potassium dicyanoaurate	0.002–0.01% aq
			PPD mix (see black rubber mix)	
	T	5	Prednisolone	1% pet
	C	5	Prilocaine hydrochloride (Propitocaine, in some caine mixes)	2.5% pet
			Primin (see 6-Methoxy-2-N-pentyl-p-benzoquinone)	
	C	5	Procaine hydrochloride (Allocaine, Neocaine, Novocaine, Syncaine, Topocaine, in some caine mixes)	1% pet
	C, T	5, 11	Promethazine hydrochloride (Phenergan, Atosil, Fenazil, Lergigan)	1% pet
		5, 10	Propargite (Omite)	1% pet
	C	10, 20	Propionic acid	3% pet
			Propitocaine (see Prilocaine hydrochloride)	
	C, T	5, 21	Propolis	10% pet
	C, T	3, 7, 21	Propylene glycol	10% aq
		4	Propylene phthalide	2% pet
	C, T	3, 21	Propyl gallate	1% pet
	C, T	3, 15	Propyl-4-hydroxybenzoate (Propyl paraben, in paraben mix)	3% pet
			Propylparaben (see Propyl-4-hydroxybenzoate)	
			Proxel (see 1,2-Benzisothiazolin-3-one)	
			PTBF (see 4-tert-Butylphenol formaldehyde resin)	
			PTD (see Dipentamethylene thiuram disulfide)	
			Pyrethrum (see Chrysanthemum cinerariaefolium)	
		3, 5	Pyridoxine hydrochloride	10% pet
		8, 12, 15	Pyrocatechol	2% pet
	T	8, 12, 17	Pyrogallol	1% pet
			Quaternium 15 (see 1-(3-Chloroallyl)-3,5,7-triaza-1-azoniaadamantane chloride)	
	C, T	3, 5	Quinine sulfate	1% pet
	C, T	5	Quinoline mix (Chlorquinaldol and Clioquinol)	6% pet
		8	Quinoline yellow	0.1% pet
			Resol (see Phenol formaldehyde resin, alkali catalyzed)	
	C, T	5, 21	Resorcinol	1% pet
	C	14	Resorcinol monobenzoate	1% pet
		8, 21	Rhodamine	10% aq

A	B	C	D	E
	C	4	Rose oil, Bulgarian	2% pet
		2, 7, 9, 17, 21	Rosin (Colophony)	20% pet
		10	Rotenone (Derris root)	1% pet
			Saligenin (see 2-Monomethylol phenol)	
	T	3, 4	Salicylaldehyde	2% pet
	C	4	Sandalwood oil (Santal oil)	2% pet
E	C	13	Sesquiterpene lactone mix (Alantolactone 0.033% + oil isolated from the Compositae plant *Saussurea lappa* containing a mix of 0.066% Costunolide and Dehydrocostus lactone)	0.1%
		1, 2, 5, 6, 12	Silver nitrate (Lapis)	1% aq
		10	Simazine	1% pet
			Skane M-8 (see 2-*N*-Octyl-4-isothiazolin-3-one)	
	C, T	3, 15	Sodium benzoate	5% pet
			Sodium ethylmercury thiosulfate (see Thimerosal)	
	C	7, 9, 15	Sodium omadine (Sodium-2-pyridinethiol-1-oxide)	0.1% aq
			Sodium thiosulfatoaurate (see Gold sodium thiosulphate)	
	C, T	21	Sorbic acid	2% pet
	C	21	Sorbitan monooleate (Span 80)	5% pet
	C, T	21	Sorbitan sesquioleate (Aracel 83)	20% pet
			Span 80 (see Sorbitan monooleate)	
		2, 3, 5	Spearmint oil	2% pet
	C	13	Spruce wood (in wood mix)	5% pet
			Staphylomycine (see Virginiamycin)	
	C	8, 21	Stearyl alcohol	30% pet
			Sterosan (see Chlorquinaldol)	
			Stovaine (see Amylocaine)	
		5	Streptomycin	1% pet
	C	4, 5	Styrax	2% pet
			Sulisobenzone (see Benzophenone-4)	
	C, T	5	Sulfanilamide	5% pet
		1, 21	Sulfonamide formaldehyde resin	5% pet
			Syncaine (see Procaine hydrochloride)	
	C	13	*Tanacetum vulgare* (Tansy)	1% pet
			Tansy (see *Tanacetum vulgare*)	
	C	13	Taraxacum Officinale (Dandelion)	2.5% pet
			TBS (see 3,4',5-Tribromsalicylanilide)	
			TCC (see 3,3,4-Trichlorocarbanilide)	
			TCSA (see 3,3',4',5-Tetrachlorosalicylanilide)	
			TOI (see Toluene diisocyanate)	
	C	13	Teak wood (in wood mix)	10% pet
			TEGMA (see Triethyleneglycol diacrylate)	
			Tegobetaine L 7 (see Cocamidopropyl betaine)	
			Tekamer 38 (see 1,3-Dibromo-2,4-dicyanobutane)	
			Terraclor (see Pentachloronitrobenzene)	
	C, T	5	Tetracaine hydrochloride (2-Dimethylaminoethyl parabutyl-aminobenzoate, in some caine mixes)	5% pet
			TETD (see Tetraethylthiuram disulfide)	
			N-(1,1,2,2-Tetrachloroethylthio)-4-cyclohexene-1,2-dicarboximide (see Captafol)	
	C, T	7, 8, 11, 15	3,3',4',5-Tetrachlorosalicylanilide (Irgasan BS 200; TCSA)	0.1% pet
	C	14	Tetraethyteneglycol dimethacrylate	2% pet
	C, T	5, 10, 16	Tetraethylthiuram disulfide (Disulfiram, TETD, Antabuse, in thiuram mix)	0.25% pet
	C	1, 2, 14	Tetrahydrofurfurylmethacrylate	2% pet
			2,2',4 4,-Tetrahydroxybenzophenone (see Benzophenone-2)	
	C	8	Tetramethylol acetylene diurea (Fixapret 140)	5% aq
	C	20	3,3,5,7-Tetramethyl benzidine	0.1% pet
	C, T	15, 16	Tetramethylthiuram disulfide (Thiram, TMTD, in thiuram mix)	1% pet
	C, T	10, 15, 16	Tetramethylthiuram monosulfide (TMTM, in thiuram mix)	1% pet
			TGIC (see Triglycidylisocyanurate)	

A	B	C	D	E
		5	Thiamine hydrochloride	10% pet
J	C, T	15	Thimerosal (Merthiolate, Sodium ethyl mercury thiosalicylate, Thiomersal)	0.1% pet
			2,2'-Thiobis(4,6-dichlorophenol) (see Bithionol)	
			Thiocarbanilide (see *N,N*-Diphenylthiourea)	
	C, T	11, 12, 14, 16	Thiourea	0.1% pet
			Thiomersal (see Thimerosal)	
			Thiram (see Tetramethyl thiuram disulfide)	
N, E, J	C, T	15, 16	Thiuram mix (Dipentamethylenethiuram disulfide, Tetraethylthiuram disulfide, Tetramethylthiuram disulfide and Tetramethylthiuram monosulfide)	1% pet
	C	2, 6, 9	Tin	2.5% pet
			Tinuvin P (see 1H-Benzotriazole)	
	C	5	Tixocortol-21-pivalate	1% pet
			TMTM (see Tetramethylthiuram disulfide)	
			TMTD (see Tetramethylthiuram disulfide)	
			TMPTA (see Trimethylol propane triacrylate)	
		5	D,L-α-Tocopherol	10% pet
		5	Tolnaftate	1% pet
			Toluene-2,5-diamine sulfate (see 4-Diaminotoluene sulphate)	
	C	14	Toluene diisocyanate (TDI)	0.1% pet
	C, T	1	Toluene sulfonamide formaldehyde resin	10% pet
	C	2, 14	4-Tolyldiethanolamine	2% alc
			TPGDA (see Tripropylene glycol diacrylate)	
			Topocaine (see Procaine hydrochloride)	
			TREGDMA (see Triethylene glycol diglycolmethacrylate)	
	C, T	10, 11, 15	3,4',5-Tribromsalicylanilide (Tribromsalan; TBS)	1% pet
			Tribromsalan (see 3,4',5-Tribromosalicylanilide)	
	C	7, 11, 15	3,3,4'-Trichlorocarbanilide (Triclocarban, TCC)	1% pet
			Triclocarban (see 3,3,4-Trichlorcarbanilide)	
			N-(Trichloromethylthio)-4-cyclohexene-1,2-dicarboximide (see Captan)	
	C, T	10, 11, 15	3,4,5-Trichlorosalicylanilide (Triclosan, Irgasan DP 300)	2% pet
			N-(Trichloromethylthio)phthalimide (see Folpet)	
			Triclosan (see 3,4,5-Trichlorosalicylanilide)	
	C, T	7, 14	Tricresyl phosphate	5% pet
	C, T	7, 21	Triethanolamine (Trolamine)	2% pet
	C	14	Triethylene glycol diacrylate (TEGMA)	0.1% pet
	C, T	2, 14	Triethylene glycol dimethacrylate (TREGDMA)	2% pet
	C, T	7, 14	Triethylenetetramine (TETA)	0.5% pet
	C	14	Triglycidylisocyanurate (TGIC)	0.5% pet
	C	14, 16	2,2,4-Trimethyl-1,2-dihydroquinoline (Flectol H, Agerite Resin D)	1% pet
		9, 14	Trimethylol propane triacrylate (TMPTA)	0.1% pet
			3,4,4-Trimethyloxazolidine (see Bioban CS 1135)	
	C, T	9, 14	Triphenyl phosphate	5% pet
		14	Triphenylmethane triisocyanate	0.1% pet
	C	12, 14	Tripropylene glycol diacrylate (TPGDA)	0.1% pet
	T	15	1,3,5-Tris(hydroxyethyl)-hexahydrotriazine	1% pet
			Tris-Nitro (see 2-Hydroxymethyl-2-nitro-1,3-propanediol)	
			Trivalent chromium (see Basic chromium sulfate)	
			Trolamine (see Triethanolamine)	
			TSS (see 4-Amino-*N,N*-diethylaniline sulfate)	
			Tulipaline A (see α-Methylene-γ-butyrolactone)	
	T	9	Turpene oil	10% pet
	C	5, 7, 9, 13	Turpene peroxides	0.3% pet
			Tween 80 (see Polyoxyethylene sorbitan monooleate)	
		21	Tween 85	2.5% pet
		5	Tylosin tartrate	5% pet
			UDEMA (see Urethane dimethacrylate)	
	C	8, 14	Urea formaldehyde resin (Kaurit 5)	10% pet

A	B	C	D	E
	C	14	Urethane diacrylate aliphatic (Ebecryl 270)	0.1% pet
	C	14	Urethane diacrylate, aromatic (Ebecryl 220)	0.05% pet
	C	2, 14	Urethane dimethylacrylate (UEDMA)	2% pet
J		13	Urushiol (Pentadecyl catechol)	0.002% pet
	C, T	11, 13	(+)-Usnic acid (in lichen acid mix)	
			Uvinyl MS-40 (see Benzophenone 4)	
			Vancide 89 (see Captan)	
	C, T	3, 4	Vanillin	10% pet
		9, 13	Venice turpentine	20% pet
			Vioform (see Clioquinol)	
		5	Virginiamycin (Staphylomycin)	5% pet
N, E, J	C, T	1, 5	Wool alcohols (Lanolin alcohols)	30% pet
			Xylocaine (see Lidocaine hydrochloride)	
	C	4	Ylang-ylang oil	2% pet
			ZBC (see Zinc dibutyldithiocarbamate)	
			ZDC (see Zinc diethyldithiocarbamate)	
	C	6	Zinc	2.5% pet
	C	10, 16	Zinc dibutyldithiocarbamate (ZBC, in carba mix)	1% pet
	C, T	10, 16	Zinc diethyldithiocarbamate (ZDC, in carba mix)	1% pet
	C, T	10, 16	Zinc dimethyldithiocarbamate (Ziram)	1% pet
	C, T	7, 10	Zinc ethylenebis(dithiocarbamate) (Zineb)	1% pet
			Zinc omadine (see Zinc pyrithione)	
		5	Zinc pyrithione (Zinc omadine)	1% pet
			Zineb (see Zinc ethylenebis(dithiocarbamate))	
			Ziram (see Zinc dimethyldithiocarbamate)	
		21	Zirconium sodium lactate	0.01% aq

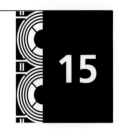

The Computer

ENRIQUE A. MULLINS, M.D.

Computers currently hold an important place in medicine, and every practitioner should have some knowledge of them.

Expenditures allotted to information technology by U.S. hospitals amount to approximately 1.5 to 2.5% of the budget, whereas in the United Kingdom the amount is 0.7 to 0.8%.[1] Even now, only a small percentage of hospital doctors use computers regularly in their institutions, but at least one-third of them have a computer on the consulting room desk, and possibly nearly all of them have one at home.

The following pages summarize the most important aspects of hardware and software from a medical point of view and provide information about how to construct a database to manage contact dermatitis and occupational dermatology.

HARDWARE

Small Computer Systems

A computer system is defined as small if it is a single unit or a group of microcomputers that have no communication with each other.

Medium-sized Computer Systems

The key attribute that allows a computer system to be called medium-sized is the ability to communicate. If microcomputers are interconnected, then the system is considered to be medium-sized.

When two or more computers are physically connected, a network is formed. To connect computers, cables, connectors, network adapters, or cards are required. A network can contain one or more workgroups; a workgroup is a set of connected computers that is organized for a particular purpose.

There are two main types of multiuser systems:

1. A central machine that communicates with various "dumb" terminals and

2. A file server, the most powerful machine of the network. It is in the file server that data and programs are stored, and it is connected to microcomputers, or workstations, with their own intelligence.

Medium-sized computer systems are the most important category of systems found in medical practice.

Large Computer Systems

A large computer system is centralized and has multiple terminals. It is usually dedicated to administration and finance rather than to clinical activities. They are made by IBM or other large manufacturers.

Input Devices

The input device is an appliance used for feeding data to the computer's central processing unit (CPU).

1. The keyboard is the standard device. It is like a typewriter in that it uses the traditional arrangement of letters (QWERTY type), but it also has special function keys and controls a cursor. It is likely that the keyboard will remain the most common device for the near future. Although using a keyboard can be a bit intimidating for new users, after a few sessions, these difficulties tend to disappear.

2. Alternative input devices include the mouse, which is usually provided with microcomputers. The mouse is a popular hand-driven device that is convenient for drawing, pointing, activating screen icons, and selecting menus.

The light pen is an input device that is used to touch sensitive screens and special keyboards.

The ultimate input device would be one that understands the human voice. Several voice recognition applications have reached the market. IBM Via Voice 98 Executive Edition, Dragon System Naturally Speaking, and Philips Free Speech 98 are some examples.[12] With these applications, you can virtually talk to the computer—via a microphone. Thus, the user can not only dictate a document, but can also give simple commands: "Open or close files," "spell check," "print documents," and so forth.

Printers

A printer is an essential complement of the computer. In medical practice it is used to print out reports, forms, insurance claims, charts, and so forth. There is a wide variety of printers, one to meet virtually every requirement. Printers most commonly used in clinical settings are of three types:

1. Dot-matrix printers were the first to appear on the market. They are very reliable and produce printouts of moderate quality with copies for a low price but they are relatively slow and noisy, which can be an important issue in a medical area.

2. Laser printers are capable of superb printing quality, and they work silently and at great speed. Color laser printers are very expensive.

3. Inkjet printers share the features of laser printers but have the additional and valuable capacity of printing color at a low price, which is useful for charts, photographs, and so forth.

Communications

One of the valuable and exciting features of computers is their ability to communicate among themselves, sharing, distributing, or getting ("downloading") the needed information from other machines' programs, such as medical databases and the Internet. This linkage can be made through a special line devoted to that purpose, like a local area network (LAN). Communications over longer distances are carried by telephone lines or special-dedicated fiber-optic cables and in most plases also via communications satellites that reach around the world.

For contacts with computers at remote sites, a modem (MOdulator DEModulator) is necessary. This device is the most indispensable add-on for the use of computers in the field of medicine. Modems have a great variety of working speeds (1,200, 2,400, 9,600, or 14,400 bits per second);

nowadays a speed of 33,600 bits per second is becoming widely used, and devices with even higher transmission speeds are available (e.g., 56,000 bits per second). Before selecting the modem speed it is vital to know the maximum velocity of data transfer the local telephone lines can accept; otherwise money may be unnecessarily spent on a high-speed device. All modems also incorporate the fax function at speeds up to 14,400 bps, so medical reports, letters, and other documents can be sent to colleagues or institutions with great ease.

The *medical Internet* is possibly the most powerful medical resource available, and it lies just beneath our fingertips on the keyboard. Doctors and other health-care professionals are rapidly joining the more than 80 million users and 20,000 networks that make up the Internet. The usual way to access to the World Wide Web is through a university or a hospital, but commercial Internet service providers are very easy to find, and fees are getting lower every day. All these providers offer electronic mail (e-mail), too, and that expands methods of communication by allowing letters and attachments, such as graphs, pictures, software, and so forth, to be sent and received worldwide at the cost of a local phone call. For a list of Internet resources dealing with dermatology, contact dermatitis, and occupational dermatology, see Table 15–1.

Choosing a Computer

The first decision to be made when buying a computer is whether to choose an IBM-compatible or an Apple Macintosh. IBM-compatible machines offer a great variety of hardware (clones) and software for a wide range of applications at reasonable prices. They are virtually the standard machines worldwide. Apple Macintosh computers have more restricted uses and higher prices for hardware and software, but they are excellent machines that have superior graphics-handling capacities, and they are very user-friendly.

The advances in technology are so rapid in this area that any suggestion given in a book would surely become irremediably obsolete in a short time. Nonetheless, as a rough guide, it would be fair to say that today a computer should have at least the following specifications:

1. IBM-compatible personal computer with pentium or higher processor (Apple equivalents can be used);

2. A hard disk of at least 3.2 gigabytes (GB);

3. SVGA or compatible display;

4. MS DOS, version 6 or later;

TABLE 15–1 • **Dermatological Internet Sites**

Electronic Address http://	Description
Contact Dermatitis and Occupation Dermatology	
www.mc.vanderbilt.edu/vumcdept/derm/contact/	Contact dermatitis homepage, a site that contains a list of allergens found in commercial patch-test kits, synonyms and uses for the allergens, background information, crossreactions, and other reactions; created by Trey Truett, M.D.
www.cdc.gov/niosh/homepage.html	National Institute for Occupational Safety and Health
www.osha.gov/	Occupational Safety and Health Administration, U.S. Department of Labor
www.ou.dk/Med/Homepages/eecdrg/egen.htm	European Environmental and Contact Dermatitis Research Group, a website that is under construction
BoDD.cf.ac.uk/	Botanical Dermatology Database, an electronic reincarnation of *Botanical Dermatology* (Mitchell J, Rook A. Vancouver, B.C., Canada: Greengrass; 1979)
uhs.bsd.uchicago.edu/uhs/topics/latex.allergy.html	University Health Services, rubber and latex allergy
Medical Organizations and Institutions	
www.aad.org/	American Academy of Dermatology, homepage
telemedicine.org/	Internet Dermatology Society
tray.dermatology.uiowa.edu/home.html	University of Iowa, Department of Dermatology, College of Medicine; contains clinical skin images and links to databases, resources, and journals
www.internets.com/smedlink.htm	Stanford Medical Center, medical databases
www.ctfa.org/	Cosmetic Toiletry and Fragrance Association; CTFA on-line database requires password
www.os.dhhs.gov/	Department of Health and Human Services
www.nih.gov/	National Institutes of Health homepage
www./fda.gov/default.htm	Food and Drug Administration homepage
www.who.int/	World Health Organization homepage
Journals	
matrix.ucdavis.edu/DOJ.html	*Dermatology On-line Journal* by Art Huntley, M.D.
www.ama-assn.org/public/journals/derm/ dermhome.htm	*Archives of Dermatology;* shows tables of contents, abstracts, selected full-text articles, and searching possibilities
www.ctv.es/dermanet/derma046.html	*Archives of Dermatology,* Spanish edition
www1.mosby.com/periodicals/temp-med.html	*Journal of the American Academy of Dermatology,* official publication of the American Academy of Dermatology
cmu.unige.ch/jid/jid.html	*Journal of Investigative Dermatology,* information and tables of contents, offical journal of the Society for Investigative Dermatology and the European Society for Dermatological Research
www.blacksci.co.uk/products/journals/bjd.htm	*British Journal of Dermatology,* journal of the British Association of Dermatologists; shows table of contents
www.elsevier.nl/locate/jeadv	*Journal of the European Academy of Dermatology and Venereology*
www-usz.unizh.ch/IJD/IJD-Contents.html	*International Journal of Dermatology;* shows table of contents; owned by the International Society of Dermatology

Table continued on following page

TABLE 15–1 • Dermatological Internet Sites *Continued*

Electronic Address http://	Description
www.derm.ubc.ca/jcms/	*Journal of Cutaneous Medicine and Surgery,* official journal of the Canadian Dermatology Association; includes tables of contents and abstracts
www.blacksci.co.uk/products/journals/xajd.htm	*Australasian Journal of Dermatology;* official journal of the Australian College of Dermatologists
www.ctv.es/dermanet/mcila.html	*Medicina Cutanea Ibero-Latinoamericana,* official publication of the Ibero-Latin-American College of Dermatologists
www.karger.ch./journals/drm/drmdes.htm	*Dermatology,* international journal for clinical and investigative dermatology, official organ of the Swiss Society for Dermatology and Syphiligraphy and of the Belgian Royal Society for Dermatology and Syphiligraphy; shows tables of contents
www.webmedlit.com/topics/DermLit.html	Hyperlinked articles and abstracts from the literature
Libraries	
www.nlm.nih.gov/	National Library of Medicine; bibliographic search, free Medline
www.healthgate.com/HealthGate/home.html	Health Gate, search Medline, Cancerlit, Bioethicsline, Health Star, Aidsline, Aidstrials, Aidsdrugs, free Medline
Clinical Images	
www.derma.med.uni-erlangen.de/bilddb/index_e.htm	Dermatology on-line atlas of the University of Erlangen, Germany; contains images linked to diagnosis (more than 2,200 images); query interface
tray.dermatology.uiowa.edu/DermImag.htm	Dermatological image database, University of Iowa, Department of Dermatology, College of Medicine
www.uiowa.edu/~oprm/AtlasHome.html	Atlas of Oral Pathology image database, College of Dentistry, University of Iowa
www.meddean.luc.edu/lumen/MedEd/medicine/dermatology/melton/content1.htm	Skin cancer and benign tumor image atlas, Dermatology Medical Education website, Loyola University, Chicago
www. kumc.edu/instruction/medicine/cont-ed/infotech/der-main.htm	Clinical Medical Education, University of Kansas Medical Center
www.tmc.edu.tw/medimage	Dermatology Image Bank, Taipei Medical College
Search of Medical Resources	
www.medmatrix.org/index.asp	Medical Matrix, guide to Internet medical resources; free registration is required to use Medical Matrix database
webcrawler.com/	Webcrawler, medical resources search
www.MedWeb.Emory.Edu/MedWeb/	Med Web, biomedical Internet resources, Emory University Health Sciences Center Library
www.ohsu.edu/cliniweb/	CliniWeb, Oregon Health Sciences University
healthweb.org/	HealthWeb
www.medsearch.com/	America's Physician Referral Service
galaxy.einet.net/galaxy/Medicine.html	Galaxy Medicine
Miscellaneous	
www.telemedicine.org/stamfor1.htm	Electronic Textbook of Dermatology, from the Internet Dermatology Society

Note: This is not intended to be a complete listing of websites related to dermatology. The address of a site may change.

5. A Microsoft mouse or other compatible pointing device;

6. Microsoft Windows 95 or later version;

7. Thirty-two megabytes (MB) of random access memory (RAM); 64 MB or more are recommended for certain programs.

Before making a final decision in this matter, it is advisable to consult computer magazines such as *PC Magazine, PC Computing, Info World,* or *Computer Shopper,* to name just a few. These publications have excellent reviews of hardware and software along with editorials relating to the most important aspects of computer technology. They are also a good source of pricing information, which changes at the same speed as computers.

It is always good to bear in mind that most computers are installed on a physician's desk or elsewhere in the office setting, where space is usually limited, so bulky machines are hard to accommodate. If this is the case, a notebook computer is a nice choice. With falling hardware costs and improving technology, very powerful machines are available at a reasonable price, although they are always higher than the desktop equivalent. Portable equipment has the extra benefit of allowing the possibility of working with them at a wide variety of sites.

SOFTWARE: COMPUTER LANGUAGES

The term "software" refers to a set of programs, procedures, and documentation associated with computers. A program is a coded set of instructions that interprets the information given to the computer by the input device (keyboard or mouse) and instructs the machine to accomplish the task.

Operating Systems

The operating system is the principal, or master, program of a computer. It is responsible for the general management of the computer and for its relationship with peripheral devices. To run any program, it is first necessary to run the operating system. Currently, the main operating systems are DOS (MS-DOS), UNIX, and Apple-Macintosh. Graphical user interface (GUI) operating systems have gained in popularity and include Microsoft Windows for DOS (version 3.11), Windows 95, and X Windows for UNIX systems.

Word Processors

The word processor (WP) is the most widely used program in medicine. This package transforms the computer into a typewriter so it is possible to create, open, fill, edit, save, and print documents. Additional features of these programs include the spelling checker and the grammar checker contained in them.

There are also electronic (CD-ROM) medical dictionaries and spelling checkers that offer great help to those in the field of medicine (Table 15–2).

Relational Database Management Systems

The most appropriate program for the computer in the medical office is the relational database management system (RDB), which is ideal for maintaining patients' records because it

1. Has screens (forms) for inputting, editing, and outputting information,

2. Allows the user to make queries or searches based on specific criteria,

3. Can create reports of all kinds, and

TABLE 15–2 • CD-ROM Medical Dictionaries and Spellcheckers

Name	Author	Publisher	Address
Electronic Medical Dictionary	Stedman	Mosby-Williams & Wilkins	351 W. Camden St., Baltimore, MD 21201-2436, USA
Spellchecker	Stedman	Mosby-Williams & Wilkins	
Word/Dermatology Dictionary	Morris Leider, Morris Rosenblum	Dermatologic Services Inc.[a]	Dept 21-8248, Chicago, IL 60678-8248, USA
Dr. Spell		Salient Software System	4 Framingham Dr., Thornhill, Ontario L3T 4H3, Canada

[a] Subsidiary of the American Academy of Dermatology.

4. Can perform data analysis using statistics and graph functions.

Various high-quality packages are available, such as Dbase IV, Access, Paradox, FoxPro, Clipper, and Dataease.

Spread Sheets

Spread sheets are oriented toward performing calculations of numeric values through the building of formulas. Statistical analysis of data and the creation of charts (graphic representations of data) are strong points of these applications. They can also create and manage simple databases, executing tasks such as finding, sorting, filtering, or subtotaling data. In general, they are powerful tools used chiefly for investigation, administration, and finance.

How to Choose Software

Choosing software can be a difficult and complex issue. The following points should be considered before a decision is made:

1. Existing personal or group experience,
2. Programs that the unit or institution already has running,
3. User-friendly interface,
4. Available support from the company's local distributor (a hotline), and
5. Price, which should be the least important issue; considering the time and effort invested in any project, it is not a wise decision to buy the least expensive application, for it could become the most expensive one in the long run.

COMPUTERS IN MEDICINE

Computers can play a role in many aspects of medical practice and may be considered part of the basic equipment. They are useful in diagnosis, treatment, administration, and education, and in the management of clinical data collection, storing, and retrieval.

The Computer Medical Record

Although the process of replacing paper with electronics has been rather slow-moving, the computer medical record (CMR) will continue its inexorable advance, and soon every patient will have some kind of electronic medical record. The CMR should be designed to handle patient care, documentation (such as reports, referral letters, and any printed information given to patients), clinical research, and accounting.

A CMR is particularly appropriate under certain circumstances:

A. For chronic problems that require long-term follow-up, such as cancer and occupational diseases and
B. For diseases or exams that have a fixed pattern of data collection, such as diabetes,[2] and the study of contact dermatitis. Extensive computer records are particularly useful in cases of contact dermatitis for several reasons:
   1. There is a great quantity of fixed data to be handled in each case:
      a. The patient's clinical history and background,
      b. Details of the physical examination, including eczema pattern, distribution, etc.,
      c. The patient's labor area and specific occupation,
      d. The patient's hobbies,
      e. Results of the patch test; a standard and an accessory tray of allergens and an open test; results of 48- and 96-hour readings, which produce nine possibilities for each reading.
   2. Written reports are necessary. Because of medical or legal reasons such as impairment or disability evaluation or if the patient is a referral, a written report of each patient studied is indispensable.
   3. Data can be stored and retrieved conveniently. Patients' histories and their responses to specific allergens, including description, distribution, and crossreactions, can be studied by means of a quick search procedure that specifies criteria such as name, sex, date, diagnosis, type of allergen, etc.
   4. The cause of scientific research is aided. Having all this information readily at hand allows it to be processed easily, and that can lead to valuable scientific conclusions.

COMPUTERIZED METHODS FOR CLINICAL MANAGEMENT OF OCCUPATIONAL DERMATOLOGY AND CONTACT DERMATITIS

To accomplish these tasks we will require the following software elements:

1. A word processor,
2. A relational database management system,
3. A programming language for building appli-

cations and customizing them to the user's needs (optional).

Preparing Reports

The principal value of a computer in the field of dermatology is its ability to deal with paperwork in a neat and efficient way with the assistance of a word processor. Thus, making a template, or form, for a patch-test (PT) report is a valuable tool for everyday work (Table 15–3). During the PT procedure, the dermatologist, nurse, or technologist can fill in the blank spaces in the template with the patient's name, age, diagnosis, occupation, additional allergens, and so forth. At the 48- and 96-hour readings, observed results are typed according to the guidelines of the International Contact Dermatitis Research Group.[3] To shorten the typing time, all the standard allergens in the template show a negative (−) response, so the operator will have to change only those that have produced positive (allergic or irritant) reactions. Through the use of word processor functions such as Autocorrect and Autotext (in MS Word for Windows),[4] preformed blocks of text containing the information for each allergen can be included in the Comments section of the form, which can be accessed by clicking a button or typing a few keystrokes followed by a space. This function also can be used for inserting letter closings, graphics, logos, or letterheads. (Of course, all this information that is to be used repeatedly has to be typed or scanned only once to store it on the computer's hard disk so the program will have access to it whenever necessary.) Thus, at the end of this procedure, you will have a customized document for each patient, referring doctor, or institution.

The Collection and Processing of Clinical Data

The second use for computers in the field of occupational dermatology is the collection of clinical data with the aid of an RDB. For this application, an integrated package called an office productivity suite can be used (Microsoft Office 97, Lotus Smartsuite 97, or Corel Office Professional 7). The extra benefits of these packages are that apart from the RDB, they also contain a WP, a spreadsheet, a presentation graphics program, and Internet tools, all linked together, which gives the user great potential for managing data by importing and exporting information among these applications. According to reports,[5] Microsoft Office 97 seems to be the best of these packages, although all of them are of good quality and are excellent choices for any medical task.

The other possibility is to have a special, customized RDB program for Windows written, for example, in Microsoft Access or Visual Basic. This solution is much more expensive and requires more time and dedication in guiding the programmers to produce the desired polished results. Chemotechnique Diagnostics AB (P.O. Box 80, Edvard Ols väg 2, S-230 42 Tygelsjö, Manlo, Sweden) released a software program called Quick Search-Daluk for Windows for the management of PT routines. The program allows the user to register patients' information, print PT records recall data, and run statistical evaluations and follow-up.

The design of the questionnaire, or database, is by far the most important work involved in the building of a CMR. A high level of medical expertise is needed, although only a little technical knowledge of computing is necessary. Generally speaking, however, it is not cost- or time-effective for a busy practitioner with no experience in database programming to try to develop such a program. The best solution for a nonexperienced user is to guide a programmer in writing the specific application. However, to provide adequate guidance, the physician should have some basic knowledge about databases.

Steps in Designing a Database[6, 7]

1. Determine the objectives of your database. This tells you what information you want from the database and how it will be used. Talk to all the people who will use the database. Various categories of medical staff are usually involved; do not assume all the users will have great medical knowledge.

2. Determine the tables in the database. Once your objectives are clear, the information has to be divided into "containers" of data about a particular topic. Each container will be a table (e.g., identification of patient, affected zone, occupation, etc.).

3. Determine the fields. Each category of information in a table is called a field. It is displayed as a column; for example, in the table "identification of patient," you should find the following fields: name, surname, age, address, and so forth.

After you name the field, the data type has to be chosen in order to allow a specific kind of value in the field. There are various data types: text, number, date/time, counter, currency, yes/no, memo, OLE object.* Each data type has its maximum size expressed in bytes; 1 byte = 1

---

*Any unit of information created in a Window-based application that supports or works with object linking and embedding (OLE).

TABLE 15–3 • Patch-test Form

NAME: (Patient's first name, middle name, and surname)

AGE:

ADDRESS[a]: (complete address)

TELEPHONE HOME:

OFFICE: EXT:

REFERRAL: (doctor's name or institution)

EVOLUTION TIME: (duration of the disease)

DIAGNOSIS:

CLINICAL DESCRIPTION: (history and physical examination with detailed description of clinical signs and anatomical distribution of lesions)

RELATION: (patient's opinion, suspicious agents in relation to the dermatitis, etc.)

TREATMENTS: (description of all past treatments)

LABOR AREA: (specify labor area, e.g., mining, fishing, industry, construction, transport, services, etc.)

OCCUPATION: (description of precise occupation, exposures to allergens or irritants, details of movements and actions during work)

PERSONAL BACKGROUND: Dermatitis (   ) Asthma (   ) Rhinitis (   )

FAMILY BACKGROUND: Dermatitis (   ) Asthma (   ) Rhinitis (   )

   Father:

   Mother:

HOBBIES:

COMMENTS:

HEALTH INSURANCE:

DATE:

TYPE OF PATCH: Finn Chamber; ALLERGEN: Trolab

Patch Test: European Standard Battery

		48 Hours	96 Hours
1. Potassium dichromate	0.5 %	—	—
2. Neomycin sulfate	20.0 %	—	—
3. Thiuram mix	1.0 %	—	—
4. Paraphenylenediamine free base	1.0 %	—	—
5. Cobalt chloride	1.0 %	—	—
6. Benzocaine	5.0 %	—	—
7. Formaldehyde	1.0 %	—	—
8. Colophony	20.0 %	—	—
9. Clioquinol	5.0 %	—	—
10. Balsam of Peru	25.0 %	—	—
11. N-Isopropyl-N-phenyl paraphenylenediamine	0.6 %	—	—
12. Wool alcohols	30.0 %	—	—
13. Mercapto mix	1.0 %	—	—
14. Epoxy resin	1.0 %	—	—
15. Paraben mix	16.0 %	—	—
16. Paratertiarybutylphenol formaldehyde resin	1.0 %	—	—
17. Fragrance mix	8.0 %	—	—
18. Ethylenediamine dihydrochloride	1.0 %	—	—
19. Quaternium 15	1.0 %	—	—
20. Nickel sulfate	5.0 %	—	—
21. Kathon CG	0.01 %	—	—
22. Mercaptobenzothiazole	2.0 %	—	—
23. Primin	0.01 %	—	—

Accessory Battery[b]

		48 Hours	96 Hours
24. Imidazolidinyl urea	2.0 %	—	—
25. Gentamicin sulfate	20.0 %	—	—
26. Chloramphenicol	5.0 %	—	—
27. Bacitracin	20.0 %	—	—
28. Thiomersal	0.1 %	—	—

⌂ TABLE 15–3 • Patch-test Form *Continued*

Accessory Battery[b] *Continued*

		48 Hours	96 Hours
29. Propylene glycol	5.0 %	—	—
30. Toluene sulfonamide formaldehyde resin	10.0 %	—	—
Sorbic acid	2.0 %	—	—
Bronopol	0.5 %	—	—
Chlorocresol	1.0 %	—	—
Methyl methacrylate	2.0 %	—	—
Benzoylperoxide	1.0 %	—	—
Sodium thiosulfatoaurate	0.25 %	—	—
Hydroquinone	1.0 %	—	—
Ammoniated mercury	1.0 %	—	—
Para-aminobenzoic acid	10.0 %	—	—
2-Ethylhexyl-p-methoxycinnamate	10 %	—	—
Oxybenzone	10 %	—	—
Methoxycinnamate	10 %	—	—
Medical cream[c]			
Shampoo[d]			
Shampoo			
Soap[d]			
Soap[d]			
Perfume[c]			
Perfume[c]			
Cologne[c]			
Cleansing cream[c]			
Moisturizer cream[c]			
Nourishing cream[c]			
Hand cream[c]			
Body cream[c]			
Nail polish[c]			
Mascara[c]			
Eyeliner[c]			
Eye shadow[c]			
Eyelid cream[c]			
Lipstick[c]			
Blush[c]			
Makeup[c]			
Deodorant[c]			
Shaving cream[d]			

Interpretation guide:
  − Negative reaction
  ? Doubtful reaction; macular erythema
  + Weak reaction; erythema, micropapules
  + + Severe reaction; vesicular, erythema, infiltration, papules
  + + + Extreme positive reaction; bulla, necrosis
  IR Irritant reaction of different types
  NT Not tested

Open Test

		48 Hours	96 Hours
1. Insert name of contactant		—	—
2.			

(Apply test substance over flexor surface of the patient's forearm twice a day for 2 days, then take the first reading. If no reaction is seen, application for 2 additional days is required.)

Comments

(Insert preformed blocks of text, including description of allergens and where they are found. Add a personalized conclusion about the specific case.)

Sincerely,

(Dermatologist), M.D.

[a] The underlined words are formatted as hidden text. This type of text is used to hide notes and comments in a document or to include any kind of information that should not appear on the printout. The text will be displayed on the screen and can be printed if necessary.
  [b] Number, delete, or include contactant, as necessary.
  [c] Insert the number and the name of the specific product.
  [d] Insert the name of the product and test if diluted 1 to 2% in water. If possible, perform an open test or check with control subjects.

TABLE 15–4 • **Relational Database: Patient Identification**

Field Name	Type	Size (Bytes)	Comments
Patient code	Numeric	9	Primary key field; use a unique number for each record.
Date of entry	Date	8	Date format
Name	Text	15	
Middle initial	Text	1	
Surname	Text	15	
Sex	Text	1	
Date of birth	Date	8	Date format
Address	Text	25	
City	Text	17	
State, Region	Text	2	
Postal code	Text	6	
Country	Numeric	3	Use international telephone coding.
Starting date	Date	8	Date of the beginning of the disease

Note: Telephone and fax numbers are on a separate form, as more than one number for each can be entered for a patient.

character For example, the text field may be allowed up to 255 bytes, the number field up to 8 bytes.

For more information, read the manual of the database to be used. In this case the RDB used is Microsoft Access, version 2.0.[8]

A record is a row in a table. You can think of fields as characteristics of a table, and each record in a table contains the same set of fields. For example, in the table "Patient ID," a record would

TABLE 15–5 • **Relational Database: Affected Zone**[a]

Field Name	Type	Size (Bytes)	Comments
Record number	Numeric	4	Primary key field
Patient code	Numeric	9	Foreign key field[b]
Site	Numeric	10	Insert code[c]

[a] A patient can have more than one principal affected zone, for example, hands, earlobes, and neck in a nickel-sensitive case. In such an instance various inputs can be made; all will have the patient's code so the RDB will gather them when they are needed.
[b] The foreign key is the primary key from a different table.
[c] Codes are linked to a coded anatomical site table.

be a specific patient, this information formed by the set of fields contained in the table such as patient code, date of entry, name, middle initial, surname, and so forth (Table 15–4).

4. Include all the information you might need; don't omit important aspects.

5. Determine the relationship among tables. Decide how the data in one table are related to the data in other tables. In the RDB, you store related data in separate tables, and then you define the relationships among the tables so the program can use the relationship to find the required information. There are three types of relationships among tables: one-to-one, one-to-many, and many-to-many.

You can find more information about this point in the manual for the program. Is a good idea to ask for assistance from an experienced database user or programmer at this point.

Structured Response–Choice from a List

Exclusive choice from a list	Inclusive choice from a list
Is the observed patch-test reaction:	What does the patient have on the affected site?
1. Allergic ☑ 2. Irritant 3. Doubtful 4. Negative	1. Erythema ☑ 2. Papules ☑ 3. Infiltration ☑ 4. Scaling 5. Vesicles
Only one choice is possible.	More than one condition can be present in the patient.

FIGURE 15–1 • Structured response types in clinical data collection.

TABLE 15–6 • Relational Database: Patient's Background[a]

Field Name	Type	Size (Bytes)	Comments
Record number	Numeric	4	Primary key field
Patient code	Numeric	9	Foreign key field
Background	Numeric	8	Insert diagnostic codes[b, c]

[a]A similar table is established for family background (not shown).

[b]One or more personal background diagnoses can be entered; they will all have the patient's unique code attached to them.

[c]Codes are linked to a coded diagnosis table.

6. Refine your design. Create forms (just like paper forms that are filled out with a pen). They provide an easy way of entering, viewing, and changing information and calculating totals. Forms are based on database tables, queries, and calculated values.

Is always good at the beginning, once the database is ready, to experiment with sample data before starting to input real information, as any mistake will be easily fixed at that time.

Clinical Data Collection

Data is collected by means of questions, known as fields in database language. Because the questions are so important, their design should be attended to with great care. It is good to have in mind the following aspects in regard to formulating questions:

A. Ask for a structured response[9] that is precise and short. Avoid questions that may lead to a discursive response (a block of free text): Does the patient have itching? Yes/No.
  1. There are three types of structured responses:
     a. A simple yes or no.
     b. An exclusive choice from a list; only one choice can be made for it excludes all others (Fig. 15–1).
     c. A Nonexclusive choice from a list from which more than one item may be chosen. It is always good to leave "none," "don't know," or "other" on the list of responses as escape clauses.
  2. Advantages of structured responses:
     a. Entering the answer is quick, requiring only the pressing of a single key.
     b. Spelling errors are avoided
     c. Ready definitions of the possible range of responses are provided.
     d. Storage is compact, saving space on the hard disk.
  3. Disadvantages of structured responses:
     a. They are difficult to design, requiring time and effort on the part of medical personnel.
     b. Sometimes it is not possible to define every possible option, so the category of "other" has to be included and it is of a discursive nature.
B. Avoid repetition and irrelevant questions.
C. Phrase questions to elicit exact data, not a personal opinion.

Principal Structures in an RDB of Occupational Dermatology

Tables. Settings up the tables in a database can be a complex aspect of the design process because the objectives of the program do not necessarily provide clues about the structure of the tables. Tables 15–5 through 15–9 show the structure of

TABLE 15–7 • Relational Database: Occupation

Field Name	Type	Size (Bytes)	Comments
Patient code	Numeric	9	Primary key field
Labor area	Numeric	10	Insert code.
Occupation	Numeric	10	Insert code.
Duration	Date	8	Date of the initiation of work
Relation to occupation	Yes/No	$1/8$[a]	Is the disease related to the patient's occupation?
Others affected	Yes/No	$1/8$[a]	Are others in the workplace affected?
Hobbies	Yes/No	$1/8$[a]	Linked with a coded hobby table.
Comments	Text	30	

[a]$1/8$ byte = 1 bit, so 8 bits = 1 byte.

TABLE 15–8 • Relational Database: European Standard Battery, 48-hour Results[a]

Field Name	Type	Size (Bytes)	Comments
Patient code	Numeric	9	Primary key field
Chromium	Numeric	1	Insert code of patch-test results.
Neomycin	Numeric	1	Insert code.
Thiuram mix	Numeric	1	Insert code.
Cobalt	Numeric	1	Insert code.
Kathon CG	Numeric	1	Insert code.
MBT	Numeric	1	Insert code.
Primin	Numeric	1	Insert code.

[a] Only some allergens are shown here. See Table 15–10 for patch-test coding.

Note: A similar table is constructed to record the results of the 96-hour reading (not shown).

TABLE 15–10 • Codes of Patch-test Results

Negative	1
Doubtful (?)	2
Weak (+)	3
Severe (+ +)	4
Extreme (+ + +)	5
IR +	6
IR + +	7
IR + + +	8
Not tested	9
Relevance	
Present	
Primary	PRP
Aggravating	PRA
Past	
Primary	PTP
Aggravating	PTA
Not relevant	NTR

the key tables of a program the author uses to manage occupational dermatology and contact dermatitis. As you can see, all the information of a specific type is categorized in one table. Each table has it own descriptive name and primary key field.

Primary Key Fields. The primary key field uniquely identifies each individual record stored in the table. It is used by the program to quickly associate data from multiple tables, for example, the patient code. Thus, each patient (each record in the RDB) has its own unique code. For this purpose the national identification number, the social security number, or the medical record num-

ber can be used. If none of those are suitable for your needs, you can use a field that simply numbers the records consecutively.

Coding. To facilitate the data input and to prevent typing errors, much of the information, such as anatomic sites, diagnosis, labor area, occupation, patient results, relevance, hobbies, and health insurance should be coded (Table 15–10). Codes can be created by arbitrary methods, or you can adhere to some of the existing international codes, such as the International Coding Index for Dermatology[10] or the International Classification of Disease.[11]

Calculations. The cost of an exam can be assessed effortlessly through a form named, for example, Statement of Account, taking the information from the fields of the tables Medical Expenses (Table 15–11) and Cost (not shown). The program

TABLE 15–9 • Relational Database: Summary

Field Name	Type	Size (Bytes)	Comments
Patient code	Numeric	9	Primary key field
Pre-PT diagnosis	Numeric	8	Insert code.[a]
Post-PT diagnosis	Numeric	8	Insert code.
Number of allergic reactions	Numeric	2	
Number of irritant reactions	Numeric	2	
Test relevance	Yes/No	1/8	
Comment	Text	30	Add any additional relevant observations.

[a] Codes are linked to a coded diagnosis table.

TABLE 15–11 • Relational Database: Medical Expenses[a]

Field Name	Type	Size (Bytes)	Comments
Code	Numeric	9	Primary key field
Referral source	Numeric	3	Insert the code of the referring doctor or institution.
Place of exam	Numeric	2	Insert code; coding required.
Health insurance	Numeric	2	Insert code; coding required.
Type of patch	Numeric	2	Insert code; a code is assigned to each brand.
Premount patch	Numeric	1	Insert code of T.R.U.E. test or similar patch.
Type of allergen	Numeric	2	Insert code; a code is assigned to each brand.
Number of allergens	Numeric	2	Enter the number used in the test.
Number of patches	Numeric	2	Enter the number used in the test.

[a]This table is linked to the Cost and Statement of Account tables.

calculates the final cost of the exam based on the types and numbers of allergens and patches used, plus other variables such as the place of exam and the referral source (sometimes there are special prices for certain institutions, e.g., 10% of the normal cost).

Important Features of the Database Design

The design of the database must include several specific elements.

A. The program must be able to register patient data, PT allergens (standard and accessory), and the results of the tests.
B. It must be able to retrieve specific data and run statistical evaluations, for example, locating all patients with allergies to chromium, listing sex, age, occupation, and principal affected zone, who have been examined during the past 5 years.
C. It must produce summaries, charts, and reports of selected information for medical, legal, or scientific purposes (see the following section, Examples of Data Processed by an RDB).
D. The program may include certain optional features which should be managed by a programmer or an experienced database builder.
   1. The system should have attractive, easy-to-read screens to eliminate eye strain.
   2. There should be a logical sequence to the screens, and it should be possible to move back and forth among them easily to modify or correct an entry.
   3. The program should contain a validation of response. This is an error trap that eliminates the typing of erroneous material and the choice of answers that are not in the

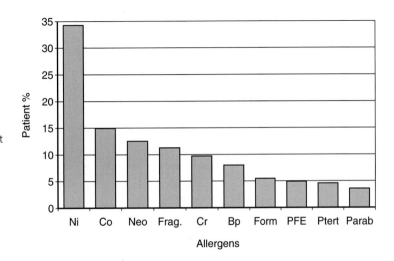

FIGURE 15–2 • The ten most frequent contact allergens in 1000 studies of contact dermatitis. (Ni, nickel sulfate; Co, cobalt chloride; Neo, neomycin sulfate; Frag., fragrance mix; Cr, potassium dichromate; Bp, balsam of Peru; Form, formaldehyde; PFE, paraphenylenediamine; Ptert, *p*-butylphenol formaldehyde resin; and Parab, paraben mix.)

TABLE 15–12 • Principal Affected Areas in 1,000 Patients with Contact Dermatitis

Area	Males % (n = 298)	Females % (n = 702)
Scalp	5.9	1.3
Face	23.5	55.6
Forehead	3.9	10.6
Eyelids	5.9	27.8
Cheeks	5.9	23.2
Nose	3.9	7.9
Lips	—	4.6
Perioral	—	11.9
Ears	2.0	5.3
Neck	7.8	21.9
Arms	11.8	6.6
Forearms	5.9	4.0
Hands	52.9	24.5
Thorax	2	9.9
Abdomen	3.9	4.6
Thighs	5.9	2.0
Legs	11.8	5.9
Feet	13.7	4.6
Genitals	—	2.0
Folds	17.6	8.6

Note: Percentages total more than 100% because some patients were affected at more than one site.

TABLE 15–13 • Causes of Occupational Dermatosis[a, b]

Cause	Number	%
Cement and derivatives	536	53.0
Rubber and derivatives	91	9.0
Petroleum and derivatives	61	6.0
Epoxy resin	51	5.0
Metals (nickel, chromium)	41	4.0
Physical agents	41	4.0
Biological agents	41	4.0
Solvents	25	2.5
Detergents	15	1.5
Others	110	11.0
Total	1,012	100.0

[a]Vera C, Mullins E, Lobos P, et al. Occupational Dermatoses. In: Honeyman J, ed. Clinical Series, Santiago Medical Society. *Advances in Dermatology* I, vol. VII, 2, Santiago, Chile: Mediterráneo; 1988: 174.

[b]This information is from the outpatient clinic of the Hospital of the Insurance Mutuality of the Chilean Chamber of Construction.

option list, which would generate error messages on the screen.

4. The program may contain specific validations that are more sophisticated audits. With these, questions applied after general validity checks are based on specific criteria; for example, more than five positive reactions in a patch test generates a warning message on the screen.

Examples of Data Processed by an RDB

One of the most important facts a dermatologist working in contact dermatitis should know is the most frequent contact allergens in a given population of patients during a certain period of time; for example, what were the 10 most frequent allergens in 1,000 consecutive patch tests during a particular 4-year period (Fig. 15–2)? The area that has been affected is also important to know (Table 15–12). This information could, of course, be crossed with other variables such as age and occupation.

It is also possible to collect data from an outpatient clinic for occupational dermatology, as in Table 15–13, which lists the causes of occupational dermatoses in descending order and the workers at risk for these diseases (Table 15–14). It is possible to investigate the prevalence of contact dermatitis in the presence of a specific allergen, for example gold in a particular group of patients (Fig. 15–3). In this case is important to know the sex and age distribution (Fig. 15–4) and the

TABLE 15–14 • Workers at Risk for Developing Occupational Dermatosis

Occupation	Number	%
Cement workers	455	45
Rubber & derivatives workers	91	9
Machinists	61	6
Painters	61	6
Other construction workers	51	5
Others	293	29
Total	1,012	100

[a]Vera C, Mullins E, Lobos P, et al. Occupational Dermatoses. In: Honeyman J, ed. Clinical Series, Santiago Medical Society. *Advances in Dermatology I,* vol VII, 2, Santiago, Chile: Mediterráneo; 1988: 175.

[b]This information is from the outpatient clinic of the Hospital of the Insurance Mutuality of the Chilean Chamber of Construction.

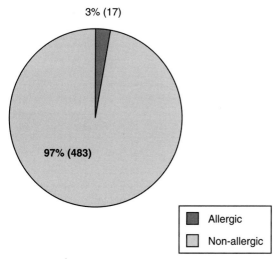

3% (17)

97% (483)

■ Allergic
□ Non-allergic

FIGURE 15–3 ● Prevalence of contact dermatitis in reaction to gold in 500 patients.

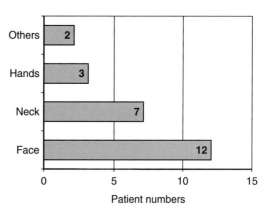

FIGURE 15–5 ● The principal affected anatomic site in 17 patients allergic to gold. The numbers add to more than 17 because some patients had more than one site affected.

anatomic site principally affected (Fig. 15–5). It is possible to retrieve data about labor area, occupation, personal background, or any other significant aspect of the problem. In addition, it is possible to begin investigating from the affected site, for example, the hands, and have the principal allergens associated with hand dermatitis listed by sex (Table 15–15). The feet and eyelids can also be investigated (Figs. 15–6 and 15–7).

Of course these are only examples, but they serve to reveal the value of working with computers equipped with adequate software.

FINAL COMMENTS

If this chapter has stimulated the reader to use computers or to deepen his or her knowledge about them, the author's goal has been fully accomplished. It is worthwhile to consider these machines valuable instruments that complement a medical practice devoted to skin disease.

Acknowledgment

The author would like to thank Robert M. Adams, M.D., for his advice and support and the interest shown this work and the medical staffs of the Department of Dermatology, Hospital del Salva-

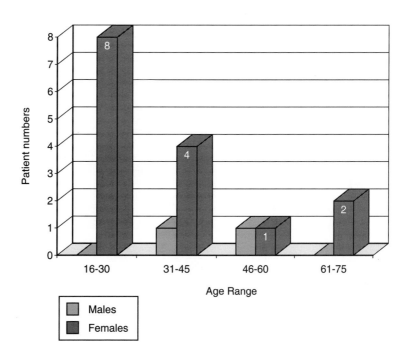

FIGURE 15–4 ● Sex and age distribution of 17 patients allergic to gold.

■ Males
■ Females

TABLE 15–15 • Principal Allergens in Patch Tests of 100 Patients with Hand Dermatitis

Allergens		Sex	
European Standard Battery Trolab		Male % (n = 52)	Female % (n = 48)
Nickel sulfate	5.0%	30.7	50.0
Potassium dichromate	0.5%	23.0	16.6
Fragrance mix	8.0%	23.0	16.6
Neomycin sulfate	20.0%	—	16.6
Thiuram mix	1.0%	—	16.6
Cobalt chloride	1.0%	—	16.6
Carba mix	3.0%	23.0	—
Quinoline mix	6.0%	23.0	8.3
Colophony	20.0%	7.7	8.3
Wood alcohols	30.0%	7.7	—
Kathon CG	0.01%	7.7	—
Formaldehyde	1.0%	—	8.3
Balsam of Peru	25.0%	—	8.3
Paraphenylenediamine free base	1.0%	—	8.3

Note: Percentages total more than 100% because some patients were affected at more than one site.

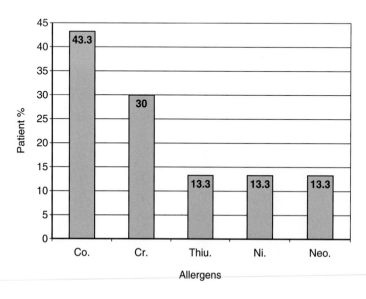

FIGURE 15–6 • Principal allergens in 50 patients with dermatitis of the feet. (Co., cobalt chloride; Cr., potassium dichromate; Thiu., thiuram mix; Ni., nickel sulfate; and Neo., neomycin sulfate.)

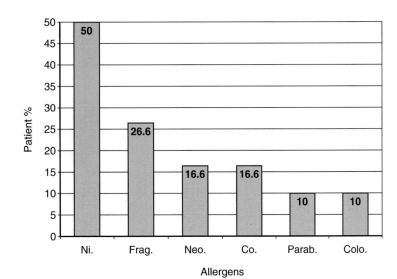

FIGURE 15–7 ● Principal allergens in 60 patients with dermatitis of the eyelids. (Ni., nickel sulfate; Frag., fragrance mix; Neo., neomycin sulfate; Co., cobalt chloride; Parab., parabene mix; Colo., Colophony.)

dor, and of the Department of Dermatology, University of Chile, Santiago, Chile, for the important contributions, suggestions, and support that have made this work possible.

References

1. Chard T. Preface. In: Chard T., Ed. *Computing for Clinicians,* 2nd ed. London: Edward Arnold; 1995.
2. Jones; RB, Hedley AJ. Methods of estimating losses to follow-up from a diabetic clinic. *Practical Diabetes* 1989; 6:129–133.
3. Wilkinson DS, Fregert S, Magnusson B, et al. Terminology of contact dermatitis. *Acta Derm Venereol* 1970; 50:287.
4. Autocorrect and Autotext. In: User's Guide, Microsoft Word, Version 6.0. *Redmond,* WA: Microsoft; 1993.
5. Miller M. Suite deals. *PC Magazine* 1997; 16:145–169.
6. Date CJ, ed. *Introduction to Database Systems,* 5th ed.: Addison-Wesley; 1990.
7. Viescas JL, ed. Running Microsoft Access. Redmond, WA: Microsoft Press; 1993.
8. User's Guide, Microsoft Access, Version 2.0. Redmond, WA: Microsoft; 1994.
9. Chard T. Computers for clinical data collection. In: Chard T, Ed. *Computing for Clinicians,* 2nd ed. London: Edward Arnold; 1995.
10. Alexander S, Shrank A. *International Coding Index for Dermatology.* Oxford: Blackwell; 1978.
11. PHO/WHO. Disease of the skin and subcutaneous tissue. In: Pan-American Health Organization/World Health Organization, ed. *International Classification of Disease.* Vol. 1. Washington, D.C.: WHO; 1978.
12. Miastkowski S, McEvoy A, McCraben H, et al. Your PC—Listen. *PC World Chile* 1998; 11:56–64.

Multiple Chemical Sensitivities

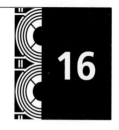

16

A B B A I . T E R R , M . D .

Multiple chemical sensitivities (MCS) is a controversial concept that holds that subjective, wide-ranging symptoms can occur in some people because of exposure to numerous environmental chemicals. The symptoms are typically multiple and various, although fatigue, pain, and problems with memory and cognition are most common. Physical findings are absent, and there are no diagnostic laboratory markers of the disease. In this respect, MCS is similar to other current syndromes such as the chronic fatigue syndrome and to somatoform illness, with the additional factor of a claimed connection to environmental exposures. It differs in that the numerous subjective symptoms are attributed to environmental chemicals, especially synthetic ones, in the air, water, soil, food, and medications. The quantity of chemical claimed to trigger symptoms may be exceedingly small, orders of magnitude below any known toxic dosage for that chemical, and the symptoms may bear no similarity to its recognized toxic effect.

The concept of MCS as a disease is unproven. It should not be confused with diseases and disease mechanisms with well-established environmental causes, particularly allergic and toxic diseases. The former are characterized by objective signs of inflammation and organ dysfunction usually localized to a particular tissue such as the skin or the nasal or bronchial mucosa, and verified testing procedures can identify the immunologically specific sensitivities. Toxic and irritant diseases are dose-dependent and cause objective signs of pathology consistent with the chemical or physical properties of the environmental chemical and the route of exposure. Building-related illnesses include a range of allergic, toxic, irritative, and infectious syndromes that similarly should also not be confused with MCS.

The MCS phenomenon has been extensively studied and critiqued. A workshop organized by the International Program on Chemical Safety of the World Health Organization recommended a new name—idiopathic environmental intolerances—because the term "multiple chemical sensitivities" makes an unsupported judgment about causation, does not refer to a clinically defined disease, and is not based on accepted theories of underlying mechanisms or validated clinical criteria for diagnosis, and because the relationship between exposures and symptoms is unproven.[1]

In this chapter, the theories and methods of diagnosis and management of patients suspected of having this condition are discussed from the perspectives of the proponents of MCS as a physical disease caused by unique sensitivity to environmental chemicals and of those with alternative explanations for these patients' symptoms.

HISTORY

In the 1950s, Theron Randolph, a practicing allergist, founded a small movement outside the conventional boundaries of medicine; he called it clinical ecology. The cornerstone of this movement was a presumed newly described disease which he named environmental illness. According to Randolph, this putative disease actually encompasses a variety of diseases of uncertain etiology, including rheumatoid arthritis, inflammatory bowel disease, asthma, and others, as well as virtually all forms of psychiatric illness. He contended in numerous publications that low levels of environmental chemicals are responsible for these diseases.[2] Over time, the concept of environmental illness centered on patients, mostly women, who complained of a large variety of symptoms suggestive of multisystem disease, but in the absence of any objective abnormalities on physical examination or by extensive laboratory testing. He and others envisioned the mechanism of disease as a failure of human adaptation to 20th-century synthetic chemicals. Interestingly, Beard, a psychiatrist, had described the same clinical condition 70 years earlier, which he ascribed to certain items and activities introduced into 19th-century living, specifically "the telegraph, the sciences, industry, the periodical-press, and female education."[3]

Randolph's name for this condition, environmental illness, held for many years, although others offered additional terminology to reflect differing views of etiology (see Table 16–1). As more and more patients claimed that their disease arose from a work-related chemical exposure, the currently popular name of multiple chemical sensitivities was proposed.[4] Other followers of the clinical ecology hypothesis have come forward with a number of alternative theories that generally focus on the immune system or the nervous system as the site of disease activity. As the number of cases has grown, investigators from many different medical specialties have critically examined these patients and the theories. There is now a strong consensus that the MCS phenomenon is best explained as a psychosocial one without evidence of an environmentally related physical cause, and that the clinical features are similar to those of other currently popular, but controversial, syndromes. Because patients with MCS attribute their symptoms and disabilities to environmental chemicals, this "diagnosis" is being used with increasing frequency in the United States as a cause of legal action against the manufacturers and marketers of many common products, especially perfumes, pesticides, and organic solvents, as well as against those responsible for the disposal of commercial toxic wastes. Many current cases bearing this diagnosis are generated within the context of such litigation.

 TABLE 16–1 • Other Names for Multiple Chemical Sensitivities

Specific adaptation syndrome
Environmental illness
Twentieth-century disease
Universal allergy
Total allergy syndrome
Cerebral allergy
Chemically induced immune deficiency
Chemical AIDS
Chemical hypersensitivity syndrome
Idiopathic environmental intolerances
Chemical sensitivity

DEFINITION

The definition of environmental illness, the former widely used term for MCS, was:

> an adverse reaction to environmental insult or excitant in air, water, food, drugs, or our habitat—domiciliary, occupational, or avocational.[5]

The term "multiple chemical sensitivities" was created to apply to environmental illness in those persons believed to have acquired the illness as a result of their work. It was defined as:

> an acquired disorder characterized by recurrent symptoms, referable to multiple organ systems, occurring in response to demonstrable exposure to many chemically unrelated compounds at doses far below those established in the general population to cause harmful effects. No single widely accepted test of physiologic function can be shown to correlate with symptoms.[4]

It is apparent that these definitions describe a subjective and therefore highly variable condition on the basis of which no objective diagnostic criteria can be named. There have been a number of other names for this phenomenon; they are listed in Table 16–1. It is apparent that definitions and theories of causation influence the terminology.

EPIDEMIOLOGY

There are no data on the prevalence of patients with the diagnosis of multiple chemical sensitivities. The diagnosis is based on a biased sample of physicians who subscribe to one of the theories of its causation. The subjective nature of MCS makes case-finding for epidemiological evaluation difficult if not impossible.

CLINICAL DESCRIPTION

In almost all published work, most of the patients diagnosed with multiple chemical sensitivities are women,[6, 7] and the most common complaints are cognitive difficulties and fatigue.[8] Somatic symptoms are numerous, including a variety of pains, mucosal irritation, weakness, nausea, headache, and paresthesias. The appearance of symptoms is always related to an incident of known or perceived exposure to environmental chemicals, although the relationship of chemical to symptom, the amount of exposure, and the latency period required for the appearance of symptoms are neither specific nor constant, and many times, the connection is made in retrospect.[9] The environ-

TABLE 16–2 • Multiple Chemical Sensitivities: Most Commonly Reported Environmental Causes

Organic solvents	Perfumes
Pesticides	Vehicle exhaust fumes
Paints	Fuels
New carpets	Newsprint
New clothing	Foods and food additives
Household detergents	Medications
Office machine fumes	Formaldehyde
Smoke	Phenol
Petrochemicals	Ammonia

mental trigger may be a specific chemical, such as formaldehyde, phenol, ethanol, or ammonia, but usually it is a familiar item encountered in everyday experience, often one that is identified as having a "chemical odor." New carpets, automobile exhaust fumes, perfume, pesticides, paints, solvents, and household cleaners are the substances most commonly mentioned (Table 16–2). These triggering substances can, for the most part, be identified by odor, which is also consistent with the subjective nature of the MCS phenomenon. No dose-response studies have been performed, although the exposure resulting in symptoms is usually reported to be at or well below ambient levels that have no ill effects on the population in general. Symptoms are also triggered by the ingestion of foods,[10, 11] food additives, and drugs, as well as by natural gas, *Candida albicans*,[12] viruses, electromagnetic fields, and even by endogenous compounds, such as progesterone, histamine, and serotonin.

Many times a patient reports that the illness began with a specific exposure—in some cases in an occupational setting—to a certain chemical; that incident is followed by reactions to many other, unrelated chemicals.[9, 13, 14]

In MCS, the complaints and their presumptive triggers are both subjective. Although symptoms often suggest significant visceral or musculoskeletal pathology, physical examinations typically reveal no objective findings that can explain the patient's subjective complaints. Extensive laboratory testing is frequently used in an effort to identify a pathognomonic finding, but without success to date. No gross or microscopic pathology has ever been associated with this condition. There are no long-term prospective studies on the course, prognosis, or outcome of MCS.

DIFFERENTIAL DIAGNOSIS

MCS is distinct from all recognized diseases that arise from environmental agents, including infections, allergies, and toxic and irritant diseases. In each of these disorders, there is objective evidence of the disease in the patient as determined by physical examination, physiological evaluation, laboratory testing, and pathologic investigation. In particular, MCS should not be confused with building-related illnesses,[15] the sick building syndrome,[16] occupational allergies, hypersensitivity pneumonitis,[17] or reactive airways dysfunction syndrome.[18]

Several investigators have pointed out the similarity between MCS and other recently described syndromes, particularly chronic fatigue syndrome. Although the clinical manifestations of MCS vary greatly among patients,[6, 9] the majority are almost indistinguishable from those with the chronic fatigue syndrome except for the attribution to the environment in MCS.

MCS THEORIES

Theories of the etiology and pathogenesis of multiple chemical sensitivities are numerous, and they frequently change. Proponents of the environmental chemical theory have hypothesized a variety of mechanisms for both etiology and pathogenesis, including allergic, immunotoxic, neurotoxic, cytotoxic, enzyme-inhibiting, hormone receptor–inhibiting, and detoxification-inhibiting processes. As new theories emerge, they often add to, rather than replace, existing theories, which results in expanding numbers of diagnostic and therapeutic measures that are recommended for these patients. On the other hand, those who do not find convincing the evidence that MCS is a physical disease caused by environmental chemicals have proposed a variety of psychological, sociological, and iatrogenic explanations. The scientifically rigorous experimental and clinical research necessary to evaluate every one of these concepts is problematic, owing to the subjective nature of the illness and the lack of a precise definition of the condition itself.

The Failure-of-Adaptation Theory

When originally proposed, the condition was presented as a failure in evolutionary adaptation to the synthetic chemicals of Western industrialization.[19] The patient's symptoms were viewed as a newly discovered form of allergy to environmental chemicals that was distinct from known allergic diseases and allergens. The increasing disability of these patients in response to an expanding number of environmental triggers was named the spreading phenomenon, a descriptive term that has never had a physiological explanation. The theory of adaptation failure has never been tested, and there is no empirical evidence for its existence.

The Allergy Theory

The presumptive allergy to environmental chemicals and foods was predicated on both IgE and IgG antibody–mediated models of symptom pathogenesis.[10, 20] Allergic diseases involving specific antibodies of one or the other of these two immunoglobulin isotypes have been well described and studied for many years. They are easily recognized and appropriately tested clinically, have well-defined objective physical findings and physiological abnormalities, and relevant experimental animal models are readily generated and have been extensively studied. There is no similar evidence of any kind to support allergy as an operative mechanism in patients with MCS.

The Autoimmune Theory

An autoimmune theory based on either a presumed molecular mimicry by environmental chemicals of unidentified native human autoantigens[21] or a toxic induction of immune dysregulation[22] appeared briefly in isolated publications. Human autoimmune diseases exist in two broad categories. Organ-specific diseases, exemplified by autoimmune thyroiditis, are caused by autoimmunity with specificity for defined antigens within the organ, pathological inflammation consistent with autoimmunity, and corresponding organ dysfunction. Multisystem diseases, exemplified by systemic lupus erythematosus, are characterized by multiple circulating antibodies with nonorgan specificity, such as the antinuclear antibodies, and these antibodies have shown little or no defined pathogenic role in the primary disease manifestations. There is a drug-induced variant of systemic lupus that differs significantly both clinically and serologically from the naturally occurring form of the disease. However, none of the currently recognized human autoimmune diseases has been traced to an environmental chemical source in the atmosphere or in foodstuffs. Furthermore, the concept of autoimmunity does not fit the purely subjective condition of MCS that has no objective sign of tissue pathology. Low autoantibody levels reported occasionally in MCS patients occur also in normal individuals of similar age and gender.

The Immunotoxic Theory

Toxic immune dysregulation by environmental chemicals causing autoimmunity or immunodeficiency has been a prevalent concept among proponents of the environmental theory of MCS.[22, 23] Presumably, this would be expressed as adverse reactions to chemicals, foods, and drugs. Support consists only of serum immunoglobulin and complement levels in selected cases,[10, 21, 24, 25] but even these are, at best, marginally abnormal. Other investigators find no consistent immunological abnormalities,[6, 26] and clinically, MCS bears no resemblance to any recognized autoimmune disease or immunodeficiency. Congenital and acquired immunodeficiencies invariably cause a typical pattern of recurrent opportunistic infections and, commonly, an increased risk of certain neoplasms. The specific humoral or cellular immune system deficit in these patients can be identified by using the facilities of the modern clinical immunology laboratory.[27]

It is unlikely that the diverse chemicals typically cited as causing MCS would have the same potential for immunotoxicity, especially since the healthy population tolerates these everyday items without suffering disease. The subjective nature of MCS is not consistent with known immunodeficiency diseases. Immune system testing in a series of MCS patients did not suggest any immunological abnormality.[28] Unfortunately, the name chemical AIDS has been suggested as a synonym for MCS, but its use clearly should be discouraged, regardless of which theory is subscribed to.

Neurotoxic Theories

The theoretical approach to MCS of neurotoxicity offers to explain the memory loss and cognitive deficits, such as difficulty in concentration, that are among the most commonly reported symptoms. Because the patient and practitioner attribute these symptoms to "chemicals," which the patient identifies because of odor, one theory postulates that MCS is caused by chemical odor–induced olfactory nerve stimulation of the limbic system and hypothalamus, resulting in symptoms that are attributed to autonomic nervous system activity. Progression of the disease—that is, additional symptoms and additional environmental triggers being identified by the patient—is explained by "limbic kindling." Although this term is borrowed from animal studies of electrically induced seizures, the application of the concept to MCS is reminiscent of the so-called spreading phenomenon.[29–31] To date, there is no experimental proof of this theory in MCS.

The Sociogenic Theory

The theory that MCS is a belief system that is based on an unfounded fear of chemicals accompanied by a distrust of the conventional medical-care system derives from patient interviews. The belief is strengthened by media reports of environmental pollution and by a strong group dynamic among patients with this disorder. MCS patients and their physicians have been described as a "medical subculture."[32]

The Conditioned Response Theory

MCS has been viewed as a behavioral conditioned response. This theory proposes that an initiating unpleasant or strong odor conditions the person to later responses to the same or different chemical exposures at lower doses.[33] In this model, even the perception of exposure, in the absence of an actual exposure, can result in a conditioned response that produces behavioral, cognitive, and somatic symptoms. There is no direct experimental proof of this theory to date.

Psychogenic Theories

Several studies have documented that patients diagnosed with MCS have a high prevalence of current and past depression, anxiety, somatization, conversion, obsessive-compulsive disorder, and panic disorders.[7, 26, 32, 34–36] As mentioned earlier, these patients typically reject any suggestion that they are psychiatrically ill. The psychiatric model of MCS proposes that patients feel less threatened if they can attribute illness to the environment than they would if they had to face unpleasant internal conflicts and stresses. One study of an occupational epidemic of MCS supports this theory. A group of workers had transient irritation resulting from phenol/formaldehyde fumes. Those with preexisting tendencies to somatization later developed MCS, whereas those without such a history did not.[37]

The symptom complex of MCS has been compared to that of somatoform illness, panic disorder,[38, 39] mass hysteria, and atypical posttraumatic stress disorder.[40] The condition has also been characterized as an adult manifestation of prior childhood abuse.[41] Several investigators have observed a high prevalence of several different psychiatric diagnoses among patients with MCS.[7, 35] Some proponents of the environmental theory of causation also recognize the presence of psychopathology in their patients, but they interpret this as the result rather the cause of the illness.[42]

Other Theories

MCS has been ascribed to the effects of oxidative damage to tissue by environmental chemicals,[43] to a newly described form of hereditary coproporphyria,[44] and to an overly sensitive state of the respiratory[45] or nasal[46] mucosa. Their are no clinical or experimental data supporting any of these views.

DIAGNOSIS

Many testing procedures have been recommended for MCS, but self-diagnosis satisfies the disease's definition.

The diagnosis of MCS is usually made on the basis of the patient's history detailing the subjective experiences as reported to the examining physician or on a standardized questionnaire. Physical examination does not reveal any diagnostic information, as stated in the definition of this condition.

Various tests are performed but none are diagnostic, and the choice of tests is dependent to some extent on the particular theory of symptom pathogenesis. Some procedures are designed to elicit symptoms from exposures. Other procedures are done to bolster the concept of a toxin as the cause. Still others are selected to confirm the idea that the patient suffers from deficits in brain functions, presumably because of environmental chemical toxicity.

Provocation-neutralization is employed by some physicians to document specific chemical sensitivities. The procedure involves administering to the patient small amounts of highly diluted solutions of chemicals or extracts of allergens in an effort to deliberately provoke symptoms, followed by further challenges to clear the symptoms (neutralization). The challenges are given by intradermal or subcutaneous injections or by sublingual drops.[47] The testing is performed without controls, and it has not been standardized.[48] A definitive double-blind, placebo-controlled study showed that MCS patients could not distinguish active from control test materials,[11] indicating that provocation-neutralization results reflect suggestion, not sensitivity.

Quantitating blood levels of immunoglobulins, complement components, immune complexes, autoantibodies, and lymphocyte subsets have all been claimed to have useful diagnostic value in MCS by those who have propounded the immunotoxic theory.[33] However, careful analysis of these results show that, although some patients may exhibit a random test result slightly outside the laboratory's reference range, there is no consistency among patients and no significant differences between groups of patients and normal controls.[33] Furthermore, MCS patients display no objective clinical evidence of known forms of immunological disease.[6, 9]

A number of practitioners rely on the quantitative measurements of pesticides, organic solvents, and other chemicals in blood and other body fluids or tissues to confirm the diagnosis. Clinical laboratories are capable of detecting and quantitating almost any chemical in biological material at exceedingly low concentrations. However, the results are of no diagnostic value, as the presence and amounts of such chemicals in the healthy population with no complaints of chemical sensitivity are, for the most part, unknown. Nevertheless, these measurements are often rationalized with the statement that no xenobiotic substance "belongs in the human body." This is, of course, a philosophical issue that has no bearing on the diagnostic value of such tests for MCS.

Antibodies to certain chemicals such as formaldehyde, aromatic organic compounds, and certain chemicals known to cause occupational allergy such as acid anhydrides[49] are sometimes recommended, even in cases without known exposure to these chemicals. Positive results in MCS cases are typically barely above the detection limits and, again, testing of an appropriate control population to assess the clinical significance of these results has not been done.

Nutritional deficiency theories of MCS are commonly combined with those invoking immunotoxicity, neurotoxicity, or cytotoxicity. For this reason, many patients diagnosed with MCS have had their blood analyzed for levels of amino acids, vitamins, minerals, and other nutrients and nutritional cofactors. The diagnostic value of such testing for MCS has never been investigated.

MANAGEMENT

Because all aspects of MCS are highly controversial, management of the patient depends upon the physician's view of the disease. The proponents of MCS as an environmental disease use certain treatment modalities based on the theory that the patient's symptoms are triggered by minute amounts of environmental chemicals from numerous sources at dosage levels that exist almost everywhere. Those who interpret MCS as a manifestation of a primary psychiatric illness or other nonenvironmental factors recommend an entirely different approach to management. A rational program of treatment is hampered by the continuing controversy over the cause of the condition, the lack of a case definition that satisfies all or even most physicians who see these patients, the heterogeneity of the clinical manifestations, the subjective nature of the illness, and the resistance of most patients to certain therapeutic recommendations because of their own interpretation of the meaning of MCS.

Management of MCS as an Environmental Illness

Environmental chemical avoidance is the linchpin of treatment recommended by physicians who diagnose MCS as an environmentally induced toxic or allergic disease. The patient must avoid even the most trivial exposure to pesticides, solvents, perfumes and all scented products, exhaust fumes from cars and trucks, synthetic clothing, plastics, and medications, at the least, as well as any other item suspected of causing symptoms. Typically, symptoms abate only transiently on such a program, leading to a wider sphere of restricted items. In the most extreme case, the patient may be required to live in a remote locale in a specially constructed building. Some practitioners recommend avoiding exposure to electromagnetic radiation from power lines and appliances. Others consider that mercury amalgam in dental fillings contributes to the illness and advise removal of the fillings. Work disability is common in MCS. No clinical trial has yet been done to establish efficacy for such extreme lifestyle changes. On the contrary, anecdotal evidence suggests that serious iatrogenic disability with progressive worsening symptomatology is the only outcome from such extreme "chemical" restrictions.[6]

Elimination of specific food items such as sugar, wheat, corn, red meats, and all additives is part of the overall regimen of chemical avoidance recommended, even if there is no history of intolerance to any foods or additives. This usually requires a rotating diet in which the same food is not eaten more often than once every 4 or 5 days. Rotation of foods in this manner is also believed to lessen the chance of developing food allergies, although there is no experimental or empirical evidence for this assertion. None of these dietary recommendations is supported by clinical trials to establish efficacy and safety.

Neutralization therapy is an extension of the diagnostic provocation-neutralization testing procedure.[50] Self-administered applications of sublingual drops or injections of extracts of foods or chemicals are used to prevent or treat symptoms. This can be done prior to a particular anticipated exposure, following exposure, during symptomatic experiences, or on a routine basis, daily or twice weekly. There have been no clinical trials to document the efficacy and safety of such neutralization therapy or to show that benefit is based on anything other than suggestion.

Some practitioners who subscribe to the MCS theory believe that this multisystem disease can be caused by (in addition to environmental chemicals) a toxin released from *Candida albicans* that is resident in the gastrointestinal or vaginal tract in the absence of clinical evidence of local infection. Others diagnose "mold allergy" as another cause of MCS, based not on evidence of allergy to mold spores, but rather on a theory that all molds in the air and in food can exacerbate MCS through an as yet undescribed mechanism. Nystatin, ketoconazole, and their congeners are prescribed to be taken orally, usually in minute doses, along with a diet free of sugar and yeast, by those who subscribe to the yeast theory. Antifungal drugs such as oral amphotericin B, again in extremely small doses, may be prescribed in accord with the latter theory.

Based on the persisting theory of MCS as an immune disorder, some clinicians have recommended intravenous gamma globulin therapy for its presumed immunomodulatory effect, but to date there are no clinical trials showing benefit in MCS. Multiple vitamin and mineral supplements, amino acids, and antioxidants are frequently prescribed for a presumed but undocumented immune-enhancing effect. Although the disease is supposed to be caused and worsened by "drugs," especially antibacterial antibiotics and corticosteroids, it is surprising how often these patients are given antifungal, antiyeast, and antiviral drugs, as well as thyroxin.

"Detoxification" as a means of reducing the body's so-called burden of foreign chemicals is recommended in a rigid program of saunas, exercise, induced sweating, induced flushing with niacin, and mobilization of toxins from fat by administration of fatty acids.[51] This regimen is carried out daily for as long as 1 month, but there are no reliable data to show that toxins are removed by this method, or that it is safe.

Other Recommendations for Management of MCS

Patients who have been diagnosed as chemically sensitive are often seen by physicians who are skeptical or disbelieving of the concept that the symptoms are in fact environmentally induced. Many studies suggest that psychological factors or psychiatric disease explains the illness, whereas others interpret the MCS phenomenon as iatrogenic or sociogenic. It is generally agreed that these patients tend to reject any suggestion that they are psychiatrically ill. All agree that the patients have strongly held opinions about the cause of their illness.

Psychopharmacology is frequently recommended as an alternative to environmental avoidance and treatment for allergy, immune dysfunction, or toxicity. The specific psychoactive drug depends on whether the patient is judged to be suffering from anxiety, depression, panic, or phobia. Although specific data on the effectiveness of these drugs in MCS is lacking, antidepressants appear to be of some use; they are now being recommended by MCS proponents, who justify their use in these patients by informing them that they are "immune-modifying" drugs, although there is no evidence that such an action occurs clinically in this group of patients. Long-term psychotherapy, even if indicated, is unlikely to be successful because the typical patient does not generally accept it. Short-term psychotherapy may be achieved, but without any assurance of benefit.[52]

Behavior modification intervenes at the symptomatic phase of the patient's experience without altering the exposure. The relationship of the environmental exposure to symptom production leads to an undesirable behavior pattern and disability. The aim of behavior modification is to achieve tolerance of symptoms through desensitization, a series of graded, controlled exposures designed to achieve behavioral tolerance. It is labor-intensive and time-consuming, and it requires the skill of a trained professional. It is also the antithesis of environment-avoidance therapy and must be accepted by the patient. A variety of methods such as visualizations, biofeedback, breathing exercises, and relaxation techniques can be used, as appropriate to the individual case. To date, success in MCS is limited to a few anecdotal reports.

A strong, supportive patient-physician relationship is consistent with good medical practice and is especially recommended for MCS, regardless of one's theory of etiology or pathogenesis. There is widespread agreement that a patient with MCS needs help from a concerned physician, and that clinical management is a long-term commitment by both patient and doctor. In each case, a workable therapeutic goal should be established. Without definitive information about the cause of MCS, it should be recognized by both the patient and the physician that management will be directed toward the alleviation or lessening of symptoms in order to eliminate or diminish the patient's disability. It is unrealistic to anticipate a "cure." Other reasonable goals are improvement in a lifestyle that has been impacted negatively by the illness and the environmental restrictions imposed by "treatment," enhancement of skills a patient can use to cope with the illness, and better understanding of the factors contributing to the illness.

CLINICAL STUDIES

The published literature on MCS includes numerous papers and books discussing theory and criticizing the current state of the environment. There is no extensive body of experimental and clinical studies by the proponents of the MCS concepts or by others. The principal studies that have appeared to date include the following.

Reports Favoring the MCS Concept

The initial publications by Randolph consist of a series of case reports published in abstract form in the 1950s. These cases contain his introductory concepts of environmental illness, which he first called cerebral allergy[53] and later named the specific adaptation syndrome.[19] He enumerated the environmental triggers: solvents, fuels, pesticides, exhaust fumes, gas and oil fumes, drugs, cosmetics, combustion products, foods, and food additives. He described the numerous symptoms, recommended "neutralization" treatment with sodium bicarbonate,[54] and suggested that psychiatric disease was in fact caused by environmental chemicals.[42] He later published several books on the subject and founded the field of clinical ecology.[2, 55] He and others[47, 56, 57] recommended provocation-neutralization testing.

Clinical descriptions of MCS have appeared subsequently in several texts.[5, 14, 58] These anecdotal reports generally agree well with those originally provided by the brief case descriptions of Randolph.

Claims of abnormal blood levels of immunoglobulins, complement components, and lymphocyte subsets are based on selected cases,[10, 20, 21] but the published abnormalities are minimal and inconsistent.[9] The usefulness of measuring blood, urine, and fat tissue levels of environmental and natural chemicals, a procedure favored by many MCS proponents today, is not supported by any published data.

The claims that MCS is caused and exacerbated by endogenous hormones (especially progesterone), electromagnetic radiation, viruses, fungi, yeast (especially *Candida albicans*), and foods also are unsupported by any published reports.

Treatment by avoidance of environmental chemicals, elimination diets, rotational diets, neutralization therapy by injected or sublingual chemicals or oral administration of salts, immune system modulation, antifungal drug, and vitamin and mineral supplements has been described and recommended on theoretical grounds,[12, 14, 58] but at this time none of these forms of treatment has yet been subjected to controlled clinical trials.[59]

Published Studies of Alternative Explanations of MCS

The basis for the diagnosis of MCS (or its various synonyms) has been examined by a number of investigators who find it to be arbitrary and predicated solely on the perception by the patient that a harmful environmental exposure had occurred and was responsible for subsequent symptoms.[6, 9, 26, 34, 60–62] The wide range of symptoms, the enormous variety of reported causative items, and the variable time spans between exposure and symptoms raise fundamental doubt that a single pathophysiological process could be responsible, especially in the absence of any objective physical or laboratory-based abnormality or pathology. The clinical pattern of symptomatology was found by some investigators to be most consistent with a somatization process, whereas others, using standardized psychological testing, uncovered objective evidence of significant preexisting and comorbid psychopathology, as was discussed more fully earlier.

Placebo-controlled, blinded testing of MCS patients has been accomplished using sublingual administration of food extracts[11] and environmental booth challenges with chemicals.[62, 63] The results of these studies show that responses by MCS patients are not reproducible when the patient is unaware of the nature of the challenge substance, demonstrating the importance of suggestion in this condition.[64]

The anecdotal reports of immunological abnormalities in MCS are unfounded when immunological testing is repeated in an unselected series of patients with proper controls.[6, 26, 65]

Position Statements

A number of major medical societies and other organizations have taken the position that MCS is not a recognized clinical syndrome and that its concepts are unscientific and lack validation.[36, 66–74]

SUMMARY

The concept of multiple chemical sensitivities as an illness caused by the toxic effects of very low concentrations of common environmental exposures is currently popular among a small group of physicians. The disease typically presents with numerous symptoms but no objective physical or laboratory-derived abnormalities. It has been known by many names, but it lacks a clear definition. Numerous theories have been offered to explain the condition—immunotoxic, allergic, autoimmune, neurotoxic, cytotoxic, metabolic, behavioral, psychiatric, iatrogenic, and sociological mechanisms.

Multiple chemical sensitivities, in the absence of its presumed association with the environment, is similar to if not identical with other controversial syndromes such as chronic fatigue syndrome. Patients with the diagnosis of MCS are commonly subjected to unproven and unnecessary diagnostic tests and to untested therapeutic modalities. In spite of the lack of physical illness and absence of pathology, MCS patients often experience extreme disability because their symptoms are triggered by common environmental exposures, and they are counseled in avoidance measures that may require extreme lifestyle changes. Studies to date do not support the theories of an environmental chemical cause of MCS or the diagnostic techniques and treatment recommendations based on those theories. Unless future studies that are scientifically sound change this assessment, clinicians should avoid recommending these diagnostic and therapeutic procedures in patients with multisymptomatic subjective complaints.

References

1. UNEP-ILO-WHO et al. Conclusions and recommendations of a workshop on multiple chemical sensitivities (MCS). *Reg Toxicol Pharmacol* 1996; 24:S188–S189.
2. Randolph TG. *Human Ecology and Susceptibility to the Chemical Environment.* Springfield, Ill.: Charles C. Thomas; 1962.
3. Beard GM. *American Nervousness, its Causes and Consequences: A Supplement to Nervous Exhaustion (Neurasthenia).* New York: GP Putnam; 1881.
4. Cullen MR. The worker with multiple chemical sensitivities: an overview. *Occup Med* 1987; 2:655–661.
5. Dickey LD, ed. *Clinical Ecology.* Springfield, Ill.: Charles C. Thomas; 1976.
6. Terr AI. Environmental illness: a clinical review of 50 cases. *Arch Intern Med* 1986; 146:145–149.
7. Black DW, Rathe A, Goldstein RB. Environmental illness: a controlled study of 26 subjects with "20th-century disease." *JAMA* 1990; 264:3166–3170.
8. Sparks PJ, Daniell W, Black DW, et al. Multiple chemical sensitivity syndrome: a clinical perspective. I. Case definition, theories of pathogenesis, and research needs. *J Occup Med* 1994; 36:718–730.
9. Terr AI. Clinical ecology in the workplace. *J Occup Med* 1989; 31:257–261.
10. Rea WJ. Environmentally triggered cardiac disease. *Ann Allergy* 1978; 40:243–251.
11. Jewett DL, Fein G, Greenberg MH. A double-blind study of symptom provocation to determine food sensitivity. *N Engl J Med* 1990; 323:429–433.
12. Crook WG. *The Yeast Connection: A Medical Breakthrough.* Jackson, Tenn.: Professional Books; 1983.

13. Cullen MR, Pace PE, Redlich CA. The experience of the Yale Occupational and Environmental Medicine clinics with multiple chemical sensitivities, 1986–1991. *Toxicol Ind Health* 1992; 8:15–9.
14. Ashford NA, Miller CS. *Chemical Exposures: Low Levels and High Stakes.* New York: Van Nostrand Reinhold; 1991.
15. Edelstein PH. Legionnaire's disease. *Clin Infect Dis* 1993;16:741.
16. Marks PJ, Daniel EB. The sick building syndrome. *Immunol Allergy Clin N Am* 1994; 14:521–535.
17. Fink JN. Hypersensitivity pneumonitis. In: Middleton E, et al., eds. *Allergy: Principles and Practices,* 4th ed. St. Louis: Mosby–Year Book; 1993:1415–1431.
18. Brooks SM, Weiss MA, Bernstein IL. Reactive airways dysfunction syndrome. *Chest* 1985; 88:376–384.
19. Randolph TG. The specific adaption syndrome. *J Lab Clin Med* 1956; 48:934.
20. McGovern JJ, Lazaroni JA, Hicks MF, Adler CJ, Cleary P. Food and chemical sensitivity: clinical and immunologic correlates. *Arch Otolaryngol* 1983; 109:292–297.
21. Rea WJ. Environmentally triggered small vessel vasculitis. *Ann Allergy* 1977; 38:245–251.
22. Levin AS, Byers VS. Environmental illness: a disorder of immune regulation. *Occup Med* 1987; 2:669–682.
23. Bell IR. *Clinical Ecology: A New Medical Approach to Environmental Illness.* Bolinas, Cal.: Common Knowledge Press; 1982.
24. Rea WJ. Environmentally triggered thrombophlebitis. *Ann Allergy* 1976; 37:101–109.
25. McGovern JJ, Lazaroni JA, Saifer P. Clinical evaluation of the major plasma and cellular measures of immunity. *Orthomolec Psychiatry* 1983; 12:60.
26. Simon GE, Daniell W, Stockbridge H, Claypoole K, Rosenstock L. Immunologic, psychological, and neuropsychological factors in multiple chemical sensitivity: a controlled study. *Ann Intern Med* 1993; 119:97–103.
27. Rich RR, ed. *Clinical Immunology: Principles and Practice.* St. Louis, Mo.: Mosby–Year Book, 1996.
28. Terr AI. "Multiple chemical sensitivities": immunologic critique of clinical ecology theories and practice. *Occup Med* 1987; 2:683–694.
29. Bell IR, Miller CS, Schwartz GE. An olfactory-limbic model of multiple chemical sensitivity syndrome: possible relationships to kindling and affective spectrum disorders. *Biol Psychiatry* 1992; 32:218–242.
30. Bell IR, Bootzin RR, Davis TP, et al. Time-dependent sensitization of plasma beta-endorphin in community elderly with self-reported environmental chemical odor intolerance. *Biol Psychiatry* 1996; 40:134–143.
31. Miller CS. Possible models for multiple chemical sensitivity: conceptual issues and role of the limbic system. *Toxicol Ind Health* 1992; 8:181–202.
32. Brodsky CM. Allergic to everything: a medical subculture. *Psychosomatics* 1983; 24:731–742.
33. Shusterman D, Balmes J, Cone J. Behavioral sensitization to irritants/odorants after acute exposure. *J Occup Med* 1988; 30:565–567.
34. Selner JC, Staudenmayer H. Neuropsychophysiologic observations in patients presenting with environmental illness. *Toxicol Ind Health* 1992; 8:145–155.
35. Stewart DE, Raskin J. Psychiatric assessment of patients with "20th-century disease" ("total allergy syndrome"). *Can Med Assoc J* 1985; 133:1001–1006.
36. Brodsky CM, Green MA, Ogrod ES. Environment illness: does it exist? *Patient Care* 1989; 23:41–59.
37. Sparks PJ, Simon GE, Katon WJ, Ayars GH, Johnson RL. An outbreak of illness among aerospace workers. *West J Med* 1990; 153:28–33.

38. Dager SR, Holland JP, Cowley DS. Panic disorder precipitated by exposure to organic solvents in the workplace. *Am J Psychiatry* 1987; 144:1056–1058.

39. Leznoff A. Provocative challenges in patients with multiple chemical sensitivity. *J Allergy Clin Immunol* 1997; 99:438–442.

40. Schottenfeld RS, Cullen MR. Occupation-induced post-traumatic stress disorder. *Am J Psychiatry* 1985; 142:198–202.

41. Staudenmayer H, Selner ME, Selner J. Adult sequelae of childhood abuse presenting as environmental illness. *Ann Allergy* 1993; 71:538–546.

42. Randolph TG. Ecologic mental illness—psychiatry externalized. *J Lab Clin Med* 1959; 54:936.

43. Levine SA, Reinhart JH. Biochemical pathology initiated by free radicals, oxidant chemicals and therapeutic drugs in the etiology of chemical hypersensitivity disease. *J Orthomolec Psychiatry* 1983; 12:166–183.

44. Hahn M, Bonkovsky HL. Multiple chemical sensitivity syndrome and porphyria. *Arch Inter Med* 1997; 157: 281–285.

45. Bascom R. Multiple chemical sensitivity: a respiratory disorder? *Toxicol Ind Health* 1992; 8:221–228.

46. Meggs WJ, Cleveland CH Jr. Rhinolaryngoscopic examination of patients with the multiple chemical sensitivity syndrome. *Arch Environ Health* 1993; 48:14–18.

47. Lee CH, Williams RT, Binkley EL. Provocative testing and treatment for foods. *Arch Otolaryngol* 1969; 90:87.

48. Grieco MH. Controversial practices in allergy. *JAMA* 1982; 247:3105.

49. Zeiss CR, Patterson R, Pruzansky JS, Miller MM, Rosenberg M, Levitz D. Trimellitic anhydride-induced airway syndromes: clinical and immunologic studies. *J Allergy Clin Immunol* 1977; 60:96–103.

50. Kailin EW, Collier R. "Relieving" therapy for antigen exposure. *JAMA* 1971; 217:78.

51. Root DE, Katzin DB, Schnare DW. Diagnosis and treatment of patients presenting subclinical signs and symptoms of exposure to chemicals that bioaccumulate in human tissue. Proceedings of the National Conference on Hazardous Wastes and Environmental Emergencies, Silver Springs, MD. 1985:150–153.

52. Haller E. Successful management of patients with "multiple chemical sensitivities" on an inpatient psychiatric unit. *J Clin Psychiatry* 1993; 54:196–199.

53. Randolph TG. Sensory aspects of cerebral allergy. *J Lab Clin Med* 1954; 44:910.

54. Randolph TG. Sodium bicarbonate in the treatment of allergic conditions. *J Lab Clin Med* 1954; 44:915.

55. Randolph TG, Moss RW. *An Alternative Approach to Allergies.* New York: Lippincott and Crowell; 1980.

56. Morris DL. Use of sublingual antigen in diagnosis and treatment of food allergy. *Ann Allergy* 1971; 27:289.

57. Willoughby JW. Provocative food test technique. *Ann Allergy* 1965; 23:543.

58. Rea WJ. Considerations for the diagnosis of chemical sensitivity. In: Talmage DW et al., eds. *Biologic Markers in Immunotoxicology.* Washington D.C.: National Academy Press; 1992.

59. Sparks PJ, Daniell W, Black DW, et al. Multiple chemical sensitivity syndrome: a clinical perspective. II. Evaluation, diagnostic testing, treatment, and social considerations. *J Occup Med* 1994; 36:731–737.

60. Brodsky CM. Multiple chemical sensitivities and other "environmental illness"; a psychiatrist's view. *Occup Med* 1987; 2:695–704.

61. Grammer LC, Harris KE, Shaughnessy MA, Sparks PJ, Ayars GH, Altman LC. Clinical and immunological evaluation of 37 workers exposed to gaseous formaldehyde. *J Allergy Clin Immunol* 1990; 86:177–181.

62. Staudenmayer H, Selner JC, Buhr MP. Double-blind provocation chamber challenges in 20 patients presenting with multiple chemical sensitivity. *Regul Toxicol Pharmacol* 1993; 18:44–53.

63. Selner JC, Staudenmayer H. The practical approach to the evaluation of suspected environmental exposures: chemical intolerance. *Ann Allergy* 1985; 55:665–673.

64. Ferguson A. Food sensitivity or self-deception? *N Engl J Med* 1990; 323:476–478.

65. Patterson R, Beltrani VS, Singal M, Gorman RW. Creating an indoor environmental problem from a nonproblem: a need for cautious evaluation of antibodies against hapten-protein complexes. *N Engl Reg Allergy Proc* 1985; 6:135–139.

66. American Academy of Allergy and Clinical Immunology Executive Committee. Position statement: clinical ecology. *J Allergy Clin Immunol* 1986; 78:269–271.

67. Black DW, Rathe A, Goldstein RB. Measures of distress in 26 "environmentally ill" subjects. *Psychosomatics* 1993; 34:131–138.

68. Brodsky CM, Green MA, Ogrod ES. Environment illness: does it exist? *Patient Care* 1989; 23:41–59.

69. American College of Physicians. Position paper: clinical ecology. *Ann Intern Med* 1989; 111:168–178.

70. Council on Scientific Affairs, American Medical Association. Clinical ecology. *JAMA* 1992; 268:1634–1635.

71. Committee on Environmental Hypersensitivities. Report of the ad hoc committee on environmental hypersensitivity disorders. Toronto, Ont.: Ministry of Health; 1985.

72. National Research Council. *Multiple Chemical Sensitivities.* Washington, D.C.: National Academy Press; 1992.

73. Board of the International Society of Regulatory Toxicology and Pharmacology. Report of the ISRTP Board. *Regul Toxicol Pharmacol* 1993; 18:79.

74. Barrett S. *MCS: Multiple Chemical Sensitivity.* New York: American Council on Science and Health; 1994.

75. Kay AB. Alternative allergy and the General Medical Council. *Br Med J* 1993; 306:122–124.

Prevention, Treatment, Rehabilitation, and Plant Inspection

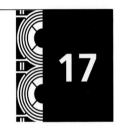

ROBERT M. ADAMS, M.D.

Since Congress passed the United States Occupational Safety and Health Act (OSHA) in 1970, the Department of Labor's Bureau of Labor Statistics (BLS)* has published annual statistics on safety and health for employees in private industry (except for workers in railroad and most mining industries, who are covered by other legislation). In 1994, there were 6.8 million job-related injuries and illnessses reported in the United States, a rate of 8.5 per 100 equivalent full-time workers, an incidence that has fluctuated within a range of 7.5 to 9.0 since 1980. Approximately 3.7 million resulted neither in workdays lost nor in restricted workdays, while 2.25 million cases involved at least 1 day away from work. Of these 515,000 were illnesses, among which manufacturing led all industries, followed by service industries. Disorders associated with repeated trauma (e.g., conditions due to repeated pressure, vibration, or motion such as carpal tunnel syndrome) comprised 332,100 cases, nearly two-thirds of the illness cases, followed by 65,700 skin diseases or disorders, of which the most frequent diagnosis was contact dermatitis.

The annual direct costs of occupational illness and injury have been estimated at $30 billion to more than $60 billion.[1] All states require physicians to report occupational injuries and illnesses to an appropriate state agency. In California, the Division of Labor Statistics and Research serves this purpose and requires that physicians file reports within 5 days of the initial examination on forms prescribed by the Division; employers must also file a report at the same time. If the condition is, or is suspected to be, caused by a pesticide, the physician must file within 24 hours and also notify the local health officer. In the California legal code, "occupational illness" is defined as "any abnormal condition or disorder caused by exposure to environmental factors associated with employment, including acute and chronic illnesses or diseases which may be caused by inhalation, absorption, ingestion, or direct contact" (Leg.H. 1994 ch. 667).

Many work injury and illness cases today are not filed on the employer's worker's compensation insurance, but filed instead with the worker's private health insurance. Long-term latent illnesses such as cancer are difficult to associate with the workplace and are also underreported. As a result, many cases of occupational skin disease are not included in the annual state and national statistical reports and consequently it is impossible to determine the incidence of occupational skin disease in the United States with any degree of accuracy.[2] In 1985, Mathias[3] estimated the annual cost in the United States of reported occupational skin disease was approximately $1 billion. Today, factoring in the inflation of the last decade, the annual cost from medical care expenses, disability payments, and lost worker productivity must be far in excess of this estimate. In 1990 in California, out of a payroll of 51,305,096 workers, compensation benefits amounted to $838,534,000, including indemnity benefits and health costs. Of these, skin diseases accounted for approximately $192 million.[4]

GOVERNMENTAL AGENCIES FOCUSING ON WORKER PROTECTION

National Institute for Occupational Safety and Health

The National Institute for Occupational Safety and Health (NIOSH) was created in 1970 by OSHA

---

*Bureau of Labor Statistics, Survey of Occupational Injuries and Illnesses, Room 3180, Massachusetts Avenue N.E., Washington, D.C. 20212

to conduct research and training and to make recommendations on prevention of work-related illnesses and injuries. It currently has a staff of about 900 as part of the Centers for Disease Control and Prevention within the Department of Health and Human Services. NIOSH provides scientific recommendations for workplace safety and health standards to OSHA, which then sets and enforces the standards. Mine Safety and Health Administration (MSHA) provides the same service for the mining industry.

The four chief functions of NIOSH are (1) surveillance, to identify hazardous working conditions; (2) laboratory research, to evaluate workplace hazards and study protective measures; (3) field research to identify potential hazards and degree of worker exposure and to establish and update criteria documents and permissible exposure limits (PELs); (4) provision of funds for educational resource centers at universities across the nation, to train occupational health professionals. Educational grants are also available. On line are NIOSH Recommended Exposure Levels (NIOSH RELS) and Immediate Dangerous to Life and Health Values (NIOSH IDLHs), with their documentation. Indexes with chemical names, synonyms and Chemical Abstract Services numbers and a useful pocket guide are also on line. So far these are prepared in English only, but availability in 24 languages is planned. A literature bibliographic database called NIOSHTIC is also available. The very useful Registry of Toxic Effects of Chemical Substances has been published for several years and also is now on line.

An international program for chemical safety is currently under development as a joint activity of three cooperating international organizations: the United Nations Environment Programme, the International Labour Office, and the World Health Organization (WHO). The chief objective of this program is to prepare and disseminate evaluations of chemicals hazardous to human health and the environment. This information will be prepared on safety cards that will provide essential health and safety information on chemicals used at the "shop floor" level by workers and employers in factories, agriculture, construction, and other workplaces. So far this information is being prepared in 24 languages, with a goal of approximately 2,000 cards by 2003. Currently on the NIOSH website, only English is available.

NIOSH also focuses on developing more affordable, simpler technologies and guidelines for industries to reduce chemical exposures, especially in small industries and businesses, by establishing closer relationships with these groups.[5]

OSHA

OSHA functions as the regulatory agency for occupational safety and health, enforcing the standards set by NIOSH, and from these standards develops PELs. The work standards it promulgates are law in the United States. It has compliance officers who inspect a workplace at any time to determine the health status of the employees, and citations can be issued for any infractions of the law. The states are permitted to formulate their own compliance programs; nearly half of them do so, and most have equivalent laws.

MATERIAL SAFETY DATA SHEETS

Because workers need information about the substances they work with, especially substances with a potential for fire or explosion, acute and chronic health effects, and measures to take in case of spills, chemical manufacturers, importers, and distributors in the United States are required to provide Material Safety Data Sheet (MSDS) (Fig. 17–1) for every chemical produced, distributed, or used in industry. All employers in Codes 20 to 39 are required to provide MSDS information to their employees and have it available at all times. Each MSDS must include the following information[6]:

- The chemical name and any common name or names are required. Although not required, the Chemical Abstract Survey Registry numbers of the hazardous substances should be included. If a chemical qualifies as a bona fide trade secret under the Hazard Communication Standard Act, its identity may be omitted. For mixtures, a list of the ingredients that are known hazards and ingredients that comprise 1% or more of the mixture must be identified; however, carcinogens comprising 0.1% or more must be listed.
- The hazards or risks associated with the hazardous substances must be named, including the potential for fire (flash point), explosion, corrosiveness, and reactivity; the acute and chronic health effects resulting from exposure, including any medical conditions that might be aggravated by exposure; the potential routes of entry (skin, ingestion, inhalation, and so on); symptoms of overexposure; the OSHA PEL; the American Conference of Governmental Industrial Hygienists threshold limit values; and any other known exposure limit.
- If the chemical is listed as a potential carcinogen by the National Toxicology Program's Annual Report on Carcinogens or by the International Agency for Research on Cancer, this also must

be noted. If it is not listed by either reference, this fact should also be noted.

- The proper precautions, handling practices, necessary personal protective clothing and equipment, and any other safety precautions in the use of, or exposure to, the hazardous substances must be listed.
- It must list the emergency procedures, including first aid treatment in the case of spills, fire, disposal, and overexposure at hazardous levels.
- The month and year that the information was compiled and the name, address, and emergency telephone numbers or number of the manufacturer responsible for preparing the information must be included.

The address and telephone number of the manufacturer are usually of the greatest importance for physicians, as the MSDS often does not include specific chemical information. Furthermore, substances (except known carcinogens) in concentrations less than 1% are not required to be listed on the MSDS,[6] while most preservatives and germicidal agents causing contact allergy are present in this concentration or below. To obtain this and other ingredient information, physicians must contact the manufacturer directly by telephone or fax number found on the front sheet. The information is usually forthcoming, but in nonemergency situations the release of specific chemical information may require a written request, with explanation of the reasons for the request and a confidentiality agreement not to use the information, which may be a trade secret, for any other purpose than a specific medical purpose. If the request is denied, a referral to OSHA for determination whether the denial is legitimate may be made. If OSHA rules that it is not, the company must reveal the information and, furthermore, may be subject to a citation and fine.

Unfortunately, many workers are unaware of the existence of the MSDS. They also are of little value if the employees are unable to read and understand the information. Furthermore, some of them are up to 50 pages in length. Since 1986, federal law has required that workers be taught in an organized training program to evaluate and benefit from the information on the MSDS. The documents must also be readily available at the worksite at all times.

Since 1986 NIOSH has been working with the WHO to develop an easily understood international MSDS, especially for use in developing countries. It consists of a two-page document that uses standard nontechnical terms and phrases. It is available in 18 languages, and a computer program has also been developed at NIOSH. International data sheets have not yet been universally accepted, but several nations have already placed the version on the Internet.

To help in identifying a specific chemical on the MSDS, the Chemical Abstract Services can be very helpful. Many chemicals are known by more than one name, and the abstract service can provide a useful cross-reference as well as additional information.

PREPLACEMENT PROCEDURES

Questionnaires

Preplacement questionnaires should attempt to reveal a skin disease that could limit a worker's employability, placement, and performance. Diseases to look for during preplacement examinations are listed in Table 17–1. Those that most commonly contribute to work-related skin disability are atopic dermatitis, psoriasis, chronic hand eczema, and specific contact allergies.[7] In its early stages, mycosis fungoides (T-cell lymphoma) may superficially resemble contact dermatitis.[8] If suspected, referral should be made for evaluation, including biopsy examination of the skin.

Examinations

The entire skin is rarely checked in preplacement physical examinations. However, a thorough examination is especially necessary before placement in occupations that have potential hazards for the skin. Nevertheless, if a skin disease is found, disruptive work preclusions must be made. They should be made with caution, however, be-

 TABLE 17–1 • Skin Diseases Important To Discover During Preplacement Examinations

Atopic dermatitis
Psoriasis
Chronic hand eczema
Chronic hypertrophic dermatosis of palms
Specific contact allergies (nickel, bichromate, rubber, epoxy, others depending on occupation)
Raynaud's phenomenon
Scleroderma, discoid and systemic lupus erythematosis, and dermatomyositis
Cold urticaria
Chronic urticaria
Necrobiosis lipoidica (in diabetics)
Severe sweating disorders
Extensive acne vulgaris
Severe actinic damage

U.S. DEPARTMENT OF LABOR Occupational Safety and Health Administration	Form Approved OMB No. 44-R1387

MATERIAL SAFETY DATA SHEET

Required under USDL Safety and Health Regulations for Ship Repairing,
Shipbuilding, and Shipbreaking (29 CFR 1915, 1916, 1917)

SECTION I

MANUFACTURER'S NAME	EMERGENCY TELEPHONE NO.
ADDRESS *(Number, Street, City, State, and ZIP Code)*	
CHEMICAL NAME AND SYNONYMS	TRADE NAME AND SYNONYMS
CHEMICAL FAMILY	FORMULA

SECTION II - HAZARDOUS INGREDIENTS

PAINTS, PRESERVATIVES, & SOLVENTS	%	TLV (Units)	ALLOYS AND METALLIC COATINGS	%	TLV (Units)
PIGMENTS			BASE METAL		
CATALYST			ALLOYS		
VEHICLE			METALLIC COATINGS		
SOLVENTS			FILLER METAL PLUS COATING OR CORE FLUX		
ADDITIVES			OTHERS		
OTHERS					

HAZARDOUS MIXTURES OF OTHER LIQUIDS, SOLIDS, OR GASES	%	TLV (Units)

SECTION III - PHYSICAL DATA

BOILING POINT (°F.)		SPECIFIC GRAVITY (H$_2$O=1)	
VAPOR PRESSURE (mm Hg.)		PERCENT, VOLATILE BY VOLUME (%)	
VAPOR DENSITY (AIR=1)		EVAPORATION RATE (_____ =1)	
SOLUBILITY IN WATER			
APPEARANCE AND ODOR			

SECTION IV - FIRE AND EXPLOSION HAZARD DATA

FLASH POINT (Method used)	FLAMMABLE LIMITS	Lel	Uel
EXTINGUISHING MEDIA			
SPECIAL FIRE FIGHTING PROCEDURES			
UNUSUAL FIRE AND EXPLOSION HAZARDS			

PAGE (1) (Continued on reverse side) Form OSHA-20
Rev. May 72

FIGURE 17-1 • A typical Material Safety Data Sheet.

SECTION V · HEALTH HAZARD DATA

THRESHOLD LIMIT VALUE

EFFECTS OF OVEREXPOSURE

EMERGENCY AND FIRST AID PROCEDURES

SECTION VI · REACTIVITY DATA

STABILITY	UNSTABLE		CONDITIONS TO AVOID
	STABLE		

INCOMPATABILITY *(Materials' to avoid)*

HAZARDOUS DECOMPOSITION PRODUCTS

HAZARDOUS POLYMERIZATION	MAY OCCUR		CONDITIONS TO AVOID
	WILL NOT OCCUR		

SECTION VII · SPILL OR LEAK PROCEDURES

STEPS TO BE TAKEN IN CASE MATERIAL IS RELEASED OR SPILLED

WASTE DISPOSAL METHOD

SECTION VIII · SPECIAL PROTECTION INFORMATION

RESPIRATORY PROTECTION *(Specify type)*

VENTILATION	LOCAL EXHAUST	SPECIAL
	MECHANICAL *(General)*	OTHER

PROTECTIVE GLOVES	EYE PROTECTION

OTHER PROTECTIVE EQUIPMENT

SECTION IX · SPECIAL PRECAUTIONS

PRECAUTIONS TO BE TAKEN IN HANDLING AND STORING

OTHER PRECAUTIONS

FIGURE 17–1 • *Continued*

cause many of these patients understand their disease and are able to avoid recurrence and disability, even in high-risk jobs. Furthermore, U.S. antidiscrimination laws must be observed.

Nevertheless, if active, widespread *atopic dermatitis* is found, a worker should not be recommended for placement where there exists heavy and frequent exposure to solvents, soaps, detergents, and grease or work environments where marked changes in temperature and humidity occur. Persons with *psoriasis* or a convincing history of this disease should not be placed in jobs where there is a likelihood of repeated trauma. Persons with severe or even moderate *acne vulgaris* should not be employed where there is heavy contact with oils and greases, particularly insoluble cutting oils in machining jobs. Workers with specific *contact allergies* should avoid work in which the allergen plays an intrinsic role in the work setting and readily and frequently contacts the skin.

Preplacement patch testing to predict the possibility of future allergic dermatitis is not recommended. However, in a situation where there is strong suspicion that a worker in the past became sensitized to a workplace allergen, testing may be done. However, it must be kept in mind that exclusion of workers with a disability, including a specific contact sensitivity, is not permissible under current U.S. law. A suggested questionnaire for use at the preplacement evaluation is given in Table 17–2.

TABLE 17–2 • Questions for Preplacement* Questionnaires

For atopic dermatitis
  Have you ever had asthma? _____
    Hay fever? _____
  Both? _____ Eczema? _____ All three? _____
  Have you ever had hives? _____
  Have any of your relatives had hay fever,
    asthma, eczema? _____ Which? _____
  Do you have food allergies? _____
    Pollen allergies? _____
  Can you wear wool clothing? _____ Does your
    skin dry and chap easily? _____
For psoriasis
  Do you have psoriasis?
  Have you ever had a persistent rash on your
    elbows, knees, or scalp?
  Do you have severe, stubborn dandruff?
  Do any of your close relatives have
    psoriasis? _____ Which? _____
For contact allergies
  Have you ever been "allergic" to any substance
    with which you worked?
  Are you "allergic" to cosmetics?
  To medications applied to your skin?
  To jewelry, watch bands, buttons, or other
    metals?
For chronic hand eczema
  Do your hands break out from time to time?
  Do you occasionally develop small itching
    blisters on your fingers and/or palms?
  Do your palms sweat a lot?

From Adams RM. High risk dermatoses. *J Occup Med* 1981; 23:829–834.

BARRIER CREAMS

Barrier creams, also known as protective ointments or "invisible gloves," are widely used as substitutes for protective clothing. Because they must be washed off before coffee breaks and meals and at the end of a shift, they encourage cleanliness, and at the same time remove workplace grease, oils, and dirt from the skin. An important requirement is that they not interfere with work performance. Many workers prefer them because they are easy to apply and in many situations are comfortable and hardly noticed during use. On the face (especially around the eyes) they may provide protection from airborne irritants. Two chief types of barrier creams are available:

Water repellent creams: Water repellent creams
  form a hydrophobic film on the skin.
  Composed of various waxes, silicones, and
  oils, they are designed for "wet work" to
  block skin contact with water-soluble
  substances such as acids, alkalis, foods, and so

on. They tend to leave a greasiness on the
  skin, which can be objectionable to many
  workers. Also when a firm grip on a tool is
  needed, the slipperiness of the cream can be
  hazardous.
Oil- and solvent-resistant creams: These creams
  contain lanolin, beeswax, tragacanth, acacia,
  and other substances that repel oils and
  solvents. They are, of course, water soluble,
  making them less effective when there is
  active perspiration. For work with water-
  miscible oils and coolants, aqueous solutions,
  acids, alkalis, salts, cement, chalk, and
  fertilizers, a barrier cream containing sodium
  bis-chlorophenyl sulfamine has been
  recommended.[9]

Water miscible creams must contain germicidal agents to prevent deterioration. These include bronopol (P), isothiazolones, quaternium 15, *p*-chloro-*m*-xylenol, *p*-chloro-*m*-cresol, and diazolidinyl urea. These agents are allergically sensitizing. Using the repetitive irritation test in animals[10]

TABLE 17–3 • Abrasives Present in Certain Industrial Skin Cleaners

Cornmeal
Wood flour
Rice hulls
Sugarbeet flour
Sand
Pumice
Silica

and humans,[9] the efficacy of these creams was evaluated. In humans, four standard irritants were studied.[11] The results of these studies brought into question the long-held dogma that oil-in-water emulsions are primarily effective against lipophilic irritants, and water-in-oil emulsions protect against hydrophilic irritants.

Wigger-Alberti et al.[12] have emphasized that, to be effective, protective creams should be applied frequently and in adequate amounts. Using the Wood's lamp, they showed that workers frequently miss many areas, especially on the dorsal aspects of the hands, the finger webs, and fingertips.

SKIN CLEANSERS

While removing dirt and grease, skin cleansers eliminate significant amounts of irritating and potentially sensitizing materials found in the work process. Industrial skin cleansers are commercially available as cakes, liquids, powders, creams, and waterless preparations. Abrasives, which are added to aid in cleaning by means of friction, are common causes of skin irritation and potential background causes of allergic sensitization; examples are listed in Table 17–3. Antibacterial agents are listed in Table 17–4.

 TABLE 17–4 • Antibacterial Agents Commonly Found in Industrial Skin Cleaners

Triclosan
Zinc pyrithione
Chlorhexidine digluconate
Zinc phenolsulfonate
Triclocarban
Chlorhexidine dihydrochloride
p-Chloro-*m*-xylenol
Chlorhexidine acetate
Sodium phenolsulfonate

PROTECTIVE CLOTHING

Protective clothing is available to meet a variety of requirements, such as heat, cold, acid, alkali, and solvent resistance, as well as mildew and fire. In about 1910 natural rubber began to be used, but it soon became obvious that it possessed many drawbacks. Synthetic materials became available in the early 1930s and rapidly became acceptable for use in many different situations. Manufacturers of protective clothing provide guidelines for selection for different exposures, and there are U.S. federal regulations for laboratory standards for evaluation. These are based on data from the American Society for Testing and Materials. In addition, for gloves used in food and pharmaceutical applications, the U.S. Government Code of Federal Regulations, 21CFR, Section 177.2600, has listed requirements. The National Fire Protective Association publishes lists of recommended garments for protection against hazardous chemicals. In 1993 the European Common Market established wide-ranging standards for personal protective equipment.

The degree of protection varies with the job and the materials contacted. For many jobs, only gloves and aprons are required, while spray painters, for example, must be completely enclosed in coveralls, gloves, hood, and respirator when painting automobile bodies and parts. In the so-called clean rooms of the semiconductor industry, workers must wear coveralls, gloves, face masks, hoods, safety glasses, and high-top boots. Pesticide sprayers must wear goggles, gloves, a respirator with pesticide vapor cartridges and filters, boots, and a heavy-duty apron, and a hooded pair of coveralls as well. Such full-body suits are usually expensive and are used repeatedly. They must be inspected prior to each use for tears and holes. Repair kits for total-body suits are available so that emergency repairs of minor punctures or tears can be made during the work.

Common materials used in the manufacture of gloves are listed in Table 17–5. Suggested requirements for other articles of protective clothing are given in Table 17–6.

TREATMENT

Because 90% of occupational skin diseases are contact dermatitis, this section is limited to a description of treatment for this condition. The basic requirement of successful treatment is removal from the cause. If the cause is unknown, the workers should be removed from the worksite for a period of time, and aggravating factors, includ-

TABLE 17–5 • Common Glove Materials

Leather
Cotton, terry cloth
Pigskin
Goatskin
Natural rubber latex
Synthetic rubber
   Neoprene (chlorprene)
   Nitrile (acrylonitrile)
   PVA (polyvinyl alcohol)
   PVC (polyvinyl chloride)
   Evon (polyethylene vinyl alcohol)
   Viton (fluor-elastomer)
   SBR (styrene-butadiene)
   EMA (ethylene/methacrylate)
   Polyamide (Kevlar)

ing irritating and/or potentially sensitizing home exposures including medications, should be eliminated. When the condition is acute, the cause is often obvious, and management is relatively simple, with wet dressings if blistering is present and topical and occasionally systemic corticosteroids. The possibility of allergic contact sensitization must be considered. Identification of a specific allergen often requires considerable time and investigation, especially in searching through numerous MSDS and inspecting the labels of workplace chemicals, cleaning agents, and the cosmetics and medications used at home.

Irritant Dermatitis

Dermatitis caused by contact with strong irritants is immediate and often severe, with blistering and pain. Treatment is the same as for a burn, with antibiotic dressings, pain medication, and systemic antibiotics. Treatment of subacute and chronic contact dermatitis consists in application of topical corticosteroids once or twice daily and advice on avoidance of additional irritation, especially from soaps and detergents, oils, greases, mechanical friction, and so on. If there are no contraindications in severe cases oral corticosteroids may be required for 7 to 14 days. After administration of an initial dosage of 40 or 60 mg, 40 mg/day can usually be continued without reduction for 7 to 10 days, followed by gradual reduction in 5 or 10 decrements every 2 or 3 days. The use of popular, so-called dose-paks is not recommended, because the dose reduction is too rapid, often resulting in recurrence, which then requires a higher dose and a longer period of treatment. Injectable corticosteroids should be used only once for initial treatment. Oral antihistamines are useful in controlling

itching, especially at night. If secondary infection is present, a short course of an oral antibiotic is indicated. Avoidance of further irritation is essential.

Allergic Contact Dermatitis

Treatment of allergic contact dermatitis is the same as for irritant dermatitis; in fact, the conditions often coexist. When contact allergy is suspected, patch testing should be done as soon as possible, but not before the effects of corticosteroid treatment have subsided, usually 3 or 4 weeks following the last treatment. Failure to find the allergen will result in recurring dermatitis and often loss of the job because of repeated absences from work. Job loss and a career change in midlife can create a major crisis for workers, requiring all the skill and assistance rehabilitation personnel and physicians can provide.

TABLE 17–6 • Suggested Requirements for Protective Clothing

Sleeves
May extend to elbow or axilla; have adjustable snaps at wrist; perforations to permit air circulation; should tear readily if caught in machinery

Shoes
Puncture and flame resistant; have plastic shoe caps; metatarsal bars and steel toes; metal or plastic inner sole; U.S. regulations require resistance to a 75-pound drop test and to a 2,500-pound compression test. Foundry shoes should fit tightly around the ankles and have elastic tops or quick-release buckles to easily remove the shoe if welding sparks or splashes of molten metal drop into the shoe

Face Shields, Goggles, and Respirators
Face shields should be constructed of lightweight plastic; drop-down and full-face shields are available. Fog-free chemical splash goggles are available; some can be worn over prescription glasses. Respirators range from half-mask air-purifying types to self-contained breathing units for entry and escape from areas designed as "IDLH" (Immediately Dangerous to Life or Health)

Clothing To Protect Against Solar Radiation
Tightly woven fabric provides greater protection; hats should be made of a fabric that blocks UVB and UVA rays, with an oversized bill and a wraparound outer flap to shade the neck and ears. Additional use of sunscreen that blocks both UVA and UVB is recommended

Other Treatment Modalities

Desensitization and Induction of Tolerance

For decades, attempts have been made to desensitize persons already sensitive to specific allergens. Kligman[13, 14] and Epstein[15] have been pioneers in these efforts, using oral administration of cashew nut shell oil and other *Rhus* extracts to desensitize or hyposensitize persons with contact allergy to poison ivy or poison oak (urushiol). Diminished patch-test reactions occur, but the results are temporary and often require up to 4 months to reach any degree of hyposensitization. Acetyl esters of urushiol were used by Watson et al.[16] and Epstein[15] for this purpose, but at present there does not appear to be a satisfactory means of desensitizing humans to any of the allergens responsible for allergic contact dermatitis.

In persons not already sensitive, however, induction of tolerance by oral administration may be partially successful, but this is controversial. There is some evidence that hardening does occur, as shown by Epstein,[17] who reported that outdoor firefighters who experience outbreaks of poison oak dermatitis in the beginning of summer, but continue to work through the end of summer, when the fires are more extensive and much more poison is burned and there is much heavier contact with the resin, the sensitized workers are able to continue working without dermatitis.

PUVA Therapy

For some patients, especially those with long-lasting, severe chronic actinic dermatitis, treatment with oral psoralens and ultraviolet A (PUVA) can be effective.[18] Other conditions responding to this treatment are chronic palmar eczema,[19] Compositae plant dermatitis,[20] and some cases of photoallergic contact dermatitis. 8-Methoxy psoralen 0.6 mg/kg is given orally 1 to 6 hours before administration of graded light exposure. Because of the risk of ultraviolet-induced cataracts, ophthalmoscopic examination must be made prior to initiating treatment and at intervals during treatment. In some cases, the results can be dramatic.[20]

Grenz Ray Treatment

From the German *die Grenz*, meaning "the border," grenz rays are low-energy ("ultrasoft") electromagnetic waves of very long wavelength, present in the electromagnetic spectrum between x-rays and ultraviolet waves. Their effects are similar to those of hard x-rays, but, because of limited penetration, they have been used for treatment of superficial dermatoses such as chronic eczematous dermatitis, allergic contact dermatitis,[21] psoriasis, lichen planus, and other chronic skin conditions. Long-term harmful sequelae, such as cutaneous malignancy, have caused this treatment to fall into disfavor. Although several dermatology textbooks do not mention this therapy today, it is still used by a few physicians.

Chelation Therapy

Disulfiram (Antabuse) has been used for decades in the treatment of recalcitrant chronic alcoholism. An interesting observation is that, when administered orally, it combines with nickel to form a tightly bound molecule.[22-24] Thus the therapy has been recommended for nickel-sensitive persons on the theory that ingestion of nickel, even in amounts found in normal diets, can cause recurrent bouts of dermatitis. Because low-nickel diets are very difficult for patients to maintain, and almost impossible for most of them, this form of chelation therapy, which renders nonallergenic oral nickel, has not been advocated. During treatment patients must avoid not only alcohol, but also medications containing alcohol, such as tinctures, elixirs, and over the counter liquid cough and cold medications, which may contain as much as 40% alcohol. The effectiveness of this therapy is not universally accepted. The treatment is contraindicated in pregnancy and in patients with impaired liver function.

Immunosuppressive Therapy

Severe chronic dermatitis, especially actinic dermatitis, may show improvement after treatment with immunosuppressive and antimetabolite drugs such as azathioprine, given in a daily dosage of up to 200 mg/day (2.5 mg/kg). The therapy is also sometimes used to reduce the dosage level of a corticosteroid ("steroid sparing"), but it has many side effects, including bone marrow depression, hepatitis, and teratogenicity. In women of childbearing age, pregnancy must be ruled out and contraceptive measures taken before, during, and for a period of time after treatment. It is also important to keep in mind that some patients with chronic actinic dermatitis have, in fact, mycosis fungoides or actinic reticuloid, and treatment with antimetabolites such as azathioprine could mask these conditions and retard correct diagnosis. Repeated biopsies are often necessary to diagnose these conditions.

Low-Nickel Diet in Treatment of Chronic Nickel Dermatitis

Following the suggestion of Christensen and Moller[25] that hand eczema could be maintained by ingestion of small amounts of nickel in foodstuffs, low-nickel diets were tried in these patients.[26] The results have been inconclusive, and the treatment has yet to be generally accepted.

REHABILITATION

Rehabilitation should restore economic and vocational usefulness in a worker who must change occupation or stop working because of a disabling injury or disease. For years, government and private agencies have provided vital services for the thousands of occupationally disabled persons. Frequently, however, the personnel of these agencies have little knowledge of skin disease and especially the role that contact allergens play in causing disability.

Many patients with a work-caused allergic contact dermatitis are good candidates for rehabilitation, because they often have satisfactory general health and also because their dermatitis develops only from contact with a single, specific chemical, which frequently can be avoided in a different job setting. The solution of course varies with the worker's age, motivation, intelligence, and other factors constituting employability. Older workers even with highly specialized skills often find it very difficult to learn a new trade and because of their age cannot find other work. Great personal expenditures may be required of these workers, often from resources already depleted by the unemployment.

In 1975, California enacted Labor Code Section 139.5, making it mandatory for worker's compensation insurance carriers to provide rehabilitation to workers who, from occupational illness or injury, cannot return to their usual occupation. The Rehabilitation Bureau provides enforcement of this law. A large number of workers are processed each year; only a small percentage of them have skin disorders.

Participation by injured workers in a rehabilitation program is compulsory. Workers are restricted to a single vocational rehabilitation plan, and it must be completed within 18 months. A $16,000 cap is placed on expenditures and is applied to all expenses, including counseling, training, personal maintenance, and vocational rehabilitation services. The fee for rehabilitation counseling is capped at $4,500, and rehabilitation counselors and insurers are prohibited from referring injured workers for evaluation, training, or rehabilitation to any entity in which they have a financial interest. In California, living expenses are provided, plus a maintenance allowance not exceeding $246 per week (which may be supplemented up to a temporary disability maximum if the medical condition has become permanent and stationary) or a temporary disability indemnity. Other states vary in their provisions for injured workers, especially in maintenance allowances.[27]

PLANT INSPECTION

A majority of workers worldwide are employed in factories and offices with fewer than 100 employees. These plants rarely have a full-time nurse or physician, and work-related disease is usually treated by nearby physicians or clinics. For this reason a plant inspection visit is often necessary, which will provide physicians a valuable opportunity to actually observe a worker at the job (Fig. 17–2).

Plant inspections usually originate either by the need to learn specific information of the work processes because of recent treatment of an employee with a work-related dermatitis or by the desire to view potential skin problems of the plant's operations. Frequently management or the worker's compensation insurance carrier will ask for a survey of a particular department or process to determine the cause of an outbreak of skin disease. Sometimes dermatologists are requested by local or state occupational health authorities, or a worker's compensation insurance carrier, for consultation on suspected dermatological hazards of a plant and recommendations for correction. This is especially likely to occur when there are increasing reports or a "minor epidemic" of occupational disease as revealed by reports filed by physicians practicing in the area.

Prior knowledge of the operation of a plant, work materials, and processes, as well as the attitudes of workers and management, make it easier to diagnose and treat occupational skin disease and recommend preventive measures and placement of workers with skin conditions that could be aggravated by a specific type of work.

Appointment for a plant visit is usually made with the personnel manager or the medical department. After arrival at the plant, a discussion with the safety personnel takes place regarding the prevalence of dermatitis in previous years, the dates of current outbreaks, the various departments and processes involved, and so forth. Management personnel usually have an opinion regarding the cause of the outbreak, and their evaluation should be carefully considered, although it may not be medically applicable. New chemicals or processes introduced to the work area, as well as preventive measures, should be learned. Information from plant personnel on the chemical aspects of a process can help the physician understand the often complicated operations and procedures.

FIGURE 17–2 • A "walk through" a plant involves much more than "a walk." Checking the worksites, as well as the general environment of the plant, the washrooms, the chemicals used, and so forth, are vital parts of the visit.

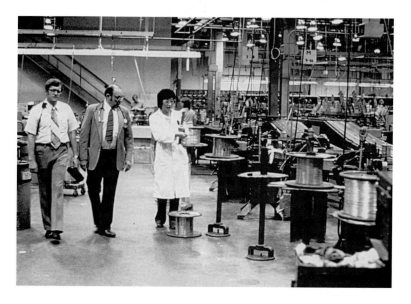

The plant physician, nurse, and industrial hygienist will provide information on the past frequency of dermatitis. The medical records of workers with skin complaints for the previous couple of years can be examined. Material Safety Data Sheets are invaluable sources of information, although frequently specific ingredient information must be obtained by direct contact with the manufacturer.

A walk-through of the plant follows, with a guide who is able to provide specific information about chemicals and processes. Plant physicians rarely have detailed information, but production superintendents, plant engineers, safety engineers, industrial hygienists, and sometimes plant chemists can usually answer specific questions.

Most plants have flow sheets describing the plant in detail, from the initial operations to the completed product(s).

A complete walk-through begins where raw materials are delivered, which should be checked for any preliminary treatment, including storage conditions. The work process in each department is then examined. Engineering controls, such as exhaust hoods, ventilation, use of protective clothing and whether it is appropriate to the tasks, and the general environment of the plant including the temperature and relative humidity should be noted. The foreman of each department, who can usually provide valuable information, should be the physician's guide.

When an actual outbreak of dermatitis is studied, a private examination and questioning of workers should be conducted. The condition of protective clothing must be noted and whether it is appropriate to the job. The use of solvents to clean the skin should be asked about, as well as whether barrier creams are available and used and their type and contents, keeping in mind that the preservatives in these creams are sometimes found to be the cause of allergic contact dermatitis. The washrooms, locker rooms, and toilet and shower facilities should be checked, as well as areas where the workers eat, rest, and congregate during breaks.

The Material Safety Data Sheets should be checked and usually help in learning the exact chemicals handled by the workers. Their ready availability at the work site is mandated by U.S. law. The company personnel, especially chemists, can also often provide additional information. A visit to the research and development laboratory will often have the plant operations in miniature, and the personnel, too, often can provide invaluable information about ingredients and processes.

Following completion of the tour, workers with suspected dermatitis can be examined. Often, further evaluation will reveal that some of the suspected workers have a nonoccupational skin condition; this especially occurs during "epidemics" of dermatitis, when many of the cases prove to be unrelated to any work exposure.

A summary report should be submitted as soon as possible. It is important for the report to recommend control and preventive measures in addition to the usual data such as the number of persons exposed and affected; their ages; sex; work description; department; materials contacted; skin regions involved; a description of the lesions; the presumed length of exposure; adequacy of washing facilities and type and use of special soaps and hand creams; personal cleanliness; control measures and protective clothing; barrier creams, and so forth. The final conclusion may be based on ingredient information obtained from manufacturers and the results of patch testing, if any.

References

1. Schmulowitz J. Workers' compensation: Coverage, benefits, and costs, 1992–1993. *Social Security Bull* 1995; 58(2):51.
2. Pollack ES, Keimig DG, eds. *Counting Injuries and Illness in the Workplace.* Washington DC: National Research Council, Panel on Occupational Safety and Health Statistics and Committee on National Statistics. National Academy Press; 1987.
3. Mathias CGT. The cost of occupational skin disease. *Arch Dermatol* 1985;121:332–334.
4. Department of Industrial Relations, State of California. *Occupational Injuries and Illnesses Survey, California, 1990.* California: Department of Industrial Relations; September 1992.
5. Hileman B. NIOSH is focusing on practical ways to protect workers. *Chemical Eng News* March 4, 1996.
6. Emmett EA. The dermatologist and the right to know. *Dermatol Clin* 1988;6:21–26.
7. Adams RM. High risk dermatoses. *J Occup Med* 1981;23:829–834.
8. Koh HK, Sharif M, Weinstock MA. Epidermal and clinical manifestations of cutaneous TC lymphoma. Hematol Oncol Clin North Am 1995;9:943–960.
9. Frosch PJ, Kurti A, Pilz B. Efficacy of skin barrier creams III: The repetitive irritation test (RIT) in humans. *Contact Dermatitis* 1993a;29:113–118.
10. Frosch PJ, Schulze-Dirks A, Hoffmann W, et al. Efficacy of skin barrier creams, I: The repetitive irritation test (RIT) in the guinea pig. *Contact Dermatitis* 1993;28:94–100.
11. Frosch PJ, Kurte A. Efficacy of Skin barrier creams, IV: The repetitive irritation test (RIT) with a set of 4 standard irritants. *Contact Dermatitis* 1994;31:161–168.
12. Wigger-Alberti W, Maraffio B, Wenli M, Elsner P. Self-application of a protective cream: Pitfalls of occupational skin protection. *Arch Dermatol* 1997;133:861–864.
13. Kligman AM. Poison ivy *(Rhus)* dermatitis. *Arch Dermatol* 1958;77:149–180.
14. Kligman AM. Hyposensitization against *Rhus* dermatitis. *Arch Dermatol* 1958;78:47–72.
15. Epstein WL. Allergic contact dermatitis to poison oak and ivy. Feasibility of hyposensitization. *Dermatol Clin* 1984;2:613–617.
16. Watson ES, Murphy JC, Elsohly MA. Immunologic studies on poisonous Anacardiaceae: Oral desensitization to poison ivy and oak urushiols. *J Invest Dermatol* 1983;80:149–155.
17. Epstein WL. Allergic contact dermatitis to poison ivy dermatitis. In: Adams RM, ed: *Occupational Skin Disease,* 2nd ed. Philadelphia: WB Saunders Co.; 1990:541.
18. Roelandts R. Chronic actinic dermatitis. *J Am Acad Dermatol* 1993;28:240–249.
19. Rosen K, Mobacken H, Swanbeck G: Chronic eczematous dermatitis of the hands: A comparison of PUVA and UVB treatment. *Acta Dermatol Venereol (Stockh)* 1987;67:48–54.
20. Burke DA, Corey G, Storrs FJ. Psoralen plus UVA protocol for Compositae photosensitivity. *Am J Contact Dermatitis* 1996;7:171–176.
21. Lindelof B, Liden S, Lagerholm B. The effect of grenz rays on the expression of allergic contact dermatitis in man. *Scand J Immunol* 1985;21:463–469.
22. Kaaber K, Menne T, Tjell JC, Neien N. Antabuse(R) treatment of nickel dermatitis. Chelation—A new principle in the treatment of nickel dermatitis. *Contact Dermatitis* 1979;5:221–228.
23. Kaaber K, Menne T, Neien N, et al. Treatment of nickel dermatitis with Antabuse(R); a double blind study. *Contact Dermatitis* 1983;9:297–299.
24. Christensen OB, Kristensen M. Treatment of disulfiram in chronic nickel hand dermatitis. *Contact Dermatitis* 1982;8:59–63.
25. Christensen OB, Moller H. Nickel allergy and hand eczema. *Contact Dermatitis* 1975;1:129–135.
26. Kaaber K, Neien NK, Tjell JC. Low nickel diet in the treatment of patients with chronic nickel dermatitis. *Br J Dermatol* 1978;98:197–201.
27. U.S. Chamber of Commerce. *Analysis of 1992 Workers' Compensation Laws.* Washington, DC: U.S. Chamber of Commerce; 1996.

Bibliography

Adams RM. Allergen replacement in industry. *Cutis* 1977;20:511–516.

Wigger-Alberti W, Elsner P: Preventive measures in contact dermatitis. Clin Dermatol 1997;15:661–665.

18

Health Risk Assessment

DENNIS PAUSTENBACH, PhD
HON-WING LEUNG, PhD
JULIE A. ROTHROCK, MS

The practice of occupational dermatology began, in its most simple form, as long ago as the work of Paracelsus (1493–1541) in his *Morbis Metallicus* when he noted the changes in skin caused by salt compounds.[173] At about the same time Agricola, in his book on the diseases of metal workers, described some of the deep ulcers he observed. In this century, the field became more sophisticated and by the 1930s was recognized as a specialty within the medical and health sciences.[173] Until the 1980s and 1990s, however, the field has not relied significantly on quantitative methods. For example, few dermatologists or occupational physicians have performed mathematical calculations in order to estimate the possible acute or chronic risks of exposure to patients whose skin has been exposed to industrial or environmental chemicals. However, it is now clear that enough is known about the specific behavior of chemicals to introduce more quantitative aspects into the daily practice of occupational dermatology.

Understanding and quantifying the penetration of chemicals into and through the skin is important in pharmacology, toxicology, and medicine. Armed with this information, the systemic dose of an agent can be estimated and possible adverse effects can be predicted. Of course, much of that information is based on the study of laboratory animals, which are used as surrogates, particularly in the field of toxicology. Appropriate use of laboratory animals necessitates a quantitative understanding of the differences among species so that the process of extrapolation to humans is meaningful.[126, 129] A substantial amount of data has been collected about the rates of transport of industrial chemicals through the skin, the amounts of these chemicals that come into contact with the skin, the

resulting blood concentrations, and the subsequent adverse effects.[128, 137, 188, 200]

Likewise, there have been a number of enhancements in the methods of estimating the degree of dermal exposure associated with various activities and of predicting systemic uptake.[26, 43, 64, 71, 105, 115, 131] Physiologically based pharmacokinetic (PB-PK) models have recently taken the field even farther, as the desk top computer now allows us to make reasonably good predictions of the actual uptake and distribution of chemicals by humans, based almost exclusively on data that can be collected from animals.[129]

The field of allergic contact dermatitis (ACD) has been well studied by dermatologists for more than 50 years and thousands of pages of research have been published about this hazard. Tens of thousands of workers each year suffer from this disease. However, the application of quantitative risk assessment methods to the study of chemicals that enter the skin and cause ACD is quite recent.[144, 157] One example of this type of research is described later in this chapter.

By and large, the process by which we bring all of this quantitative information into the environmental and occupational health sciences is called health risk assessment. Risk assessment can be defined in a number of ways, but for purposes of this discussion, it is the process of integrating toxicological and epidemiological information with data about human exposure so that the likelihood of an adverse health effect can be quantitatively predicted.[140, 141, 159] One reason that the field of risk assessment obtained such rapid acceptance by regulatory agencies and the public is that it introduced a relatively objective procedure for predicting safe levels of exposure, contrary to his-

291

torical approaches that relied on professional judgment, or what some called a "black box." This chapter discusses the field of health risk assessment as it applies to occupational dermatology. The goal is to better prepare physicians to tackle many of the challenges associated with low-level dermal exposure to industrial chemicals.

FUNDAMENTALS OF HEALTH RISK ASSESSMENT

Risk assessment has been broadly defined as the methodology that predicts the likelihood of numerous unwanted events, including industrial explosions, workplace injuries, natural catastrophes, and injury or death due to an array of voluntary activities (such as skiing and sky diving), diseases (such as cancer and developmental toxicity caused by chemical exposures), natural causes (such as heart attack and cancer), lifestyle choices (such as smoking, alcoholism, and diet), and so forth.[159]

Health risk assessment, just one specialty within the field of risk analysis, is the process through which toxicological data collected from animal studies, data from human epidemiology studies, and theories about the dose-response relationship are combined with information about the degree of exposure to predict quantitatively the likelihood that a particular adverse response will be seen in a specific human population.[140] Some aspects of the risk assessment methodology have been used by regulatory agencies for almost 40 years, most notably within the U.S. Food and Drug Administration (FDA).[112] In the 1950s, 1960s, and 1970s many activities that now are part of the risk assessment field were generally considered to be part of the practice of toxicology. The transition from toxicology to risk assessment can be traced to the late 1970s, when regulatory agencies adopted low-dose extrapolation models to estimate the cancer risk at extremely low doses.[40] The use of these models, coupled with more complex and quantitative methods of measuring or estimating exposure and the absorbed dose, represents the origin of the field of risk assessment (as separate from toxicology). The art of risk assessment differentiated itself from toxicology one step farther in the 1980s and 1990s as more complex computer-assisted exposure assessment methods and Monte Carlo techniques used to quantify uncertainty were integrated into the risk estimation calculations.[62, 131]

With the emergence of numerous quantitative methods and a significant increase in the amount of toxicological data, future risk assessments should be better able to estimate the likelihood that a specific adverse effect will occur over a wide range of doses[167] than were those conducted in the past. The increased confidence in the risk assessment process that has existed since 1980 explains why so many environmental regulations and occupational health standards are now, at least in part, based on this methodology. For example, risk assessment methods have been used to set standards for pesticide residues, contaminated soil, drinking water guidelines, water discharges and air emissions, sediment quality, and ambient air, as well as for exposure limits for contaminants found in indoor air, consumer products (such as plumbing fixtures, baby pacifiers, hair dyes, and foods), and other media.[151] Risk managers rely increasing on the results of risk assessments to decide which risks are significant and which are trivial—an important task because, for example, there are approximately 5,000 chemicals routinely used in industry.

Since 1975, nearly 60 guidance documents (encompassing more than 5,000 pages) on how these assessments should be conducted have been written by the U.S. Environmental Protection Agency (EPA). Regrettably, as the various U.S. agencies institutionalized the risk assessment process through regulation, the recommended procedures and methods often became inflexible and, as a result, these guidelines did not keep pace with achievements in our scientific understanding. For example, it has been and continues to be difficult to incorporate information on the mechanism of action or other biological information into regulatory risk assessments. As a result, over the years, the agencies' predictions of the risks posed by various contaminated sites or media were often overstated.[159] Furthermore, most attempts by the agencies to standardize health risk assessment methods introduced a significant level of conservatism by relying on default assumptions that could significantly overestimate the true risks.

The ultimate goal of risk assessment is to characterize the magnitude of a specific risk so that decision-makers can conclude whether the potential hazard is sufficiently great that it should be managed or regulated. If regulation is desired, the assessment can be used to identify the proper level of controls. Therefore, before deciding to conduct such analyses, it is important that all concerned parties (e.g., stakeholders), either implicitly or explicitly, accept that some level of risk can be deemed safe or insignificant; that is, there has to be agreement that a risk-benefit balance can be found.[181]

Health risk assessments are separated into four parts: hazard identification, dose-response assessment, exposure assessment, and risk characterization (Fig. 18–1).[140] Hazard identification is the first and most easily recognized step in risk assessment. It is the process of determining whether or not exposure to an agent can (at any dose) cause an adverse health effect (cancer, birth defects, sensitization, and so forth). Dose-response evaluations define the relationship between the dose of an agent and the incidence of a specific adverse effect. Exposure assessment estimates the magnitude of uptake from the environment by any combination of oral, nasal, and dermal routes of exposure. The last and perhaps most important step, risk characterization, integrates and interprets the information collected during the previous steps and, to the extent that is practical, describes or quantifies the uncertainty or variability in the risk estimates.[57, 141] Although this description has evolved as a result of environmental and occupational regulatory history, the same approach can and should be used in the evaluation of many clinical situations.

The Four Cornerstones

Hazard Identification

Hazard identification involves gathering and evaluating data about the types of health injury or disease that may be produced by a chemical and about the conditions of exposure under which injury or disease occurs.[140] It may also involve characterization of the behavior of a chemical within the human body and its interactions with organs, cells, or macromolecules. This biological information can be useful in determining if the kinds of adverse effects known to be produced by a chemical agent in one population group or in a particular experimental setting are likely to be produced in the human population group of interest. To a large degree, the hazard identification process is dominated by data provided by toxicologists, epidemiologists, and occupational physicians about whether a certain dose of a chemical can cause adverse effects within a given population. However, risk—that is, the probability of occurrence—is not judged at this stage of the assessment. Instead, the hazard identification is conducted to determine whether and to what degree it is scientifically correct to infer that toxic effects observed in one setting will occur in another; for example, are chemicals found to be carcinogenic, teratogenic, or neurotoxic in experimental animals likely to produce similar effects at the same dose in humans?[41, 86, 94]

Data about the toxicity of a chemical may come from several sources. The most relevant data come from studies of humans. During the early years of

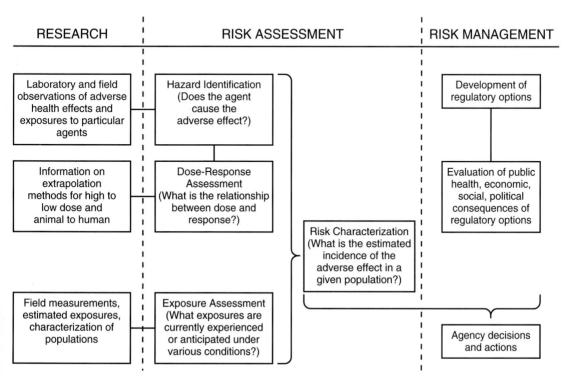

FIGURE 18–1 ● A schematic that illustrates the four components of a risk assessment. (From the National Academy of Sciences, *Science and Policy in Risk Assessment.* Washington, D.C.: National Academy Press; 1994.)

toxicology, from 1920 to 1960, a large body of data was derived from the observation of adverse effects in workers.[6, 98] More recently, however, most toxicological information has come from experiments with laboratory animals. It is necessary to be cautious in extrapolating animal toxicology data to humans, because many assumptions about the biological similarity of mammalian species have not been verified. The assumptions concerning the applicability of toxicity test conditions (such as exposure route and doses) to human exposure conditions, as well as some quantitative understanding about the appropriateness of the scale-up procedure, must be carefully considered.[141] Fortunately, methods are now available that did not even exist 10 years ago.

Although there is a substantial body of evidence showing that the results of animal studies are, with the appropriate qualifications, generally applicable to humans, there are important exceptions to this broad assertion. Nonetheless, in an effort to err on the side of safety, unless there are data from human studies that refute a specific finding in animals, or unless there are other biological reasons to consider certain types of animal data irrelevant to humans (e.g., α_{2u}-globulin-mediated nephropathy in male rats), it is generally assumed that the human response can be inferred from observations in experimental animals.[3] The assumption that all forms of adverse health effects observed in experimental animals could also be observed in humans is a conservative assumption that is accepted for reasons of prudent public health policy or regulatory mandate. However, the bulk of the evidence indicates, and most experts believe, that animal data alone are not sufficient to conclude that an agent will cause specific types of effects in humans exposed to a particular dose.

Dose-Response Assessment

A dose-response assessment describes the quantitative relationship between the amount of chemical that is administered (the applied dose) and the incidence of toxic injury or disease. Data are usually collected from animal studies or, less frequently, from studies of exposed human populations. There may be many different dose-response relations for a chemical agent, depending on the condition of exposure (e.g., single vs. repeated exposures), the route of administration (oral, dermal, or nasal), and the response (e.g., cancer, dermatitis, systemic toxicity) being considered.

When applying data derived from experiments with animals to estimate the risks to humans, at least two major extrapolations are required: (1) interspecies adjustments for differences in size, lifespan, and basal metabolic rate and (2) extrapo-

lation of the dose-response relation observed at doses used in animal experiments and the lower doses to which humans are likely to be exposed (Fig. 18–2). Models have been developed that attempt to estimate the results because, in general, the responses at these low doses (e.g., those that were less than a 10 to 20% response) cannot be observed or measured.[80, 95, 109]

Interspecies adjustments of dose, often called interspecies scaling factors, are necessary to compensate for differences between humans and laboratory animals in size, lifespan, and basal metabolic rate.[4, 10, 11, 76, 190, 191] Because most studies involve oral dosing, the most commonly used measures of dose are milligrams of chemical per kilogram of body weight of the animal per day (mg/kg-day) and milligrams of chemical per square meter of body surface area per day (mg/m^2-day). There are numerous other measures of dose (dose metrics) that can be used, and it is becoming clear that one method cannot be used as the basis for interspecies extrapolation for all adverse effects, such as liver toxicity, neurotoxicity, developmental effects, irritation, or cancer. Rather, the proper dose metric depends on the mechanism of action, the specific biological effect, and the pharmacokinetics of the chemical.[14]

For carcinogenic compounds, several different scaling factors have been used by different risk assessors and by different federal agencies. For example, the EPA originally used mg/m^2-day which is the more conservative scaling factor because it tends to give higher risk estimates per unit of dose. In contrast, the FDA uses mg/kg-day. In 1996, the EPA suggested that mg/kg-day to the 0.66 or 0.75 power might be a better predictor of risk. For some carcinogens, like the persistent organohalogens that produce their effects through nongenotoxic mechanisms, peak concentrations in a tissue times the amount of time above that concentration is probably the most relevant dose metric.[14] Comparison of risk estimates generated from human data and animal data on a number of chemical carcinogens indicates that the use of body weight provides good agreement for some of them, whereas surface area is better for others. A significant amount of research effort is needed to determine the appropriate scaling factor approach for specific chemicals and toxic effects.

With rare exception, for any given chemical and route of exposure, the severity and frequency of the effect (that is, the response) decreases with decreasing dose. In addition, the type of effect may also change with dose. For example, anesthetic gases may cause death at high doses, induce sleep at moderate doses, produce headaches or lethargy at low doses, and produce no detectable

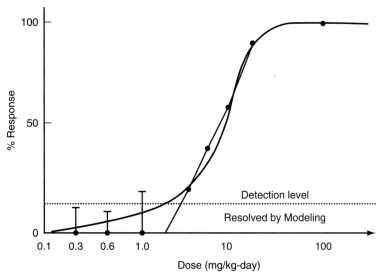

Dose (mg/kg-day)

FIGURE 18–2 • A dose-response curve from an exceptionally thorough (eight dose groups) carcinogenicity study. The solid line is a best fit of the eight data points identified in the test. The three lowest points indicate that at these doses, no increased incidence in tumors was observed in the test animals. The error bars on the three lowest doses indicate the statistical uncertainty in the test results because a limited number of animals were tested at each dose (*n* = 100). In an effort to derive risk estimates that are unlikely to underestimate the risk, the models most frequently used by regulatory agencies in the United States to estimate risk are based on the upper bound of the plausible response rather than on the best estimate. (From Paustenbach DJ. The practice of health risk assessment in the United States (1975–1995): how the U.S. and other countries can benefit from that experience. *Hum Ecol Risk Assess* 1995; 1:29–79.)

effect at even lower doses.[148] Clearly, an understanding of any dose-response relationship and its effect is critical to describing the human health hazard. To the extent that this relationship is not well defined, uncertainty about the estimated risk at various doses exists and, accordingly, the uncertainty is greater as attempts are made to predict effects far below the doses tested. An example of a dose-response curve and the different results that can occur as a result of applying different extrapolation models is presented in Figure 18–3.

For purposes of risk assessment, chemicals are usually divided into two categories—carcinogens and noncarcinogens—because somewhat different methods are used for estimating the risks at various levels of exposure to each of these classes of chemicals. Most carcinogens can also produce noncarcinogenic effects, but for virtually all chemicals, the doses needed to minimize the cancer hazard are so low that the noncarcinogenic effects are generally not a concern. Therefore, the term "noncarcinogen" is strictly operational—a term that is useful to describe a situation rather than an inherent biological property. For example, the term is used to describe chemicals that have not been shown to be carcinogenic by epidemiological or experimental studies and chemicals that have not been evaluated for carcinogenic potency. The term is used only for convenience and it is recognized that future studies may suggest carcinogenic

activity. Noncarcinogenic toxic effects include such diverse responses as sensory irritation; damage to specific organs, such as the kidney, heart, liver, or nervous system; and birth defects.

Noncarcinogenic effects are generally thought not to occur until some minimum (threshold) level of exposure is reached.[5] In contrast, carcinogens are thought by many scientists to pose a finite risk at all exposure levels. This "no-threshold" assumption has been adopted by federal agencies for most carcinogens as a prudent practice to protect public health. This assumption may not be true for some classes of carcinogens because they appear to act through mechanisms that require a threshold dose to be exceeded prior to initiation of the carcinogenic process.[31–33, 204] Functionally, in light of the fact that human diets are abundant with carcinogens, there must be a practical threshold below which we would call a dose "safe."[8] In recent years, there seems to have been growing agreement in the scientific community that not all carcinogens pose a hazard at all doses. This is reflected in the 1996 EPA draft carcinogen assessment guidelines,[55] which acknowledge that many chemicals that are carcinogens at high doses in animals may not pose a risk to humans at much lower doses—that is, they have a practical threshold.

As noted previously, scientists have developed several mathematical models to estimate low-dose

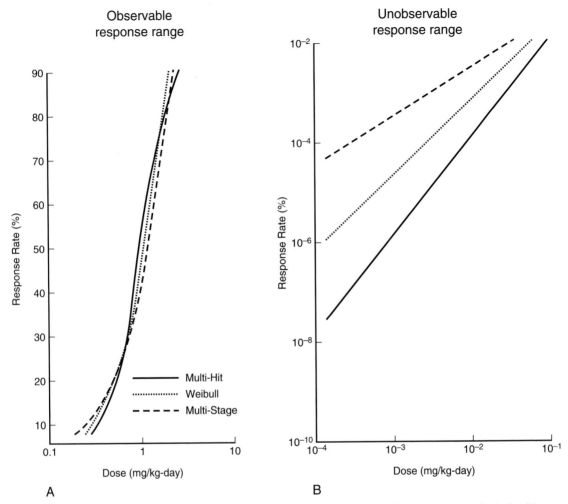

Observable response range

Unobservable response range

A

B

FIGURE 18–3 • *A* and *B*. The fit of most dose-response models to data in the observable range is generally similar *(A)*. However, due to the differences in the assumptions and equations upon which the models are based, the risk estimates at low doses can vary dramatically among the different models *(B)*. (From Paustenbach DJ. The practice of health risk assessment in the United States (1975–1995): how the U.S. and other countries can benefit from that experience. *Hum Ecol Risk Assess* 1995; 1:29–79.)

carcinogenic risks based on observed high-dose responses.[40, 88, 110] Such models describe the expected quantitative relationship between risk and dose and are used to estimate a value for the risk at the dose of interest. For example, if it is known that there was a 20% increased incidence of tumors in rodents exposed to 100 μg/kg-day, and a 50% increased incidence at 1,300 μg/kg-day, what is the risk to humans who ingest 1.0 mg/kg-day? The accuracy of the projected risk at the dose of interest is a function of how accurately the mathematical model describes the true, but unmeasurable, relation between dose and risk at the low dose. Although most of the available models fit the experimental, high-dose data, the predicted risks at low doses may vary significantly (see Fig. 18–3). In general, because of the spread in the various risk estimates among the various models at low doses, and because science cannot be sure which model is likely to be accurate, most U.S. regulatory agencies rely upon the most conservative method—the linearized multistage model developed by Crump et al.[40]

Exposure Assessment

An exposure assessment describes the nature and size of the various populations exposed to a chemical agent and the magnitude and duration of their exposures.[53, 56] The evaluation can concern past, current, or future anticipated exposures.[140, 141]

Exposure assessments determine the degree of contact a person has with a chemical and estimate the absorbed dose. Several factors affect the prediction of absorbed dose, including the duration of the exposure, the route of exposure, the bioavailability of the chemical from the contaminated media (for example, soil), and, sometimes, the unique characteristics of the exposed population (e.g., the workers may have chronic dermatoses which facilitate dermal penetrations).

The duration of exposure is the period of time over which a person is exposed. An acute exposure generally involves one contact with the chemical, usually for less than a day. An exposure is considered chronic when it covers a substantial portion of the person's lifetime. Exposures of intermediate duration are called subchronic.

Knowledge of the concentration of a chemical in an environmental medium is essential for determining the magnitude of the absorbed dose. This information is usually obtained by analytical measurements of a sample of the medium, such as soil, groundwater, or sediment. Estimates can also be made using certain mathematical models, such as models relating air concentrations at various distances from a point of release such as a smoke stack to factors including release rate, weather conditions, distance, and the stability of the chemical agent.

To determine the dose, it is also necessary to know the magnitude of intake of, or contact with, the contaminated medium per unit of time. For example, knowledge of the number of liters of contaminated water ingested per day is the intake information necessary to estimate the dose received from this medium. Similarly, knowledge of the amount of soil coming into contact with the skin each day is necessary to estimate the dose received from this medium. Note that intake or contact with a given medium may occur by more than one route—soil may contact the skin or be ingested, dust may be inhaled.

Absorption rates of a chemical agent through the lungs, skin, or gastrointestinal tract also must be known in order to estimate dose. The fraction of the agent absorbed by way of a given route is a function of many complex variables and often is not known with accuracy. In fact, the toxicity of a particular substance depends not only on the magnitude of the systemic dose but also on the behavior of the dose after it enters the body.

The bioavailability of the chemical in the medium of interest is a factor that has begun to be studied.[92, 180] Bioavailability is the percentage of the agent in a medium that is accessible for absorption. For example, only a small fraction of the lead in the ash or aggregate of incinerators can be removed (by extraction using many different solvents). It is now known that there is a correlation between extraction by acidified water or solvents and the percent of gastrointestinal uptake by

animals or humans. It follows, therefore, that if the aggregate is in the soil and is eaten by children or wildlife, the majority of the lead is not absorbed and passes unchanged through the gastrointestinal tract.

Risk Characterization

Risk characterization involves integration of the data and analyses involved in the other three steps of risk assessment to determine the likelihood that the human population of interest will experience any of the various forms of toxicity associated with a chemical (under its known or anticipated conditions of exposure).[140] In risk characterization, all information is combined to generate a statement of risk, which is generally characterized by the presence or absence of a cancer hazard.

Noncarcinogens. Potential noncarcinogenic adverse health effects are usually characterized by comparing predicted doses to established regulatory criteria. It is generally accepted that noncarcinogenic health effects are not expected to occur until after a threshold dose is reached. Regulatory agencies have established reference doses (RfDs) for many "threshold chemicals," those chemicals for which an oral dose exists below which no adverse health effects are expected to occur, even in sensitive individuals. The RfD is normally set near the value of 1/100th of the no observed adverse effect level (NOAEL) seen in animals.

In order to evaluate the acceptability of a particular dose relative to this reference criterion, the data are analyzed using the hazard quotient approach.[54] The hazard quotient (HQ) is the ratio of the predicted average daily dose (ADD) to the RfD:

$$\text{Hazard Quotient} = \text{ADD/RfD} \qquad \text{(Equation 1)}$$

If the potential exposure is through ingestion, the oral RfD is used to characterize risk. If the potential exposure is through inhalation, risk is characterized using the inhalation RfD. Usually, inhalation exposure is evaluated using the inhalation reference concentrations (RfCs) or, when these are not available, it is possible to convert the dose into an oral uptake and then compare it to the oral RfD, if a route-to-route extrapolation of this type is determined to be appropriate.

The EPA has not established RfDs for dermal exposure; therefore, in general, the risks due to dermal uptake are predicted using the oral RfD. Oral toxicity criteria are adjusted by incorporating appropriate dermal absorption factors (ABFs) into the dose equation. Because most substances are typically absorbed less efficiently by the dermal route than by the oral route, dermal ABFs are used to account for the likelihood that a smaller fraction of the substance will be absorbed following dermal contact than if the substance were ingested. Guidance is available for using dermal ABFs.[44]

A hazard quotient less than or equal to 1 indicates that adverse health effects are not expected to occur. An HQ greater than 1 indicates only that further evaluation is required; it does not mean that effects will occur. The possible effects due to potential exposure to multiple chemicals are addressed by calculating a hazard index (HI). This is a screening approach in which all substances are conservatively assumed to act in an additive manner. This approach, by design, overstates the potential for noncarcinogenic health effects, but it can be used as a rapid screening tool to eliminate those exposure scenarios that do not pose a noncarcinogenic hazard.

The HI is calculated as follows:

$$\text{Hazard Index} = \Sigma \text{ Hazard Quotients}$$

$$= \Sigma \frac{ADD_i}{RfD_i} \qquad \text{(Equation 2)}$$

Example Calculation 1: Noncarcinogenic Hazard from Multiple Chemical Exposure

Assume that a female construction worker is exposed to chlorobenzene and PCBs in subsurface soils at ADD levels of 4.2×10^{-7} and 1.5×10^{-4} mg/kg-day, respectively. What is the hazard index that describes these levels of exposure? Chlorobenzene has an RfD of 2×10^{-2} mg/kg-day, and PCBs have an RfD of 5×10^{-5} mg/kg-day.[87, 96]

Using Equation 1:

$$\begin{aligned}
HQ_{chlorobenzene} &= ADD/RfD \\
&= (4.2 \times 10^{-7} \text{ mg/kg-day})/ \\
&\quad (2 \times 10^{-2} \text{ mg/kg-day}) \\
&= 2.1 \times 10^{-5}
\end{aligned}$$

$$\begin{aligned}
HQ_{PCBs} &= ADD/RfD \\
&= (1.5 \times 10^{-4} \text{ mg/kg-day})/ \\
&\quad (5 \times 10^{-5} \text{ mg/kg-day}) \\
&= 3
\end{aligned}$$

Using Equation 2:

$$\begin{aligned}
HI &= \Sigma (HQ_{chlorobenzene}, HQ_{PCBs}) \\
&= (2.1 \times 10^{-5} + 3) \\
&= 3
\end{aligned}$$

Carcinogens

For carcinogens, the risk to humans is estimated by multiplying the lifetime average daily dose (LADD) by the risk per unit of dose predicted by the dose-response modeling. A range of risks might be produced using different models and assumptions about dose-response curves and the information available on the relative susceptibilities of human and animals.

In these calculations, the theoretical excess cancer risk is based on the total incremental LADD of the chemical of interest received as a result of the exposure averaged over a 70-year lifetime. Once the dose has been calculated, the cancer risk is predicted as follows:

$$\text{Estimated Cancer Risk by Inhalation Route} = \text{Inhalation LADD}_i \times Sf_{inhalation, I} \quad \text{(Equation 3)}$$

$$\text{Estimated Cancer Risk by Oral Route} = \text{Oral LADD}_i \times Sf_{oral, I} \quad \text{(Equation 4)}$$

$$\text{Estimated Cancer Risk by Dermal Route} = \text{Dermal LADD}_i \times Sf_{oral, I} \quad \text{(Equation 5)}$$

where Sf = slope factor.

The total cancer risk estimate is calculated by summing the predicted carcinogenic risk for each chemical, across all routes and media (e.g., indoor air). This approach overestimates the actual risk because different substances generally have different mechanisms of action and different target organs relative to the cancer hazard. In addition, this approach assumes that exposure to carcinogens at any dose will present some risk. Although it is not known to be true for numerous categories of carcinogenic substances, additivity is currently assumed, at least for regulatory purposes, until better data are available.

Example Calculation 2: Cancer Risk from Inhalation Exposure

A utility worker is exposed to PCB particles in soils at an LADD of 6.4×10^{-7} mg/kg-day. What is his cancer risk, assuming that PCBs have an inhalation slope factor of 2 $(\text{mg/kg-day})^{-1}$?

Using Equation 3:

$$\begin{aligned}
\text{Cancer Risk} &= \text{Inhalation LADD} \times SF_{inhalation} \\
&= (6.4 \times 10^{-7} \text{ mg/kg-day}) \\
&\quad (2 \text{ mg/kg-day}^{-1}) \\
&= 1.3 \times 10^{-6}
\end{aligned}$$

In this example, the increased cancer risk is 1.3 in one million. It can be inferred that this level of exposure raises the risk from a background level of 25% to no greater than 25.0001%.

A key trait of a high-quality risk characterization is the accurate and unbiased discussion of the significance of the data. Often, regulatory agencies and the press have claimed or implied that the results of low-dose models actually predict the increased cancer risk for exposed individuals. As discussed by Dr. Frank Young,[208] a former commissioner of the FDA, this was not the intent of such estimates:

> The risk level of one in one million is often misunderstood by the public and the media. It is not an actual risk, i.e., we do not expect one out of every million people to get cancer if they drink decaffeinated coffee. Rather, it is a mathematical risk based on scientific assumptions used in risk assessment.
>
> FDA uses a conservative estimate of risk to ensure that the risk is not understated. We interpret animal test results conservatively and we are extremely careful when we extrapolate risks to humans. When FDA uses the risk level of one in one million, it is confident that the risk to humans is virtually nonexistent.

The hallmark of an exceptional risk characterization is a discussion of the uncertainties in the risk estimates. Several papers have discussed how uncertainty analyses can be conducted.[27, 62, 132, 189]

Like other health professionals, occupational physicians would benefit from knowing how to describe the significance of model-estimated cancer risks in an understandable fashion for patients and for the public at large. This is a significant challenge to the professional who does not routinely work with and apply risk assessment methods. For example, how does one explain why the cancer risks to which workers are permitted to be exposed are so much greater than those allowed for the general public? Specifically, the theoretical or plausible risks associated with exposure to the threshold limit values (TLVs) are relatively high (Table 18–1). For example, the theoretical cancer risk associated with exposure to the TLV for ethylene dichloride is 1 in 1,000, while EPA's maximum contaminant levels (MCLs) for ethylene dichloride in drinking water attempt to limit the maximum plausible cancer risk to about 1 in 100,000.[152, 153]

To most persons, both of these incremental risks might be considered insignificant because the background cancer risk to the general population is currently about 25%. Therefore, a 1 in 100,000 incremental risk is equivalent to ensuring that the lifetime cancer risk for any person exposed to this level of contamination is not greater than 250,010 in 1,000,000 (25.001%), rather than 250,000 in 1,000,000 (25%). The standard of care or protectiveness that the United States chooses to be "acceptable" for its workers as opposed to that for the general public is a complicated issue that will

TABLE 18–1 • Estimated Lifetime Risks of Death from Cancer per 1,000 Persons Associated with Occupational Exposure at Pre-1989 and Proposed Post-1989 OSHA-Permissible Exposure Limits (PELs) for Selected Substances

Substance	Cases/1,000 at Previous PEL	Cases/1,000 at Revised PEL
Inorganic arsenic	148–767	8
Ethylene oxide	63–109	1–2
Ethylene dibromide (proposal)	70–110	0.2–6
Benzene (proposal)	44–152	5–16
Acrylonitrile	390	39
Dibromochloropropane (DBCP)	—	2
Asbestos	64	6.7

From Paustenbach DJ. Health risk assessment and the practice of industrial hygiene. *Am Ind Hyg Assoc J* 1990;51:339–351.

receive a good deal of discussion in the coming years.[80, 148]

THE ROLE OF SKIN UPTAKE IN HEALTH RISK ASSESSMENT

One of the most common routes of exposure to chemicals, especially in the work environment, is the skin, that is, dermal or percutaneous absorption. The skin is a complex organ consisting of several organized layers, and it has been well characterized anatomically and morphologically.[50, 123] An understanding of the processes that affect the transport of compounds across the skin enables health risk assessors to use physical or chemical data, such as the permeability of the skin (expressed as a permeability coefficient, K_p) or the n-octanol/water partition coefficient (K_{ow}) of the chemical, to estimate the rate at which a chemical will be absorbed.[52, 115]

FATE OF COMPOUNDS APPLIED TO THE SKIN

Numerous environmental pollutants are known to permeate the skin's diffusional barriers and to enter the systemic circulation via capillaries at the dermo-epidermal junction. Therefore, percutaneous absorption can be regarded as the translocation of a chemical from the skin surface through the various strata of the epidermis and a small portion of underlying dermis that contains papillary capillaries where the chemical enters the bloodstream. Some portion of the chemical may be metabolized during its movement through the living epidermis.

The fates of compounds that come into contact with skin are as follows: (1) evaporative loss from the skin surface; (2) uptake into the stratum corneum with reversible or irreversible binding followed by loss through sloughing of the stratum corneum; (3) penetration into the viable epidermis, followed by possible metabolism; or (4) absorption into the systemic circulation. In many of the studies used to generate K_p values, the extent of skin absorption has been estimated by measuring the loss of compound from the skin surface. However, if loss processes such as those presented in Figure 18–4 are occurring, an overestimation of the extent and rate of skin sorption is possible. Therefore, the risk assessor must consider these sorption and loss processes together to use the K_p values effectively.

Percutaneous absorption is highly influenced by the microstructure and biochemical composition of the skin. The skin is composed of two layers, each of which is layered as well: (1) the epidermis, a nonvascular layer about 100 μm thick, and (2) the dermis, a highly vascularized layer about 500 to 3,000 μm thick. The stratum corneum, the outermost layer of the epidermis, is approximately 10 to 40 μm thick and is composed of dead, keratinized, and partially desiccated epidermal cells. Michaels et al.[135] describe the stratum corneum as a heterogeneous structure containing about 40% protein (primarily keratin), 15 to 20% lipids, and 40% water. It is thought to be the major rate-limiting diffusional barrier to most compounds; thus, it limits the extent of skin absorption.

Transport Processes in the Skin

The molecules of a chemical can follow an intercellular or a transcellular route through the stratum corneum, depending on their relative solubility and their partitioning in each phase of the stratum corneum's two-phase structure. Michaels et al.[135] offer evidence for the existence of separate pathways for hydrophilic and lipophilic molecules.

An alternative to the transport of a compound through transcellular or intercellular pathways in the stratum corneum is its penetration via skin appendages, such as hair follicles, sebaceous glands, and sweat glands. These appendages can serve as diffusional shunts through rate-limiting barriers, thereby facilitating the skin absorption of topically applied chemicals. However, because they occupy less than 1% of the skin surface of humans, their role as transport channels is usually negligible.

The purpose of understanding the skin transport mechanism in chemical hazard assessment is to be able to predict the absorbed dose and the resulting toxicity. Systemic toxicity refers to the absorption and distribution of a toxicant from its entry point to a distant site at which adverse effects are produced. Most chemicals, except for reactive materials and primary irritants, produce systemic effects. Most of these chemicals causing systemic toxicity produce adverse effects in only one or two organs of the body, referred to as target organs. The most frequent target organ of systemic toxicity is the central nervous system, followed by the circulatory system, the blood and hematopoietic system, and visceral organs such as the kidneys, lungs, liver, and skin.[5]

DERMAL EXPOSURE PATHWAYS

People routinely expose their skin to a variety of contaminated media through a wide range of activities. These media include water (e.g., bathing, swimming), soil (e.g., outdoor recreation, gardening, construction), sediment (e.g., wading, fishing), liquids (e.g., use of commercial prod-

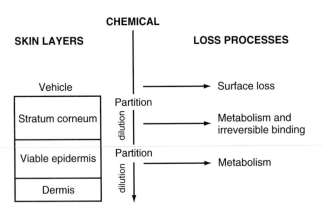

FIGURE 18–4 • Transport-loss processes occurring in the skin. (From Environmental Protection Agency. *Dermal Exposure Assessment: Principles and Applications.* EPA 600/8-91/011B. Washington, D.C.: EPA; 1992.)

ucts), vapors (e.g., use of paints, cleaning agents), and indoor dust (e.g., children playing on floors). However, the primary and possibly most significant modes of dermal exposure are contact with liquids and contact with soils or house dust. Populations experiencing dermal exposure to groundwater or surface water contaminants can be identified through geographically defined sources of recreational surface waters or through public water supply systems; few of these will present a significant chemical hazard. Children who play at contaminated sites and adults who are construction workers or gardeners can be exposed to appreciable concentrations of chemicals in soils.[104, 158]

The use of agricultural pesticides can result in the contamination of water, soil, and air. The chlorinated hydrocarbons (e.g., DDT, chlordane, and other cyclodienes) were the first class of compounds to be recognized as significant environmental pollutants. This recognition, along with a growing public awareness spurred by Rachel Carson's *Silent Spring*,[37] resulted in the phasing-out of such pesticides. Organophosphates and *N*-methylcarbamates were substituted for the chlorinated hydrocarbons; however, even though these pesticides are biodegradable and usually pose little hazard to the environment, they are still dermally toxic and can pose a genuine hazard to applicators. The use of these pesticides can result in high exposure of the skin of agricultural workers reentering treated fields or groves to harvest fruits and vegetables.[105]

Over the past 20 years, scientists have been working with physicians to develop exposure and risk assessment methods that will evaluate the hazards resulting from dermal uptake. The so-called reentry periods are the time intervals after which it is considered safe for workers to enter a sprayed field to harvest crops following the application of pesticides. The sheer numbers of field workers (approximately 300,000 annually), crops (e.g., 692,000 acres of grapes, 175,000 acres of citrus fruits), and organophosphorus and N-methylcarbamate pesticides used in California alone (approximately 1.5 million pounds per year) are enough to illustrate the potential magnitude of the problem.[105]

Pesticides are probably the primary hazard to the skin of nonagricultural workers as well, because of their ubiquitous application to residential lawns, schoolyards, and other public areas. For example, the professional lawn-care industry treats an estimated 11% of all single-family households in the United States, and approximately 67 million pounds of active chemical ingredients are applied to lawns annually. Though many studies in this area have focused on chemical residue measure-ments after treatment, no standard methodology has yet been established to measure dislodgeable residues from turf.[22, 39, 82, 105] These residues are present for contact with those who work with crops.

FACTORS AFFECTING DERMAL ABSORPTION

The skin behaves as a rate-limiting barrier and, in general, allows only a relatively slow penetration of chemicals. The stratum corneum is largely responsible for this barrier function.[125] As discussed above, the stratum corneum is typically lipoidal in nature,[166] which facilitates the accumulation of fatty chemicals there. The stratum corneum behaves as a storage site and releases these chemicals slowly, over a long period of time, a phenomenon known as the reservoir effect.[197] The living cells of the epidermis, however, are more permeable and do not act as rate-limiting barriers under most circumstances. Although sweat glands and hair follicles may facilitate the passage of chemicals—the transappendageal route—their total area in humans is small, and for most chemicals, absorption through the general skin surface—the transepidermal route—is the preferred route.[93] In short, for humans, hairy skin may be no more permeable than nonhairy skin. However, rodent skin hair appears to contribute significantly to overall percutaneous absorption.[101] It is, therefore, necessary to account for these and other potential species differences when extrapolating animal data to predict human responses.

The greatest potential for skin absorption occurs when a high concentration of a chemical is spread over a large area of the body's surface area.[131, 202] Depending on the chemical, the relationship between its concentration and the efficiency of its absorption may not be linear. In addition, absorption of a chemical can often be significantly increased with repeated application. This enhanced absorption may be related to an alteration in the barrier function of the stratum corneum that has been induced by the chemical, among other factors.[203] Damage to the skin, through disease and through occupational factors that occlude or defat it, increases its hydration and temperature, prevents evaporative loss, and thereby enhances the absorption of chemicals.[192]

The site of application of a chemical can also be a factor that affects the rate of percutaneous absorption. For example, the skin over the abdomen and the dorsa of the hands of an average human are twice as permeable as the palm and forearm, whereas the scalp, angle of the jaw, and the forehead are four times as permeable, and the scrotum is almost twelve times as permeable.[120]

Metabolism of a chemical can occur during penetration of the skin, and the resulting metabolite may or may not affect the chemical's toxicity. Nonetheless, this is an issue that must be accounted for when evaluating data from rodents. For example, the skin contains many of the same metabolic enzymes as are found in the liver, although the quantity is only about 2% of the amount.[149] Skin absorption of a chemical can be affected by metabolism because the metabolites are absorbed through the skin at different rates as a result of differences in physicochemical properties. The more slowly a chemical is absorbed through the skin, the greater the opportunity for some metabolism by the skin; however, in most cases, the metabolism will be too small to be worthy of consideration.

The ability of a chemical in a medium like soil or dust to be absorbed by the skin is influenced by its capacity to adhere to the skin surface. Soil adherence, or loading, is affected by such characteristics as soil type, particle size, moisture level, and the chemical contaminant itself.[65] For example, Kissel et al.[106] found that adherence varies inversely with soil grain size under dry (less than 2% moisture) conditions. Additionally, increasing adherence of soil to hands with increasing moisture has been frequently observed at moistures up to approximately 30%.[106] Most contaminants are present in the soil at such low concentrations that they are unlikely to influence adherence. However, petroleum hydrocarbons, often found in contaminated soils at relatively high concentrations, have been found to moderately increase dermal adherence of soil at high concentrations.[89] The significance of increased soil adherence lies in the corresponding increase in the reservoir of the contaminant on the skin, e.g., the potential dose. The conditions of exposure determine whether greater skin uptake is a likely consequence of greater dermal loading.

Finley et al.[65] developed a "standard" soil adherence probability density function (PDF) for use in Monte Carlo analysis based on a review of all published soil adherence studies. Data were examined with respect to study design, results interpretation, and the influence of certain key variables, such as age, sex, and soil particle size. The soil adherence PDFs were developed separately from adult and child data and were found to resemble one another closely in terms of the central tendency (mean = 0.49 and 0.63 mg-soil/cm²-skin, respectively) and 95th percentile values (1.6 and 2.4 mg-soil/cm²-skin, respectively). The proposed standard PDFs, 50th and 95th percentiles

(0.25 and 1.7 mg-soil/cm²-skin, respectively) based on the combined adult and child data are quite similar to the EPA's average and upper bound values of 0.2 and 1.0 mg-soil/cm²-skin, respectively. Because soil adherence under typical conditions is minimally influenced by age, sex, soil type, or particle size,[65] the proposed PDF can be considered applicable to all settings and conditions. Finley et al.[67] suggest that standard PDFs be developed for all variables unlikely to be significantly influenced by site-specific conditions. The utility of Monte Carlo analysis is such that even if less than perfect standard PDFs are initially developed for some variables used in health risk assessments, the results are still more informative and useful than those obtained by point estimate methods.[66]

DERMAL ABSORPTION STUDIES

Percutaneous absorption of neat chemicals had historically been studied in humans until the late 1970s.[47, 59, 60, 163, 186] Because of the potential toxicity of many chemicals and improved laboratory techniques, in vivo human studies have been largely supplanted by experiments with laboratory animals and athymic rodents grafted with human skin.[107] In general, the penetration of chemicals through the human skin is similar to that in the pig or monkey and much slower than that in the rat and rabbit.[18]

Starting in the 1980s, in vitro studies using human skin began to be conducted on a more routine basis. In these studies, a piece of excised skin is attached to a diffusion apparatus with a top chamber to hold the applied chemical and a temperature-controlled bottom chamber containing saline or other fluids, plus a sampling port to withdraw fractions for analysis.[75] Although human forearm skin is optimal, it is difficult to obtain, so abdominal or breast skin is commonly used. Generally, a properly conducted in vitro test can be a reasonably good predictor of the absorption rate in vivo.[24, 174] However, because of the fragile nature of the technique, these studies must be carefully interpreted.[17] Often, depending on the conditions of the test, the results are not applicable to humans.

After neat liquids, dermal exposures occur most frequently through soil or dust-bound contaminants.[160] A few studies[43, 65, 105, 113, 165, 179] have directly estimated soil loading on human skin. Although they contain sufficient data to generate point estimates of soil adherence and perhaps can provide a reasonable PDF for most persons, the degree to which the data are representative of the general population is unknown.[65] Recently, a more specific study was conducted to measure the adherence of soil to multiple skin surfaces under genuine occupational and recreational conditions.[106] Measured skin surfaces included the hands, forearms, lower legs, faces, and feet. Dermal loading on hands was found to vary over five orders of magnitude and to be dependent on the type of activity. Differences between pre- and postactivity adherence demonstrated the episodic nature of dermal contact with soil. However, because of the activity-dependent nature of soil exposure, data from these studies must be interpreted for their relevance to the type of activity, frequency, duration, and otherwise site-specific nature of exposure.

A reasonable level of research has been undertaken to investigate exposure to house dust. The basis for the concern has been increasing evidence that controlling exposure to house dust, especially in homes that are located in proximity to sites with considerable surface soil contamination, is more important for reducing the overall health hazard than is remediating soil.[160] Of particular interest is the work in developing standardized approaches to wipe sample collection and to estimate the amount of dust-loading on the skin.[117, 118] Although dermal absorption of toxicants in house dust will almost always pose an insignificant dermal uptake hazard, the research is of interest to occupational dermatologists who may want to draw on these procedures to assess dermal contact with a number of media.

QUANTITATIVE DESCRIPTION OF DERMAL ABSORPTION

The benefit of incorporating risk assessment methods into the field of occupational or environmental dermatology is to produce quantitative estimates of skin uptake. For the purposes of risk assessment, percutaneous absorption is defined as the transport of externally applied chemical through the cutaneous structures and the extracellular medium and into the bloodstream. The simplest way to describe the rate of skin absorption is to apply Fick's first law of diffusion at steady-state[199]:

$$J = dQ/dt = D \cdot k\nabla C/e \approx K_p \cdot C \quad \text{(Equation 6)}$$

where:

$J = dQ/dt$ = chemical flux or rate of chemical absorbed (mg/cm²-h),
D = diffusivity in the stratum corneum (cm²/h),
k = stratum corneum/vehicle partition coefficient of the chemical (unitless),

∇C = concentration gradient (mg/cm³),
e = thickness of the stratum corneum (cm),
K_p = permeability coefficient (cm/h), and
C = applied chemical concentration (mg/cm³).

The concentration gradient is equal to the difference between the concentration above and below the stratum corneum. Because the concentration below is small compared to the concentration above, ∇C can be approximated as being equal to the applied chemical concentration. From Equation 6 it can be seen that the rate of absorption is directly proportional to the applied concentration. The diffusivity represents the rate of migration of the chemical through the stratum corneum. Because the stratum corneum has a nonnegligible thickness, there is a period of transient diffusion (lag time) during which the rate of transfer rises to reach a steady state. In these studies, the steady state is maintained indefinitely thereafter, provided the system remains constant. Depending on the type of chemical, the lag time can range from minutes to days.[115] From the standpoint of exposure assessment, if the exposure duration is shorter than the lag time, it is unlikely that there will be any significant systemic absorption.[73, 78]

The partition coefficient in Equation 6 illustrates the importance of solubility characteristics in the ability of a chemical to penetrate the skin.[13, 188] Fatty chemicals tend to accumulate in the stratum corneum. Conversely, the stratum corneum is an effective barrier for hydrophilic substances which tend to have low skin absorption rates. Because stratum corneum/vehicle partition coefficients are difficult to measure, the three parameters, D, k, and e, are combined to give an overall permeability coefficient, K_p. It must be emphasized that Equation 6 only approximates most in vivo exposure situations in which true steady-state conditions are rarely attained. In spite of its limitations, this equation has yielded satisfactory estimations of the actual absorption rates of chemicals in most situations.

RECOGNIZED SYSTEMIC DERMAL HAZARDS

Almost all occupational exposure limits (OELs), such as the TLVs of the American Conference of Governmental Industrial Hygienists (ACGIH) and the Permissible Exposure Limits of the U. S. Occupational Safety and Health Administration (OSHA), are criteria for acceptable exposure to chemicals through inhalation. However, it is well known that skin contact is also an important portal of entry for many industrial chemicals used in the workplace.[72, 81, 84, 130, 154, 172] When certain chemicals are judged to have a significant potential to be absorbed from skin contact, a skin notation is appended to the OEL. For example, the ACGIH TLV booklet[7] states:

> Listed substances followed by the designation "skin" refer to the potential significant contribution to the overall exposure by the cutaneous route, including mucous membranes and the eyes, either by contact with vapors or, of probable greater significance, by direct contact with the substance. Vehicles present in solutions or mixtures can also significantly enhance potential skin absorption. It should be noted that while some materials are capable of causing irritation, dermatitis, and sensitization in workers, these properties are not considered relevant when assessing a skin notation.

Clearly, this definition is rather loose and lacks a precise criterion for deciding if a chemical warrants a skin notation. The inclusion or exclusion of the skin notation is largely a process of subjective judgment by the deliberating standard-setting committees, and that results in many inconsistencies.[71, 88, 172, 205] In order to bring some consistency to the skin notation process, a quantitative criterion for the biological significance of dermal absorption should be established, and several approaches for doing so follow.

ESTIMATING THE SKIN UPTAKE OF CHEMICALS IN AQUEOUS SOLUTION

The first criterion for identifying chemicals that deserve skin notations was proposed by Hansen,[85] who based his proposal on the swelling of psoriasis scales. More recently, Fiserova-Bergerova et al.[71] proposed another scheme which is toxicologically based and is more consistent with ACGIH's definition. In this approach, the dermal absorption potentials of the industrial chemicals, as defined by fluxes predicted from physicochemical properties, are compared with certain defined reference values referred to as critical fluxes. Berner and Cooper[21] proposed the following model for calculating the fluxes:

$$J = (C/15) (0.038 + 0.153 K_{ow}) e^{-0.016 MW}$$
(Equation 7)

where:

J = flux
C = saturated aqueous solution of the chemical
K_{ow} = octanol-water partition coefficient
MW = molecular weight of the chemical

Critical fluxes are determined by comparing the skin uptake rate under specified exposure conditions with the inhalation uptake rate during exposure to the time-weighted average TLV at steady-state conditions. The specified exposure condition for the critical flux can be calculated assuming exposure of 2% of the body surface area (equivalent to the stretched palms and fingers) to a saturated aqueous solution of the chemical. Two reference values have been recommended as criteria for using the skin notation[72]: dermal absorption potential and dermal toxicity potential. If the dermal absorption (flux) of a chemical exceeds the critical flux by 30%, the chemical should be classified as possessing "dermal absorption potential." If the flux of a chemical exceeds three times the critical flux, the chemical should be classified as possessing "dermal toxicity potential" and should carry a skin notation. Based on this scheme, a dermal absorption potential was predicted for 122 chemicals, of which only 43, as of 1991, carry a skin notation with their TLVs.[72] A significant dermal toxicity potential was indicated for 77 chemicals, of which only 40 had skin notations (Table 18–2).

TABLE 18–2 • Chemicals with Dermal Absorption Potential Only*	
Acetone	Isopropyl alcohol
n-Amyl acetate	Methoxychlor
Atrazine	Methyl acetate
1,3-Butadiene	Methyl n-amyl ketone
n-Butyl acetate	Methyl chloroform
p-ter-Butyltoluene	Methyl ethyl ketone
Cumene†	Methyl isoamyl ketone
Cyclohexanone†	Methyl isobutyl ketone
o-Dichlorobenzene	Methyl propyl ketone
1,1-Dichloroethane	Metribuzin
1,2-Dichloroethylene	Naphthalene
Diethyl ketone	Nitromethane
Diuron	Pentaerythritol
Enflurane	n-Propyl acetate
Ethanol	Propylene dichloride
Ethyl acetate	Strychnine
Ethyl benzene	Styrene†
Ethyl ether	Toluene
Ethyl formate	1,2,4-Trichlorobenzene
Halothane	Trichloroethylene
n-Heptane	Trimethyl benzene
Hexachloroethane	o-Xylene
n-Hexane	m-Xylene
Isoamyl alcohol	p-Xylene

*Lists only chemicals that pass through the skin.
†Skin notation appears in 1987–1988 TLV-BEI booklet.
From Fiserova-Bergerova V, Pierce JT, Droz PO. Dermal absorption potential of industrial chemicals: criteria for skin notation. *Am J Ind Med* 1990;17:617–635.

In general, whenever dermal uptake is potentially significant, biological monitoring of the individuals involved is recommended. In cases of chemicals classified as possessing dermal toxicity potential, biological monitoring should be instituted because measurement of airborne concentrations alone may not yield enough information to protect potentially exposed workers. Physicians and others should be aware that, generally, a skin notation is not used for chemicals whose TLVs are based on skin irritation. This is because the threshold for systemic toxicity is usually higher than that for irritation, and the critical fluxes for chemical irritants are likely to be underestimated.

The percutaneous permeability coefficients for some common industrial chemicals in aqueous media have been determined experimentally in humans (Table 18–3). The corresponding K_p values for the chemicals were calculated using Equation 7 (see Table 18–3). Comparison of the observed and calculated permeability coefficients suggests that there is a general concordance—the lower the observed value, the lower the predicted value and vice versa. However, the accuracy of the calculated values was rather poor. Specifically, the model equation grossly overpredicted the dermal penetration rates. For example, of the 43 chemicals, the permeability coefficients of only 12 were predicted within a factor of 5. Thus, although this model is useful as a qualitative screening tool to classify organic chemicals in aqueous media according to their skin absorption potential, it should not be used for precise determination of dermal absorption rates.

PHARMACOKINETIC MODELS FOR ESTIMATING THE UPTAKE OF CHEMICALS IN AQUEOUS SOLUTION

A four-compartment pharmacokinetic model to describe the percutaneous absorption of chemicals has been proposed.[83] This model describes, using first-order rate constants, a chemical moving through the compartments representing the various skin structures. The model has been used successfully to predict the disposition of chemicals in the skin and plasma as a function of their physicochemical properties, and when an input rate constant to the skin surface is added to the model, it can be used to assess vehicle effects. A similar model that treats the barrier membrane as a series of spaces filled with immiscible liquids has also been developed[209]; its advantage is that it allows the examination of nonsteady-state conditions in which Fick's law does not apply.

In an infinite-dose situation in which the amount of a chemical lost by penetration is too small to alter the applied concentration, such as when swimming, the rate of absorption is essentially linear once the steady state has been reached. In the finite-dose system, however, the chemical solution is applied as a thin film such as would occur in the case of a splash, and the concentration decreases as penetration proceeds. All other model parameters being the same, penetration is reduced under finite-dose conditions. This is because the chemical concentration is continuously reduced over time, resulting in a decrease in the gradient across the stratum corneum. These modeling results indicate that the mechanism by which fluxes are affected must be considered when extrapolating to nonsteady-state conditions.

Although classic pharmacokinetic modeling like that described by Guy et al.[83] can provide a good mathematical description of the disposition of chemicals, it does not depict exactly the biological processes in the intact animal. Fortunately, because of recent increases in the availability of computer hardware and software, pharmacokinetic methods based on physiological principles are now feasible alternatives for analysis of in vivo skin penetration studies. These PB-PK approaches realistically describe the disposition of the chemical in the intact animal in terms of rates of blood flow, permeability of membranes, and partitioning of chemicals into tissues.[10, 129] Characterizing dermal absorption in terms of actual anatomical, physiological, and biochemical parameters facilitates extrapolations to the species of real interest, humans.

In 1991, a PB-PK model was developed to describe the percutaneous absorption of volatile organic contaminants in dilute aqueous solutions.[177] The exposure scenario modeled was either hand or full-body immersion into a vessel of solute-contaminated water. Modeling results suggest that the uptake of chemicals in aqueous solutions is most markedly influenced by epidermal blood-flow rates followed by epidermal thickness and lipid content of the stratum corneum. In general, thicker and fattier skin provides a better barrier to dermal penetration of chemicals than does thinner less fatty skin. These are precisely the principles on which barrier creams offer their protection—increasing the effective thickness and lipophilicity of the skin. This model also predicts that the dose of some volatile organic chemicals in water absorbed through the skin during a 20-minute bath may be equivalent to the amount inhaled.[177]

The most complex and perhaps the best validated of the various models of dermal uptake of liquids is that developed by McDougal et al.[129]

TABLE 18–3 • Human Cutaneous Permeability Coefficient Values for Some Industrial Chemicals in Aqueous Medium

	MW	K_{ow}	Observed	Calculated[a]
Organic Chemicals				
2-Amino-4-nitrophenol	154.13	21.38	0.00066	0.019
4-Amino-2-nitrophenol	154.13	9.12	0.0028	0.0081
Aniline	93.12	7.94	0.041[b]	0.019
Benzene	78.11	134.90	0.11	0.39
p-Bromophenol	173.02	389.05	0.036	0.25
Butane-2,3-diol	90.12	0.12	<0.00005	0.0009
n-Butunol	74.12	7.59	0.0025	0.024
2-Butanone	72.10	1.94	0.0045	0.007
Carbon disulfide	76.14	100.	0.54[b]	0.3
Chlorocresol	142.58	1,258.93	0.055	1.31
S-Chlorophenal	128.56	147.91	0.033	0.19
p-Chlorophenal	128.56	257.04	0.036	0.34
Choroxylenal	156.61	1,621.81	0.059	1.35
m-Cresol	108.13	100.	0.015	0.18
o-Cresol	108.13	100.	0.016	0.18
p-Cresol	108.13	85.11	0.018	0.15
Decanol	158.28	37,153.52	0.08	30.11
2,4-Dichlorophenol	163.01	1,995.26	0.06	1.5
1,4-Dioxane	88.10	0.38	0.00043	0.0016
Ethanol	46.07	0.49	0.0008	0.0036
2-Ethoxyethanol	90.12	0.29	0.0003	0.0013
Ethylbenzene	106.16	1,412.54	1.215[b]	2.65
Ethylether	74.12	6.76	0.016	0.022
p-Ethylphenol	122.17	549.54	0.035	0.79
Heptanol	116.20	257.04	0.038	0.41
Hexanol	102.17	107.15	0.028	0.21
Methanol	32.04	0.17	0.0016	0.0026
Methyl hydroxybenzoate	152.15	91.2	0.0091	0.082
β-naphthol	144.16	691.83	0.028	0.7
3-Nitrophenol	139.11	100.00	0.0056	0.11
4-Nitrophenol	139.11	81.28	0.0056	0.09
Nitrosodiethanolamine	134.13	0.13	0.0000055	0.0005
Nonanol	144.26	2,951.21	0.06	2.99
Octanol	130.22	933.25	0.061	1.19
Pentanol	88.15	36.31	0.006	0.091
Phenol	94.11	32.36	0.0082	0.074
Propanol	60.09	2.00	0.0017	0.0088
Resorcinol	110.11	6.03	0.00024	0.011
Styrene	104.14	891.25	0.635[b]	1.72
Thymol	150.21	1,995.26	0.053	1.84
Toluene	92.13	489.78	1.01	1.15
2,4,6-Trichlorophenol	197.46	2,344.23	0.059	1.02
3,4-Xylenol	122.16	169.82	0.036	0.25
Inorganic chemicals				
Cobalt chloride	129.84		0.0004	
Lead acetate	325.29		0.0000042[b]	
Mercuric chloride	271.50		0.00093	
Nickel chloride	129.60		0.0001	
Nickel sulfate	154.75		<0.000009	
Silver nitrate	169.87		<0.00035[b]	
Sodium chromate	161.97		0.0021[b]	

[a]Permeability coefficients calculated using Equation 7.
[b]All the observed permeability coefficients were obtained by using in vitro techniques except those denoted with superscript b, which were determined in vivo.
From Leung HW, Paustenbach DJ. Techniques for estimating the percutaneous absorption of chemicals due to occupational and environmental exposure. *Appl Occup Environ Hyg* 1994;9:187–197.

This group has successfully predicted dermal uptake rates for humans for nearly a dozen chemicals, based on animal and physical chemistry data. One advantage of dermal PB-PK models over traditional in vivo methods is their ability to describe accurately nonlinear biochemical and physical processes. For example, describing skin penetration based on blood concentrations or excretion rates as "percent absorbed" assumes that all processes have a simple linear relationship with the exposure concentration. This is often not the case. The kinetics become non-linear when the absorption, distribution, metabolism or elimination of a chemical is saturated at high exposure concentrations and this can be accounted for by using a PB-PK model.

MODELS FOR ESTIMATING UPTAKE OF CHEMICALS IN SOIL

A model to estimate the amount of a chemical in soil that crosses the stratum corneum into the underlying tissue layer has been developed.[131] To differentiate this absorptive process from bioavailability, which also includes transport into blood, McKone refers to the percentage of the available chemical as an uptake fraction. The approach is based on the concept of fugacity, which measures the tendency of a chemical to move from one phase to another. Because the skin has a fat content of about 10% and soil has an organic carbon content of 1 to 4%, lipophilic chemicals in soil placed on the skin will move from the soil to the underlying adipose layers of the skin. However, this transfer depends on the period of time between deposition on the skin and removal by evaporative processes. It is the mass-transfer coefficients of the soil-to-skin layer and the soil-to-air layer that define the rate at which these competing processes occur.

Results of this model suggest that the uptake fraction of a chemical in soil varies with the duration of exposure, the soil deposition rate, and the physical properties of the chemical, and is particularly sensitive to the values of the K_{ow}, and the mass or depth of soil deposited on the skin. When the amount of soil on the skin is low (< 1 mg/cm^2), a high uptake fraction, approaching unity in some cases, is predicted. With higher soil loading (20 mg/cm^2), an uptake of only 0.5% is predicted. Because of the diverse variations in the uptake fraction with soil loading, results obtained from experiments with a single soil loading should be applied with caution to human soil-exposure scenarios.

The dermal uptake of chemicals in soil is a complex process, but its behavior is predictable if the controlling factors are accounted for and quantified. In situations involving a relatively thin layer of a chemical on the skin, a few generalizations can be made. First, for chemicals with a high K_{ow} and a low air to water partition coefficient, it is reasonable to assume 100% uptake in 12 hours. Second, for chemicals, with an air to water partition coefficient greater than 0.01, the uptake fraction is unlikely to exceed 40% in 12 hours. Third, for chemicals with an air to water partition coefficient greater than 0.1, less than a 3% uptake is likely in 12 hours. In most occupational settings, contaminated soil is rarely in contact with the skin for more than 4 hours before it is washed off. Consequently, this should be accounted for when attempting to predict systemic uptake.

FACTORS USED IN EXPOSURE CALCULATIONS

At least 10 different factors have to be quantitatively accounted for in order to estimate the likely systemic uptake of a chemical that comes into contact with the skin, either as a liquid or when present in soil or dust.

Bioavailability

The typical media of concern for assessing cutaneous contact with environmental chemicals, in contrast with occupational exposure, are house dust, soil, fly ash, and sediment. A number of parameters can influence the degree of cutaneous bioavailability of chemicals in complex matrices. These may include aging (time following contamination), soil type (silt, clay, or sand), type and concentration of cocontaminants (e.g., oil and other organics), and the concentration of the chemical contaminant in the media. The bioavailability of a chemical in soil is usually affected by its physicochemical properties. Chemicals of high molecular weight tend to bind to soil and be less water-soluble, whereas smaller molecules are commonly water-soluble, less tightly bound, and relatively bioavailable.[131] The cutaneous bioavailability of various chemicals in soils has been determined in animals.[119, 180, 183, 193, 194, 201] These studies show that different media and different chemicals can yield dramatically different cutaneous bioavailabilities. The results of these studies, for example, range from 0.01 to 3.0% for chemicals in soil.

Skin Surface Area

The rule of nines may be used for estimating the surface area of the human body[184]: the head and neck are 9%; upper limbs are 9% each; lower limbs are 18% each; and the front and back of the trunk are 18% each. The EPA[53] has estimated an exposed surface area (arms, hands, legs, and feet) of 2,900 cm² for children up to 2 years old; 3,400 cm² for children 2 to 6 years old; and 2,940 cm² for adults (an adult is assumed to wear pants, an open-necked, short-sleeved shirt, shoes, and no hat or gloves). Most of the necessary surface area information can be found in the EPA Exposure Factors Handbook.[53] Table 18–4 presents the skin surface areas commonly used when conducting exposure assessments.

Soil-Loading on the Skin

Soil-to-skin adherence rates of 0.5 to 0.6 mg/cm² and 0.2 to 2.8 mg/cm² have been reported for adults and children, respectively.[35, 43, 150, 165] Recent work by Finley et al.[65] and Kissel et al.[105] has built on those studies and has shown that dermal load-ing can vary significantly. The EPA[52] has sug-gested a default soil-to-skin adherence rate of 0.2 mg/cm² (median) and 1.0 mg/cm² (95th percentile) for an adult exposed to contaminated soil.

CALCULATING DERMAL UPTAKE

To estimate the uptake of a chemical, it is neces-sary to know the percutaneous absorption rate, the area of exposed skin, the concentration of the chemical, and the duration of exposure.[151] One scenario is when there is a thin film of chemical on the skin. For this finite-dose scenario:

$$\text{Uptake (mg)} = (C)(A)(x)(f)(t) \qquad \text{(Equation 8)}$$

where:

C = concentration of the chemical (mg/cm²),
A = skin surface area (cm²),
x = thickness of the film layer (cm)
f = absorption rate (%/h), and
t = duration of exposure (h).

Another scenario is when there is an excessive amount of a chemical on the skin, an infinite dose. In this case, the thickness of the chemical layer is not calculated and steady-state kinetics are as-sumed. For a chemical in aqueous or gaseous me-dia:

$$\text{Uptake (mg)} = (C)(A)(K_p)(t) \qquad \text{(Equation 9)}$$

For a neat liquid chemical:

$$\text{Uptake (mg)} = (A)(J)(t) \qquad \text{(Equation 10)}$$

where:

K_p = permeability coefficient (cm/h) and
J = flux of chemical (mg/cm²-h).

Skin Uptake of Chemicals in Soil

The EPA has suggested the use of the following equation to estimate the percutaneous absorption of chemicals in soil[52, 54]:

$$\text{Uptake (mg)} = (C)(A)(r)(B) \qquad \text{(Equation 11)}$$

where:

C = concentration of the chemical in soil (mg/g),
A = skin surface area (cm²),
r = soil-to-skin adherence rate (g/cm²), and
B = cutaneous bioavailability (unitless).

TABLE 18–4 • Representative Surface Areas of the Human Body (Adult Male)

Body Portion	Area (cm²)
Whole body	18,000
Head and neck	1,620
Head	1,260
Back of head	320
Neck	360
Back of neck	90
Torso	6,480
Back	2,520
Chest	2,520
Sides	1,440
Upper limbs	3,240
Upper arms (elbow-shoulder)	1,440
Lower arms (elbow-wrist)	1,080
Hands	720
Palms	360
Upper arms (back of)	360
Lower arms (back of)	270
Lower limbs	6,480
Thighs	3,240
Lower legs (knee-ankle)	2,160
Feet	1,080
Soles of feet	540
Thighs (back of)	810
Lower legs (back of)	540
Perineum	180

Data adapted from Snyder WS. *Report of the Task Group on Reference Man*. International Commission on Radiological Protection Pub. No. 23. New York: Pergamon Press; 1975.

Example Calculation 3: Skin Uptake of a Chemical in Soil

A man gardens with soil contaminated on average with 250 ng dioxin per gram of soil (250 ppb). Assuming that both hands and lower arms are in contact with the soil and that the cutaneous bioavailability of dioxin in soil is 1%,[180] what is the plausible uptake of dioxin by this person (using Equation 11)? Assume that he washes his hands every 4 hours.

$$\text{Uptake (ng)} = (C)(A)(r)(B)$$

where:

C = 250 ng/g
A = 1,800 cm² (see Table 18–4)
r = 0.2 mg/cm²[52]
B = 0.01[180]

By substitution,

$$\text{Uptake} = \left(\frac{250 \text{ ng TCDD}}{1 \text{ g soil}}\right) \left(\frac{0.2 \text{ mg soil}}{\text{cm}^2 \text{ skin}}\right) \left(\frac{1 \text{ g}}{10^3 \text{ mg}}\right) (1{,}800 \text{ cm}^2 \text{ skin}) (0.01) = 0.9 \text{ ng TCDD}$$

Note: A preferred method of performing this calculation is to use a flux rate (ng/cm²-hour) for the chemical:

$$\text{Uptake (ng)} = (C)(J)(A)(t)$$

where:

J = 500 ng/cm²-hr
t = 4 hours

By substitution,

$$\text{Uptake} = \left(\frac{250 \text{ ng TCDD}}{1 \text{ g soil}}\right) \left(\frac{1 \text{ g}}{10^9 \text{ ng}}\right) (1{,}800 \text{ cm}^2 \text{ skin}) (4 \text{ hours}) \left(\frac{500 \text{ ng}}{\text{cm}^2 - \text{hr}}\right) = 0.9 \text{ ng}$$

Uptake of Chemicals in an Aqueous Matrix

Several studies have estimated the possible dermal uptake of low concentrations of chemicals in water by humans. For example, the amount of chlordane absorbed through the skin by a man swimming for 4 hours in water containing 1 ppb chlordane has been estimated to be about 0.036 µg.[175] Similarly, the amount of chloroform absorbed by a boy swimming for 3 hours in water containing 0.5 ppm chloroform has been calculated to be about 1.65 mg.[20] Approximately 0.5 µg and 3.3 µg, respectively, can be absorbed through the skin during a 10-minute shower and a 20-minute bath in water containing 1 ppb 1,1,1-trichlorethane.[34] Comparisons have been made of the chloroform concentration in exhaled breath after a shower to that after an inhalation-only exposure.[100] The concentration after showering is about twice that after inhalation-only exposure, indicating that the absorbed dose from skin absorption is approximately equivalent to that from inhalation absorption. With better limits of detection in our analytical procedures, it is likely that this topic will continue to be studied and that the estimates will increase in precision.

Example Calculation 4: Skin Uptake of a Chemical From Water

A person has filled his swimming pool with shallow well water contaminated with 0.002 mg/mL (2 ppb) toluene. What is the plausible dermal uptake of toluene while swimming in the contaminated water for half an hour? From Equation 9:

$$\text{Uptake} = (C)(A)(K_p)(t)(d)$$

where:

C = 0.002 mg/mL
A = 18,000 cm² (see Table 18–4)
K_p = 1.01 cm/h (see Table 18–3)
t = 0.5 h
d = distribution factor (1 mL of water covers 1 cm³)

By substitution,

uptake = (0.002 mg/mL) (18,000 cm²) (1.01 cm/h)(0.5 h)(1 mL water/1 cm³)
uptake = 18 mg

Percutaneous Absorption of Liquid Solvents

The percutaneous absorption of chemical solutes generally proceeds by simple diffusion, but the skin uptake of neat chemical liquids is not necessarily exclusively governed by Fick's law. Consequently, the uptake of neat liquid through the skin has to be estimated using direct in vivo skin contact techniques. Table 18–5 presents the percutaneous absorption rates of some neat industrial liquid solvents as they have been determined for humans.

Example Calculation 5: Skin Uptake of a Neat Liquid Chemical

Due to carelessness or a leak, the inside of a glove gets contaminated with 2-methoxyethanol. How much can be absorbed if a worker wears the contaminated glove on one hand for half an hour? From Equation 10:

$$\text{Uptake} = (A)(J)(t)$$

where:

A = 360 cm² (see Table 18-4)
J = 2.82 mg/cm²-h (see Table 18-5)
t = 0.5 h

By substitution,

uptake = (360 cm²) (2.82 mg/cm²-h) (0.5 h)
uptake = 508 mg

To understand the relative hazard from skin exposure vs. inhalation exposure, the dose of 2-methoxyethanol absorbed by the same worker via inhalation for 8 hours (10 m³ of air inhaled) at the TLV of 16 mg/cm³ can be estimated. Assume an 80% inhalation uptake efficiency.

TABLE 18–5 • Absorption Rates of Some Neat Industrial Liquid Chemicals in Human Skin in Vivo

Chemical	Absorption Rate (mg/cm²-h)
Aniline	0.2–0.7
Benzene	0.24–0.4
2-Butoxyethanol	0.05–0.68
2-(2-Butoxyethoxy) ethanol	0.035
Carbon disulfide	9.7
Dimethylformamide	9.4
Ethylbenzene	22–23
2-Ethoxyethanol	0.796
2-(2-Ethoxyethoxy) ethanol	0.125
Methanol	11.5
2-Methoxyethanol	2.82
2-(2-Methoxyethoxy) ethanol	0.206
Methyl butyl ketone	0.25–0.48
Nitrobenzene	2
Styrene	9–15
Toluene	14–23
Xylene (mixed)	4.5–9.6
m-Xylene	0.12–0.15

From Leung HW, Paustenbach DJ. Techniques for estimating the percutaneous absorption of chemicals due to occupational and environmental exposure. *Appl Occup Environ Hyg* 1994; 9:187–197.

Inhalation uptake = (16 mg/m³)(10 m³)(0.8)
= 128 mg

Thus, the uptake of 2-methoxyethanol following half an hour of skin exposure in a single hand can be as much as four times that resulting from inhalation for 8 hours at the TLV concentration, a presumably safe level of exposure. From this example, it is clear that the cutaneous route of entry can, in some situations, significantly contribute to the total absorbed dose, especially in the occupational setting.

Percutaneous Absorption of Chemicals in the Vapor Phase

Until the 1990s, it was generally assumed that the dose attained by chemical vapors absorbed through the skin was too low to pose a hazard. Only a few studies have examined this issue.[102, 139] A few clinical reports have encouraged some limited in vitro research to evaluate the absorption of several chemicals in the gaseous phase through the human skin (Table 18–6). A chamber system to measure the whole-body percutaneous absorption of chemical vapors in rats has been described by McDougal et al.,[128] and this work has produced some interesting results.[126] In this system, the flux

TABLE 18–6 • **Percutaneous Absorption Rates for Chemical Vapors in Vivo**

Chemical	Skin Uptake in Combined Exposure[a] (%)	Permeability Coefficient K_p (cm/h)	
		Rat	*Human*
Styrene	9.4	1.75	0.35–1.42
m-Xylene	3.9	0.72	0.24–0.26
Toluene	3.7	0.72	0.18
Perchloroethylene	3.5	0.67	0.17
Benzene	0.8	0.15	0.08
Halothane	0.2	0.05	
Hexane	0.1	0.03	
Isoflurane	0.1	0.03	
Methylene chloride		0.28	
Dibromomethane		1.32	
Bromochloromethane		0.79	
Phenol			15.74–17.59
Nitrobenzene			11.1
1,1,1-Trichloroethane			0.01

[a]In combined exposure, rats are simultaneously absorbing chemical vapors by inhalation and by whole-body absorption through the skin.

Rat data from McDougal JN et al. Dermal absorption of organic chemical vapors in rats and humans. *Fundam Appl Toxicol* 1990;14:229–308.

of a chemical across the skin is determined from the chemical concentration in blood during exposure by using a PB-PK model. In most cases, the absorption of vapors through the skin amounts to less than 10% of the total dose received from a combined skin and inhalation exposure (see Table 18–6). There is good agreement between the rat and human in the relative ranking of the permeability coefficients among the chemicals studied, but for an individual chemical, the rat skin appears to be two to four times more permeable than is the human skin. This observation is consistent with previously reported data.[24, 163]

It is generally not necessary to account for the contribution of percutaneous uptake of vapors when the OEL is used as a guideline for acceptable exposure, because uptake via this route is usually inherent in the data used to derive it; that is, the animals or humans from whom the data were collected were usually exposed via inhalation (whole body) as dermal uptake occurred. However, although good work practices and the law require that certain situations not occur, sometimes an air line respirator or self-contained breathing apparatus is worn in environments containing chemical concentrations tenfold to 1,000-fold greater than the TLV. In these cases, it is important to account for the uptake of vapor through both exposed and covered skin.

Although nearly all data on the absorption of vapors involve bare skin, the role of clothing in preventing skin uptake has occasionally been eval-uated. For example, a study of workers wearing denim clothing indicated no decreased uptake of phenol vapors[162] but found a 20% and a 40% reduction in the uptake of nitrobenzene[161] and aniline[46] vapors, respectively. Although standard clothing may slightly decrease the amount of a chemical transferred from air through the skin, it can be a significant source of continuous exposure if the clothing has been contaminated by liquids from spills.

Example Calculation 6: Skin Uptake of a Chemical Vapor

Assuming that a person wears an airline respirator for a half hour in a room containing 250 mg/m³ nitrobenzene (50 times the current TLV), how much nitrobenzene might be absorbed through the skin?

The head, neck, and upper limbs are assumed to be exposed (surface area = 4,860 cm²), and the rest of the body (surface area = 13,140 cm²) is covered with clothing (see Table 18–4). The percutaneous K_p of nitrobenzene is 11.1 cm/h (see Table 18–6), and clothing reduced the skin uptake rate of vapors by about 20%.[161] From Equation 9:

$$\text{Uptake} = (C)(A)(K_p)(t)$$

Uptake through exposed skin = (250 mg/m³)
(4860 cm²)(11.1 cm/h) (0.5 h) (1 m³/10⁶ cm³)
= 6.74 mg

Uptake through clothing $= (250$ mg/m^3)(13,140
cm^2)(11.1cm/
h)(0.8)(0.5 h)
(1 m^3/10^6 cm^3)
$= 14.59$ mg

Total uptake $= 21.33$ mg

From this example, it is clear that if one enters an environment that contains a high concentration of airborne contaminant, even if a supplied-air respirator is worn, the degree of skin uptake of the vapor may be worthy of evaluation to ensure that the worker is protected.

INTERPRETING WIPE SAMPLES

In some workplaces, wipe-sampling has been conducted to assess the degree of surface contamination. Hospitals were among the first occupational settings, as long ago as 1940, to rely on this method to determine microbial levels in operating rooms. In pharmaceutical manufacturing, wipe-sampling has been used as an indicator of hygienic conditions since the 1960s. The health physics profession has utilized wipe samples extensively as an indicator of the need for better housekeeping, and has performed most of the early work in quantifying the relationship of wipe samples to air concentrations.[25, 36, 48, 49, 61, 127] When the primary effect of a chemical is skin discoloration, ACD, or chloracne, wipe-sampling is often a preferable approach to air-sampling for assessing the acceptability of the workplace. Recently, wipe samples have been collected within office buildings contaminated with dioxins and furans after electrical transformer fires to estimate the potential human exposure.[103, 136]

Although wipe-sampling data have been used as an indicator of cleanliness,[36] these data can also be used to estimate systemic uptake of a contaminant if the degree of skin contact with the contaminated surfaces is known. Although this exposure assessment methodology is rather imprecise, it can be useful in obtaining a rough estimate of the possible exposure that may be refined later with other means such as biological monitoring.

If it is known that wipe-sampling results are representative of what comes into contact with the hands—what is actually able to be absorbed—then the procedures for converting wipe-sampling data to estimates of systemic uptake are straightforward. For example, if one knows the number of times a surface (for example, a valve handle, instrument controller, or drum) is handled, the surface area of the hand touching these items (usually the palm), and the percutaneous absorp-

tion rate of the chemical, then the uptake can be estimated using wipe-sample information. One of the most thorough evaluations that relies on wipe-sample data and time-motion studies was conducted by the National Institute for Occupational Safety and Health (NIOSH) to examine the amount of dioxins absorbed by chemical operators in a 2,4,5-T manufacturing plant.[124] In general, most of the historical wipe-sample data collected by industry over the past 40 years have not been published. Perhaps the most robust data sets in the chemical industry are those collected by Dow Chemical and Monsanto during the 1950s when they were trying to understand the cause of the chloracne observed in workers.

Until recently, no standardized approaches existed for conducting wipe-sampling. Differences in the use of wetting agents (acetone, methylene chloride, water, saline, isopropanol, or ethanol) and sampling media (paper, cotton, or synthetic fibers) produced drastically different results. In some procedures, especially those that used methylene chloride (in which the paint was stripped by the solvent), the chemical in the paint matrix was assumed to be bioavailable (a highly unlikely situation). In addition, much of the previous work that involved the aggressive scrubbing of the contaminated surfaces with solvent did not reflect a realistic exposure scenario. Standard techniques that attempt to mimic the conditions in which a hand comes into contact with a contaminated surface have been developed.[127] Even more sophisticated work to standardize the procedure has been conducted by researchers at Rutgers University, and their wipe-sampling procedure and device have been patented.[117] They have also developed a dry-contact sampling device.[118] The implications of the recent wipe-sampling research are that (1) a minimum number of samples is necessary to have statistical confidence; (2) the pressure applied to the cloth during sample collection should be standardized and later techniques address this issue; (3) neat solvent should not be used; (4) the size of the sample area should be sufficient to collect enough contaminant for quantification; and (5) the technique should be validated by using glove analyses.

Sample Calculation 7: Using Wipe-Sample Data to Estimate Skin Uptake

Wipe samples have been collected in office buildings where electrical transformers containing PCBs have caught fire and the smoke has been distributed through the ventilation system and deposited on the carpets, furniture, and walls. What dose of dioxin due to skin contact with contaminated building surfaces might be plausible if the dioxin concentration in the wipe samples is 10 pg/cm² (using Equation 11)?

$$Uptake = (C)(A)(r)(B)$$

In applying this equation to wipe-sampling, C = concentration of chemical in contaminated surface (mg/cm²), A = surface area of one palm (cm²), r = removal efficiency of chemical from contaminated surface by skin (unitless), and B = cutaneous bioavailability (unitless). The chemical concentration in the wipe samples (C_{wipe}) is a measure of the surface contamination and is related to the removal efficiency (R_{wipe}) of the particular wiping procedure, that is, $C = C_{wipe}/R_{wipe}$. Thus,

$$Uptake = (C_{wipe})(A)(r)(B)(R_{wipe})$$

where:

C_{wipe} = 10 pg/cm²,
A = 180 cm² (see Table 18–4),
r = 10%,
B = 1%[(180)], and
R_{wipe} = 50%.

Using substitution,

$$uptake = (10 \text{ pg/cm}^2) (180 \text{ cm}^2) (0.10) (0.01)/(0.50)$$
$$= 3.6 \text{ pg}$$

ASSESSING THE RISKS OF DERMAL SENSITIZERS

Eczematous dermatitis is defined as inflammation of the skin consisting of erythema, vesiculation, oozing, and crusting.[42] Contact dermatitis, a type of eczematous dermatitis, is caused by contact with a particular material or substance. Contact dermatitis can be divided into two distinct groups: (1) irritant contact dermatitis (ICD) and (2) ACD (mentioned previously).

ICD is caused by exposure to a substance that has a damaging effect on the normal barrier function of the epidermis and may occur in both sensitized and unsensitized individuals (prior exposure to the substance is not required). Therefore, to varying degrees and in varying concentrations, everyone is susceptible to ICD. However, persons with histories of atopic dermatitis and those considered to have hyperirritable skin have been shown to be predisposed to ICD.[176] The propensity to induce a rapid response (minutes to hours) and the development of a response within a defined topical location on the skin are characteristic of ICD.[198] The clinical morphological characteristics

of ICD range from mild scaling to an eczematous dermatitis indistinguishable from ACD.[77] If there is no further contact with the irritant, ICD will resolve rapidly.[169] Additionally, a response may be diagnosed as a "delayed irritant response."[198] Delayed irritancy has been demonstrated in human experiments to have a latency period of 12 to 24 hours before the first signs appear.[198] The clinical significance and prevalence of delayed irritancy are not fully understood.[198] However, it is thought that a strong irritant causes an immediate response and a weak irritant causes a delayed response.

One of the most common occupational diseases is contact dermatitis that results from exposure to industrial chemicals.[2, 121] Although contact dermatitis is not a life-threatening disease, it can be a persistent condition and can be debilitating in severe cases. Once sensitized to a chemical, an individual is at risk of dermatitis whenever exposed to the same or to an antigenically cross-reactive chemical. Table 18–7 presents some examples that illustrate the wide spectrum of chemicals that are known or suspected to cause ACD.[51]

CROSS-SENSITIZATION

Cross-sensitization refers to the phenomenon in which an allergic sensitization engendered by one chemical compound extends to one or more other compounds.[19] For example, some persons sensitized to poison ivy can also become concurrently sensitized to poison oak. The chemical causing the primary reaction is referred to as the primary sensitizer or allergen. Secondary allergens are compounds that can cause cross-sensitization and are, in general, chemically related to the primary allergen.[45] Systematic studies of cross-sensitization involving iodinated and methylated compounds were initially performed by Bloch.[23] Subsequent studies by other investigators have resulted in the establishment of the critical role of chemical function similarities in cross-sensitization.[114]

Skin sensitizers are generally believed to show both dose-response and threshold characteristics.[170] In order to define the risk properly, one must consider not only the inherent properties of the chemical sensitizer, but also the degree and extent of exposure. The key factors in exposure assessment for skin sensitization include chemical dose, concentration, dose/unit surface area, duration, body location, presence of any skin penetration aid or vehicle, primary skin irritation potential, and extent of occlusion of the exposed skin.

TABLE 18–7 • Selected Allergic Contact Sensitizers

Metals
Nickel and nickel salts
Chromium salts
Cobalt salts
Organomercurials

Plant Sensitizers
Toxicodendron genus: pentadecylcatechols and
    other catechols
Primula obconica: a-methylene-y-butyrolactone
Compositae family: sesquiterpene lactones

Rubber Additives
Mercaptobenzothiazole
Thiuram sulfides
p-Phenylenediamine and derivatives
Diphenylguanidine
Resorcinol monobenzoate

Others
Epoxy oligomer (M.W. 340)
Methyl methacrylate and other acrylic monomers
Pentaerythritol triacrylate and other multifunctional
    acrylates
Hexamethylenediisocyanate
p-Tertiary butyl phenol
Ethylenediamine, hexamethylenetetramine, and
    other aliphatic amines
Formaldehyde
Neomycin
Benzocaine
Captan

From Emmett A. Toxic responses of the skin. In: Klaassen CD, Amdur MO, Doull J, eds. *Casarett and Doull's Toxicology: The Basic Science of Poisons,* 3rd ed. New York: MacMillan; 1986:412–431.

CONTROLLING SKIN EXPOSURE TO ALLERGENS

Health professionals are faced with significant challenges in devising practical ways to reduce the risk of inducing contact allergic response in naïve individuals and to prevent its elicitation in previously sensitized persons. It has been suggested that scientific groups should consider setting limits on the concentration of the allergen in a specific medium for given exposure periods such as an 8-hour work shift, akin to a TLV recommended by the ACGIH for airborne exposures. Information with respect to the dose of the allergen on the skin (mg/cm^2) over a time-weighted average exposure period would be needed to establish such limits. This would be similar to an airborne exposure standard in that it would be based on exposure level, not absorbed dose. Unlike ambient standards for which personal or area

air is monitored, a method of measuring the dose of allergen applied to the skin would be necessary for these limits to be useful. A drawback to establishing such standards is the lack of an acceptable quantitative method to measure such exposures. Some possible hand-wash and wipe-sample methods are being evaluated.[38, 39, 61, 105, 127, 133, 134, 196]

RISK ASSESSMENT METHODS AND ACD

The surface area of exposure to an allergen and the dose per unit area are the two exposure factors that determine whether or not ACD will be elicited.[9, 143, 195] The risk assessment approaches to quantifying the hazards of ACD have been illustrated by two case studies.[155, 156, 178] Both evaluated the hazard posed by hexavalent chromium (Cr(VI)) contaminated soil.

A CASE STUDY: DETERMINING THE ELICITATION THRESHOLD OF Cr(VI)

This case study presents the methodology by which a minimum elicitation threshold (MET) for Cr(VI) in solution was identified in humans.[144] It describes perhaps the most complex and sophisticated human study of an environmental ACD hazard. The MET is the minimum concentration to which an already sensitized person is likely to respond, that is, develop the characteristic papules and redness.[63] The goal of the work was to identify soil clean-up criteria that would protect citizens who are already sensitized to chromium (which typically occurs due to occupational exposure).

Background

Several million tons of chromite ore were processed in Hudson County, N.J. between 1897 and 1971.[58] This procedure involved roasting a chromium-rich ore in a kiln with soda ash or lime and then leaching it with water. The remaining material contained from 2 to 5% total chromium, primarily in two forms—hexavalent chromium (Cr(VI)) and trivalent chromium (Cr(III)).[58] Between 1905 and 1960, approximately 3 million tons of this chromite-ore processing residue (COPR) were used to fill in low-lying areas of Hudson County and provide base material for industrial building pads and parking lots, for tank dikes, and for backfill following demolition activities. Total chromium concentrations, both Cr(VI) and Cr(III), in the COPR measured at these sites ranged from 5 to approximately 70,000 ppm, and

Cr(VI) concentrations ranged from < 0.5 to approximately 7,000 ppm[58, 178] In recent years, there has been a significant amount of discussion among regulatory authorities and health risk assessors regarding the nature and extent of the health hazards posed by the COPR and the need for health-based cleanup standards for Cr(III) and Cr (VI).[15, 145, 155–157, 178, 185]

Cr(VI) is one of the most common dermal sensitizers in occupational settings and accounts for about 5% of clinically reported cases of ACD in the United States.[122] Cr(VI)-related ACD, which has been reported in chromium plating workers,[28, 29] lithographers,[116] diesel-repair-shop workers,[206] and leather workers,[138] is known as a type IV, delayed, or cell-mediated allergic reaction.[2, 28, 121] The localized biological response of ACD is similar to a poison oak hypersensitive reaction and elicits the standard symptoms of erythema, edema, and small vesicles.[1, 2, 121] Type IV allergic dermatitis reactions are most often not life-threatening and their effects are generally limited to the skin. Epidermal contact with high concentrations of Cr(VI) can also produce ICD, a nonimmunological response.[99, 111, 171]

Several patch-testing studies were conducted in the 1950s and 1960s to determine the MET of Cr(VI) in sensitized persons.[12, 30, 79, 164, 182, 210] In those studies, people known to be Cr(VI)-sensitive were tested with patches containing serial dilutions of Cr(VI), usually as potassium dichromate ($K_2Cr_2O_7$) in petroleum jelly, water, or acid-glycine. The New Jersey Department of Environmental Protection (NJDEP) evaluated these historical studies in an effort to establish a soil concentration that would prevent elicitation of ACD in Cr(VI)-sensitized individuals who might come in contact with the Cr(VI)-impacted soils. They suggested that an elicitation threshold of approximately 10 ppm Cr(VI) could be derived from the dose-response data[16, 146] and proposed a 10 ppm Cr(VI) soil standard.

However, the data upon which NJDEP relied were collected before the improved and standardized diagnostic criteria for contact dermatitis were developed.[147] It is likely that some irritant reactions were scored erroneously as allergic responses in these earlier studies. Also, these reports often failed to disclose information regarding the diagnostic criteria used to determine allergy, duration of patch application, and the analytical methods used to validate the chromium concentration and valency state. Furthermore, it is known that the patch preparation methods were inconsistent and that interpatch variability of the amount of Cr(VI) applied could be as high as an order of magnitude.[69]

Paustenbach et al.[157] and Stern et al.[185] evaluated the historical data and attempted to identify the patch concentration they believed to represent a MET. However, the exercise proved to be fruitless for the purposes of setting ACD-based soil standards because the patch concentrations were always reported in terms of mass of Cr(VI) per mass of patch (i.e., ppm) and not in terms of mass per unit area (mg-Cr(VI)/cm²-skin), which is the standard dose metric for quantifying dermal exposure. As described by Horowitz and Finley,[90] area-based elicitation thresholds (mg-Cr(VI)/cm²-skin) are necessary to properly estimate a soil concentration of Cr(VI) that will not elicit ACD.

In order to generate the appropriate data for establishing an area-based MET for solubilized Cr(VI), a patch-test study was conducted. Under the direction of the North American Contact Dermatitis Group (NACDG), a group of human volunteers known to be sensitized to Cr(VI) were patch-tested with serial dilutions of Cr(VI). The NACDG is a group of about 20 academic dermatologists who conduct original research on contact allergens. To reduce the variability inherent in earlier patch preparation methods, TRUE Test patches were manufactured specifically for use in this study.[144]

Potassium dichromate ($K_2Cr_2O_7$) was chosen as the test Cr(VI) compound because it is one of the most penetrating and potentially reactive species. Patches were prepared by mixing $K_2Cr_2O_7$ with a wet hydroxylpropyl cellulose gel. The $K_2Cr_2O_7$ was mixed to a specified mass of Cr(VI) per unit area and dried to a thin film. TRUE Test patches are specifically designed to hydrate by perspiration when taped to the skin under occlusion. The hydrated gel, occluded by adhesive backing and plastic, ensures maximal contact with the skin, thus enabling high allergen bioavailability.[168] With this approach, the allergen is evenly distributed over the test area, and the quantitative dose of allergen is accurately controlled.[68, 69, 207] This provides a significant advantage over other current techniques, such as the Finn chamber, in which the mass of allergen loaded onto the skin may vary by up to an order of magnitude from patch to patch.[69]

Dermatologists identified 113 persons from more than 6,000 patient files, of which 102 eventually took part in the study. All were believed to be Cr(VI)-sensitized based primarily on previous clinical patch tests performed by these physicians. Table 18–8 presents some of the demographics of this initial study population. People taking immunosuppressive or steroidal medications and pregnant women were excluded from the study. Subjects with eczema at the scheduled time of testing were not tested until the dermatitis subsided, and

TABLE 18–8 • Description of Cr(VI)-Sensitized Volunteers Who Participated in the Study

Sex	Number Originally Patch-Tested	Number Who Qualified and Participated	Range of Ages (y)	Average Age (y (SD))
Men	78	39	24–74	45.6 (12.6)
Women	24	15	25–59	29.6 (10.3)

From Nethercot JH et al. A study of chromium-induced ACD with 54 volunteers: implications for environmental risk assessment. *Occup Environ Med* 1994;51:371–380.

it was requested that topical steroids not be used for 2 weeks before testing. All volunteers provided their respective dermatologists with written consent to participate in the study.

Before initial testing, each patient filled out a medical and occupational history questionnaire. The medical history included questions about incidence, type, and duration of past and present dermatitis and other known allergies, including asthma, and any other skin problems or sensitivities. The questionnaire also asked for a history of jobs held and their durations, as well as any known or potential exposure to Cr in the workplace. Use of over-the-counter medications and vitamins was also recorded. Information on allergic and atopic dermatitis was available to all 102 subjects. Past atopic dermatitis was present in 15% of those who completed the study (8 people), and 22% of the volunteers worked in the construction industry or a related field. A significant number of participants had no known previous occupational exposure to Cr(VI).

In each round of testing, all patches were applied to the upper sides of the back for total occlusion, with each patient serving as his or her own control. The patches remained in place for 48 hours, at which time they were removed, and readings were taken at that time and at 96 hours, according to the following scale:

1 = Weak (no vesicular) reaction: erythema, infiltration, papules (+)

2 = Strong (edematous or vesicular) reaction (++)

3 = Extreme (spreading, bullous, ulcerative) reaction (+++)

4 = Doubtful reaction, macular erythema only (?)

5 = Irritant morphology

6 = Negative reaction (−)

7 = Not tested

Of the 102 people who were initially selected for the study, only 54 responded positively (+, ++, or +++) to the diagnostic Cr(VI) patch (4.4 mg-Cr(VI)/cm²). This response rate (53%) was far less than the projected estimate of 80% but still yielded enough people (54) to provide statistically significant results. The 54 subjects who proceeded to round two of the study consisted of 39 men (72%) and 15 women (28%). In round two, testing was performed with very low doses to prevent an "excited skin" response, so that future responses to the challenge would yield representative results. In this round, 4 of 54 subjects (7%) responded positively to 0.088 mg-Cr(VI)/cm², but not to 0.018 mg-Cr(VI)/cm². Accordingly, an MET of 0.088 mg-Cr(VI)/cm² was recorded for these 4 people and they were not required to complete round three. Only 1 of 54 (2%) responded positively to both 0.018 mg-Cr(VI)/cm² and 0.088 mg-Cr(VI)/cm²; an MET of 0.018 mg-Cr(VI)/cm² was recorded for this person, and he was not required to complete round three. Of the 54 subjects, 49 did not respond to either concentration and, therefore, proceeded to round three. In round three, 1 of the 49 subjects responded to both 0.88 and 0.18 mg-Cr(VI)/cm². The MET for this person was recorded as 0.18 mg-Cr(VI)/cm². Also, 22 subjects responded to 0.88 mg-Cr(VI)/cm² but not to 0.18 mg-Cr(VI)/cm²; therefore, 0.88 mg-Cr(VI)/cm² was recorded as the MET for those subjects. Of

TABLE 18–9 • Cumulative Dermal Response of 54 Cr(VI)-Sensitized Participants to Various Concentrations of Cr(VI)

Cr(VI) (μg/cm²)	Minimum Elicitation Threshold Response (%)	Cumulative Response (%)
0.018	1/54 (2)	1/54 (2)
0.088	4/54 (7)	5/54 (9)
0.18	5/54 (9)	10/54 (19)
0.88	22/54 (41)	32/54 (59)
4.4	22/54 (41)	54/54 (100)

From Nethercot J et al. A study of chromium-induced ACD with 54 volunteers: implications for environmental risk assessment. *Occup Environ Med* 1994;51:371–380.

the volunteers tested in round three, 22 had no response to either concentration. Because these volunteers did not respond to any patch concentration lower than the diagnostic patch, the MET recorded for them was 4.4 mg-Cr(VI)/cm². Table 18–9 presents the MET and cumulative frequency of responses for Cr(VI).

Interestingly, almost half of the sensitized volunteers in this study did not respond to a diagnostic concentration lower than 4.4 mg-Cr(VI)/cm². Many of these subjects were thought to be sensitive because of earlier positive responses to 0.5% $K_2Cr_2O_7$ in petroleum jelly or to 0.25% $K_2Cr_2O_7$ in TRUE Test matrix. Many dermatologists in North America believe that the use of 0.25% $K_2Cr_2O_7$ minimized or eliminated the incidence of irritant reactions.[187] It is likely that many of those volunteers who initially reacted to 0.5% $K_2Cr_2O_7$ exhibited an irritant (false-positive) reaction in earlier testing and that the 0.25% $K_2Cr_2O_7$ patch used in this study failed to produce the irritant response. It is also possible that some of these subjects actually are Cr(VI)-sensitive but have a threshold greater than 0.25% $K_2Cr_2O_7$. If this is true, then the results of this study could be considered to relate only to worst-case scenarios, as only the hypersensitive volunteers represented the typical population of sensitized persons. The results of this study indicate that the 10% MET for Cr(VI)-induced ACD is approximately 0.089 mg-Cr(VI)/cm². No significant correlations among age, sex, or occupation were found at any of the tested concentrations.

Marks et al.[122] recently reported that the prevalence of Cr(VI)-related ACD in a large clinical population was approximately 1%. The prevalence rate in the general population is certain to be much lower. Therefore, if Cr(VI)-sensitized subjects are less than 1% of the general population, an ACD-based soil clean-up criterion that is protective of 90% of the Cr(VI)-sensitized population should be protective of about 99.9% of the general population.

It is noteworthy that there is some uncertainty associated with reading a patch-test response as an allergic vs. an irritant reaction. Nethercott[142] has reported that the incidence of misread test sites can be as high as 20%, especially by those dermatologists who do not specialize in research involving patch-testing. Because the patch-test reactions in this study were interpreted by members of the NACDG, this rate should be much lower, as the interpretation of patch tests is a routine part of their practice. Because it is more common to misread irritant reactions as allergic than to discount an allergic reactions as irritant ones,[70] the MET estimated from this study can be considered conservative (no less than predicted here).

CALCULATING AN ACD-BASED SOIL CONCENTRATION FOR Cr(VI)

$$\text{Soil Concentration(mg allergen / kg soil)} = \frac{\text{MET} \left(\dfrac{\text{mg allergen}}{\text{cm}^2 \text{ skin}} \right) \times \text{CF} \left(\dfrac{100 \text{ mg soil}}{\text{kg soil}} \right)}{\text{SA} \left(\dfrac{\text{mg soil}}{\text{cm}^2 \text{ skin}} \right) \times \text{BVA (unitless)}} \qquad \text{(Equation 12)}$$

As described by Horowitz and Finley,[91] a concentration of allergen in soil that should protect 99.9% of the population (at least for Cr(VI), because 1% of the population may be sensitized) can be derived as above: where MET = the minimum elicitation threshold determined from patch-test data (10%); CF = conversion factor; SA = soil adherence factor; and BVA = bioavailability. If the leachability of the allergen from soil to skin is less than 100%, then the soil concentration must be adjusted upward accordingly.

The 10% MET for Cr(VI) in sensitized people, as identified in the patch-testing study, was 0.089 mg-Cr(VI)/cm²-skin. As discussed previously, a threshold derived from a 48-hour, occluded patch-test study is highly conservative (health-protective) with respect to realistic environmental exposures. Accordingly, to remain consistent with the EPA's reasonable maximal exposure philosophy of risk assessment (wherein average and upper-bound values are combined to give a reasonable estimate, rather than simply compounding worst-case assumptions), it is appropriate to use an average value to represent soil adherence. The EPA's suggested average value of 0.2 mg soil/cm²-skin was used for this analysis. Other values for soil adherence to skin can be found in Finley et al.[65] and Kissel et al.[106]

With these values for the MET and soil adherence factor, it was estimated that a concentration of 445 mg Cr(VI)/kg soil (e.g., 445 ppm in soil) should not pose an ACD hazard. Hence, even if it were conservatively assumed that all Cr(VI) in soil adhering to skin was able to leach into skin moisture and cross the skin barrier, this concentration in soil should protect the vast majority of the Cr(VI)-sensitized population from the ACD hazard.

CONCLUSIONS

As recently as 1985, the fields of clinical dermatology and quantitative toxicology infrequently had reason to interact. Now that significant interest has been placed on the role of dermal uptake and skin diseases as they relate to exposure to environmental chemicals, there is a genuine need for the two disciplines to work more closely together. Although significant contributions to our quantitative understanding of the uptake of chemicals through the skin have been made by a number of researchers over the past 2 decades, it can be anticipated that maximal benefit from future work will be attained because of a better understanding of how the data will be constructively used by risk assessors. The information presented in this chapter addressed some of the areas of mutual interest to dermatologists, occupational physicians, toxicologists, and risk assessors. It is hoped that this will stimulate more focused research that will lead to an increase in the precise prediction of the dermal uptake of chemicals and thus to accurate estimation of the probability of producing adverse health effects in exposed individuals.

References

1. Ackerman AB. *Histologic Diagnosis of Inflammatory Skin Disease*. Philadelphia: Lea & Febiger; 1978:233–236.
2. Adams RM. ACD. In: Adams RM, ed. *Occupational Skin Disease*, 2nd ed. Philadelphia: W.B. Saunders; 1990:26–31.
3. Albert RE. Carcinogen risk assessment in the U.S. *Crit Rev Toxicol* 1994; 24:75–85.
4. Allen BC, Crump KS, Shipp AM. Correlation between carcinogenic potency of chemicals in animals and humans. *Risk Anal* 1988; 8:531–544.
5. Klaassen CK. *Casarett and Doull's Toxicology: The Basic Science of Poisons*, 5th ed. New York: Pergamon Press; 1996.
6. American Conference of Governmental Industrial Hygienists (ACGIH). *Documentation of the Threshold Limit Values*. Cincinnati: ACGH; 1995.
7. American Conference of Governmental Industrial Hygienists (ACGIH). *1997 TLVs and BEIs: Threshold Limit Values for Chemical Substances and Physical Agents and Biological Exposure Indices*. Cincinnati: ACGIH; 1997.
8. Ames BN, Magaw R, Gold LS. Ranking possible carcinogenic hazards. *Science* 1987; 236:271–273.
9. Andersen K, Linden C, Hansen J, et al. The degree of nickel allergy and the enhancing effect of multiple reactions evaluated by dose-response testing in allergic patients. In: *Proceedings of the First Congress of the European Society of Contact Dermatitis*. Amsterdan: 1992.
10. Andersen ME, Clewell HJ, Gargas ML, Smith FA, Reitz RH. Physiologically based pharmacokinetics and the risk assessment for methylene chloride. *Toxicol Appl Pharmacol* 1987; 8:185–205.
11. Andersen ME, Clewell HJ, Kirshnan K, et al. Tissue dosimetry, pharmacokinetic modeling, and interspecies scaling factors. *J Risk Anal* 1995; 95:533–537.
12. Anderson FE. Cement and oil dermatitis: the part played by chrome sensitivity. *Br J Dermatol* 1960; 72:108–117.
13. Anderson BD, Higuchi WI, Raykar PV. Heterogeneity effects on permeability: partition coefficient relationships in human stratum corneum. *Pharm Res* 1988; 5:566–573.
14. Aylward LL, Hays S, Karch NJ, Paustenbach DJ. Evaluation of the relative susceptibility of animals and humans to the cancer hazard posed by 2,3,7,8-Tetrachlorodibenzo-p-dioxin (TCDD) using internal measures of dose. *Environ Science Tech* 1996; 30:3534–3543.
15. Bagdon RE. *Dermal Absorption of Selected Chemicals under Experimental and Human Exposure Conditions to Facilitate Risk Assessment and the Development of Standards for Soil. I. Chromium*. Trenton, N.J.: New Jersey Department of Environmental Protection; 1989.
16. Bagdon, RE, Hazen RE. Skin permeation and cutaneous hypersensitivity as a basis for making risk assessments of chromium as a soil contaminant. *Environ Health Perspect* 1991; 92:111–119.
17. Barber ED, Teetsel NM, Kolberg KF, et al. A comparative study of the rates of in vitro percutaneous absorption of eight chemicals using rat and human skin. *Fundam Appl Toxicol* 1992; 19:493–497.
18. Bartek MJ, LaBudde JA, Maibach HI. Skin permeability *in vivo*: comparison in rat, rabbit, pig and man. *J Invest Dermatol* 1972; 58:114–123.
19. Bayer RL. Cross-sensitization phenomena. In: MacKenna RMB, ed. *Modern Trends in Dermatology*, 2nd series. London: Butterworth Publishing; 1954:232–258.
20. Beech JA. Estimated worst-case trihalomethane body burden of a child using a swimming pool. *Med Hypoth* 1980; 6:303–307.
21. Berner B, Cooper ER. Models of skin permeability. In: Kydonieu AF, Berner B, eds. *Transdermal Delivery of Drugs*, Vol. 2. Boca Raton, Fla.: CRC Press; 1987:107–130.
22. Black KG, Fenske RA. Dislodgeability of chlorpyrifos and fluorescent tracer residues on turf: comparison of wipe and foliar wash sampling techniques. *Arch Environ Contam Toxicol* 1996; 31:563–570.
23. Bloch B. Experimentelle studien uber das wesen der jodoformidiosynkrasie. *Z Exper Pathol Ther* 1911; 9P:509–538.
24. Bronaugh RL, Stewart RF, Congdon ER, et al. Methods for in vitro percutaneous absorption studies: I. Comparison with in vivo results. *Toxicol Appl Pharmacol* 1982; 62:474–480.
25. Brouwer DH, Van Hemmen JJ. *Elements of a Sampling Strategy for Dermal Exposure Assessment*. Brussels, Belgium: International Occupational Hygiene Association, First International Scientific Conference; 1992 [abstract].
26. Burmaster DE, Maxwell NI. Time and loading-dependence in the McKone model for dermal uptake of organic chemicals from a soil matrix. *Risk Anal* 1991; 11:491–497.
27. Burmaster DE, von Stackelberg K. Using Monte Carlo simulations in public health risk assessments: estimating

and presenting full distributions of risk. *J Expo Anal Environ Epidemiol* 1991; 1:491–521.

28. Burrows D. Adverse chromate reactions on the skin. In: Burrows D, ed. *Chromium: Metabolism and Toxicity.* Boca Raton, Fla.: CRC Press; 1983.

29. Burrows D, Adams RM. Metals. In: Adams RM, ed. *Occupational Skin Disease*, 2nd ed. Philadelphia: W.B. Saunders; 1990:349–386.

30. Burrows D, Calnan CD. Cement dermatitis II: clinical aspects. *Trans St. John Hosp Dermatol Soc* 1965; 51:27–39.

31. Butterworth BE, Slaga T. *Nongenotoxic Mechanisms in Carcinogenesis: Banbury Report 25.* New York: Cold Spring Harbor Press; 1987.

32. Butterworth BE. Consideration of both genotoxic and nongenotoxic mechanisms in predicting carcinogenic potential. *Mutat Res* 1990; 239:117–132.

33. Butterworth B. *A Review of Mechanisms of Carcinogenesis.* Boca Raton, Fla.: CRC Press; 1993.

34. Byard J. Hazard assessment of 1,1,1-trichloroethane in groundwater. In: Paustenbach DJ, ed. *The Risk Assessment of Environmental and Human Health Hazards: A Textbook of Case Studies.* New York: John Wiley; 1989: 331–334.

35. California Department of Health Services. *The Development of Applied Action Levels for Soil Contact: A Scenario for the Exposure of Humans to Soil in a Residential Setting.* Sacramento, Cal.: CDHS; 1986.

36. Caplan K. The significance of wipe samples. *Am Ind Hyg Assoc J* 1993; 54:70–75.

37. Carson R. *Silent Spring.* Boston: Houghton Mifflin; 1962.

38. Cherrie JW, Robertson A. Biologically relevant assessment of dermal exposure. *Ann Occup Hyg* 1995; 39:387–392.

39. Chester G. Revised guidance document for the conduct of field studies of exposure to pesticides in use. In: PB Curry, S Iyengar, P Maloney, M Maroni, eds. *Methods of Pesticide Exposure Assessment* New York: Plenum Press; 1995.

40. Crump KS, Hoel DG, Langler CH, et al. Fundamental carcinogenic processes and their implications for low-dose risk assessment. *Cancer Res* 1976; 36:2973–2979.

41. Dourson ML, Stara JF. Regulatory history and experimental support of uncertainty (safety factors). *Regul Toxicol Pharmacol* 1983; 3:224–238.

42. Dorland I, Newman WA. *Dorland's Illustrated Medical Dictionary.* Philadelphia: W.B. Saunders; 1994.

43. Driver JH, Konz JJ, Whitmyre GK. Soil adherence to human skin. *Bull Environ Contam Toxicol* 1989; 17:1831–1850.

44. Department of Toxic Substances Control, California. *Guidance on Dermal Absorption Factors.* Environmental Protection Agency; 1994.

45. Dupuis G, Benezra C. *Allergic Contact Dermatitis to Simple Chemicals: A Molecular Approach.* New York: Marcel Dekker; 1982.

46. Dutkiewicz T, Piotrowski J. Experimental investigations on the quantitative estimation of aniline absorption in man. *Pure Appl Chem* 1961; 3:319–323.

47. Dutkiewicz T, Tyras H. A study of the skin absorption of ethylbenzene in man. *Br J Ind Med* 1967; 24: 330–332.

48. ECETOC. *Strategy for Assigning a "Skin Notation."* Revised ECETOC Document No. 31. Brussels: European Centre for Ecotoxicology and Toxicology of Chemicals; 1993.

49. ECETOC. *Percutaneous Absorption.* Monograph No. 20. Brussels: European Centre for Ecotoxicology and Toxicology of Chemicals; 1993.

50. Elias PM, Feinghold KR, Menon GK, et al. The stratum corneum two-compartment model and its functional implications. In: Shroot B, Schaefer F, eds. *Pharmacology and the Skin: Skin Pharmacokinetics*, Vol. 1. Basel, Switzerland: Karger; 1987.

51. Emmett A. Toxic responses of the skin. In: Klaassen CD, Amdur MO, Doull J, eds. *Casarett and Doull's Toxicology: The Basic Science of Poisons*, 3rd ed. New York: MacMillan; 1986:412–431.

52. Environmental Protection Agency. *Dermal Exposure Assessment: Principles and Applications.* EPA 600/8-91/011B. Washington, D.C.: EPA; 1992.

53. Environmental Protection Agency. *Exposure Factors Handbook*, Vol. LI. EPA/600/P-95/002B. Washington, D.C.: EPA; 1996.

54. Environmental Protection Agency. *The Risk Assessment Guidance for Superfund, Human Health Evaluation Manual.* Washington, D.C.: EPA; 1989.

55. Environmental Protection Agency. *Proposed Guidelines for Carcinogen Risk Assessment.* EPA/600/P-92/003C. Washington, D.C.: EPA; 1996.

56. Environmental Protection Agency. *Superfund Exposure Assessment Manual.* EPA 540/I-88/001. Washington, D.C.: EPA; 1988.

57. Environmental Protection Agency. *Guidance for Risk Characterization.* Washington, D.C.: EPA; 1995.

58. Environmental Science and Engineering. *Remedial Investigation for Chromium Sites in Hudson County, New Jersey.* Trenton, N.J.: New Jersey Department of Environmental Protection; 1989.

59. Feldmann RJ, Maibach HI. Percutaneous absorption of steroids in man. *J Invest Dermatol* 1969; 52:89–94.

60. Feldmann RJ, Maibach HI. Percutaneous penetration of some pesticides and herbicides in man. *Toxicol Appl Pharmacol* 1974; 28:126–132.

61. Fenske RA. Dermal exposure assessment techniques. *Ann Occup Hyg* 1993; 37:687–706.

62. Finley BL, Paustenbach DJ. The benefits of probabilistic exposure assessment: three case studies involving contaminated air, water, and soil. *Risk Anal* 1994; 14:53–73.

63. Finley BL, Paustenbach DJ. Using applied research to reduce uncertainty in health risk assessment: five case studies involving human exposure to chromium in soil and groundwater. *J Soil Contamination* 1997; 6:649–705.

64. Finley BL, Mayhall DA. Airborne concentrations of chromium due to contaminated interior building surfaces. *Appl Occup Environ Hyg* 1994; 9:433–441.

65. Finley BL, Scott PK, Mayhall DA. Development of a standard soil-to-skin adherence probability density function for use in Monte Carlo analyses of dermal exposure. *Risk Anal* 1994; 14:555–569.

66. Finley BL, Scott P. Response to letter by Kissel. *Risk Anal* 1998; 18:9–12.

67. Finley BL, Price P, Proctor DM, Scott PK, Paustenbach DJ. Standard probability density functions for routine use in probabilistic health risk assessment. *Risk Anal* 1994; 14:533–553.

68. Fischer TI, Maibach HI. Amount of nickel applied with a standard patch test. *Contact Dermatitis* 1984; 11:285–287.

69. Fischer TI, Maibach HI. The Thin Layer Rapid Use Epicutaneous Test (TRUE Test™), a new patch test method with high accuracy. *Br J Dermatol* 1985; 112: 63–68.

70. Fischer TI, Maibach HI. Easier patch testing with TRUE Test™. *J Am Acad Dermatol* 1989; 20:447–453.

71. Fiserova-Bergerova V, Pierce JT, Droz PO. Dermal absorption potential of industrial chemicals: criteria for skin notation. *Am J Ind Med* 1990; 17:617–635.

72. Fiserova-Bergerova V. Relevance of occupational skin exposure. *Ann Occup Hyg* 1993; 37:673–685.

73. Flynn GL. Physicochemical determinants of skin absorption. In: Gerrity TR, Henry CJ, eds. *Principles of Route-to-Route Extrapolation for Risk Assessment*. New York: Elsevier Science; 1990:93–127.

74. Food Safety Council. Quantitative risk assessment. In: *Food Safety Assessment*. Washington, D.C.: FSC;1980.

75. Frantz SW. Instrumentation and methodology for in vitro skin diffusion cells. In: Kemppainen BW, Reifenrath WG, eds. *Methods for Skin Absorption*. Boca Raton, Fla.: CRC Press; 1990:35–59.

76. Freedman DA, Zeisel H. From mouse to man: the quantitative assessment of cancer risk. *Stat Sci* 1988; 3:3–56.

77. Frosch P, Wissing C. Cutaneous sensitivity to ultraviolet light and chemical irritants. *Arch Dermatol Res* 1992; 272:263–278.

78. Gargas M, Burgess RJ, Voisaro GE, et al. Partition coefficients of low molecular weight volatile chemicals in various liquids and tissues. *Toxicol Appl Pharm* 1989; 98:87–99.

79. Geiser JD, Jeanneret JP, Delacretaz T. Eczema au ciment et sensibilization au cobalt. *Dermatologica* 1960; 121:1–7.

80. Gough M. How much cancer can EPA regulate, anyway? *Risk Anal* 1990; 10:1–6.

81. Grandjean P, Berlin A, Gilbert M, Penning W. Preventing percutaneous absorption of industrial chemicals: the "skin" notation. *Am J Ind Med* 1988; 14:97–107.

82. Grandjean P. *Skin Penetration: Hazardous Chemicals at Work*. London: Taylor & Francis; 1990.

83. Guy RH, Hadgraft J, Maibach HI. A pharmacokinetic model for percutaneous absorption. *Int J Pharm* 1982; 11:119–129.

84. Hakkert BC, Stevenson H, Bos PMJ, Van Hemmen JJ. Methods for the establishment of health-based recommended occupational exposure limits for existing substances. Zeist: TNO. Report V96.463; 1996:1–16.

85. Hansen CM. *The Absorption of Liquids into the Skin*. Report T3-82. Horsholm, Denmark: Scandinavian Paint Painting Ink Research Institute; 1982.

86. Hart WL, Reynolds RC, Krasavage WJ, et al. Evaluation of developmental toxicity data: a discussion of some pertinent factors and a proposal. *Risk Anal* 1988; 8:59–70.

87. HEAST. *Health Effects Assessment Summary Tables: Fiscal Year 1997 Update*. EPA-540-R-97-036. Washington, D.C.: Environmental Protection Agency, Office of Solid Waste and Emergency Response; 1997.

88. Holland CD, Sieklen RL Jr. *Quantitative Cancer Modeling and Risk Assessment*. Englewood Cliffs, N.J.: Prentice Hall; 1993.

89. Holmes KK, Kissel JC, Richter KY. Investigation of the influence of oil on soil adherence to skin. *J Soil Contam* 1996; 5:301–308.

90. Horowitz SB, Finley BL. Using human sweat to extract chromium from chromite ore processing residue: applications to setting health-based cleanup levels. *J Toxicol Environ Health* 1994: 40:585–599.

91. Horowitz SB, Finley BL. Setting health protective soil concentrations for dermal contact allergens: a proposed methodology. *Regul Toxicol Pharmacol* 1994; 19:31–47.

92. Hrudey SE, Chen W, Rousseaux C. *Bioavailability*. New York: CRC Lewis; 1996.

93. Hueber F, Wepierre J, Schaefer H. Role of transepidermal and transfollicular routes in percutaneous absorption of hydrocortisone and testosterone: *in vivo* study in the hairless rat. *Skin Pharmacol* 1992; 5:99–107.

94. Huff J, Haseman J, Rall D. Scientific concepts, value, and significance of chemical carcinogenesis studies. *Ann Rev Pharmacol Toxicol* 1991; 31:621–652.

95. International Life Sciences Institute. *Low-dose Extrapolation of Cancer Risks: Issues and Perspectives*. Washington D.C.: ILSI Press; 1995.

96. Integrated Risk Information System. *Chemical Search for Polychlorinated Biphenyls*. Cincinnati, OH and the Bethesda, Md.: National Library of Medicine; 1996.

97. Integrated Risk Information System. *Chemical Search for Chlorobenzene*. Cincinnati, OH and the Bethesda, Md.: National Library of Medicine; 1997.

98. Irish D. *Patty's Industrial Hygiene and Toxicology*, Vol. II. New York: John Wiley; 1959.

99. Jackson EM, Goldmen R, eds. *Irritant Contact Dermatitis*. New York: Marcel Dekker; 1990.

100. Jo WK, Weisel CP, Lioy PJ. Routes of chloroform exposure and body burden from showering with chlorinated tap water. *Risk Anal* 1990; 10:575–580.

101. Kao J, Hall J, Helman G. In vitro percutaneous absorption in mouse skin: influence of skin appendages. *Toxicol Appl Pharmacol* 1988; 94:93–103.

102. Kezic S, Mahieu K, Monster AC, de Wolff FA. Dermal absorption of vapors and liquid 2-methoxyethanol and 2-ethoxyethanol in volunteers. *Occup Environ Med* 1997; 54:38–43.

103. Kim N. *An Evaluation of the Human Health Risks of PCB Soot Following a Transformer Fire*. Albany, N.Y.: New York State Department of Health; 1983.

104. Kimbrough RD, Falk H, Stehr P, Fries GF. Health implications of 2,3,7,8-tetrachlorodibenzo-*p*-dioxin (TCDD) contamination of residential soil. *J Toxicol Environ Health* 1984; 14:47–93.

105. Kissel JC, Richter KY, Fenske RA. Field measurement of dermal soil loading attributable to various activities: implications for exposure assessment. *Risk Anal* 1996; 16:115–125.

106. Kissel JC, Richter KY, Fenske RA. Factors affecting soil adherence to skin in hand-press trails. *Bull Environ Contam Toxicol* 1996; 56:722–728.

107. Klain GJ, Black KE. Specialized techniques: congenitally athymic (nude) animal models. In: Kemppainen BW, Reifenrath WG, eds. *Methods for Skin Absorption*. Boca Raton, Fla.: CRC Press; 1990:165–174.

108. Knaak JB, Iwata Y, Maddy KT. The worker hazard posed by reentry into pesticide-treated foliage: development of safe reentry times, with emphasis on chlorthiophos and carbosulfan. In: Paustenbach DJ, ed. *The Risk Assessment of Environmental Hazards: A Textbook of Case Studies*. New York: John Wiley; 1989:797–842.

109. Krewski D, Murdock D, Withey JR. Recent developments in carcinogenic risk assessment. *Health Physics* 1989; 571:313–325.

110. Krewski D, Brown C, Murdoch D. Determining "safe" levels of exposure: safety factors or mathematical models. *Fundam Appl Toxicol* 1984; 4:383–394.

111. Lammintausta KH, Maibach HI. Contact dermatitis due to irritation. In: Adams RM, ed. *Occupational Skin Disease*, 2nd ed. Philadelphia: W.B. Saunders; 1990:1–3.

112. Lehmann AJ, Fitzhugh G. 100-fold margin of safety. *Q Bull Assoc Food Drug Off US* 1954; 18: 33–35.

113. Lepow ML, Bruckman L, Gillette M, et al. Investigations into sources of lead in the environment of urban children. *Environ Res* 1975; 10:415–426.

114. Leung HW, Auletta CS. Evaluation of skin sensitization and cross-reaction of nine alkylene amines in the guinea pig maximization test. *J Toxicol Cut Ocular Toxicol* 1997; 16:189–195.

115. Leung HW, Paustenbach DJ. Techniques for estimating the percutaneous absorption of chemicals due to occupational and environmental exposure. *Appl Occup Environ Hyg* 1994; 9:187–197.

116. Levin HM, Brunner NJ, Ratner LT. Lithographer's dermatitis. *JAMA* 1959; 169:566–569.

117. Lioy PJ, Wainman T, Weisel C. A wipe sampler for the quantitative measurement of dust on smooth surfaces: laboratory performance studies. *J Exp Anal Environ Epidemiol* 1993; 3:315–320.

118. Lioy PJ, Yiin LM, Adgate J, et al. The effectiveness of a home cleaning intervention strategy in reducing potential dust and lead exposures. *J Exp Anal Environ Epidem* [in press].

119. Lucier GW, Rumbraugh RC, McCoy Z, et al. Ingestion of soil contaminated with 2,3,7,8-tetrachlorodibenzo-*p*-dioxin (TCDD) alters hepatic enzyme activities in rats. *Fundam Appl Toxicol* 1986; 6:364–371.

120. Maibach HI, Feldmann RJ, Milby TH, et al. Regional variation in percutaneous penetration in man. *Arch Environ Health* 1971; 23:208–211.

121. Marks JG, DeLeo VA. *Contact and Occupational Dermatology.* St. Louis: Mosby-Year Book; 1992.

122. Marks J, Belsito D, DeLeo V, et al. North American Contact Dermatitis Group standard tray patch test results (1992–1994). *Am J Contact Derm* 1995; 6:160–165.

123. Marks RM, Barton SP, Edwards C, eds. *The Physical Nature of the Skin.* Lancaster, Pa.: MTP Press; 1988.

124. Marlow D, Sweeney MH, Fingerhut M. *Estimating the Amount of TCDD Absorbed by Workers Who Manufactured 2,4,5-T.* Bayreuth, Germany: Tenth Annual International Dioxin Meeting; 1990.

125. Marzulli FN, Tregear RT. Identification of a barrier layer in the skin. *J Physiol* 1961; 157:52–53.

126. Mattie DR, Bates GD, Jepson GW, et al. Determination of skin:air partition coefficients for volatile chemicals: experimental method and applications. *Fundam Appl Toxicol* 1994; 22:51.

127. McArthur B. Dermal measurement and wipe sampling methods: a review. *Appl Occup Environ Hyg* 1992; 7:599–606.

128. McDougal JN, Jepson GW, Clewell HJ, et al. Dermal absorption of organic chemical vapors in rats and humans. *Fundam Appl Toxicol* 1990; 14:229–308.

129. McDougal JN. Physiologically based pharmacokinetic modeling. In: Marzulli FN, Maibach HI, eds. *Dermatotoxicology.* Washington, D.C.: Taylor & Francis; 1996.

130. McDougal JN, Grabau JH, Dong L, et al. Inflammatory damage to skin by prolonged contact with 1,2-dichlorobenzene and chloropentafluorobenzene. *Microsc Res Tech* 1997; 37:214–220.

131. McKone TE. Dermal uptake of organic chemicals from a soil matrix. *Risk Anal* 1990; 10:407–419.

132. McKone TE, Bogen KT. Predicting the uncertainties in risk assessment. *Environ Sci Technol* 1991; 25:16–74.

133. Methner MM, Fenske RA. Pesticide exposure during greenhouse applications. I. Dermal exposure reduction due to directional ventilation and worker training. *Appl Occup Environ Hyg* 1994; 9:560–566.

134. Methner MM, Fenske RA. Pesticide exposure during greenhouse applications. II. Chemical permeation through protective clothing in contact with treated foliage. *Appl Occup Environ Hyg* 1994; 9:567–574.

135. Michaels AS, Chandrasekaran SK, Shaw JE. Drug permeation through human skin: theory and *in vitro* experimental measurement. *AIChE* 1975; 19:985–996.

136. Michaud JM, Huntley SL, Sherer RA, et al. PCB and dioxin re-entry criteria for building surfaces and air. *J Expo Anal Environ Epidemiol* 1994; 4:197–227.

137. Morgan DL, Cooper SW, Carlock, DL, et al. Dermal absorption of neat and aqueous volatile organic chemicals in the Fischer 344 rat. *Environ Res* 1991; 55:51–63.

138. Morris GE. Chrome dermatitis: a study of the chemistry of shoe leather with particular reference to basic chromic sulfate. *Arch Dermatol* 1958; 78:612–618.

139. Mraz J, Nohova H. Percutaneous absorption of N,N-dimethylformamide in humans. *Int Arch Occup Environ Health* 1992; 64:79–83.

140. National Academy of Sciences. *Risk Assessment in the Federal Government: Managing the Process.* Washington, D.C.: National Academy Press; 1983.

141. National Academy of Sciences. *Science and Policy in Risk Assessment.* Washington, D.C.: National Academy Press; 1994.

142. Nethercott JR. Practical problems in the use of patch testing in evaluation of patients with contact dermatitis. In: Westin W, ed. *Current Problems in Dermatology.* St. Louis: Mosby-Year Book; 1990:101–123.

143. Nethercott J, Finley B, Horowitz S, et al. Safe concentrations of dermal allergens in the environment. *N J Med* 1994; 91:694–697.

144. Nethercott J, Paustenbach D, Adams R, et al. A study of chromium-induced ACD with 54 volunteers: implications for environmental risk assessment. *Occup Environ Medicine* 1994; 51:371–380.

145. New Jersey Department of Environmental Protection. *Derivation of a Risk-Based Chromium Level in Soil Contaminated with Chromite-Ore Processing Residue in Hudson County.* Trenton, N.J.: NJDEP; 1990.

146. New Jersey Department of Environmental Protection. *Risk Assessment of the ACD Potential of Hexavalent Chromium in Contaminated Soil—Derivation of an Acceptable Soil Concentration.* Trenton, N.J.: NJDEP; 1992.

147. North American Contact Dermatitis Group. Preliminary studies of the TRUE Test™ patch test system in the United States. *J Am Acad Dermatol* 1984; 21:841–843.

148. Ottoboni MA. *The Dose Makes the Poison: A Plain Language Guide to Toxicology,* 2nd ed. New York: Van Nostrand Reinhold; 1991.

149. Pannatier A, Jenner B, Testa B, et al. The skin as a drug-metabolizing organ. *Drug Metab Rev* 1978; 8:319–343.

150. Paustenbach DJ, Shu HP, Murray FJ. A critical examination of assumptions used in risk assessment of dioxin-contaminated soil. *Regul Toxicol Pharmacol* 1986; 6:284–307.

151. Paustenbach DJ. A survey of health risk assessment. In: Paustenbach DJ, ed. *The Risk Assessment of Environmental and Human Health Hazards: A Textbook of Case Studies.* New York: John Wiley; 1989:27–124.

152. Paustenbach DJ. Occupational exposure limits: their critical role in preventive medicine and risk management—a guest editorial. *Am Ind Hyg Assoc J* 1990; 51:332–336.

153. Paustenbach DJ. Health risk assessment and the practice of industrial hygiene. *Am Ind Hyg Assoc J* 1990; 51:339–351.

154. Paustenbach DJ. Occupational exposure limits, pharmacokinetics, and unusual work schedules. In: Harris RL, Cralley LJ, Cralley LV, eds. *Patty's Industrial Hygiene and Toxicology,* 3rd ed. New York: John Wiley; 1994: 191–348.

155. Paustenbach DJ, Rinehart WE, Sheehan PJ. The health hazards posed by chromium-contaminated soils in residential and industrial areas: conclusions of an expert panel. *Regul Toxicol Pharmacol* 1991; 13:195–222.

156. Paustenbach DJ, Sheehan PJ, Lau V, et al. An assessment and quantitative uncertainty analysis of the health risks to workers exposed to chromium contaminated soils. *Toxicol Ind Health* 1991; 7:159–196.

157. Paustenbach DJ, Sheehan PJ, Paull JM, et al. Review of the ACD hazard posed by chromium-contaminated soil: identifying a safe concentration. *J Toxicol Environ Health* 1992; 37:177–207.

158. Paustenbach DJ, Wenning RJ, Lau V, Harrington NW, Rennix DK, Parsons AH. Recent developments on the hazards posed by 2,3,7,8-tetrachlorodibenzo-*p*-dioxin in soil: implications for setting risk-based cleanup levels at residual and industrial sites. *J Toxicol Environ Health* 1992; 36:103–148.

159. Paustenbach DJ. The practice of health risk assessment in the United States (1975–1995): how the U.S. and other countries can benefit from that experience. *Hum Ecol Risk Assess* 1995; 1:29–79.

160. Paustenbach DJ, Finley BL, Long TF. The critical role of house dust in understanding the hazards posed by contaminated soils. *Int J Toxicol* 1997; 16:339–362.

161. Piotrowski JK. Further investigations on the evaluation of exposure to nitrobenzene. *Br J Ind Med* 1967; 24:60–65.

162. Piotrowski J. Evaluation of exposure to phenol: absorption of phenol vapor in the lungs and through the skin and excretion of phenol in urine. *Br J Ind Med* 1971; 28: 172–178.

163. Piotrowski J. *Exposure Tests for Organic Compounds in Industrial Toxicology.* Cincinnati: National Institute for Occupational Safety and Health; 1977.

164. Pirila V. On the role of chromium and other trace elements in cement eczema. *Acta Derm Venereol* 1954; 34:137–143.

165. Que Hee SS, Peace B, Scott CS, et al. Evolution of efficient methods to sample lead sources, such as house dust and hand dust, in the homes of children. *Environ Res* 1985; 38:77–95.

166. Raykar PV, Fung M, Anderson BD. The role of protein and lipid domains in the uptake of solutes by human stratum cornum. *Pharm Res* 1988; 5:140–150.

167. Reitz RH, Gargas ML, Andersen ME, et al. Predicting cancer risk from vinyl chloride exposure with a physiologically based pharmacokinetic model. *Toxicol Appl Pharmacol* 1996; 137:253–267.

168. Rietschel RL, Marks JG, Adams RM. Preliminary studies of the TRUE™ patch test system in the United States. *J Am Acad Dermatol* 1989; 21:841–843.

169. Rietschel RL, Fowler JF. *Fisher's Contact Dermatitis*, 4th ed. Baltimore: Williams & and Wilkins; 1995.

170. Robinson MK, Stotts J, Danneman PJ. A risk assessment process for allergic contact sensitization. *Food Chem Toxicol* 1989; 27:479–489.

171. Rook A, Wilkinson DS, Ebling FJ, et al. *Textbook of Dermatology.* Oxford: Blackwell Scientific; 1986.

172. Scansetti G, Piolatto G, Rubino GF. Skin notation in the context of workplace exposure standards. *Am J Ind Med* 1988; 14:725–732.

173. Schwartz L, Tulipan L, Peck SM. *Occupational Diseases of the Skin.* Philadelphia: Lea & Febinger; 1947.

174. Scott RC, Batten PL, Clowes HM, et al. Further validation of an in vitro method to reduce the need for in vivo studies for measuring the absorption of chemicals through rat skin. *Fundam Appl Toxicol* 1992; 19:484–492.

175. Scow K, Wechsler AE, Stevens J, et al. *Identification and Evaluation of Waterborne Routes of Exposure from Other than Food and Drinking Water.* EPA-440/4-79-016. Washington, D.C.: Environmental Protection Agency; 1979.

176. Seidenari S. Skin sensitivity, interindividual factors: atopy. In: Pieter GM, van der Valk J, eds. *The Irritant Contact Dermatitis Syndrome.* New York: CRC Press; 1996.

177. Shatkin JA, Brown HS. Pharmacokinetics of the dermal route of exposure to volatile organic chemicals in water: a computer simulation model. *Environ Res* 1991; 56:90–108.

178. Sheehan P, Meyer DM, Sauer MM, et al. Assessment of the human health risks posed by exposure to chromium-contaminated soils at residential sites. *J Toxicol Environ Health* 1991; 32:161–201.

179. Sheppard SC, Evenden WG. Contaminant enrichment and properties of soil adhering to skin. *J Environ Qual* 1994; 23:604–613.

180. Shu HP, Teitelbaum P, Webb AS, et al. Bioavailability of soil-bound TCDD: dermal bioavailability in the rat. *Fundam Appl Toxicol* 1988; 10:648–654.

181. Silbergeld EK. Risk assessment: the perspective and experience of the US environmentalists. *Environ Health Perspect* 1993; 101:100–104.

182. Skog E, Wahlberg JW. Patch testing with potassium dichromate in different vehicles. *Arch Dermatol* 1969; 99: 697–700.

183. Skrowronski GA, Turkall RM, Abdel-Rahman MS. Soil adsorption alters bioavailability of benzene in dermally exposed male rats. *Am Ind Hyg Assoc J* 1988; 49:506–511.

184. Snyder WS. *Report of the Task Group on Reference Man.* International Commission on Radiological Protection, Pub. No. 23. New York: Pergamon Press; 1975.

185. Stern AH, Freeman NCG, Plesan P, et al. Residential exposure to chromium waste--urine biological monitoring in conjunction with environmental exposure monitoring. *Environ Res* 1992; 58:147–162.

186. Stewart RD, Dodd HC. Absorption of carbon tetrachloride, trichloroethylene, tetrachloroethylene, methylene chloride, and 1,1,1-trichloroethane through the human skin. *Am Ind Hyg Assoc J* 1964; 25:439–446.

187. Storrs FJ, Rosenthal LE, Adams RM, et al. Prevalence and relevance of allergic reactions in patients patch tested in North America: 1984 to 1985. *J Am Acad Dermatol* 1989; 20:1038–1044.

188. Surber C, Wilhelm KP, Maibach HI, et al. Partitioning of chemicals into human stratum corneum: implications for risk assessment following dermal exposure. *Fundam Appl Toxicol* 1990; 15:99–107.

189. Thompson KM, Burmaster DE, Crouch EAC. Monte Carlo techniques for quantitative uncertainty analysis in public health risk assessments. *Risk Anal* 1992; 12:53–63.

190. Travis CC, White RK. Interspecies scaling of toxicity data. *Risk Anal* 1988; 8:119–125.

191. Travis CC, White RK, Ward RC. Interspecies extrapolation of pharmacokinetics. *J Theoret Biol* 1990; 142:285–304.

192. Treffel P, Muret P, Muret-DAniello P, et al. Effect of occlusion on *in vitro* percutaneous absorption of two compounds with different physicochemical properties. *Skin Pharmacol* 1992; 5:108–113.

193. Umbreit TH, Hesse EJ, Gallo MA. Acute toxicity of TCDD-contaminated soil from an industrial site. *Science* 1986; 232:497–499.

194. Umbreit TH, Hesse EJ, Gallo MA. Comparative toxicity of TCDD-contaminated soil from Times Beach, Missouri, and Newark, New Jersey. *Chemosphere* 1986; 15:2121–2124.

195. Upadhye M, Maibach HI. Influence of area of application of allergen on sensitization in contact dermatitis. *Contact Dermatitis* 1992; 27:281–286.

196. Van Hemmen JJ, Brouwer DH. Assessment of dermal exposure to chemicals. *Sci Total Environ* 1995; 168:131–141.

197. Vickers CFH. Existence of reservoir in the stratum corneum. *Arch Dermatol* 1963; 88:20–23.

198. Wahlberg JE. Clinical overview of irritant dermatitis. In: Pieter GM, van der Valk J, eds. *The Irritant Contact Dermatitis Syndrome.* New York: CRC Press; 1996.

199. Wepierre J, Marty JP. Percutaneous absorption of drugs. *Trends Pharmacol Sci* 1979; 1:23–26.

200. Wester RC, Maibach HI. Percutaneous absorption of organic solvents. In: Maibach HI, Marzulli F, eds. *Occupational and Industrial Dermatology*, 2nd ed. Chicago: Yearbook Medical Publishers; 1987.

201. Wester RC, Maibach HI, Sedik L, et al. Percutaneous absorption of pentachlorphenol from soil. *Fundam Appl Toxicol* 1993; 20:68–71.

202. Wester RC, Noonan PK. Relevance of animal models for percutaneous absorption. *Int J Pharm* 1980; 7:99–110.

203. Wester RC, Noonan PK, Maibach HI. Percutaneous absorption of hydrocortisone increases with long-term administration. *Arch Dermatol* 1980; 116:186–188.

204. Williams GM, Weisburger JH. Chemical carcinogenesis. In: Amdur MD, Doull JD, Klaassen CD, eds. *Casarett and Doull's Toxicology: The Basic Science of Poisons*, 4th ed. New York: Pergamon Press; 1991:127–236.

205. Wilschut A, Ten Berge WF, Robinson PJ, McKone TE. Estimating skin permeation: the validation of five mathematical skin permeation models. *Chemosphere* 1995; 30:1275–1296.

206. Winston JR, Walsh EN. Chromate dermatitis in railroad employees working with diesel locomotives. *JAMA* 1951; 147:1133–1134.

207. Wright RW. Evaluation of contact dermatitis using the TRUE™ patch test. *J Ark Med Soc* 1991; 88:271–272.

208. Young FA. Risk assessment: the convergence of science and the law. *Regul Toxicol Pharmacol* 1987; 7:179–184.

209. Zatz JL. Computer simulation using multicompartmented membrane models. In: Bronaugh RL, Maibach HI, eds. *Percutaneous Absorption: Mechanisms, Methodology, Drug-Delivery*, Vol. 6. New York: Marcel Dekker; 1985:165–181.

210. Zelger J. Zur klinik und pathogenses dis chromate ekzems. *Arch Clin Exper Dermatol* 1964; 18:499–542.

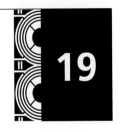

Workers' Compensation

JOSEPH LADOU, M.D.

Virtually all countries provide some form of entitlements to workers or their survivors to assist them in the event of an occupational injury or illness. Workers' compensation is the form of social insurance broadly accepted in the industrially developed countries. Most commonly, workers' compensation is embedded in a country's social security system. In the United States, however, the workers' compensation insurance system has almost no linkages with the social security system.[1] U.S. employers incur more than $60 billion in direct workers' compensation costs each year, triple the amount spent a decade earlier. Counting other costs—production delays, damage to equipment, and recruiting and training replacement workers—the total cost is about $350 billion.[2]

Workers' compensation systems are designed to ensure the injured worker prompt but limited benefits and to assign to the employer sure and predictable liability. There are many important differences in workers' compensation laws between the several federal and state systems in the United States.[3] Physicians and other health care professionals who render care for work-related injuries and illnesses must understand the goals and requirements of their state's workers' compensation system and provide the necessary medical services to ensure that workers receive the appropriate level of benefits.

WORKERS' COMPENSATION LAW

The financial responsibility of the employer for the injury or death of an employee in the workplace was first established under Bismarck in Germany in 1884. Great Britain followed in 1897 with legislation requiring employers to compensate employees or their survivors for an injury or death regardless of who was at fault. Thus, workers' compensation laws are the result of a historic compromise wherein the employee gave up the right to sue the employer for negligence in exchange for the employer's agreement to pay the cost of medical care and to compensate the worker for time lost from work. At the turn of the century, all European countries had workers' compensation laws. The workers' compensation movement did not begin in the United States until 1908, when a forerunner of the Federal Employees' Compensation Act was passed. In 1911, the first states enacted their laws. These initial workers' compensation systems were far from the array of programs that deal with disability income loss, medical care, accident prevention, and vocational rehabilitation that characterize contemporary workers' compensation programs.[4]

One of the major deficiencies in workers' compensation law is that its roots are in the past century at a time when occupational disease was not recognized. The system operates with relative success in the recognition and compensation of work-related injuries. But far less than half of all occupational disease is compensated under workers' compensation systems, and its reporting by government agencies is also woefully inadequate. This is particularly true for chronic diseases (e.g., occupational cancer). Consequently, preventive measures aimed at occupational diseases receive less attention than those directed at the causes of occupational injury.[5]

The Occupational Safety and Health Administration (OSHA) requires the reporting of skin conditions on OSHA 200 logs. Thus, occupational dermatoses are an important exception to the underreporting of occupational illnesses under workers' compensation. This mandatory requirement to report all skin conditions, however, creates the impression that occupational dermatoses are a major cause of occupational illness. This, with rare exception, is not the case.

Compensability

To be compensable, an injury usually must "arise out of and in the course of employment (AOE/COE)." A work injury that activates or aggravates a preexisting condition also is compensable. Recurrence of an earlier compensable injury is compensable as well. Depending on the jurisdiction, judicial action may be necessary to resolve questions of liability for self-inflicted injuries and suicidal acts. Similar determinations may be necessary for injuries occurring under the influence of alcohol or drugs or during an entirely personal activity (not AOE/COE) or fights at work.

Occupational diseases are the direct result of work or exposure to toxic substances or infectious agents in the workplace. Occupational disease claims have increased in recent decades. In some states, this situation occurs because of judicial interpretation. In other jurisdictions, the increase is the result of "presumptions" that lead to the automatic acceptance of workers' compensation liability for certain diseases in designated worker groups. An example is the presumption in California law that heart disease in police and fire personnel, and in some other uniformed services, is work related and will receive workers' compensation benefits. In all areas of the United States, occupational disease claims are increasing as physicians become more familiar with the discipline of occupational medicine and more confident of their diagnoses of occupational diseases or causality of multifactorial diseases.[6]

Many states recognize cumulative injury claims as occupational illnesses when the worker has sustained repeated small physical or psychic injuries that eventually result in a disability. These broadened interpretations of illness and disability open workers' compensation systems to numerous claims of occupational stress. They also bring many new cases of repetitive motion disorders, cardiovascular diseases, hearing loss, and emotional disturbance into the system. Dermatoses caused or aggravated by stress may be recognized by workers' compensation jurisdictions as work-related diseases. Dermatologists and specialists in occupational medicine play key roles in many states where their medical opinions are necessary to resolve issues surrounding compensability of contentious cases. Many physicians devote their practices to such forensic activities.

Worker Benefits

The objectives of workers' compensation systems are to provide injured employees with an income following an injury and during recovery, to ensure injured workers a competitive position in the employment market, and to avoid lengthy and costly legal action. In the event of death, dependents are compensated for the loss of their income provider.[7] An injured employee is entitled to medical treatment and compensation, whether the incident is the fault of the employee or the employer. The cost of workers' compensation benefits is considered to be a cost of doing business and is passed on to purchasers of the product or service. In the case of governmental workers' compensation systems, the costs are included in the taxes collected by federal and state governments.

Benefits to workers or their families are of several types: (1) permanent total disability, (2) temporary total disability, (3) permanent partial disability, (4) temporary partial disability, (5) survivors' benefits, and (6) vocational rehabilitation benefits.

Permanent Total Disability

Permanent total disability covers those workers who are so disabled that they will never be able to successfully compete in an open labor market and for whom further treatment offers no hope of recovery. Most states compensate such individuals with two-thirds of average wages (since benefits are not taxed, this amounts to about 85 to 90% of take-home wages), and some also provide additional funds for dependents. Although some states limit the duration of payments, others provide compensation for the remainder of the injured worker's life. These payments are governed by guidelines that stipulate minimum and maximum payments.

Temporary Total Disability

The majority of injured workers experience a period of temporary total disability classification—that is, the worker is expected to recover with treatment but is unable to work for a time.[8] Benefits are paid during the recovery period on the basis of average earnings, again with a minimum and a maximum of two-thirds of gross or 80% of take-home wages, until the individual is able to return to work or reaches maximum recovery. There is a waiting period for this type of compensation, but it is paid retroactively if the worker cannot work for a certain number of days or if hospitalization is necessary. The waiting period serves as an incentive to return to work after less serious injuries. Thus, it is like a deductible provision in other forms of health insurance.

Permanent Partial Disability

Permanent partial disability occurs when an injured worker is disabled to the point that he or she has lost some ability to compete in the labor market. In some jurisdictions, benefits compensate the injured worker for losses in future earnings and are divided into two categories: (1) scheduled injuries (e.g., loss of a limb, an eye, or hearing) and (2) nonscheduled injuries (e.g., back injury, tenosynovitis). The first is paid according to a schedule fixed by statute. Under this category, benefits are paid whether or not the individual is working. Payment is usually provided for a specified number of weeks, the length of which depends on which part of the body is damaged. Benefits are based on a percentage of earnings at the time of injury and again are subject to a minimum and a maximum amount. Nonscheduled injuries receive weekly benefit payments based on a wage-loss replacement percentage. The percentage is derived from the difference between wages earned before and after injury. In some states, however, nonscheduled permanent partial disabilities are compensated as a percentage of the total disability cases.

Temporary Partial Disability

Temporary partial disability occurs when a worker is injured to the degree that he or she cannot perform his or her usual work but is still capable of working at some job during convalescence. Modified duty is viewed by many insurers and employers as a critical element of the treatment plan and rehabilitation of these injured workers. Under this category, the injured worker is compensated for the difference between wages earned before the injury and wages earned during the period of temporary partial disability, usually at two-thirds of the difference. Modified duty may save the worker from wage differentials by stopping the temporary partial disability payment.

Survivors' Benefits

Dependent survivors of employees killed on the job are paid death benefits under workers' compensation. The method and size of payments vary widely among the various states, but all systems provide for a death benefit and some reimbursement for burial expense.

Vocational Rehabilitation

Some level of rehabilitation is provided in all states even if unspecified by statute. Vocational and psychological counseling or retraining and job placement assistance are typical benefits, with the goal of returning the injured worker to suitable, gainful employment.

Benefits from Other Sources

A number of benefits are available to workers from other sources.

Social Security Disability Insurance

Social Security supplements workers' compensation with monthly benefits for disability. Such benefits are available only after a 5-month waiting period and are calculated as if the disabled individual had reached Social Security retirement age. To be considered disabled, the injured person must be unable to work in substantial gainful employment. Furthermore, the disability must be expected to last more than 1 year or to result in premature death. Social Security Disability Insurance (SSDI) combined with workers' compensation cannot exceed 80% of the worker's average earnings or the total family benefit under Social Security before the injury. If this is the case, SSDI benefits are reduced accordingly, although some states will reduce workers' compensation benefits by all or part of the SSDI payments. Annual expenditures for SSDI rose by 80% between 1982 and 1992, from $17.3 billion to $31.1 billion.[9]

Second Injury Funds

Second injury funds compensate workers for injuries that are exacerbated by a subsequent injury. Other states' second injury funds compensate workers for flare-ups that do not necessarily lead to total disability. These funds are established and maintained by most states in the hope that the outcome will encourage employers to hire the handicapped or previously injured workers. Payments are made for the second injury by the employer's compensation carrier, and the fund reimburses the carrier for the additional costs.

Employers' Responsibilities

Employers are responsible for providing medical treatment and compensation benefits for employees injured at work or made ill from exposure to the workplace environment. The system is based on a premise of liability without fault—that is, regardless of whether the worker, the employer, or neither is at fault, the employer is still responsible for providing medical treatment and compensation benefits to the injured employee.

Workers' compensation insurance coverage is compulsory for most private employment except in New Jersey, South Carolina, and Texas. In those states, employers may decline coverage, but, in turn, they lose the customary defenses against suits filed by employees (the "exclusive remedy" is the quid pro quo under which the employer enjoys tort immunity in exchange for accepting absolute liability for workers' compensation benefits). Employees most likely to be exempted from coverage include domestic workers, agricultural workers, and casual laborers. Coverage is also incomplete among workers in small companies having fewer than six (varies by state) employees, nonprofit institutions, and state and local governments. About 87% of all wage and salary workers are covered in accordance with prevailing law.

Unless exempted by the law, employers must demonstrate their ability to pay workers' compensation benefits. There are three ways of accomplishing this: (1) insurance with a state fund, (2) insurance through a private carrier, or (3) self-insurance.

State Insurance Funds

The states have adopted two methods of meeting the problem of workers' compensation coverage. Some states require that employers insure through a state fund that operates as the exclusive provider of insurance. Other states operate their funds in competition with private carriers. A few states do not permit an employer to be self-insured.

Private Insurance Carriers

Private workers' compensation insurance contracts have two purposes: (1) to satisfy the employer's obligation to pay compensation and (2) to ensure that the injured employee receives all the benefits provided by law. Once the contract is signed, the insurer is responsible for compensating the injured worker. The carrier's liability is not relieved by either the insolvency or death of the employer or by any argument the carrier may have against the employer. Most state funds are similarly restricted.

Self-Insurance

Large employers may decide to serve as their own insurers. This approach includes the responsibility for adjusting claims and paying benefits, although it is possible to contract these tasks out to companies that provide such services. To qualify as a self-insurer, a company must demonstrate that it has the financial ability to pay all claims that may reasonably be expected. The state agency requires that a bond or other security be posted. Because this form of insurance is both time-consuming and requires financial reserves, smaller companies can seldom self-insure.

Companies choose to self-fund to reduce costs and to maximize cash flows. Because costs of benefits, claim reserves, litigation, and attendant administrative costs have spiraled in recent years, many companies have concluded that they could do as well as independent carriers while saving the cost of commissions and premium taxes and take advantage of greater cash flow and increased investment income rates. Self-insured employers are more likely to contest injury and illness claims than are privately insured employers and state insurance funds. This tendency to litigate may erase some of the cost savings that are realized by self-insurance.

Penalties for Not Having Insurance

Employers occasionally fail to provide workers' compensation insurance coverage for their employees. The cost of even one serious injury can deplete a company's entire annual income or even bankrupt it. Consequently, all but three states make workers' compensation insurance mandatory. Otherwise, a company could be out of business even before a seriously injured employee is fully recovered.

There are heavy penalties for uninsured employers. They can be subject to fines, loss of common-law defenses, increases in the amount of benefits awarded, and payment of attorneys' fees. The biggest financial deterrent is suit at common law. A number of states will force closure of an uninsured business. All states have established uninsured employers' funds to which the injured employee can apply for benefits. Applying to such a fund does not preclude the individual from also bringing action against the employer for penalties and legal fees. The uninsured employer may also be required to reimburse the fund for benefits paid the injured worker.

The cost of workers' compensation insurance is rate adjusted for all but the smallest employers—a process known as *experience rating*. When fewer injuries and illnesses occur, the employer pays lower workers' compensation insurance costs. Experience modification provides an automatic financial incentive for employers to provide their employees a work environment free from hazards that may result in compensation claims. There are conflicting economic studies on the value of experience rating and numerous problems in the interpretation of available data. Nonetheless, it is a hallowed provision of workers' compensation systems. Most large employers are experience rated, whereas small employers are typically insured in groups of similar companies. As the definitions of compensable injury are broadened, the intent and the benefits of experience rating are diluted.[2]

About three-fourths of all compensable claims for workers' compensation benefits and one-fourth of all cash payment benefits involve temporary total disability. Permanent total disability occurs in less than 1% of all compensable workers' compensation claims. Benefits paid in cash compensation are nearly equaled by medical and hospitalization benefits.

State and federal funds and self-insured employers each pay about one-fifth of all regular benefits, while private insurance companies pay the remaining three-fifths. The total costs to employers include the expenses of policy writing, claims investigation and adjustment, allocation to reserves to match increases in accrued liabilities, payroll auditing, commissions, premium taxes, and other administrative expenses and profit.

Employers are required to provide medical treatment as well as compensation benefits. The injured or ill employee is required to report the injury or illness as soon as possible. There is typically a statute of limitation that limits the employer's liability when an injury or illness is not promptly reported. It is considered that the requirement has been met if the employer is informed by someone other than the injured individual. The employer must then provide all medical care reasonably required to alleviate the problem. In fact, the law allows for treatment even when recovery is not possible—that is, palliative care that does not cure but only relieves.

In most states, there are no statutory limitations on the length of time or the cost of treatment, although a number of cost containment strategies are now being implemented by states and private insurers. These include (1) utilization review of inpatient and outpatient care, (2) hospital bill auditing of inpatient services, (3) medical bill auditing of practitioner and other services, and (4) preferred provider networks for inpatient care (where fees are discounted) and outpatient care (where the emphasis is on optimization of outcome measures). Some jurisdictions are considering the disallowance of services provided by physicians who own facilities where patients are referred for testing or treatment.

THE ROLE OF THE OCCUPATIONAL HEALTH PROFESSIONAL

Health professionals are involved in many of the required activities of workers' compensation systems because medical treatment involves the services of physicians and nurses and, frequently, that of physical therapists. Hospitalization, medicines, prosthetic appliances, and surgical supplies are all paid for by workers' compensation. Many states also allow treatment by licensed psychologists, dentists, optometrists, podiatrists, osteopaths, and chiropractors. Some states even permit treatment by acupuncturists, naturopaths, and Christian Science practitioners.

Workers in many states are permitted by state workers' compensation regulations to choose their own physicians. The choice may be any licensed physician or may be made from a list maintained by the employer or the state workers' compensation agency. Regardless of how the physician is chosen, the worker must submit to periodic examinations by a physician of the employer's choice. If either the employer or the worker is dissatisfied with the progress under the chosen physician's treatment, he or she can request and often be allowed to change doctors. Typically, an employee is permitted one such change for subjective reasons alone. In contrast, the employer can be required to prove to the state agency that a change is needed. Reasons for discharging a physician include incompetence, lack of reasonable progress toward recovery, inadequate or insufficient reporting by the physician, or inconvenience of the physician's practice location. If the employer selects the physician, an employee who is not satisfied with the treatment and progress may be permitted consultation with another physician at the employer's expense.

Although the employer must provide medical treatment for the injured employee, if the employee refuses reasonable treatment or surgery without justifiable cause, the employer is relieved of responsibility for any benefits related to injuries caused by the delay in or refusal of any treatment. The worker's refusal is usually considered justified when the suggested treatment or surgery entails a significant risk.

When a compensation case results in litigation, occupational health professionals and, on occasion, dermatologists become important witnesses in settling disputes. They serve as forensic experts for trial or settlement.

Claims Disputes

Differences of opinion often arise over workers' compensation claims. Such disputes often result from issues of insurance coverage, work relatedness of the injury or illness, provision of medical treatment, the worker's earnings capacity, and the extent of the disability. The last is the most common cause of disputes that require the physician to provide expert medical opinion. Although the system was designed to be "no fault," a large number of claims are subject to disputes among the employer, the insurance carrier, and the worker. Because adjudication is cumbersome, costly, and time consuming, tribunals have been established to hear claims disputes in the minimum time possible and at the least cost.

In most states, the initiation of a claim is by the worker, and the initial review is by the insurer. When there is a disagreement on the result, either party can apply for a hearing before the workers' compensation agency or court. If there is still dissatisfaction with the hearing officer's decision, an appeal can be made.

The states vary widely in their methods of hearing disputes, but the most commonly used methods are (1) a court-administered system, (2) a wholly administrative system, and (3) a combination of the two. The last is rapidly becoming almost as unwieldy as the common-law approach that it was designed to replace.

The Court-Administered System

The court-administered system is closest to common-law procedure and is based on the hypothesis that the parties of a dispute are more likely to receive justice from a court than from a referee or commission.

In this type of system, the employer may be covered either by a carrier or by self-insurance. All injuries or illnesses resulting in more than 6 days of disability must be reported within 14 days, usually accompanied by a physician's report. (In this discussion, time periods, exact procedures, fee percentages, and so on are drawn from one state for the purposes of example.) The state Department of Labor, through its workers' compensation division, decides whether the worker should receive compensation other than medical treatment. A form letter is then sent to the worker informing him or her of rights in case additional benefits are decided upon. Unless there is a complaint, the compensation agency takes no further action to ensure prompt payment, but the carrier must file notice when the claim is first paid. The system also requires that a settlement agreement be filed even if the worker refuses to sign it. A trial court reviews that agreement to determine whether the worker is receiving the correct benefits. If so, the agreement is approved and payments are made accordingly.

The employer has 10 days thereafter to file with the division certified copies of all relevant documents from the worker's file. If the division decides that the agreement does not provide sufficient benefits to the worker, the insurance carrier is required to adjust the agreement and have the court order modified. If the carrier refuses, the division advises the worker to take court action. Once a settlement has been approved by the court, it is binding on all parties if not contested within 30 days. However, the worker may go to trial court to contest the settlement at any time within 1 year of the injury. Compensation cases receive priority attention and are usually completed within 10 weeks. The case is heard by a trial judge and may be appealed to a circuit court and even to the state supreme court if the judge's finding is

unacceptable to the worker. The attorney may receive 20% of the award for his or her services.

The Wholly Administrative System

Under a wholly administrative system, the workers' compensation board pays benefits from assessments made against covered employers on the basis of payroll. Injuries must be reported as soon as possible, and benefits or the denial of benefits is determined by a claims adjudicator of a board located closest to the worker's home (again, using one state's system as an example). If the claim is denied, the worker is informed of the reason for denial and how to appeal. Either the government, without charge, or the worker's union assists in the appeal. Judgments can be appealed, in turn, to a board of review in all cases except those related to a rehabilitation decision.

The review boards are part of the Department of Labor but are totally dissociated from the workers' compensation division. They consist of a chairman and two members, one chosen by an employers' group and the other by an organization of workers in this state's example.

The claimant must make an appeal within 90 days after the claims adjudicator's report has been received. The appeal may be in the form of a letter stating the claimant's objections, or it may be submitted on a two-page form used for that purpose. The review board studies the workers' compensation board file and any new information the board obtains in the course of its decision-making. There is no hearing on the matter unless the claimant requests it, and such a request will be denied if the board decides that an appeal is not justified. If the board agrees to a hearing, it is held at a location convenient for the worker. The worker may have an attorney, but the appeals process does not include payment of the attorney's fees, that being the responsibility of the worker.

Although the decision of the review board is usually binding, it can be appealed further to the commissioners of the workers' compensation board within 60 days by a labor union on behalf of the injured worker or by an organization of employers on behalf of the injured worker or employer. If the chairman of the review board believes that an important principle underlies the appeal, he or she may allow the worker to make an appeal within 30 days. Furthermore, if the decision of the review board is not unanimous, the worker is permitted to appeal to the commissioners on his or her own behalf within 60 days. The decision of the commissioners is binding and may not be appealed to the courts.

A medical review panel exists for purely medical issues. This panel consists of a chairman appointed by the government and two physicians, one selected by the worker and one by the employer. Decisions by this panel are final. Many states sponsor less formal panels of physicians who interview and examine the claimant and then render opinions on disability, work restrictions, treatment, and prognosis.

The Combination System

The workers' compensation agency under the combination system consists of a seven-member appeals board that is responsible only for reviewing appeals and an administrative director who is responsible for the administrative functions of the agency. In California, for example, seven individuals are appointed by the governor and confirmed by the state senate.

First reports of worker injury or illness must be filed with the state Division of Labor Statistics and Research by both the employer and the attending physician. They are usually submitted through the employer's compensation carrier or adjusting agent and constitute the initiation of a claim. Furthermore, within 5 days of the injury the employer must inform the injured worker in simple terms not only about the benefits he or she is entitled to but also about the services available from the state Division of Workers' Compensation. The employer is further required to inform the compensation system administrator, as well as the worker, concerning commencement and termination dates of benefits, nonpayment of benefits, or rejection of claims. The worker is informed of his or her rights. The worker must also be informed that he or she can obtain an attorney, if desired. The worker must further be advised that any action must be taken promptly to avoid loss of compensation.

Most claims are paid automatically. There are penalties for the unwarranted rejection of compensation. The Division of Workers' Compensation becomes involved only if either the employer or the employee seeks adjudication from the workers' compensation appeals board. Such adjudication is initiated by the filing of a simple one-page form. The application must be filed within 1 year of the injury or by the date of the termination of benefits, whichever is longer. If the adjudication claim is related to further trauma resulting from the original injury, the application requirement is 5 years from the date of the original injury.

Although the system anticipates that a hearing will be held within 30 days after the application, that is seldom possible because of backlog. The hearings are conducted at several locations throughout the state and are assigned to a workers'

compensation judge who makes the decision. Usually, each judge reviews about 90 cases a month.

The hearings are designed to be informal, but often they cannot be distinguished from a nonjury court trial. The judges are knowledgeable in the workers' compensation process and are required to develop additional information if the evidence provided by the parties is inadequate. Medical information is usually presented in written reports. Once all the evidence is presented, the judge must present a written decision within 30 days.

If the employer or the employee is unhappy with the decision, he or she may file an appeal. This appeal is called a *petition for reconsideration* and must be filed within 20 days of the posting of the original decision. It is heard by a panel of three members of the appeals board. The panel is authorized to approve or deny reconsideration, issue a different decision on the original evidence, or seek additional information, including consultation with an independent medical specialist.

The decision of this panel is final unless the dissatisfied party seeks a review by an appellate court within 45 days by submitting a petition for a writ of review to the appeals court. The court is empowered to deny the review without explanation. If a review is permitted, the appeals court studies the evidence, hears oral arguments, and presents a written decision. If the party bringing the appeal is still dissatisfied, he or she may petition the state supreme court for a further hearing. However, the supreme court will rarely accept more than a few workers' compensation cases each year.

In the great majority of contested cases, both parties are represented either by attorneys or by expert lay representatives. On average, those representing the worker receive 9 to 15% of the award.

Reopening of Claims

Workers' compensation proceedings differ from civil law suits in one important aspect—the body that originally decided the award may alter its decision if the worker's condition changes or there is other reasonable cause. This process may be limited under certain conditions by state compensation laws, and most states establish a time limit beyond which a modification cannot be made. If the requirements of the law cannot be met, final decisions in compensating cases are as binding as those in any judicial proceeding.

There is a wide divergence among states as to benefit amounts, conditions that are compensable, processing of claims, settlement of disputes, and the general economics of each system. Consequently, physicians who expect to be treating occupational injuries and illnesses are well advised to learn how the workers' compensation system operates in the state in which they are practicing.

THE PHYSICIAN'S EXAMINATION

Impairment and Disability

Medical judgment is necessary to resolve workers' compensation cases. The physician evaluates the degree of "impairment" (measured by anatomical or functional loss) and supplies an opinion to disability raters, workers' compensation judges, commissioners, or hearing officers. These nonmedical people make the decision as to "disability." Unlike impairment, disability depends on the job and one's ability to compete in the open job market.

Impairment does not necessarily imply disability. For example, the loss of the distal phalanx of the second digit on the left hand results in the same impairment rating in a concert violinist and a roofer, but the disability would be much greater for the musician. It is important to discuss impairment and disability separately. An individual with carpal tunnel syndrome may be disabled when considered for a job with repetitive hand movements, but not for a job that does not require extensive use of the hands.

Insurers frequently ask the physician to determine work restrictions (e.g., no further exposure to sensitizing chemicals in the case of a contact dermatitis, limited exposure to trauma in the case of Koebner's phenomenon, and so forth) in order to match the impairment to specific jobs.

When an impairment evaluation is requested, the examining physician should utilize the most current AMA *Guides to the Evaluation of Permanent Impairment*[10] or the guides utilized in the physician's jurisdiction.[11] Standards for disability evaluation can be found in the AMA *Guides* and in schedules provided by the Social Security Administration and the Veterans Administration and some states.[12] Physicians who perform impairment evaluations should make sure that they know which schedule is applicable in each case.[13] Many states will send medical examiners their recommended guidelines for general medical and psychiatric assessments.

A handicap, under the Americans with Disabilities Act definition, is "an impairment that substantially limits one or more of life's activities" but also includes the individual who "has a record of such an impairment or is regarded as having such an impairment."[14] Therefore, an individual who has a documented contact dermatitis could be considered handicapped even though he or she has no symptoms away from exposure and would have neither an impairment rating nor a disability.[15]

Addressing the issue of employability is complex, but not usually a part of a medical disability evaluation. Does the medical condition preclude traveling to and from work, being at work, or performing required essential functions of the job? Motivation is a factor in determining return to work status, but not for the purpose of determining employability.

Written Report

Physicians who are experienced with submission of current status and progress reports to employers and insurance companies can expand their experience to include impairment evaluations. Physicians who treat injured workers should develop the experience and confidence to undertake impairment and disability evaluations. The physician who has been asked to do an impairment evaluation should understand exactly what the requesting party wants to know. Copies of all relevant medical records, reports, and test results should be obtained and reviewed completely. In a workers' compensation case, the patient will probably see reports written by the physician. All details should be presented in unambiguous terms and in appropriate detail. Use of abbreviations and other time savers is not appropriate in this form of medical record. Be sure to explain technical terms for the benefit of nonmedical readers.

History

The history of the injury or exposure to toxic materials at work should be detailed, and there should be a complete and careful description of the activities of the job. All historical information should be obtained by the physician and not by office personnel. The history should also include information about all previous employment and all nonwork activities, with particular attention to factors that might have some relation to the present complaints. An example occurs in claims of toxic exposure where the claimant has a cognitive deficit corroborated by neuropsychological testing. In these cases, individuals may have had preexisting problems secondary to head injuries, hypoxia at birth, and so forth, and it may be necessary to review school records as well as previous medical history.

The history of the illness or injury should include all preexisting conditions. The injured employee's complaints and symptoms should be listed. Many examiners quote these verbatim, without comment, to capture the flavor of the words and avoid misinterpretation. Be precise about temporal relationships between work and the injury or between exposures and the illness. The history of all former medical treatment and treatment outcomes should be obtained in detail.

Occupational History. In obtaining the occupational history, physicians may need to have additional information than that contained in the medical file. This may be requested from the workers' compensation judge or the appropriate governmental agency (e.g., the Division of Industrial Accidents in the state). Additional medical reports and other evidence can often be obtained. The physician may need to talk with the claimant's family and with coworkers and friends. Beware the legal implications of telephone calls to or from the claimant's representatives, as well as supervisors or company management. Allegations of collusion between management and occupational physicians are not infrequent in workers' compensation actions.

The history should be as complete as necessary, yet as brief as possible. In the occupational history, summarize all jobs and note any work-related illnesses and injuries chronologically. Discuss required activities in the last job, including hours worked, shiftwork or other assignments that might have caused excessive fatigue or a circadian dysrhythmia (desynchronosis), changes in work routine that might interfere with safety and hygiene practices, and chemical and other toxic exposures in great detail. If industrial hygiene measurements are available to determine dose of exposure, these are vital to the evaluation of the health risk to the employee.

It is important to mention any preexisting condition that limited the ability to work or to compete in the job market, including work limitations or preclusions imposed by a physician. The job title is less useful information than a detailed description of the work activity and its duration. Formal job descriptions are often available and can be very useful in documenting the occupational history. Are other workers affected by the same working conditions? Does the company provide personal protective equipment? The dermatologist is primarily interested in skin exposures to trauma, radiation, metals and chemicals, and infectious agents. These are often difficult exposures to document in the best of circumstances. Some toxic agents have long latent periods, and it may be necessary to go back 25 or 30 years in taking the history.

Past Medical History. The past medical history should include relevant previous as well as concurrent conditions, or complaints if there are no physical findings. List medications taken for these conditions. The social and family history should always include information on use of alcohol, cigarettes, and family history of similar or related problems when relevant. Workers' compensation claims and settlements data can and should be obtained. In some instances, historical data on major medical insurance utilization may be relevant as well. In the review of systems, list pertinent positives and negatives without resorting to long lists.

Differences between the histories obtained by various physicians should be noted and explained. List and summarize the relevant reports reviewed to document having read them.

Physical Examination

When examining patients, the physical examination requires precise, objective measurements of impairment. The ultimate rating of disability will reflect the findings more exactly if nonmedical raters are presented with terms that are readily understandable. Physicians who know the rating system are much better able to properly assist the rater to translate the medical condition into ratable terms. Physicians often learn through the mentoring of disability raters, attorneys, and other physicians experienced in workers' compensation.

Conclusions

Draw no medical conclusions that are not reasonably supported by the medical record. Conclusions should include the following:

Diagnoses: Differential diagnoses should not be included in the report. References, unless they are critical to your conclusions, should not be cited. When stating the diagnosis, the opinions should be logically and adequately conveyed.

Causation: Is there a causal relationship between the condition(s) found and the claimed injury or occupational exposure? In this and in other answers give reasons for the opinion and be as definite as possible. "Possibly" or "maybe" are not helpful terms. "Probably" or "more likely than not" is appropriate phrasing if it applies. In determining causation in workers' compensation, if the condition found would not now exist *but for* the occupational injury or exposure—even though there may have been other contributing nonoccupational causes—the occupational injury or exposure will be considered to be the cause of the condition.[16] Nonetheless, do not attempt to make legal determinations. Do not say, "impairment is due to an industrial injury." Say, "impairment is more likely than not the result of the chemical exposures described occurring over (the following time period)."

Disability: During what periods of time was the injured employee unable to work as a result of the medical conditions found? Temporary disability requires careful attention to questions of when and how long.

Are the condition(s) "permanent and stationary" and on what date did they become so? A practical working definition of permanent and stationary is "the condition is not going to get significantly better or worse with further medical treatment." In some states, a person has reached "permanent and stationary" or "maximum medical improvement" if the condition has been stable for 6 months and additional therapy will not significantly change the impairment rating. If the worker is not permanent and stationary, when will the condition become so? What medical treatment(s) are recommended, and what are the anticipated benefits? Psychiatric factors may also have to be considered.

Summarize the factors of impairment, listing subjective symptoms and objective losses and limitations. In California, disabling symptoms such as pain should be referred to as "minimal," "slight," "moderate," or "severe," which are defined as follows: *Minimal* constitutes an annoyance, but causes no handicap in the performance of the particular employment activity. *Slight* can be tolerated but would cause some handicap in the performance of the employment activity bringing about the pain. *Moderate* can be tolerated but would cause marked handicap in the performance of the employment activity precipitating the pain. *Severe* would preclude the employment activity precipitating the pain.

Some other words often have special meaning.[17] California, *occasional* means 25% of the time, *termittent* means 50% of the time, *frequent* means 75% of the time, and *constant* means 100% of the time.

In giving an opinion, do not use "guess" or "speculate." Instead, say, "Based on my experience, my opinion is. . . ." In this circumstance, the physician is the expert medical authority and should be confident of his or her opinion.

Work restrictions should be stated in no uncertain terms. If the injured employee should not do certain things at work, this should be stated emphatically. It is very important that work restrictions be understood.

Apportionment: Some jurisdictions request the physician to determine apportionment. Apportionment is a legal method for distributing financial responsibility. It is intended to ensure that employers are only responsible for those injuries or illnesses caused in their workplace. Apportionment applies only to permanent disability. The examining physician does not apportion causation, disease, or pathology. The person being examined may have a disability other than that resulting from the work injury or illness. There may be disability resulting from congenital defects, from previous work- or nonwork-related injuries, from aging, from subsequent injuries, or from the natural progression of preexisting disease.

When physicians address apportionment, there is a relatively simple way to do it that avoids legal complications. The physician should write two paragraphs. The first should describe the existing impairment factors (objective and subjective) and work restrictions. The second paragraph should describe the impairment factors and work restrictions that would exist in the absence of the occupational injury or illness. The hearing officer can then decide the extent of the impairment represented by each of the two paragraphs and, by subtraction, can decide the level of impairment caused by the employment environment. Do not attempt to figure out the percentage of impairment that is represented by either of the paragraphs. The judge and trained raters will do this.

Medical Treatment: Further medical treatment is an important consideration. Many workers' compensation cases are settled with "continuing medical treatment" provided either within limits or as a lifelong benefit. The opinion as to the value of continued medical treatment and for what purpose it is to be rendered should be stated, along with recommendations for current treatment should it be different from treatment already rendered the employee by other physicians.

Vocational Rehabilitation: Vocational rehabilitation may be recommended for employees who cannot return to their former job. The treating physician's opinion is very important here. If the employee is unable to perform the former job, the physician should say so. The physician may be of the opinion that vocational rehabilitation services will benefit the worker in a possible return to the former job. The physician's role here is to state that vocational rehabilitation should be considered. It should be left to vocational rehabilitation specialists to determine whether the worker will benefit from such services. If conclusions about the extent of impairment have been stated clearly, experts on the physical requirements of various occupations will be able to make an appropriate decision regarding rehabilitation.

Specialized Medical Examiners

When the employer or the worker objects to the treating physician, many jurisdictions provide the opportunity for the worker to be seen by an "agreed medical evaluator" selected by the employer and the worker's attorney. If the parties do not agree to a permanent disability rating based on the treating physician's evaluation, specialized medical examiners with documented experience and background in workers' compensation medicine, often referred to as *qualified medical evaluators*, are specified by the jurisdiction, and/or selected from a panel by the employee, and provide an evaluation that settles the contested issue of impairment. As usual, the names and qualifications of these specialized evaluators vary widely between jurisdictions.

Occupational Dermatology

A number of review articles address the topic of occupational dermatology and workers' compensation. Adams[18] presents clinical examples of the dermatologist's participation in the settlement of workers' compensation claims. Ross[19] reviews the literature of workers' compensation and skin disease. In his discussion of liability, he points out that there is reasonable concern that occupational skin disease can be overdiagnosed. His study of 250 workers from a background of 14 different industries showed that only 127 (51%) had skin findings consistent with workplace exposure. Holness and Nethercott[20] discuss work outcome with occupational skin disease. They studied the employment outcomes of 230 workers with a diagnosis of occupational skin disease who were at least 2 years postdiagnosis. Seventy-eight percent of the workers were working, but 57% of those working had changed jobs because of their skin disease, while 35% had lost at least 1 month of work. Forty-three percent had applied for workers' compensation benefits, and 87% of those who had applied were successful in their claims. Those who had changed their jobs tended to have a better outcome with respect to active dermatitis, though they had lost more time from work and had more often applied for workers' compensation benefits. Cooley and Nethercott[21] review the literature on prognosis of occupational skin disease. They point out that the prognosis in occupational skin disease, which is largely irritant and allergic contact dermatitis, is guarded.

A large proportion of workers developing such disease do not improve with present methods of secondary preventive intervention and treatment. Although cases of allergic contact dermatitis may do better when a specific cause can be found and avoided, as when allergic contact dermatitis is due to the metals nickel and chromium, they have a poor prognosis. Moreover, job changes appear to be of equivocal value. Early diagnosis and intervention are associated with a better prognosis for cure. Greater attention to primary prevention through regulation of exposure to irritants and sensitizers, combined with more effective measures for control of industrial hygiene, offers the possibility of more effective management.

TREATMENT GUIDELINES FOR CONTACT DERMATITIS

Contact dermatitis is the most common form of occupational skin disease. Eligibility for coverage under workers' compensation requires only reasonable probability that the dermatitis directly resulted from, or was aggravated by, employment.[22] Because so many cases of contact dermatitis are diagnosed and treated by primary care physicians, the State of California developed a Treatment Guideline for the diagnosis and treatment of the disease.[23] It can be assumed that many more occupational illnesses will be strictly defined and the care they receive be monitored in this way by workers' compensation jurisdictions. The American Academy of Dermatology's Committee on Guidelines of Care has also developed a useful Guideline of Care for Contact Dermatitis.[24]

References

1. Barth PS. Compensating workers for occupational disease: An international perspective. *Int J Occup Environ Health* 1995; 1(2):147.
2. Schmulowitz J. Workers' compensation: Coverage, benefits, and costs, 1992–93. *Social Security Bull* 1995; 58(2):51.
3. *State Workers' Compensation Laws.* U.S. Department of Labor, Employment Standards Administration, Office of Workers' Compensation Programs, Branch of Workers' Compensation Studies, January 1997.
4. Greenwood J, Taricco A, eds. *Workers' Compensation Health Care Cost Containment.* Horstman PA: LRP Publications; 1992.
5. U.S. Chamber of Commerce. *Analysis of Workers' Compensation Laws.* Washington, DC: US. Chamber of Commerce; 1999.
6. National Council on Compensation Insurance. *Issues Report, 1997.* Boca Raton, FL: NCCI; 1997.
7. Larson A: *The Law of Workmen's Compensation.* New York: Matthew Bender; 1999.
8. Bureau of Labor Statistics. *Occupational Injuries and Illnesses in the United States by Industry, 1996.* Washington, DC: Bureau of Labor Statistics, U.S. Department of Labor; 1997.
9. Hennessey JC, Muller LS. Work efforts of disabled-worker beneficiaries: Preliminary findings from the new beneficiary followup survey. *Social Security Bull* 1994; 57(3):42.
10. American Medical Association. *Guides to the Evaluation of Permanent Impairment,* 4th ed, rev. Chicago: American Medical Association; 1993.
11. Babitsky S, Sewall HD. *Understanding the AMA Guides in Workers' Compensation.* Colorado Springs: Wiley Law Publications; 1992.

12. Carey TS, Hadler NM. The role of the primary physician in disability determination for Social Security Insurance and workers' compensation. *Ann Int Med* 1986; 104:706–710.

13. Crook PL. Worker's compensation. In: Tollison A, ed. *Handbook of Chronic Pain Management.* Baltimore: Williams & Wilkins; 1989:644–653.

14. Schramm D, Sridhar VV. Assessment of impairment and disability. In: Ashburn MA, Rice LJ, eds. *The Management of Pain.* New York: Churchill Livingstone; 1998:63–74.

15. Davies NF, Rycroft RJG. Dermatology. In: Cox RAF, ed. *Fitness for Work: The Medical Aspects.* New York: Oxford University Press; 1995:102–112.

16. LaDou J. Workers' compensation law. In: LaDou J, ed. *Occupational and Environmental Medicine,* 2nd ed. Stamford, Conn: Appleton & Lange; 1997.

17. Engelberg AL, Matheson LN. Impairment, disability, and functional capacity. In: Rom WN, ed. *Environmental and Occupational Medicine.* Philadelphia: Lippincott-Raven; 1998:67–78.

18. Adams RM: The dermatologist and workers' compensation: Theory and practice. *Dermatol Clin* 1994; 121(3):583.

19. Ross JB. Workers' compensation for skin disease. *Occup Med* 1994; 9(1):25.

20. Holness DL, Nethercott JR. Work outcome in workers with occupational skin disease. *Am J Ind Med* 1995; 27(6):807.

21. Cooley JE, Nethercott JR. Prognosis of occupational skin disease. *Occup Med* 1994; 9(1):19.

22. Mathias CGT. Association, causation of work-related contact dermatitis. *Clin Care Update* 1997; 3(14):3.

23. Industrial Medical Council. *Treatment Guidelines for Contact Dermatitis.* Labor Code Section 139(e)(8). Department of Industrial Relations, State of California; 1996.

24. Committee on Guidelines of Care, American Academy of Dermatology. Guidelines of care for contact dermatitis. *J Acad Dermatol* 1995; 32:109.

Industrial Processes Commonly Associated with Skin Disease

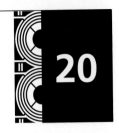

20

JAMES R. NETHERCOTT, M.D.*
D. LINN HOLNESS, M.D.

The world of work is complex and ever changing. Service industries have slowly enlarged in the 20th century to become the largest employers rather than manufacturers. Some predict that work as we currently know it will change dramatically over the next few decades as we move from an industrially based age to the information age.[1] Nonetheless, currently primary and secondary industry continue to produce a variety of products, and these, in addition to certain types of service work, are principal sources of many occupational dermatoses.

There are a number of sources from which information regarding the frequency of contact dermatitis arising from various operations can be obtained. Government statistics (including workers' compensation) are one source, but these may be subject to a number of biases. Statistics for lost-time dermatitis claims in the Province of Ontario from 1988 to 1995 are presented in Table 20–1.[2] This demonstrates that while there is a decreasing absolute number of lost-time dermatitis claims, their proportion relative to all lost-time claims has remained relatively stable, suggesting an overall trend in decreasing compensation claims as opposed to a relative decrease in dermatitis claims.

Another source of information on the sources of occupational dermatitis is the contact dermatitis literature. A review of the content of journals related to contact dermatitis is helpful in gaining an understanding of some of the current issues. The contents of the *American Journal of Contact Dermatitis* from its inception in 1990 to the end of 1997 were reviewed. Articles were classified as to whether they had occupational content and then

further whether the work was related to a population-based study (clinic based or industry based), case reports, or neither. There were over 400 articles published in the *American Journal of Contact Dermatitis* during this interval. Approximately 20% dealt with occupational issues. Thirty percent were based on clinic- or industry-based populations, approximately 55% on case reports, and 15% reviews of other topics related to occupational dermatology (e.g., NIOSH prevention strategy, workers' compensation). Of the population-based articles, 50% were based on industry populations and 50% on clinic populations.

The articles that were based on populations were reviewed to determine the industry sectors and agents studied. The industry sectors that were represented in more than one article included agriculture, hairdressing, automotive (parts manufacturing), plastics and resin manufacture, and health care. The agents that were the subject of study in more than one publication included plants, plastics

TABLE 20–1 • Lost-Time (LT) Dermatitis Claims, Province of Ontario

Year	LT Dermatitis Claims	Overall LT Claims	% Dermatitis Claims
1988	606	208,499	0.29
1989	530	200,967	0.26
1990	475	184,444	0.26
1991	502	155,475	0.32
1992	377	136,940	0.28
1993	343	125,122	0.27
1994	314	125,644	0.25
1995	260	118,814	0.22

*Deceased.

and resins, and metal-working fluids. This provides one measure of areas of continuing activity in occupational contact dermatitis.

Furthermore, a perusal of the topics covered in this text should quickly lead one to the realization that certain occupations present greater risks. While there are many different industrial processes, a knowledge of at least a few basic ones is essential to understanding the exposure that may have produced a patient's dermatosis and to establishing an occupational association. Without such basic information, it is difficult to intelligently approach the problem of work-related skin disease or, often, to manage it effectively.

Patient management in the occupational setting not only involves the treatment of the patient's skin affliction but also offers the challenge of primary prevention.[3, 4] The clinician is faced with trying to mitigate the effects of the workplace environment on the skin disease that is already present in his or her patient. The protection of other workers who are not affected but are potentially at risk is a further encumbrance beyond the management of one's own patient that differentiates occupational dermatological management from many other aspects of dermatological practice.

Minimizing or eliminating the industrial exposure that led to the patient's disease, to the degree that this can be accomplished consistent with the worker remaining on the job (i.e., the practicality of implementing the use of personal protective equipment, engineering controls, substance substitution), is often dependent on an understanding of the industrial process in which the worker participates. Compliance with suggestions in this regard, not unlike compliance with the use of prescribed medications, is often largely determined by the practicality of the suggestions.

A knowledge of industrial processes is also vital if primary preventive measures are to be taken to protect other workers who may be at risk. The cause of many cutaneous diseases is unknown, and the dermatologist has no ability to prevent them. In contrast, many occupational skin disorders can be related to a given chemical (e.g., epoxy resin, p-phenylenediamine, tetramethyl thiuram disulfide), to physical agents (e.g., ultraviolet light, thermal injury, vibration), or to a combination of such agents (e.g., phytophotodermatitis, photoallergic contact dermatitis). By recognizing the hazard, steps may be taken to minimize exposure and reduce or eliminate the risk of inducing skin disease in workers not yet affected. Understanding the process is essential if practical solutions are to be found in such situations.

The purpose of this chapter is to give the reader a brief introduction to industrial processes that are associated with skin disease. Eight categories have been chosen for discussion. For more detailed information, a number of references are available.[5–8]

MIXING, BLENDING, AND GRINDING

Many workers in the chemical industry mix combinations of ingredients to yield formulations for specific uses. Liquid raw materials may be blended for mixtures for products such as liquid shoe polish, intravenous solutions, and paint strippers. Liquids and solids (e.g., plasticizers, pigments, drugs) may be mixed to produce finished products like sealants, varnishes, adhesives, and pharmaceuticals.

Such mixing activity is not unlike working a large kitchen mixer. Materials are weighed or measured by volume and are placed in the mixer (Fig. 20–1). The worker uses a recipe or batch card that outlines how much of each ingredient is to be added. The various components are then mixed, sometimes with the addition of heat, for a defined time. The finished mixture is then transferred to a finished packaging format, which could be anything from a small bottle to entire tank cars of the product. The hazard to the worker depends on the components mixed. Cutaneous contamination may occur from the raw materials or from the final formulation in which a reaction product formed in the mixing, a single ingredient, or the entire formulation may be a skin hazard.

Cement is manufactured in this fashion by the addition of gravel and water to produce Portland cement. Skin contamination during the mixing or pouring, or from dry cement dust, may cause allergic contact dermatitis from bichromate.

When pigments are added to a mixture to make products such as paint, ink, and cosmetics, the pigment has to be dispersed so that when the finished product is applied to a surface it will produce a constant color. The steps in this process are illustrated in Figure 20–2.[9] It is accomplished by grinding the mixture to disperse the pigment, using a roller mill, rod mill, or ball mill in a manner that is similar to using a rolling pin to spread dough. The mashing device may consist of metal rods, metal balls, or opposing cylinders that compress the product. Depending on the batch size processed, such mills may be relatively small or as large as a boxcar. Skin contamination may be a problem for a worker operating a milling machine.

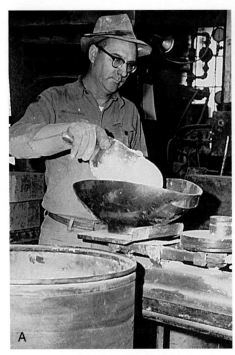

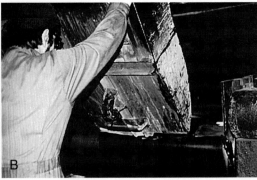

FIGURE 20–1 • *A,* Worker weighing the various ingredients to be added to a rubber stock in the Banbury mixer. *B,* Worker dumping the stock and additives into the mixer.

PAINTING, COATING, AND PRINTING

In the processes of painting, coating, and printing, a film is applied to a stock, which may be metal, plastic, paper, and so on. Paints are colored liquids that will opacify the surface to which they are applied and impart a color. The liquid is made up of a vehicle, fillers, and additives (Table 20–2).[10] The most commonly used resins in the vehicle component are listed in Table 20–3.[5]

Many pigments are used as opacifiers and to impart color (Table 20–4).[5] Solvents are used to alter the viscosity of paints in different operations and in clean-up work (Table 20–5).[5] These paint components may result in contact dermatitis.

Paint may be transferred to a surface by spraying. In such operations, a mist is generated, which is directed toward the surface to be coated. Some bounces off and misses the object, which is referred to as the *overspray*. The remainder adheres to the surface. Local exhaust is often used to draw air from behind the worker spraying the paint to entrain the mist, thereby reducing the operator's exposure (Fig. 20–3). Some contamination of the worker and the workplace still occurs. There is a problem of skin contamination for maintenance mechanics, often called *millwrights,* who must repair the equipment and service the ventilation system.

An electrostatic charge may be applied to the spray particles, with an opposite charge given to the object to be painted. This results in better adhesion to the object painted through the electrostatic effect, reducing the overspray. Powdered paints have been developed that are applied with a spray gun and adhere to the coated surface, after which heat is applied to produce the liquid coating. This reduces the operator's exposure to active ingredients like epoxy resins. Such spray painting operations may be fully automated in a large operation, such as a car assembly plant in which robotic devices may spray a vehicle in a totally enclosed area. Not infrequently, though, touch-up painting is carried out in an open work area without local ventilation, which leads to airborne contact with the paint components. Once again, millwrights are at risk when servicing such equipment.

Coatings are applied to a large number of surfaces to seal them or to give an adhesive surface. The film is often applied from a bath, with the surface passing into contact with it as sheets or as a continuous roll of material. This procedure may be used to apply paint to articles rather than spray painting them. This process is commonly used to coat things such as paper products (e.g., glossy coatings on magazine covers, wax paper, wallpaper, adhesive tape), metal articles (air conditioning casings, furniture, machines), and plastic equipment (computer cases, handles, moldings). The coating material may pose a skin hazard (e.g., rosin in paint, acrylic monomers in coatings). Coatings may also be applied by spraying or dip-

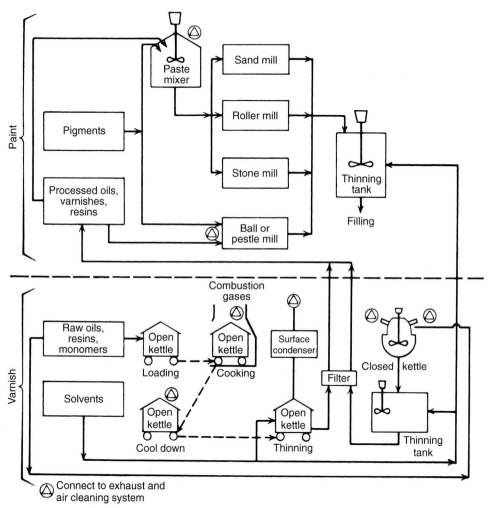

FIGURE 20–2 • Flow diagram for paint and varnish operations. (From American Conference of Governmental Industrial Hygienists, Cincinnati, 1973.)

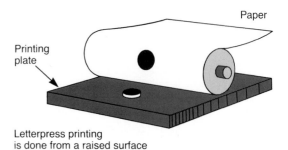

Letterpress printing
is done from a raised surface

FIGURE 20–4 • Letterpress printing. (From The World Book Encyclopedia. Chicago: Field Enterprises; 1973.)

TABLE 20–2 • Basic Paint Ingredients		
Major Component	**Constituents**	**Purposes**
Vehicle	Binder	Resin that forms film
	Thinner	Thinner for adjustment of viscosity
Filler	General filler	Hiding ability, body, color
	Pigment	Opaqueness, color
	Extender	Fillers that build body
Additives	Driers	Speed drying or curing
	Biocide	Prevent growth of mold and fungus
	Flatting agents	Provide low luster
	Stabilizers	Protect against heat and ultraviolet radiation
	Antiskinning	Prevent skin formation in can

From Murphy J. *Surface Preparations and Finishes for Metals.* New York: McGraw-Hill; 1971.

Letterpress (Fig. 20–4)[11] is the oldest form and involves the transfer of the image from a raised surface to which ink has been applied to another surface to which the image is applied under pressure. The image may be on a flat surface, and the stock is applied to it from another flat surface

ping the object into the coating material (e.g., armature wire).

Printing is a specialized form of coating. Ink is a varnish containing a pigment, and it may be thought of as a specialized form of paint. It is applied to a surface in a pattern. This may involve one of four processes: letterpress, offset, gravure, and silkscreen printing.[11, 12]

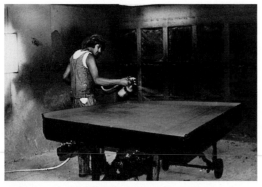

FIGURE 20–3 • In spray painting, protective clothing and exhaust systems are very important. In the operation shown here, these precautions are not used.

TABLE 20–3 • Common Paint Resins	
Resin	**Method of Manufacture**
Alkyd	Reaction product of dicarboxylic acid with polylols; alkyd resin may react with soybean oil, linseed oil, or phenolic resin
Modified alkyd	Reaction of alkyd resin with styrene, vinyl chloride, allyl alcohol, or urea formaldehyde resin
Phenols	Reaction of phenol or substituted phenols with an aldehyde to produce acidic or alkaline resins
Acrylic	Polymerization of esters of acrylic or methacrylic acid
Vinyl	Vinyl polymers and copolymers
Amino resins	Reaction of amino resins of urea or melamine with formaldehyde
Epoxy	Reaction of phenol (bisphenol A) and an epoxy (epichlorhydrin); frequently mixed with amino or phenolic resins
Polystyrene	Styrene in ethyl benzene with catalyst (benzoyl peroxide)
Polyurethanes	Polyurethane prepolymer reacted with alcohols and amines
Cellulose	Esters or ethers of cellulose such as nitrocellulose

From Burgess WA. *Recognition of Health Hazards in Industry—A Review of Materials and Processes.* New York; John Wiley & Sons; 1981.

TABLE 20–4 • Commonly Used Paint Pigments and Extenders		

White Pigments
White lead
   Basic carbonate
   Basic sulfate
   Basic silicate
Zinc oxide
Lead zinc oxide
Titanium dioxides
Lithopone
Antimony oxide
 	
Iron Oxide
Red and brown iron oxides
   Natural
   Synthetic
Yellow iron oxide
   Synthetic
Ochre
Raw and burnt siennas
Raw and burnt umbers
Black iron oxide
	Green Pigments
	Chrome green
	Chromium oxide
	Phthalocyanine green
	
	Blue Pigments
	Iron blue
	Ultramarine blue
	Indanthrene blue
	Others
	
	Red Pigments
	Cadmium red
	Cadmium-mercury red and
	   orange
	Toluidine red
	Para red
	Toners
	
	Yellow and Orange
	Chrome yellow
	Chrome orange
	Molybdate orange
	Zinc yellow
	Cadmium yellow and orange
	Hansa yellow
	Orange toner
		Metallic and Other
		Aluminum powders
		Bronze powders
		Zinc dust
		Lead powder and flake
		Nickel flake
		Stainless steel
		Cuprous oxide
		
		Extenders
		Barytes
		Blanc fixe
		Calcium carbonate
		Amorphous silica
		Diatomaceous silica
		Talc
		China clay
		Mica
		Bentonite
		Asbestos

From Murphy J. *Surface Preparations and Finishes for Metals.* New York; McGraw-Hill; 1971.

(platen press), or a rotating drum may carry the stock, impressing it on a flat surface carrying the image (flat bed cylinder press).

Offset lithography involves the transfer of the image from a plate to a rubber "blanket" and from the blanket to the surface to be printed up (Fig. 20–5).[11] The offset plates are made of etched metal or photoreactive acrylic materials, and workers making the plates may experience problems with dermatitis caused by metals or acrylic monomers.[13] The use of light-sensitive acrylic printing plates has become common. The uncured plate has reactive acrylic monomers in it, and skin contact with the monomers is possible in the conversion to the finished plate. Contact may occur either when the uncured monomers are dissolved to yield the relief image or in the handling of the uncured plates.

Large-scale printing, such as newspaper printing, is carried out with two cylindrical surfaces, one of which carries the stock as the impression cylinder, whereas the other carries the image (ro-

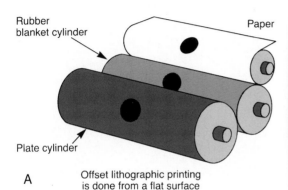

Offset lithographic printing
is done from a flat surface

A

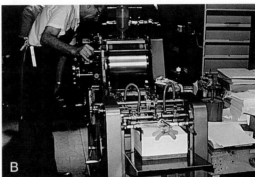

B

FIGURE 20–5 • *A,* Offset lithography. (From The World Book Encyclopedia. Chicago: Field Enterprises; 1973.) *B,* A typical offset printing press used for small products such as calling cards and stationery.

TABLE 20–5 • Commonly Used Paint Solvents and Thinners

Aromatic	Chlorinated	Acetates
Benzene	Methyl chloride	Ethyl
Toluene	Chlorothene	Isopropyl
Xylene	Carbon	*n*-Propyl
Aromatic	tetrachloride	*n*-Butyl
naphthas	Ethylene	Trichloroethylene
Aromatic	dichloride	**Ketones**
petroleum	Perchloroethylene	Acetone
solvents		Methylethyl
Amyl	**Terpenes**	ketone
Aliphatics	Turpentine	Methylacetone
Petroleum	Dipentene	Methylisobutyl
ether	Pine oil	ketone
VM and P	**Alcohols**	Diacetone
naphtha	Methanol	Cyclohexanone
Mineral	Ethanol	Isophorone
spirits	Isopropanol	Diisobutyl ketone
Kerosene	*n*-Propanol	
High-flash	*n*-Butanol	
naphthas	Amyl alcohol	
Glycol Ethers	Cyclohexanol	
Various		

From Murphy J. *Surface Preparations and Finishes for Metals.* New York: McGraw-Hill; 1971.

tary press). Such presses may have single sheets of paper fed into them (sheet fed) or may operate with a continuous roll of paper (web fed).

Gravure printing involves the transfer of an image using an engraved plate in which the ink is inspissated in wells on the plate. The excess is squeezed off by a blade, called a *doctor blade,* and is then transferred to the surface as minute dots (Fig. 20–6).[11]

Silk screening involves the application of ink to the surface using a template through which the ink is pressed to transfer the image to the printed surface (Fig. 20–7).

Workers in printing plants are exposed to solvents used in cleaning the presses (Fig. 20–8), and

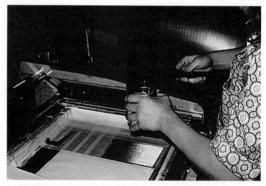

FIGURE 20–7 • In silk screening, the application of ink can be a source of dermatitis.

gravure and flexographic inks are themselves high in solvent content. The wearing of personal protective equipment, such as gloves, may pose a safety hazard in terms of catching one's hand in a press while cleaning it. When presses are run at high speed, an ink mist may be generated, which may lead to airborne contact.

DYEING

Dyes are commonly applied to various materials such as leather and textiles. In the case of leather products, the hides are treated with formaldehyde as a mordant and chromium to make the leather impervious to wear. In a tannery, this is done in a large mixer that is similar to a batch mixer. Contact with the dyes and other raw materials may result in irritant or allergic contact dermatitis.

The dyeing of textiles is similar and might be likened to washing clothing in a slowly agitating washing machine in which the dye has been added to the washing solution. The clothing may be soaked in a solution containing a formaldehyde-

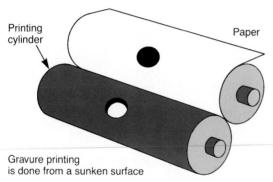

Printing cylinder

Paper

Gravure printing is done from a sunken surface

FIGURE 20–6 • Gravure printing. (From The World Book Encyclopedia. Chicago: Field Enterprises; 1973.)

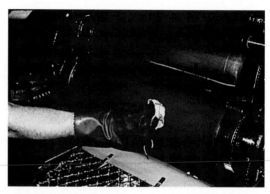

FIGURE 20–8 • In operating a printing press, the roller must be regularly wiped clean of ink using a volatile solvent.

based resin to make it wrinkle resistant and may then be heat cured. Cotton is commonly mercerized by soaking it in formaldehyde.

PLASTIC PROCESSING

Plastics are in very wide use. Problems with these materials usually occur from direct contact with chemically reactive compounds in the product.

One of the most common industrial processes used in plastic manufacturing is called *extrusion molding*. Beads of solid plastic, such as polypropylene or polyvinyl, are placed under pressure and heat using an auger. As the auger compresses the thermoplastic resin and heat is added, a liquid plastic is produced, which is then forced into a mold. The mold may be like a cake tin or cookie tray, or it may be a die or mandrel through which the resin is extruded to produce a continuous object like a tube or piece of molding. The extruded material may, for instance, be applied continuously to the outside of a wire cable to yield a plastic-coated electrical wire. After the mold cools, the plastic molding is removed. The rough edges are trimmed, and the product is ready for use. Such thermoplastic products are inert unless reactive cross-linking agents (e.g., dicumyl peroxide in electrical cables) are added to give rigidity in special applications. Beads of pigment are mixed with the colorless plastic beads to impart color to the finished product.

Phenolic plastics, like urea formaldehyde resin and phenol formaldehyde, are commonly used laminates. In this case, the plastic is applied to two surfaces that are pressed together to cause occlusion (e.g., arborite applied to plywood). Multiple layers may be joined at one time in a press to give a multilayered laminate like plywood. Phenol formaldehyde resin is used in waterproof plywood and particle board, as it is not affected by water. Plywood for indoor use is made with urea formaldehyde resin, as water exposure will lead to resin decomposition, making it unsuitable for outside use.

A liquid plastic, such as polymethylmethacrylate and methylmethacrylate monomer may be cast to make a product like a denture or an eyeglass frame. The liquid is poured into a casting mold with a catalyst such as benzoyl peroxide (Fig. 20–9). Skin contact is common, and sensitization to methylmethacrylate is not an infrequent occurrence in workers such as dental mechanics. Related acrylates are also used in dental work to coat teeth for esthetic reasons or to prevent caries. In these instances, ultraviolet light is used to provide the energy necessary for curing (Fig. 20–10).

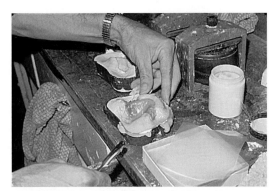

FIGURE 20–9 ● Dental plate manufacturing is often performed in small establishments where there can be considerable contact with the plastic materials, usually acrylates, catalysts, and solvents.

Orthodontists use acrylics to fix braces to teeth, as do orthopedic surgeons in the placement of artificial joints. Such health care workers are at risk of sensitization, as appropriate personal protective equipment is not feasible in these applications. Heat may be applied to facilitate polymerization of the plastic to its final thermoset form.

In the last 20 years, radiation curing of plastics has become a common method of inducing cross-linkage between reactive acrylic monomers and oligomers (e.g., epoxy acrylate, urethane acrylate) to produce thermoset resins. This procedure has been used with acrylic materials extensively. With this method one can dry or cure a coating on metal, cardboard, paper, plastic, or other surface almost instantaneously by imparting energy to the coating in the form of intense ultraviolet light or a beam of electrons.

Epoxy chemistry is very widely used in adhesive coating and electrical insulation work. It involves the mixture of an epoxy resin and a curing agent such as a primary amine, polyamine, or

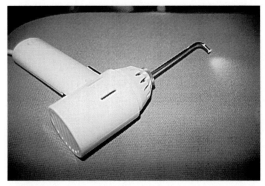

FIGURE 20–10 ● This handheld ultraviolet light is a source of light for curing the polyfunctional acrylates used in dentistry.

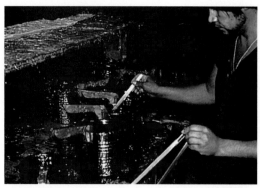

FIGURE 20–11 • Polyester resins are widely employed for manufacture of auto and truck accessories, such as pickup tops, as shown here. The worker is stirring a mixture of resin and catalyst in a very disordered, messy working environment.

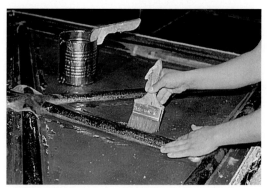

FIGURE 20–13 • Hand lay-up is a common operation in the plastics industry. Here the worker is applying a resin mixture over a fabric in successive layers. The potential for skin contact is great.

anhydride. These substances are often mixed by hand by adding the curing agent to the resin as a liquid (Fig. 20–11). In small operations (e.g., laying an epoxy floor, gluing a cabinet together), the risk of skin contact is substantial (Fig. 20–12). When larger quantities are being used, mixing devices that minimize skin contact can be practically used to minimize skin exposure. The risk of skin contact in large facilities that make the raw

materials is less, but is still present in the transfer of the reactive materials to packaging containers.

Fiberglass enclosures are made using cloth woven of fiberglass over cloth that is applied by hand to a mold, following which a polyester resin solubilized in styrene, usually activated by methyl ethyl ketone peroxide, is applied. Successive layers are placed over each other in this "hand lay-up operation" until the desired thickness is reached (Fig. 20–13).

Significant skin exposure to the resin, catalyst, and styrene may occur. Styrene inhalation may occur. The resin may sensitize the worker. Styrene and the catalyst are potent irritants. Fiberglass fibers may induce physical injury to the skin, which in dermatographic individuals may cause an intolerable disability.

RUBBER COMPOUNDING

There are many similarities between the manufacture of rubber and that of plastics. The latex is either natural or synthetic. The polymer is cross-linked by the addition of a sulfur-containing accelerator, such as a thiuram, a carbamate, a mercapto compound, or other like material. The latex is mixed in a special batch mixer called a Banbury mixer (Fig. 20–14). Additives such as carbon black and antioxidants are placed in the mixer with slabs of latex. The mixture is then transferred to either an extruding machine to be processed through a die for a given shape (e.g., a wiper blade, a car molding) or is applied to a woven material using a calendaring process (Fig. 20–15). The latter involves the apposition of one side of a sheet of material to a bath containing a coating to be applied to a stock (e.g., paper, cloth). The stock comes in contact with the bath and is coated; then it is fed into a web or roller to produce a roll of

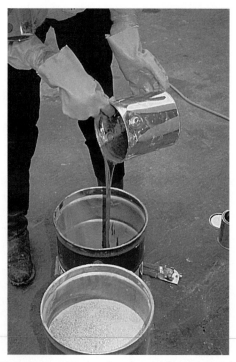

FIGURE 20–12 • Epoxy resins when cured are extremely hard and resistant to many kinds of stresses. They are shown here mixed with grout for laying a floor.

FIGURE 20–14 • Rubber stock is dumped into the mouth of the mixing machine, called the Banbury, a batch-type internal mixing machine. A plunger at the entrance opening rides on top of the batch to furnish pressure to achieve proper mixing. Various additives such as accelerators and antioxidants are added. The Banbury is also used for plastic molding powders. Following thorough mixing, the load is discharged through a gate located below the mixing chamber onto a hamper on the floor below.

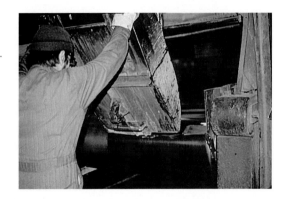

coated material (e.g., adhesive tape, coated table-cloth, rolls of mastic material). A form may be dipped into the latex to produce a coating on it that can subsequently be separated to produce the finished product (e.g., rubber gloves, condoms). Manufacturing the latex involves grinding to disperse components in the matrix, as in paint and ink manufacturing; a two-roller mill is used to accomplish this.

Once the rubber is the desired shape, it is cured and cross-linked by heating it with steam or electrically generated thermal energy or by immersing it in a salt bath, usually of potassium or sodium nitrate or nitrite, at 150° to 250°C.

The mixing operation involves exposure to raw materials that may induce allergic contact dermatitis. Both the reactive stock (i.e., with accelerators added), which is called *green rubber,* and the vulcanized rubber may induce or elicit allergic contact dermatitis. Green rubber poses the greater risk.

MINING

Mining involves removing ore from seams in the rock below the earth's surface. This may be done by creating an open pit and quarrying the ore from the pit. More commonly, a shaft is drilled to a level below the surface, and the ore is removed from the seams below ground in an area called a *stope.* In either instance, holes are drilled into the rock face using a diamond drill. For small operations, a jackleg drill is used, and the operator is exposed to hand and arm vibration as well as to noise. In larger operations, instruments called *jumbo drills,* which have several diamond drills attached to them, are used. There is no direct hand–arm vibration involved, but noise exposure is considerable. The use of wet drilling methods has reduced dust exposure in such operations, but in the past the risk of silica exposure could be considerable, depending on the quartz content of the rock. Workers carrying out such work are

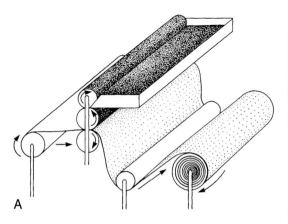
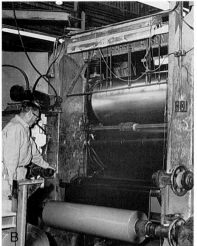

FIGURE 20–15 • *A, B,* Calendering. Note how the coating material is applied to one surface of the stock using an interposed roller system.

at risk for vibration-induced white finger disease (occupational Raynaud's disease).

METAL FABRICATION

Metal products are made from molten metal that is poured into ingots of different sizes or into casting molds (Fig. 20–16).[14] They are then converted into shapes called *slabs, blooms,* or *billets* (Fig. 20–17).[5] Slabs, either hot or cold, are first rolled to form plates in a rolling mill. The metal is rolled into plates and may be modified at high temperatures, and the crystals in the metal structure become fluid and are changed into a new shape. This may involve smashing or pressing the metal into a shape, which is called *forging*. As with plastics, the hot metal can be extruded to form objects like tubing. Tubing may be drawn through dies to modify its diameter. In all these processes, cutting oils, consisting principally of mineral oil, are sprayed onto the metal surfaces to reduce damage to the tools and facilitate the shaping of the metal. The resulting sheets of metal may be used in a cold state. In this instance, they are bent, squeezed (as in swaging), drawn, or extruded. Once in the cold state, the metal is worked, and its crystalline structure does not change. Lubricants are essential to these operations also. As in hot metal-working situations, dies may be used to provide the shape.

Metal may also be machined to produce given shapes for particular uses. In such operation (lathing, milling, drilling), mineral oil–based cutting fluids and soluble oils are used. Synthetic oils are occasionally used in grinding operations. These products have myriad trade names. The soluble oils are primarily water with a small amount of mineral oil plus an emulsifier and other additives (e.g., rust inhibitors, high-pressure additives). The synthetic materials are low in mineral oil and contain surfactants, synthetic oils, corrosion inhibitors, and biocides; when diluted, they are primarily water. Table 20–6 summarizes the usual compositions of these lubricants, and Table 20–7 lists the common additives in them.[15, 16]

The machining of metal consists of many operations. Cutting metal to a defined shape using a press is a basic process. Once a cutout or blank is produced, it may be modified by notching, perforating, slitting, and so on. The edges are usually smoothed after cutting. Metal may be sawed, drilled, or ground to yield the final metal article.

Solid metal pieces are milled, lathed, and

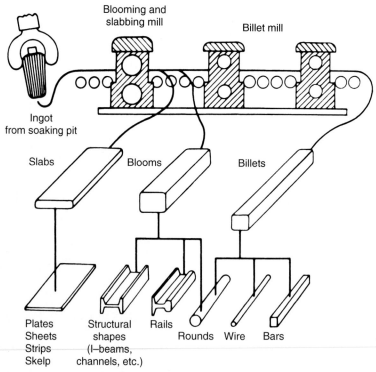

FIGURE 20–16 ● Process for the production of slabs, blooms, and billets. (From Burgess WA: Recognition of Health Hazards in Industry. New York: John Wiley & Sons; 1981.)

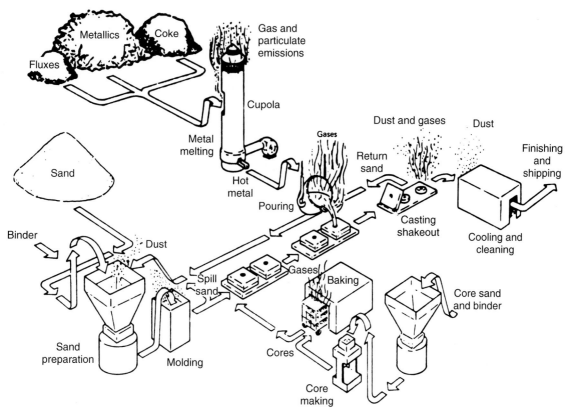

FIGURE 20–17 • Process drawing for a foundry illustrating the production of molten metal, the production of green sand molds, and the conversion to finished castings. (From U.S. Environmental Protection Agency, Research Triangle Park, NC, 1971.)

planed using machines in which a cutting tool removes part of the metal while either the metal or the tool moves. The surfaces are then smoothed by processes such as honing, lapping, and finishing. These latter techniques involve altering the surface by using either a rotating metal tool or an abrasive in a closed container, moving the parts around in contact with it to remove rough edges.

The finished pieces may then be welded or coated with a metal by electroplating. Prior to either of these steps, the surface has to be cleaned. Cutting or soluble oil can be removed with solvents, often by immersing the object in a solvent bath, which is called *degreasing* (Fig. 20–18).[10] It may be necessary to sandblast a surface with silica to remove debris to allow welding, plating, or the application of a coating.

Electroplating involves placing the object in a bath of electrolyte solution, often cyanide, as a cathode.[5] A metal, such as nickel (Fig. 20–19), chrome, or gold, is then activated as the anode. The anode metal is deposited on the metal object,

which is the cathode. This is how bumpers are chrome plated and how jewelry is plated. It is also the process used to recover copper in copper refining. In addition, it is used in reverse in jewelry work in which a fashioned metal object, for instance, has its surface removed, acting as the anode to provide a smooth-finished surface. There is a risk of exposure to metal salts by direct contact with the metal or plating solution and through airborne contact with the mist generated in such operations. Chemical burns from the bath solution are also a risk.

Clean surfaces may be welded either with oxy-acetylene or arc welding methods. There is a potential for airborne metal fume exposure and rosin contact in these operations, as the rods may contain both, depending in the application. Flux used in welding contains diverse chemicals (Table 20–8),[17] which may result in skin disease. Corneal injury due to flash burns through inadvertent direct exposure to the ultraviolet light generated is a significant risk in this occupation, as is ultraviolet-induced skin erythema or thermal burns, de-

TABLE 20–6 • Composition of Cutting Fluids

Mineral Oil
  Base: paraffinic or naphthenic oils (60–100%)
  Polar additives
    Animal and vegetable oils, fats, waxes
    Synthetic boundary lubricants such as esters, fatty oils, fatty acids, polyols, and complex alcohols
  Extreme Pressure Lubricants
    Sulfur free or combined as sulfurized mineral oil or fat
    Chlorine—in the form of a chlorinated wax or ester
    Combination—sulfochlorinated mineral or fatty oil
    Phosphorus—as organic or metallic phosphate
  Germicides

Soluble Oil
  Base
    Mineral oil (50–90%)
    Diluted with water in a ratio of 1:5 to 1:50
  Emulsifiers
    Petroleum sulfonates, amine and rosin soaps, naphthenic acids
  Polar additives—sperm or lard oil and esters
  Extreme pressure lubricants
  Corrosion inhibitors
  Germicides
  Dyes

Synthetics
  Base
    50–80% water
    Diluted with water in a ratio of 1:10 to 1:200
    True synthetics contain no oil, but semisynthetics may have up to 25% mineral oil in the concentrate
  Corrosion inhibitors
    Inorganic—borates, nitrates, nitrites, phosphates
    Organic—amines, nitrites
  Surfactants
  Lubricants
  Dyes
  Germicides

From O'Brien D, Frede JC. *Guidelines for the Control of Exposure to Metalworking Fluids.* Publ. No. (NIOSH) 78–165. Cincinnati: Department of Health, Education, and Welfare; 1978.

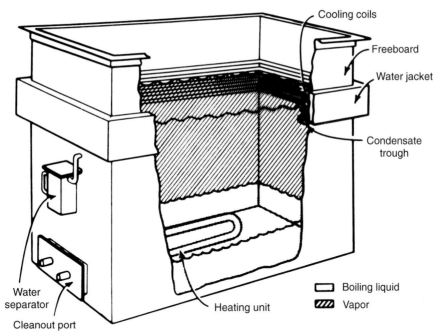

FIGURE 20–18 • Typical construction of a solvent degreasing tank. (From Murphy J: Surface Preparations and Finishes for Metals. New York: McGraw-Hill; 1971.)

pending on the emission spectrum of the welding device (Fig. 20–20).[18]

WOODWORKING

The conversion of trees to lumber involves cutting the trunks to defined lengths and then cutting the trunks lengthwise to produce finished planks. There is exposure to turpentine generated in the cutting. Direct and airborne contact with the oleoresin of the wood, and sesquiterpene lactones from

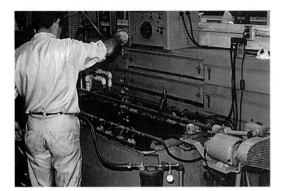

FIGURE 20–19 • In nickel plating there is considerable opportunity for skin contact with the solution of nickel salts, although nickel allergy in these workers is not widely reported.

liverwort on the bark during debarking operations, may be a risk.

The manufacture of wood articles involves exposure to urea formaldehyde and phenol formaldehyde resins in plywood and particle board, as well

 TABLE 20–7 • Additives Common to Lubricants, Coolants, and Cutting Fluids

Extreme pressure additives
    Tricresyl phosphate
    Zinc dithiophosphate
    Chlorinated paraffins
    Chlorinated diphenyls
Antioxidant and anticorrosion inhibitors
    Zinc alkyl
    Aryl dithiophosphate
    Methyl ditertiary butyl phenol
    p-Phenylenediamine
    Chrome and sodium nitrite
Detergents and dispersants
    Methylalkyl sulfonates
    Alkyl phenolates
Bacteriocides
    Phenolic agents
    Quaternary ammonium compounds
    Isothiazolin derivatives

Modified from Boothroyd G. *Fundamentals of Metal Machining and Machine Tools.* Washington, DC: Scripta/McGraw-Hill; 1975.

TABLE 20–8 • Common Flux Materials

Inorganic	Halogens
Acids	Aniline hydrochloric
Hydrochloric	Glutamic acid hydrochloric
Hydrofluoric	Bromine derivatives of
Orthophosphoric	Palmitic acid
Salts	Hydrazine hydrochloric
Zinc chloride	Hydrazine hydrobromide
Ammonium chloride	Amines and amides
Tin chloride	Urea
Gases	Ethylenediamine
Hydrogen-forming gas	Monoethanolamine
Dry hydrochloride	Triethanolamine
Organic—Not Rosin-based	**Rosin-based Organics**
Acids	Rosin with or without activators for specific uses
Lactic	
Oleic	
Stearic	
Glutamic	
Phthalic	

From Manko HH. *Solders and Soldering.* New York: McGraw-Hill; 1979.

as the formaldehyde that is released. Rare woods (e.g., teak, mahogany, ebony) may cause allergic contact dermatitis. Adhesives such as epoxy resins are commonly used and may also constitute a cutaneous hazard.

CONCLUSION

In this brief discussion, we have endeavoured to cover a number of industrial processes that are associated with occupational skin disease. Many

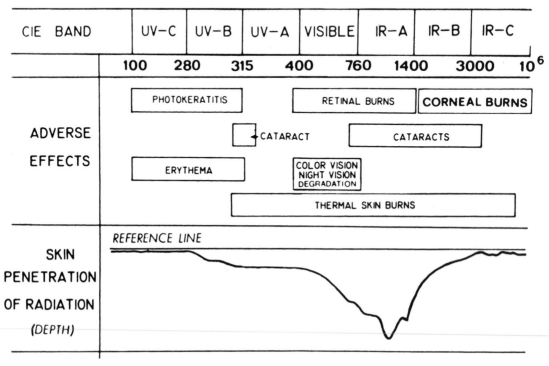

FIGURE 20–20 • The biological effects of various components of the light spectrum emitted in welding operations. (From Sliney D, Wolbarsht M: Safety with Lasers and Other Optical Sources. New York: Plenum Publishing; 1980.)

other processes are important. In the final analysis, the best way to gain an understanding of the work a given worker performs is to visit his or her workplace. The time taken is rewarded not only by a gratified patient but often also by the possibility of preventive intervention and a greater enlightenment as to the nature of industrial processes.

References

1. Rifkin J. *The End of Work.* New York: G.P. Putnam's Sons; 1995.
2. Workers' Compensation Board. *Statistical Supplement to the 1995 Annual Report.* Toronto: Ontario Workers' Compensation Board; 1996.
3. The Prevention of Occupational Skin Disorders: A Proposed National Strategy for the Prevention of Dermatological Conditions. Part 1. *Am J Contact Dermatitis* 1990; 1:56–64.
4. The Prevention of Occupational Skin Disorders: A Proposed National Strategy for the Prevention of Dermatological Conditions. Part 2. *Am J Contact Dermatitis* 1990; 1:116–125.
5. Burgess W. *Recognition of Health Hazards in Industry: A Review of Materials and Processes.* New York: John Wiley & Sons; 1981.
6. Cralley LV, Cralley LJ. *Industrial Aspects of Plant Operations, vol I, Process Flows.* New York: Macmillan Book Co.; 1982.
7. Cralley LV, Cralley LJ. *Industrial Aspects of Plant Operations, vol II, Unit Operations and Product Fabrication.* New York: Macmillan Book Co.; 1984.
8. Clayton GD, Clayton FE. *Patty's Industrial Hygiene and Toxicology, vol III, Theory and Rationale of Industrial Hygiene Practice.* New York: John Wiley & Sons; 1982.
9. American Conference of Governmental Industrial Hygienists (ACGIH). *Process Flow Diagrams and Air Pollution Emission Estimates.* Cincinnati: ACGIH; 1973.
10. Murphy J. *Surface Preparations and Finishes for Metals.* New York: McGraw-Hill; 1971.
11. Triebe EJ. Printing. In: *The World Book Encyclopedia.* Chicago: Field Enterprises Educational Corporation; 1973:700–708b.
12. Nethercott JR. Dermatitis in the printing industry. *Dermatol Clin* 1988; 6:61–66.
13. Nethercott JR. Skin problems associated with multifunctional acrylic monomers in ultraviolet curing inks. *Br J Dermatol* 1978; 98:541–555.
14. U.S. Environmental Protection Agency. *Systems Analysis of Emission and Emission Control in the Iron Foundry Industry, vol 2. Exhibits.* Research Triangle Park, NC: Environmental Protection Agency; 1971.
15. O'Brien D, Frede JC. *Guidelines for the Control of Exposure to Metalworking Fluids.* Publ. No. (NIOSH) 78–165. Cincinnati: Department of Health, Education, and Welfare; 1978.
16. Boothroyd G. *Fundamentals of Metal Machining and Machine Tools.* Washington, DC: Scripta/McGraw-Hill; 1975.
17. Manko HH. *Solders and Soldering.* New York: McGraw-Hill; 1979.
18. Sliney D, Wolbarsht M. *Safety with Lasers and Other Optical Sources.* New York: Plenum Publishing Co.; 1980.

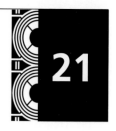

21

Soaps and Detergents

C.G. TOBY MATHIAS, M.D.

HISTORY

The earliest historic evidence of soap manufacturing was discovered during the excavation of ancient Babylon, where inscriptions on clay cylinders (dated approximately 2800 B.C.E.) described the boiling of animal fats with ashes but did not state how the resulting product was actually used. The Ebers Papyrus, a medical document dated about 1500 B.C.E., indicates that the ancient Egyptians combined animal and vegetable oils with alkaline salts to form a soap-like material and used it for bathing and to treat various skin diseases. The Phoenicians manufactured soap from goat tallow. The ancient Germans and Gauls made soap from animal fat and plant ashes and called this product *saipo*.

In Roman times, soap was manufactured from mutton tallow and wood ashes. According to Roman legend, soap got its name from Mount Sapo, a place where animals were ritualistically sacrificed. Rain washed a mixture of melted animal fat and wood ashes down from the mountain into the Tiber River, where women found that it made washing clothes easier and got them cleaner. As Roman civilization advanced, the popularity of bathing increased. The first Roman bath was built about 312 B.C.E. These baths were very luxurious and contributed further to an enthusiasm for bathing. By the second century C.E., the Greek physician Galen was recommending the use of soap for cleansing and medicinal purposes.

In the eighth century C.E., small soap factories appeared in Italy and Spain. The original Castile soap, made from olive oil, wood ashes, and perfume, was a product of this period. About the year 1200, a thriving French soap and perfume industry began with the opening of a soap plant in Marseilles.

When community bathing was common practice during the Middle Ages, bathhouses were important centers of social and business activities. In the late 13th century, the Church attempted to close these establishments because communal bathing was then considered sinful and unhealthy. By the time the great epidemics of bubonic plague began to sweep over Europe in 1346, most bathhouses had been closed by governmental decree, which undoubtedly contributed to the severity of the epidemics.

Soap was not manufactured on a significant scale in England until after 1622, when King James I granted a monopoly to a soapmaker in return for about $100,000 per year. Soap became a luxury item, affordable only by the wealthy. The Crown suppressed its sale for years by steadily increasing excise and luxury taxes, some of which remained on the statute books until as late as 1853. When the tax was finally repealed, the British treasury lost more than 1 million pounds in revenue annually, but cheaper soap became available to ordinary people and cleanliness standards improved.

Until about 1800, soap-making in the United States was exclusively a household art, but by the mid-19th century, advances in chemistry made its manufacture possible on a large scale. In 1791, the French chemist Nicholas Leblanc developed and patented a process for making soda ash (sodium carbonate) from common salt. This process yielded large quantities of inexpensive, high-quality material that could be readily combined with animal fat to make soap. About 20 years later, another French chemist, Michel-Eugène Chevreul, discovered the chemical relationship of fats, glycerin, and fatty acids, the basis for fat and soap chemistry. Ernest Solvay, a Belgian chemist, discovered how to make even cheaper soda ash by treating table salt with an ammonia process. These technologies could be easily used in America's new factories, and by 1850 soapmaking was one of its fasting growing industries. The advent of World War I and World War II spurred the development of synthetic chemical detergents. Today, 50 to 60% of soaps and detergents manufactured in the United States are used in industrial and institutional cleaning products, 25 to 30% are used in household cleaners, and the remainder are used in skin-care products or shampoos and toilet soaps.

COMPOSITION OF SOAPS AND DETERGENTS

Soaps and detergents are composed of numerous additives that contribute to the cleaning process.[42a, 133] All contain surface-active agents (surfactants), which facilitate surface wetting and soil removal. Additional ingredients—such as builders, corrosion inhibitors, antiredeposition agents, superfatted materials, optical whiteners, suds-controlling agents, special enzymes, abrasives, germicidal agents, solvents, perfumes, dyes, and pigments—may be present to serve the special purposes for which the specific detergent product was designed.

Surfactants

Surfactants in true soaps are carboxylates, that is, salts of fatty acids formed by the interaction of naturally occurring fatty oils and alkali. The most common starting material is tallow oil, obtained from cattle, horses, or sheep.[60] This oil is blended with other fatty oils, such as coconut, olive, palm, or palm-kernel oils. Some common toilet or laundry soaps may be 80% tallow and 20% coconut oil. The fatty acids contained in these oils are chiefly lauric, oleic, palmitic, stearic, and myristic, containing from 12 to 20 carbon atoms. All except oleic acid are saturated fatty acids. Other oils sometimes include rosin, fish, whale, corn, soya, castor bean, cottonseed, sunflower, peanut, and sesame oils. Rosin and tall oil, from the cellulose and paper industries, are important in soap manufacture. Rosin is found in yellow laundry soap, less expensive toilet soaps, and certain specialty soaps in concentrations up to 25%.[18] Saddle soap, used for cleaning leather, may also contain rosin. Tall oil from wood pulp is used in some liquid soaps, for example, Murphy's oil soap.

Although the first synthetic surfactant, sulfonated castor oil (also known as turkey red oil and still used in textile and leather manufacture), was introduced in 1851 as a cleanser and carrier in the rug-dyeing industry, the first serious attempts to develop soap substitutes were made in Germany during World War I. The earliest were alkyl sulfates and sulfonated fatty acid esters, which were derived from natural fats and were employed almost entirely in cleaning and dyeing textiles. Since the mid-1930s, the surfactants in synthetic detergents have been manufactured from petroleum rather than from natural fats and have replaced conventional soaps to the extent that in 1967 more than 55% of the world production of soap products belonged to this class.[42a] Synthetic surfactants derived exclusively from petroleum include olefin sulfonate, alkyl-ether sulfates, alkyl-benzene sulfonates, ethoxylates, and propoxylates.

Synthetic surfactants (synthetic detergents, syndets) differ from carboxylates in several important ways: (1) they do not form lime soaps in hard water, (2) they have a neutral pH in solution, and (3) they may produce suds at various pH levels. Although their surface-active properties are similar, the chemical properties of synthetic surfactants make them far more versatile than the carboxylates in ordinary soap. For example, a chemist can juggle and balance the spatial position of polar groups or change the head group to obtain soaps with varying properties.[60] Depending solely upon the position of the hydrophilic moiety on the chain, detergents can be made that are soluble in inorganic solvents or that have excellent wetting ability but low detergent action. Others have low wetting ability but a superior detergent action. This adaptability gives such products much wider application than ordinary soap. Most liquid soaps for personal use are made from synthetic detergents.

Alkalies

Great quantities of sodium hydroxide are used as alkalies by the soap industry each year in the manufacture of hard soaps. Potassium hydroxide, as stated previously, is used for soft and liquid soaps. Combinations of these alkalies are often used to obtain the desirable features of both. Shampoos use ammonium hydroxide and mono-, di-, and triethanolamine. There is little free alkali in most soaps intended for skin cleansing. More than 0.1% of free sodium hydroxide alkali is considered excessive by most authorities.[124] The pH of most toilet bar soaps in solution ranges from 9 to about 11.

Builders

Builders are alkaline materials that are added to certain soaps to increase their cleaning action. They are not used to cheapen the product, as is commonly believed. The most important builders are sodium carbonate, trisodium phosphate, pyrophosphates, sodium silicate, and ethylenediaminetetraacetate (EDTA). They act as sequestering agents, combining with unwanted metallic ions, such as calcium and magnesium, to soften the water, thus preventing scum formation while holding dirt and grease in solution. They cannot be employed in soaps designed for cleaning fine fabrics, such as woolens, silks, and synthetic fibers, and are therefore used mostly in heavy-duty laundry soaps. Builders contribute significantly to the alkalinity of the product during use. Phosphates have fallen somewhat in popularity, as they nourish plant growth and have contributed to pollution of our waterways. Builders are used most frequently in laundry detergents.

Perfumes

Toilet soaps contain 0.2 to 2.0% perfume.[122] Common perfumes found in soap are the natural oils of anise seed, bitter almond, carnation, citronella, eucalyptus, geranium, lavender, peppermint, rosemary, sweet orange, and thyme,[124] as well as numerous artificial fragrances.

The perfume itself may contain up to 100 ingredients, substances derived not only from plants but also from animal sources, such as musk from the preputial follicles of the musk deer and ambergris from the intestinal tract of the sperm whale. Both are used as perfume fixatives; that is, they retard evaporation of the perfume and equalize the evaporation of the solvent. Perfumes are used not only to enhance the cosmetic appeal of soaps but also to mask any offensive base odor.

Dyes and Pigments

Dyes and pigments for soaps include eosin, rhodamine, fuchsin, cinnabar, ultramarine green, chlorophyll, ultramarine blue, orange II, caramel, ochre,[124] chromium oxide, and others. Even though D & C Yellow No. 11, a quinoline dye used for toilet soaps and shampoos, is a potent experimental contact allergen, allergic reactions to the use of commercial soaps and detergents containing this color are exceedingly rare.

Superfat

When more fat than necessary is added during manufacture, an excess known as superfat results. Fatty materials commonly used are lanolin, cold cream, and mineral oil. Superfat makes the product somewhat less alkaline than ordinary soap and less irritating to the skin.

Germicidal Agents

Until about 1950, common disinfectants incorporated into soaps included phenol, thymol, cresol, mercuric iodide, and organic mercurials. Subsequently, agents such as hexachlorophene (G-11), bithionol, and halogenated salicylanilides were employed. Although uncommon, photodermatitis has been reported from use of soaps containing these substances (see further on). Bithionol was removed from commercial products in the United States in 1967, and the halogenated salicylanilide tribromosalan (TBS) was prohibited for use in cosmetics by the Food and Drug Administration (FDA), effective October 31, 1975. The use of hexachlorophene also has been considerably restricted and is banned from use in over-the-counter soaps. The chief germicidal agents used today in cosmetic soaps are triclocarban (TCC) and triclosan. The former has occasionally showed cross-reaction with the halogenated salicylanilides in patch-testing but probably does not initiate allergic photosensitization itself. Special disinfectant soaps marketed for food handlers and hospital personnel contain chlorhexidine, povidone iodine, or other similar germicidal agents. Detergents for disinfecting hard surfaces may contain a variety of phenolic compounds and quaternary ammonium compounds, such as benzalkonium chloride, formalin, or ammonia. Germicidal agents employed as preservatives in liquid or cream soaps are similar to those used in cosmetics.

Additional Ingredients of Soaps and Detergents

Corrosion Inhibitors. A protective film is formed around metal parts and surfaces by corrosion inhibitors, which protect those parts from the corrosive effects of detergents and washing solutions. They are usually added to laundry detergents. Sodium silicate is the most common.

Antiredeposition Agents. Soil and grime removed by washing is prevented from settling back onto the cleaned surface by antiredeposition agents. Carboxymethylcellulose is most commonly employed for this purpose.

Optical Whiteners. Optical whiteners (brighteners) are compounds that absorb invisible ultraviolet light and convert it into visible light, enhancing brightness. They are usually found in laundry detergents for both domestic and industrial use. Most are derivatives of stilbene or coumarin.

Suds-controlling Agents. Suds-controlling agents are added to increase or decrease the sudsing action of the detergent as needed. Suds enhancers (foaming agents) include the mono- and diethanolamides of C10 to C16 fatty acids. Suds depressants (antifoamers) may include nonionic detergents such as ethoxylated fatty alcohols and long-chain C16 to C22 fatty acids.

Enzymes. Enzymes may be added to detergents to assist in removing difficult stains. Proteases derived from bacterial strains of *Bacillus subtilis* or *Bacillus licheniformis* break down protein-aceous stains, whereas amylases break down carbohydrate material.

Abrasives. Substances may be added to some products to produce mechanical friction and agitation to assist in the removal of difficult dirt and grease stains. Commonly used abrasives are inorganic minerals (borax, sand, pumice) or hard plant substances (sawdust or other ground vegetable matter). They may be found in scouring powders, particularly those used for cleaning cookware, and are popular additives in soaps used by mechanics. The abrasive action may be assisted by applying the detergent with brushes, steel wool, scouring pads, or other devices.

Solvents. Solvents may be combined with detergents for specialized cleaning operations, such as dry cleaning. Petroleum distillates are added to waterless hand cleansers marketed for mechanics. Although they are technically not soaps or detergents, a variety of industrial solvents (acetone, alcohol, petroleum distillate) are often used alone for cleaning hard surfaces soiled with oily substances.

MANUFACTURING PROCESS

The manufacture of synthetic detergents is a relatively simple process, basically involving only the combination of raw materials. The manufacture of true soap (carboxylates), on the other hand, is a more complex process.

Boiling Process

In the boiling method of making soap, the entire manufacturing process takes place in a huge kettle, which may contain from 100,000 to 100 million pounds per charge, making it one of the largest single pieces of equipment used in the chemical industry. First, a solution of sodium hydroxide (caustic soda) is pumped into the kettle, followed by melted fats. The mixture is boiled by direct heat from steam entering through a perforated coil at the bottom of the kettle; agitation is also supplied by the jets of steam. Gradually saponification (i.e., the formation of fatty acid salts) occurs, requiring several days for completion.

The contents of the kettle separate into layers:

an upper layer of melted, impure soap; a middle layer known as niger, consisting of soap (approximately 30%), water, and various impurities; and a bottom layer consisting of glycerin and a small amount of alkali. Adding more alkali and boiling longer cause any traces of unsaponified fat to react. Glycerin is drawn off the bottom of the kettle and treated for recovery; the soap is then passed through a brine solution to remove any traces of unreacted alkali. Further boiling in water causes the soap to separate into a viscous upper layer known as neat soap, containing about 50% water, and a lower layer of niger, containing the remaining impurities. The neat soap is then drawn off, bleached with absorbent earth, processed by the incorporation of various additives, and finally packaged into a wide assortment of commercial products.

Continuous Hydrolyzer Process

In the continuous hydrolyzer process of making soap, the fat is placed in a tall, vertical autoclave under high temperature and pressure. It is first split into fatty acids and glycerin in the presence of a catalyst. The fatty acids are continually drawn off and treated with alkali and water to produce neat soap. The entire process can be completed in a few hours, whereas the boiling method demands up to 14 days. Such greater speed of production, improved soap quality, need for less factory space, and better production control have influenced the soap industry in recent years to convert almost universally to this method of soap manufacture.

CLASSIFICATION

Based on the ionizing properties of their principal surfactants, soaps and detergents may be classified into four general categories: (1) anionic detergents, (2) cationic detergents, (3) nonionic detergents, and (4) amphoteric detergents.

Anionic Detergents

Anionic detergents contain surfactants composed of salts of fatty acids, organic sulfonates, or sulfates in which the lipophilic portion of the molecule becomes a negative ion when dissolved in water. Many hundreds of anionic agents have been developed, the most common being dodecylbenzene sulfonate. Other common examples are sodium lauryl sulfate, sodium cetyl sulfate, lauryl ether sulfates, and lignin sulfonate and its derivatives.

Cationic Detergents

Cationic detergents are strong electrolytes. The surface-active portion, which is lipophilic, is positively charged. The anionic agent is generally a chloride or bromide ion. These surfactants are incompatible with anionic detergents because the two oppositely charged ions combine to form an insoluble precipitate. Cationic detergents are expensive and thus account for a relatively small percentage of the total synthetic detergent production of the United States. They are most useful as germicidal agents in surgical soaps, surface disinfectants, washes for bar and restaurant glassware, and fabric softeners. Salts of quaternary ammonium compounds and long-chain amines are the most common cationic agents used today.

Nonionic Detergents

Nonionic detergents do not ionize in aqueous solution; their entire molecule is considered surface-active. They usually have a long, oxygenated side chain, which is hydrophilic. The oil-soluble groups are commonly amides or ether or ester linkages. By suitable adjustment of the molecular structure and proper choice of side chain, the wetting, detergent, and foaming characteristics can be varied considerably. Detergents of this type are not altered by acids or mild alkalies and are compatible with both anionic and cationic types of detergents. As a result, they have numerous industrial uses as stabilizers, antifoam agents, and viscosity reducers. They are excellent dispersing agents for deep-fat frying, for example. Examples are polyoxyethylene derivatives of fatty acids and ethoxylate derivatives of alcohol and glycols.

Amphoteric Detergents

Amphoteric detergents contain both anionic and cationic groups and, depending upon the pH of the solution, have either a negative or a positive charge. They are cationic in acid media and anionic in alkaline media. The nonpolar constituent is a hydrocarbon moiety of variable molecular size and complexity. Amphoteric detergents have both cleaning (anionic) and antibacterial (cationic) properties. They may be used for special purposes in shampoos and cosmetics and in electroplating.

MECHANISM OF ACTION

Soaps and detergents are designed to remove soil and stains from a variety of surfaces in a four-step process. First, the surface to be cleaned must be wetted. Soaps and detergents are traditionally dispersed in water to accomplish this objective. Detergents and other added surfactants decrease the surface tension of water, thereby facilitating the spread and penetration of the soap into uneven or recessed portions of the soiled surface. Second, a layer of soap or detergent must be absorbed at the interface of the cleaning solution and the surface to be cleaned. All soaps and detergents dispersed in water have chemical structures that impart properties of water solubility (hydrophilia) at one end of the molecule and lipid solubility (hydrophobia) at the other end. The hydrophobic portion of the molecule attaches itself at the interface onto the soil to be removed, whereas the hydrophilic end remains solubilized in the water portion of the detergent solution. Third, the soil must be removed and dispersed into the detergent solution. This is facilitated by agitation, elevated temperature of the washing solution, and foaming agents. Special chemical additives, such as enzymes or sodium hydroxide, may be required to break down and remove certain types of soil or stain, such as proteinaceous or burned organic material. Fourth, the soil or dirt must be prevented from becoming deposited on the cleaned surface again once it has been removed. Emulsifiers and antiredeposition agents may be added to the soap to accomplish this.

The physical properties of soaps and detergents enable them not only to solubilize and remove soil from contaminated surfaces but also to change the pH of the skin surface from acidic to alkaline and to remove important lipids and proteins from the outermost protective layer of skin, the stratum corneum. Occupational exposure to these products may cause contact dermatitis through excessive delipidization and destruction of cutaneous tissue cell walls, with subsequent release of lysosomal enzymes and pursuant inflammation.

USES

Personal Cleaning

Products for personal cleaning include bar soap, gels, liquid soaps, shampoos, and heavy-duty hand cleaners. Bar soaps and gels are formulated for cleaning the hands, face, and body. Fat-based bar soaps still command the major part of the bar soap market, but a few of the newer syndet-based bar soaps such as Dove and Oil of Olay, which contain less than 15% true soap and have a neutral pH, enjoy some popularity. Some bar soaps are formulated to moisturize as well as clean; these are superfatted soaps. Others may contain additives to inhibit odor-causing bacteria (deodorant soaps). Specialty bars include transparent glycerin-based products, soaps based on oatmeal fat, and medicated soaps. Liquid soaps and shampoos are synthetic-based; all contain an antimicrobial preservative to prolong shelf-life, and some contain stronger germicidal agents for killing disease-causing bacteria on the skin surface. Heavy-duty hand cleaners are available as bars, liquids, powders, and creams. Products formulated for removing stubborn grease may contain an abrasive (e.g., pumice soap) or a petroleum-based solvent (e.g., waterless hand cleaner).

Laundry Detergents

Laundry detergents are formulated to remove soil and stains from fabric under varying water, temperature, and use conditions. They are most often formulated as liquids or powders but may also be manufactured as gels, sticks, sprays, sheets, or bars. General-purpose detergents are suitable for all washable fabrics, whereas light-duty detergents are used for washing lightly soiled or delicate fabrics.

Laundry aids, which provide special functions beyond simple cleaning, are often added to laundry detergents, but may also be formulated and used separately. Bleaches whiten and brighten fabrics by converting soils into colorless soluble particles which can then be removed by detergents. Oxygen bleach is gentler on fabric than chlorine (sodium hypochlorite) bleach and does not fade fabric. Bluing agents contain a blue dye or pigment which absorbs the yellow portion of the light spectrum and counteracts the natural yellowing of many fabrics. Boosters enhance soil and stain removal. Enzymes may be used to accelerate and facilitate removal of difficult proteinaceous soil and stains. Fabric softener may be added to the final rinse or placed in the dryer to decrease static cling and wrinkling and to make ironing easier. Starches and fabric finishes may also be added to the final rinse or applied after drying to give body to fabrics and to make them more soil- and stain-resistant. Water softeners inactivate hard minerals; because detergents are more effective in soft water, they increase cleaning power.

Dishwashing Products

Dishwashing products are formulated for either hand or machine washing. They are available in liquids, powders, and gels. Hand dishwashing products provide longer lasting suds which indicate how much cleaning power is left in the wash water. Automatic dishwasher detergents produce almost no suds, which could interfere with the washing action of the machine and suppress foam from proteinaceous food soil. Rinse agents lower the surface tension of water and improve draining from dishes and utensils. Film removers remove hard water film and cloudiness from dishes and minimize spotting.

Household Cleaners

Household cleaning products are available in a wide range of formulations and are used extensively, both at home and in the workplace. No single product can provide optimum cleaning for all surfaces and for all types of soiling. Although all-purpose cleaners are available for general use, many others work best only for specialized uses. Abrasive cleaners contain small mineral or metallic particles that facilitate the removal of heavy soil accumulation. Numerous specialty cleaners perform a variety of functions; there are glass cleaners, tub and sink cleaners (which often contain chlorine bleach), metal cleaners and polishers, oven cleaners (which usually contain sodium hydroxide), rug and upholstery cleaners, toilet bowl cleaners and drain openers (which may contain acids, alkalies, enzymes, or bacteria).

Oil Drilling

Detergents are employed in the process of drilling for oil to inhibit the formation of waxes on pipes, and the use of foaming agents greatly increases the petroleum recovery from wells. Surfactants prevent the sludging of drilling muds.

Textile Manufacturing

The textile industry consumes a large part of the output of soaps and detergents used in scouring, removing sizing, and wetting fabrics. They help penetrate dyes and act as leveling agents. Non-ionic detergents function as spreading agents and carriers in resin-treating textiles for mildew resistance, water repellence, and so on.

Food Industry

The food industry uses large quantities of soap to keep workers and clothing clean and to wash equipment and areas in which food is stored and prepared. Many specialty cleaning compounds are available today that are specially tailored with selected surfactants, builders, and germicidal agents to provide required properties. Detergents are used to remove surface dirt and insecticides from fruits, vegetables, eggs, and other foods.

Nonionic surfactants are valuable dispersing agents in food processing for shortening, salad dressing, bakery goods, and prepared food mixes.

Additional Uses of Soaps and Detergents

Dry Cleaning. In combination with organic solvents, detergents are important in many dry cleaning operations.

Sewage Treatment. Detergents, especially cationic ones, are employed as both surfactants and germicidal agents in sewage treatment.

Paper Manufacture. Synthetic detergents are used in the manufacture of paper to emulsify oil-water products, to make paper sizing, finishes, and coatings, to remove resins from pulp, and wash the huge woolen belts of paper machines.

Metal Cleaning. Prior to plating, painting, or enameling, metal surfaces must be completely free of dirt and grease. Large amounts of nonionic surfactants are employed for this purpose.

Ore Flotation. Detergents are used to modify the surface of minerals and to prevent frothing and corrosion.

Agricultural Uses. Detergents are used to clean livestock and work areas and to disperse the chemical agents in pesticide sprays. They are also used to prevent fertilizer from caking.

Synthetic Manufacturing. Sodium tallow soaps and detergents are employed in the manufacture of butadiene rubber to emulsify the ingredients during processing.

Paint Manufacturing. Detergents emulsify synthetic resins in aqueous media for the manufacture of water-based paints.

Lubricants. Detergents are used in hydraulic oils to prevent sludging in engine parts. Most heavy-duty greases are composed of heavy metals and nonionic detergents.

Cutting Oils. In water-soluble types of cutting oils, detergents are used as emulsifiers, and cationic detergents are used as germicidal agents.

Plastics Manufacturing. Polymerization of plastics takes place more rapidly in detergent solutions, and soaps were the first surfactants used to mass-produce vinyl polymers.

Miscellaneous Uses. Detergents are also used in printing inks, in waterproofing solutions for wood and concrete, in degreasing solutions used in the leather industry prior to dyeing, in furniture cleaners and polishes, in wetting solutions used as antifog agents, in fire-fighting foams, as dust preventive agents, and as antistatic agents. The list grows longer and more impressive each year and, in fact, there are few industrial processes in which soaps or detergents are not used in some way.

CONTACT DERMATITIS CAUSED BY SOAPS AND DETERGENTS

Occupational contact dermatitis resulting from soaps and detergents usually arises from skin irritation that occurs in one of the following circumstances: excessive skin washing with products marketed for skin cleaning, inappropriate skin contact with products intended solely for industrial cleaning during the course of their normal use, and the inappropriate use as skin cleansers of products marketed for industrial cleaning. Rarely, a contact or photocontact allergy may occur. Cutaneous depigmentation from phenolic germicides in disinfectant soaps has also been reported.

Workers in the soap and detergent industry may get contact dermatitis from handling strong alkalies and rancid oils, but this is very uncommon today because closed systems are used almost exclusively. In addition, most of the companies that manufacture soaps and detergents are among the most safety-conscious manufacturers in the United States.

In other industries, however, cleaning agents cause a significant amount of contact dermatitis each year. Schwartz[123] ranked the causes of occupational dermatitis among 41,628 workers, and cleaning agents were among the leading ones. Klauder[68] summarized the "actual causes of certain occupational dermatoses" in 3,229 workers from 1943 to 1962 and reported that water, soap, and alkaline detergents were responsible for 796 cases—more than 24% of the total. Soaps, detergents, and industrial cleaners are the third most frequent cause of occupational contact dermatitis in California, ranking behind only poison ivy and solvents.[20] Kanerva et al.[66] found that detergents caused 37.8% of all cases of occupational irritant contact dermatitis observed over a 10-year period. Contact dermatitis resulting from soaps and detergents is a significant cause of occupational skin disease among health-care professionals and hospital personnel. Hansen[59] found a 15.3% prevalence rate of occupational skin diseases among 541 employees of a hospital cleaning department. Irritant contact dermatitis accounted for 75% of cases, most of which were caused by detergents. Meding[93] found that hand eczema was more common among people reporting occupational skin exposures, with detergents among the list of most harmful exposures. Aggravation of existing skin disease by the use of soaps and detergents is an additional factor not usually accounted for in such statistics. The incidence of occupational dermatitis caused by soaps is probably the same today as it was 25 years ago.

Surfactants

Irritant contact dermatitis caused by soaps and detergents is usually attributable to the principal surfactant contained in the product. Most products marketed for skin cleaning have a primary irritant effect when used excessively or repetitively. Patrizi et al.[110] have reported a peculiar form of irritant diaper dermatitis in infants that is caused by excessive washing of the diaper area with liquid detergents. Patterson[111] reported a case of hand dermatitis in a cleaning-products salesman that was caused by his cleaning his hands with a waterless cleaner numerous times daily to demonstrate the product's effectiveness. However, under conditions of ordinary usage, normal skin is not irritated. Soap solutions have an average pH of approximately 9.5, and when soap is used repeatedly over several days, the skin pH rises to about 8 and remains there as long as cleaning is continued.[69] Surfactants designed for cleaning surfaces other than the skin tend to be harsher, more alkaline, and more irritating to skin than those designed for skin cleaning. Mathias[86] reported a case of severe irritant facial contact dermatitis caused by undiluted dishwashing liquid used as a vehicle for face paint at a school carnival. Furthermore, such detergents often contain a variety of other potentially irritating additives. Workers who usually contact large amounts of soap and detergents include dishwashers, bartenders, cannery workers, textile workers, janitors, maids, cooks, food handlers, typists, mimeograph operators, nurses, physicians, dentists, and dental assistants. Dermatitis is common in these individuals.

Surfactant concentration is the most important factor to influence the development of irritant contact dermatitis, with irritancy increasing at higher concentrations, but other factors contribute too. Irritancy increases as the temperature of the washing solution increases.[11, 26, 101] Warren et al.[141] have shown that water hardness increases detergent irritancy. Bettley[13] has pointed out the role of repetitive exposures to low concentrations of detergent, insufficient to provide irritation following a single exposure, in producing clinical irritant contact dermatitis. This has been supported by experimental studies documenting continued deterioration of the parameters of skin function (e.g., transepidermal water loss) with repeated exposures to sodium lauryl sulfate.[55, 77] Atopic individuals (those with personal or family histories of atopic dermatitis, asthma, allergic conjunctivitis, or rhinitis) possess an increased clinical susceptibility to the irritating effects of soaps and detergents. Irritant hand dermatitis occurred in approximately two-thirds of hospital employees with atopic diatheses who performed wet work, presumably attributable to soaps, detergents, and disinfectants.[74] The Anionic content of the detergent is also important. Bettley[12] found that the anionic detergent potassium laurate was more irritating than potassium octanoate or palmitate. Clarys et al.[26] also found that increasing the anionic content of the detergent increased irritancy. Prottey and Ferguson[116] have noted the role of mechanical trauma and friction in predisposing to irritancy resulting from soaps and detergents. In some cases, factors other than the detergent concentration may be the most important determinant. Suskind et al.[131] removed patients with chronic hand eczema from work and subjected them to daily immersions of one hand into alkaline detergent solution and of the other hand into water of the same temperature without detergent; both hands improved in a parallel fashion.

With the exception of a unique epidemic of allergic contact dermatitis resulting from sultones, contact allergy caused by anionic surfactants is very rare. Dermatitis resulting from sultones first occurred in Norway in 1966 and was associated with the use of a dishwashing liquid.[81] Some of the patients had systemic symptoms, such as nausea, fever, and a peculiar kind of mental depression. The causative agent was not discovered at first, but it was soon found from patch-testing that the substance was a component of the surfactant (lauryl ether sulfate) fraction. The total number of cases reached approximately 1,000 of an estimated exposed population of 200,000 to 500,000 individuals. The cutaneous reaction was severe, and the hands and arms were most severely affected, with papules, vesicles, and often purpura. Some patients required hospitalization. A similar outbreak occurred in Denmark in 1971.[132] The allergen was later found to be unrelated to lauryl ether sulfate; it was an accidental contaminant formed during manufacturing: 1-dodecene-1,3-sultone and 2-chloro-1,3-dodecane sultone and their C-14 homologs.[27] The sensitizing properties of these sultones were found to be even stronger than 1-chloro-2,4-dinitrobenzene (DNCB), which is one of the most potent contact sensitizers known.[119] The problem of allergic contact dermatitis resulting from sultones has been reviewed by Lindup and Nowell.[79] Foussereau et al.[47] and Dooms-Goossens and Blockeel[38] have reported cases of allergic contact dermatitis caused by sodium lauryl sulfate (SLS); however, the patch-test concentrations of SLS used to confirm the diagnoses (5.0% and 0.5%, respectively) would be considered definite and marginal irritants by most authorities. A laundry detergent containing 6% SLS was associated with an outbreak of contact dermatitis in Sweden,[100] presumably due to contact irritation. In the United States, dermatitis occurring on skin surfaces covered by clothing is sometimes blamed on laundry detergent, but supporting evidence is circumstantial and has never been substantiated by patch-testing or provocation testing. Orlandini et al.[103] have reported a case of allergic conjunctivitis resulting from airborne exposure to a detergent containing lauryl alkyl sulfonate patch-tested at a 0.1% aqueous concentration. Anionic surfactant derivatives are generally less irritating than pure anionic surfactants but have occasionally been implicated as causes of contact allergy. Emmett and Wright[42] and Dooms-Goosens and Blockeel[38] have reported cases of contact allergy from triethanolamine (TEA) cocohydrolyzed protein in skin cleansers and shampoos. Reynolds and Peachey[118] described cases of allergic contact dermatitis caused by sodium ricinoleic monoethanolamine sulfosuccinate in a hand cleanser, tested at 0.5% and 5.0% in petrolatum. Andersen et al.[5] reported a case of contact dermatitis from triethanolamine (TEA)-polyethyleneglycol (PEG)-3-cocamide sulfate in a shampoo, tested at 1% aqueous.

Cationic surfactants, often used as foam-enhancing agents, have rarely been implicated as causes of contact allergy. Lauryldimethylamine oxide in a surgical scrub has been implicated as a contact allergen in hospital personnel.[38, 95, 120] Lachapelle and Tennstedt[73] have reported five cases of allergic contact dermatitis from lauryloxypropylamine in a soap used in a food distribution company. DeGroot and Liem[36] reported contact allergy to the cationic surfactant oleamidopropyl dimethylamine used as an emulsifier in a cosmetic body lotion. Subsequent investigations established crossreactivity to four other cationic surfactants: ricinoleamidopropyl dimethylamine lactate, tallowamidopropyl dimethylamine, lauramidopropyl dimethylamine, and myristamidopropyl dimethylamine.[35]

Nonionic surfactants are frequently used in shampoos and liquid detergents. Nethercott and Murray[98] and Meding[92] have reported cases of allergic contact dermatitis from nonoxynol-6 (nonylphenol ethoxylate) in industrial waterless hand cleansers. Dooms-Goosens et al.[40] described a case of allergic contact dermatitis from nonoxynol-10 in a liquid household detergent. Nonoxynols may be tested at a 1 or 2% aqueous concentration, but the latter may sometimes produce slight irritant reactions. Cocamide diethanolamine (DEA) and lauramide DEA have excellent foam-enhancing properties and are often used in shampoos and

liquid hand soaps. DeGroot et al.[34] have reported contact allergy from shampoos containing these substances. Pinola et al.[115] described three cases of contact allergy from cocamide DEA in a liquid hand soap and a metalworking fluid containing this surface active agent.

Amphoteric detergents contain both an anionic and a cationic component. These substances are often used when both a cleaning (anionic) function and a disinfecting (cationic) function are desired. Dodycyldi(aminoethyl)glycine and related compounds ("Tego" compounds) were first reported as contact sensitizers in hospital operating room personnel by Bowers[17] and by Fregert and Dahlquist.[50] Additional cases have subsequently been observed where they are used as sanitizers for food and dairy machinery and for swimming pool areas.[38, 72, 127, 136, 148] Tego compounds are tested at a 1% aqueous concentration. Cocamidopropyl betaine, another amphoteric detergent with relatively low irritancy potential, has been extensively used in shampoos since 1970. Andersen et al.[5] reported the first case of allergic sensitization resulting from a shampoo. Subsequently, it has been shown to be an important potential contact allergen among hairdressers.[10, 70] Fowler[48] found 12 cases among 210 patients routinely tested over a 15-month period, suggesting this could be an important shampoo allergen in patients with otherwise unexplained head and neck dermatitis. Contact dermatitis of the eyelids from its use in contact lens cleaning solutions has also been reported.[24, 125] The allergenic properties of cocamidopropyl betaine are thought to be caused by residual amine impurities[114] which possibly could be removed during the manufacturing process. Cocobetaine, a closely related compound, has also caused allergic sensitization and may crossreact with cocamidopropyl betaine.[137]

Optical Whiteners

In 1968 and 1969, an outbreak of allergic contact dermatitis in 167 patients in Denmark was reportedly caused by a recently introduced optical brightener, a mixture of 2-pyrazoline derivatives.[104, 106, 109] All patients had positive patch-test results to the brightener at 0.1 and 1.0% in yellow petrolatum. Pruritus was prominent, especially at night, and the eruption was similar to that seen in textile dermatitis, appearing in places such as the inner aspect of the upper arm, the axillae, and the volar forearms. An unusual reticulate pigmentation was seen in some patients.[105] Around the same time, a similar outbreak of contact dermatitis, attributable to the same optical brightener, occurred in 103 patients in Spain (cited in

Fisher[45]). The offending brightener was withdrawn from the world market and has not been used since. Today, the usual optical brighteners are stilbene derivatives. Although Gloxhuber and Bloching[53] did not feel that stilbene or its derivatives were contact allergens, the Spanish outbreak included 12 patients who apparently were also sensitized to stilbene.

Proteolytic Enzymes

Dermatitis caused by enzyme additives was reported in the late 1960s and early 1970s.[41, 63, 126] Contact allergy has been reported rarely[135]; contact irritation accounts for virtually all cases. Extensive studies of oral toxicity, cutaneous sensitization potential, and skin and eye irritant effects were conducted in the late 1960s without findings of adverse effects.[56] However, Okamota and coworkers[102] found them to be irritating to rabbit eye and skin. McMurrain[90] and Zachariae and coworkers[152] analyzed large groups of occupationally exposed workers and found the effect to be irritant in nature but not allergic, as had been suspected. Occupational asthma caused by immediate hypersensitivity reactions to these enzymes has occurred among workers exposed to high concentrations of detergent dusts containing these enzymes during manufacture.[46, 54, 99, 112, 150] Both skin irritation and pulmonary hypersensitivity have, for the most part, disappeared as occupational diseases among workers in the detergent manufacturing industry because of implementation of superior control technologies. However, exposure to these enzymes in other industries without adequate exposure controls may still cause contact dermatitis.[128] The role of proteolytic enzymes in modern detergents as an explanation of consumer complaints of dermatitis is controversial. White et al.[145] investigated complaints of dermatitis among 225 consumers who had used a washing powder containing the enzyme alcalase. Of 80 persons who agreed to be evaluated, no cases attributable to the enzyme-containing detergent could be confirmed by patch, prick, or use tests (the wearing of jackets washed with the laundry detergent, both with and without the enzyme). Furthermore, Pepys et al.[113] did not find that enzyme-containing laundry detergent could induce allergic pulmonary sensitization in consumers, although respiratory irritation could still be a possibility.

Perfumes

In his study of balsams, Hjorth[62] found that 50% of Scandinavian patients found to be sensitive to balsam of Peru on patch-testing were also sensitive to perfumes in soap. Rotenburg and Hjorth[122] later expanded this study and used patch-testing for 1,943 patients over a 17-month period. Of these individuals, 78 were found to be sensitive to toilet-soap perfume, most frequently benzyl salicylate. Of these 78 patients, 64% had dermatitis of the hands, forearms, and face; 46% showed simultaneous reactions to wood tars; and 23% reacted to balsam of Peru. All perfumes were used in patch tests at a concentration of 5% in petroleum. Hjorth[62] stressed that the concentration of perfume in soap is so low that patch-testing with a solution of soap misses sensitivity unless the sensitivity level is very high. Cooke and Kurwa[28] have reported a case of allergic contact dermatitis from colophony in a bar soap which cleared when the patient switched to a colophony-free soap.

Dyes and Pigments

Contact dermatitis resulting from inorganic pigments used as coloring agents in soaps and detergents is rare. Mathias[87] reported contact allergy from chromic hydroxide in a green toilet soap. Calnan[21] first reported allergic contact dermatitis from D & C Yellow No. 11 (C.I. No. 47000, also called Solvent Yellow 33) from a blush stick (color stick) and later from a lipstick.[22] D & C Yellow No. 11 is 2(2-quinolyl)-1,3-indandione.

Larsen[76] described a similar eruption from a rouge and mentioned its use in soaps and shampoos. A simultaneous reaction of D & C Yellow No. 11 and D & C Yellow No. 10 (C.I. 47005, also called Food Yellow No. 13 or Acid Yellow No. 2; it is used in drugs and soft drinks) suggests cross-sensitivity.[15]

The presence of D & C Yellow No. 11 in a popular yellow toilet soap in the United States was reported by Jordan.[64] A 42-year-old woman had showered using this soap, after which a generalized dermatitis developed. Jordan's investigation of this patient showed that the induction-elicitation levels of D & C Yellow No. 11 were very low, indicating a high sensitization index for this dye. This has been confirmed by Rapaport,[117] who induced contact sensitization in 14 of 56 subjects using the human repeated-insult patch-testing procedure. Fisher[44] has described a similar case of allergic contact dermatitis caused by D & C Yellow No. 11 in a shampoo.

Fabric Softeners

Liquid fabric softeners have been used for years, especially in textile manufacturing. They usually contain cationic surfactants such as tallow dimethylammonium chloride.[147] A fabric softener consisting of sheets of nonwoven nylon with two softening agents and a perfume was introduced in the United States in 1973. Although there was some initial concern that these agents could induce allergic sensitization, so far, all but one of the suspected cases have proved unrelated to use of the product. In 8 years of study, only one instance of sensitization resulted from the perfume, and it involved a woman who was already perfume-sensitive.[144]

Metallic Salts

Trace amounts of nickel, chromium, and cobalt are present in many soaps and detergents. The sources can probably be traced to the raw materials used to formulate the final product during the manufacturing process. The clinical significance of these trace amounts in provoking eczema in metal-sensitive individuals remains disputed. Almost certainly, clothing laundered in detergents contaminated with trace amounts of metals poses no risk. Soaps and detergents marketed for use on human skin are rinse-off products that are diluted with water (further reducing the concentration of the trace metals) and that contact the skin in an open, nonoccluded manner for only a brief time. The presence of chelating agents in the formulated detergent may decrease the concentration of bioavailable metal even further. Menne and Calvin[94] failed to find definite allergic reactions to open applications of aqueous solutions of nickel chloride, also containing 4% sodium lauryl sulfate, in nickel-sensitive subjects at concentrations of 100 p.p.m. or below. However, Basketter et al.[8] feel that concentrations as low as 1 p.p.m. might provoke reactions in highly sensitized individuals if skin has been damaged with surface active agents prior to exposure. Exceptions may occur when metals are deliberately added to the final cleaning product, obviously raising concentrations above simple trace contamination. Javel water, a bleach containing sodium chromate as a stabilizer and coloring agent, caused many cases of allergic contact dermatitis in reaction to chromate in Belgium.[71] Mathias[87] reported a case of pigmented cosmetic contact dermatitis resulting from a contact allergy to chromium oxide that had been added to a toilet soap as a coloring agent.

Superfats

Lanolin may be added to hand soaps, especially lotion soaps, to "enrich" them and make them milder. Pecquet et al. (cited in Dooms-Goossens and Blockeel,[38]) reported four cases of generalized dermatitis traced to a soap containing lanolin. This author has seen at least one case of occupational hand dermatitis associated with a contact allergy to lanolin in a lotion soap used in the workplace. Calzavara-Pinton et al.[23] reported a case of chronic protein contact dermatitis of the face, hands, and arms in a pizza maker; the dermatitis worsened after contact with wheat flour and an oatmeal-containing detergent. Prick and RAST testing to oats and wheat flour were both positive.

Corrosion Inhibitors

Corrosion inhibitors form a protective film around metal parts to protect them from the corrosive effects of detergents. Baadsgaard and Jorgensen[7] reported a case of allergic contact dermatitis in a cleaning woman to butin-2-diol 1,4, a corrosion inhibitor in one of her cleaning products. Andersen[4] reported a case of occupational hand dermatitis in a janitor caused by diethylthiourea in an acidic detergent.

Germicidal Agents and Preservatives

Allergic contact dermatitis and photocontact dermatitis have been caused by germicidal agents that have been added to soaps and detergents. Although TCC may crossreact with related halogenated bacteriostatic agents such as dibromosalicylanilide, Maibach and coworkers[82] found the potential for allergic contact dermatitis to be minimal following use of bar soaps containing it. Freeman and Knox[49] studied photocontact dermatitis resulting from the halogenated salicylanilides and related compounds and found only one patient whose test results were positive on photo patch-testing to TCC alone. Since then, no other cases of primary photosensitization to TCC have been reported.[29] However, TCC has occasionally been described as a contact allergen in antiperspirants used in Europe.[2, 58, 107] Allergic contact dermatitis from the germicidal agent triclosan has been reported from a liquid toilet soap.[153]

Chlorhexidine, an antiseptic used in surgical liquid soaps, has rarely caused allergic contact dermatitis, considering its extensive use. Wahlberg and Wennersten[140] reported several cases and suspected photosensitivity. Ljunggren and Moller[80] described allergic sensitization in a 78-year-old man with a stasis ulcer from a topical preparation containing chlorhexidine. Patch-test results to a 0.5% concentration in alcohol and to a 0.05% solution in water were positive, but tests in a petrolatum vehicle gave negative results. Osmundsen[108] patch-tested 551 patients with chlorhexidine gluconate (1% in water) and found 14 relevant allergic reactions; on this basis, he estimated that contact allergy was probably more common than is generally believed.

Formaldehyde and formaldehyde releasers have been used extensively as preservatives in water-based shampoos, dishwashing liquids, hand lotions, and various skin cleansing products. Cases of contact allergy have occasionally been reported; Zemstov et al.[154] reported a case of allergic contact dermatitis caused by formaldehyde in a liquid soap. The ability of formaldehyde to provoke allergic contact dermatitis in rinse-off products such as shampoos probably depends on the degree of sensitivity of the individual, the length of contact time, and the condition of the skin with which it is in contact. It rarely causes reactions in shampoos, even in strongly sensitized subjects.[19] The use of formaldehyde per se in soaps, shampoos, and cosmetics in general has declined significantly and has been replaced by formaldehyde releasers and other classes of germicidal agents. Like formaldehyde, formaldehyde releasers in soaps and detergents, rinse-off products, rarely cause allergic contact dermatitis, even in formaldehyde-sensitive individuals.

Quaternium-15 is a potent skin sensitizer in its own right as well as a formaldehyde releaser. Tosti et al.[134] described two cases of occupational allergic hand eczema in hair dressers that had been caused by this preservative in shampoos. Marren et al.[84] reported nail dystrophy resulting from allergic contact dermatitis to quaternium-15 in a liquid soap. Imidazolidinylurea and diazolidinylurea are not considered very strong sensitizers. In most cases in which positive reactions to these formaldehyde releasers are considered relevant, concomitant sensitization to formaldehyde has also occurred. Zaugg and Hunziker[153] reported a case of allergic sensitization to diazolidinylurea in a liquid soap.

Isothiazolinone derivatives are important contact sensitizers. The mixture of methylisothiazolinone and methylchloroisothiazolinone (Kathon CG) is used extensively as a preservative in shampoos and liquid soaps. Although most cases of allergic contact dermatitis have occurred from leave-on cosmetics containing this preservative, a few cases have been reported from rinse-off shampoos.[31] Others have described cases of perianal dermatitis from contact sensitization to this preservative in moistened paper pads used for perianal cleansing.[32, 37]

Phenolic germicidal agents are also important contact allergens. Allergic contact dermatitis as well as vitiligo-like leukoderma has been caused by p-tertiary butylphenol and amylphenol in hospital sanitizing cleansers.[65] Sonnex and Rycroft[129] reported a bartender with allergic contact dermatitis caused by orthobenzyl parachlorophenol in a drinking glass cleanser. Libow et al.[78] reported a case of allergic contact dermatitis from chloroxylenol (para-chloro-meta-xylenol, PCMX) in a disinfectant soap. This author has personally observed several cases of allergic contact dermatitis caused by chloroxylenol in waterless hand cleaners used by machinists and mechanics.

Storrs et al.[130] have reported an outbreak of allergic contact dermatitis among mechanics using a waterless hand cleanser containing glutaraldehyde.

Chloroacetamide in a liquid hand soap caused allergic contact dermatitis in a hospital nurse.[39]

The mixture of dibromodicyanobutane (methyldibromoglutaronitrile) and phenoxyethanol is an important emerging allergen.[33] This preservative may be found in some lotion hand soaps, but cases of contact allergy from its use in soaps has not yet been reported.

Abrasives

Abrasives work by mechanically stripping soil or grime from skin or an inert surface, particularly when combined with vigorous agitation. Irritant dermatitis is common when soaps containing abrasives are used excessively to clean skin. Allergic dermatitis caused by nickel has been reported from the use of metal fiber scouring pads.[30]

Solvents

Irritant contact dermatitis caused by waterless hand cleansers (mechanics' soap) may occur because of excessive use or occlusion on skin beneath protective work clothing such as gloves. Irritation most likely results from a hydrocarbon solvent incorporated into a cream base in concentrations up to 20%. The irritant effect may be enhanced if the waterless hand cleanser formulation incorporates an alkaline detergent as well.[14] Although contact allergy to solvents is extremely rare, Gaioch and Forsyth[52] have reported a case of allergic contact dermatitis in a litho printer that was caused by orange turpene oil in a solvent-based blanket wash.

Miscellaneous

Meding[91] reported two cases of contact allergy in goldsmiths that was caused by diethylenetriamine in a detergent used for ultrasonic cleaning of jewelry.

PHOTOCONTACT DERMATITIS

Although photocontact dermatitis (see also Chapter 10) was known to have resulted from contact with coal tar, bergamot oil, and certain plants and medications for many years, it was not until 1960 that a major outbreak of photodermatitis occurred in Great Britain. The clinical appearance resembled an exaggerated sunburn and ultimately affected more than 10,000 individuals. Through clever detective work, Wilkinson[146] found the causative agent to be a photosensitizing germicidal substance, tetrachlorosalicylanilide, contained in a commonly used soap. This agent is no longer used in toilet soaps made in the United States or Great Britain but has been superseded by closely related compounds such as other halogenated salicylanilides and carbanilides. Bithionol was used for a period of time, but it was removed from the market in 1967. Because of its toxicity when absorbed through denuded skin,[67] the use of hexachlorophene has been severely restricted, and a prescription is now required. Although banned for use in toilet soaps, tetrachlorosalicylanilide may still be found as a disinfectant in industrial detergents used to clean inert surfaces and in first-aid cream used in the workplace to treat burns and other injuries. Fentichlor, chemically related to bithionol, may also be found in soaps and detergents marketed for industrial use, although it is not used in household soaps for personal cleaning. A case of photocontact allergy to fentichlor in a French industrial liquid hand soap has been reported (cited in Dooms-Goossens and Blockeel[38]).

Germicidal agents in common use in toilet soaps today are TCC and triclosan (Irgasan). Irgasan DP 300 is widely used in soaps, shampoos, and other items of personal use such as foot powders and deodorants. Marzulli and Maibach[85] showed no sensitization or photosensitization on predictive testing using the Draize test, and contact allergy to this substance has proved to be quite rare. Roed-Petersen and colleagues[121] reported contact sensitization from its use in a deodorant stick and in a foot deodorant powder. Hindson[61] described sensitivity to triclosan from its presence in a deodorant-antiperspirant spray. Of 1,100 patients tested using a 2% concentration in petroleum jelly, Wahlberg[139] found sensitivity in two patients. Both had contracted dermatitis from using deodorants containing this substance.

The accidental contamination of chloro-2-phenylphenol (Dowicide 32) in a liquid soap resulted in photodermatitis in four school gardeners in 1971 and 1972.[1] Dowicide 32 is used as a disinfectant in soaps, a fungicide in textile manufacturing, and a mold inhibitor in gaskets for machinery.

Yates and Finn[151] reported a case of photosensitivity induced by the germicidal agent zinc pyrithione in an antidandruff shampoo.

The ability of optical whiteners added to laundry detergents to cause clinical photoallergy is debatable. Dooms-Goossens and Blockeel[38] state that a number of cases of photoallergy, confirmed by positive patch tests, have been caused by stilbene derivatives used in washing powder.

In addition to germicidal agents, various fragrances added to soaps may cause photosensitization. Shall and colleagues[125a] reported allergic photocontact dermatitis from musk ambrette added to a toilet soap.

The wavelengths of light responsible for photodermatitis are chiefly those greater than 320 nm. Dermatitis may, therefore, result from exposure to sunlight filtered through window glass and occasionally from exposure to fluorescent light. Possible industrial sources of the ultraviolet light necessary for the development of photocontact dermatitis are welding, silk screening, lithography, and magnaflux. Willis and Kligman[149] showed that photosensitizing chemicals are decomposed by light to haptens and that the reaction is simply allergic contact dermatitis. In their view, the sole role of light is to transform the photosensitizer into a more potent contact allergen.

Photodermatitis is usually limited initially to sun-exposed areas, such as the face, the posterior neck, the V of the anterior chest, the extensor surfaces of the forearms, the dorsal surfaces of the hands, and the anterior surfaces of the lower legs and feet. Eyelids, submental areas, and regions of the body covered by clothing and jewelry are spared. Widespread involvement may occur later, probably because of autosensitization. Persistence for months or years is common. Although the morphological characteristics of the dermatitis are similar to those of other types of contact dermatitis, lichenification and hyperpigmentation are usually pronounced.

Other conditions likely to be considered in a differential diagnosis include airborne contact dermatitis, atopic dermatitis, and photoallergic drug sensitivity. Types of airborne contact dermatitis that most closely resemble allergic contact photodermatitis include ragweed oleoresin contact dermatitis and cement (dichromate) dermatitis. Airborne contact dermatitis, however, tends to be concentrated in moist body folds, such as the creases of the neck, the antecubital and popliteal areas, the axillae, and the folds of the eyelids, areas that are typically spared in photodermatitis. Allergic contact dermatitis caused by pollens or ragweed oleoresin usually demonstrates a seasonal occurrence, and results of patch-testing with the appropriate antigens are positive.

Photoallergic drug eruptions are very difficult to differentiate from allergic contact photodermatitis because of the great similarity in appearance and distribution. A careful drug history, however, should help in differentiation. Contact phototesting results are normal in almost all cases, but the eruption can be reproduced by repeated administration of the minimal erythema dose, using a carbon arc lamp,[43] or in the case of demeclocycline hydrochloride (Declomycin) and perhaps other drugs, by natural sunlight filtered through a thin sheet of mylar plastic.[83] It must be remembered, however, that the action spectra of different drugs vary. Artificial light sources may not produce sufficient radiation in the appropriate action spectrum for the drug in question, in which case falsely negative results are obtained. For this reason, phototesting for drug sensitivity is best left to physicians with special knowledge and equipment in this field.

Other diseases that should be considered in the differential diagnosis are polymorphic light eruption, lupus erythematosus, pellagra, dermatomyositis, and the porphyrias.

PIGMENTARY DISTURBANCES

Kahn[65] reported depigmentation of the skin in five workers in one hospital and seven workers in another that was caused by phenolic germicides found in detergent preparations used to clean and sanitize floors, walls, and equipment. The hands and forearms were affected in all patients, and distant sites in two employees also showed depigmentation. Repigmentation was very slow and incomplete and often did not occur at all. The phenolics found and studied in this study included o-benzyl-p-chlorophenol, p-tert-butylphenol, p-tert-amylphenol, and p-phenylphenol; p-tert-amylphenol and p-tert-butylphenol were found to cause depigmentation without also causing irritation, but Kahn's work, which included animal studies with guinea pigs, suggested that any moderately irritating phenolic compound, including hexachlorophene, can cause depigmentation of the skin.[65]

Soaps and detergents may sometimes cause hyperpigmentation. Mathias[87] reported pigmental facial cosmetic dermatitis caused by contact allergy to chromium oxide used as a green pigment in a toilet soap. Some of the Danish cases of contact dermatitis caused by optical whiteners, reported by Osmundsen,[105] were associated with a peculiar reticulated hyperpigmentation.

PREVENTION

Soaps and detergents in the workplace are not only primary causes of contact dermatitis; they also may aggravate preexisting dermatitis. Prevention is most appropriately accomplished before dermatitis occurs.[88, 89]

Soaps and detergents should be used only for the purposes intended by the manufacturer. Only products intended for skin cleaning should be used for personal hygiene. Frequent hand-washing during the workshift (between 10 and 20 times) should be discouraged except when absolutely necessary. Liberal use of a skin moisturizer or even petrolatum should be encouraged after washing to combat the skin-drying effects of detergents. Regular use of moisturizers has been shown to decrease clinical irritation caused by daily exposure to detergents among cleaners and kitchen workers.[57] Solvents or products marketed for cleaning inert industrial surfaces should never be used for skin cleaning. The water temperature of detergent solutions should be no hotter than necessary for the cleaning operation when skin contact is unavoidable.

Specialized skin cleansers such as abrasives and waterless hand cleansers may actually cause dermatitis unless used correctly. Abrasive use should be limited to thick palmar skin, since the relatively thinner skin of the dorsal parts of the hands and arms is less resistant to irritation. Waterless hand cleansers should be removed from the skin after application by gentle washing with a mild toilet soap, as the solvent contained in any residual film is a potential cause of dermatitis. Neither abrasives nor waterless hand cleansers should be used to clean skin that is already inflamed because they are likely to aggravate the dermatitis.

Appropriate protective clothing should be worn or barrier creams used for dirty work whenever feasible; this minimizes skin soiling and the need for skin cleaning in the first place. The clinical protective value of barrier creams against direct irritation from industrial soaps and detergents is still questionable. Experimentally, some barrier creams have prevented irritation from sodium lauryl sulfate.[9, 51] Waterproof gloves or other clothing should be worn whenever industrial detergents must be used. If gloves must be worn for long periods, removable cotton liners are advisable to reduce mechanical irritation caused by sweating and the rubbing of gloves against the skin. Prolonged glove-wearing may aggravate preexisting dermatitis and should be avoided by workers with dermatitis. Industrial cleansers should not be stored with protective clothing, as accidental spillage or leakage may contaminate their interiors and cause contact dermatitis. If industrial cleansers get inside work gloves while an individual is working, he or she should promptly remove them, thoroughly rinse and dry the hands, and put on a dry pair of gloves. If gloves develop holes or tears, they should be immediately discarded.

References

1. Adams RM. Photoallergic contact dermatitis to chloro-9-phenylphenol. *Arch Dermatol* 1972; 106:711–714.
2. Agren-Jonsson S, Magnusson B. Sensitization to propantheline bromide, trichlorcarbanilide and propylene glycol in an antiperspirant. *Contact Dermatitis* 1976; 2:79–80.
3. American Chemical Society and National Science Foundation. *Chemistry in the Economy.* Washington, D.C.: ACS, NSF; 1973:202.
4. Andersen KE. Diethylthiourea contact dermatitis from an acidic detergent. *Contact Dermatitis* 1983; 9:146.
5. Andersen KE, Roed-Petersen J, Kamp P. Contact allergy to TEA-PEG-3-Cocamide sulfate in a shampoo. *Contact Dermatitis* 1984; 11:192–193.
6. Aust LB, Maibach HI. Modified Draize sensitization test with D & C yellow No. 10 in combination dye systems. *Contact Dermatitis* 1981; 7:357.
7. Baadsgaard O, Jorgensen J. Contact dermatitis to butin-2-diol 1,4. *Contact Dermatitis* 1985; 13:34.
8. Basketter DA, Briatisco-Vangosa G, Kaestner W, et al. Nickel, cobalt, and chromium in consumer products: a role in allergic contact dermatitis? *Contact Dermatitis* 1993; 28:15–25.
9. Barnes EG, Jenkins HL. Barrier cream protection against detergent solutions. *Contact Dermatitis* 1990; 23:296.
10. Beck MH. Allergic contact dermatitis of the hands in hairdressers. *Contact Dermatitis* 1990; 23:240.
11. Berardesca E, Vignoli GP, Distante F, et al. Effects of water temperature on surfactant-induced skin irritation. *Contact Dermatitis* 1995; 32:83–87.
12. Bettley FR. The irritant effect of soap in relation to epidermal permeability. *J Dermatol* 1963; 75:113–116.
13. Bettley FR. The irritant effect of detergents. *Trans St John's Hosp Derm Soc* 1972; 58:65–74.
14. Birmingham DJ, Perone VB. Waterless hand cleaners. *Ind Med Surg* 1957; 28:361–368.
15. Bjorkner B, Magnusson B. Patch test sensitization to D & C yellow no. 11 and simultaneous reaction to quinoline yellow. *Contact Dermatitis* 1981; 7:1–4.
16. Bolam RM, Hepworth R, Bowerman LT. In-use evaluation of safety to skin of enzyme containing wash products. *Br Med J* 1971; 2:449–501.
17. Bowers RE. Tego (dodecyl aminoethyl glycine hydrochloride). *Contact Dermatitis Newsletter* 1988; 4:78.
18. Brady CS, Clauser HR. *Materials Handbook.* 11th ed. New York: McGraw-Hill; 1977:718.
19. Brunzeel DP, van Ketel WG, de Haan P. Formaldehyde contact sensitivity and the use of shampoos. *Contact Dermatitis* 1984; 10:179–180.
20. California Division of Labor Statistics. *Occupational Skin Disease in California.* San Francisco: California Department of Industrial Relations; 1982.
21. Calnan CD. Allergy to D & C red 17 and D & C yellow 11. *Contact Dermatitis Newsletter* 1973; 14:405.
22. Calnan CD. Quinazoline yellow SS in cosmetics. *Contact Dermatitis* 1976; 2:180–186.
23. Calzavara-Pinton PG, Tosoni C, Carlino A, et al. Contact eczematous dermatitis caused by wheat and oats. *G Ital Dermatol Venereol* 1989; 124: 289–291.
24. Camelli NJ, Tosti G, Venturo N, et al. Eyelid dermatitis due to cocamidopropylbetaine in a hard contact lens solution. *Contact Dermatitis* 1991; 25:261–262.
25. Carter RO, McMurrain KD. Consumer safety of enzyme detergents. *JAMA* 1970; 211:2017.
26. Clarys P, Manon I, Barel AO. Influence of temperature on irritation in the hand/arm immersion test. *Contact Dermatitis* 1997; 36:240–243.
27. Conner DS, Ritz H, Ampulski RS, et al. Identification of certain sultones as the sensitizers in an alkyl ethoxy sulfate. *Fette Seifen Anstrichmittel* 1975; 77:25–29.
28. Cooke MA, Kurwa AR. Colophony sensitivity. *Contact Dermatitis* 1975; 1:192–193.
29. Cronin E. *Contact Dermatitis.* London: Churchill Livingstone; 1980:435.
30. Dawber R, Sonnex T. Nickel dermatitis due to steel fibre and soap cleaning pads. *Contact Dermatitis* 1982; 8:342.
31. DeGroot AC. Kathon CG: a review. *J Am Acad Dermatol* 1988; 18:350–358.
32. DeGroot AC, Baar TJM, Terpstra H, et al. Contact allergy to moist toilet paper. *Contact Dermatitis* 1991; 24:135–136.
33. DeGroot AC, Bruynzeel DP, Coenraads PJ, et al. Frequency of allergic reactions to methyldibromoglutaronitrile (1,2-dibromo-2,4-dicyanobutane) in the Netherlands. *Contact Dermatitis* 1991; 25:270–271.
34. DeGroot AC, DeWit FS, Bos JD, et al. Contact allergy to cocamide DEA and lauramide DEA in shampoos. *Contact Dermatitis* 1987; 16:117–118.
35. DeGroot AC, Jagtman BA, Van Der Meeren HLM, et al. Cross-reaction pattern of the cationic emulsifier oleamidopropyl dimethylamine. *Contact Dermatitis* 1988; 19:284–289.
36. DeGroot AC, Liem DH. Contact allergy to oleamidopropyl dimethylamine. *Contact Dermatitis* 1984; 11:298–301.
37. Dooms-Goossens A. A patient bothered by unexpected sources of isothiazolinones. *Contact Dermatitis* 1990; 23:192.
38. Dooms-Goossens A, Blockeel I. Allergic contact dermatitis and photoallergic contact dermatitis due to soaps and detergents. *Clin Dermatol* 1996; 14:67–76.
39. Dooms-Goosens A, Degreef H, Vanhee J, et al. Chlorocresol and chloroacetamide: allergens in medications, glues, and cosmetics. *Contact Dermatitis* 1981; 7:51–52.
40. Dooms-Goossens A, Deveylder H, deAlam AG, et al. Contact sensitivity to nonoxynols as a cause of intolerance to antiseptic preparations. *J Am Acad Dermatol* 1989; 21:723–727.
41. Ducksbury CFJ. Dave VK. Contact dermatitis in home helps following the use of enzymes detergents. *Br Med J* 1970; 1:535–539.
42. Emmett EA, Wright RC. Allergic contact dermatitis from TEA-cocohydrolysed protein. *Arch Dermatol* 1976; 112:1008–1009.
42a. Soaps and Detergents. In: *Encyclopedia Britannica*, vol. 16. Chicago: Encyclopedia Britannica Inc., 1980:916–919.
43. Epstein JH. Photosensitivity testing procedures. In: Rees RB, ed.: *Dermatoses Due to Environmental and Physical Factors.* Springfield, IL.: Charles C Thomas; 1962.
44. Fisher AA. Allergic reactions to D&C Yellow No. 11 Dye. *Cutis* 1984; 34:344–346, 350.
45. Fisher AA. *Contract Dermatitis*, 3rd ed. Philadelphia: Lea & Febiger; 1986:312–313.
46. Flindt MLH. Pulmonary disease due to inhalation of derivatives of *Bacillus subtilis* containing proteolytic enzymes. *Lancet* 1969; 1:1177–1180.
47. Foussereau J, Petitjean J, Lantz JP. Allergy to sodium lauryl sulphate. *Contact Dermatitis Newsletter* 1974; 15:433.

48. Fowler JF. Cocamidopropyl betaine: the significance of positive patch test results in twelve patients. *Cutis* 1993; 52:281–284.
49. Freeman RG, Knox JM. The action spectrum of photo contact dermatitis caused by halogenated salicylanilide and related compounds. *Arch Dermatol* 1968; 97:130–138.
50. Fregert S, Dahlquist I. Allergic contact dermatitis from Tego. *Contact Dermatitis Newsletter* 1969; 5:103.
51. Frosch PJ, Kurte A, Pilz B. Efficacy of skin barrier creams. III. The repetitive irritation test (RIT) in humans. *Contact Dermatitis* 1993; 29:113–118.
52. Gaioch JJ, Forsyth A. Allergic contact dermatitis from "Varn Ecol-Oj Wash" in a litho printer. *Contact Dermatitis* 1988; 19:229.
53. Gloxhuber CH, Bloching H. Toxicologic properties of fluorescent whitening agents. *Clin Toxicol* 1978; 13:171–203.
54. Gothe CJ, Nilzen A, Holmgren A, et al. Medical problems in the detergent industry caused by proteolytic enzymes from *Bacillus subtilis*. *Acta Allergolica* 1972; 27:63–88.
55. Grunewald AM, Gloor M, Gehring W, et al. Damage to the skin by repetitive washing. *Contact Dermatitis* 1995; 32:225–232.
56. Griffith JF, Weaver JE, Whitehouse HS, et al. Safety evaluation of enzymes detergents: oral and cutaneous toxicity, irritancy and skin sensitization studies. *Food Cosmet Toxicol* 1969; 17:581–593.
57. Halkier-Sorensen L, Thestrup-Pedersen K. The efficacy of a moisturizer (Locobase) among cleaners and kitchen assistants during everyday exposure to water and detergents. *Contact Dermatitis* 1993; 29:266–271.
58. Hannuksela M. Allergy to propantheline in an antiperspirant (Ecoril lotion). *Contact Dermatitis* 1975; 1:244.
59. Hansen KS. Occupational dermatoses in hospital cleaning women. *Contact Dermatitis* 1983; 9:343–351.
60. Harris JC. Soap and synthetic detergents. In: Kent JA, ed. *Riegel's Industrial Chemistry*. New York: Reinhold; 1962.
61. Hindson TC. Irgasan DP-300 in a deodorant. *Contact Dermatitis* 1975; 1:328.
62. Hjorth N. *Eczematous Allergy to Balsams*. Copenhagen: Munksgaard; 1961:112–123,137–140.
63. Jensen NE. Severe dermatitis and "biological" detergents. *Br Med J* 1970; 1:299.
64. Jordan WP. Contact dermatitis from D & C yellow dye #11 in a toilet bar soap. *J Am Acad Dermatol* 1981; 4:813–814.
65. Kahn C. Depigmentation caused by phenolic detergent germicides. *Arch Dermatol* 1970 102:177–187.
66. Kanerva L, Estlander T, Jolanki R. Occupational skin disease in Finland: an analysis of 10 years of statistics from an occupational dermatology clinic. *Int Arch Occup Environ Health* 1988; 60:89–94.
67. Kimbrough RD. Review of toxicity of hexachlorophene. *Arch Environ Health* 1971; 25:119–122.
68. Klauder JV. Actual causes of certain occupational dermatoses. *Arch Dermatol* 1962; 85:441–454.
69. Klauder JV, Gross BA. Actual causes of certain occupational dermatoses. *Arch Dermatol* 1951; 63:1–23.
70. Korting HC, Parsch EM, Enders F, et al. Allergic contact dermatitis to cocamidopropyl betaine in shampoo. *J Am Acad Dermatol* 1992; 27:1013–1015.
71. Lachapelle JM, Lauwerys R, Tennstedt D, et al. Eau de Javel and prevention of chromate allergy in France. *Contact Dermatitis* 1980; 6:107–110.
72. Lachapelle JM, Reginster JP. Occupational contact dermatitis from an ampholytic soap (TEGO). *Contact Dermatitis* 1977; 3:211–212.
73. Lachapelle JM, Tennstedt D. Occupational soap dermatitis: contact allergic reactions to lauryloxypropylamine. *Contact Dermatitis* 1975; 1:260–261.
74. Lammintausta K, Kalimo K. Atopy and hand dermatitis in hospital wet work. *Contact Dermatitis* 1981; 7:301–308.
75. Lamson SA, Kong BM, DeSalva SJ. D B C yellow nos. 10 and 11: delayed contact hypersensitivity in the guinea pig. *Contact Dermatitis* 1982; 8:200–203.
76. Larsen WG. Cosmetic dermatitis due to a dye (D & C yellow no. 11). *Contact Dermatitis* 1975; 1:61.
77. Lee CH, Maibach HI. Study of cumulative irritant contact dermatitis in man utilizing open application on subclinically irritated skin. *Contact Dermatitis* 1994; 30:271–275.
78. Libow LF, Ruszkowski AM, Deleo VA. Allergic contact dermatitis from para-chlorometa-xylenol in Lurosep soap. *Contact Dermatitis* 1989; 20:67–68.
79. Lindup WE, Nowell PT. Role of sultone contaminants in an outbreak of allergic contact dermatitis caused by alkyl ethoxysulfates: a review. *Food Cosmet Toxicol* 1978; 6:59–62.
80. Ljunggren B, Moller H. Euematous contact allergy to chlorhexidine. *Acta Derm Venereol* 1972; 52:308–310.
81. Magnusson B, Gilje O. Allergic contact dermatitis from a dish-washing liquid containing lauryl ether sulfate. *Acta Derm Venereol* 1973; 53:136–140.
82. Maibach HI, Bandmann J-H, Calnan CD, et al. Triclocarban: evaluation of contact dermatitis potential in man. *Contact Dermatitis* 1978; 4:282–288.
83. Maibach HI, Sams WM, Epstein JH. Screening for drug toxicity by wavelengths greater than 3100 A. *Arch Dermatol* 1967; 95:12–15.
84. Marren P, DeBerker D, Dawber RPR, et al. Occupational contact dermatitis due to quaternium-15 presenting as nail dystrophy. *Contact Dermatitis* 1991; 25:253–255.
85. Marzulli FN, Maibach HI. Antimicrobials: experimental contact sensitization in man. *J Soc Cosmet Chem* 1973; 24:399–421.
86. Mathias CGT. Contact dermatitis in children due to face paints. *Cutis* 1980; 26:584–585.
87. Mathias CGT. Pigmented contact dermatitis from contact allergy to a toilet soap containing chromium. *Contact Dermatitis* 1982; 8:29–31.
88. Mathias CGT. Contact dermatitis: when cleaner is not better. *Occup Health Safety* 1984; 53:45–50.
89. Mathias CGT. Contact dermatitis from use or misuse of soaps, detergents and cleansers in the workplace. *Occup Med State Art Reviews* 1986; 2:205–218.
90. McMurrain KD. Dermatologic and pulmonary responses in the manufacturing of detergent enzyme products. *J Occup Med* 1970; 12:416–418.
91. Meding B. Allergic contact dermatitis from diethylenetriamine in a goldsmith shop. *Contact Dermatitis* 1982; 8:142.
92. Meding B. Occupational contact dermatitis from nonylphenolpolyglycolether. *Contact Dermatitis* 1985; 13:122–123.
93. Meding B, Swanbeck G. Occupational hand eczema in an industrial city. *Contact Dermatitis* 1990; 22:13–23.
94. Menne T, Calvin G. Concentration threshold of non-occluded nickel exposure in nickel-sensitive individuals and controls with and without surfactant. *Contact Dermatitis* 1993; 29:180–184.
95. Muston HL, Boss JM, Summerly R. Dermatitis from Ammonyx LO, a constituent of a surgical scrub. *Contact Dermatitis* 1977; 3:347–348.
96. Nelson LS, Stoesser AV. Cleansing agents—irritating and non-irritating to the skin. *Am Allergy* 1953; 11:572–579.

97. Nester U, Hausen BM. Berufsbedingtes Kantakrtekzem durch gelben Chinophthalonfarbstoff (Solvent yellow 33: C.I. 47000). *Hautarzt* 1978; 29:153–157.

98. Nethercott JR, Murray JL. Allergic contact dermatitis due to nonylphenol ethoxylate. *Contact Dermatitis* 1984; 10:235–239.

99. Newhouse ML, Tagg B, Pocock SJ, et al. An epidemiological study of workers producing enzyme washing powders. *Lancet* 1970; 1:689–693.

100. Nilzen A. Some aspects of synthetic detergents and skin reactions. *Acta Derm Venereol* 1958; 38:104.

101. Ohlenschlaeger J, Friberg J, Ramsing D, Agner T. Temperature dependency of skin susceptibility to water and detergents. *Acta Derm Venereol* 1996; 76:274–276.

102. Okamota K, et al. Skin irritation and allergy inductivity due to alkaline protease. *Eisei Kagaku* 1972; 8:304–308.

103. Orlandini A, Viotti G, Martinoli C, et al. Allergic contact conjunctivitis from synthetic detergents in a nurse. *Contact Dermatitis* 1990; 23:376–377.

104. Osmundsen PE. Contact dermatitis due to an optical whitener in washing powders. *Br J Dermatol* 1969; 81:799–803.

105. Osmundsen PE. Pigmented contact dermatitis. *Br J Dermatol* 1970; 83:296–301.

106. Osmundsen PE. Contact dermatitis from an optical whitener in washing powders. *Cutis* 1972; 10:59–66.

107. Osmundsen PE. Concomitant contact allergy to propantheline bromide and TCC. *Contact Dermatitis* 1975; 1:251–252.

108. Osmundsen PE. Contact dermatitis to chlorhexidine. *Contact Dermatitis* 1982; 8:81–83.

109. Osmundsen PE, Alani MD. Contact allergy to an optical whitener. "CPY," in washing powders. *Br J Dermatol* 1971; 85:61–66.

110. Patrizi A, Neri I, Marzaduri S, et al. Pigmented and hyperkeratotic napkin dermatitis: a liquid detergent irritant dermatitis. *Dermatology* 1996; 193:36–40.

111. Patterson AH. Hand dermatitis in a hand cleanser salesman. *Contact Dermatitis* 1993; 28:119–120.

112. Pepys J, Hargreave FE, Longbottom JL, et al. Allergic reactions of lungs to enzymes of *B. subtilis. Lancet* 1969; 1:1181.

113. Pepys J, Mitchell J, Hawkins R, et al. A longitudinal study of possible allergy to enzyme detergents. *Clin Allergy* 1985; 15:101–115.

114. Pigatoo PD, Bigardi AS, Cusano F. Contact dermatitis to cocamidopropyl betaine is caused by residual amines: relevance, clinical characteristics, and review of the literature. *Am J Contact Dermatitis* 1995; 6:13–16.

115. Pinola A, Estlander T, Jolanki R, et al. Occupational allergic contact dermatitis due to coconut diethanolamine (cocamide DEA). *Contact Dermatitis* 1993; 29:262–265.

116. Prottey C, Ferguson T. Factors which determine the skin irritation potential of soaps and detergents. *J Soc Cosmet Chem* 1975; 26:29–35.

117. Rapaport MJ. Allergy to D & C yellow dye no. 11. *Contact Dermatitis* 1980; 6:364–365.

118. Reynolds NJ, Peachey RDG. Allergic contact dermatitis from a sulfosuccinate derivative in a hand cleanser. *Contact Dermatitis* 1990; 22:59–60.

119. Ritz HL, Conner DS, Sauter ED. Contact sensitization of guinea pigs with unsaturated and halogenated sultones. *Contact Dermatitis* 1975; 1:349–358.

120. Roberts DL, Summerly R, Byrne JPH. Contact dermatitis due to constituents of Hibiscrub. *Contact Dermatitis* 1981; 7:326–328.

121. Roed-Petersen J, Auken G, Hjorth N. Contact sensitivity to Irgasan DP-300. *Contact Dermatitis* 1975; 1:293–294.

122. Rotenburg HW, Hjorth N. Allergy to perfumes from toilet soaps and detergents in patients with dermatitis. *Arch Dermatol* 1968; 91:417–421.

123. Schwartz L. *The Prevention of Occupational Skin Disease.* New York: Association of American Soap and Glycerine Products; 1955.

124. Schwartz L, Tulipan L, Birmingham DI. *Occupational Diseases of the Skin.* Philadelphia: Lea & Febiger; 1957:252.

125. Sertoli A, Lombardi P, Palleschi GM, et al. Tegobetaine in contact lens solutions. *Contact Dermatitis* 1987; 16:111–112.

125a. Shall L, Reynolds AJ, Holt PJA. Photosensitivity to musk ambrette in a toilet soap and hair gel. *Contact Dermatitis* 1986; 14:324.

126. Shapiro RS. Sensitivity to proteolytic enzymes in laundry detergents. *J Allergy* 1971; 47:74–77.

127. Sinclair S, Hindson C. Allergic contact dermatitis from dodecyldiaminoethyl glycine. *Contact Dermatitis* 1988; 19:320.

128. Smith DJ, Mathias CGT, Greenwald DI. Contact dermatitis from *B. subtilis*-derived protease enzymes. *Contact Dermatitis* 1989; 20:58–59.

129. Sonnex TS, Rycroft RJG. Allergic contact dermatitis from orthobenzyl parachlorophenol in a drinking glass cleanser. *Contact Dermatitis* 1986; 14:247–248.

130. Storrs FJ. Personal communication; 1996.

131. Suskind RR, Meister MM, Scheen SR, et al. Cutaneous effects of household synthetic detergents and soaps. *Arch Dermatol* 1963; 88:117–124.

132. Sylvest B, Hjarth N, Magnuson B. Lauryl ether sulfate dermatitis in Denmark. *Contact Dermatitis* 1975; 1:359–362.

133. Symposium on skin cleaning. *Trans St Johns Hosp Dermatol Soc* 1965; 51:133–252.

134. Tosti A, Piraccini BM, Bardazzi F. Occupational contact dermatitis due to Quaternium-15. *Contact Dermatitis* 1990; 23:41–42.

135. Valer M. Skin irritancy and allergy to laundry detergents containing proteolytic enzymes. *Berufsdermatosen* 1975; 23:16–30.

136. Valsecchi R, Cassina GP, Migliori M, et al. Tego dermatitis. *Contact Dermatitis* 1985; 12:230.

137. Van Haute N, Dooms-Goossens A. Shampoo dermatitis due to cocobetaine and sodium lauryl ether sulfate. *Contact Dermatitisc* 1983; 9:169.

138. Wahlberg JE. Percutaneous absorption from chromium (51Cr) solutions of different pH 1.4-12.8. *Dermatologica* 1969; 137:17–25.

139. Wahlberg JE. Routine patch testing with Irgasan DP-300. *Contact Dermatitis* 1976; 2:292.

140. Wahlberg JE, Wennersten G. Hypersensitivity and photosensitivity to chlorhexidine. *Dermatologica* 1971; 143:376–379.

141. Warren R, Ertel KD, Bartolo RG, et al. The influence of hard water (calcium) and surfactants on irritant contact dermatitis. *Contact Dermatitis* 1996; 35:337–343.

142. Weaver JE. Personal communications, 1981. Cincinnati: Procter & Gamble.

143. Weaver JE. Dose-response relationships in delayed hypersensitivity to quinoline dye. *Contact Dermatitis* 1983; 9:309–312.

144. Weaver JE, Hermann KW. Evaluation of adverse reaction reports for a new laundry product. *J Am Acad Dermatol* 1981; 4:577–583.

145. White IR, Lewis J, Alami AE. Possible adverse reactions to an enzyme-containing laundry powder. *Contact Dermatitis* 1985; 13:175–179.

146. Wilkinson DS. Photodermatitis due to tetrachlorosalicylanilide. *Br J Dermatol* 1961; 73:213–219.

147. Wilkinson RN. Detergents. In: Considine DM, ed. *Chemical and Process Technology Encyclopedia*. New York: McGraw-Hill; 1974:347–348.

148. Wilkinson SM, Schouten P, English JSC. Allergic contact dermatitis from Tego 51. *Contact Dermatitis* 1991; 24:74–75.

149. Willis I, Kligman AM. The mechanism of photoallergic contact dermatitis. *J Invest Dermatol* 1988; 51:378–384.

150. Wuthrich B, Ott F. Industrial asthma caused by proteases in the detergent industry. *Swiss Med J* 1969; 99:1584.

151. Yates VM, Finn OA. Contact allergic sensitivity to zinc pyrithione followed by the photosensitivity dermatitis and actinic reticuloid syndrome. *Contact Dermatitisc* 1980; 6:349–350.

152. Zachariae H, Thomsen K, Gowertz Rasmussen O. Occupational enzyme dermatitis. *Acta Derm Venereol* 1973; 53:145–148.

153. Zaugg T, Hunziker T. Germall II and Triclosan. *Contact Dermatitis* 1987; 17:262–263.

154. Zemstov A, Taylor JS, Evey P, et al. Allergic contact dermatitis from formaldehyde in a liquid soap. *Cleve Clin J Med* 1990; 57:301–303.

Cosmetics

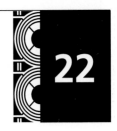

JAMES G. MARKS, JR., M.D.

The U. S. Food and Drug Administration (FDA) broadly defines cosmetics as topical agents for personal grooming that influence appearance and improve self-image. If they have an active ingredient, such as the aluminum salts found in antiperspirants or the para-aminobenzoic acid (PABA) found in sunscreens, they are classified as over-the-counter drugs. The division between cosmetics and over-the-counter drugs, is not, however, always clear. By legal definition, cosmetics are not supposed to affect the structure or function of the skin. They are intended to be rubbed, poured, sprinkled, or sprayed on, or otherwise applied to the human body for cleaning, beautifying, or altering its appearance. New biologically active ingredients in cosmetics, particularly those aimed at altering the aging process, have created problems with this definition. The European Union (EU) and Japan have significant differences from the United States in their definitions and regulations of cosmetics that make these issues even more complex.

The cosmetics industry in the United States is regulated primarily by two federal laws, the Federal Food Drug and Cosmetic Act of 1938, with its color additive amendment of 1962, and the Fair Packaging and Labeling Act of 1966. These laws are enforced by the FDA and the Federal Trade Commission (FTC). The cosmetics industry, however, is primarily a self-regulated industry that uses three FDA-industry voluntary programs: (1) the Cosmetic Product Ingredient Statement filing (CPIS), (2) the Cosmetic Establishment Registration Program for plants (CERP), and (3) the Product Experience Registration program for adverse reactions (PER).[1, 2]

Drugs are intended to treat or prevent disease or otherwise affect the structure and function of the skin. Some products are considered cosmetics even though they have, by strict definition, the

properties of a drug. For example, antidandruff shampoos are sold to treat and prevent seborrheic dermatitis. Antiperspirants affect the function of the body, resulting in decreased sweating. Sunscreens protects against sunburn and skin cancer. There is no statutory requirement that cosmetic products or ingredients be proved safe, as is the case with new drugs or food additives.

To remove a cosmetic from the marketplace, the FDA must demonstrate that the cosmetic may be harmful to consumers under customary conditions of use. This requires adequate toxicological and epidemiological data. Fortunately, the cosmetics industry has removed ingredients on its own when potential harm has been identified. For example, acetyl ethyl tetramethyl tetralin (AETT), a synthetic fragrance, was at one time present in many cosmetics. Topical application to rats produced neurotoxicity and blue discoloration of internal organs. The industry voluntarily discontinued the use of AETT after these findings became known. There were no reports of human toxicity from this ingredient.[3] Nor does the cosmetic product's labeling have to be substantiated prior to introduction. The proliferation of skincare products that claim to be antiaging and wrinkle-preventing is an example of controversial labeling. The burden of proof that a product is unsafe or deceptively packaged rests with the FDA and FTC. Removal of a cosmetic from the marketplace can occur when the product is deemed harmful by the FDA or when labeling is deemed misleading or false by the FTC.

Literally millions of individuals use cosmetics each and every day without problems. Most manufacturers, realizing that a large number of consumers use their products and that adverse reactions could harm sales, do extensive premarket testing. This includes testing for irritancy and allergenicity, ingredient and product stability, microbiological preservation and contamination with microbials such as bacteria and fungi, and systemic toxicity. The cosmetic industry is large, profitable, complex, and sophisticated. It is a blend of art and science. Approximately 8,000 raw materials and fragrance ingredients are used in the making of cosmetic products.[4]

As a class of consumer products, cosmetics include toiletries, skin-care products, makeups, and fragrances. Soaps, shampoos, hair rinses and conditioners, hair dressings, sprays, and setting lotions, hair colorings, hair waving and straightening agents, deodorants, antiperspirants, and sun-protective agents are examples of toiletries. Skin-care products include shaving agents, cosmetic cleaners, astringents, toners, moisturizers, masks, night creams, and bath products. Makeup products are found in the form of foundations (liquid makeups), eye shadows, eyebrow pencils and eyeliners, mascaras, lipsticks, rouges, blushers, and nail polishes. Perfumes, colognes, toilet waters, aftershave lotions, body silks, and bath powders are examples of cosmetics that contain fragrances.[5]

The psychological, emotional, and social benefits of the improved appearance of the skin, hair, and nails must be balanced by the potential adverse reactions or risks of the intentional and unintentional use of cosmetic preparations. Fortunately, cosmetics are remarkably safe. Their mass public use, however, has resulted in adverse reactions, such as burning or irritation of the skin, allergic contact dermatitis, photoallergic and phototoxic reactions, acne, contact urticaria, hypo- and hyperpigmentation, and hair and nail dystrophy and discoloration.

Most of the information concerning adverse cutaneous reactions to cosmetics is gleaned from individual case reports published in the medical literature, from consumer reactions reported to cosmetics manufacturers or the FDA, and from the collective experience of patch-testing clinics. This must be put into perspective: it probably represents the tip of the iceberg, as these individuals have had reactions significant enough to result in their seeking medical care. Surely, the vast majority of individuals with minor reactions simply tolerate them or stop using the suspected cosmetic and switch to another product.

Certain generalizations may be made about the occurrence of contact dermatitis in response to cosmetics in the general population: (1) 4 to 5% of patch-testing clinic patients had contact dermatitis as a reaction to a cosmetic; (2) frequently, neither the patient nor the physician was aware that a cosmetic was the causative agent of the dermatitis prior to testing; (3) most of the reactions were associated with skin-care and hair-care

products; (4) most reactions occurred in adults, with women being predominantly affected; (5) the face and periorbital regions were the most commonly involved areas; and (6) fragrances and preservatives were the most common causes of cutaneous reactions.[6, 7] In the United States, regulations require that all ingredients be declared on the cosmetic's label, making it easier for the consumer to avoid known allergens.

Two industrial groups have been instrumental in reviewing the safety of cosmetics' ingredients: (1) the Cosmetic Ingredient Review (CIR), 1110 Vermont Ave., N.W., Suite 800, Washington, D.C. 20005; and (2) the International Fragrance Association (IFRA), 800 rue Charles-Humbert, CH-1205, Geneva, Switzerland. Manufacturers, suppliers, and testing laboratories, which number more than 500 members and account for more than 90% of all the cosmetic products in the United States, make up the Cosmetic, Toiletry, and Fragrance Association (CTFA). The CTFA publishes the *CTFA Dictionary*, which lists more than 3,800 cosmetic ingredients, and the booklet *The Cosmetics Industry on Call*, which provides the names, addresses, and telephone numbers of key individuals in cosmetics companies who can provide technical data and patch-testing samples.

Two investigations, one in North America and the other in Europe, helped to identify which products (Table 22–1) and ingredients (Table 22–2) are the most common causes of cutaneous reactions to cosmetics.[6, 7] The following discussion focuses first on occupational contact dermatitis caused by cosmetics and then on cosmetic products and the individual ingredients that cause dermatitis.

OCCUPATIONAL SKIN DISEASE CAUSED BY COSMETICS

Hairdressers and manicurists are the workers at highest risk for developing occupational skin disease that results from cosmetics. Occupational skin disease in workers who manufacture cosmetics must be uncommon, as there are few reports in the literature,[8] and personal communications with toxicologists in the cosmetics industry fail to reveal significant problems or outbreaks. This is probably the result of a combination of factors, including good manufacturing processes that reduce skin contact (most major companies manufacture cosmetic products according to the FDA's Good Manufacturing Practice Regulations for Drug Products), and that ensure that whatever contact does occur involves normal skin rather than skin with dermatitis. The following discussion, therefore, deals predominantly with cosme-

TABLE 22–1 • Cutaneous Reactions to Cosmetic Products[a]

	North America[b]	Netherlands[c]
Skin-care products	28%	52%
Hair products	25%	7%
Facial makeup	10%	1%
Nail preparations	8%	8%
Fragrance	7%	3%
Hygiene products	6%	—
Eye makeup	4%	4%
Shaving preparations	4%	8%
Other cosmetics	13%	17%

[a]Irritant and allergic contact dermatitis
[b]North American Contact Dermatitis Group; 713 patients[6]
[c]De Groot A; 75 patients[7]

tologists—beauticians, hair stylists, and manicurists.

Hairdressers

Contact dermatitis of the hands is the main occupational hazard for hairdressers.[9, 10] Prior to becoming a licensed hairdresser, required schooling teaches the biological and pathological features of the scalp and hair, the chemistry of compounds used, and the technique and art of hair cleaning, conditioning, cutting, waving, styling, and coloring.

In contrast to some industries that are regionally located, hairdressers are found universally, and all physicians who treat occupational skin disease

TABLE 22–2 • Cosmetic Ingredients Causing Cutaneous Reactions[a]

	North America[b]	Netherlands[c]
Fragrance	30%	45%
Preservative	28%	21%
p-Phenylenediamine	8%	4%
Lanolin	5%	6%
Glycerol monothioglycolate	5%	—
Propylene glycol	5%	—
Toluene sulfonamide formaldehyde resin	4%	7%
Sunscreens and ultraviolet absorbers	4%	6%
Acrylates	1%	—
Others	10%	11%

[a]Irritant and allergic contact dermatitis
[b]North American Contact Dermatitis Group; 713 patients
[c]De Groot A; 75 patients

will see these workers. The U.S. National Hairdressers and Cosmetologists Association found that 50% of 405 respondents had experienced dermatitis caused by shampoos, permanent wave solutions, or hair bleaches. Of the 203 hairdressers with dermatitis, 63 had been seen by a dermatologist,[11] and 20 had chronic dermatitis. As with other occupationally induced hand dermatitis, a history of atopic dermatitis puts the hairdresser particularly at risk. Hairdressing, therefore, is one of those occupations that would be a poor career choice for atopic individuals.

Apprentices, who do the most shampooing, are at greater risk for contracting irritant contact dermatitis. This makes the development of allergic contact dermatitis and chronic, self-perpetuating dermatitis an even greater risk for them in the future. The prognosis of chronic dermatitis is guarded, even in the experienced hairdresser. Topical therapy, allergen avoidance, and the wearing of gloves, although helpful, may not prevent its self-perpetuation.

The most common causes of allergic contact dermatitis in hairdressers are p-phenylenediamine in permanent hair dyes, glyceryl thioglycolate in acid permanent waving solutions, rubber chemicals in gloves (Fig. 22–1), nickel in tools, and ammonium persulfate in hair bleach.

A study of 100 hairdressers with hand eczema by James and Calnan[12] revealed 23 individuals who had allergic contact dermatitis. Of the 100, 61 had irritant dermatitis and 16 had atopic dermatitis complicated by irritant contact dermatitis. The most common allergen was p-phenylenediamine causing allergic contact dermatitis in 12 hairdressers, whereas 10 reacted to ammonium thioglycolate. Because patch-testing with ammonium thioglycolate is difficult, these 10 cases were probably irritant reactions rather than allergic contact dermatitis. Only 5 individuals had a sensitivity to the rubber gloves they had worn for protection.

Calnan and Schuster[13] described several hairdressers who had urticaria and dermatitis secondary to the ammonium persulfate found in bleaches. Bleaches are most universally based on hydrogen peroxide, which destroys the pigment of the hair. Ammonium hydroxide is added to activate the bleaching activity of hydrogen peroxide. The hydrogen peroxide-ammonia bleach combination is accelerated or boosted with ammonium or potassium persulfate. Contact urticaria and severe anaphylactic reactions have been produced in some patients. Therefore, testing with ammonium persulfate must be done cautiously.[14] Kellet and Beck[15] found ammonium persulfate to be a relatively common sensitizer in hairdressers. Using a 2.5% concentration in petrolatum and in aqueous

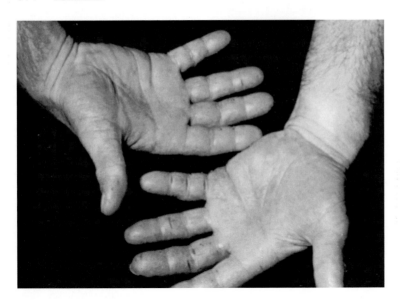

FIGURE 22–1 • Allergic contact dermatitis to thiuram in the rubber gloves worn by this hairdresser. He also had irritant contact dermatitis from shampooing as well as atopic hand dermatitis. He eventually quit his job.

solution, 12 of 49 hairdressers had positive reactions, whereas only 1 of 118 control subjects reacted positively. Because of degradation, the allergen samples should be replaced every 6 months.

Wahlberg[16] studied 35 hairdressers with hand eczema and found that 29 of them had positive patch-testing results in response to substances found in the standard tray or to the products in their salons, or to both. Of these individuals, 14 reacted to nickel, 9 reacted to hair dyes, and 10 reacted to rubber chemicals. The high prevalence of nickel allergy was attributed to wet work in combination with the use of nickel-containing tools such as scissors, clips, pins, rollers, and rods.

When Marks and Cronin[17] studied 60 English hairdressers with hand dermatitis, 70% were found to have positive patch-test results in response to at least one allergen, and the longer the duration of eczema, the greater the chance of sensitivity.

The experience of the St. John's Contact Dermatitis Clinic[18] is similar to that of others. Of 84 hairdressers tested, 48 had positive patch-test reactions. The most common cause of allergic contact dermatitis was hair dyes; this was true in 27 individuals (32%). p-Phenylenediamine, p-toluenediamine, and orthonitroparaphenylenediamine were the dyes tested. Ammonium persulfate caused positive reactions in 15 individuals and may have been either irritant or allergic. Nickel sulfate caused 16 positive reactions, and rubber chemicals caused 2 positive reactions.

Cronin and Kullavanijaya[19] studied 107 employees at a hairdressing salon in a large London store. Of 33 junior hairdressers, 30 had hand dermatitis. They had a dry irritant dermatitis of the hands caused by frequent shampooing, and it disappeared when the shampooing stage of their training was over. Only 1 of 25 stylists had dermatitis.

Hannuksela and Hassi[20] studied 30 women hairdressers from small salons and 2 barbers. They found 12 subjects with hand dermatitis; 3 of them had allergic contact dermatitis, 1 to p-phenylenediamine and 2 to nickel.

Lynde and Mitchell[21] patch-tested 66 hairdressers with the North American Contact Dermatitis Group Standard Screening Tray or with a Hairdressing Screening Tray. Of the 66, 48 subjects had one or more positive reactions: 30 reacted to p-phenylenediamine, 18 to nickel sulfate, and 6 to glyceryl thioglycolate. All 10 patients who had positive reactions to para derivatives (p-aminophenylamine, orthonitroparaphenylenediamine, and p-toluenediamine sulfate) had positive reactions to p-phenylenediamine, making it an excellent screening compound for hair dye sensitivity. Selected other chemicals produced positive reactions in 4 patients.

Nethercott and coworkers[22] reported on 18 cases of hand dermatitis in hairdressers seen in Toronto, Canada. p-Phenylenediamine and related hair dyes were the predominant cause of allergic contact dermatitis in younger hairdressers, whereas formaldehyde allergy was the cause in those who were older. The hand dermatitis often resulted in the worker's being unable to continue in the hairdressing trade.

Matsunaga and coworkers[23] patch-tested 13 beauticians with hand dermatitis and found the causes of allergic contact dermatitis in Japan to be similar to those in North America and Europe. Of the 13, 12 individuals had positive reactions to p-phenylenediamine and 3 had positive reactions to ammonium thioglycolate that were considered to be allergic in nature. All their subjects were young female novice beauticians or were in training. Of the 12 individuals, 5 continued in the occupation. However, 4 individuals had persistent hand dermatitis despite protective measures. Of the 7 beauticians who quit, the dermatitis healed in 5 of them, whereas 2 continued to have atopic hand dermatitis.

Reviewing these and more recent studies of hairdressers reveals the following common conclusions: (1) hairdressers are at significant risk of developing occupationally induced hand dermatitis, particularly hairdressers with a history of atopic dermatitis; (2) the allergens present on standard patch-testing trays provide an excellent screening series for hairdressers, with the exception of glyceryl thioglycolate and ammonium persulphate; (3) contact urticaria occurs in response to latex, ammonium persulfate, and other styling products; (4) once dermatitis occurs, it is important to reduce its severity and clear it as quickly as possible to prevent self-perpetuation despite the affected individual's leaving work.[24–32]

The prevention and management of hand dermatitis in hairdressers can be difficult. Van der Walle[33] suggested several preventive measures, including: (1) washing infrequently, (2) frequently using moisturizers, (3) wearing disposable vinyl gloves for shampooing, bleaching, and dying, (4) avoiding nickel in tools and jewelry, and (5) keeping the workplace clean and tidy. Once contact dermatitis develops, identifying the putative chemical and avoiding exposure to it is the obvious, but not always easy, solution.

Manicurists and Nail Artists

Manicurists are cosmetologists who specialize in the care of fingernails and toenails. They shape, trim, clean, and polish the nail plate, trim and remove the cuticle, remove and apply nail enamels, and mend and apply artificial nails. There are no epidemiological surveys of occupational skin disease among manicurists, and few case reports.[33–37] Cleaning the nails in soapy water and removing enamels with solvents exposes manicurists to primary irritants. Sensitization may occur, as was reported in a manicurist in whom allergic contact dermatitis of the right hand developed secondary to an orangewood stick used for applying cuticle remover.[38] Sensitization may occur as a result of exposure to the toluene sulfonamide formaldehyde resin in nail polish, the cyanoacrylic glues used to mend nails and to apply press-on nails, and the acrylic monomers used to make artificial sculptured nails.[39] Toluene sulfonamide formaldehyde resin seems to be a problem for the client rather than for the manicurist. A more likely cause of allergic contact dermatitis among manicurists is sensitization to the acrylic monomers in sculptured nails and the cyanoacrylate glue used to repair fractured nail plates and to apply press-on, preformed plastic plates. An illustrative case is a manicurist seen at the Hershey Medical Center Patch Test Clinic who applied artificial sculptured nails using acrylic plastics that were self-cured and ultraviolet light-cured. Patch tests revealed positive reactions to multiple methacrylate monomers, and upon discontinuation of her work as a manicurist, her hand dermatitis cleared (Fig. 22–2). Another manicurist had hand dermatitis for 8 months. She was trained as a hairdresser and manicurist but limited her work to the care and enhancement of fingernails. Her job entailed all the routine functions of a manicurist, including the application of press-on fingernails as well as mending nails with cyanoacrylate glue. Despite the use of topical and systemic steroids, the hand dermatitis resulted in loss of work. Her

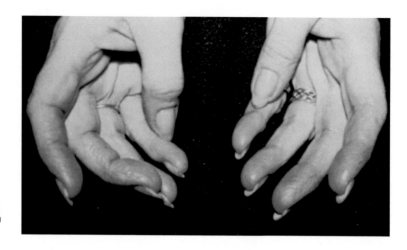

FIGURE 22–2 • Allergic contact dermatitis to artificial sculptured nails, which this manicurist applied on clients. Her hands cleared when she stopped this work.

hand dermatitis persisted even after a 2-month absence from the salon. After a positive open test to cyanoacrylic glue, she realized that she was continuing to mend her own fingernails with the glue two or three times a week. She had negative patch-test results to methacrylate monomers and to toluene sulfonamide formaldehyde resin.

For manicurists to be patch-tested appropriately, a few additional chemicals besides the standard allergens should be used. They include toluene sulfonamide formaldehyde resin for nail polish sensitivity, cyanoacrylate glue, and acrylic monomers to screen for sensitivity to artificial nails.[40] Five acrylates have been identified as screening allergens for reactions to artificial nails: ethyl acrylate, 2-hydroxy ethyl acrylate, ethylene glycol dimethacryate, ethyl α cyanoacrylate, and triethylene glycol diacrylate.[41] If the screening of acrylic monomers produces negative results, further testing must be done with the specific nail preparation, as there may not be total crossreactivity among these chemicals.

FRAGRANCES

Perfumes are complex mixtures of fragrance ingredients that are of organic (derived from animal or plant sources) and synthetic origin. Many of these aromatic chemicals are used as both fragrances and flavorings. Cinnamic aldehyde, for example, is found commonly in perfumes, household deodorizers, detergents, soaps, and toothpastes and also in soft drinks, candy, chewing gum, and ice cream. The North American Contact Dermatitis Group's (NACDG) prospective study of cosmetic reactions identified fragrances as the leading cause of allergic contact dermatitis.[6] This was confirmed by others.[7] Although photodermatitis, contact urticaria, irritation, and depigmentation are occasionally seen, the most common reaction is allergic contact dermatitis.[42–49] The maximum concentration of fragrances allowed in various products is as follows: masking perfumes, 0.1% or less; cosmetics, 0.5%; colognes, 4.0%; toilet water, 5.0%; and perfumes, 20.0%. Several groups have been formed to evaluate the safety of fragrance materials, including the Research Institute of Fragrance Materials (RIFM) and the International Fragrance Association (IFRA). Based on the results of the scientific advisory committee reviews, as well as on information from industrial laboratories and academic research, these groups provide guidelines for ingredient usage.[50]

Perfumery is both a science and an art. The perfumer combines the biochemistry of the fragrance ingredients with the artistry of blending aromas to produce the final product. Creative perfumers have an extensive odor memory based upon which they able to create pleasing and harmonious perfumes that have identity and character. They write a formula almost like a recipe, listing the exact amounts of various ingredients to be included in the mixture. A typical fragrance formula contains 200 to 300 individual ingredients, and some perfumes can contain up to 800 ingredients. Once blended together, the perfumer adjusts the mixture to fit his or her mental image by adding or deleting ingredients. Although it may appear simple, it is not. The creative perfumer has to have not only the chemical background but also a highly developed odor memory, an instinct for odor harmony, and an ability to balance fragrance formulations to achieve a pleasing and distinctive fragrance.[51]

Approximately 1,500 ingredients are used to formulate most fragrances, although up to 5,000 to 6,000 have been cited in the literature. Fewer than 100 of these ingredients appear to have significant toxicity, and most of these offenders are contact allergens.[52–54] Carcinogens and neurotoxins are extremely rare in fragrance ingredients at present.

The 5-year study of cosmetic reactions conducted by the North American Contact Dermatitis Group from 1977 to 1983 identified 161 reactions to fragrances.[6] Most were from unspecified fragrances (67 reactions). Individual fragrances, identified in decreasing order of frequency, were cinnamic alcohol, 17 reactions; musk ambrette, 17 reactions; hydroxycitronellal, 11 reactions; isoeugenol, 10 reactions; geraniol, 8 reactions; cinnamic aldehyde, 4 reactions; coumarin, 4 reactions; and eugenol, 4 reactions.

Although these individual cosmetic ingredients are sensitizing, this potential may be reduced by a phenomenon known as quenching.[55] For example, allantoin has been shown to reduce the irritant and allergenic potential of PABA, and cinnamic aldehyde mixed with eugenol appears to reduce the sensitizing potential of both these fragrances. Some investigators, however, doubt the quenching phenomenon.[56] Other methods of reducing the sensitization potential include reducing the concentration of sensitizers, increasing the purity and standardization of both natural and synthetic products, and using antioxidants, sequestering agents, neutralizers, and quenching agents.

Cinnamic Alcohol and Cinnamic Aldehyde

Cinnamic alcohol (cinnamyl alcohol) and cinnamic aldehyde (cinnamaldehyde) are used as both flavoring agents and fragrances. They are found in beverages, chewing gum, mouthwashes, soaps, and toothpastes, as well as in cosmetics.

Cinnamic alcohol is found in the free state or as an ester in cinnamon leaves, hyacinth, and essence of daffodil flowers. It is prepared by the reduction of cinnamic aldehyde. The usual concentration of cinnamic alcohol varies from 0.05% in soaps and creams to 0.30% in perfumes.[57] Because of its sensitizing capacity, the IFRA recommends that cinnamic alcohol be used in a concentration of less than 4%.

Cinnamic aldehyde is found in cinnamon leaves and bark and in the essential oils of hyacinth and myrrh. It is manufactured by the condensation of acetaldehyde with benzaldehyde. Its concentration varies from 0.003% in creams to 0.100% in perfumes.[58] Cinnamic aldehyde is a skin irritant and a strong sensitizer. Schorr found positive patch-test results to this fragrance in 3% of 34 males and 9% of 55 females with contact dermatitis of unknown cause.[59] The NACDG found 62 allergic reactions to cinnamic aldehyde in 1,048 patients tested between January 1984 and May 1985. Tolerance of perfumes containing cinnamic aldehyde in a patient known to be sensitive to it has been reported, suggesting a quenching phenomenon. The IFRA recommends cinnamic aldehyde be used with an equal proportion by weight of eugenol to prevent sensitization. Cinnamic alcohol and cinnamic aldehyde crossreact, and along with contact dermatitis, they have caused hypo- and hyperpigmentation and contact urticaria.[59–61]

Eugenol and Isoeugenol

Eugenol and isoeugenol do not necessarily crossreact. Eugenol is isolated from the essential oils of the clove bud and leaf and the cinnamon leaf. Its usual concentration varies from 0.03% in creams and lotions to 0.40% in perfumes. Eugenol is used in over-the-counter medications such as inhalants and antiseptics.[62]

Isoeugenol is found in the oils of clove, ylang ylang, and jonquil, and is manufactured by the isomerization of eugenol. Because of its sensitizing capacity, it has been recommended that isoeugenol be used at no more than a 1% concentration in fragrance compounds.[63]

Oak Moss Absolute

Oak moss absolute is derived from the tree lichen oak moss, or *Evernia prunasti*. It is commonly used in aftershave lotions. Allergic contact dermatitis in response to lichen substances has usually been reported in occupational settings in which individuals such as foresters, gardeners, and lichen pickers are exposed during work. Allergy to oak moss absolute, however, does occur in response to aftershave lotions and less commonly to perfumes. Oak moss contains atranorin, evernic acid, and fumarprotocetaric acid, among other chemicals, as the potential allergens.[64–66]

Hydroxycitronellal

Hydroxycitronellal is widely used in perfumes, antiseptics, and insecticides. It is a synthetic compound prepared by hydration of citronellal and is not found in nature. Its usual concentration is 0.02% in creams and lotions and 0.20% in perfumes. The IFRA recommends it not be used at a level of more than 5.0% in fragrance compounds.[67]

Musk Ambrette

Musk ambrette causes allergic and photoallergic contact dermatitis (Fig. 22–3). This synthetic chemical is found in fragrances, soaps, detergents, creams, lotions, and dentifrices. In all patients who are photosensitive to musk ambrette, the der-

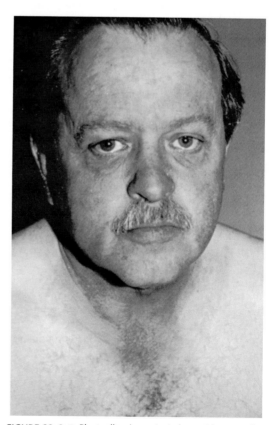

FIGURE 22–3 • Photoallergic contact dermatitis to musk ambrette in an aftershave lotion.

matitis initially begins in the sun-exposed areas of the face, neck, and arms, but with chronic photodermatitis, it may become generalized and cause persistent light sensitivity. The IFRA recommends that musk ambrette not be used in a concentration greater than 4% as a fragrance ingredient and not be used in compounds for cosmetics, toiletries, and other products that normally involve skin contact.[68, 69]

Balsam of Peru

Balsam of Peru is included in standard patch-test series as a screen for fragrance sensitivity. Many of the allergens found in fragrances are ingredients of balsam of Peru or are chemically related. They include benzyl alcohol, benzyl acetate, cinnamic alcohol, cinnamic aldehyde, cinnamic acid, eugenol, isoeugenol, and other coniferyl alcohols. The IFRA recommends that balsam of Peru not be used as a fragrance ingredient. Balsam of Peru is obtained from trees *(Toluifera perriae)* that grow in El Salvador. It is a natural product that is a thick brown liquid containing a mixture of resin compounds and having an aroma of vanilla and cinnamon. Balsam of Peru is used by the pharmaceutical, cosmetic, and flavoring industries. Although approximately half of patients sensitive to fragrances react to balsam of Peru, if perfume sensitivity is suspected, it is necessary that the fragrance mixture, as well as the specific perfume to which the subject is exposed, be tested.[70, 71]

PRESERVATION OF COSMETICS

Preservatives are the most common cosmetic ingredient to cause contact dermatitis. The need for preservation to prevent the growth of microorganisms is twofold. First, contamination of the cosmetic with bacteria or fungi can result in spoilage, preventing its sale and use. Second, microorganisms in the contaminated cosmetic could cause infection in consumers. The potential of harmful health effects on users became evident when staphylococcal infections were reported in hospitals because of the use of contaminated hand creams and hand lotions.[73] In addition, some eye infections that occurred during the 1970s appeared to be associated with the use of contaminated mascaras,[74] and more recently, an outbreak of invasive mycoses was caused by a contaminated skin lotion.[75] Thus, the cosmetic preservative should be sufficient to prevent spoilage as well as to prevent the growth of inadvertently added microorganisms under conditions of normal use. With this goal in mind, it would seem that one

need only choose a chemical that will kill the microorganisms and add it to the cosmetic. There has to be a balance, though, between the desired preservation of the cosmetic and the potential harm it may cause to the consumer—for example, allergic contact dermatitis.

Despite there being hundreds of chemicals that have germicidal actions, only a few of them are used. The use of preservatives in cosmetics formulas is disclosed by cosmetic manufacturers when they voluntarily register their product formulations with the FDA under the CPIS program. The 10 most commonly used preservatives are listed in Table 22–3.[76] The limited number is a reflection of the compound's safety and effectiveness when placed in the final cosmetic product. In contrast to the perfumer who has hundreds of compounds to choose from, the cosmetic microbiologist has relatively few compounds to choose from. The ideal preservative should have (1) broad antimicrobial activity, (2) effectiveness over a wide range of pH, (3) effectiveness for the entire shelf-life of the product, (4) antimicrobial activity in both oil and water vehicles, (5) compatibility with the other cosmetic ingredients, (6) nontoxic and nonirritating qualities, and (7) low cost.

Cosmetics systems incorporating a formula with more than a single preservative were developed to meet these requirements to cover a wide spectrum of microbial organisms. Cosmetics, generally, are not sterile products and are made from raw materials that are not sterile. They are not sterilized during manufacture and are usually in multiple-use containers that allow contamination by the consumer. When sufficient water is present, aqueous cosmetics will support the growth of microorganisms unless preservatives are added. Anhydrous materials, such as petrolatum and powders, may be temporarily contaminated with repeated

TABLE 22–3 • Preservatives: Frequency of Use in Cosmetic Formulas, 1996

Preservative	1996
Methylparaben	7,731
Propylparaben	6,278
Imidazolidinyl urea	2,498
Butylparaben	1,991
Ethylparaben	1,240
Phenoxyethanol	1,143
DMDM hydantoin	955
Methylchloroisothiazolinone/ methylisothiazolinone	808
Sodium sulfite	789
Quaternium-15	704

use, but will not support the growth of microorganisms unless water is present. The microorganisms may be either pathogens or nonpathogens. If *Pseudomonas aeruginosa* or *Staphylococcus aureus* contaminates the product, there is a possibility that skin infection will result. The presence of nonpathogens, although not a health hazard, may result in spoilage.[77]

Parabens

The parabens are the most commonly used preservatives in cosmetics today. They are the alkyl esters of parahydroxybenzoic acid. The methyl, propyl, and butyl parabens are the most widely used. The properties that make them ideal cosmetic preservatives are that they are colorless, odorless, nonvolatile, stable, effective over a wide range of pH, and have low cost and a relatively broad spectrum of antimicrobial activity. Each ester has a different antimicrobial range, but in general they are more effective against fungi than against bacteria and are more effective against gram-positive bacteria than against gram-negative bacteria. They are usually used in combination rather than singly, and because of their poor activity against gram-negative bacteria, especially *Pseudomonas aeruginosa*, they are often used in combination with other types of preservatives. The parabens are believed to be among the safest of all cosmetic preservatives, considering their widespread use and low incidence of adverse reactions. When used in cosmetics on normal skin, they are virtually nonsensitizing. When incorporated into topical medications to be used on skin with dermatitis, however, the potential for sensitization is greater. The parabens are commonly used in cosmetics at a concentration of 0.1 to 0.8%. The combination of parabens with other preservatives, specifically imidazolidinyl urea or quaternium-15, increases the antimicrobial spectrum of activity, allows a lower concentration of the independent preservative components, reduces potential toxic reactions, and prevents the development of resistent organisms.[78]

Paraben esters are not strong sensitizers. Predictive testing as well as years of use in cosmetics confirm this. Parabens used in cosmetics can cause sensitization when applied to normal skin.[79, 80] Most of the reports concerning paraben sensitivity, however, have involved the use of topical medicines used to treat eczematous skin or stasis ulcers.[81] Because of this, a number of topical medicinal formulations were changed to exclude parabens. There are several aspects of patch-testing and allergic contact dermatitis in response to parabens that produce conflicting or paradoxic

results.[82] One such paradox is the individual who is sensitized to parabens in topical medications, but who can continue to use cosmetics that contain parabens. One explanation for this paradox is that normal skin can tolerate exposure to small concentrations of parabens in cosmetics, whereas skin with dermatitis has reduced threshold for paraben-induced allergic contact dermatitis caused by a topical medicament. Another contradictory phenomenon is a false-negative patch-test result from a paraben-containing medicament that caused allergic contact dermatitis. One of several reasons for this conflicting result is that the medication is being used on skin with dermatitis, whereas patch-testing takes place on normal skin. Thus, the concentration of the paraben for patch-testing on normal skin must be increased to produce a positive reaction. Another explanation is that if the parabens are contained in a corticosteroid preparation, the anti-inflammatory effects of the steroid may suppress the elicitation of allergic contact dermatitis in normal skin.

In summary, parabens are the most commonly used preservatives in cosmetics. Although allergic contact dermatitis caused by parabens does exist, the risk of sensitization is low and does not constitute a significant hazard to the public.[83–85]

Imidazolidinyl Urea (Germall 115)

Imidazolidinyl urea was the first of a family of substituted imidazolidinyl urea compounds that became available after 1970. It was particularly timely, as the cosmetics industry needed new cosmetics preservatives following observations in Europe and the United States of gram-negative bacterial contamination of topical medications and cosmetics. Imidazolidinyl urea is a stable, odorless, white compound with high water solubility. Alone or in combination, it acts steadily and effectively against a wide range of organisms and has the stability to last over a long period. A sample preservative system that has been successful in numerous cosmetic products is 0.3% imidazolidinyl urea, 0.2% methyl paraben, and 0.1% propyl paraben. Imidazolidinyl urea is active primarily against bacteria, with less activity against fungi. It acts against *Pseudomonas aeruginosa*, with few strains having resistance. The combination of parabens and imidazolidinyl urea forms a very effective preservative system, covering both gram-positive and gram-negative bacteria, along with fungi.[86, 87]

Imidazolidinyl urea has been found to be widely accepted in the cosmetic industry because of its high degree of safety. Although imidazolidinyl urea is in the family of formaldehyde-releasing preservatives, only small amounts of formaldehyde are available, and most formaldehyde-sensitive patients do not react to this preservative. Repeated insult test with 10% imidazolidinyl urea on human subjects revealed neither irritation nor sensitization.[87] Widespread use, though, has resulted in some cases of allergic contact dermatitis.

A new member of the imidazolidinyl urea family, diazolidinyl urea (Germall II), has been introduced and is commercially available in cosmetic products. It resembles imidazolidinyl urea in physical, chemical, and toxicologic properties. However, it has greater activity against *Pseudomonas* and fungi. A drawback may be that it has greater sensitizing potential than does imidazolidinyl urea.[88–91]

Quaternium-15 (Dowicil 200)

The cosmetics preservative that caused the greatest number of allergic reactions in the North American Contact Dermatitis Group clinics was quaternium-15 (Fig. 22–4).[92] Quaternium-15 is a broad-spectrum antimicrobial that is used mainly in cosmetics, providing antimicrobial activity against bacteria and fungi. It is particularly effective against *Pseudomonas aeruginosa*. It is highly water soluble, being most effective in the water phase of formulations where it is needed. It is commonly used in cosmetic products at a concentration between 0.02 and 0.03%. Quaternium-15 is among the family of formaldehyde-releasing preservatives, which includes bronopol, DMDM hydantoin, imidazolidinyl urea (Germall-115), and diazolidinyl urea (Germall II). Although quaternium-15 does release small amounts of formaldehyde, not all patients who are allergic to quaternium-15 are allergic to formaldehyde and vice versa. The concentration of formaldehyde released by quaternium-15 is less than the threshold reactivity of formaldehyde-sensitive individuals in most cases. Thus, many formaldehyde-sensitive individuals can use products containing quaternium-15 without having allergic contact dermatitis develop.[93–96]

Formaldehyde

Formaldehyde is a colorless gas at room temperature. It is commonly sold as an aqueous solution, formalin, which contains 37 to 50% formaldehyde by dry weight. It was first used as a biological preservative in 1868.

Allergic contact dermatitis resulting from formaldehyde has been reported to be caused by permanent press clothing, paper, nail hardeners, coolants, photographic chemicals, carpet and fabric resins, air fresheners, and cosmetics. Formaldehyde sensitivity presents a significant problem because exposure is so widespread.[97] Its greatest use in cosmetics is in shampoos. Patients who have formaldehyde sensitivity can usually tolerate shampoos preserved with this chemical because it is quickly diluted and then washed away. Allergic contact dermatitis of the scalp or face rarely comes from this source. Formaldehyde showed significant sensitizing potential in predictive testing, but despite that, and probably because it is used mainly in products that wash off, it appears to be a relatively uncommon cause of cosmetically induced dermatitis. Studies by Jordan and coworkers[98] indicate that the threshold limit of 30 p.p.m. aqueous formaldehyde can be tolerated by formaldehyde-sensitive individuals if repeatedly applied to normal skin. The formaldehyde-releasing preservatives can be greater than or less than this threshold-eliciting response, explaining the varied patch-test reactions seen with these preservatives.[95, 96]

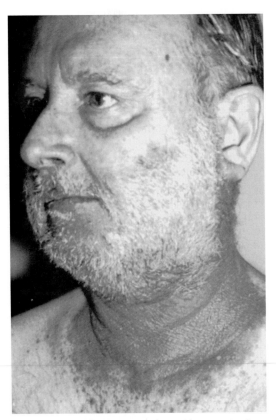

FIGURE 22–4 • Allergic contact dermatitis to quaternium-15 found in several moisturizers used by the patient. He also was sensitive to isoeugenol.

2-Bromo-2-nitro propane-1,3 diol (Bronopol)

Bronopol is an antimicrobial agent that is used in many cosmetics, including shampoos, hair conditioners, makeup, eye pencils and eyeliners, and cleansing lotions. It is an odorless, colorless to pale yellow compound that is soluble in water and has a broad spectrum of antibacterial action, especially against gram-negative organisms. Irritant and allergic contact dermatitis in animals and humans has been reported (Fig. 22–5).[99] Cosmetics contain bronopol concentrations of 0.01 to 0.20%. When that concentration is raised to 1% or more, it may be a considerable irritant.[100] There are data that suggest the possibility that when absorbed, bronopol may contribute to the endogenous formation of nitrosoamines or nitrosamides in humans and thus can be a potential carcinogen.[101]

Because it is a potential formaldehyde-releasing agent, it is not surprising that Fisher found that three of four formaldehyde-sensitive patients had positive results on bronopol patch-testing. He also had three patients with allergic contact dermatitis in response to bronopol found in cosmetics who reacted to patch-testing with formaldehyde.[102] Storrs and Bell[103] reported seven patients in whom allergic contact dermatitis developed after they used a bronopol-preserved moisturizing cream (Eucerin) on previously inflamed skin for periods varying from several weeks to a couple of years. None of these patients was allergic to formaldehyde or other formaldehyde-releasing preservatives. However, patients who became sensitized to bronopol in other cosmetics had previously been sensitive to formaldehyde and often to other formaldehyde releasers.

Methylchloroisothiazolinone/ Methylisothiazolinone (Kathon CG)

Kathon CG is a mixture of 5-chloro-2-methyl-4-isothiazolin-3-one and 2-methyl-4-isothiazolin-3-

one (MCI/MI). It has a wide range of compatibility with cosmetics ingredients and a broad spectrum of activity against bacteria and fungal organisms. Its recommended concentration in cosmetic and toiletry formulations, shampoos, hair conditioners, hair and body gels, skin creams, and lotions ranges from 0.02 to 0.10% (3 to 15 p.p.m. active ingredient).[104]

A rapid increase in allergic contact dermatitis caused by this chemical was noted in Europe in contrast to the experience in North America.[105, 106] In Europe, MCI/MI was used in maximum concentrations of 50 p.p.m. of active ingredient, and this may be one of the reasons for the increased reports of sensitivity. There are contradictory results and opinions in the literature regarding the proper patch-testing concentration. Therefore, different investigators have used varying concentrations for patch-testing. The highest nonirritating and nonsensitizing concentration of aqueous MCI/MI appears to be 100 p.p.m. Most cases of allergic contact dermatitis in response to MCI/MI were caused by moisturizing creams used on injured skin. Rinse-off products do not seem to be a significant cause of contact dermatitis.[107]

Methyldibromo Glutaronitrile Phenoxyethanol (Euxyl K-400)

Methyldibromo glutaronitrile phenoxyethanol is a 1:4 mixture of 1,2-dibromo-2,4-dicyanobutane and 2-phenoxy-ethanol. It has a broad spectrum of antibacterial activity against bacteria, fungi, and yeast and was introduced in Europe in 1985 and in the United States in 1990 for the preservation of cosmetics and personal care products.

The main preservative action is provided by 1,2-dibromo-2,4-dicyanobutane, which is a pow-

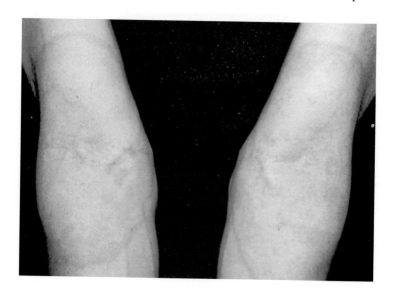

FIGURE 22–5 • Allergic contact dermatitis to bronopol, which was used to preserve a common moisturizer.

der and is mixed with the liquid phenoxyethanol for ease of use. Allergic contact dermatitis in response to the mixture has been reported to result from the use of a number of products, including ultrasonic gel, cucumber eye gel, cosmetic creams, and moist toilet papers. The sensitization rates of response to this preservative mixture in European contact dermatitis clinics range from 0.5 to 2.8%.

Methyldibromo glutaronitrile is the main allergen in this mixture, with phenoxyethanol having very little sensitizing potency. The Cosmetic Ingredient Review panel of experts concluded that methyldibromo glutaronitrile is safe if used in rinse-off products (concentrations in formulations range from 0.0075 to 0.0600%) and is safe in concentrations of up to 0.025% in leave-on products. Although methyldibromo glutaronitrile phenoxyethanol is available commercially for patch-testing at 0.5% in petrolatum, a 1.0% concentration may be preferable, and some investigators prefer a 2.5% concentration; however, the latter concentration may cause irritant reactions.[108–110]

NAIL PREPARATIONS

Nail polishes are varnishes or lacquers that are coated onto the nail plate. They include enamels, top coats, and base coats, which are similarly composed of a film former, a resin, a plasticizer, solvents, and colors. The film former is predominantly nitrocellulose and is used because it is hard and waterproof. Resins are added to improve the gloss and adhesion of the polish to the nail plate. The most commonly used resin is toluene sulfonamide formaldehyde resin. Plasticizers (camphor, dibutyl phthalate, and tricresyl phosphate) are added to prevent wrinkling and increase ease of applicability. Major ingredients in nail polishes are solvents, which account for about three-quarters of the product. They include acetates, acetones, methyl ethyl ketone, xylene, toluene, and alcohols. The solvents keep the nitrocellulose, resins, and plasticizers in a liquid state prior to application. Numerous colors are added, mostly insoluble pigments.

Nail mending or wrapping kits repair fractured nails with cyanoacrylate glue reinforced with wrapping materials such as paper, linen, or silk. Nail wrapping is done on the free edge of the nail that has splintered. Preformed, plastic press-on nails are used to cover the nail plate. They are glued in place with a cyanoacrylate glue. Another way of adding to or altering the nail plate is by using sculptured artificial nail kits, which contain a template, a liquid monomer, and a powdered polymer that is either self-curing or requires ultraviolet light polymerization. The natural nail plate is roughened and the artificial nail is then constructed by painting the liquid plastic on the nail plate immediately after mixing the liquid monomer with the powdered polymer prior to its hardening (Figs. 22–6 and 22–7).

Other preparations used for the care of nails include buffing creams to polish the nail plate; hardeners, which formerly contained formaldehyde; enamel removers; cuticle removers; and conditioners. The following discussion is limited to the most common causes of contact dermatitis resulting from use of nail preparations: toluene sulfonamide formaldehyde resin, acrylic nails, and cyanoacrylates glues.[111–113]

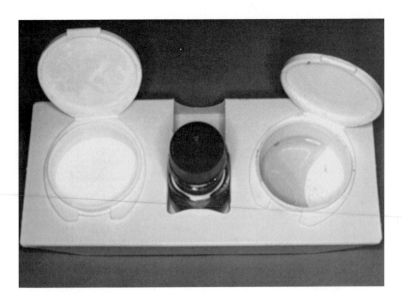

FIGURE 22–6 • Acrylic artificial nails setup with powdered monomer and liquid polymer in separate wells.

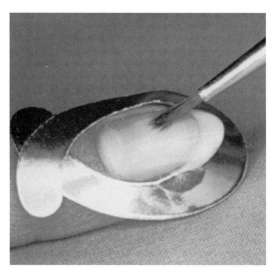

FIGURE 22–7 • Application of an acrylic artificial nail.

Toluene Sulfonamide Formaldehyde Resin

Toluene sulfonamide formaldehyde resin (tosylamide/formaldehyde resin) is added to nail polish to improve the gloss and the adhesion of the film. The pattern of allergic contact dermatitis to nail polish containing toluene sulfonamide formaldehyde resin characteristically involves the face, particularly the eyelids, and the sides of the neck. Less commonly, it can cause otitis externa, cheilitis, and generalized dermatitis. The dermatitis distant from the fingernails is a result of inadvertently transferring the resin from the nail plate to the skin, regardless of whether the nail polish is still wet. Besides periungual allergic contact dermatitis, toluene sulfonamide formaldehyde resin has caused onycholysis.[114–116]

Acrylic Artificial Nails

Acrylic plastics derive their basic structure from acrylic acid. They can combine with themselves or with other monomers or polymers. Acrylic compounds are widespread in cosmetics and in medical and industrial products. Exposure occurs through contact with dental plates, surgical prostheses, sealants, printing plates, coatings of glass, rubber, textile fibers, and artificial sculptured nails. Methyl methacrylate plastics are clear, colorless, and rigid, making them good substrates for artificial nail plates. The monomer is stable if an inhibitor (hydroquinone) is added, or if air and light are prohibited. Polymerization can be initiated by ultraviolet light, heat, oxygen, or peroxides. The powdered polymer is manufactured by adding benzyl peroxide to the liquid monomer as a catalyst. Despite polymerization, residual monomer persists, and in 1957 Fisher and coworkers[117] described four subjects who had allergic reactions to the methyl methacrylate in their acrylic plastic fingernails. In subsequent regulation by the FDA, methyl methacrylate was removed as an ingredient of artificial nails, but allergic contact dermatitis was reported in reaction to other monomers such as ethyl methacrylate.[118] Although cross-sensitization occurs, screening with only one acrylic plastic, such as methyl methacrylate, does not pick up all cases of acrylate sensitivity.[41, 119, 120] Besides allergic contact dermatitis, onycholysis, nail dystrophy, paronychia, and permanent nail loss have also been reported to result from use of these artificial nails.[121]

Cyanoacrylate Glues

Cyanoacrylate adhesives (Krazy Glue) are used to mend broken nails or apply preformed plastic nails. At one time it was believed that cyanoacrylates were not sensitizers, but this has proved to be untrue. The use of cyanoacrylates is widespread throughout industry because they polymerize rapidly at room temperature and have superb adhesive qualities for virtually any substance. These glues are composed of ethyl cyanoacrylate, hydroquinone, organic sulfonic acid, and polymethylmethacrylate. Paronychia, onychia, nail dystrophy, eyelid dermatitis, and a generalized dermatitis resembling parapsoriasis have been reported to occur as a result of hypersensitivity to cyanoacrylate glue used on the fingernails. Patch-testing can be performed with the glue by applying it to the skin and allowing it to dry prior to placing a patch over it in a manner similar to testing fingernail polish.[34, 122, 123, 124]

HAIR PRODUCTS

Shampoos

Shampoos are a common cause of irritant contact dermatitis in hairdressers, particularly in apprentices who shampoo clients' hair many times daily (Fig. 22–8). The surfactants in shampoos remove surface grease, dirt, and skin debris from the hair and scalp. They also remove protective skin lipids and have a drying action on the hands of the cosmetologist. After repeated exposure to water and surfactant action on the skin, the irritant contact dermatitis develops in the operators. Shampoos contain a number of other ingredients, including thickeners, opacifiers, preservatives,

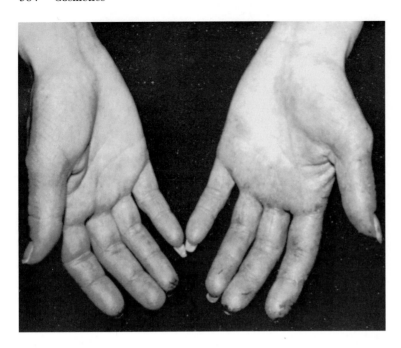

FIGURE 22–8 • Irritant contact dermatitis of a beautician's hands from shampooing. She also had atopic dermatitis.

colors, perfumes, and antidandruff agents, which rarely cause allergic contact dermatitis in the client or the beautician.

Hair Colorings

Paraphenylenediamine

It is estimated that 40% of the women in the United States use hair colorings. These preparations can be temporary, semipermanent, or permanent in nature, with the latter being the most commonly used.[125] Permanent hair colorings, the most important, are used in salons as well as at home. They require three types of chemicals: (1) base or primary intermediates, which include paraphenylenediamine (PPD) and related chemicals, (2) couplers or modifiers, and (3) an oxidizing agent, which is usually hydrogen peroxide. These dyes are particularly popular because of the variety of natural colors that can be achieved with them and the permanence of the color. The primary intermediate, PPD, is oxidized by hydrogen peroxide and coupled within the hair shaft, which causes permanence. Other hair dye products that are less commonly used because of their temporary or semipermanent nature include vegetable and metallic dyes and synthetic rinses.

Virtually all PPD sensitivity is secondary to hair dyes. Crossreactions occur in response to other related hair dyes, such as *p*-toluenediamine, *p*-aminodiphenylamine, 2,4-diaminoanisole, and o-aminophenol. In the client, PPD produces acute dermatitis involving the scalp, eyelids, face, and hairline. In the hairdresser, the most common region affected is the hands, but dermatitis may also involve other exposed areas such as the forearms and face (Fig. 22–9). PPD was banned in Europe because of the hazard of allergic contact dermatitis, and paratoluenediamine (PTD) was substituted. Whether or not PTD is a weaker allergen is controversial. Guinea pig sensitization tests have indicated that both are strong sensitizers, with PTD causing more allergy than PPD. In contrast to the guineas pig findings, Epstein and Taylor, using the maximization test, found PPD to sensitize 44% of their subjects (15 of 34), whereas PTD sensitized none (0 of 31).[126] The St. John's experience would tend to support the concept that PPD was the stronger allergen, but when 45 patients with hair dye dermatitis were tested with both PPD and PTS, 43 patients had positive reactions to PPD, whereas 21 patients had positive reactions to PTD. Similar findings occurred with hairdressers.[127] PPD-sensitive patients may also have crossreactions to azo and aniline dyes, paba esters, and local anesthetics. Once the dye has become fully oxidized inside the hair it is not an allergen; thus, dyed hair does not cause dermatitis. This is particularly important, as hairdressers frequently handle dyed hair.

Permanents

Glyceryl and Ammonium Thioglycolate

Salon hairdressers use either ammonium thioglycolate (ATG), for alkaline permanents, or glyceryl thioglycolate (GTG) for acid permanents, to alter the curvature of the hair. This is accomplished by breaking the disulfide bonds within the keratin structure of the hair shaft to allow a softening and the assumption of a new shape. Once the new shape is achieved, it is permanently held by re-bonding the disulfide bonds. Chemically, ATG or GTG reacts with cystine, producing two molecules of cysteine that disrupt the keratin chains. The hair shaft is manipulated to the desired configuration and hydrogen peroxide is added, causing oxidation of cysteine back to cystine, reforming disulfide bonds and assuring the structural change needed for a permanent wave. It is well known that ATG is an irritating chemical that causes irritant contact dermatitis in the client and the hairdresser if there is prolonged or repeated contact with the skin. Although there have been reports that allergic contact dermatitis can result from ATG, the difficulty in performing patch tests with ATG makes these reactions questionable.

The acid permanents using GTG have been found to be significant sensitizers in cosmetologists and patrons. Storrs[128] reported eight hair-

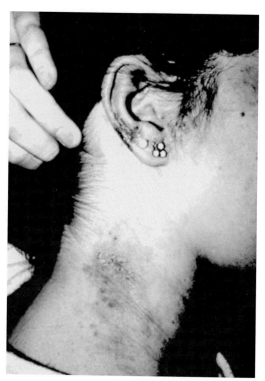

FIGURE 22–10 • Allergic contact dermatitis to glyceryl thioglycolate in a client who had an acid permanent. The dermatitis lasted for months after the permanent was done.

dressers and four clients who were allergic to the GTG found in the acid permanents they had used. GTG easily penetrates rubber gloves and either it or its by-products remain in the hair shaft for months, causing persistent dermatitis in the client or recurrent allergic contact dermatitis in the hairdresser (Fig. 22–10).[129]

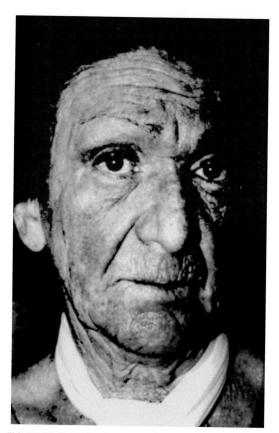

FIGURE 22–9 • Allergic contact dermatitis of a beautician's face from paraphenylenediamine found in permanent hair colorings.

References

1. Marks JG, DeLeo VA. *Contact and Occupational Dermatology*, 2nd ed. St. Louis: C.V. Mosby; 1997:162–170.
2. Steinberg DC. What is a cosmetic? (regulatory review). *Cosmet Toiletries* 1997; 112:27–29.
3. Eiermann HJ. Regulatory issues concerning AETT and 6-MC. *Contact Dermatitis* 1980; 6:120–122.
4. Eiermann HJ, Larsen W, Maibach HI, et al. Prospective study of cosmetic reactions: 1977–1980. *J Am Acad Dermatol* 1982; 6:909–917.
5. Brauer EW. The states of cosmetics in society. In: Frost P, Horwitz SN, eds. *Principles of Cosmetics for the Dermatologists*. St. Louis: C.V. Mosby; 1982:1–2.
6. Adams RM, Maibach HI. A five-year study of cosmetic reactions. *J Am Acad Dermatol* 1985; 13:1062–1069.
7. De Groot AC. Contact allergy to cosmetics: causative ingredients. *Contact Dermatitis* 1987; 17:226–234.
8. Ancona-Alayon A, Jimenez-Castilla JL, Gomez-Aluarez EM. Dermatitis from epoxy resin and formaldehyde in shampoo packers. *Contact Dermatitis* 1976; 2:356–364.

9. Marks JG, DeLeo VA. *Contact and Occupational Dermatology*, 2nd ed. St. Louis: Mosby; 1997; 326–329.

10. Marks JG. Occupational skin disease in hairdressers. *Occup Med Rev* 1986; 1:273–284.

11. Stovall GK, Levin L, Oler J. Occupational dermatitis among hairdressers: a multifactor analysis. *J Occup Med* 1983; 25:871–878.

12. James J, Calnan CD. Dermatitis of the hands in lady's hairdressers. *J Trans St John's Hosp Dermatol Soc* 1959; 42:19–42.

13. Calnan CD, Shuster S. Reactions to ammonium persulfate. *Arch Dermatol* 1963; 88:812–815.

14. Fisher AA, Dooms-Goosens A. Persulfate hair bleach reactions. *Arch Dermatol* 1976; 112:1407–1409.

15. Kellet JK, Beck MH. Ammonium persulphate sensitivity in hairdressers. *Contact Dermatitis* 1985; 13:26–28.

16. Wahlberg JE. Nickel allergy and atopy in hairdressers. *Contact Dermatitis* 1975; 1:161–165.

17. Marks R, Cronin E. Hand eczema in hairdressers. *Aust J Dermatol* 1977; 18:123–126.

18. Cronin E. *Contact Dermatitis*. Edinburgh: Churchill Livingstone; 1980:134–139.

19. Cronin E, Kullavanijaya P. Hand dermatitis in hairdressers. *Acta Dermatol Venereol* Suppl (Stockh) 1979; 85:47–50.

20. Hannuksela M, Hassi J. Hairdresser's hand. *Dermatosen* 1980; 28:149–151.

21. Lynde CW, Mitchell JC. Patch test results in 66 hairdressers, 1973–1981. *Contact Dermatitis* 1982; 8:302–307.

22. Nethercott JR, MacPherson M, Choi BC, et al. Contact dermatitis in hairdressers. *Contact Dermatitis* 1986; 14:73–79.

23. Matsunaga K, Hosokawa K, Suzuki M, et al. Occupational allergic contact dermatitis in beauticians. *Contact Dermatitis* 1988; 18:94–96.

24. Guerra L, Tosti A, Bardazzi F, et al. Contact dermatitis in hairdressers: the Italian experience. *Contact Dermatitis* 1992; 26:101–107.

25. Frosch PJ, Burrows D, Camarasa JG, et al. Allergic reactions to a hairdressers' series: results from 9 European centres. *Contact Dermatitis* 1993; 28:180–183.

26. Pilz B, Frosch PJ. Hairdressers' eczema. In: Menne T, Maibach HI, eds. *Hand eczema*. Boca Raton, Fla.: CRC Press; 1994:179–188.

27. Sutthipisal N, McFadden JP, Cronin E. Sensitization in atopic and non-atopic hairdressers with hand eczema. *Contact Dermatitis* 1993; 29:206–209.

28. Van der Walle HB, Brunsveld VM. Dermatitis in hairdressers. I. The experience of the past 4 years. *Contact Dermatitis* 1994; 30:217–221.

29. Van der Walle HB, Brunsveld VM. Latex allergy among hairdressers. *Contact Dermatitis* 1995; 32:177–178.

30. Katsarou A, Koufou B, Takou K, et al. Patch test results in hairdressers with contact dermatitis in Greece (1985–1994). *Contact Dermatitis* 1995; 33:347–361.

31. Conde-Salazar L, Baz M, Guimaraens D, Cannavo A. Contact dermatitis in hairdressers: patch test results in 379 hairdressers (1980–1993). *Am J Contact Dermatitis* 1995; 6:19–23.

32. Majoie IML, Bruynzeel DP. Occupational immediate-type hypersensitivity to henna in a hairdresser. *Am J Contact Dermatitis* 1996; 7:38–40.

33. Van der Walle HB. Dermatitis in hairdressers. II. Management and prevention. *Contact Dermatitis* 1994; 30:265–270.

34. Belsito DV. Contact dermatitis to ethyl-cyanoacrylate-containing glue. *Contact Dermatitis* 1987; 17:234–236.

35. Kanerva L, Lauerma A, Estlander T, et al. Occupational allergic contact dermatitis caused by photobonded sculptured nails and a review of (meth) acrylates in nail cosmetics. *Am J Contact Dermatitis* 1996; 7:109–115.

36. Freeman S, Lee MS, Gudmundsen K. Adverse contact reactions to sculptured acrylic nails: 4 case reports and a literature review. *Contact Dermatitis* 1995; 33:381–385.

37. Fitzgerald DA, Bhaggoe R, English JSC. Contact sensitivity to cyanoacrylate nail-adhesive with dermatitis at remote sites. *Contact Dermatitis* 1995; 32:175–176.

38. Fisher AA. *Contact Dermatitis*, 3rd ed. Philadelphia: Lea & Febiger; 1986:383–384.

39. Rosenzweig R, Scher RK. Nail cosmetics: adverse reactions. *Am J Contact Dermatitis* 1993; 4:71–77.

40. Marks JG, DeLeo VA. *Contact and Occupational Dermatology*, 2nd ed. St. Louis: C.V. Mosby; 1997:179–185.

41. Koppula SV, Fellman JH, Storrs FJ. Screening allergens for acrylate dermatitis associated with artificial nails. *Am J Contact Dermatitis* 1995; 6:78–85.

42. Larsen WG. Perfume dermatitis. *J Am Acad Dermatol* 1985; 12:1–9.

43. Emmons WW, Marks JG. Immediate and delayed reactions to cosmetic ingredients. *Contact Dermatitis* 1985; 13:258–265.

44. Marks JG. Contact urticaria. *Cosmetics Toiletries* 1986; 101:59–62.

45. McDaniel WR, Marks JG. Contact urticaria due to sensitivity to spray starch. *Arch Dermatol* 1979; 115:628.

46. VonKrogh G, Maibach HI. The contact urticaria syndrome: an update review. *J Am Acad Dermatol* 1981; 5:326–342.

47. Guin JD. History, manufacturer, and cutaneous reaction to perfumes. In: Frost P, Horwitz SN, eds. *Principles of Cosmetics for the Dermatologist*. St. Louis: C.V. Mosby; 1982:111–129.

48. Santucci B, Cristaudo A, Cannistraci C, et al. Contact dermatitis to fragrances. *Contact Dermatitis* 1987; 16:93–95.

49. De Groot AC. Contact allergy to cosmetics: causative ingredients. *Contact Dermatitis* 1987; 17:226–234.

50. Hostynek JJ. Safeguards in the use of fragrance chemicals. *Cosmetics Toiletries* 1997; 112:47–54.

51. Calkin RR, Jellinek JS. *Perfumery: Practice and Principles*. New York: Wiley-Interscience; 1994.

52. De Groot AC, Frosch PJ. Adverse reactions to fragrances: a clinical review. *Contact Dermatitis* 1997; 36:57–86.

53. Scheinman PL. Allergic contact dermatitis to fragrance: a review. *Am J Contact Dermatitis* 1996; 7:65–76.

54. Frosch PJ, Pilz B, Andersen KE, et al. Patch testing with fragrances: results of a multicenter study of the European Environmental and Contact Dermatitis Research Group with 48 frequently used constituents of perfumes. *Contact Dermatitis* 1995; 33:333–342.

55. Dooms-Goossens A. Reducing sensitizing potential by pharmaceutical and cosmetic design. *J Am Acad Dermatol* 1984; 10:547–553.

56. Basketter DA, Allenby CF. Studies of the quenching phenomenon in delayed contact hypersensitivity reactions. *Contact Dermatitis* 1991; 25:160–171.

57. Research Institute of Fragrance Materials: cinnamic alcohol. *Food Cosmetics Toxicol* 1974; 12:855–856.

58. Research Institute of Fragrance Materials: cinnamic aldehyde. *Food Cosmetics Toxicol* 1979; 17:253–258.

59. Schorr WF. Cinnamic aldehyde allergy. *Contact Dermatitis* 1975; 1:108–111.

60. Nate JP, DeJong MCJM, Baar AJM, et al. Contact urticarial skin responses to cinnamaldehyde. *Contact Dermatitis* 1977; 3:151–154.

61. Guin JD. Cinnamic aldehyde. In: Guin JB, ed. *Practical Contact Dermatitis: A Handbook for the Practitioner*. New York: McGraw-Hall; 1995.

62. Opdyke DLJ. Eugenol. *Food Cosmetics Toxicol* 1975; 13:545–547.

63. Opkyke DLJ. Isoeugenol. *Food Cosmetics Toxicol* 1975; 13:815–817.

64. Solberg PT, McFadden N, Staerfelt F, et al. Perfume allergy due to oak moss and other lichens. *Contact Dermatitis* 1982; 8:396–400.

65. Held JL, Ruszkowski AN, Deleo VA. Consort contact dermatitis due to oak moss. *Arch Dermatol* 1988; 124:261–262.

66. Calnan CD. Perfume dermatitis from the cosmetic ingredients oak moss and hydroxycitronellal. *Contact Dermatitis* 1979; 5:194.

67. Research Institute of Fragrance Materials. Hydroxycitronellal. *Food Cosmetics Toxicol* 1974; 12:921.

68. Raugi GJ, Storrs FJ, Larsen WG. Photoallergic contact dermatitis to men's perfumes. *Contact Dermatitis* 1979; 5:251–260.

69. Fisher AA. Perfume dermatitis: photodermatitis to musk ambrette and 6-methylcoumarin. *Cutis* 1980; 26:549–552.

70. Hjorth N. Skin reaction to balsams and perfumes. *Clin Exp Dermatol* 1982; 7:1–9.

71. Hausen BM, Simatupang T, Bruhn G, et al. Identification of new allergenic constituents and proof of evidence for coniferyl benzoate in balsam of Peru. *Am J Contact Dermatitis* 1995; 6:199–208.

72. Larsen W, Nakayama H, Lindberg M, et al. Fragrance contact dermatitis: a worldwide multicenter investigation. I. *Am J Contact Dermatitis* 1996; 7:77–83.

73. Morse LJ, Schornbeck LF. Hand lotions: a potential nosocomial hazard. *N Engl J Med* 1968; 278:376–378.

74. Wilson LA, Kuehne W, Hall SW, et al. Microbial contamination in occular cosmetics. *Am J Ophthalmol* 1971; 71:1298–1302.

75. Orth B, Frei R, Itin PH, et al. Outbreak of invasive mycoses caused by *Paecilomyces liacinus* from a contaminated skin lotion. *Ann Intern Med* 1996; 125:799–806.

76. Steinberg DC. Frequency of use of preservatives. *Cosmetics Toiletries* 1997; 112:57–65.

77. Kabara JJ. *Cosmetics and Drug Preservation: Principles and Practice.* New York: Marcel Deckker; 1984:339–356.

78. Haag TE, Loncrini DF. Esters of para-hydroxybenzoic acid. In: Kabara JJ, ed. *Cosmetics and Drug Preservation: Principles and Practice.* New York: Marcel Dekker; 1984:63–77.

79. Cronin E. *Contact Dermatitis.* Edinburgh: Churchill Livingstone; 1980:665–667.

80. Fisher AA. *Contact Dermatitis*, 3rd ed. Philadelphia: Lea & Febiger; 1986:238–241.

81. Schorr WF, Mohajerin AH. Paraben sensitivity. *Arch Dermatol* 1966; 93:721–723.

82. Fisher AA. The paraben paradox. *Cutis* 1973; 12:830.

83. Lorenzetti OJ, Wernet TC. Topical parabens: benefits and risks. *Dermatologica* 1977; 154:244–250.

84. Cosmetic ingredient review: final report on the safety assessment of methyl paraben, ethyl paraben, propyl paraben, and butyl paraben. *J Am Coll Toxicol* 1984; 3:147–209.

85. Hansen J, Mollgaard B, Avnstorp C, Menne T. Paraben contact allergy: patch testing and in vitro absorption/metabolism. *Am J Dermatitis* 1993; 4:78–86.

86. Rosen WE, Berke PA. Germal-115 a safe and effective preservative. In: Kabara JJ, ed. *Cosmetic and Drug Preservation: Principles and Practice.* New York: Marcel Dekker; 1984:191–205.

87. Cosmetic ingredient review: final report of the safety assessment for imidazolidinyl urea. *J Environ Pathol Toxicol* 1980; 4:133–146.

88. Dooms-Goossens A, de Boulle K, Dooms M, et al. Imidazolidinyl urea dermatitis. *Contact Dermatitis* 1986; 14:322–324.

89. Kantor KR, Taylor JS, Ratz JL, et al. Acute allergic contact dermatitis from diazolidinyl urea (Germall II) in a hair gel. *J Am Acad Dermatol* 1985; 13:116–119.

90. Jackson EM. Diazolidinyl urea: a toxicologic and dermatologic risk assessment as a preservative in consumer products. *J Toxicol Cutan Ocular Toxicol* 1995; 14:3–21.

91. Hectorne KJ, Fransway AF. Diazolidinyl urea: incidence of sensitivity, patterns of cross-reactivity and clinical relevance. *Contact Dermatitis* 1994; 30:16–19.

92. Marks JG, Belsito DV, DeLeo VA, et al. North American Contact Dermatitis Group standard tray patch test results: 1992 to 1994. *Am J Contact Dermatitis* 1995; 6:160–165.

93. Marouchoc R. Dowicil-200 preservative. In: Kabara JJ, ed. *Cosmetic and Drug Preservation: Principles and Practice.* New York: Marcel Dekker; 1984:143–164.

94. Cosmetic ingredient review: final report on the safety assessment of quaternium-15. *J Am Coll Toxicol* 1986; 5:61–101.

95. Fransway AF, Schmitz NA. The problem of preservation in the 1990s. I. Statement of the problem, solution(s) of the industry, and the current use of formaldehyde and formaldehyde-releasing biocides. *Am J Contact Dermatitis* 1991; 2:6–23.

96. Fransway AF, Schmitz NA. The problem of preservation in the 1990s. II. Formaldehyde and formaldehyde-releasing biocides: incidences of cross-reactivity and the significance of the positive response to formaldehyde. *Am J Contact Dermatitis* 1991; 2:78–88.

97. Cosmetic ingredient review: final report on the safety assessment of formaldehyde. *J Am Coll Toxicol* 1984; 3:157–184.

98. Jordan WP, Sherman WT, King SE. Threshold responses in formaldehyde-sensitive subjects. *J Am Acad Dermatol* 1979; 1:44–48.

99. Shaw S. Patch-testing bronopol. *Cosmetics Toiletries* 1997; 112:67–73.

100. Croshaw B, Holland VR. Chemical preservatives: use of bronopol as a cosmetic preservative. In: Kabara JJ, ed. *Cosmetic and Drug Preservation: Principles and Practice.* New York: Marcel Dekker; 1984:31–62.

101. Cosmetic ingredient review: addendum to the final report on the safety assessment of 2-bromo-2-nitropropane-1,3-diol. *J Am Coll Toxicol* 3:139–155.

102. Fisher AA. Cosmetic dermatitis: reactions to some commonly used preservatives. *Cutis* 1980; 26:136–137,141–142,147–148.

103. Storrs FJ, Bell DE. Allergic contact dermatitis to 2-bromo-2-nitropropane-1,3-diol in hydrophilic ointment. *J Am Acad Dermatol* 1983; 8:157–170.

104. Law AB, Moss JN, Lashen ES. Kathon CG: a new single-component, broad-spectrum preservative system for cosmetic and toiletries. In: Kabara JJ, ed. *Cosmetics and Drug Preservation: Principles and Practice.* New York: Marcel Dekker; 1984:129–141.

105. Marks JG, Moss JN, Parno JR, et al. Methylchloroisothiazolinone/methylisothiazolinone (Kathon CG) biocide: U. S. multicenter study of human skin sensitization. *Am J Contact Dermatitis* 1990; 1:157–161.

106. Marks JG, Moss JN, Parno JR, et al. Methylchloroisothiazolinone/methylisothiazolinone (Kathon CG) biocide: second U. S. multicenter study of human skin sensitization. *Am J Contact Dermatitis* 1993; 4:87–89.

107. De Groot AC, Weylan JW. Kathon CG: a review. *J Am Acad Dermatol* 1988; 18:350–358.

108. De Groot AC, van Ginkel JW, Weijland JW. Methyldibromoglutaronitrile (Euxyl K 400): an important "new"

allergen in cosmetics. *J Am Acad Dermatol* 1996; 35:743–747.

109. Aalto-Korte K, Jolanki R, Estlander T, et al. Occupational allergic contact dermatitis caused by Euxyl K 400. *Contact Dermatitis* 1996; 35:193–194.

110. Tosti A, Vincenzi C, Trevisi P, et al. Euxyl K 400: incidence of sensitization, patch test concentration and vehicle. *Contact Dermatitis* 1995; 33:193–195.

111. Scher RK. Cosmetics and ancillary preparations for the care of nails: composition, chemistry, and adverse reactions. *J Am Acad Dermatol* 1982; 6:523–528.

112. Baran R. Pathology induced by the application of cosmetics to the nail. In: Frost P, Horwitz S, eds. *Principles of Cosmetics for the Dermatologist*. St. Louis: CV Mosby; 1982:181–184.

113. Rosenzweig R, Scher RK. Nail cosmetics: adverse reactions. *Am J Contact Dermatitis* 1993; 4:71–77.

114. Tosti A, Guerra L, Vincenzi C, et al. Contact sensitization caused by toluene sulfonamide-formaldehyde resin in women who use nail cosmetics. *Am J Contact Dermatitis* 1993; 4:150–153.

115. Hausen BM, Milbrodt M, Koenig WA. The allergens of nail polish. I. Allergenic constituents of common nail polish and toluenesulfonamide-formaldehyde resin (TS-F-R). *Contact Dermatitis* 1995; 33:157–164.

116. Paltzik RL, Enscroe I. Onycholysis secondary to toluene sulfonamide formaldehyde resin used in a nail hardener mimicking onychomycosis. *Cutis* 1980; 25:647–648.

117. Fisher AA, Franks A, Glick H. Allergic sensitization of the skin and nails to acrylate plastic nails. *J Allergy* 1957; 28:84–88.

118. Marks JG, Bishop ME, Willis WF. Allergic contact dermatitis to sculptured nails. *Arch Dermatol* 1979; 115:100.

119. Jordan WO. Cross-sensitization patterns in acrylate allergies. *Contact Dermatitis* 1975; 1:13–15.

120. Hemmer W, Focke M, Wantke F, et al. Allergic contact dermatitis to artificial fingernails prepared from UV light-cured acrylates. *J Am Acad Dermatol* 1996;35:377–380.

121. Fisher AA. Permanent loss of fingernails from sensitization and reaction to acrylate in a preparation designed to make artificial nails. *J Dermatol Surg Oncol* 1980; 6:70–71.

122. Fisher AA. Allergic reactions to cyanoacrylate "Krazy Glue" nail preparations. *Cutis* 1987; 40:475–476.

123. Shelley ED, Shelley WB. Chronic dermatitis simulating small-plaque parapsoriasis due to cyanoacrylate adhesive used on fingernails. *JAMA* 1984; 252:2455–2456.

124. Tomb RR, Lepoittevin JP, Durepaire F, et al. Ectopic contact dermatitis from ethyl cyanoacrylate instant adhesives. *Contact Dermatitis* 1993; 28:206–208.

125. Wilkinson JB, Moore RJ. *Harry's Cosmeticology*. New York: Chemical Publishing; 1982.

126. Epstein WL, Taylor MK. Experimental sensitization to paraphenylenediamine and paratoluenediamine in man. *Acta Derm Venerol Suppl (Stockh)* 1979; 59:55–57.

127. Cronin E. *Contact Dermatitis*. Edinburgh: Churchill Livingstone; 1980:115–126.

128. Storrs FJ. Permanent wave contact dermatitis: contact allergy to glyceryl monothioglycolate. *J Am Acad Dermatol* 1984; 11:74–85.

129. Morrison LH, Storrs FJ. Persistence of an allergen in hair after glyceryl monthioglycolate-containing permanent wave solutions. *J Am Acad Dermatol* 1988; 19:52–59.

Corticosteroids

A. GOOSSENS, R.PHARM., Ph.D.
M. MATURA, M.D., Ph.D.

Contact allergy in response to corticosteroids is now a well-established phenomenon, and cases from all over the world have been reported in the literature. The incidence of the reactions observed, however, varies and depends on several factors, including the nature and amount of corticosteroids used in each country, the prescription habits, the awareness among the medical profession of the importance of corticosteroid sensitivity, the selection of the patients and their referral to test centers, the routine testing of screening agents for corticosteroid sensitivity as well as of all the corticosteroids used by the patient, and the testing and reading methods used. See Dooms-Goossens for a review.[1-4]

CHARACTERIZATION OF THE CORTICOSTEROID-ALLERGIC PATIENT

The typical patient at risk for a corticosteroid allergy suffers from a chronic eczema that may originally have started as an irritant or allergic dermatitis of the hands, a seborrheic or contact dermatitis of the face (where sometimes other side effects such as rosacea also may have occurred; see Figure 23–1), a stasis dermatitis, chronic otitis, anal pruritus, or an atopic dermatitis, even in children (Fig. 23–2). In fact, any place on the body to which corticosteroids (often many) have been applied is apt to give rise to contact-allergic reactions to them. When such sensitivity is present, the dermatitis is generally not aggravated by the use of corticosteroids; it just does not respond to them.

Indeed, the allergenic and simultaneous anti-inflammatory effects of topical corticosteroids cause a nonspecific, self-supporting eczematous condition that is rarely recognized as a potentially iatrogenic sensitivity.[5] In rare cases—and this has been observed particularly with contact allergy to budesonide—a more acute and even erythema-multiforme–like reaction may constitute the clinical picture (Fig. 23–3).

Although infrequent relative to the large scale of their use, allergic reactions may also arise in

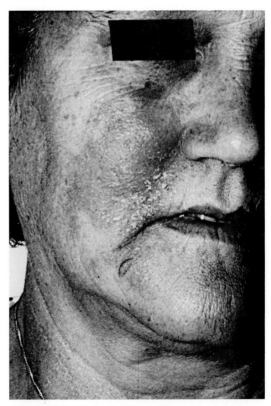

FIGURE 23–1 • Patient with steroid rosacea on the face as well as a contact allergy to multiple pharmaceutical ingredients, including corticosteroids.

389

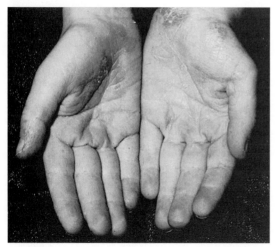

FIGURE 23–2 • Atopic hand dermatitis in a 6-year-old boy complicated by a corticosteroid contact allergy.

response to the corticosteriods administered by inhalation in the treatment of rhinitis or bronchial asthma.[6] The clinical symptoms appear as eczema on the face, mainly the eyelids and in the perioral and perinasal areas (Fig. 23–4), but sometimes also on distant body sites. A severe flare-up of previous eczematous lesions as well as a systemic contact-dermatitis–type of reaction may also occur. In some cases, there is associated endonasal intolerance and bronchial constriction. The symptoms generally commence as soon as 2 to 5 days after the first administration, which indicates a previously existing, but often undetected, corticosteroid sensitivity. Indeed, inhalation corticosteroids rarely induce primary sensitization.

Generalized reactions may, of course, also occur after systemic administration (oral, intravenous, or intra-articular). The lesions may manifest themselves as eczema, exanthema, purpura, urticaria,

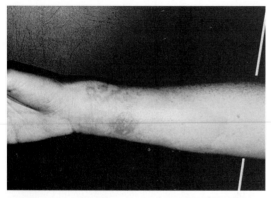

FIGURE 23–3 • EEM-like contact dermatitis after primary sensitization by a skin preparation containing budesonide.

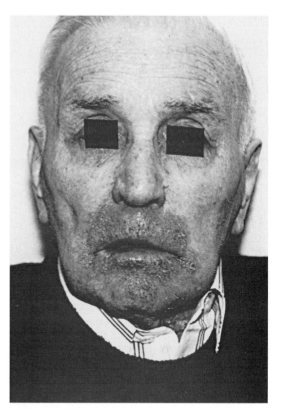

FIGURE 23–4 • Dermatitis on the face due to an inhalation corticosteroid.

and so on.[7, 8] For example, Figures 23–5 and 23–6 show a patient who developed a strongly itching, symmetric, maculopapular eruption on the trunk and all the limbs after intramuscular injection of a methylprednisolone preparation in the right shoulder to alleviate joint pain at that site. The reaction persisted for 10 days. The patient's sensitivity to this corticosteroid was caused by the local application of the same corticosteroid to stasis dermatitis and the sensitivity had been diagnosed 15 years previously.

TESTING FOR CORTICOSTEROID SENSITIVITY

Although severe patch-test reactions may occur (see Figure 23–7, which illustrates sensitivity to tixocortol pivalate), because of their anti-inflammatory effect, corticosteroids often mask not only the clinical signs of a contact allergy to corticosteroids but also the patch-test reactions to the corticosteroid preparations and the corticosteroid molecules themselves. A weak concentration of a corticosteroid in a pharmaceutical product in which skin penetration and hence bioavailability

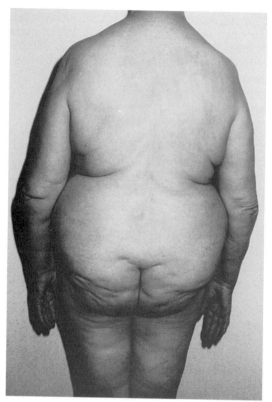

FIGURE 23–5 • Generalized systemic contact-dermatitis–type eruption (maculopapular) due to an intramuscular injection of methylprednisolone in a previously sensitized patient.

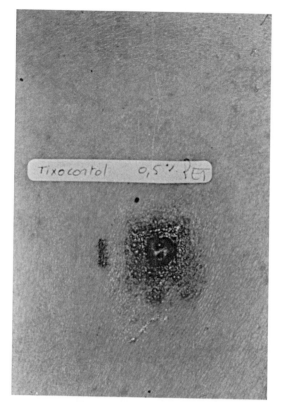

FIGURE 23–7 • Strong positive patch-test reaction to tixocortol pivalate (0.5% pet = petrolatum).

have been optimized may cause a contact dermatitis on the treated eczema site but no reaction on the intact skin of the back when patch tested, particularly when a vehicle like petrolatum is used. However, in contrast to noninflammatory agents, the concentration cannot be too high, lest the suppressive effect dominate. For budesonide, for example, preliminary results have shown the

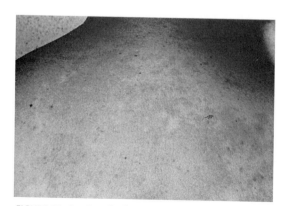

FIGURE 23–6 • Detail of the eruption on the upper back.

superiority of test concentrations lower than 0.1% for revealing contact allergy to it.[9]

Along with false-negative reactions, corticosteroids may also produce particular patch-test reactions such as the edge effect in which, at early readings, the eczematous reaction is apparent only on the outer edge of the patch-test site, where a small amount of the corticosteroid has probably diffused into the surrounding skin, and not in the middle, where the concentration is the highest. At later readings, though, the entire patch-test site becomes eczematous; the allergenic effect prevails over the anti-inflammatory effect. Figures 23–8 and 23–9 illustrate this phenomenon.

Other frequently occurring phenomena are vasoconstrictive, or blanching, effects and reactive vasodilation, which are due to the intrinsic pharmacological activity of corticosteroids. These responses occur in only some of the patients tested because of the individual variability in response to local corticosteroids. Weak erythematous reactions, however, must certainly be checked, as they could well indicate the beginning of an allergic reaction. Indeed, it is common for patients to react to corticosteroids only 5 to 7 days after their application.

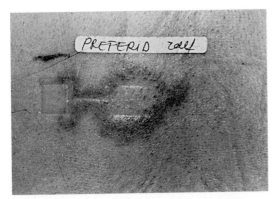

FIGURE 23–8 • The edge effect at day 2. The reaction was obtained with 0.025% budesonide skin ointment tested as such with a Van der Bend chamber. Note that the test substance has "contaminated" the linking plastic material between two chambers to produce a fish-like appearance.

Difficulties in patch testing have led some authors such as Wilkinson and English[10] to use intradermal testing to screen for allergies to certain corticosteroids. However, one must keep in mind that the results of intradermal testing are not always relevant to the patient's allergic skin condition and that side effects like atrophy and even systemic reactions may occur.

In many countries, two or three screening corticosteroids have been added to the standard series: tixocortol pivalate (1.0% pet.), budesonide (0.1% pet.), and sometimes also hydrocortisone-17-butyrate (1.0% ethanol). Because the clinical picture of a potential corticosteroid-sensitive patient—a nonresponding dermatitis—almost never suggests the possibility of a corticosteroid sensitivity, most contact allergies are missed if corticosteroids are not routinely tested for.

Moreover, as corticosteroid sensitivity is found

to be particularly common among patients who have used many topical pharmaceutical products, all other ingredients should be tested in addition to the corticosteroids themselves in order to detect concomitant allergenic ingredients. In most cases, up to 80% of corticosteroid-allergic patients react to other, mainly iatrogenic allergens, such as, for example, neomycin and propylene glycol.[5]

CLINICAL AND THERAPEUTIC CONSEQUENCES OF CROSSREACTIONS OBSERVED WITH CORTICOSTEROIDS

Most corticosteroid-sensitive patients react to several corticosteroids. This may be in part because most of them have used large numbers of corticosteroids and would thus be vulnerable to concomitant sensitization. However, irrefutable proof of the existence of crossreactions is provided by reactions to substances to which the patient has never been exposed.

Cross-sensitivity studies are valuable from the scientific point of view as they can provide information about the molecular structure of antigenic determinants. They also can have practical consequences involving the identification of screening agents and advice regarding which topical and systemic corticosteroids the corticosteroid-sensitive patient can safely use. Our own studies have led us to suggest the following four groups of crossreacting molecules (Fig. 23–10):[11, 23]

1. Group A, hydrocortisone type: no substitution on the D ring except a short chain ester on C17 or C21 or a thioester on C21, e.g., tixocortol pivalate;

2. Group B, triamcinolone acetonide type: C16, C17-cis-ketal or -diol structure;

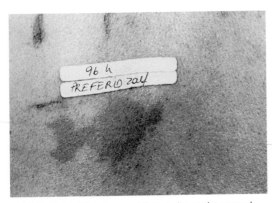

FIGURE 23–9 • The same patch-test site at the second reading (day 4).

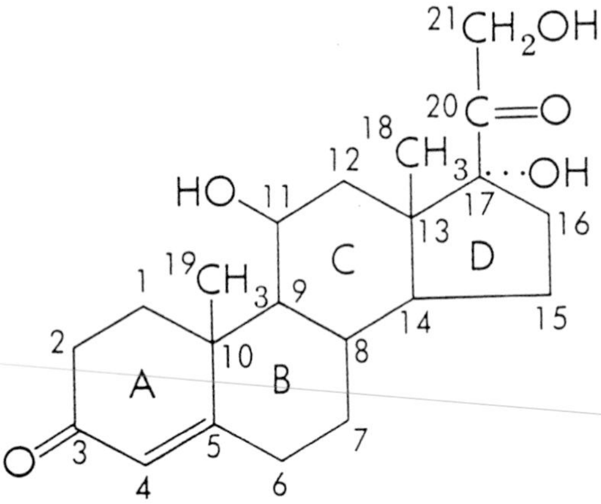

FIGURE 23–10 • The chemical structure of hydrocortisone.

3. Group C, betamethasone type: C16-methyl substitution;

4. Group D1, betamethasone dipropionate type: methylsubstitution on C16 and halogenation, long side chain ester on C17, often also on C21.

5. Group D2, methylprednisolone aceponate type: no methylsubstitution on C16, no halogenation, long side chain ester on C17, possibly side chain on C21.

Clinical observations identified tixocortol pivalate as a good screening agent for group A, which has also been confirmed by other authors.[12, 13] Budesonide was found to be a marker for a variety of corticosteroids, not only for other acetonides (group B, to which it theoretically belongs), but also for certain esters (group D), such as hydrocortisone-17-butyrate, prednicarbate, and alclometasone dipropionate.

These clinical observations were fully supported by conformational analysis of the electronic shape of the corticosteroids involved.[14] Groups A, B, and D were found to be highly homogeneous within each group in terms of molecular structures, and significant differences were observed among the groups. The special behavior of the budesonide can be attributed to its unique molecular structure, that is, its acetal function that allows the molecule to mimic both the group B and the group D molecular shape. Although conformational analysis did not detect group-specific characteristics of volume and shape for molecules of group C, it is still clinically important to maintain this group, as it seems that its members do not crossreact with other corticosteroid groups.

Membership in a certain group, however, does not indicate the sensitizing potential of a given molecule. For example, when testing group D molecules, contact-allergic reactions are much more frequently observed with substances such as hydrocortisone-17-butyrate, methylprednisolone aceponate, and prednicarbate. They are now classified as group D2 corticosteroids. Indeed, not only the molecular configuration but also other factors such as the presence of certain substituents, the solubility in the vehicle used, skin penetration, and skin metabolization seem to be critical for the sensitization and cross-sensitization potential of individual corticosteroids. For instance, Wilkinson and coworkers[15] have attached a great deal of importance to the presence of a substitution at the C6 or C9 position of the corticosteroid structure, whereas Oh-i,[16] who based his findings on only 38 Japanese case reports, also classified corticosteroids into four groups, but they differ somewhat from those that emerged from our study. Besides grouping the acetonide and betamethasone types,

he classifies clobetasol propionate and clobetasone butyrate separately because of the presence of the chlormethyl ketone residue, which is an alkyl side chain at the C17 position. In our experience, these molecules rarely cause sensitivity. As regards the influence of the skin metabolization of corticosteroids, patch test results (data to be published) have shown that, for instance, positive reactions to the more recently developed molecules such as prednicarbate and methylprednisolone aceponate correlate significantly with reactions obtained with group A corticosteroids ($p < 0.01$). Prednicarbate and methylprednisolone aceponate are highly lipophilic esters that penetrate the skin easily; prednicarbate[17] is then hydrolyzed to form prednisolone-17-ethylcarbonate and then slowly to form prednisolone, whereas methylprednisolone aceponate[18] is metabolized to form methylprednisolone-17-propionate, which in turn is rapidly converted to methylprednisolone. The metabolites bind more strongly to the corticosteroid receptors than do the other molecules, which, in fact, are "prodrugs." The higher penetration ability of these molecules together with their skin-metabolization properties might account for the reactions observed. Such a mechanism might also account for crossreactions that have been observed between hydrocortisone and hydrocortisone-17-butyrate,[15] the latter being able to be converted to hydrocortisone-21-butyrate, which is rapidly hydrolyzed to form hydrocortisone.[19] However, individual skin-metabolization characteristics certainly influence the cross-sensitivity patterns observed.

Furthermore, certain molecules are extremely rare sensitizers such as betamethasone and its esters, including valerate and dipropionate, diflucortolone valerate, diflorasone diacetate, and also the newer mometasone furoate. They are now classified as group D1 corticosteroids. The precise reasons why this is the case are still unclear, except perhaps for mometasone furoate, which differs significantly in electronic shape from the other "esters."[20] In addition, it penetrates poorly into the skin.

Cross-sensitivity studies have practical consequences for the treatment of corticosteroid-allergic patients. For patients with a contact allergy to some corticosteroids, the outcome of patch testing with an extended series of corticosteroids has been extremely helpful in finding other, safer alternatives for local and also systemic treatment.[21] For example, we recently observed two patients with generalized skin reactions after systemic corticosteroid administration who were successfully treated with corticosteroids that had given negative patch-test results: one had had a contact-dermatitis–type reaction to an intramuscular injection of methylprednisolone (this patient is shown in Figures 23–5 and 23–6) and was successfully treated with betamethasone orally; the other suffered a generalized skin reaction after administering a budesonide aerosol to her child to treat its asthma and became symptom-free with methylprednisolone tablets. Similar observations have been reported in the literature.[22] Bircher and coworkers, in a review of this subject, conclude with regard to delayed allergic reactions to systemically administered corticosteroids that the cross-sensitivity patterns are generally the same as in contact-allergic reactions. They also state that the identification of safe corticosteroids for systemic application is often possible by means of patch testing but that, in some cases, intradermal tests are necessary to improve diagnostic certainty, although false-negative reactions with patch and intradermal testing may occur.

RECOMMENDATIONS

Patients with contact allergy to corticosteroids generally present with a chronic dermatitis that is not exacerbated by but fails to respond to corticosteroid therapy. In such cases, all topical treatment should be stopped. If corticosteroid therapy is absolutely necessary, one of the "safer" corticosteroids such as mometasone furoate, betamethasone, or diflucortolone esters could be used, and then only in a paraffin base in order to avoid other pharmaceutical allergens. For systemic use, betamethasone or dexamethasone derivatives may be appropriate. The patient should be patch tested in order to screen for corticosteroid allergy. Should a corticosteroid sensitivity be detected, more extensive corticosteroid series should be tested to determine crossreactivity patterns so that appropriate advice for the future can be given.

References

1. Dooms-Goossens A. Sensitization to corticosteroids: consequences for anti-inflammatory therapy. *Drug Saf* 1995; 13:123–129.
2. Dooms-Goossens A, Andersen KE, Brandao FM, et al. Corticosteroid contact allergy: EECDRG Multicentre Study. *Contact Dermatitis* 1996; 35:40–44.
3. Matura M. Prevalence of corticosteroid contact allergy in Hungary. *Contact Dermatitis* 1998; 38:225–226.
4. Dooms-Goossens A, Meinardi MMHM, Bos J, et al. Contact allergy to corticosteroids: the results of a two-centre study. *Br J Dermatol* 1994; 130:42–47.
5. Dooms-Goossens A, Morren M. Results of routine patch testing with corticosteroid series in 2073 patients. *Contact Dermatitis* 1992; 26:182–191.
6. Dooms-Goossens A. Allergy to inhaled corticosteroids: a review. *Am J Contact Dermat* 1995; 6:1–13.
7. Uter W. Allergische Reaktionen auf Glukokorticoide. *Derm Beruf Umwelt* 1990; 38:75–90.
8. Lauerma AI, Reitamo S. Allergic reactions to topical and systemic corticosteroids. *Eur J Dermatol* 1994; 5:354–358.
9. Isaksson M, Bruze M, Matura M, et al. Patch testing with low concentrations of budesonide detects contact allergy. *Contact Dermatitis* 1997; 37:241–242.
10. Wilkinson SM, English JSC. Patch tests are poor detectors of corticosteroid allergy. *Contact Dermatitis* 1992; 36:67–68.
11. Coopman S, Degreef H, Dooms-Goossens A. Identification of cross-reaction patterns in allergic contact dermatitis from topical corticosteroids. *Br J Dermatol* 1989; 121:37–34.
12. Wilkinson SM, English JSC. Hydrocortisone sensitivity: a prospective study of the value of tixocortol pivalate and hydrocortisone acetate as patch test markers. *Contact Dermatitis* 1991; 25:132–133.
13. Lauerma AI, Tawainen K, Förström L, et al. Contact hypersensitivity to hydrocortisone-free alcohol in patients with allergic patch test reactions to tixocortol pivalate. *Contact Dermatitis* 1993; 28:10–14.
14. Lepoittevin J-P, Drieghe J, Dooms-Goossens A. Studies in patients with corticosteroid contact allergy: understanding cross-reactivity among different steroids. *Arch Dermatol* 1995; 131:31–37.
15. Wilkinson SM, Hollis S, Beck M. Reaktionen auf andere Kortikosteroide bei Patienten mit allergischer Kontaktdermatitis infolge Hydrocortison. *Z Haut Geschlechtskr* 1995; 70:368–372.
16. Oh-i T. Contact dermatitis due to topical steroids with conceivable cross-reactions between topical steroid preparations. *J Dermatol* 1996; 23:200–208.
17. Barth J, Lehr KH, Derendorf H, et al. Studies on the pharmacokinetics and metabolism of prednicarbate after cutaneous and oral administration. *Skin Pharmacol* 1993; 6:179–186.
18. Töpert M, Olivar A, Optiz D. New developments in corticosteroid research. *J Dermatol Treat* 1990; 1(suppl 3): S5–S9.
19. Täuber U. Dermatocorticosteroids: structure, activity, pharmacokinetics. *Eur J Dermatol* 1994; 4:419–429.
20. Dooms-Goossens A, Lepoittevin J-P. Studies on the contact allergenic potential of mometasone furoate: a clinical and molecular study. *Eur J Dermatol* 1996; 5:339–340.
21. Lepoittevin J-P, Basketter D, Goossens A, et al. Practical therapeutic consequences of classifying corticosteroids. In: *The Practical Approach, Allergic Contact Dermatitis: A Molecular Basis*. Berlin: Springer-Verlag; 1998.
22. Bircher AJ, Levy F, Langauer S, et al. Contact allergy to topical corticosteroids and systemic contact dermatitis from prednisolone with tolerance of triamcinolone. *Acta Derm Venereol* 1995; 75:490–493.
23. Matura M, Goossens A, Lepoittevin J-P. Not all corticosteroid esters have the same allergenic potential. Presentation at the 4th Congress of the European Society of Contact Dermatitis, Helsinki, July 8–11, 1998.

Metals

24

DESMOND BURROWS, M.D.
ROBERT M. ADAMS, M.D.
G.N. FLINT, F.R.S.C., F.I.M.

ALUMINUM

The second most abundant of all elements, aluminum, occurs in the earth's crust as a mineral aggregate known as *bauxite,* in which the aluminum occurs largely as hydrated oxides with silica. The process of making aluminum oxide (anhydrous alumina) from bauxite is known as the Bayer process, after the German chemist Karl Joseph Bayer, who patented it in 1888.

In the Bayer process, refined alumina (Al_2O_3) is obtained by digestion of the bauxite with caustic soda, from which aluminum metal is recovered by electrolytic reduction of the alumina dissolved in molten cryolite (Na_3AlF_6). There may be considerable dust in plants where alumina is processed. Although it is often considered a nuisance dust, the fine powdered alumina can cause an irritant dermatitis associated with considerable itching. In factories that use recycled aluminum, Johannessen and Bergan-Skar[1] reported pruritus, but not contact dermatitis, from the dust among potroom workers.

The excellent combination of properties available in aluminum and its alloys ensures their extensive use throughout industry and in everyday household articles. These properties are high strength–weight ratio, resistance to corrosion, high thermal and electrical conductivity, and good fabricability.

Aluminum salts have been included in lists of sensitizers by several authors,[2, 3] but allergic sensitivity is exceedingly rare, especially considering the amount of aluminum contact—for example, among persons who use antiperspirants. Hall,[4] who first reported allergy to aluminum, examined 202 workers with suspected occupational dermatitis in an aircraft manufacturing plant, four of whom had persistent positive patchtests to aluminum filings. However, Clemmensen and Knudsen[5] were the first to record a well-documented case of aluminum sensitivity. This appeared to be due to aluminum precipitated allergens used for hyposensitization injections. Their patient showed positive reactions to aluminum disks used in patchtesting and to various aluminum allergens as well: 2% aluminum chloride in water, aluminum subacetate, 1% in water, and aluminum powder. When the injections were discontinued, the eczema disappeared.

Others have since reported cases of suspected sensitivity: Bohler-Sommeregger and Lindemayr[6]; Veien and coworkers[7]; Cox and Moss[9]; Tosti and colleagues.[10] In Tosti's report, a marble worker was exposed to an abrasive powder that consisted mainly of aluminum oxide used for burnishing the surface of the marble. Most of the reported cases, however, have been granulomatous reactions to antiperspirants.[11] Reports of reactions to the Finn chamber used in patchtesting have also been reported.[12, 13] It should be remembered that the aluminum in Finn chambers can react with mercury, and occasionally with nickel and cobalt.[14] Most cases of aluminum sensitivity in childhood contacted through vaccination seem to disappear, as evidenced by the nonreactivity of adults to the aluminum in Finn chambers used for patchtesting. Dwyer and Kerr[15] described two brothers who reacted to aluminum Finn chambers when patchtested and who then reacted with sensitivity when patchtested with aqueous aluminum chloride. Hemmer's group[16] found moderate reactions in four of 1,922 patients tested to an aluminum test series, but the reactions could not be reproduced on further testing. They concluded that,

TABLE 24–1 • Irritating and Corrosive Aluminum Salts Commonly Used in Industry

Aluminum borohydride: jet fuel additive
Aluminum bromide: catalyst
Aluminum iodide: organic chemical synthesis
Aluminum phosphate: ceramics, dental cements, cosmetics, paints, varnishes, pharmaceuticals, pulp and paper
Aluminum phosphide: insecticides, fumigants
Aluminum pictrate*: explosives
Aluminum sulfide: manufacture of hydrogen sulfide
Anhydrous aluminum chloride: catalyst dye intermediate, butyl rubber and petroleum refining
Anhydrous aluminum fluoride: fluxes, especially for aluminum brazing, ceramics, enamels

*May also be an allergic contact sensitizer.

while contact sensitization to aluminum may be a clinically relevant complication of persisting vaccine-induced subcutaneous nodules, positive patchtest reactions to aluminium are extremely rare and any reactions should be reassessed, using a series of aluminum compounds to exclude false-positive reactions.

Many salts of aluminum are irritating to the skin (Table 24–1). The corrosion resistance of aluminum products, and thus their appearance, can be improved by anodizing, an electrolytic process in which a thin oxide film is formed on the surface in a bath of sulphuric or chromic acid and then sealed by steam treatment. This process provides excellent resistance to corrosion. A cold sealing process using nickel acetate is also used that requires thorough rinsing of the surface of the product after anodizing; otherwise, nickel ions might remain on the surface and cause nickel contact dermatitis during subsequent handling of the product.[17]

ANTIMONY

Antimony, a hard, brilliant metal, is useless in its pure state but extremely valuable when combined with other metals. Approximately half of all antimony is used in alloys. Typical compositions of alloys of antimony are given in Table 24–2. Because antimony imparts a hard, smooth surface to soft metal alloys it has been used for years in the manufacture of pewter utensils.

Antimony trioxide, the principal compound of antimony, is used in paint pigments, ceramics, and as a fire retardant in paper, textiles, and plastics. At one time the sulfides of antimony were used as

rubber accelerators; today their main application is in making red pigments. Workers at the smelting furnaces are exposed to considerable heat and dust and must wear heavy protective gear. The powder is extremely fine and readily penetrates clothing. With sweating, a highly pruritic eruption results that consists of small, erythematous papules and pustules called *antimony spots,* which are largely limited to the arms, legs, and trunk.[18] The dermatitis does not result from allergic sensitization but from the irritating effects of the antimony salt combined with sweat. The condition is usually short lived unless secondary infection develops. Preventive measures include protective clothing and daily showers.[18]

A lichenoid contact dermatitis was reported by Paschoud[19, 20] in two workers after contact with antimony trioxide powder. Because patchtesting was done with the undiluted powder, the results were likely caused by irritation rather than allergic sensitization.

Antimony salts have been recognized as skin irritants in the rubber and textile industries, in ore extraction, and in smelting. Conjunctivitis, rhinitis, and pneumonitis have also been reported.[20–26] White and Mathias[27] reported a case of a brazing rod–manufacturing operator who developed a generalized eruption of follicular papules and pustules. The work included breaking up antimony and melting the pieces in a crucible, tasks that exposed the worker to antimony dust and antimony oxide fumes. The authors stated that the existing Occupational Safety and Health Administration (OSHA) permissible exposure limits (PELs) were inadequate to prevent the cutaneous effects of the antimony exposure.

ARSENIC

Metallic arsenic is found almost everywhere. Over 150 arsenic-bearing minerals are known. It occurs in trace amounts in freshwater and saltwater and in many foodstuffs and metal ores. Its chief commercial form, white arsenic or arsenic trioxide, is a byproduct of the smelting of copper, lead, cobalt, and nickel. During the smelting process, the white arsenic collects in the flues of the smelter furnaces and is trapped by electrostatic precicitators designed to prevent contamination of the environment.

Arsenic trioxide is the form most often used to manufacture arsenic compounds, which are marketed as insecticides, herbicides, and rodenticides. They are also used as growth stimulants for poultry and swine, as defoliants, and in the manufacture of glass and ceramics. Wood preservatives

TABLE 24–2 • Typical Compositions of Alloys Containing Antimony

Alloy	Composition (%)				
	Sb	Sn	Pb	Cu	Other
Electrotype	2.5	2.5	95		
Stereotype	14	6	80		
Lead base bearing alloy	9	5	85	0.5	
Tin base bearing alloy	6	87	3	4	
Cable sheathing	0.5		99.5		
Pewter	1–8	bal		0–3	
Storage battery plates	1.5–06	0.25–1	bal		
Antimonial naval brass	0.05	0.5–1			60, bal Zn

Key: Sb, antimony; Sn, strontium; Pb, lead; Cu, copper; bal, balance; Zn, zinc.

may contain as much as 25% sodium arsenate, with salts of copper and chromium. Alloyed with metals such as gallium, arsenic is an important ingredient in silicon wafers used in the semiconductor industry. In 1979, the National Institute of Occupational Safety and Health (NIOSH)[28] estimated that approximately 900,000 workers in the United States were daily exposed to some form of arsenic.[28] Arsenic dermatitis is usually irritant and most often occurs in smelter workers, who are exposed when cleaning the flues and dust collectors and loading and transporting the flue dust.[3] The fine dust collects in the clothing and under the face pieces of respirators; it mixes with sweat and can cause marked dermatitis. Initially, the lesions consist of perifollicular erythema accompanied by burning and itching. Later, papular and vesicular lesions appear, which sometimes progress to widespread pustular folliculitis.

In a study of several copper-smelting works in Sweden, Holmquist[29] found arsenic dermatitis in a large number of workers. The dermatitis was localized chiefly to areas of greatest exposure, such as the face, neck, forearms, wrists, and hands, but the scrotum, thighs, upper chest, back, and lower legs were also affected. Patchtesting with arsenic trioxide and other arsenic compounds resulted in eczematous and follicular reactions, which Holmquist considered to be allergic in nature; however, the test concentration of arsenic trioxide was not stated, so allergic sensitization was not proven.

In a study of arsenic contamination in a mining community in Utah, Birmingham and colleagues[30] described an eczematous, follicular eruption in smelter workers, two of whom showed perforation of the nasal septum. Several children of the workers were also affected as a result of contact with arsenic-laden dust in the environment. In some cases, the dermatitis closely resembled atopic dermatitis. Patchtesting with arsenic trioxide gave negative results.

Fisher[2] listed several arsenic compounds as potential allergens and stated that patchtesting with these compounds frequently resulted in irritant pustular reactions. It seems likely that inorganic arsenic compounds are chiefly irritants, but there have been reports that organic arsenic compounds may be allergic sensitizers.[31, 32] Contact dermatitis in glass workers was reported by Barbaud's and Goncalo's groups.[33, 34] In the factory described by Goncalo's group, three of the workers in contact with the arsenic trioxide developed dermatitis, which appeared to be irritant rather than allergic because patchtesting with dilutions of 5%, 2%, and 1% was negative whereas testing with the undiluted arsenic compound produced a reaction. The pattern of dermatitis in Goncalo's cases is similar to that described by Birmingham and colleagues.[30] Barbaud and coworkers[33] described one worker, a truck driver for a crystal factory, who in contact with sodium arsenate developed erythematous and vesicular dermatitis on the hands, arms, and legs. Patchtesting to 1% aqueous sodium arsenate was positive at 2 and 4 days. As with the patients of Goncalo and coworkers,[34] the dermatitis in each of these cases cleared when the source was withdrawn.

The cutaneous manifestations of chronic arsenic poisoning include pigmentary changes and keratotic lesions of the skin. The transverse white striae in fingernails, termed Mees' lines[35] were once considered characteristic of arsenic poisoning. Now they are known also to be associated with numerous other chemicals and diseases.[36] Other signs of arsenic poisoning are polyneuritis and alopecia. After years of exposure, keratotic lesions appear on the palms and soles, some of which may evolve into cutaneous carcinomas, a phenomenon first observed by Sir Jonathan Hutchinson in 1887.[37] The association between previous arsenic exposure and the later development of pulmonary and cutaneous malignancy, including Bowen's disease, was reconfirmed by Miki's group.[38]

Auto batteries contain lead and antimony alloys to which arsenic is added as a corrosion inhibitor. During recycling and melting of the batteries, calcium arsenite may be formed, which releases arsine gas in the presence of water. Because inhaled or ingested arsine gas breaks down to inorganic arsenic, chronic arsenic poisoning can result when small amounts are inhaled repeatedly over long periods.[28]

BERYLLIUM

Beryllium is a light, ductile, stable metal. The beryllium ores of most significance are beryl ($3BeO \cdot Al_2O_3 \cdot SiO_2$) found in Brazil, and vertrandite ($4BeO \cdot SiO_2 \cdot H_2O$) the latter occurring in Utah and being the principal source of beryllium in the Western world. Until 1920 beryllium was considered a curiosity, but by 1932 it had begun to assume importance in nuclear science and technology. Today beryllium is used as a hardening agent in metallurgy and in many space and nuclear applications. It has been used in x-ray windows for transmission of rays and to filter out electrons.

In contact with the skin the ore itself is innocuous, but during extraction from its ore, skin contact with soluble beryllium salts such as beryllium chloride and fluoride can cause ulceration and necrosis as well as systemic disease.[39] Besides eye, nose, and throat irritation, tracheobronchitis, and pneumonitis, granulomatous pulmonary disease, and skin ulcerations and granulomas occur. Accidental implantation of insoluble beryllium salts such as beryllium oxide in the skin can result in localized ulceration,[40] followed by the formation of granulomas, not only in skin but also in the regional lymphatics. Later, systemic granulomatous disease of the lungs and other organs may occur.[41] The granulomatous lesions resemble those of sarcoidosis and probably represent delayed hypersensitivity reactions.[40] The latent period between exposure and systemic disease is long, and individual susceptibility is varied.

Contact allergic sensitization from beryllium compounds was first described by Curtis,[42] who investigated 13 cases of dermatitis among workers in two beryllium extraction plants and found beryllium fluoride to have the greatest capacity to sensitize the skin. He considered the beryllium ion itself to be the allergen. Vilaplana and associates[43] reported two cases of beryllium contact allergy in

dental patients wearing beryllium-containing dental prostheses but noted no reactions on testing the dental personnel. Zissu and coworkers[44] found that persons sensitized to beryllium may also react to copper and aluminum beryllium alloys containing as little as 2%—or less—beryllium. For patchtesting, beryllium sulfate, 1% in petrolatum, has been recommended.[43, 45]

BORON

Boron, a metal closely resembling silicon, is a metalloid element occurring in bedded deposits and lake brines in the United States, Russia, and Turkey. Borax ($Na_2B_4O_7 \cdot 10H_2O$) and kernite ($Na_2B_4O_7 \cdot 4H_2$) are its chief mineral sources. It is used in the manufacture of glass, such as textile Fiberglas, glazes, coatings, enamels, soaps, and cleansers. Jet fuel propellants and additives in gasoline also use boron compounds. It is an important dopant for semiconductor devices. Boric acid has been used medically for decades as a topical antiseptic. Paint and soap manufacturers, glass workers, and welders may be exposed to this metal.

Allergic sensitization to boron and its compounds has not been reported, but several boron compounds are strong irritants. Diborane, a colorless gas used for synthesis of other boron compounds and as a catalyst for ethylene, is very irritating and can cause acute respiratory irritation and pulmonary edema. Exposure to pentaborane may induce severe central nervous system effects, including encephalopathy, seizures, and coma. The boron halides are strong irritants that cause eye, skin, and respiratory tract irritation.[46] Decaborane, used as a fuel additive, propellant, and rubber accelerator, is highly toxic and readily absorbed through the skin. Boron carbide is used as an abrasive for grinding and lapping. When inhaled, it is very irritating to the respiratory tract. Boron trifluoride is used mainly as a metallic catalyst for rapid-cure epoxy resins, but it is also found in soldering fluxes, as a fire retardant, and for gas brazing. It is very irritating to the skin and mucous membranes.

CADMIUM

Cadmium is present in the ores of zinc, lead, and copper and is rarely extracted from greenockite, the chief cadmium mineral, which, however, contains mostly cadmium sulfide. Its chief use is in electroplating, where it imparts corrosion resistance to steel, iron, and other metals intended for use in automotive and aircraft parts, marine equipment, and industrial machinery. It is also used in semiconductors, in photoelectric cells,[47] scintillation counters, fluorescent paint, and x-ray screens, among others. Cadmium sulfide and cadmium selenide are popular yellow pigments. Cadmium succinate is used as a fungicide.

Inhalation of cadmium oxide fumes has accounted for several industrial fatalities. Welders working in silver brazing are at risk, but cadmium poisoning also occurs in workers smelting zinc and remelting metal scraps that may not be suspected to contain cadmium, especially by persons who melt cadmium-nickel storage batteries during recycling.[48] There is often a delay of several hours after exposure before symptoms of sore throat, headache, myalgias, nausea, and a metallic taste appear (so-called metal fume fever). In severe cases, fuminant chemical pneumonitis with pulmonary edema and death can result. Chronic exposure has produced renal disease, Fanconi's syndrome, emphysema, and osteomalacia. Cadmium is also considered a lung carcinogen.

Cadmium has only rarely been reported as a contact allergen.[49] Wahlberg,[50] patchtesting 1,502 patients with eczema, found only 25 persons (1.7%) with $1+$ or $2+$ reactions to cadmium chloride, and in no subject could relevance be found. He thus concluded that the reactions must have been irritant. Later Wahlberg and Boman[51] were unable to demonstrate contact allergic sensitivity to cadmium using the guinea pig maximization method. Kaaber and associates (1982) tested 21 denture-wearers who complained of burning mouth sensations, with both cadmium chloride and cadmium sulfate, 2% in water.[8] Of these, 29 showed positive test results. When 17 were retested after 3 months, however, only seven showed definite positive reactions, and Kaaber concluded that they probably were allergic to cadmium. Six of the seven were heavy cigarette smokers, and Kaaber and his coworkers reported that a high concentration of cadmium is present in cigarettes and that cigarette smokers have twice the concentration of cadmium in their kidneys as nonsmokers.

Gebhardt and Geier[52] patchtested 42 dental technicians exhibiting contact dermatitis with cadmium chloride, 1% in petrolatum. Weak positive reactions were obtained in four, but the authors were unable to find relevance and concluded that the reactions probably represented irritant reactions.

When cadmium sulfide is used as the yellow pigment for tattoos, phototoxic reactions can result from sun exposure.[53] Trace amounts of yellow cadmium sulfide may also be present in red tattoos, along with mercuric sulfide, and photosensitivity may result. Sarcoidlike granulomas also may develop.[54]

CHROMIUM

Chromite ($FeOCr_2O_3$) is the principal ore of chromium and one of the most widely distributed of all metals. Chromium is the 13th most common element and occurs naturally almost entirely in trivalent form, usually combined with magnesium and aluminium oxides. Beside the earth's crust and saltwater, chromium is found in minute quantities in most foods and in freshwater. It has been recognized as an essential trace element in humans, particularly for glucose metabolism.[55] Human intake is small, about 60 μg per day.

Industrial uses for chromium were found soon after its discovery in 1797 by the French chemist Louis-Nicholas Vauquelin. By 1820 potassium dichromate was widely employed as a mordant in textiles. Because textile dyeing at that time was performed mostly by hand, the toxic properties of chromium soon became apparent. The Scottish physician William Cumin[56] in 1827 described "chrome holes" on the hands and forearms of dyers working in the Barrowfield Dye Works near Glasgow. By the mid-19th century, leather tanning with chromic acid had been introduced, and in 1879 chromite ore began to be used in refractory furnace bricks, because of its great heat resistance. By 1910, the importance of chromium as an alloy with other metals was well recognized. After World War I, chrome plating was introduced, and it found extensive application in the growing markets for automobiles and household appliances.

About 85% of all chromium produced is used in the metallurgy industries, principally for stainless steels, the most common variety of which contains 18% chromium. Other extensive uses are for low-alloy engineering steels to provide hardness; in nickel and cobalt alloys to provide high-temperature strength and corrosion resistance; and in cast irons for hardness, toughness, wear, and corrosion resistance. Minor applications in alloys are aluminium, zirconium, and zinc. Typical chromium alloys are listed in Table 24–3.

About 8% of the chromium produced is used in chemical applications. Leather tanning and timber preservation consume large amounts. Also, chromium pigments are used in paints, inks, and plastics to give green and yellow colors. Zinc and strontium chromates are corrosion inhibitors in primer paints. Other uses are as catalysts, in drilling muds, for anticorrosion in water treatment,

TABLE 24–3 • Types of Chromium Alloys

| Composition (%) | | | | | | Application |
Cr	Ni	Co	Fe	Mo	Other	
1			bal			Low alloy steel: engineering
17			bal			Stainless steel: domestic/industry
30			bal		1.5C	Chromium cast iron: engineering
12	12		bal			Stainless steel: watch cases
18	9		bal			Stainless steel: domestic/industry
18	9		bal		>0.155	Stainless steel: free machining
17	12		bal	2½		Stainless steel: domestic/industry
25	20		bal			Heat resisting steel
28	1	bal		6		Surgical implant alloy
26	14	bal		4		Surgical implant alloy
15	bal		8			High temperature alloy
20	bal				.05 Ti	Wrought jet engine alloy
18	bal	19		4	3A1, 3Ti	Cast jet engine alloy
16	bal		5	16	4W	Corrosion-resistant alloy

Key: Cr, chromium; Ni, nickel; Co, cobalt; Fe, iron; Mo, molybdenum; bal, balance.

electroplating, chromating passivation treatment, and for textile dyes.

Another major use of chromium occurs in refractories, which consume about 7% of total production. The chromium ore, often blended with magnesium, is used as refractory lining for furnaces and converters in the steel, copper, and other metal industries and for rotary kilns in the cement industry. Chromite foundry molding sands have the advantage of high heat conductivity. Major chromium compounds and their uses are shown in Table 24–4. In 1976 NIOSH[57] estimated that 175,000 workers in the United States were exposed to chromium.

Chromium exists in each of the oxidation states from −1 to +6, but only the ground states of 0, +2, +3, and +6 are common. Of these, only the trivalent and hexavalent salts are sufficiently stable to act as haptens. The bivalent compounds are unstable and have no industrial uses. The trivalent forms predominate in industry; they are generally less irritating than the hexavalent compounds and only rarely induce allergic sensitization. The hexavalent compounds are corrosive and destructive to the skin and are strong allergic sensitizers. It is important to emphasize that only the salts of chromium act as haptens and induce sensitization; the chromium molecule itself is not a sensitizer.

Irritant Chromate Dermatitis

The classic chromium lesion is the chrome ulcer (chrome hole or chrome sore), which results from contact with chromic acid, sodium or potassium chromate or dichromate, or ammonium dichromate. Ulceration is enhanced when these compounds contact moist surfaces such as the nasal septum and conjunctivae or abrasions or puncture wounds. The ulcers often appear over the joints of fingers, on the anterior areas of the legs, in periungual regions, on the eyelids, and anywhere the skin is broken.[3] In 1902 Legge described them on the tonsils, palate, and larynx. They are small, punched-out, relatively painless lesions with firm, rolled borders (Fig. 24–1). They invade cartilage, but not bone, and range in diameter from 2 to 4 mm.[58] They heal very slowly and leave scars. Secondary bacterial infection is common, but malignant change never occurs.[59] There is no relationship between chrome ulcers and allergic sensitization.[60]

Ulceration and perforation of the anterior nasal septum are caused by persistent irritation of the nasal mucous membranes by dusts or mists containing chromic acid, sodium or potassium dichromate, or ammonium chromate. Accompanied by surprisingly little discomfort, the necrosis of the cartilage ceases after healing of the mucous surface.

In the past chrome ulcers were common in textile dyers and finishers, leather tanners, chromium ore smelters, electroplaters, and other industrial workers. They are less common today, but still occur in smelters and electroplaters.[3, 61] In 1978 Burrows found the incidence in the United Kingdom to be approximately 100 cases per year, mostly in electroplaters, almost the same frequency that was reported during the 1930s.

The incidence of chrome ulcers is directly related to contamination of the workplace. Dornan[62]

TABLE 24-4 · Chromium Compounds Commonly Used in Industry

Analytic Standards Reagents
Potassium

Batteries
Barium chromate (fused-salt batteries for the space
  program)
Calcium chromate (fused-salt batteries)
Sodium dichromate (dry cells)
Zinc chromate (dry cells)

**Catalysts (for Hydrogenation, Oxidation, and
  Polymerization)**
Chromic acid
Chromic chloride
Magnesium dichromate
Nickel chromate
Silver chromate
Zinc chromate

Ceramics
Aluminum chromate
Chrome oxide green
Chromic acid
Chrome sulfate
Chromium potassium sulfate
Cobalt chromite
Manganese chromate
Pyridine dichromate

Corrosion Inhibitors
Calcium chromate
Lithium chromate
Lithium dichromate
Magnesium chromate
Morpholine chromate
Sodium and potassium dichromates
Strontium chromate
Zinc chromate

Chromate Surface Treatments
Ammonium dichromate
Chromic acid
Potassium dichromate
Sodium dichromate

Drilling Muds
Chromium lignosulfonates (from sodium dichromate
  using lignosulfate waste)

Electroplating
Chromic acid
Chromic chloride

Engraving
Chromic acid

Explosives
Chromic nitrate

Fire Retardant
Chromatized zinc chloride

Magnetic Tapes
Chromium dioxide

Milk Preservatives
Potassium dichromate

Paints and Varnishes
Barium potassium chromate
Calcium chromate
Chromic acid
Chromic hydroxide
Chromic phosphate
Chromic sulfate
Chromium naphthenate
Chromium oxide green
Lead chromate
Lead silicochromate
Mercuric chromate
Mercurous chromate
Strontium chromate
Zinc chromate
Zinc tetroxychromate

Paper
"Chromic cake" (sodium sulfate and sodium
  dichromate)

Photography
Chromium phosphate sulfate
Sodium and potassium dichromate

Roofing
Chromic oxide green

Surgical Sutures
Ammonium dichromate (catgut)
Potassium dichromate (silk)

Tanning Leather
Basic chromic sulfate
Chromic acetate
Chromic acid
Chromic formate
Chromic sulfate
Chromium ammonium sulfate

Television Screens
Ammonium chromate

Textile Mordants and Dyes
Chromium acetate
Chromic acid
Chromic chloride
Chromic formate
Chromic sulfate
  Chromium ammonium sulfate
  Chromium potassium sulfate
  Chromium ammonium sulfate
  Sodium potassium dichromate

Wood Preservatives
Chromated copper arsenate
Fluorochrome-arsenic phenol

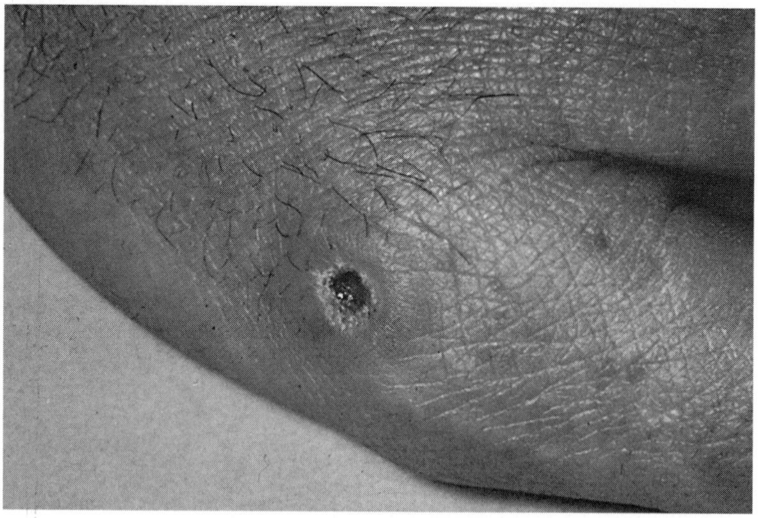

FIGURE 24–1 • A typical chrome hole in a common location. The lesion is a shallow, punched-out ulcer that is relatively painless. (Photograph courtesy of Dr. Alan Lyell.)

visited 27 firms in England that did chrome plating and examined 150 chrome platers. Nine workers had either nasal or skin ulcers. An active health education program was established and chromate in the environment was reduced, and a repeat survey 3 years later revealed no new cases of chrome ulceration.

Allergic Chromate Dermatitis

Parkhurst[63] in 1925 was the first to report chromium contact allergy based on skin testing in a blueprint processor who had eczematous dermatitis on the forearms, wrists, and neck. Open testing on the thigh with a 0.5% aqueous solution of potassium dichromate produced a papulovesicular reaction in 24 hours. The Prussian blue method of blueprinting was used by Parkhurst's patient: a dilute solution of potassium dichromate was used as a fixative. Several of the steps in the process were done by hand. With a procedure that Prosser-White[64] had previously recommended, Parkhurst succeeded in keeping the patient free of dermatitis by having her rinse her hands and arms in a concentrated solution of sodium bisulfite, which acted as a reducing agent. So long as she used this solution every hour or so, she remained free of dermatitis.

A few years later, Smith observed a patient with chromate sensitivity from occupational contact with ammonium chromate.[65] Patchtesting with a 1% aqueous solution produced a positive, probable irritant, result; intradermal testing with a 0.5% concentration, however, resulted in a severe, generalized eruption.

Chromate dermatitis in lithography was first described in 1931 by Englehardt and Mayer,[66] who found 25 workers with chromate dermatitis and positive patchtest results to 0.5% potassium dichromate. None of these patients reacted to testing with trivalent chromium. Kesten and Laszlo[67] also in 1931, described a printer who developed severe, widespread dermatitis from contact with a 0.1% solution of sodium dichromate. Patchtesting produced a reaction.

In 1939 Bonnevie[68] reviewed a large number of patients with eczema and found that 5.5% reacted to patchtesting with potassium dichromate. Schwartz and Dunn[69] reported chrome dermatitis in workers in woolen mills and air-conditioning services.[69] They showed a rising incidence of sensitivity as increasing concentrations of chromium were used in the workplace; when the concentration was raised from 0.5% to 3%, many workers who had not previously been sensitive became so.

During World War II numerous cases of chrome dermatitis occurred in the aircraft industry, especially from contact with zinc chromate primer paints.[4] Hall emphasized the severity and persistence of chrome dermatitis and cautioned against using chrome in preemployment patchtesting.

In 1949, Pirila and Kilpio[70] found chrome sensitivity in workers in 41 different jobs, including lithography, cement work (Fig. 24–2), radio repair, chrome plating, painting, and dyeing among others. In each, patchtesting with 0.5% potassium dichromate produced results. The authors stressed the persistence of chrome dermatitis and the long duration of disability. Ten cement workers were sensitive to dichromate, but the significance of this finding eluded the authors. They implicated the interaction of alkaline cement with chrome-tanned leather gloves releasing chromate ions onto the skin, rather than the presence of chromate ion in the cement.

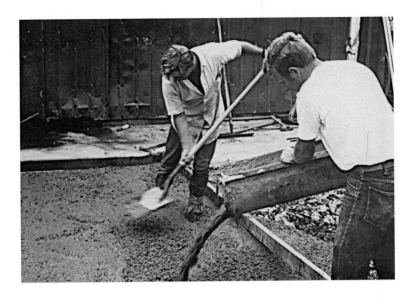

FIGURE 24–2 • Cement contains variable amounts of hexavalent chromium, which can cause a chronic, persistent, disabling dermatitis.

It was at a congress of Swiss dermatologists in 1950 that Jaeger and Pelloni[71] reported their important work on the significance of chromium in cement as a cause of dermatitis.[71] In describing 32 cement workers, of whom 30 had positive patchtest reactions to chromium, they demonstrated the presence of minute amounts of hexavalent chromium in cement and concluded that it was the cause of cement sensitivity dermatitis. The results of testing with trivalent chromium produced negative results in three patients. The relationship of chromate sensitivity to cement dermatitis has since been confirmed by numerous investigations worldwide.

Because of their potent anticorrosion properties, potassium and sodium dichromate found wide application in the cooling systems of diesel locomotives. Winston and Walsh[72] were the first to recognize that locomotive repair shop workers with severe, incapacitating dermatitis required hospitalization; each one had a positive patchtest reaction to 0.25% sodium dichromate. The final concentration of sodium dichromate in the radiator and cooling system water was approximately 0.08%. The workers at greatest risk were those who prepared and poured the solutions; those who cleaned and repaired the motors received less exposure. In 1952 Schwartz[73] reported additional cases of chrome dermatitis in railroad roundhouses and machine shops, and Calnan and Harman[74] further studied diesel coolant dermatitis resulting from chromates. Chromates are still used in some coolant systems because they are very effective and do not form insoluble deposits, but because of concerns about carcinogenicity, their use has been much curtailed in recent years.

Chromium Metals and Alloys

Considerable exposure to chromium metal occurs because of its use as a decorative coating on nickel plating of steel, brass, and zinc alloys. It is highly resistant to atmospheric corrosion and to many aqueous solutions and thus is an unlikely cause of contact allergy; however, thin coatings tend to be porous and those thicker than about 0.6 μm tend to be cracked. Thus, chromium coatings do not always provide consistently effective protection from allergy arising from corrosion of the nickel undercoat.

Chromium is an extremely important alloying element, providing strength, toughness, hardness, and especially corrosion resistance, to iron-, nickel-, and cobalt-based alloys. Stainless steels contain 10% to 30% chromium, but at the lower end of the range their passivitiy is suspect, owing to the presence of a surface film of chromium oxide. Under adverse environmental conditions of acidity and a high chloride content, especially in crevices, the oxide film can break down and permit corrosion to occur. The corrosion products formed are trivalent chromium, unless an oxidizing agent is present, in which case hexavalent chromium could be produced. The formation of hexavalent chromium ions from body implants has been reported[75]; however, determination of chromium release from low-chromium stainless steels and a nickel-based alloy in synthetic sweat or in saline solution showed only the formation of trivalent chromium. Hexavalent chromium could not be detected (detection limit 0.003 μg/mL) (Carter, personal communication). Accordingly, it may be deduced that should dermatitis occur as a result of corrosion of stainless steel in contact with the skin, it is more likely to be caused by the formation of nickel ions than by the presence of hexavalent chromium.

Since the early 1950s allergic contact dermatitis from chromium has been reported from numerous occupational sources and processes, including lithography;[76, 77] galvanized sheet metal;[78] primer paints[79, 80] (Fig. 24–3); chrome-tanned leather shoes and gloves[81–83]; boiler linings[84]; welding fumes[85]; green felt covers for gambling tables[87]; military uniforms[88]; tattoos[89, 90]; match heads[91, 92]; auto assembly[93] (Fig. 24–4); magnetic tapes[94]; paper pulp manufacture[95–97]; cutting fluids[98]; tire fitters[99]; milk testers[100, 101]; food laboratories[102]; machine oils[103–105]; pigment in soap[106]; aircraft workers in contact with resin hardeners containing large amounts of chromate[107]; and many others.

Incidence of Chromate Dermatitis

Men are more likely than women to become sensitized to chromate because of the type of work men traditionally, at least in the past, performed.[108, 109] Nethercott, reviewing the world literature on routine patchtesting for dichromate (17,021 cases), found an incidence of 7.9% positivity to potassium dichromate.[110] The true incidence of chromate allergy is probably considerably lower, however. The question arises whether potassium dichromate, 0.5% in petrolatum, which has been the standard patchtest dilution for chromate, produces a number of irritant, false-positive, reactions. In the United States 0.25% is the standard test concentration for patchtesting dichromate, and 0.5% is used in Europe. Burrows,[111] in a multicenter study, showed that testing with 0.5% potassium dichromate detects more allergic reactions than 0.25% challenge, but it also results in more irritant

reactions; 0.25% misses some true positives but shows fewer irritant responses. A compromise at 0.375% produced a similar result (Burrows et al, 1989).[111a] Samsoen and associates[112] have suggested that 0.25% might be a better percentage for patchtesting. Whichever patchtest concentration is used, one must keep in mind that 0.5% produces a number of irritant reactions that can be mistaken for positives, and testing at 0.25% misses some positive reactions. Burrows,[113] on retesting patients with positive patchtest results within 6 months later, found that only 36% had a positive reaction with a single chromate patchtest. Fischer and Rystedt[114] (1985) considered that only 40% of their positive chromium patchtest results were accurate, and Peltonen and Fraki[115] found only 1.7% positive patchtest results in selected clinic patients. It is possible that sensitization can occur to bichromate without obvious (or remembered) skin disease. Burrows and Calnan[116] found two healthy cement workers, each with positive patchtest results to chromate, but it was months later when one of them developed severe dermatitis. Peltonen and Fraki[115] found a higher incidence of positive patchtest results (even in workers without skin disease) in those exposed to chromate, for instance, lithographers. Decaestecker and coworkers[117] found the same phenomenon in workers in a chromate pigment factory, 1.7% of whom had a positive patchtest to dichromate although they had no evidence of dermatitis. Goh and coworkers[118] found that 2.9% of workers in a prefabrication construction factory also had asymptomatic chromate sensitivity.

Positive patchtests to chromate persist long. Thormann and coworkers[119] showed that, even after 4 to 7 years, 79% of the chromate-sensitive subjects still tested positive. Keczkes' group[120]

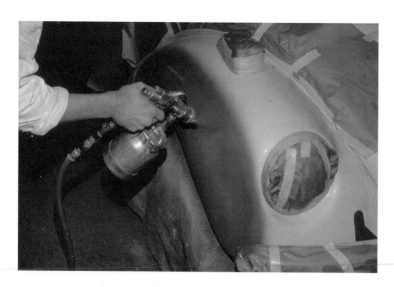

FIGURE 24–3 • Some primer paints contain small amounts of hexavalent chromium as a preservative. In body and fender painting there can be considerable exposure to the spray.

FIGURE 24–4 • *A* and *B*: Radiator cleaning solutions as well as carburetor cleaners may contain dichromate to inhibit rusting.

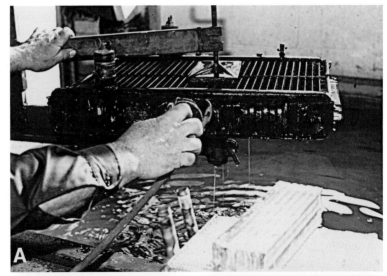

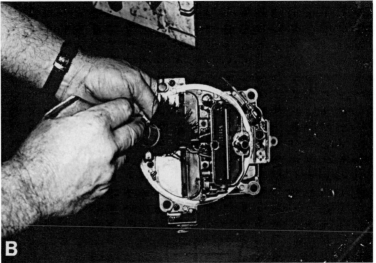

confirmed this, demonstrating that 100% of their patients with a positive patchtest to potassium dichromate were still positive even 10 years later.

Allergic contact dermatitis caused by chromium is eczematous, often widespread, very persistent, and may exhibit a pattern resembling nummular eczema.[108, 119] Often, lichenification and marked dryness resemble atopic dermatitis. Relapse occurs repeatedly after exposure, and after each recurrence the condition becomes more extensive, severe, and difficult to treat.

Photosensitivity has been said to be associated with chrome dermatitis. Feuerman[120a] considered photosensitivity common in these patients and attributed the increased incidence to the amount of sunlight in the regions where the workers lived and worked. Wahlberg and Wennersten[121] tested 25 patients with chrome allergy and showed more intense reactions in sites irradiated with short-wave length ultraviolet light; however, it has not been proved that there is any connection between ultraviolet light sensitivity and chromate dermatitis except what could be expected in subjects with irritable, sun-damaged skin who are tested with a mild irritant. White and Rycroft (personal communication) were unable to find an increased incidence of chromate sensitivity in patients with photosensitivity. Wall,[122] from Western Australia, reported a single case of a person with long-standing dichromate allergy who developed a severe degree of photosensitivity later in life. Because the distribution of widespread chromate dermatitis often is not entirely characteristic of contact dermatitis, its appearance on exposed areas of skin, and its superficial resemblance to photodermatitis, it is easy to confuse the two conditions. Goh[123] has shown, however, that there was little chromate in the atmosphere of a Singapore cement construction factory, or in a busy city center.

Still to be explained is the consistent finding of a high incidence of unexplained positive patchtest reactions in women.[111, 114] Goh[125] reported that only 25.6% of patchtest reactions remained unexplained in men, but 66.7% were unexplained in women. There are two possible explanations for this.

The first is the chromate content of detergents. In 1969 Feuerman[126] reported that many household detergents contain small amounts of dichromate. In some European countries certain commonly used bleaches contain dichromate as a coloring and stabilizing agent.[127] Burrows[113] also demonstrated that several detergents contain minute amounts of chromate.

Allenby and Goodwin[128] found that 13 of 14 patients did not react to less than 885 ppm of dichromate, although one patient reacted to as little as 1 ppm. Basketter and coworkers[129] showed an analysis of various detergents that the chromium concentration was less than 5 ppm, levels that the authors considered too low to cause initial sensitization, especially considering the typically brief exposures. Dermatitis could not be excluded, however, in a presensitized person. Furthermore, considering the dilution with water, patients would be unlikely to contact more than 0.3 ppm, which would be unlikely to cause sensitization. Nethercott and associates[130] reported that persons previously sensitized to dichromate developed inflammation of sweat ducts after dipping their forearms in a solution containing 25 μg/mL of chromate for 30 minutes. Thus, it is not likely that detergents can be ruled out as a cause of contact dermatitis in persons sensitive to dichromate. Other sources of exposure have been suggested, such as chromate remaining on cloths used to clean metal, and perhaps exposure even to cigarette ash.[131]

The second possibility is women also have a higher incidence of positive patchtest results to several other substances, for example, nickel.[132a] If testing with 0.5% potassium dichromate causes numerous irritant reactions, is it possible that the reaction to dichromate in women is simply an example of the so-called angry back phenomenon, in which marginal irritants (such as dichromate) become positive in the presence of other genuine positive reactions (e.g., nickel)?

The marked and unusually chronic nature of chrome dermatitis is a major problem for patients and dermatologists. In contrast to patients with other chemical dermatitides, many chrome-sensitive patients fail to improve even after years of no contact with chromium.[133] Burrows[134] has shown that although 20% of persons with occupational dermatitis from various sources are free of dermatitis after 10 to 13 years, only 6% of chromate-sensitive cement workers are asymptomatic. In a study of 1,152 patients with occupational dermatitis in the building, metal, and tanning industries, Fregert[108] found that 2 or 3 years after diagnosis and treatment, only 10% of those responding to a follow-up questionnaire reported complete freedom from dermatitis.

Although the reasons for persistence of chrome dermatitis are not known, a common explanation is that the abundance of unrecognized chromium in the environment makes daily contact rather common. Nater[135] found trace amounts in many articles of daily life and in many workplaces. Minute quantities are found in food, water, and even cigarettes.[136] There has been speculation that oral ingestion may precipitate recurrences in sensitive patients,[137, 138] but so far this has not been proven.[139, 140]

In hospital cleaning personnel, Hansen[132] found a low incidence of chromate dermatitis. Chrome-tanned leather has also been suggested as a source of continuing dermatitis. While it is true that trivalent chrome is used mostly in leather tanning, potassium dichromate has been considered the most reliable chemical for diagnostic patchtesting for chrome sensitivity to leather in shoes.[39]

Another explanation is that chromium may persist in human tissues for a long time, especially after heavy exposure. A worker who died of maxillary and lung cancers after having been exposed at work to hexavalent chromium for more than 30 years was found at autopsy to have much more chromium content in his lungs and other organs than did normal healthy controls.[141]

The Chromate Content of Cement

There is much variation in the hexavalent chromium content of finished cement ready for use. In British cement, for example, Johnston and Calnan[142] found the chromate content to range from none to 1,200 μg/L in 24 samples. In the United States, Perone's group[143] could find only 18 of 42 cement samples to have measurable amounts of soluble chromate, which varied from 0.1 to 5.4 μg. Other studies also show great variation in chrome content, from zero to 40 μg to 0.2%.[144, 145] Brun in Switzerland,[146] Meneghini and colleagues in Italy,[147] and Wahlberg's group in Sweden[148] studied the soluble hexavalent content of the cement of their respective countries and showed variations in chromium content. Ellis and Freeman,[149] analyzing Australian cement, found that water-soluble hexavalent chromate content varied from less than 1 to 124 ppm, the majority of samples having less than 10 ppm. It is important to remember that the water-soluble fraction is the most important in causing dermatitis and that it does not necessarily correlate with the total chromium content.

There has always been difficulty reconciling the small amounts of hexavalent chromium in cement with the much higher concentrations required to induce positive patchtest results. Pirila,[150] testing chrome-sensitive patients with various dilutions, found only one patient who reacted to testing at 0.001%, whereas 25 patients reacted to 0.1%. The cement with which these workers were in contact had a concentration of only 0.0001%! The lowest dilution of potassium dichromate to which workers reacted in a study by Geiser and coworkers[151] was 0.01%. In a similar study, Anderson[152] found nearly identical results. Possible explanations for this discrepancy are that (1) the alkalinity of cement contributes greatly to percutaneous absorption of the soluble chromate ion and (2) dermatitis from cement usually develops on skin already damaged by irritation caused by the cement's alkalinity and abrasiveness. Patchtesting, on the other hand, is performed on normal skin, and a much stronger concentration is required for penetration of the allergen.

Hexavalent Versus Trivalent Chromium as Allergens

Can trivalent chromium compounds induce allergic sensitization? In 1966 Kligman,[153] using the maximization test, showed that both valence forms have the ability to sensitize and suggested that the reason why trivalent forms rarely induce sensitization is their poor solubility. In fact, most trivalent chromium compounds are insoluble and penetrate the epidermal barrier only with difficulty. Hexavalent chromium compounds are freely soluble and pass readily through the skin's barrier.[154] When the barrier is bypassed by intradermal injection, however, trivalent chromium readily induces delayed hypersensitivity reactions in sensitized subjects.[155] Using standard patchtest techniques, Fregert and Rorsman showed that, if the concentration of trivalent chromium is high enough and exposure time sufficiently prolonged, positive patchtest results occur.[155]

Samitz and Katz[154] showed that 1 g of skin was able to reduce 1.06 mg of hexavalent chromium to the trivalent form. This trivalent chromium then combines with protein.

Polak,[156] patchtesting guinea pigs, demonstrated

that there was no difference in eliciting an allergic response when sensitizing with either hexavalent or trivalent chromium. The same percentage of guinea pigs reacted to hexavalent and trivalent chromates, whether sensitized with one or the other. In both cases, a much smaller percentage of them reacted to trivalent chromium. Polak's conclusion was that the difference was in the eliciting rather than in the sensitizing. It has been shown that lymphocytes of guinea pigs sensitized to two different antigens and repeatedly stimulated in vitro with one of them lose their capacity to respond to the other.[157] Siegenthalar and coworkers[158] found that lymphocytes from animals sensitized with potassium dichromate did not lose their ability to respond to chromium chloride (trivalent), even after repeated stimulation in vitro with potassium dichromate. These results present strong evidence for existence of a single, common determinant. Polak and colleagues[157] demonstrated that patchtest results with chromium compounds depend more on solubility than on valence. They claimed that any chromium compound, even the relatively insoluble lead chromate, can be allergenic under certain conditions.

Chrome Dermatitis from Oral Ingestion

Fregert[137] and others[138, 159, 160] have suggested that oral ingestion of minute amounts of chromates can provoke flare-ups of chrome dermatitis. The difficulties of performing a controlled study of this type using volunteers, not to mention the medicolegal issues, are considerable. McMillan[161] was unable to confirm that ingestion of chromate made any difference to chromate dermatitis, whether it was fed with or without ascorbic acid. Veien and colleagues[160] have repeated their studies, which consisted in placebo-controlled oral challenge. They found that 17 of 30 patients reacted to oral chromate but not to placebo, two reacted to both chromate and placebo, and four reacted to placebo but not to dichromate. Seven patients had no reaction.

Treatment of Chrome Dermatitis

Chrome ulcers can be prevented by immediate, prolonged flushing with large amounts of water followed by application of an antibiotic ointment. Immersion of the hands and arms in a reducing solution such as 10% aqueous ascorbic acid, which converts the hexavalent chromium to trivalent, was suggested by Samitz.[162] For maximum effectiveness, treatment must begin immediately after chromium exposure and be repeated frequently. When chromate exposure ceases, the lesions heal in 4 to 6 weeks.

Prevention of Chromate Dermatitis

Prevention of chrome ulcers depends almost entirely on the personal cleanliness of the worker and the use of protective clothing. Adequate ventilation to remove mists and dusts is also essential; electroplating tanks, especially, must be equipped with functioning exhaust ventilation. Respirators should be only those approved by OSHA and should be checked daily for contamination and properly functioning valves. Bimonthly examination of the skin and nose to detect the early signs of irritation is advisable, as is a yearly physical examination, including a chest radiograph.

Chromate-sensitive persons should have some knowledge of the many other environmental sources of chromium. Although a lengthy list of substances that may contain chromium could confuse and unduly alarm patients, workers should know which occupations carry the greatest risk for producing chrome dermatitis. Table 24–5 is a list of the workers who may be at risk of chromium dermatitis.

Unfortunately, changing occupations does not always ensure healing of dermatitis, and some physicians have suggested that workers with mild or moderate dermatitis be encouraged to remain at work and to use precautions. Indeed, many highly motivated workers will want to do so. In the initial stages, however, chromate dermatitis often clears on removal from the source of contact, and if a change of occupation can be arranged, the prognosis may be much better. Lips and coworkers[163] found that a change of occupation and strict avoidance of all contact with cement and other sources of chromium result in a much better prognosis for these workers; 72% had healed in the first few years. Substitution for the aggravating allergen is sometimes possible for leather gloves, work shoes, printing materials, and anticorrosion agents, among others. Substitution of trivalent chromium for hexavalent chromium in electroplating baths could greatly reduce toxicity and allergic contact dermatitis.[164] Occasionally, a plant can find acceptable substitutes for hexavalent chromium in the manufacturing process.

Barrier creams containing various substances that may reduce hexavalent chromium to the trivalent form have been tested in patients who are allergic to chromate. Among the substances believed to reduce the hexavalent chromium are ascorbic acid[165]; ascorbic acid with ethylenediamine tetraacetic acid (EDTA),[166] dithionate,[167] tartaric acid plus glycine,[166] and sodium metabisul-

 TABLE 24–5 • Workers Potentially Exposed to Chromium

Abrasive makers	Laboratory workers
Acetylene purifiers	Leather finishers
Adhesive workers	Lithographers
Alloy makers	Match makers
Aluminum anodizers	Metal cleaners
Anodizers	Milk preservers
Battery makers	Oil drillers
Biologists	Oil purifiers
Boiler scalers	Painters
Candle makers	Paper waterproofers
Cement workers	Pencil makers
Ceramic workers	Perfume makers
Chemical workers	Photoengravers
Chromate workers	Photographers
Chromate alloy workers	Platinum polishers
Chromium-alum workers	Porcelain decorators
	Pottery frosters
Chromium platers	Pottery glazers
Copper etchers	Printers
Copper plate strippers	Refractory brick makers
Corrosion inhibitor workers	Rubber makers
	Shingle makers
Drug makers	Silk screen makers
Dye makers	Smokeless powder makers
Dyers	
Electroplaters	Soap makers
Enamel workers	Sponge bleachers
Explosives makers	Steel workers
Fat purifiers	Tanners
Fireworks makers	Textile workers
Fur processors	Wax workers
Glass frosters	Welders
Glassmakers	Wood preservative workers
Glue makers	
Histology technicians	Wood stainers
Jewelers	

Adapted from Milby TH, Key MM, Gibson RL, et al: Chemical hazards. In: Occupational Hazards: A Guide to Their Recognition, publ 1097, U.S. Dept. of Health, Education, and Welfare. Washington, U.S. Public Health Service, 1964.

fite.[116] Romaguera has also found effective in a clinical trial a preparation containing silicone, glyceryl lactate, glycine, and tartaric acid.[166]

Should Ferrous Sulfate Be Added to Cement?

The rationale for adding ferrous sulfate to cement is to change the hexavalent chromium to trivalent, which has less potential for causing dermatitis.[168] In 1971 Burckhardt[169] found that ferrous sulfate combines with hexavalent chromium in cement to form an insoluble trivalent compound. Iron sulfate ($FeSO_4 \cdot 7H_2O$), 0.3% weight for weight, is sufficient to reduce 20 μg of hexavalent chromium per gram of dry cement. The resulting concrete is not altered in any way. Fregert and colleagues[168] have recommended that the iron sulfate be added to the cement immediately before mixing, when contact with the skin is most likely to occur; however, others have advocated adding it at the time of manufacture. The purpose is to decrease the content of hexavalent chromium to less than 2 ppm. It has been shown that ferrous sulfate does indeed do this, and patchtesting with such cement in chromate-allergic patients does not produce an allergic reaction.

The addition of ferrous sulfate to cement became mandatory in Denmark in 1983, in Finland in 1987, and in Sweden in 1989. Follow-up studies have shown a considerable reduction in allergic dermatitis in all three countries[170]; in Denmark, irritant dermatitis decreased as well. In Finland the results were striking: a reduction in the average number of chromate cases decreased from 23 per year before introduction of ferrous sulfate to an average of 6.5 cases afterward.[171] Avnstorp's study showed a considerable reduction in cement dermatitis in cement fabrication plants, a result also observed in Finland (Table 24–6).[170] The problems of worldwide acceptance of this remarkable preventive procedure are these:

1. Many countries that have not added ferrous sulfate to cement also report decreases in chrome dermatitis.[172–174]

2. Chromate allergy was already decreasing significantly before the introduction of ferrous sulfate.[173]

3. Contact allergic dermatitis due to chromium has been described from cement to which ferrous sulfate had been added.[175] It has been suggested that this could be due to the relatively short shelf life of the ferrous sulfate.[171]

4. The incidence of chromate dermatitis is decreasing in other industries as well, such as the pottery industry.

5. Contact dermatitis to chromate in Scandinavian countries is decreasing in females as well, suggesting factors other than cement.[176] It is possible that the reduction in the presumed incidence of chrome dermatitis could result from more rigorous criteria for reading patchtest results, and not considering results allergic when, in fact, they were irritant.

6. It may be that other substances such as cobalt are involved in cement dermatitis.[177] Irvine and coworkers[178] found a high incidence of cobalt dermatitis in underground workers during construction of the tunnel under the English Channel (the Chunnel). It is possible that cobalt is a significant allergen in cement and of course would not be eliminated by the addition of ferrous sulfate.

7. One of the greatest deterrents to the general use of ferrous sulfate is its cost. In a country the size of Britain the cost would be approximately £20 million per year, with a capital cost of £3 million. Is this cost effective? It might be considered that, in the case of a disease that produces only about six cases per million per year (in Finland), a better use might be found for this expenditure.

8. The incidence of chromate dermatitis could be expected to decrease because of changes in cement manufacture: certain gas and coal-fired kilns with magnesium-chrome refractories are currently being changed to magnesium aluminate (spinel) refractories.[179] Also, there is likely to be increasing use of slag (a clinker substitute) from iron blast furnaces, which contain little or no chromate.[180] These changes will likely significantly decrease the chromate content of cement. It is well-recognized that large differences in chromate content of cement already exist throughout the world,[181] and the effect of using ferrous sulfate in countries where there is normally a low level may not prove as effective, or even as desirable, as in countries where levels are high.

COBALT

Cobalt was discovered in the 16th century by miners in Saxony, and for many years it was discarded as an impurity, although oxides of cobalt have been used as pigments for more than 2,000 years. Cobalt is the 33rd element in order of abundance in the earth's crust and is essential for

TABLE 24–6 • Iron Sulfate Method of Reducing Hexavalent Chromium to the Trivalent, Nonsensitizing State

Prepare a solution of crystalline ferrous sulfate by dissolving 1 kg (2.2 lb) of crystalline ferrous sulfate in 3 L (3 quarts) of water. Keep the solution in a dark plastic container. Do not prepare more than 3–4 days' supply at one time. If the solution turns brown, it is inactive. Crystalline ferrous sulfate is hygroscopic, and containers must be closed and kept dry.

Add the solution to concrete as follows: 1.3 L (approx. 1⅓ quarts) to each 100 kg (220 lb) of cement.

The preparation does not alter the characteristics of the concrete in any way when used in the above concentration.

all animal life, being the central constituent of vitamin B_{12}. Cobalt is usually a co-product from nickel and copper ores and is obtained in two forms, ingot and powder. As a result, nickel frequently occurs as a minor element in cobalt alloys and compounds. Cobalt is a silvery metal having many properties similar to those of iron and nickel. Its main use as an individual metal is as a binder for cemented carbide tools, but its major application is in alloys with iron, nickel, chromium, and molybdenum. Compounds of cobalt are used as pigments, as driers in paints and inks, catalysts, in adhesives, and in agriculture and medicine.

Until World War II the glass and ceramics industries used much of the world's supply as a blue pigment. Since then, metallic cobalt has been used chiefly for various high-temperature, high-strength alloys required for machining and cutting functions and for jet and rocket parts. Cobalt salts, especially cobalt naphthenate and cobalt oleate, are employed as driers for lacquers, varnishes, paints, printing inks, pigments, and enamels. Cobalt is also used as a catalyst in polyester resin systems, as an oxidizing agent, in automobile exhaust control, in electroplating to brighten nickel-plated objects, and in lamp filaments. It may also be found in small quantities in European cement but probably not to any extent in cement made in the United States (Table 24–7).[143]

Like nickel, cobalt is everywhere and can be detected by atomic absorption in minute quantities in soil, water, plants, and animal tissues. It is not highly reactive but does oxidize in air on heating. It reacts with many acids to form divalent salts. The major use of the metal is as a very fine powder mixed with tungsten or other carbides in the production of sintered carbide parts. Cobalt metal reacts slowly with sweat to form cobalt ions, and, as a result, prolonged direct contact may cause contact allergy. However, domestic exposure to cobalt metal is extremely rare, and in consequence the occurrence of contact dermatitis due to cobalt is much less frequent than that due to nickel.

The major alloys and their applications are listed in Table 24–8, together with an assessment of the likelihood of their behaving as cobalt metal does and of having the potential for causing contact dermatitis. The cobalt atom can exist in oxidation states of 0, +1, +2, and +3. The commonest are +2 and mixed +2/+3; +1/+2 occurs in only a few complex compounds. Soluble salts are used in electroplating, in animal feed, and in catalysts used for production of terephthalate plastics. Oxide catalysts are used extensively in the oil industry for desulfurization. Cobalt oxides,

TABLE 24–7 • Major Cobalt Compounds Used in Industry

Adhesives for bonding steel cable to rubber in tires
  Cobalt naphthenate
  Cobalt stearate
  Cobalt boro-acrylate complexes
Additives for animal feed
  Cobalt sulfate
Catalysts
  For hydro-treating, desulfurization: cobalt oxide
    plus molybdenum oxide
  For production of terephthalic acid: cobalt
    acetate plus manganese
  For hydroformylation: cobalt metal, oxide,
    hydroxide, inorganic salts
Driers in oil-based paints, varnishes, inks
  Cobalt oleate
  Cobalt ethylhexanoate
  Cobalt naphthenate
  Cobalt linoleate
Electroplating
  Cobalt sulfate
  Cobalt chloride
  Cobalt sulfamate
Pigments for ceramics
  Cobalt oxide (Co_3O_4) combined with oxides
    (e.g., of Cr, chromium, manganese, iron,
    aluminum, magnesium, zinc, silicon)
Pigments for paints
  Cobalt oxide (CoO) combined with oxides of,
    e.g., aluminum, silicon

mixed and calcined with other oxides, are used to provide blue, green, and yellow colors to ceramics, paints, and glass. Organic compounds of cobalt are used in paints, varnishes, and inks as driers and also in steel-braced radial tires for bonding the brass-plated steel to rubber.

Schwartz and colleagues[182] described occupational allergic contact dermatitis caused by metallic cobalt dust in a factory that made tungsten carbide alloys. The abrasive character of the dust was thought to contribute to sensitization. In 1953, Pirila[183] studied 641 workers in a Finnish pottery factory and found 12 persons with positive cobalt patch tests who had an eczematous dermatitis involving flexural areas and the dorsa of the hands. Workers in the clay shops were especially affected because of their constant exposure to cobalt in the wet, alkaline clay. In 1964, Pirila and Geiser[184] found 56 workers in a china-manufacturing plant to be sensitive to cobalt in the porcelain dyes. Marcussen[185] and Bandmann and Fuchs[186] studied cobalt sensitivity in large groups of persons and found the greatest number of positive reactions among bricklayers, metal workers, and cement masons. Bandmann and Fuchs[186] also found eight

TABLE 24–8 • Major Industrial Cobalt Alloys

Composition (%)						Probability of Contact Allergy*	Application
Co	Ni	Cr	Fe	Mo	Other		
49	–	–	49	–	2V	A	Soft magnetic alloy
24	–	–	76	–	–	A	Soft magnetic alloy
5	21	–	62	–	12A1	A	Permanent magnet alloy
29	15	–	39	–	7A1	A	Permanent magnet alloy
15	60	10	–	3	5A1, 5Ti	B	High-temperature superalloy
19	52	18	–	4	3A1, 3Ti	C	High-temperature superalloy
40	22	22	3	–	14W	C	High-temperature superalloy
46	2	32	2	–	13W	C	Wear-resistant coating
9	–	4	62	7	6W, 6V	B	High-speed steel
62	1	30	–	5		C	Surgical implant alloy
49	10	20	3	–	15W	C	Surgical implant alloy
5	31	–	63	–		A	Low-expansion alloy
8	18	–	70	3	–	A	High-hardness steel
35	35	20	–	10	–	C	Corrosion-resistant alloy

*A, Likely to behave as cobalt or nickel does; B, reacts only slowly with sweat and is unlikely to cause contact allergy; C, reacts with sweat only in exceptional circumstances and is most unlikely to cause contact allergy.

Key: Co, cobalt; Ni, nickel; Cr, chromium; Fe, iron; Mo, molybdenum; V, vanadium; Al, aluminum; Ti, titanium; W, tungsten.

cases of allergic cobalt dermatitis among persons who came into contact with black ink, such as printers, bank employees, and judges. Cobalt compounds are added to animal feeds as mineral supplements,[187] and allergic sensitization has been reported in the manufacture of these foodstuffs[188] and in farmers, from contact with cobalt as a feed additive.[189] The place of cobalt sensitivity in cement dermatitis is controversial, but it may be a factor.[190] In European studies of patients with cement dermatitis, cobalt sensitivity occurs in a large percentage. In Spain, Conde-Salazar and associates,[177] who studied 449 construction workers, found that 20.5% were allergic to cobalt, and chromate was positive in 42.1% of these cases. During construction of the Chunnel, Irvine found as many people sensitized to cobalt as to chromate among workers who developed dermatitis.

Kligman,[153] using the human maximization test, sensitized 10 to 25 volunteers to cobalt and awarded their reactions a grade of 3 (the highest possible grade was 5). Wahlberg and Boman,[190a] using the guinea pig maximization test, found cobalt to be a strong allergic sensitizer and reported it to have a grade of 5 on a scale of 1 to 5, in which grade 1 was the weakest sensitizer. All of the animals were sensitized.

Rystedt[191] reported 287 (7.1%) of 4,034 eczema patients with positive patchtest reactions to cobalt. Of the total, only 50 (1.2%) had isolated cobalt reactions. A study of 36 of these persons suggested that another contact sensitivity, or even another skin disease, is a prerequisite for the de-

velopment of cobalt allergy; however, cobalt allergy associated with other contact sensitivities, excepting that to nickel, is rare. If the cases of cobalt-positive patchtest results are separated from those to nickel and chromium, the incidence is actually quite low.

Fischer and Rystedt[192] found an incidence of about 2.5% cobalt sensitivity in a nickel factory. Of the 39 sensitive persons, only nine also had nickel sensitivity, and all were women. It has been said that intercurrent nickel and cobalt allergies tend to produce more severe dermatitis.[193]

Marcussen[185] also emphasized the frequency with which sensitivity to cobalt and to nickel is associated. Patients who are allergic to nickel are 20 times more likely also to be allergic to cobalt than are those who are not allergic to nickel, and patients with a strong positive patchtest reaction to nickel have a 50-fold greater chance of a strong cobalt-positive reaction than do those who test negative to nickel.[194] Occasionally, patients with a dermatitis that looks like nickel allergy show sensitivity only to cobalt on patchtesting. For this reason Marcussen recommended that both nickel and cobalt be included in patchtesting for all metal allergies.

It must be emphasized that simultaneous patchtest reactions to cobalt and nickel may be a manifestation of cross-sensitivity but result from the presence of both metals in alloys. During the manufacture of these alloys, it is impossible completely to separate the two metals; however, Lammintausta and colleagues[195] showed that guinea pigs sensitized to nickel were more readily sensitized to cobalt, and conversely.

An interesting case in which cobalt and nickel sensitivity occurred simultaneously and were equally important was reported by Deisler and Sheets.[196] A dental patient had stomatitis from a new denture and was found on patchtesting to be sensitive to nickel. A new denture was made without nickel, but the same reaction occurred on the gums. Patchtesting to cobalt revealed a strong reaction, and the new denture was found to contain cobalt. When this metal was also removed, the stomatitis completely disappeared. Cobalt may also be an important allergen in dermatitis due to orthopedic stabilizing plates. Vilaplana and colleagues[197] found cobalt to be the second most common allergen in patients with dental problems, nickel being most common. Tilsey and Rotstein[198] reported a patient who had a weeping, eczematous dermatitis over a vitallium bone plate containing cobalt, chromium, and managnese. A top screw had perforated the skin, and the patient had a patchtest reaction to cobalt. The authors attributed the eczematous dermatitis to cobalt sensitivity. Cases of photosensitivity dermatitis caused by cobalt have been reported by Romaguera and coworkers.[199]

Cobalt is an essential part of the vitamin B_{12} molecule. Fisher[200] described a patient with cobalt sensitivity who developed a pruritic eruption at the site of an injection of vitamin B_{12}. The area also flared up when the vitamin was taken orally. The patient had a strong patchtest reaction to cobalt chloride and delayed scratch and intradermal reactions to vitamin B_{12}. In 1951, Rostenberg and Perkins[201] reported a young man with positive nickel and cobalt patchtest reactions who also had a delayed tuberculin-type reaction to vitamin B_{12}.

COPPER

Copper is one of the most important metals, valued especially for its toughness and superior electrical conductivity. The bulk is used in electrical apparatus; the remainder, in combination with other metals as alloys for pipes, roof sheeting, and bronze, among other uses. The main copper ores are composed of oxides or sulfides, often in association with other metals, from which the metal is recovered by smelting and electrolytic refining. Unalloyed copper finds extensive use in electrical equipment, especially for transmissions, and in heat exchangers, because of high electrical and thermal conductivities combined with good ductility and resistance to corrosion. The most widely used alloys are those with zinc, tin, and nickel,

but those with aluminum, beryllium, or silicon have specialized and important uses.

Copper dust imparts a greenish black color to the hair, skin, and teeth of copper workers. This was once though to be evidence of copper poisoning but has since been shown to have no association with systemic disease.[202] A dermatitis termed *copper itch* is caused by fine, airborne particles of arsenic trioxide, which contaminate copper ore[3] and pose a distinct risk of systemic poisoning. Copper salts such as sulfates, oxides, and cyanides may produce skin irritation.

In 1977, Forstrom and colleagues[203] reported a welder with recurring dermatitis on his right hand, in which he had been holding a copper-covered welding wire. Patchtesting with copper sulfate in concentrations of 2%, 1%, and 0.1% in petrolatum produced delayed reactions at 96 hours.

Allergic contact dermatitis to copper is said to be rare[39]; however, the metal is seldom tested, so the incidence may be higher than is generally believed. Karlberg and coworkers[204] added 2% copper sulfate to routine patchtesting; 13 of 1,190 eczema patients showed reactions, but none could be considered relevant. Walton[205] tested 354 patients routinely with 5% copper sulfate; six patients had a positive reaction, and all of them were also allergic to nickel. Karlberg's group,[204] in a review of all the reported cases, considered that many of them should be regarded as uncertain or irrelevant. Only four cases were considered relevant, and perhaps another 20 were considered *possibly* relevant. Some of the positive results may have been false-positive reactions from metal impurities, especially nickel, in the copper used for testing.

Van Joost and coworkers[206] did not consider contamination of copper sulfate with nickel to be the cause of positive patchtest results. Patchtesting patients with known nickel allergy with 5% aqueous copper sulfate did not produce positive results. They described two other cases of copper allergy, one to jewelry and one to an intrauterine contraceptive device; both patients had positive test reactions to nickel. Most cases in the literature, however, have not been convincing.[207–209] One of the few convincing reports was by Saltzer and Wilson,[209] who described a single case of allergic contact dermatitis to jewelry containing copper. Patchtesting with copper sulfate, 1.25%, 2.5%, and 5% in water, and with a copper penny, was positive.

A systemic type of eczematous dermatitis has been reported on several occasions from copper-containing intrauterine devices.[210–212] Patchtesting in these patients with copper sulfate, 2% and 5%, produced positive results. Dhir and colleagues[213] reported allergic dermatitis in 10 furniture polishers, all of whom showed positive patchtest reactions to 5% aqueous copper sulfate, whereas 15 controls were negative. Dhir and colleagues[213] found that copper sulfate may be added to commercial alcohol and that it is also used as a coloring agent for furniture polish. Among compounds of copper that have been considered potential allergic sensitizers are copper 8-quinolinolate and copper resinate (from rosin).

A flulike illness, termed *metal fume fever,* that lasts approximately 24 to 48 hours and is accompanied by chills, fever, aching muscles, and headache, may result from inhalation of fine particles of copper oxide.[214] Several studies have shown an increased incidence of lung cancer in copper smelter workers, which, however, may more likely be due to inhalation of inorganic arsenic.[215]

GOLD

Gold is an extremely dense but soft and malleable metal that is found widely in nature, either as elemental gold or in combination with sulfides in igneous rocks and ores. The element is extremely stable and nonreactive. Table 24–9 lists the gold compounds commonly used in industry.

Gold is used principally in jewelry and as a decorative surface on china and glass, and it also has numerous industrial uses. In the electrical and electronics industries gold is used as fine wires or thin film coatings to provide stable contacts of low resistance on phosphor bronze or nickel silver for contact springs on silicon transistors and integrated circuits. It is also used to protect etched printed circuit boards during storage. Other uses are as thin films on glass for selective light filters, for lining chemical equipment, and for thermal limit fuses.

Alloys used in jewelry contain copper and silver, and sometimes also nickel and zinc. White golds are either gold-nickel-copper or gold-palladium alloys. White gold containing more than 2% nickel and less than 58% gold (18 karat) can cause nickel contact dermatitis.

High-temperature solders are generally gold-copper, gold-silver, or gold-silver-copper alloys, but some also contain nickel, chromium, or palladium. Gold alloys used in dentistry may contain silver, platinum, palladium, iridium, copper, nickel, tin, iron, or zinc. The cast alloys contain principally gold, silver, and copper.

Rings made of 18-karat gold contain copper and silver, whereas 14-karat gold contains small amounts of nickel, copper, and zinc. White gold is hardened by the addition of platinum and nickel and can cause dermatitis in persons allergic to nickel. It must also be remembered that when gold is used for plating, particularly on silver, it requires a nickel interliner. The gold plate is often very thin and porous, and dermatitis to nickel can occur in allergic persons. In most cases the allergy may appear to be caused by gold when the culprit is actually nickel.

Although gold in ores is usually in a free state, small quantities of other metals are also present. During refining and extraction, workers are exposed to hydrocyanic acid and sulfur monochloride, both highly irritating to the eyes, mucous membranes, and skin.[216] Systemic administration of gold salts by injection occasionally results in a slate-colored, bluish gray discoloration of the skin termed *chrysiasis*. This condition was described first by Hansborg[217] and later by Schmidt.[218] Today it most often results from the treatment of rheumatoid arthritis with gold salts. To assist in the diagnosis of this condition, Cox[219] described a method of identifying gold particles in the dermis that entails using a laser microprobe in emission spectroscopy. In two patients examined by this method, the gold had been in the skin for more than 20 years.

Systemic gold therapy has been used to treat pemphigus and psoriatic arthritis. Penneys[220] provides a review of its toxicity. Systemic administration of gold salts may produce severe, widespread dermatitis, usually preceded by pruritus of several days' or weeks' duration. These manifestations of gold toxicity usually do not appear until approximately 400 mg of gold has been administered. If administration continues, the eruption becomes

TABLE 24–9 • Gold Compounds Commonly Used in Industry

Gold hydroxide: gilding liquids and gold plating for porcelain

Gold oxide: gilding liquids and gold plating for porcelain

Gold potassium cyanide: electrolyte in electroplating

Gold-silver alloy: semiconductors

Gold-sodium thiomalate: medication for rheumatoid arthritis

Gold solder: "jeweler's gold"

Gold stannate: ruby glass, colored enamels, porcelain painting

Gold tin purple: glass and porcelain manufacture, "purple of Cassius"

Gold tribromide: analysis of alkaloids and seminal fluid in forensic medicine

Gold trichloride: photography, gold plating inks, ceramics, glass

progressively worse, often becoming a generalized exfoliative dermatitis.[221]

Allergic contact dermatitis to gold has in the past been considered unusual, although Kligman,[153] using the human maximization test, found that gold chloride possesses much potential for sensitization—a grade of 4 on a scale of 1 to 5. He explained that the insolubility of gold and its inertness account for the observed infrequency of contact allergy. Bjorkner could find only eight reports containing 10 patchtest–positive cases from the earliest report in 1949.[222, 223]

Most reported cases of contact sensitivity to gold are associated with jewelry. In some of the reports, the patchtest reactions were probably irritant, resulting from testing with gold chloride in an irritant concentration. Contact dermatitis to gold has also been described in photographers,[3] from gold ball orbital protheses[223] and dentures,[224–227] and in electroplaters (Fig. 24–5).[228]

Patchtesting is best done with gold sodium thiosulfate (GST), 0.5% in petrolatum.[229] Gold trichloride may irritate, and gold leaf and jewelry often produce negative results, probably because of the insolubility of metallic gold. Fowler[229] reported two cases of gold allergy. Bjorkner's group[222] has

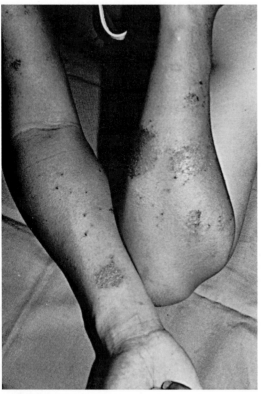

FIGURE 24–5 • Contact dermatitis due to gold in an electroplater. The patchtest reactions persisted for nearly 3 months.

reported that more than 8% of 832 patients on routine patchtesting had positive reactions. These patients also had positive patchtests to potassium dicyanoaurate but were negative on testing to gold sodium thiomalate, and metallic gold. Only patients who were reactive also had a positive intradermal test to GST, and the authors were certain that these reactions did, indeed, represent gold allergy. Many physicians consider it strange that such a large percentage of persons could be allergic to gold without significant relevance such as a history of reactions to jewelry or gold fillings. They also question why it was not discovered long before. However, the findings described have been confirmed by McKenna and colleagues,[230] who found 4.6% positive reactions to GST on routine patchtesting. A high incidence of GST allergy, 12.4%, has also been found in dental patients,[231] and in addition, a large percentage of women were affected (99%), many of whom complained of cutaneous symptoms from jewelry. Marcussen,[232] in a study of persons with subjective mouth symptoms, found a much higher percentage of gold allergy: 23% as compared with 8% on routine patchtesting of eczematous patients. Some 46% of patients allergic to GST studied by Bruze and coworkers[233] gave a history of rashes related to wearing jewelry. One could have considered this relevant to gold allergy, but most of the patients with this history were also allergic to nickel. Bruze's group[233, 233a] reported that a large percentage of the gold reactions are long lasting and that 35 of their patients developed late reactions, which has been a common finding with gold contact allergy. Sabroe and associates[234] confirmed these findings and discovered that 13% of 100 consecutive patchtest patients reacted to GST. Most of the reactive patients were female, and their dermatitis was on the neck. Among the reactive group, most of the patients seemed to wear more gold jewelry.

Gold patchtest results must be considered true allergic reactions for the following reasons: (1) many of the reactions are long lasting and appear late. (2) The reactions are reproducible. (3) Dilutions show a gradually diminishing response. (4) There is no increase in the incidence of atopic dermatitis in the positive group, who would be most likely to show nonspecific irritant responses. (5) Studies in vitro have confirmed the response as allergic.

Currently, the significance of positive patchtests to GST remains somewhat unclear; however, Bruze's group[235] found an increased number of patients with a positive patchtest to gold who also had gold dental fillings, as compared with a group of controls. There is no doubt that on routine patchtesting a large percentage of people react positively to GST; whether this indicates true gold allergy is not absolutely clear. Currently, it appears that these reactions are true positives, but their significance is not always clear. As a result, it is questionable whether one should give any specific advice to patients, particularly that they discard their gold jewelry or remove their gold fillings. Further studies will be required to understand the true significance of these findings, and routine testing with gold is not yet indicated. Few, if any, of the cases of positive patchtests to gold described in the reports cited above can be considered occupational.

MERCURY

Mercury is well-known for its use in barometers, thermometers, dental amalgams, electrical switches, and other devices. Large amounts formerly were used in extracting gold from its ore, but the practice has been discontinued owing to environmental and health concerns. An important industrial use remains the electrolytic preparation of chlorine and caustic soda, although this process is gradually being replaced by other processes less damaging to the environment. Compounds of mercury are widely used as fungicides, bactericides, catalysts, and pharmaceuticals as well as in antifouling paints and pulp and paper manufacture (Table 24–10).

Mercury fungicides have been used to prevent mildew on stored seeds, and human ingestion of seeds intended only for crops has resulted in sporadic reports of deaths from mercurialism.[236] Although dentists are generally aware of the toxic nature of mercury and avoid handling it when preparing amalgams, they are undoubtedly exposed to higher levels in their environment than are many others,[237] especially when removing old dental amalgam restorations.[238] More than 1 kg of metallic mercury is used each year in the average dental surgical practice, mostly in the preparation of amalgam fillings. Surveys indicate that at least 10% of dental surgeries in the United States have an ambient mercury vapor level in excess of 0.05 mg/m^3, and a similar percentage of dental personnel have high mercury levels in their hair and urine.[239] In a study of 298 dentists in the fifth decade of life, 13% were found to have blood mercury levels in excess of controls'. Those with the highest levels were compared with those with the lowest, and about 20% of the group with high mercury levels appeared to show changes in nerve conduction. Psychological and IQ tests did not show changes, however, with the exception perhaps of some visual graphic dysfunction and a greater level of anxiety about their health.

Whether mercury amalgam fillings in the mouth can release mercury is a matter of considerable controversy, and if so, whether this can be toxic. Several investigators found an increased level of mercury in blood and mouth air on chewing.[240–242] Two previous studies did not show this correlation, however.[243, 244] Nevertheless, this is especially important today, as suitable alternatives to mercury amalgam are available for dental fillings.

For more than two centuries, systemic mercury poisoning was associated with carroting of fur in the manufacture of felt. In 1941, a U.S. Public Health study revealed that more than 10% of felt workers in the United States had chronic mercury poisoning.[245] Today, mercury is seldom used anywhere in the world for manufacturing felt, having been replaced years ago with compounds that are much less toxic.

Most systemic mercury poisoning in industry today results from contamination of the workplace by accidental breakage of mercury thermometers, barometers, or gauges.[246, 247] Metallic mercury vaporizes readily at room temperature, and the vapor produces no warning signs.[248] When spilled, metallic mercury rapidly disperses in the form of droplets, and great care must be used in removing it.

Systemic mercury poisoning has also resulted from using metallic mercury to form a gold-mercury amalgam in the process of removing gold from its ore in a do-it-yourself home refining method. The ore is heated with mercury, often in an open pan on a kitchen stove, forming amalgam. The resulting fumes of mercury can cause symptoms of poisoning as soon as 30 minutes after the heating begins.[249]

Metallic mercury itself rarely causes contact allergic sensitization. Vickers[250] reported a generalized eruption in a woman who had come into contact with the mercury of a broken thermometer. She gave a history of having been sensitized several years earlier by a topical mercury medication. White and Smith[251] reported 28 cases from the world literature, including one of their own, in which affected persons experienced rashes attributed to mercury dental fillings. A large proportion of them had known contact and previous sensitization to mercury from other sources, as from vaccination for instance, but evidence of an associated flare-up caused by the fillings was strong, in that most of the cases either cleared up spontaneously within a few days of the new fillings' being inserted or else shortly after the old fillings were removed. Kanerva and Komulainen[252] described two cases of occupational allergic contact derma-

TABLE 24–10 • Mercury Salts Commonly Used in Industry

Analytic Reagents
Mercuric barium iodide
Mercuric chloride
Mercuric cuprous iodide
Mercuric silver iodide
Mercurous nitrate

Antiknock Compounds
Mercuric naphthenate

Batteries
Mercuric chloride
Mercuric sulfate
Mercurous sulfate
Red mercuric oxide

Catalysts
Mercuric chloride
Mercuric sulfate

Denaturants (for ethanol)
Phenylmercuric benzoate
Phenylmercuric hydroxide

Disinfectants and Pesticides
Mercuric chloride
Mercuric cyanide
Mercuric dimethyldithiocarbamate
Mercuric lactate
Mercuric stearate
Mercurous chloride
Phenylmercuric acetate
Phenylmercuric benzoate
Phenylmercuric chloride
Phenylmercuric ethanolammonium acetate and lactate
Phenylmercuric hydroxide
Phenylmercuric napthenate
Phenylmercuric oleate
Red mercuric oxide
Yellow mercuric oxide

Embalming Fluids
Mercuric chloride

Engraving
Mercuric chloride

Herbicides
Phenylmercuric acetate

Lithography
Mercuric chloride

Metallurgy
Mercuric chloride

Mirror Manufacture
Mercuric potassium cyanide

Paints
Mercuric arsenate
Mercuric naphthenate
Mercuric oleate
Mercuric oxide
Mercuric sulfide
Phenylmercuric acetate
Phenylmercuric naphthenate
Phenylmercuric oleate
Phenylmercuric propionate

Photography
Mercuric chloride
Mercuric cyanide
Mercuric thiocyanate

Seed Disinfectants
Methylmercury acetate
Methylmercury cyanide
Methylmercury 2,3-dihydroxy propylmercaptide
Methylmercury quinolinolate
Phenylmercuric formamide
Phenylmercuric salicylate
Phenylmercuric urea

Tanning
Mercuric chloride

Textiles
Mercuric chloride
Mercuric nitrate

Wood Preservatives
Mercuric chloride
Phenylmercuric naphthenate

titis from metallic mercury, one caused by amalgam and the other by mercury in a thermometer.

For many years, mercuric chloride was used in patchtesting to detect mercury sensitivity. Yet mercuric chloride, 1% aqueous, is corrosive to the skin,[253] and even with a concentration of 0.5% irritant reactions are common. Consequently, the many false-positive results have caused dermatologists and other physicians to view with skepticism much of the past literature on mercury sensitivity. Patchtesting with a concentration of 0.05% in water is more reliable. To avoid confusing results using mercury salts, the North American

Contact Dermatitis Group (NACDG) recommended using ammoniated mercury to test for mercury sensitivity.[254] Handley and coworkers,[255] however, believe that both metallic mercury and ammoniated mercury should be used, to avoid missing some reactions.

Great care must be used in interpreting patchtest reactions to all mercury compounds. The organic mercurials in particular, such as phenyl mercuric compounds and thimerosal (Merthiolate), may cause confusing results.[256] Most of them are both irritating and sensitizing.[257] Patchtesting with thimerosal frequently results in bizarre, intense, but clearly allergic reactions, bringing into question the usefulness of the test. If sensitization to thimerosal is suspected, it is better to patchtest with the two constituents of thimerosal, mercury and thiosalicylic acid. Goncalo and associates[258] showed that a large number of patients were sensitive to either mercury or thiosalicylic acid, and not to the thimerosal itself. Ethyl mercuric chloride appeared to provoke a larger percentage of positive reactions than did ammoniated mercury. Today most mercury patchtest reactions signify latent sensitivity from some past use of mercury-containing medications, especially antiseptics such as merbromin (Mercurochrome), thimerosal (Merthiolate), and other medications that until recently were present in every medicine cabinet. Mercury is still found in wedding rings, and in some cosmetics,[259] as an antifungal agent,[260] antiseptics, depigmenting creams, and in certain shampoos. It is important to remember that local applications not only can sensitize and cause contact dermatitis locally but also can be absorbed, causing systemic reactions and even poisoning.[261] The association of mercury allergy with lichenoid lesions of the mouth has been well-recognized and described by many authors. The incidence varies between 9% and 62%, the higher frequency being found when amalgam comes in intimate contact with the lesions.[262]

An often overlooked source of mercury sensitization is tattooing: the red pigment is usually cinnabar (mercuric sulfide). When allergic sensitization develops, the red areas become raised, eczematous, and very pruritic. Keiller and Warin[263] reported dermatitis spreading from a tattoo site to the face, trunk, and limbs. Patchtesting with mercury was positive.

During World War II contact dermatitis occurred in workers in munitions factories from contact with mercury fulminate (mercuric cyanate), a powder valued for its great explosive potential. The powder is very irritating, especially in contact with abraded or lacerated skin and in moist areas such as the nasal mucosa and conjunctivae. Schwartz and colleagues[3] described it as a cause of allergic sensitization in a large number of munitions workers. Mercury fulminate is still used today in manufacture of caps and detonators, but almost always in closed systems.

Systemic administration of mercurial medications to persons sensitive to mercury can result in an explosive, generalized eczematous dermatitis.[2] First demonstrated by Josef Jadassohn in 1895, the finding led to Jadassohn's discovery of the patchtest. Such reactions were common when mercury compounds were used as injections to treat syphilis and as creams to treat pediculosis pubis and other benign skin conditions. Reactions can still occur from intramuscular administration of mercurial diuretics. Slate-gray pigmentation of the skin can result from prolonged use of topical mercury preparations, especially commercial bleaching creams sold to eradicate "age spots" on the face and hands. These topical preparations, which contain ammoniated mercury, were widely available until about 1970. Lamar and Bliss[264] described pigmentation on the face of a woman who had used a mercury-containing ointment as a moisturizer for more than 50 years. Even with less prolonged use, a grayish brown hyperpigmentation usually develops, especially on the eyelids and adjacent skin.[265] Mercury is still present in certain local medications and cosmetics and can cause systemic toxicity.[266] Sarcoidlike granulomas may result from penetration into the dermis of metallic mercury from broken thermometers.[267] Similar lesions have been observed in the peritoneum from ruptured Miller-Abbott suction tubes in which metallic mercury was used in a condom as a weight.[268, 269]

NICKEL

As early as 200 B.C., the Chinese used nickel as an alloy with copper and later exported it as far away as Europe. During the Middle Ages miners in Saxony mistook ore containing nickel for copper ore; when the refined ore yielded only a brittle, slaglike material, they gave it the derogatory name of *kupfernickel* after Old Nick. The term *nickel* was applied to the metal by the Swedish mineralogist and chemist A. F. Cronstedt, who first isolated it in 1751. It is the 24th element in order of abundance in the earth's crust and is found in mineral ores in combination with arsenic, cobalt, iron, oxygen, silicon, sulfur, and especially copper. Valuable byproducts of nickel mining include platinum, gold, silver, selenium, and tellurium. During the mid-19th century, the value of nickel as an undercoat for silver electroplating led to its use as a base for electrolytic deposition of other metals. Today almost all chromium- and gold-plated articles are first nickel-plated. Canada and Russia produce most of the world's supply.

Until World War II, nickel was refined by the Orford process, but today more efficient processes are used, the choice depending on the type of ore and its origin. In Canada, ore flotation, which uses the different magnetic properties of the constituents, is now used to separate nickel from other ingredients such as iron, silica, copper, and gold. The carbonyl process for recovering nickel of high purity was discovered at a refinery in Clydach,

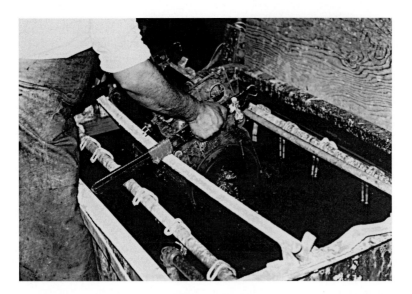

FIGURE 24–6 • Electroplating solutions containing nickel sulfate may induce nickel sensitivity in operators.

Wales. After the impure sulfide ore is roasted, a finely divided metal is formed, which is then treated with carbon monoxide to produce volatile nickel carbonyl. At high temperatures, this gas decomposes to yield pure nickel in small pellets. Worldwide restrictions have been imposed on this process because of the highly toxic properties of nickel carbonyl.

Most of the nickel in the United States is used for stainless steel and other high-nickel alloys that are strong and corrosion resistant. It is also used in electroplating (Fig. 24–6), in certain catalysts and other chemicals, and in coinage. Nickel powders are used for vacuum tubes and semiconductors. Its chief industrial uses are shown in Table 24–11.

Commercially available nickel is a silvery white metal with a melting point of 1435°C and a density of 8.9 g/cm³. It is ferromagnetic with a Curie point in the range of 350° to 360°C. It has good resistance to corrosion by water and the atmosphere, but in moist atmospheres containing sulfur dioxide a polished surface slowly fogs as a coating of basic sulfate develops. Approximately 65% of nickel produced is used for stainless steel.

Nickel metal reacts slowly with sweat to form nickel ions that cause contact allergy. Transient contact is rarely the cause of contact dermatitis, but prolonged, direct contact can induce an allergic reaction. Contact with pure nickel articles is infrequent except in countries whose coins are pure. Most contact occurs with coated articles, of

---

TABLE 24–11 • Nickel Compounds Used in Industry

Antioxidant	Fungicides
Nickel dibutyldithiocarbamate	Nickel chloride
Catalysts	Nickel sulfate
Nickel carbonate	Pigments
Nickel formate	Nickel azo yellow
Nickel hydroxide	Nickel dimethylglyoxime
Nickel hydroxy carbonate	Nickel oxide
Nickel nitrate	Storage batteries
Nickelocene	Nickel nitrate
Ceramics	Nickel hydroxide (active mass)
Nickel oxide (green)	Textiles
Nickel sulfate	Nickel acetate
Electronics	Nickel ammonium chloride
Nickel ammonium sulfate	Nickel sulfate
Nickel hydroxide	
Nickel hydroxy carbonate	
Nickel chloride	
Nickel sulfamate	
Nickel sulfate	

which numerous ones today are nickel plated: tools, keys, toys, nuts and bolts, household tools, and so on. Often the nickel coating is provided with a topcoat, which reduces but does not prevent formation of nickel ions. A common topcoat is chromium. At a thickness of about 0.1 μm it tends to be porous, whereas coats thicker than 0.6 μm tend to become fissured because of brittleness and stress in the deposit. Thus, coatings of about 0.2 μm may provide optimal protection from sensitization by the nickel undercoat.[270] Coatings of gold or silver on nickel are often used in jewelry. Such topcoats are often thin and porous or can become so with use, and thus permit release of nickel.

Nickel alloys can be broadly divided into three classes, according to their propensity to react with sweat to generate nickel ions (Table 24–12). Three groups of alloys are likely to find domestic use and require special mention.

Nickel Silvers. Nickel silver contains 55% to 63% copper, 10% to 25% nickel, and zinc and are used for jewelry, small items such as keys, and architectural components such as handles, knobs, and decorative items. The alloy behaves much as nickel does and can cause nickel contact dermatitis.

White Gold. Widely used in jewelry, this alloy can vary greatly in composition and can contain up to 12% nickel plus copper, lead, zinc, and other metals, the balance being gold. The release of nickel in sweat solutions depends on the nickel and gold content. White golds containing more than about 2% nickel and less than about 58% gold may be regarded as likely to cause an allergic reaction on prolonged and direct contact with the skin.

Stainless Steels and Heat-Resistant Alloys. The term *stainless steel* covers a range of alloys containing 12% to 30% chromium, up to 35% nickel, up to 7% molybdenum, plus iron, making alloys with widely different properties. The most common stainless steels contain 16% to 20% chromium and 6% to 14% nickel. The excellent corrosion resistance of stainless steels depends on the formation of a surface oxide film that prevents release of nickel. At the lower levels of chromium and when the sulfur content is high (e.g., 0.15%), the oxide film is less stable and can break down,[271] especially in chloride solutions. Where crevices are formed, the nickel-chromium, heat-resistant alloys behave similarly. Thus, the alloy containing 77% nickel, 15% chromium, and 8% iron was shown to release little nickel when freely exposed to synthetic sweat, but it failed in a patchtest that effectively provided crevice exposure for 48 hours.[272] Higher grades of stainless steel (e.g., those containing molybdenum) should be used in applications involving continuous, direct contact with the skin, such as watch bands, for example.

Soluble nickel compounds such as nickel chloride and -sulfate, are well-known causes of nickel contact dermatitis in industry. Accordingly, work

---

TABLE 24–12 • Major Industrial Nickel Alloys

Element	Typical Concentration (%)	Probability of Causing Contact Allergy*	Applications
Al	35	B	Raney nickel catalyst
Au	37–75	B†	White gold jewelry
Be	2	A	Springs
Co	25	A	Magnet alloys
Cr	15–20	C†	Heat-resistant alloys
Cr/Fe	18/72	C†	Stainless steels
Cu	30–90	A	Marine uses, coinage
Cu/Zn	65/20	A†	Architecture, domestic goods
Fe	64	A	Low-expansion alloy
Mn	3	A	Electronics
Mo	28	B	Corrosion-resistant alloy
Si	13	B	Corrosion-resistant alloy
Sn	65	B	Corrosion-resistant coating
Ti	45	C	Shape-memory alloy
Zn	88	B	Corrosion-resistant coating

*A, Behaves similarly to nickel metal; B, reacts only slowly with sweat and is unlikely to cause contact allergy; C, will react with sweat only in exceptional circumstances and is most unlikely to cause contact allergy.

†See text.

Key: Al, aluminum; Au, gold; Be, beryllium; Co, cobalt; Cr, chromium; Fe, iron; Cu, copper; Zn, zinc; Mn, manganese; Mo, molybdenum; Si, silicon; Sn, strontium; Ti, titanium.

practices have been adopted that eliminate contact. Insoluble compounds such as green nickel oxide do not provide nickel ions, but others may be sufficiently soluble in acid sweat to release nickel ions and present a potential problem. The chief industrial uses for nickel metal are shown in Table 24–13.

Allergic Nickel Dermatitis

Incidence

Nickel is today one of the most common contact allergens. The incidence of positive patchtests to nickel has been increasing each year. Recently, Dotterud and coworkers[273] found 14.9% of schoolchildren to be allergic to nickel (21.9% of girls, 8.5% of boys). A history of ear piercing significantly increases the number of positive patchtests to nickel—in girls, for example, from 16.3% to 30.8%. Larsson-Stymne and Widstrom[274] found the prevalence of nickel allergy among girls with pierced ears to be 13% but among girls without pierced ears, only 1%.

It was suggested previously that patients with nickel sensitivity have a higher incidence of atopy,[275, 276] but this was not confirmed by others.[277] Nickel allergy is not closely associated with any of the antigens of the HLA B or C series or the D or DR antigens.[278–280] Menne and Holme,[281] in a study of twins, concluded that nickel allergy probably was not due to common genetic predisposition.

In 1960, Marcussen[282] declared that nickel allergy appeared to be disappearing from the major industries; however, today more women are working outside the home, so exposure to nickel in the workplace has assumed greater importance. Furthermore, many new sources of nickel exposure have appeared; for example, cold impregnation of aluminum with nickel is more widespread.[17] Many workers may be affected—not only cashiers, hairdressers, jewelers, dental technicians, and homemakers but also nickel-sensitive persons who handle nickel-plated hand tools in their work. It should be emphasized that it is unlikely that nickel sensitivity is initiated from these contacts, but in persons already sensitized (from ear piercing, for example) dermatitis on the fingers and hands from working with nickel-plated hand tools sometimes causes disability or requires changing jobs. Other possible sources of occupational nickel dermatitis include mining and extraction, refining, electroplating, casting, grinding, polishing, metallurgy, alloys, nickel-cadmium batteries, chemicals, electronics, computers, food processing, and nickel waste disposal and recycling processes.[283]

There are few reports in the medical literature of occupational nickel dermatitis. In 1976, however, Reichenberger and colleagues[284] reported 239 cases of nickel allergy from Germany, 26 in men and 213 in women. All the men, but only 20 of the women, were considered to have been sensitized at work. Among the men were 12 metal workers, six construction workers, three office workers, two who worked in mining, and one each in baking, meat cutting, and painting. Of the women, 19 were employed in metal working and one in photography. Nickel-containing cutting fluids used in machining and coolants have been assumed to be responsible for allergic contact dermatitis by Arndt,[285] Gellin,[286] and Hodgson,[287] but Samitz and Katz[283] failed to demonstrate available nickel by spot testing machinery, wipe rags, workbenches, and lathe scrap. Samitz and Katz reported that on visits to factory sites they found direct contact with machinery metal to be unlikely as cause of nickel allergy. For example, no cases of nickel dermatitis occurred among approximately 800 workers employed in one plant studied. This conclusion was confirmed by Coenraads and colleagues[288] who from examination of 751 workers found only two cases of nickel dermatitis in 34 persons with dermatitis, and six cases among 213

TABLE 24–13 • Major Industrial Uses of Nickel Metal

Form	Applications
Primary nickel (cathode, pellet, rondelles, briquettes)	Alloy production, anodes in electroplating, production of compounds
Wrought and cast nickel	Anodes in electroplating and electroforming, cathode grids, TV tubes, tanks, tubes, pumps, valves for use in strong alkalies, magnetostrictors, coinage
Nickel powder	Alkaline batteries and fuel cells, sintered metal components, welding rods, sintered magnets and carbide tools, conducting paints, metal seals, thermal spraying, compounds

controls. Fischer and Rystedt[114] found 5% of 853 hard metal workers to be allergic to nickel. More recent evidence has suggested that metal workers[289] and auto mechanics[290] have higher incidences of nickel allergy, which may play an important role in their dermatitis. Workers who may be exposed to nickel shown in Table 24–14.

Wahlberg[291] reported 14 or 35 hairdressers to be allergic to nickel. An association with atopy was not confirmed, and serum immunoglobulin E (IgE) determinations failed to help differentiate between hairdressers who tested positive and those who tested negative. Other investigators have found the following percentages of nickel allergy in hairdressers: Cronin, 19%[292]; Hannuksela and Hassi, 67%[293]; Lindemayr, 44.7%[294]; Lynde and Mitchell, 27%[295]; Marks and Cronin, 44%.[296] One of the problems with the significance of these findings is that a majority of the entrants to hairdressing are already allergic to nickel. Majoie and colleagues,[297] for example, found that 27% of young hairdressers had a positive patchtest to nickel on entering the profession.

Nickel Dermatitis in Hand Eczema

There is considerable controversy about whether nickel dermatitis is more common among women with hand eczema and whether people with nickel allergy are more prone to develop hand dermatitis. And if so, is their prognosis worse? Studies have revealed varying results; for example, nickel dermatitis has been reported to be more common in women with hand eczema.[68, 108, 281, 298–300] Other researchers found no difference[132, 301] (personal communication). Whether it occurs more or less frequently in atopic persons is also controversial.[302–305] It is generally believed that nickel allergy not only predisposes to hand eczema but makes the prognosis worse. In a literature review, Wilkinson and Wilkinson[306] declared, "Previous or concomitant nickel sensitivity also appears to worsen the prognosis somewhat."

Confirming evidence has always been difficult to obtain. Nilsson and Knutsson[307] studied 800 patients referred from a dental clinic for patchtesting. Evaluating patients with all types of hand eczema (dry, chapped skin, itching, red macular and papular lesions, small vesicles, ruptured vesicles, and rough skin with cracks), they predicted a probability of hand eczema of 39% among all persons who were "nickel negative" and of 47% for those who were "nickel positive." This was not statistically significant, but when the presence of small, ruptured vesicles was the criterion, the probability increased from 14% to 28% in nickel-negative subjects and 9.7% to 21% in the nickel-positive ones—a statistically significant result. A more important factor, however, in predicting probability for hand eczema was a history of atopic dermatitis. The probability for hand eczema in women who were nickel sensitive was 38%, and in those who were nickel negative, that is who had no history of atopic dermatitis, it was 47%. For the nickel negative with a history of atopic dermatitis the probability was 81%, and for the nickel negative 86%.

Shah and colleagues[289] could find no difference in the prognosis for metal workers who were allergic to nickel as compared to those who were not; whereas Susitaival and Hannuksela[308] found the prognosis in agricultural workers to be worse in the presence of metal, and they associated this with persistent hand dermatitis. They concluded, however, that metal allergy in chronic hand dermatitis is a *parallel* skin reactivity phenomenon, since there was no evidence of an interrelationship. One of the few prospective studies available, which would show whether sensitive persons are actually more prone to dermatitis, was done by Majoie and associates.[297] In their attempt to define whether persons with nickel allergy should be excluded from jobs such as hairdressing, they found no difference between nickel-positive and nickel-negative subjects. In fact, 55% of subjects who tested negative developed hand eczema, as compared with 30% of those with a positive nickel test.

Nickel sulfate was reported as a cause of allergic asthma in a metal polisher by Block and Yeung.[309] A positive immediate-prick skin test and bronchial challenge by occupational exposure established the diagnosis. Patchtesting results, however, were negative.

 TABLE 24–14 • Workers Who May Be Exposed to Nickel

Auto mechanics
Cashiers
Ceramic makers and workers
Dyers
Electronics workers
Electroplaters
Hairdressers
Ink makers
Jewelers
Nickel catalyst makers
Production workers for hand tools
Spark plug makers
Storage battery makers
Rubber workers
Textile dyers and mordanters

Clinical Appearance of Nickel Dermatitis.
Nickel dermatitis tends to be widespread, chronic, and very persistent. Spreading from the primary site, it often is bilateral and symmetric, a phenomenon termed the *wandering effect* by Fischer[310] and *metastatic eczema* by Barranco and Solomon.[311] A similar pattern is seen in chrome dermatitis. Polak and Turk[312] suggested that such distal flare-ups are produced by humoral antibodies. In "atopic" persons, it frequently assumes a dry, diffuse character[212] that closely resembles atopic dermatitis. The original eruption may be small and insignificant, but because of marked pruritus, secondary dermatitis results from rubbing and scratching and from application of irritating or sensitizing medications. The pattern of dermatitis may conform to the design of the contactant—watch straps, buttons, rings, necklaces—especially at sites of maximum friction and pressure. The palmar aspects of the fingers and distal parts of the palm are commonly affected; this is known as the *apron pattern.* Kaaber and colleagues[313] considered an eruption on the elbow to be typical of nickel and chromate dermatitis. Eyelid dermatitis has been reported from nickel-contaminated cosmetics.[314]

Nickel Dermatitis from Oral Ingestion
The idea that nickel dermatitis could develop from systemic or local contact has been debated for decades. It was first reported in animal studies by Walthard,[315] and has been confirmed on many occasions since then. A comprehensive report was published by Christensen's group.[316] This concept is not without controversy, however, and the arguments for and against have been reviewed by Burrows.[317] The current, and generally accepted, belief is that daily oral ingestion of 5 mg nickel can exacerbate dermatitis but that persons consuming an ordinary diet are not at all likely to take in this much nickel. It was suggested that large amounts of nickel could be chelated from cooking utensils, but Flint and Packirisamy[318] demonstrated that this does not occur.

Dermatitis from Implanted Metals
A related question is the safety of hip implants containing nickel in patients who are nickel sensitive. Patients' reactions to hip implants may perhaps provide a clue to the varying opinions about the causes of systemic flares in contact-allergic patients. Old prostheses consisting of a metal head on a metal cup were responsible for a significant number of rejections from sensitization[319–321]; however, the new prostheses with a metal head and a plastic cup have not so far been found to cause sensitization, flare-ups of dermatitis, or rejection of prostheses.[322–326] Plates screwed into bones,

however, occasionally produce sensitization and dermatitis. Reviewing the literature, Dujardin and associates[327] found 54 cases, but they expressed uncertainty that the dermatitis was indeed caused by the implant in all cases. Current information suggests that although large doses of nickel given orally or systemically may aggravate nickel dermatitis, small doses and the amount found in ordinary diets are unlikely to do so.

Patchtesting for Nickel Sensitivity

For many years 5% nickel sulfate in water was used for patchtesting. Sulzberger[328] claimed that nickel sulfate in aqueous solution up to 5% caused no reaction on normal skin unless the patient was allergic to nickel. In recent years, however, to avoid occasional irritant reactions, the concentration was reduced to 2.5% and the vehicle changed to petrolatum. Because experience has shown that this concentration misses some positive reactions, however, it is now common practice to use 5% in Europe and 2.5% in the United States. Schmiel[329] showed that the two concentrations caused essentially the same reaction, and Fischer and Rystedt[114] found that 83% of positive patchtest reactions with 5% nickel were accurate, based on repeat patchtesting and history.

Because nickel sensitivity is common and the patchtest reactions often severe, Mitchell[330] recommended deleting nickel from the routine battery of test substances, to avoid what he termed the *angry back,* a state of skin hyperreactivity caused by very strong allergic reactions at other test sites.

There are two reasons for retaining nickel as a routine test substance. First, a significant percentage of people with a history of nickel allergy do not react to patchtest,[331–335] and even when intradermal testing is used, complete correspondence between the two does not always occur. Even pretreatment of the skin with an irritant does not produce 100% positives.[336] In a recent study of Norwegian school children, Dotterud and Falk[273] found metal allergy from patchtesting in only 34.2% of children who had a history of metal dermatitis. Second, a negative history of nickel allergy (i.e., no irritation from jewelry) does not ensure that the patient will not have a positive patchtest reaction.[337] Dotterud and Falk[273] found that 13.3% of those with no history of metal sensitivity had a positive patchtest to one or more metals. Thus, it appears that a history of "allergy to metals" does not necessarily mean that nickel is the cause, and it is important, medicolegally to confirm sensitivity by patchtesting. Furthermore, Lammintausta and Kalimo[338] showed that a positive test reaction to nickel on a routine test battery does not increase positive reactions to other test agents, thus causing the angry back.

Treatment of Nickel Dermatitis

The only certain way to prevent recurrence of nickel dermatitis is to avoid contact with objects containing nickel, although casual contacts with keys, coins, and other articles—without concomitant sweating or pressure—is safe. Reducing sweating with antiperspirants can sometimes prevent recurrences. Substitution of aluminium keys for nickel-plated ones and covering the handles of tools with plastic or polyurethane paint also are sometimes effective measures. It is important to be able to identify metals that contain or release substantial amounts of nickel. The dimethylglyoxime (DMG) test has been used extensively for this purpose. Originally described by Feigel,[339] it is performed by placing 1 drop each of a solution of 1% DMG in ethanol and ammonia on the object and rubbing with a cotton-tipped applicator. A pink color immediately appears and shows the presence of available nickel. The test is accurate only when more than 10 μg of nickel is released[340] or when, in an aqueous solution, 10 μg/g of nickel is released (author's unpublished data). How much nickel must be present in an object before the skin reacts depends on many factors, such as the amount of sweating, the alkalinity of the surface, electrical forces, the presence of other elements (chromium, for example), whether the patient is allergic to metal or the skin is inflamed, the volume of nickel present, and its concentration. These factors have all been reviewed by Gawkrodger.[341] Allenby and Basketter[342] showed that in a person allergic to nickel the back will react to 10 ppm, a normal forearm to 5 ppm, and an irritated forearm to 0.5 ppm. Andersen and coworkers[343] found four of 286 nickel-allergic persons reacted to 10 ppm but none reacted to lower levels. A nickel release rate of 0.5 μg/cm^2 per wk is generally considered safe, but some patients react to lower levels.[344] Thus, the DMG test, accurate to 10 ppm, may not be quite sensitive enough but still is valuable for most patients.

Some stainless steels are known to release more nickel than others.[271] Some 14% of persons allergic to nickel react to a patchtest of a high-sulfur stainless steel (grade 303), but steels with nickel but no sulfur elicit no reaction. Nickel-containing 304 and 316 steels should be safer than type 303. Liden and colleagues[270] studied various kinds of metal by patchtesting and found that many of them elicited reactions, including gold-plated silver and white gold. The former releases nickel because in the plating process an interface of nickel is laid down to facilitate adhesion and because the gold is plated so thinly the coating may be porous. The only effective method of reducing the incidence of nickel allergy to any substantial degree is either to stop ear piercing (unlikely) or to legally limit how much nickel ear-piercing equipment and jewelry may contain, so that they do not induce sensitization (or dermatitis in those already sensitized). In Europe legislation is in place that will accomplish this:

Summary of Nickel Directive (94/27/ED): Nickel may not be used:

(Part 1): In post assemblies used during epithelialization, unless they are homogeneous and the concentration of nickel is less than 0.05%.

(Part 2): In products intended to come in direct and prolonged contact with the skin such as earrings, necklaces, wristwatch cases, watch straps, buttons, tighteners, and zippers, if nickel release is greater than 0.5 μg/cm per week.

(Part 3): In coated products in Part 2, unless the coating is sufficient to ensure that the nickel release will not exceed 0.5 μg/cm per week after 2 years of normal use.

Unfortunately, rubber gloves do not afford protection from nickel, which has been demonstrated to penetrate them.[122] The chief treatment of nickel dermatitis is judicious use of topical steroids and avoidance of further contact. Consideration should also be given to barrier creams that chelate nickel.[345, 346] EDTA barrier gels may give protection, but Gawkrodger's group[346] in a literature review found 5-chloro-7-iodoquinoline-8-ol to be most effective. It is surprising that this product is not yet commercially available. The chief therapy for nickel dermatitis continues to be topical corticosteroids and avoidance of further contact.

PALLADIUM AND PLATINUM

Palladium and platinum are commonly found associated with copper and nickel and collect in residues formed during extraction and refining of these metals. Both are silvery white metals characterized by exceptional resistance to corrosion and of useful catalytic properties.

Palladium

Palladium is used (1) as a catalyst in hydrogen reduction processes (e.g., removal of residual oxygen from furnace atmospheres); (2) for contacts in electrical relays and switching systems in telecommunications equipment; (3) in dental alloys; (4) in high-temperature solders; and (5) in jewelry, often as a constituent of white gold.

There are few reports of suspected palladium allergy, and none were occupational.[347–350] Mouth problems are usually considered dental problems.[350] Marcussen[232] found a larger percentage of persons (8%) with a positive patchtest to palladium among patients who had subjective symptoms related to dental restoration materials.

Routine patchtesting with palladium chloride 1% in petrolatum produces a significant number of positive reactions. Todd and Burrows[352] found 2.4% reactive patients in their routine patchtesting but found no positive reactions to metallic palladium. Koch and Baum[351] also found this result. It is not possible to find significance for any of these positive reactions, and nearly all "reactors" also react to nickel. Explanations for this have suggested that in nature palladium may be found in close association with nickel, and therefore during simultaneous exposure, allergy to both would be expected, as is the case with cobalt and nickel. Nickel and palladium, both in group VII of the periodic table, may possess similar chemical characteristics and may cross-react in patchtesting.[353] That contamination of the patchtest material with small amounts of nickel can occur has been demonstrated by Eedy and associates.[354] The levels of nickel may not be sufficient to produce a positive patchtest reaction, but it is possible that a combination of the two allergens could induce a more pronounced reaction than either one alone.[355] In spite of studies on the subject, no satisfactory explanation has yet been found.[354] Indeed, negative patchtests using pure palladium foil cast doubt on whether palladium is an allergen.[352]

In Germany and Austria, palladium has begun to replace traditional amalgam in dental fillings, not only because of the dangers of mercury but also because palladium is less costly than gold.[356] Recent controversies have arisen, however, over possible adverse biological effects from palladium in dental alloys. For example, the carcinogenic potential of palladium is still unclear, although there is some evidence that it is capable of acting as a mutagen. Nevertheless, there are no documented cases of adverse reactions to metallic palladium. Wataha and Hanks[357] expressed the opinion that the risks of using palladium in dental casting alloys is extremely low, because of the low rate of formation of palladium ions from these alloys. The basic problem with patchtesting with palladium is similar to that with gold: few cases of relevant clinical palladium allergy have been reported, and the significance of the positive reactions is not fully understood.

Platinum

Contact dermatitis to platinum compounds in the workplace has been reported several times,[292] but there are no recent reports of platinum as a cause of occupational dermatitis. Koch and Baum[351] recently described a patient with an eruption on the oral mucosa at the sites where metal bridges had been inserted. The patient showed a positive patchtest reaction to ammonium tetrachloroplatinate, 0.25% in petrolatum, in addition to a positive reaction to palladium chloride, but the possibility of contamination must be considered.

Platinum salts, especially the chloroplatinates, can cause skin and eye irritation and asthma.[358] Dermatitis from chloroplatinic acid in jewelry manufacture was reported by Sidi and Hinkey.[359] Parrot and Saindelle[360] described dermatitis in seven workers in a platinum refinery. Although the dermatitis appeared to be work related, an allergic reaction could not be proved conclusively. The chief drawback in patchtesting with these compounds is their irritancy and capacity for inducing contact urticaria. The appropriate concentration for patchtesting is not known.[361] Testing refinery workers known to be sensitized to hexachloroplatinates showed that the compounds capable of eliciting reactions were confined to a very small group of ion complexes containing reactive halogen ligands.[362] Neutral complexes and those containing more strongly bound ligands were found to be totally inactive. Avoidance of chloroplatinates eliminated platinum sensitization at one refinery. It must be concluded that platinum metal is still in doubt as a cause of contact allergic sensitization. The salts of platinum may also be encountered in chemical analyses, electroplating, and photography.

TIN

Contact allergy to tin has never been proved; however, Menne and coworkers[344] reported 10 positive reactions to metallic tin in 73 nickel-sensitive patients. They believed that these reactions could not have been irritant or occlusive ones and that their findings indicate that tin is a common sensitizer in nickel-sensitive patients. Further investigation is needed for confirmation. Irritant reactions from tin are very well-recognized, especially when it is used as an antifouling agent in paint, specifically bis-tributyl tin oxide.[57, 363]

TITANIUM

Neither allergic nor irritant reactions have been described from titanium, even with exposure to massive amounts.[364]

ZINC

The main applications for zinc are coatings to protect iron and steel from corrosion; zinc alloys for die castings; and alloys with copper such as brass and nickel silver. Zinc coatings produced primarily by hot-dip galvanizing, by electroplating, or by powder spraying account for nearly half of all zinc consumption. This has resulted from increasing use by the automotive and construction industries in air-conditioning and ventilation ducts. Alloys containing 4% aluminium, 1% copper, and small amounts of magnesium are used for pressure-die casting, a rapid process for making components for a variety of surface finishes. Die castings of zinc are widely used in automobile production for components such as handles, locks, carburetors, and fuel pumps, and for domestic uses such as bathroom fittings, handles, locks, and toys. Of the compounds of zinc, zinc oxide is the most important, used as a white pigment in tires, paints, and ceramics and pharmaceutical applications. Zinc chloride is an extremely caustic salt used as flux in soldering, in the manufacture of dental fillings, and as a preservative and fire-proofing agent for timber. Irritating to the skin, it produces ulcers and perforation of the nasal septum. "Zinc pox" is an eruption caused by zinc oxide dust found especially in moist areas of the body such as axillas and groins. Secondary infection can occur.[3]

Allergic sensitization to zinc is extremely rare. Inhalation of fumes of zinc oxide causes an influenza-like illness (metal fume fever), which can also occur from other metals.[48] Calnan[365] described it in a welder who galvanized water pipes by dipping the metal into molten zinc at 475°C, releasing a vapor containing fine particles of zinc.

ZIRCONIUM

Most zirconium is used in alloys and in superconductors, surgical implants, vacuum tube parts, and nuclear reactors. Common uses of the metal are shown in Table 24–15. Zirconium, like beryllium, causes hypersensitive granulomas resembling sarcoid granulomas. They were first described from the use of stick deodorants containing soluble zirconium lactate.[366] Granulomas were also reported by Epstein and Allen from insoluble zirconium oxide present in poison ivy lotions.[367] Epstein and Allen recommended diagnosis by intradermal injection of 0.1 mL of a 1:100 suspension of zirconium lactate. A positive result consists of a granulomatous nodule measuring 2 to 4 mm in diameter that appears in about 3 to 4 weeks and that on biopsy shows an organized epithelioid cell tuber-

 TABLE 24–15 • Some Common Uses for Zirconium

Coating nuclear fuel rods
Alloys for corrosion resistance
Metal-to-glass seals
Photoflash bulbs (foil)
Pyrotechnics
Special welding fluxes
Vacuum tubes
Primers for explosives
Acid manufacturing
Deoxidizer and scavenger in steel manufacture
Laboratory crucibles

cle resembling sarcoid granuloma. Fisher[2] found that zirconium hypersensitivity can also be diagnosed by rubbing a zirconium preparation onto an area of scarified skin and covering it for 2 days. A positive reaction consists of discrete, reddish brown papules that appear in approximately 4 weeks and on biopsy specimens show a granulomatous reaction pattern similar to that of cutaneous sarcoid. Cronin[292] has recommended intradermal testing with aqueous zirconium salts at a concentration of 1:100 or greater, to avoid nonspecific false-positive reactions.

Zirconium granulomas occur after contact with both soluble and insoluble zirconium salts. Those produced by soluble salts usually disappear within a few months, whereas those caused by the insoluble salts persist for years and are markedly resistant to treatment. Zirconium granulomas have been reported in a worker handling heated zirconium alloys.[368] In this case, however, the eruption resembled lupus miliaris disseminatus faciei.

References

1. Johannessen H, Bergan-Skar B. Itching problems among potroom workers in factories using recycled aluminium. *Contact Dermatitis* 1980; 6:42–43.
2. Fisher AA. *Contact Dermatitis,* 2nd ed. Philadelphia: Lea & Febiger; 1973.
3. Schwartz L, Tulipan L, Birmingham DJ. *Occupational Disease of the Skin,* 3rd ed. Philadelphia: Lea & Febiger; 1957.
4. Hall AF. Occupational contact dermatitis among aircraft workers. *JAMA* 1944; 125:179–185.
5. Clemmensen OJ, Knudsen HE. Contact sensitivity to aluminium in a patient hyposensitized with aluminium precipitated grass pollen. *Contact Dermatitis* 1980; 6:305–308.
6. Bohler-Sommeregger J, Lindemayr H. Contact sensitivity to aluminium. *Contact Dermatitis* 1986; 15:278–281.
7. Veien NK, Hattel T, Justensen O, et al. Aluminium allergy. *Contact Dermatitis* 1986; 15:295–297.
8. Kaaber S, Cramers M, Jepsen FL. The role of cadmium as a skin sensitizing agent in denture and non-denture wearers. *Contact Dermatitis* 1982; 8:308–313.

9. Cox NH, Moss C, Forsyth A. Allergy to non-toxoid constituents of vaccines and implications for patch testing. *Contact Dermatitis* 1988; 18:143–146.

10. Tosti A, Vincenzi C, Peluso AM. Accidental diagnosis of aluminium sensitivity with Finn chambers. *Contact Dermatitis* 1990; 23:48–49.

11. Fischer T, Rystedt I. A case of contact sensitivity to aluminium. *Contact Dermatitis* 1982; 8:343.

12. Kotovirta M-L, Salo OP, Visa-Tolvanen K. Contact sensitivity to aluminium. *Contact Dermatitis* 1984; 11:135.

13. Meding B, Augustsson A, Hansson C. Patch test reactions to aluminium. *Contact Dermatitis* 1984; 10:107.

14. Fischer T, Maibach H. Aluminium in Finn chambers reacts with cobalt and nickel salt in patch test materials. *Contact Dermatitis* 1985; 12:200–202.

15. Dwyer CM, Kerr RE. Contact allergy to aluminium in two brothers. *Contact Dermatitis* 1993; 29:36–38.

16. Hemmer W, Wantke F, Focke M, et al. Evaluation of cutaneous hypersensitivity to aluminium by using routine patch testing with AlCl$_3$. *Contact Dermatitis* 1996; 34:217–218.

17. Liden C. Cold-impregnated aluminium—a new source of nickel exposure. *Contact Dermatitis* 1994; 31:22–24.

18. Stevenson CJ. Antimony spots. *Trans St John's Hosp Derm Soc* 1965; 51:40–45.

19. Paschoud J-M. Two cases of lichenoid contact eczema closely resembling lichen planus. *Dermatologica* 1963; 127:99–107.

20. Paschoud J-M. Notes cliniques au sujet des eczemas de contact professionelles par l'arsenic et l'antimonie. *Dermatologica* 1964; 129:410–415.

21. Chou Y-H, Hsiang H, Chung-Lua Ya Fang I: Antimony induced dermatitis. *Hsuch Tsa Chih* 1980; 13:228.

22. McCallum RI. The work of an occupational hygiene service in environmental control. *Am Occup Hyg Assoc J* 1963; 6:55–60.

23. Renes LE. Antimony poisoning in industry. *Arch Ind Hyg Occup Med* 1953; 7:99–108.

24. Prosser-White R. *Occupational Affections of the Skin,* 4th ed. London: W K Lewis; 1934:96.

25. Oliver T. The health of antimony oxide workers. *Br Med J* 1933; I:1094–1095.

26. Quinby RS. Health hazards in the rubber industry. *J Indust Hyg* 1926; 8:103–112.

27. White GP, Mathias CGT. Dermatitis in workers exposed to antimony—a smelting process. *J Occup Med* 1993; 35:392–395.

28. NIOSH. *Current Intelligence: Arsine Poisoning. Bulletin 32.* Washington: US Dept of Health, Education and Welfare. Public Health Service, 1979:4.

29. Holmquist I. Occupational arsenical dermatitis. *Acta Derm Venereol* 1951; 31[Suppl 26]:7–214.

30. Birmingham DJ, Key MM, Holaday DA, et al. An outbreak of arsenical dermatoses in a mining community. *Arch Dermatol* 1965; 91:457–464.

31. Jones WR. Arsenical sensitization induced previous to arsphenamine therapy. *Urol Cult Rev* 1940; 44:452–453.

32. Sulzberger MB. Hypersensitiveness to neoarsphenamine in guinea pigs. *Arch Dermatol* 1929; 20:669–697.

33. Barbaud A, Mougeolle JM, Schmutz JL. Contact hypersensitivity to arsenic in a crystal factory worker. *Contact Dermatitis* 1995; 33:272–273.

34. Goncalo S, Silva MS, Toncalo H, et al. Occupational contact dermatitis to arsenic trioxide. In: Frosch PJ, Dooms-Goossens A, LaChapelle JM, et al, eds. *Current Topics in Contact Dermatitis.* Berlin: Springer-Verlag; 1989: 333–336.

35. Mees RA. Nails with arsenical polyneuritis. *JAMA* 1919; 72:1337.

36. Daniel CR, Osment LS. Nail pigmentation abnormalities: their importance and proper examination. *Cutis* 1980; 25:595–607.

37. Hutchinson J. Arsenic cancer. *Br Med J* 1887; 2:1280–1281.

38. Miki Y, Kawatsu T, Matsuda K, et al. Cutaneous and pulmonary cancers associated with Bowen's disease. *J Am Acad Dermatol* 1982; 6:26–31.

39. Cronin E. Clothing and textiles. In: *Contact Dermatitis.* Edinburgh: Churchill-Livingstone; 1980:70.

40. Hanifin JM, Epstein WL, Cline MJ. In-vitro studies of granulomatous hypersensitivity to beryllium. *J Invest Dermatol* 1970; 5:284–288.

41. Jones WW. The beryllium granuloma. *Proc R Soc Med (Lond)* 1971; 64:22–24.

42. Curtis CH. Cutaneous hypersensitivity to beryllium. *Arch Dermatol* 1951; 64:470–482.

43. Vilaplana J, Romaguera C, Grimalt F. Occupational and non-occupational allergic contact dermatitis from beryllium. *Contact Dermatitis* 1992; 26:295–298.

44. Zissu D, Binet S, Cavelier C. Patch testing with beryllium alloy samples in guinea pigs. *Contact Dermatitis* 1996; 34:196–200.

45. Habermann AL, Pratt M, Storrs FJ. Contact dermatitis from beryllium in dental alloys. *Contact Dermatitis* 1993; 28:157–162.

46. Proctor NH, Hughes JP, Fischman ML. *Chemical Hazards in the Workplace,* 2nd ed. Philadelphia: JB Lippincott, 1988:100–101.

47. Lewis R. Metals. In: LaDou J, ed. *Occupational Medicine* Norwalk, Conn: Appleton-Lange; 1990:302–303.

48. Stokinger HE. The metals. In: Patty FA, ed. *Industrial Hygiene and Toxicology,* 2nd ed, Vol 2. New York: Interscience; 1963:1011.

49. Fregert S, Hjorth N. Contact dermatitis. In: Rook A, Wilkinson DS, Ebling RJC, eds. *Textbook of Dermatology,* 3rd ed. Oxford: Blackwell; 1979.

50. Wahlberg JE, Bowman A. Sensitization and testing of guinea pigs with cobalt chloride. *Contact Dermatitis* 4; 128–132, 1978.

51. Wahlberg JE, Boman A. Guinea pig maximization test method—cadmium chloride. *Contact Dermatitis* 1979; 5:405.

51a. Kaaber K, Nielsen AO, Veien NK. Vaccination granulomas and aluminium allergy: course and prognostic factors. *Contact Dermatitis* 1986; 26:304–306.

52. Gebhardt M, Geier J. Evaluation of patch test results with denture material series. *Contact Dermatitis* 1996; 34:191–195.

53. Bjornberg A. Reactions to light in yellow tattoos from cadmium sulfide. *Arch Dermatol* 1963; 88:267–271.

54. Goldstein N. Mercury-cadmium sensitivity in tattoos. A photoallergic reaction in red pigment. *Ann Int Med* 1967; 67:984–989.

55. Mertz W. Chromium occurrence and function in biological systems. *Physiol Rev* 1969; 49:163–239.

56. Cumin W. Remarks on the medicinal properties of madar and on the effects of bichromate of potash on the human body. *Med Surg J (Edin)* 1827; 28:295–302.

57. NIOSH. *Criteria document: recommendation for an occupational exposure standard for inorganic compounds.* Washington, DC: US Dept of Health, Education and Welfare; 1976.

58. Senear FE. Chrome holes: a case report. *Arch Dermatol* 1951; 63:163–164.

59. Birmingham DJ. *Chromium: Skin Effects.* Washington, DC: National Academy of Sciences; 1974:64.

60. Edmundson WF. Chrome ulcers of the skin and nasal septum and their relationship to patch testing. *J Invest Dermatol* 1951; 17:17–19.

61. Burrows D. Chromium and the skin. *Br J Dermatol* 1978; 99:587–595.

62. Dornan JD. Occupational dermatoses amongst chrome platers in the Sheffield area 197701980. *Contact Dermatitis* 1981; 7:354–355.

63. Parkhurst JH. Dermatosis industrialis in blueprint workers due to chromium compounds. *Arch Dermatol* 1925; 12:253–256.

64. Prosser-White R. *Occupational Affections of the Skin*, 4th ed. London: WK Lewis; 1920:96.

65. Smith AR. Chrome with manifestations of sensitization: report of a case. *JAMA* 1931; 97:95–98.

66. Englehardt WE, Mayer RL. Uber Chromekzema im graphischen Gewerge. *Arch Gewebepath Hyg* 1931; 2:140–168.

67. Kesten B, Laszlo E. Dermatitis due to sensitization to contact substances. Dermatitis venenata occupational dermatitis. *Arch Dermatol* 1931; 23:221–237.

68. Bonnevie P. *Etiology and Pathogenesis of the Eczemas.* Copenhagen: A Busck; 1939.

69. Schwartz L, Dunn JE. Dermatitis occurring in a woolen mill. *Indust Med Surg* 1942; 11:432–435.

70. Pirila V, Kilpio O. On dermatoses caused by bichromates. *Acta Derm Venereol* 1949; 29:550–563.

71. Jaeger H, Pelloni E. Tests epicutanes aux bichromates positifs dans l'eczema au ciment. *Dermatologica* 1950; 100:207–216.

72. Winston JR, Walsh EN. Chromate dermatitis in railroad employees working with diesel locomotives. *JAMA* 1951; 147:1133–1134.

73. Schwartz L. Skin hazards in railroad roundhouses and machine shops. *Indust Med Surg* 1952; 21:482–484.

74. Calnan CD, Harman RRM. Studies in contact dermatitis XIII: diesel coolant chromate dermatitis. *Trans St. John's Hosp Derm Soc* 1961; 46:13–21.

75. Merritt K, Brown SA. Release of hexavalent chromium from corrosion of stainless steel and cobalt chromium alloys. *J Biomed Mater Res* 1995; 29:627–633.

76. Levin HM, Brunner MJ, Rattner H. Lithographer's dermatitis. *JAMA* 1959; 169:566–569.

77. Samitz MH, Shrager J. Prevention of dermatitis in the printing and lithographing industries. *Arch Dermatol* 1966; 94:307–309.

78. Fregert S, Gruvberger B, Heijer A. Chromium dermatitis from galvanized sheets. *Berufsdermatosen* 1970; 18:254–260.

79. Adams RM, Fregert S, Gruvberger B, et al. Water solubility of zinc chromate primer paints used as antirust agents. *Contact Dermatitis* 1976; 2:357–358.

80. Engle HO, Calnan CD. Chromate dermatitis from paint. *Br J Ind Med* 1963; 20:192–198.

81. Morris GE. "Chrome" dermatitis: a study of the chemistry of shoe leather with particular reference to basic chromic sulfate. *Arch Dermatol* 1958; 78:612–618.

82. Samitz MH, Gross S. Extraction by sweat of chromium from chrome tanned leathers. *J Occup Med* 1960; 2:12–14.

83. Mancuso G, Reggiani M, Berdondini RM. Occupational dermatitis in shoemakers. *Contact Dermatitis* 1996; 34:17–22.

84. Rycroft RJG, Calnan CD. Chromate dermatitis from a boiler lining. *Contact Dermatitis* 1977; 3:198.

85. Fregert S, Ovrum P. Chromate in welding fumes with special reference to contact dermatitis. *Acta Derm Venereol* 1963; 43:119–124.

86. Shelley WB. Chromium in welding fumes as cause of eczematous hand eruption. *JAMA* 1964; 189:772–773.

87. Fisher AA. "Blackjack disease" and other chromate puzzles. *Cutis* 1976; 18:21–35.

88. Fregert S, Gruvberger B, Goransson K, et al. Allergic contact dermatitis from chromate in military textiles. *Contact Dermatitis* 1978; 4:223–224.

89. Cairns RJ, Calnan CD. Green tattoo reactions associated with cement dermatitis. *Br J Dermatol* 1962; 74:288–294.

90. Loewenthal LJA. Reactions in green tattoos: the significance of the valence state of chromium. *Arch Dermatol* 1960; 82:237–243.

91. Fregert S. Chromate eczema and matches. *Acta Derm Venereol* 1961; 41:433–440.

92. Fregert S. Book matches as a source of chromate. *Arch Dermatol* 1963; 88:546–547.

93. Newhouse MLA. A cause of chromate dermatitis among assemblers in an automobile factory. *Br J Ind Med* 1963; 20:194–203.

94. Krook G, Fregert S, Gruvberger B. Chromate and cobalt eczema due to magnetic tapes. *Contact Dermatitis* 1977; 3:60–61.

95. Conner B. Chromate dermatitis and paper manufacture. *Contact Dermatitis Newslett* 1972; 11:265.

96. Fregert S, Gruvberger B, Heijer A. Sensitization to chromium and cobalt in processing of sulfate pulp. *Acta Derm Venereol* 1972; 52:221–224.

97. Pirila V, Kilpio O. On occupational dermatoses in Finland: a report of 1752 cases. *Acta Derm Venereol* 1954; 34:395–402.

98. Calnan CD. Chromate in coolant water of gramophone record presses. *Contact Dermatitis* 1978; 4:246–247.

99. Burrows D. Chromium dermatitis in a tyre fitter. *Contact Dermatitis* 1981; 7:55–56.

100. Huriez C, Martin P, Lefebvre M. Sensitivity to dichromate in a milk analysis laboratory. *Contact Dermatitis* 1975; 1:247–248.

101. Rogers S, Burrows D. Contact dermatitis in milk testers. *Contact Dermatitis* 1975; 1:387–388.

102. Pedersen NB. Chromate in a food laboratory. *Contact Dermatitis* 1977; 3:105.

103. Calnan CD. Chromate dermatitis from soluble oil. *Contact Dermatitis* 1978; 4:378.

104. Einarsson O, Kylin B, Lindstedt G, Wahlberg JE. Chromium and cobalt in nickel used in cutting fluids. *Contact Dermatitis* 1975; 1:182–183.

105. Oleffe J, Roosels D, Vanderkell J, et al. Presence du chrome dans l'environment de travail. *Derm Beruf Umwelt* 1971; 19:57.

106. Mathias CGT. Pigmented cosmetic dermatitis from contact allergy to a toilet soap containing chromium. *Contact Dermatitis* 1982; 8:29–31.

107. Handley J, Burrows D. Dermatitis from hexavalent chromate in the accelerator of an epoxy sealant (PR1422) used in the aircraft industry. *Contact Dermatitis* 1994; 30:193–196.

108. Fregert S. Occupational dermatitis in a 10 year material. *Contact Dermatitis* 1975; 1:96–107.

109. Fregert S, Hjorth N, Magnusson B, et al. Epidemiology of contact dermatitis. *Trans St John's Hosp Derm Soc* 1969; 55:17–35.

110. Nethercott JR. Results of routine patch testing of 200 patients in Toronto, Canada. *Contact Dermatitis* 1982; 8:389–395.

111. Burrows D. Comparison of 0.25% and 0.5% potassium dichromate in patch testing. *Boll Dermatol Allergol Profess* 1987; 2:117–120.

111a. Burrows D, Andersen KE, Camarasa JG, et al. Trial of 0.5% versus 0.375% potassium dischromate. *Contact Dermatitis* 1989; 21:351.

112. Samsoen M, Stampf JL, Lefievre G, et al. Patch testing with hexavalent chromium salts in different vehicles with nickel and cobalt in petrolatum. *Derm Beruf Umwelt* 1982; 31:181.

113. Burrows D, ed. *Chromium: Metabolism and Toxicity.* Boca Raton, Fla: CRC; 1983.

114. Fischer T, Rystedt I. False positive follicular and irritant patch test reactions to metal salts. *Contact Dermatitis* 1985; 12:93–98.

115. Peltonen L, Fraki J. Prevalence of dichromate sensitivity. *Contact Dermatitis* 1983; 9:190–194.

116. Burrows D, Calnan CD. Cement dermatitis. II: Clinical aspects. *Trans St John's Hosp Derm Soc* 1965; 51:27–39.

117. Decaestecker AM, Marez T, Jdaini J, et al. Hypersensitivity to dichromate among asymptomatic workers in a chromate pigment factory. *Contact Dermatitis* 1990; 23:52–53.

118. Goh CL, Gan SL, Ngui SJ. Occupational dermatitis in a prefabrication construction factory. *Contact Dermatitis* 1986; 15:235–240.

119. Thormann J, Jespersen NB, Joensen HD. Persistence of contact allergy to chromium. *Contact Dermatitis* 1979; 5:261–264.

120. Keczkes K, Basheer AM, Wyatt EH. The persistence of allergic contact sensitivity: a 10-year follow-up of 100 patients. *Br J Dermatol* 1982; 197:461–465.

120a. Feuerman EJ. Chromates as the cause of contact dermatitis in housewives. *Dermatologica* 1971; 143:292–297.

121. Wahlberg JE, Wennersten G. Light sensitivity and chromium dermatitis. *Br J Dermatol* 1977; 97:411–416.

122. Wall LM. Nickel penetration through rubber gloves. *Contact Dermatitis* 1980; 6:461–463.

123. Goh CL, Wong PH, Kwok SF, et al. Chromate allergy: total chromium and hexavalent chromium in the air. *Derm Beruf Umwelt* 1986; 34:132–134.

124. Veien NK, Hattel T, Laurberg G. Patch test results from a private dermatologic practice for two periods of 5 years with a 10-year interval. Am J *Contact Dermatitis* 1992; 3:189–192.

125. Goh CL. Chromate sensitivity in Singapore. *Int J Dermatol* 1985; 24:514–517.

126. Feuerman EJ. Housewives' eczema and the role of chromates. *Acta Derm Venereol* 1969; 49:288–293.

127. Lachapelle JM, Cauwerys R, Tennstedt D, et al. Eau de Javel and prevention of chromate allergy in France. *Contact Dermatitis* 1980; 6:107–110.

128. Allenby CF, Goodwin BFS. Influence of detergent washing powders on minimal eliciting patch test concentration of nickel and chromium. *Contact Dermatitis* 1983; 9:491–499.

129. Basketter DA, Briatico-Vangosa G, Kaestner W, et al. Nickel, cobalt and chromium in consumer products: a role in allergic contact dermatitis? *Contact Dermatitis* 1993; 28:15–25.

130. Nethercott J, Fowler J, Kauffman L, et al. Human response to repetitive hexavalent chromium challenge at 25 μg/ml in water. Jadassohn Centenary Congress, London, October 9–12, 1996.

131. Clemmensen OJ, Jorgensen J, Jons O, et al. Exposure to chromium from hospital cleaning. *Derm Beruf Umwelt* 1981; 3:31–54.

132. Hansen KS. Occupational dermatoses in hospital cleaning women. *Contact Dermatitis* 1983; 9:343–351.

132a. Contact allergy in an adult Danish population. The Allergy Study, The Population Studies in Glostrub. *Ugeskr Laeger* 1994; 156:3471–3474.

133. Breit R, Turk RBM. The medical and social fate of the dichromate allergic patient. *Br J Dermatol* 1976; 94:349–351.

134. Burrows D. Prognosis in industrial dermatitis. *Br J Dermatol* 1972; 87:145–148.

135. Nater JP. Possible causes of chromate eczema. *Dermatologica* 1963; 126:160–166.

136. Schroeder HA, Balassa JC, Tipton IH. Abnormal trace metals in man: chromium. *J Chronic Dis* 1962; 15:941–964.

137. Fregert S. [quoted] In: Cronin E: *Contact Dermatitis.* Edinburgh: Churchill Livingstone; 1980:311.

138. Kaaber K, Veien NK. The significance of chromate ingestion in patients allergic to chromate. *Acta Derm Venereol* 1977; 57:321–323.

139. McMillen C. Oral chromate. In: *International Symposium on Contact Dermatitis,* June 1983.

140. Burrows D. Chromate dermatitis. In: Maibach H, Gellin GA, eds. *Occupational and Industrial Dermatology,* 2nd ed. Chicago: Year Book; 1987:406–421.

141. Hyodo K, Suzuki S, Furuya N, et al. An analysis of chromium, copper, and zinc in organs of a chromate worker. *Int Arch Occup Environ Health* 1980; 46:141–150.

142. Johnston AJM, Calnan CD. Cement dermatitis. I. Chemical aspects. *Trans St. John's Hosp Derm Soc* 1958; 41:11–25.

143. Perone VB, Mofitt AE, Possick PA, et al. The chromium, cobalt, and nickel content of American cement and their relationship to cement dermatitis. *Am Ind Hyg Assoc J* 1974; 35:301–306.

144. Fregert S, Gruvberger B. Chemical properties of cement. Berufsdermatosen 1972; 20:238–248.

145. Engebrigsten JK. Some investigations on hypersensitiveness to bichromate in cement workers. *Acta Derm Venereol* 1952; 32:462–468.

146. Brun RM. Contribution a l'étude des chromates du ciment: nouvelle technique pour le test epicutane au cement. *Dermatologica* 1963; 129:79–88.

147. Meneghini CL, Rantuccio F, Petruzzelli V. Hexavalent chromium content in cements. *Contact Dermatitis Newslett* 1969; 5:108.

148. Wahlberg JE, Lindstedt G, Einarsson O. Chromium, cobalt, and nickel in Swedish cement, detergents, mould and cutting oils. Berufsdermatosen 1977; 25:220–228.

149. Ellis V, Freeman S. Dermatitis due to chromate in cement. I: Chromate content in cement in Australia. *Aust J Dermatol* 1986; 27:86–90.

150. Pirila V. On the role of chrome and other trace elements in cement eczema. *Acta Derm Venereol* 1954; 34:136–143.

151. Geiser JD, Jeanneret JP, Delacretaz J. Eczema au ciment et sensibilisation au cobalt. *Dermatologica* 1960; 121:1–7.

152. Anderson FE. Cement and oil dermatitis: the part played by chrome sensitivity. *Br J Dermatol* 1960; 72:108–117.

153. Kligman AM. The identification of contact allergens by human assay. III: The maximization test, a procedure for screening and rating contact sensitizers. *J Invest Dermatol* 1966; 47:393–409.

154. Samitz MH, Katz SA. A study of the chemical reaction between chromium and skin. *J Invest Dermatol* 1964; 43:35–43.

155. Fregert S, Rorsman H. Allergy to trivalent chromium. *Arch Dermatol* 1964; 90:4–6.

156. Polak L. Immunology of chromium. In: Burrows D, ed. *Chromium: Metabolism and Toxicity.* Boca Raton, Fl: CRC; 1983:51–136.

157. Polak L, Turk JL, Frey JR. Studies on contact hypersensitivity to chromic compounds. *Progr Allerg* 1973; 17:145–226.

158. Siegenthaler U, Laine A, Polak L. Studies on contact sensitivity to chromium in the guinea pig. The role of valence in the formation of the antigenic determinant. *J Invest Derm* 1983; 80:44–47.

159. Schleiff P. Provokation des Chromatekzems zu Test-

wecken durch interne Chromzufuhr. *Hautarzt* 1968; 19:209–210.

160. Veien NK, Hattel T, Laurberg G. Chromate: allergic patients challenged orally with potassium dichromate. *Contact Dermatitis* 1994; 31:137–139.

161. McMillan C. Eighth International Symposium on Contact Dermatitis. Cambridge, 1985.

162. Samitz MH. Prevention of occupational skin diseases from exposure to chromic acid and chromates: use of ascorbic acid. *Cutis* 1974; 13:569–574.

163. Lips R, Rast H, Elsner P. Outcome of job change in patients with occupational chromate dermatitis. *Contact Dermatitis* 1996; 34:268–271.

164. Burrows D, Cooke MA. Trivalent chromium plating. *Contact Dermatitis* 1980; 6:222.

165. Valsecchi R, Cainelli T. Chromiuim dermatitis and ascorbic acid. *Contact Dermatitis* 1984; 10:252–253.

166. Romaguera C, Grimalt F, Vilaplana J, et al. Formulation of a barrier cream against chromate. *Contact Dermatitis* 1985; 13:49–52.

167. Wall LM. Chromate dermatitis and sodium dithionite. *Contact Dermatitis* 1982; 3:291–293.

168. Fregert S, Gruvberger B, Sandahl E. Reduction of chromate in cement by iron sulfate. *Contact Dermatitis* 1979; 5:39–42.

169. Burckhardt W. Abschwachung der ekzematogener Wirkung des Zements durch Ferrosulfat. *Dermatologica* 1971; 142:271–273.

170. Avnstorp C. Follow-up of workers from the prefabricated concrete industry after the addition of ferrous sulphate to Danish cement. *Contact Dermatitis* 1989; 20:365–371.

171. Roto P, Sainio H, Reunala T, et al. Addition of ferrous sulfate to cement and risk of chromium dermatitis among construction workers. *Contact Dermatitis* 1996; 34:43–50.

172. GISBAU. *Chromatarme Zemente und das Zementekzem experten Gesprach.* Frankurt am Main: Arbeitsgemeinschaft der Bau-Berufgenossenschaften, 1992.

173. Farm G. Changing patterns in chromate allergy. *Contact Dermatitis* 1986; 15:298–310.

174. Gailhofer G, Lundvan M. Zur Anderung des Allergenspekturums bei Kontaktekzemen in den Jahren 1975–1984. *Derm Beruf* 1987; 35:12.

175. Bruze M, Bruvberger B, Hradil E. Chromate sensitization and elicitation with iron sulfate. *Acta Derm Venereol (Stockh)* 1990; 70:160–162.

176. Veien NK, Hattel T, Laveberg G. Patchtest results from a private dermatologic practice for two periods of 5 years with a 10-year interval. *Am J Contact Dermatitis* 1992; 3:189–192.

177. Conde-Salazar L, Guimaraens D, Villegas C, et al. Occupational allergic contact dermatitis in construction workers. *Contact Dermatitis* 1995; 33:226–230.

178. Irvine C, Pugh CE, Hansen EJ, et al. Cement dermatitis in underground workers during construction of the Channel tunnel. *Occup Med* 1994; 44:17–32.

179. Tandon R, Aarts B. Chromium, nickel and cobalt contents of some Australian cements. *Contact Dermatitis* 1993; 28:201–205.

180. Goh CL, Gan SL. Change in cement manufacturing process: a cause for decline in chromate allergy? *Contact Dermatitis* 1996; 34:51–54.

181. Turk K, Rietschel RL. Effect of processing cement to concrete on hexavalent chromium levels. *Contact Dermatitis* 1993; 28:209–211.

182. Schwartz L, Peck SM, Blair KE, et al. Allergic dermatitis due to metallic cobalt. *J Allerg* 1945; 16:51–53.

183. Pirila V. Sensitivity to cobalt in pottery workers. *Acta Derm Venereol* 1953; 33:193–198.

184. Pirila V, Geiser L. Uber Kobaltallergie bei Porzellanarbeitern. *Hautarzt* 1964; 15:491–493.

185. Marcussen PV. Cobalt dermatitis: clinical picture. *Acta Derm Venereol* 1963; 43:231–234.

186. Bandmann HJ, Fuchs G. Uber die Kobaltkontaktallergie, ihre Beziehung zur Bichromat und Nickelkontaktallergie, sowie ihre gewerbedermatologische Bedeutung. *Hautarzt* 1963; 14:207–210.

187. Burrows D. Contact dermatitis in animal feed mill workers. *Br J Dermatol* 1975; 92:167–171.

188. Breuker G, Hoefs W. Kobalthaltiges Futtermittel fur Widerkauer als berufliches Ekzematogen. *Derm Wochenschr* 1966; 152:528–530.

189. Tuomi ML, Rasanen L. Contact allergy to tylosin and cobalt in a pig farmer. *Contact Dermatitis* 1995; 33:285.

190. Garcia J, Armisen A. Cement dermatitis with isolated cobalt sensitivity. *Contact Dermatitis* 1985; 12:52.

190a. Wahlberg JE, Boman A. Sensitization and testing of guinea pigs with cobalt chloride. *Contact Dermatitis* 1978; 4:128–132.

191. Rystedt I. Evaluation and relevance of isolated test reactions of cobalt. *Contact Dermatitis* 1979; 5:233–238.

192. Fischer T, Rystedt I. Cobalt allergy in hard metal workers. *Contact Dermatitis* 1983; 9:115–121.

193. Rystedt I, Fischer T. Relationship between nickel and cobalt sensitivity in hard metal workers. *Contact Dermatitis* 1983; 9:195–210.

194. van Joost T, van Everdingen JJ. Sensitization to cobalt associated with nickel allergy: clinical and statistical studies. *Acta Derm Venereol (Stockh)* 1982; 62:525–529.

195. Lammintausta K, Pitkanen OP, Kalimo K, et al. Interrelationship of nickel and cobalt contact sensitization. *Contact Dermatitis* 1985; 13:148–152.

196. Deisler KJ, Sheets GR. Contact stomatitis due to a denture in a metal sensitive patient. *Calif West Med* 1942; 57:354–355.

197. Vilaplana J, Romaguera C, Cornellana F. Contact dermatitis and adverse oral mucous membrane reactions related to the use of dental prostheses. *Contact Dermatitis* 1994; 30:80–84.

198. Tilsey DA, Rotstein H. Sensitivity caused by internal exposure to nickel, chromium, and cobalt. *Contact Dermatitis* 1980; 6:175–178.

199. Romaguera C, Leach M, Gramalt F, et al. Photocontact dermatitis to cobalt salts. *Contact Dermatitis* 1977; 8:383–388.

200. Fisher AA. Contact dermatitis at home and abroad. *Cutis* 1972; 10:719.

201. Rostenberg A, Perkins AJ. Nickel and cobalt dermatitis. *J Allerg* 1951; 22:466–474.

202. Browning E. *Toxicity of Industrial Metals,* 2nd ed. London: Butterworth; 1969:149.

203. Forstrom L, Kiistala R, Tarvainen K. Hypersensitivity to copper verified by test with 0.1% copper sulfate. *Contact Dermatitis* 1977; 3:280–281.

204. Karlberg AT, Boman A, Wahlberg JE. Copper—a rare sensitizer. *Contact Dermatitis* 1983; 9:134–139.

205. Walton S. Investigation into patch testing with copper sulphate. *Contact Dermatitis* 1983; 9:89–90.

206. van Joost T, Habets JMW, Stolz I. The meaning of positive patch test to copper sulphate in nickel allergy. *Contact Dermatitis* 1988; 8:101–102.

207. Gaul LE. Dermatitis from metal spectacles. Demonstration of nickel and copper compounds from corrosion of earpieces. *Arch Dermatol* 1958; 78:475–478.

208. Morris GE. Industrial dermatitis due to contact with brass. *N Engl J Med* 1952; 246:366–368.

209. Saltzer EI, Wilson JW. Allergic contact dermatitis due to copper. *Arch Dermatol* 1968; 98:375–376.

210. Barranco VP. Eczematous dermatitis caused by internal exposure to copper. *Arch Dermatol* 1972; 106:386–387.

211. Franz G, Teilum D. Cutaneous eruptions and intrauterine contraceptive copper device. *Acta Derm Venereol* 1980; 60:69–71.

212. Romaguera C, Grimalt F. Contact dermatitis from a copper-containing intrauterine contraceptive device. *Contact Dermatitis* 1981; 7:163–164.

213. Dhir GG, Rao DS, Mehrotra MP. Contact dermatitis caused by copper sulfate used as coloring material in commercial alcohol. *Ann Allerg* 1977; 39:204.

214. Proctor NH, Hughes JP. *Chemical Hazards in the Workplace.* Philadelphia: JB Lippincott; 1978:126.

215. Committee on Biological Effects of Atmospheric Pollutants. *Copper.* National Academy of Sciences, Division of Medical Sciences, National Research Council, 1977:55–58.

216. Milby TH, Key MM, Gibson RL, et al. Chemical hazards. In: *Occupational Diseases: A Guide to Their Recognition,* Publication 1097. US Dept of Health, Education and Welfare, Public Health Service, 1964.

217. Hansborg H. Chrysiasis: Ablagerung von Gold in vivo. *Acta Tuberc Scand* 1928; 4:124–132.

218. Schmidt O. Chrysiasis. *Arch Dermatol* 1941; 44:446–452.

219. Cox AJ. Gold in the dermis following gold therapy for rheumatoid arthritis. *Arch Dermatol* 1973; 108:655–657.

220. Penneys NS. Gold therapy: dermatologic uses and toxicities. *J Am Acad Dermatol* 1979; 1:315–320.

221. Freyberg RH. Gold therapy for rheumatoid arthritis. In: Hollander JL, ed. *Arthiritis and Allied Conditions: A Textbook of Rheumatology,* 8th ed. Philadelphia: Lea & Febiger; 1972:469.

222. Björkner B, Bruze M, Moller H. High frequency of contact allergy to gold sodium thiosulfate. An indication of gold allergy? *Contact Dermatitis* 1994; 30:144–151.

223. Forster HW, Dickey RF. A case of sensitivity to gold-ball orbital implant. *Am J Ophthalmol* 1949; 132:659–662.

224. Fregert S, Kollander M, Poulson J. Allergic contact stomatitis from gold dentures. *Contact Dermatitis* 1979; 5:63–64.

225. Klashka F. Contact allergy to gold. *Contact Dermatitis* 1975; 1:264–265.

226. Wiesenfeld D, Ferguson MM, Forsyth A, et al. Allergy to dental gold. *Oral Surg* 1984; 57:158–160.

227. Young E. Contact hypersensitivity to metallic gold. *Dermatologica* 1974; 149:294–298.

228. Schmollack E. Berufliche Kontaktekzema durch Kaliumgoldzyanid. *Dermatol Monatsschr* 1971; 157:821–824.

229. Fowler JF. Selection of patch test materials for gold allergy. *Contact Dermatitis* 1987; 17:23–25.

230. McKenna KE, Dolan O, Walsy YM, et al. Contact allergy to gold sodium thiosulfate. *Contact Dermatitis* 1995; 32:143–146.

231. Rasanen L, Kalimo K, Laine J, et al. Contact allergy to gold in dental patients. *Br J Dermatol* 1996; 134:673–677.

232. Marcusson JA. Contact allergies to nickel sulfate, gold sodium thiosulfate and palladium chloride in patients claiming side-effects from dental alloy components. *Contact Dermatitis* 1996; 34:320–323.

233. Bruze M, Bjorkner B, Moller H. Skin testing with gold sodium thiomalate and gold sodium thiosulfate. *Contact Dermatitis* 1995; 32:5–8.

234. Sabroe RA, Sharp LA, Peachy RDG. Contact allergy to gold sodium thiosulfate. *Contact Dermatitis* 1994; 34:345–348.

235. Bruze M, Hedman H, Bjorkner B, et al. The development and course of test reactions to gold sodium thiosulfate. *Contact Dermatitis* 1995; 33:386–391.

236. Lundgren KD, Swenson A. Occupational poisoning by alkyl mercury compounds. *J Ind Toxicol* 1949; 31:190–199.

237. Nixon GS, Rowbotham TC. Mercury hazards associated with high-speed mechanical amalgamators. *Br Dent J* 1971; 131:308–311.

238. Richards JM, Warren PJ. Mercury vapour released during the removal of old amalgam restorations. *Br J Dent* 1985; 159:231–232.

239. Ship IL, Shapiro IM, Miller WD: Mercury poisoning in dental practice. *Compend Contin Educ Dent* 1983; 4:107–110.

240. Svare CW, Peterson LC, Reinhardt JW, et al. Effect of dental amalgams on mercury levels in expired air. *J Dent Res* 1981; 60:1668–1671.

241. Vimy MJ, Lorsheider FL. Intra-oral air mercury released from dental amalgams. *J Dent Res* 1985; 64:1069–1071.

242. Abraham JE, Svare CW, Frank CW. The effect of dental amalgam restoration on blood mercury levels. *J Dent Res* 1984; 63:71–73.

243. Kronke A, Ott K, Petschelt A, et al. Mercury concentrations in the blood and urine of people with or without amalgam fillings. *Dtsch Zahnaertzl* 1980; 35:803–808, [English abstract].

244. Ott K, Kronke A. Mercury concentrations in the blood and urine of patients with or without amalgam fillings. *J Dent Res* Special Issue B 1981; 60:1210.

245. Neal DA, Grey AS. *Mercurialism and Its Control in the Felt Hat Industry.* Bulletin 263, Federal Security Agency. Washington, DC: US Public Health Service; 1941.

246. Patty FA. In: Fassett DW, ed. *Industrial Hygiene and Toxicity,* 2nd ed, Vol 2. New York: Interscience; 1963: 872.

247. Faria A, De Freitas C. Systemic contact dermatitis due to mercury. *Contact Dermatitis* 1992; 27:110–111.

248. Hygiene Guide Series. Mercury and its inorganic compounds. *Am Ind Hyg Assoc J* 1966; 27:310–312.

249. Snodgrass W, Sullivan JB, Rumach BH, et al. Mercury poisoning from home gold ore processing. *JAMA* 1981; 246:1929–1931.

250. Vickers CFH. Mercury sensitivity. *Contact Dermatitis Newslett* 1967; 2:20.

251. White IR, Smith BGN. Dental amalgam dermatitis. *Br Dent J* 1984; 156:259–260.

252. Kanerva L, Komulainen M, Estlander T, et al. Occupational allergic contact dermatitis from mercury. *Contact Dermatitis* 1993; 28:26–28.

253. Sollman T. *Manual of Pharmacology.* Philadelphia: WB Saunders; 1957:1310.

254. North American Contact Dermatitis Group (NACDG). Task Force on Contact Dermatitis of the American Academy of Dermatology. *Arch Dermatol* 1973; 108:537–540.

255. Handley J, Todd D, Burrows D. Mercury allergy in contact dermatitis clinic in Northern Ireland. *Contact Dermatitis* 1993; 29:258–261.

256. Koby GA. Phenylmercuric acetate as primary irritant. *Arch Dermatol* 1972; 106:129.

257. Ladd AC, Goldwater LJ, Jacobs MB. Absorption and excretion of mercury in man. V. Toxicity of phenylmercurials. *Arch Environ Health* 1964; 9:43–52.

258. Goncalo M, Figueiredo A, Goncalo S. Hypersensitivity to thimerosal: the sensitizing moiety. *Contact Dermatitis* 1996; 34:201–203.

259. Kawai K, Zhang X-M, Nakagawa M, et al. Allergic contact dermatitis due to mercury in a wedding ring and a cosmetic. *Contact Dermatitis* 1994; 31:330–331.

260. Barrazza V, Meuner P, Escande JP. Acute contact dermatitis and exanthematous pustulosis due to mercury. *Contact Dermatitis* 1998; 38:361.

261. Koch P, Nickolaus G. Allergic contact dermatitis and exanthem due to mercury chloride in plastic boots. *Contact Dermatitis* 1996; 34:405–409.

262. Koch P, Bahmer FA. Oral lichenoid lesions, mercury hypersensitivity and combined hypersensitivity to mercury and other metals: histologically proven reproduction of the reaction by patch testing with metal salts. *Contact Dermatitis* 1995; 33:323–328.

263. Keiller FES, Warin RP. Mercury dermatitis in a tattoo: treated with dimercaprol *Br Med J* 1957; 1:687.

264. Lamar LM, Bliss BO. Localized pigmentation of skin due to topical mercury. *Arch Dermatol* 1966; 93:450–453.

265. Kern AB. Mercurial pigmentation. *Arch Dermatol* 1969; 99:129–130.

266. Bourgeois M, Dooms-Goossens A, Knockaert D, et al. Mercury intoxication after topical application of a metallic mercury ointment. *Dermatologica* 1986; 172:48–51.

267. Kresbach H, Kerl H, Wawschinch O. Cutaneous mercury granuloma. *Berufsdermatosen* 1971; 19:173–186.

268. Crikelair GF, Hiratzka T. Intraperitoneal mercury granulomas. *Ann Surg* 1953; 137:272–275.

269. Hopf G, Winkler A. Foreign body granuloma from metallic mercury. *Derm Wochenschr* 1957; 136:1273–1279.

270. Liden C, Menne T, Burrows D. Nickel containing alloys and platings and their ability to cause dermatitis. *Br J Dermatol* 1996; 134:193–198.

271. Haudrechy P, Foussereau J, Mantout B, et al. Nickel release from nickel-plated metals and stainless steels. *Contact Dermatitis* 1994; 31:249–255.

272. Menne T, Branrup F, Thestrup-Pedersen K, et al. Patch test reactivity to nickel alloys. *Contact Dermatitis* 1987; 16:255–259.

273. Dotterud LK, Falk ES. Metal allergy in north Norwegian schoolchildren and its relationship with ear piercing and atopy. *Contact Dermatitis* 1994; 31:308–313.

274. Larsson-Stymne B, Widstrom L. Ear piercing—a cause of nickel allergy in schoolgirls. *Contact Dermatitis* 1985; 13:289–293.

275. Moorthy TT, Tan GH. Nickel sensitivity in Singapore. *Int J Dermatol* 1986; 25:307–309.

276. Rudski E, Rebandel P, Napiorkowska T, et al. Alergia na nikiel. *Przegl Dermatol* 1984; 71:431–435, [English abstract].

277. Gawkrodger DJ, Vestey JP, Wong W-K, et al. Contact clinic survey of nickel sensitive subjects. *Contact Dermatitis* 1986; 14:165–169.

278. Braathen LR, Haavelsrub O, Thorsby E. HLA antigens in patients with allergic contact sensitivity to nickel. *Arch Dermatol Res* 1983; 275:355–356.

279. Karvonen J, Silvennoinen-Kassinen S, Ilonen J, et al. No significant association between HLA and nickel contact sensitivity. *Tissue Antigens* 1979; 14:459–461.

280. Silvennoinen-Kassinens S, Tiilikainen A. No significant HLA haplotype association in nickel contact sensitivity: a family study. *Tissue Antigens* 1980; 15:455–457.

281. Menne T, Holm NV. Hand eczema in nickel sensitive female twins. Genetic predisposition and environmental factors. *Contact Dermatitis* 1983; 9:289–296.

282. Marcussen PV. Ecological considerations on nickel dermatitis. *Br J Ind Med* 1960; 17:65–68.

283. Samitz MH, Katz SA. Skin hazards from nickel and chromium salts in association with cutting oil operations. *Contact Dermatitis* 1975; 1:158–160.

284. Reichenberger M, Ebke M, Petiri C. Zur Nickel Sensibilisierung bei Frauen und ihre Relevanz zur beruflichen Tätigkeit. *Berufsdermatosen* 1976; 24:91–99.

285. Arndt KA. Cutting fluids and the skin. *Cutis* 1969; 5:143–147.

286. Gellin GA. Cutting fluids and skin disorders. *Intensive Med* 1970; 39:65–67.

287. Hodgson G. Cutaneous hazards of lubricants. *Trans Soc Occup Med* 1969; 19:9–15.

288. Coenraads PJ, Foo SC, Phoon WO, et al. Dermatitis in small-scale metal industries. *Contact Dermatitis* 1985; 12:155–160.

289. Shah M, Lerwis FM, Gawkrodger DJ. Prognosis of occupational hand dermatitis in metalworkers. *Contact Dermatitis* 1996; 34:27–30.

290. Meding B, Barregard L, Marcus K. Hand eczema in car mechanics. *Contact Dermatitis* 1994; 30:129–134.

291. Wahlberg JE. Nickel allergy and atopy in hairdressers. *Contact Dermatitis* 1975; 1:161–165.

292. Cronin E. Metals. In *Contact Dermatitis*. Edinburgh: Churchill-Livingstone, 1980:284.

293. Hannuksela M, Hassi J. Hairdressers' hand. *Derm Beruf Umwelt* 1980; 28:149–151.

294. Lindemayr H. Friseurekzem und Nickelallergie. *Hautarzt* 1984; 35:292–297.

295. Lynde CW, Mitchell JC. Patch test results in 66 hairdressers 1973–1981. *Contact Dermatitis* 1982; 8:302–307.

296. Marks R, Cronin E. Hand eczema in hairdressers. *Aust J Dermatol* 1977; 18:123–126.

297. Majoie IML, von Blomberg BME, Bruynzeel DP. Development of hand eczema in junior hairdressers: an 8-year follow-up study. *Contact Dermatitis* 1996; 34:243–247.

298. Calnan CD. Nickel dermatitis. *Br J Dermatol* 1956; 68:229–236.

299. Peltonen L. Nickel sensitivity in the general population. *Contact Dermatitis* 1979; 5:27–32.

300. Wagmann B. Beitrag zur Klinik des Nickelekzems. *Dermatologica* 1959; 119:197–210.

301. Singgih SI, Lantinga H, Nater JP, et al. Occupational hand dermatosis in hospital cleaning personnel. *Contact Dermatitis* 1986; 14:14–19.

302. Caron PA. Nickel sensitivity and atopy. *Br J Dermatol* 1964; 76:384–387.

303. Dobson RL. Discussion [of report by Vandenberg JJ, of Epstein WL: Experimental nickel contact sensitivity in man]. *J Invest Dermatol* 1963; 41:416.

304. Epstein S. Contact dermatitis due to nickel and chromium: observations on dermal delayed (tuberculin-type) sensitivity. *Arch Dermatol* 1956; 73:236–255.

305. Marcussen PV. Spread of nickel dermatitis. *Dermatologica* 1957; 115:596–607.

306. Wilkinson DS, Wilkinson JD. Nickel allergy and hand eczema. In: Maibach HI, Menne T, eds: *Nickel and the Skin: Immunology & Toxicology*. Boca Raton, Fla: CRC; 1989:133–164.

307. Nilsson EJ, Knusson A. Atopic dermatitis, nickel sensitivity and xerosis as risk factors for hand eczema in women. *Contact Dermatitis* 1995; 33:401–406.

308. Susitaival P, Hannuksela M. The 12 year prognosis of hand dermatosis in 896 Finnish farmers. *Contact Dermatitis* 1995; 32:233–237.

309. Block GT, Yeung M. Asthma induced by nickel. *JAMA* 1982; 247:1600–1602.

310. Fischer AA. Contact Dermatitis, 2nd ed. Philadelphia: Lea & Febiger, 1973.

311. Barranco VP, Solomon H. Eczematous dermatitis from nickel. *JAMA* 1972; 220:1244.

312. Polak L, Turk JL. Studies on the effect of systemic administration of sensitizers in guinea pigs with contact sensitization to inorganic metal compounds. II: The flare-up of previous test sites of contact sensitizations and the development of a generalized rash. *Clin Exp Immunol* 1968; 3:253–262.

313. Kaaber E, Sjolin KE, Menne T. Elbow eruptions in nickel and chromate dermatitis. *Contact Dermatitis* 1983; 9:213–216.

314. van Ketel WG, Liem DH. Eyelid dermatitis from nickel contaminated cosmetics. *Contact Dermatitis* 1981; 7:217.

315. Walthard B. Die Erzeugung experimentaller Nickelidiosynkrasie bei Laboratoriumstieren. *Schweiz Med Wochnschr* 1926; 16:603.

316. Christensen OB, Beckstead JG, Daniels TE, et al. Pathogenesis of orally induced flare-up reactions at old patch sites in nickel allergy. *Acta Derm Venereol (Stockh)* 1985; 65:298–304.

317. Burrows D. Is systemic nickel important? *J Am Acad Dermatol* 1992; 26:632–635.

318. Flint GN, Packirisamy S. Systemic nickel: the contribution made by stainless steel cooking utensils. *Contact Dermatitis* 1995; 32:218–224.

319. Christiansen KJ. Correlation between prosthesis failure and metal sensitivity as determined by new immunological techniques. *J Bone Joint Surg* 1979; 61B:240.

320. Elves MW, Wilson JN, Scales JT, et al. The incidence of metal sensitivity in patients with total joint replacements. *Br Med J* 1975; 4:376–378.

321. Carlsson AS, Moller H. Implantation of orthpaedic devices in patients with metal allergy. *Acta Derm Venereol (Stockh)* 1989; 69:62–66.

322. Burrows D, Creswell S, Merrett JD. Nickel hand and hip prostheses. *Br J Dermatol* 1981; 105:437–444.

323. Carlsson AS, Magnusson B, Moller H. Metal sensitivity in patients with metal to plastic total hip arthroplasties. *Acta Orthop Scand* 1980; 51:57–62.

324. Deutman R, Mulder TJ, Brian R, et al. Metal sensitivity before and after total hip arthroplasty. *J Bone Joint Surg* 1977; 59A:862–865.

325. Rooker GD, Wilkinson JD. Metal sensitivity in patients undergoing hip replacement: a prospective study. *J Bone Joint Surg* 1980; 62B:502–505.

326. Hindson M, Carlsson AS, Moller H. Orthopaedic metallic implants in extremity fractures and contact allergy. *J Eur Acad Derm Venereol* 1993; 2:22–26.

327. Dujardin F, Fevrier V, Lecorvaisier C, et al. Dermatoses d'intolerance aux implants metalliques en chirurgie orthopedique. *Rev Chir Ortho Reparatrice Appar Mot* 1995; 81:473–484.

328. Sulzberger MB. Dermatitis eczematous (contact-type) due to nickel. *Arch Dermatol* 1940; 41:815.

329. Schmiel G. Haufigkeit von Nickel-Kontaktallergien am unausgewahlten Patientgut im Raum Munchen. *Derm Beruf Umwelt* 1985; 33:92–95.

330. Mitchell JC. The angry back syndrome: "eczema creates eczema." *Contact Dermatitis* 1975; 1:193–194.

331. Kieffer M. Nickel sensitivity: relationship between history and patch test reaction. *Contact Dermatitis* 1979; 5:398–401.

332. Menne T. Nickel allergy: reliability of patch test evaluated in female twins. *Derm Beruf Umwelt* 1981; 29:156–160.

333. Lantinga H, Nater JP, Coenraads PJ. Prevalence, incidence and course of eczema on the hands and forearms in a sample of the general population. *Contact Dermatitis* 1984; 10:135–139.

334. Todd DJ, Burrows D, Stanford CF. Atopy in subjects with a history of nickel allergy but negative patch tests. *Contact Dermatitis* 1989; 21:129–133.

335. Mendelow AY, Forsyth A, Florence AT, et al. Patch testing for nickel allergy. The influence of the vehicle on the response rate to topical nickel sulfate. *Contact Dermatitis* 1985; 13:29–33.

336. Seidenari S, Manzini BM, Belletti B. Pretreatment of the test area with 1-day occlusion improves the response rate to NiSO$_4$ 5% pet patch tests in subjects with a positive history of nickel allergy. *Contact Dermatitis* 1995; 33:152–156.

337. Nilsson E. Individual and experimental risk factors for hand eczema in hospital workers. *Acta Derm Venereol* 1986; [Suppl 128].

338. Lammintausta K, Kalimo K. Do positive nickel reactions increase nonspecific patch test reactivity? *Contact Dermatitis* 1987; 16:160–163.

339. Feigel F. *Spot Test in Inorganic Analysis.* New York: Elsevier; 1958:150.

340. Fischer T, Fregert S, Gruvberger B, et al. Nickel release from ear piercing kits and earrings. *Contact Dermatitis* 1984; 10:39–41.

341. Gawkrodger DJ. Nickel dermatitis: how much nickel is safe? *Contact Dermatitis* 1996; 35:267–271.

342. Allenby CF, Basketter DA. An arm immersion model of compromised skin (II). Influence on minimal eliciting patch test concentrations of nickel. *Contact Dermatitis* 1993; 28:129–133.

343. Andersen KE, Liden C, Hansen J, et al. Dose response testing with nickel sulfate using TRUE test in nickel sensitive individuals. *Br J Dermatol* 1993; 192:50–59.

344. Menne T, Andersen KE, Kaaber K, et al. Tin: an overlooked sensitizer. *Contact Dermatitis* 1987; 16:9–10.

345. Fullerton A, Menne T. In vitro and in vivo evaluation of the effect of barrier gels in nickel contact allergy. *Contact Dermatitis* 1995; 32:100–106.

346. Gawkrodger DJ, Healy J, Howe AM. The prevention of nickel contact dermatitis. A review of the use of binding agents and barrier creams. *Contact Dermatitis* 1995; 32:257–265.

347. Munro-Ashman D, Munro DD, Highes TH. Contact dermatitis from palladium. *Trans St. John's Hosp Derm Soc* 1969; 55:196–197.

348. Sheard C. Contact dermatitis from platinum and related metals: report of a case. *Arch Dermatol* 1955; 71:357–360.

349. van Ketel WG, Niebber C. Allergy to palladium in dental alloys. *Contact Dermatitis* 1981; 7:331.

350. van Loon LA, van Elsas PW, van Joost T, et al. Contact stomatitis and dermatitis to nickel and palladium. *Contact Dermatitis* 1984; 11:294–297.

351. Koch P, Baum H-P. Contact stomatitis due to palladium and platinum in dental alloys. *Contact Dermatitis* 1996; 34:253–257.

352. Todd DJ, Burrows D. Patch testing with pure palladium metal in patients with sensitivity to palladium chloride. *Contact Dermatitis* 1992; 26:327–331.

353. Kranke B, Aberer W. Multiple sensitivities to metals. *Contact Dermatitis* 1996; 34:225.

354. Eedy DH, Burrows D, McMaster D. The nickel content of certain commercially available metallic patch test materials and its relevance in nickel-sensitive subjects. *Contact Dermatitis* 1991; 24:11–15.

355. McClelland J, Shuster S. Contact dermatitis with negative patch tests: the additive effect of allergens in combination. *Br J Dermatol* 1990; 122:623–630.

356. Aberer W, Holub H, Strohal R, et al. Palladium in dental alloys—the dermatologist's "responsibility to warn." *Contact Dermatitis* 1993; 28:163–165.

357. Wataha JC, Hanks CT. Biological effects of palladium and risk of using palladium in dental casting alloys. *J Oral Rehab* 1996; 23:309–320.

358. Hunter D, Milton R, Perry K. Asthma caused by the complex salts of platinum. *Br J Med* 1945; 2:92–98.

359. Sidi E, Hinkey M. Problems d'actualite concernment les dermatoses professionelles. *Rev Fr d'Allerg* 1965; 5:198–209.

360. Parrot JL, Saindelle HR. Platinum and platinosis. *Arch Environ Health* 1969; 19:686–691.

361. Levene GM. Platinum sensitivity. *Br J Dermatol* 1971; 85:590–593.

362. Cleare MJ, Hughes EG, Jacoby B, et al. Immediate (Type I) allergic responses to platinum compounds. *Clin Allerg* 1976; 6:183–195.

363. Lewis PG, Emmett EA. Irritant dermatitis from tributyl tin oxide and contact allergy from chlorocresol. *Contact Dermatitis* 1987; 17:129–132.

364. Revell PA, Lalor PA. Massive exposure to titanium, but without sensitization [Letter and comment]. *Acta Orthop Scand* 1995; 66:484.

365. Calnan CD. Metal fume fever. *Contact Dermatitis* 1979; 5:125.

366. Shelley WB, Hurley HJ. Allergic origin of zirconium deodorant granulomas. *Br J Dermatol* 1958; 70:75–101.

367. Epstein WL, Allen JR. Granulomatous hypersensitivity after use of zirconium-containing poison oak lotions. *JAMA* 1964; 190:940–942.

368. Palmer L, Walton W. Lupus miliaris disseminatus faciei: zirconium hypersensitivity as possible cause. *Cutis* 1967; 7:744–748.

Bibliography

Elgart ML, Higdon RS. Allergic contact dermatitis to gold. *Arch Dermatol* 1971; 103:649–653.

Legge TN. The lesions resulting from the manufacture and uses of potassium and sodium dichromate. In: Oliver T, ed. *Dangerous Trades,* London: J Murray; 1902.

Morgan LG, Flint GN. Nickel alloys and coatings: release of nickel. In: Maibach HI, Menne T, eds. *Nickel and the Skin: Immunology and Toxicology.* Boca Raton, Fla: CRC; 1989:51.

Wahlberg JE, Boman A. Sensitization and testing of guinea pigs with cobalt chloride. *Contact Dermatitis* 1978; 4:128–132.

Wall LM. Chromate dermatitis and sodium dithionite. *Contact Dermatitis* 1982; 8:291–293.

Plastic Materials

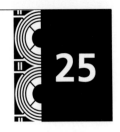

25

BERT BJÖRKNER, M.D., Ph.D.

One of the most important branches of the chemical industry is the polymer industry, which uses a wider variety of chemicals than any other. Everyone is using plastic materials in daily living, more than ever before. Plastics comes from oil, and 5% of all oil produced in the world is used by the polymer industry. Commercially important plastics today number more than 50. Application areas for plastics are many and varied: the construction industry, packaging, electronics, recreation, and medical, among others. Some 30% of all plastics are used for packaging and 20% in the construction industry.

There are several ways of classifying polymeric materials. Chemically, they are very large molecules (polymers) formed by the linking of small molecules (monomers) into large chainlike units. When only one type of monomer is involved in forming the polymer, it is called a *homopolymer*. When two or more different types are involved, it is called a *copolymer*.

The words *plastic* and *resin* are often used interchangeably; however, strictly speaking, plastics are synthetic macromolecular end products, whereas *resin* denotes all low–, medium–, and high–molecular weight intermediate synthetic substances from which plastics are made. Natural rubbers and cellulose do not fit into these definitions because their starting material is of natural origin and not synthetic.

When the monomers that form a final polymer product simply link up into long chains by joining bonds and nothing is eliminated in the process, the polymerization is called an *addition reaction*. When two or more different monomers react with each other, thereby eliminating a simple molecule such as water, the polymerization is called a *condensation reaction*.

Traditionally and practically, plastics can be divided into three major categories: thermoplastic, thermosetting, and elastomer. The thermoplastic resins are characterized by softening when exposed to heat, and when soft they can be made to flow and assume various shapes. When cooled, they become hard again. Thermoplastic resins have only long molecular chains, not connected with each other. When heated, the molecular chains becomes moveable and plastic material melts and starts floating and turns into liquid. Thus, thermoplastic resins have different characteristics at different temperatures.

The thermosetting resins have chemical bonds between the long molecular chains. When heated for the first time, they undergo further chemical reactions in which cross-links develop between polymer chains, holding them rigid in the desired position. They do not soften on reheating as the original polymer did. Examples of thermoplastic resins are polyethylene, polystyrene, polyvinyl chloride, and saturated polyesters. Examples of thermosetting resins are phenol formaldehyde resins, epoxy resins, polyurethanes, unsaturated polyesters, and acrylates. Synthetic rubbers are examples of elastomers.

The final plastic products, when completely cured or hardened, are generally considered to be inert and not hazardous to the skin. Skin problems from plastics are related almost exclusively to ingredients such as monomers, hardeners, and other additives, or to degradation products of low molecular weight.[1]

EPOXY RESIN SYSTEMS

Epoxy (or ethoxylin) resins contain at least two epoxy groups (also called *oxirane* or *epoxide* groups) in their molecules. The epoxy group is formed when two carbon atoms and one oxygen atom bind chemically. The term *epoxy resin* is commonly used to indicate the resins in both thermoplastic (uncured) and thermoset (cured) states.[2] Commercially, the most important epoxy resins are produced by polycondensation of compounds that process at least two reactive hydrogen atoms (polyhydroxy compounds) with epichlorohydrin.[2] About 75 to 90% of epoxy resins are diglycidyl ethers of the bisphenol A (DGEBA) type formed by combining epichlorohydrin and biphenol A (2,2-bis(4-hydroxyphenyl)propane).[1, 2] Epoxy resins of the DGEBA type were first synthesized in the late 1930s. When the proportions of epichlorohydrin and bisphenol A are varied during the manufacturing process, different amounts of low– and high–molecular weight resins are formed. The chemical structure of the final epoxy resin is shown in Figure 25–1.

The repeated part of the resin molecule has a molecular weight of 284. When $n = 0$, a monomeric DGEBA of molecular weight 340 is obtained. Low–molecular weight epoxy resin is semisolid or liquid and has an average molecular weight of less than 900 and contains a large amount of the oligomer of molecular weight 340. Resins with an average molecular weight of more than 900 are solids, but may contain more than 15% DGEBA of molecular weight 340. Commercial epoxy resins are thus mixtures of oligomers of different molecular weights: 340 ($n = 0$), 624 ($n = 1$), 908 ($n = 2$), 1192 ($n = 3$), etc. Also, other components, such as colorants, fillers, tar, ultraviolet (UV) light absorbers, flame retardants, solvents, reinforcement agents, and plasticizers can be added to the raw materials. Epoxy resins can also be blended with formaldehyde resins based on phenol, urea, and melamine.

Of the total world production of epoxy resins of more than 500,000 tons a year, about 45% is used in coatings and the remainder (55%) in structural applications. In the casting of models, epoxy resin is used as a glue for metal, rubber, plastics and ceramics, electrical insulation, floor covering (Fig. 25–2), anticorrosion protection of metals, mending of cracks in concrete, laminates and composites, and adhesives (Fig. 25–3). Most epoxy resins are used for paints and coatings (Fig. 25–4). High–molecular weight solid epoxy resins in various solvents and solventless low–molecular weight liquid epoxy resins are used for painting. Solid resins in powder paints are used for electrostatic hard coating of metal.

When great strength is required, fibers from carbon glass, nylon, and the like, impregnated with epoxy resin systems are increasingly used as composite materials. Difficulties are encountered, however, in getting carbon fibers to adhere to epoxy resins of the bisphenol A type. Non-DGEBA–type epoxy resins for the epoxy composites have thus been developed: tetraglycidyl-4,4'-methylenedianiline (TGMDA), triglycidyl derivative of p-aminophenol (TGPAP), and o-diglycidyl phthalate. Preimpregnated glass fibers ("pre-preg") are used as materials in the plastics and aircraft industries and in electronic circuit boards.[3–5] Diglycidyl ether of tetrabromobisphenol A (4Br-DGEBA) is often used as a flame retardant in these systems.

Instead of bisphenol A, other polyhydroxy compounds can be used in the epoxy resin system, (e.g., resorcinol, glycerol, ethylene glycol, and bisphenol F). The diglycidyl ether of bisphenol F (DGEBF) is the simplest of the phenol epoxy novolaks. Aliphatic non-DGEBA epoxy resins are constituents of paints. Epoxy acrylates, usually obtained by reacting epoxy resin with acrylic acid, are commonly used as prepolymers in ultraviolet-curable printing inks and coatings. Both aromatic and aliphatic epoxy acrylates are available, as are acrylated epoxydized oils.

Hardeners

The thermoplastic epoxy resins can be cross-linked using a variety of curing agents (hardeners) to form thermoset plastics with insoluble three-dimensional structures. When epoxy resins are used in two-component products, the hardeners are added to the resins immediately before the application, and the subsequent cross-linking occurs either at an ambient temperature or with

MW	n
340	0
624	1
908	2
1192	3

FIGURE 25–1 • Diglycidyl ether of bisphenol A (DGEBA) epoxy resin.

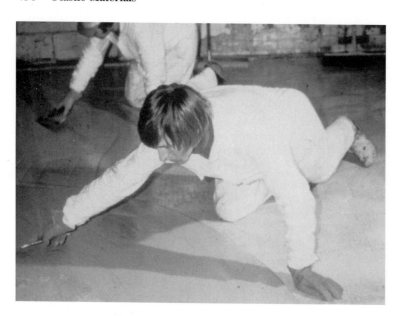

FIGURE 25–2 • Epoxy resins are important for their use as floor adhesives.

heating. One-component products contain latent curing agents that are inactive at normal storage temperatures but that initiate the cross-linking when heated. Examples of one-component epoxy products include powder paints and special adhesives.

There are many curing agents on the market. The hardeners used in cold curing are mostly

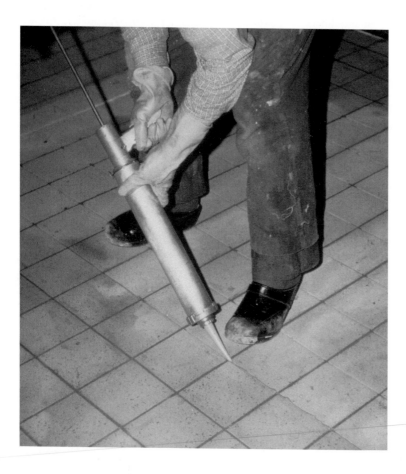

FIGURE 25–3 • Epoxy grout is used in laying floor tiles.

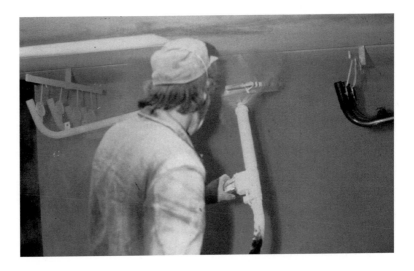

FIGURE 25–4 • When high–molecular epoxy resins are used in spray paint, the risk of sensitization is small.

polyamines, polyamides, or isocyanates, and those used for thermal curing are carboxylic acids and anhydrides or aldehyde condensation products (e.g., phenol-formaldehyde resins, melamine-formaldehyde resins, and urea-formaldehyde resins). The hardeners most commonly used for the DGEBA resin system are listed in Table 25–1.

Aliphatic and cycloaliphatic amines are low-viscosity liquids that react readily with epoxy resins at ambient temperatures; less reactive aromatic amines require heat for curing.[2] Common hardeners for composite epoxy resins are diaminodiphenylsulphone (DDS), methylenedianiline, boron-trifluorine-monoethylamine complex, and dicyandiamide.[4] Accelerators such as tertiary amines can be added to speed up polymerization of epoxy resins.

Epoxy Reactive Diluents

Reactive diluents are used to modify epoxy resins, principally by reducing their viscosity. Reactive diluents containing one or more epoxide groups react with the hardener at approximately the same rate as the resin. Most of the reactive diluents on the market are used in the cold curing process. They are blended in commercial epoxy resin at concentrations of 10% to 30%.[6, 7] The epoxy reactive diluents are generally glycidyl ethers, sometimes glycidyl esters of aliphatic or aromatic structure. Aliphatic diluents include such compounds as *n*-butyl glycidyl ether (BGE), allyl glycidyl ether, and other alkyl glycidyl ethers with longer (8 to 14) carbon chains (e.g., Epoxide 7 and Epoxide 8).[1] Examples of aromatic reactive diluents are phenyl glycidyl ether (PGE) and cresyl glycidyl ether (CGE).

Skin Hazards from Epoxy Resin Systems

Epoxy resin compounds are some of the most frequent causes of occupational allergic contact dermatitis in some countries.[7, 8] Most cases have been allergic contact dermatitis induced by DGEBA-type epoxy resins. Alkaline hardeners were blamed for most cases of dermatitis and sensitization observed during the handling of components of the epoxy system in the 1950s, but later the resin was identified as the main cause.[9, 10] Gaul[11, 12] suspected that bisphenol A was the sensitizing structure in the resin, whereas Calnan[13] believed that the epoxy group of epichlorhydrin was more likely responsible for contact allergy. Thorgeirsson and Fregert[14] finally confirmed that the main sensitizer was DGEBA-based epoxy resin oligomer with a molecular weight of 340. The guinea pig maximization test oligomer with a molecular weight of 624 was also a sensitizer, but a weaker one than the molecular weight 340 oligomer. The sensitizing capacity of epoxy resin decreases as the average molecular weight increases.[14–16] In many cases, allergic epoxy dermatitis develops after accidental contact with epoxy resin, and frequent agents of epoxy dermatitis are paints and the raw materials for paints.[8] However, it is not unusual to find a positive patchtest reaction to epoxy resin in which the cause of the sensitization is unknown. Dermatitis caused by the epoxy resin system is localized mostly to the hands and forearms, but sometimes the face is also involved. If the face and eyelids are involved, dermatitis may be caused by airborne sensitization to hardeners or to reactive diluents. These compounds are very volatile as compared with epoxy resin.[17] High–molecular weight epoxy resin in sol-

TABLE 25–1 • Most Common Hardeners in Diglycidyl Ethers of Bisphenol A–Type Resin Systems

Aliphatic Polyamines
  Ethylenediamine (EDA)
  Diethylenetriamine (DETA)
  Triethylenetetramine (TETA)
  Dipropylenetriamine (DPTA)
  Tetraethylenepentamine (TEPA)
  Diethylaminopropylamine (DEAPA)
  Trimethylhexamethylenediamine (TMDA)

Aromatic Amines
  N,N-dimethylbenzylamine
  p,p'-Diaminodiphenylmethane (DDM) = bis(4-aminophenyl)methane (MDA)
  m-Phenylenediamine (MPDA)
  p,p'-Diaminodiphenylsulphone (DDS) = bis(4-aminophenylsulfone)
  2,4,6-tris(N,N-dimethylaminomethyl)phenol

Adducts
  Based on the reaction between aliphatic or aromatic amines and epoxy resin, epoxy-reactive diluents, ethylene oxide, etc.

Acid Anhydrides
  Phthalic anhydride (PA)
  Maleic anhydride (MA)
  Methylbicyclo(2,2,1)heptene-2,3-dicarboxylic anhydride
  1,2-Cyclohexanedicarboxylic anhydride

Polymercaptanes

Cycloaliphatic Polyamines
  Isophorone diamine (IPD)
  N-aminoethylpiperazine
  3,3'-Dimethyl-4,4-diaminodicyclohexylmethane
  Cyclohexane-1,2-diamine
  Menthanediamine = (4-(2-aminopropane-2-yl)-1-methylcyclohexane-1-amine)

Polyaminoamides
  Based on polyamines (e.g., TEPA, TETA)

Amidopolyamines
  Based on amines (e.g., DETA and difunctional acids)

Dicyandiamide (DICY)
Isocyanates
  Di- and polyisocyanates

Polyphenols
Other Hardeners
  Phenolic novolaks
  Cresol novolaks
  Thiols

---

vents for painting and epoxy resin powder for electrostatic coating of metals rarely cause sensitization because of the small proportion of molecular weight 340 oligomer.

Even when an epoxy resin is believed to be cured, as much as 25% of it can remain unhardened, particularly when it is cured at room temperature.[3] When DGEBA epoxy resins are cured by polyamine-bearing hardeners at room temperature, the amounts of unreacted DGEBA or polyamine decrease rapidly within 1 or 2 days, but thereafter the decrease is slow. Nevertheless, after 1 week's cure, amounts of 0.02% to 12% free DGEBA and 0.01% to 1% free diethylenetriamine (DETA) were observed in six different epoxy resin products experimentally cured with DETA.[7] Contact dermatitis may thus be elicited in previously sensitized persons. Traces of unhardened epoxy resin have been found in twist-off caps, film cassettes, furniture, metal pieces, signboards, textile labels, stoma pouches, polyvinylchloride (PVC) plastic, nasal cannulas, hemodialysis sets, cardiac pace-

makers, Fiberglas, brass doorknobs, and tool handles, among other products.[18] Methods for detecting epoxy resins of the bisphenol A type have been described by Fregert and Trulsson.[18, 19]

Non-DGEBA epoxy resins, polyamine hardeners, and reactive diluents are also potential causes of allergic contact dermatitis. Thus, resins based on bisphenol F are also sensitizers. They probably cross-react with resins based on bisphenol A.

The composite epoxy resins based on o-diglycidylphthalate, tetraglycidyl-4,4'-methylenedianiline (TGMDA), and diglycidyl ether of tetrabromobisphenol A (4Br-DGEBA) are considered strong sensitizers of humans.[5, 16] Contact allergy to the composite epoxy resin is not revealed by testing with DGEBA epoxy resin. DGEBA, TGMDA, and o-diglycidylphthalate do not cross-react.[5, 20]

The hardeners have usually been found to be responsible for fewer than 10% of allergic contact dermatitis cases related to epoxy compounds.[21] The most potent sensitizers among the hardeners are the aliphatic polyamines (see Table 25–1).[3, 21, 22] The cycloaliphatic polyamines (e.g., isophoronediamine, *N*-aminoethylpiperazine) are also strong sensitizers.[21, 23–27] Hardeners of the polyaminoamide type are not sensitizers; however, polyaminoamides may contain aliphatic amines. The adducts are nonsensitizing, provided they do not contain free amine. The aliphatic polyamines are also strong skin irritants.[26, 28]

Reports of contact allergy to bisphenol A are controversial. In a few studies a high incidence of bisphenol A allergy was found among those sensitized to epoxy resin,[12 29] but these results have not been confirmed by other investigators.[30–32] A rather high risk of sensitization to epichlorohydrine has been reported for workers in epoxy resin manufacturing.[31–33] Contact urticaria caused by the epoxy resin hardeners methylhexahydrophthalic anhydride and methyltetrahydrophthalic anhydride has been reported as well as by aliphatic polyamine hardeners.[8, 34, 35]

Photosensitivity has been reported in relation to the heating of DGEBA epoxy resin[36] and the use of epoxy powder paints.[37] Allen and Kaidbey[36] considered the photosensitivity to be probably due to bisphenol A in the resin. They observed persistent light reactivity among the patients. Similar persistent light reactivity has been found in mice photosensitized by bisphenol A.[38]

Patchtesting with Epoxy Resin Systems

Approximately 90% of contact allergy caused by epoxy resin systems is due to epoxy resin of the bisphenol A type (DGEBA). A patchtest with the low–molecular weight epoxy resin containing a large proportion of oligomer molecular weight 340 is adequate in most cases. It is recommended to patchtest with epoxy resin, 1% in petrolatum, and this allergen is included in most standard series. Patients should also be tested with their "own" resins in corresponding concentrations. There are too many hardeners and reactive diluents on the market for all to be used in routine testing; however, if sensitivity to the hardeners or reactive diluents is suspected, it is necessary to get samples from the manufacturer and information on the ingredients and to test them separately. The recommended test concentrations for hardeners and reactive diluents is 0.1% to 1% in petrolatum, acetone, or ethanol.

Precautions for Handling Epoxy Resin Systems

Workers who handle epoxy compounds should be informed of the risk of skin sensitization. Concur-

rent use of irritant chemicals (e.g., organic solvents, amine hardeners) increases the risk of sensitization. The highly alkaline amine hardeners can be replaced by polyaminoamides or amine-epoxy adducts; this reduces the irritability of the epoxy resin system. Management as well as workers who come in contact with the epoxy resin system should be advised to avoid skin contact. Proper personal protective measures, especially careful hand protection and regular cleaning and maintenance of all contaminated equipment, are imperative. Epoxy resins penetrate plastic and rubber gloves (Fig. 25–5). Only heavy-duty vinyl gloves provide sufficient protection.[39] Multilayered glove material of folio type ("4H gloves") has nevertheless been shown to give even better protection against epoxy resins and the compounds typically used with them.[40] Also, barrier creams have been reported to protect against epoxy resins for minutes to some hours.[41–43] To reduce the allergenic properties of epoxy compounds it is best to use the molecular weight 340 oligomer in the lowest possible concentration and to use high–molecular weight reactive diluents. However, high–molecular weight epoxy resins should also be regarded as potential sensitizers, and they should be marked with labels specifying the amount of molecular weight 340 oligomer. In some countries workers are required to be educated before they may work with epoxy resin systems.

ACRYLIC RESINS

Acrylic resins are thermoplastic type of resins, formed by the derivatives of acrylic acid (CH_2=CH–COOH). The acrylic group itself is a vinyl group (CH_2=CH–). The monomers in acrylic resins are acrylic acids and methacrylic acids and their esters, cyanoacrylic acid and its esters, acrylamides, and acrylonitrile. Many different acrylic monomers thus exist, and as a result a multitude of different polymers and resins are produced.

The polymerization of acrylic monomers is an addition-type reaction and is obtained either at room temperature or by heating. The process is usually accelerated by adding initiators, accelerators, and catalysts. Polymerization or curing can also be achieved by ultraviolet light, visible light, or electron beams, for none of which are initiators necessary.[1]

Monoacrylates and Monomethacrylates

Mono(meth)acrylates (monoacrylates and monomethacrylates) are used in the production of a

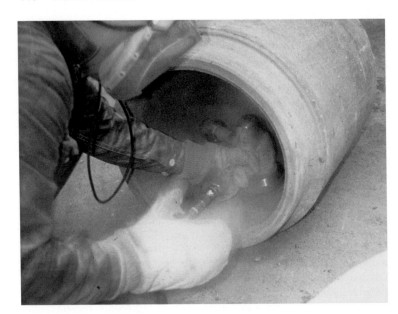

FIGURE 25–5 • This worker developed dermatitis from spraying epoxy to seal cracks in this pipe.

great variety of polymers. Polymethyl methacrylate is the most important plastic in the group of the acrylics with the following repeating unit: $\{CH_2-CH(CH_3)COOCH_3\}_n$. This plastic has excellent transparency and is thus used in products such as skylights, housewares, watch "crystals," bags, lamp housings, and windshields. A two-component system is used in the manufacture of dentures (Fig. 25–6), hearing aids, noise protectors, and bone cement for orthopedic implants. The first component is a prepolymer powder of polymethyl methacrylate with benzoyl peroxide as initiator. The second component is a monomeric liquid of methyl methacrylate containing an accelerator such as N, N-dimethyl-p-toluidine.

Other polymers of the mono(meth)acrylate type are used mostly in industry. Leather finishes, adhesives, paints, printing inks, and coatings are example of practical applications. Butyl acrylate is sometimes used in spectacle frames. 2-Ethylhexyl acrylate is often used in the manufacturer of pressure-sensitive adhesives, but a wide range of other acrylates also have this application.

The acrylic monomers preferred for preparation of UV-curable inks and coatings or in the photoprepolymer printing plate procedure are 2-hydroxyethyl acrylate (2-HEA), 2-hydroxypropyl acrylate (2-HPA), 2-hydroxypropyl methacrylate (2-HPMA), 2-hydroxyethyl methacrylate (2-HEMA; Fig. 25–7), and 2-ethylhexyl acrylate (2-EHA) (Fig. 25–8). 2-HPMA is also used in light-sensitive compositions for dental fissure seal-

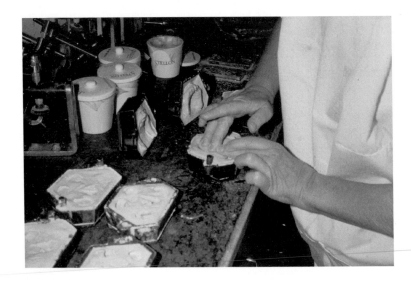

FIGURE 25–6 • In dentistry, methyl methacrylate is commonly used for construction of dental plates, a context in which there can be considerable skin contact.

FIGURE 25–7 • A common bonding material in dentistry is hydroxyethyl methacrylate, a potential skin sensitizer.

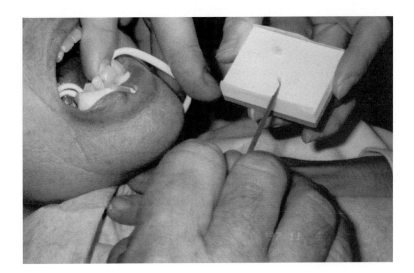

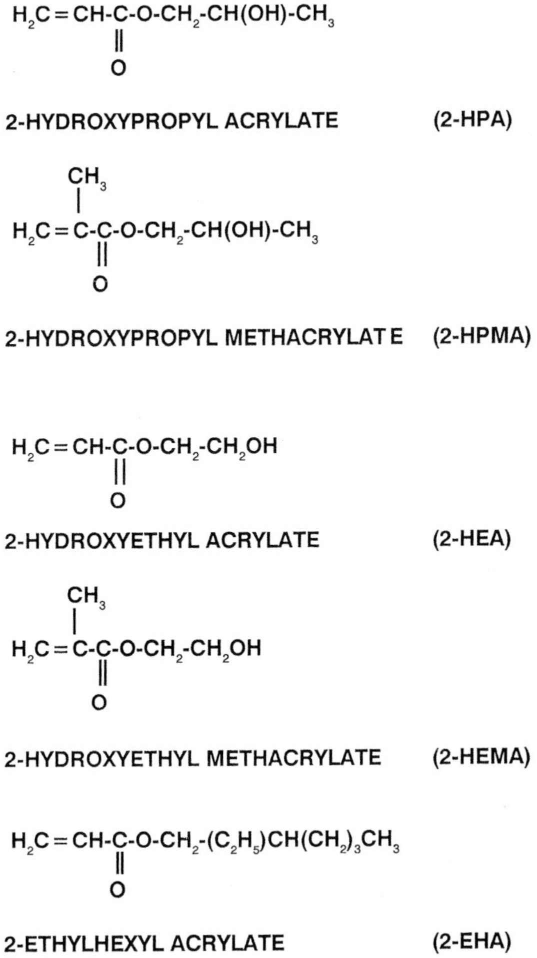

$$H_2C = CH\text{-}C\text{-}O\text{-}CH_2\text{-}CH(OH)\text{-}CH_3$$
$$\overset{\parallel}{O}$$

2-HYDROXYPROPYL ACRYLATE   **(2-HPA)**

$$\overset{\overset{\displaystyle CH_3}{|}}{H_2C = C\text{-}C\text{-}O\text{-}CH_2\text{-}CH(OH)\text{-}CH_3}$$
$$\overset{\parallel}{O}$$

2-HYDROXYPROPYL METHACRYLAT E   **(2-HPMA)**

$$H_2C = CH\text{-}C\text{-}O\text{-}CH_2\text{-}CH_2OH$$
$$\overset{\parallel}{O}$$

2-HYDROXYETHYL ACRYLATE   **(2-HEA)**

$$\overset{\overset{\displaystyle CH_3}{|}}{H_2C = C\text{-}C\text{-}O\text{-}CH_2\text{-}CH_2OH}$$
$$\overset{\parallel}{O}$$

2-HYDROXYETHYL METHACRYLATE   **(2-HEMA)**

$$H_2C = CH\text{-}C\text{-}O\text{-}CH_2\text{-}(C_2H_5)CH(CH_2)_3CH_3$$
$$\overset{\parallel}{O}$$

2-ETHYLHEXYL ACRYLATE   **(2-EHA)**

FIGURE 25–8 • Chemical formulas of some monofunctional acrylate compounds in UV-curable acrylate-based paints and lacquers.

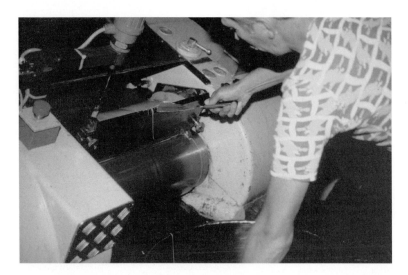

FIGURE 25–9 • Printing inks use UV-curable acrylates in the photoprepolymer printing plate procedure.

ants, adhesives, or bonding preparations and in Napp printing plates (Fig. 25–9). Various mono-(meth)acrylates can be used in water-based acrylic (latex) paints. Plastic dispersions of acrylic polymers are used as binders or thickeners in paints and in cosmetic creams. The monomer content is usually less than 0.3%.[1]

Multifunctional Acrylates

Acrylates with at least two reactive acrylic groups are called *multifunctional acrylates*. Examples are di(meth)acrylate esters of dialcohols or triacrylate and tetraacrylate esters of polyalcohols. Multifunctional acrylates are used in formulations for UV-curable inks (Fig. 25–10) and coatings, where they act as cross-linking agents and reactive diluents and on UV exposure become a part of the

final coating. The multifunctional acrylates are also important acrylic compounds in photopolymers, flexographic printing plates, and photoresists (an etch resist for printed circuit boards). The multifunctional acrylate esters are useful in acrylic glues, adhesives, and anaerobic sealants, as well as in artificial fingernail preparations (Fig. 25–11). Some of the more common multifunctional acrylates used for artificial nail preparations are ethylene glycol dimethacrylate (EGDMA), diethylene glycol dimethacrylate (DEGDMA), and trimethylol propane trimethacrylate (TMPTMA). The various acrylates used in acrylic nail preparations are listed in Table 25–2.[44–48]

Most of the dental composite resin materials and denture base polymers are "diluted" with the less viscous "difunctional" acrylates. These are the methacrylic monomers of which EGDMA,

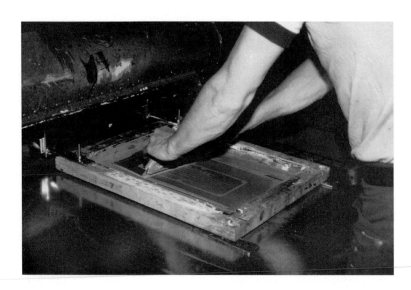

FIGURE 25–10 • In silk screening, UV-cured acrylates are commonly used. Here the worker is at risk because of failure to wear gloves.

FIGURE 25–11 • Artificial fingernails use a multifunctional acrylate which may induce allergic sensitization in customers.

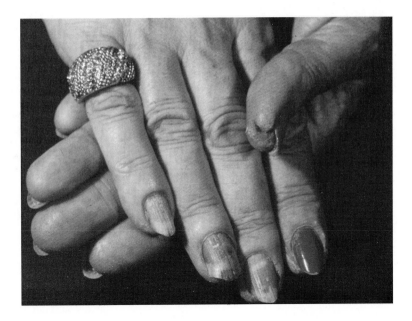

DEGDMA, triethylene glycol dimethacrylate (TREGDMA) (Fig. 25–12), and 1,4-butanediol dimethacrylate (BUDMA; Fig. 25–13) are the ones most widely used (Table 25–3). Acrylates used in dentistry are an expanding field. Some are "new" to dermatologists, but some are well-known sensitizers.[1, 49, 50] 1,6-Hexanediol diacrylate (HDDA), also used as a dental acrylate, is a known sensitizer in printing inks and coatings.

The simplest UV-curable ink or coating formulations consist of only three components. In practice, however, typical industrial formulations contain many more ingredients. The three *essential* components are a UV-reactive prepolymer that provides most of the desired properties, a diluent system composed of multifunctional acrylate es-ters (and at times monofunctional acrylic esters), and a photoinitiator system. The most commonly used multifunctional acrylate in a UV-curable ink or coating formulation is an acrylic acid ester of pentaerythritol (PETA), TMPTMA, or HDDA (Fig. 25–14).

During the past 15 to 20 years, the use of UV-

TABLE 25–2 • Acrylates Used in Acrylic Nail Preparations

Methyl methacrylate
Ethyl methacrylate
Ethyl acrylate
2-Hydroxyethyl acrylate
Butyl methacrylate
Isobutyl methacrylate
Methacrylic acid
Tetrahydrofurfuryl methacrylate
Ethyleneglycol dimethacrylate
Diethyleneglycol dimethacrylate
Triethyleneglycol dimethacrylate
Trimethylolpropane trimethacrylate
Urethane methacrylate
Tripropyleneglycol acrylate

TABLE 25–3 • Acrylic Compounds Used in Dental Materials

Methyl methacrylate
Triethyleneglycol dimethacrylate
Urethane dimethacrylate
Ethyleneglycol dimethacrylate
Bis-GMA
Bis-MA
Bis-EMA
Bis-PMA
2-(Dimethylamino)ethyl methacrylate
Butyl methacrylate
2-Hydroxyethyl methacrylate
1,6-Hexanediol diacrylatae
1,10-Decanediol dimethacrylate
1,4-Butanediol dimethacrylate
1,12-Dodecanediol dimethacrylate
Trimethylolpropane trimethacrylate
Phenylsalicylate glycidylmethacrylate
Tetrahydrofurfuryl methacrylate
Benzaldehyde glycol methacrylate
N-tolylglycine-glycidylmethacrylate
1,3-Butyleneglycol diacrylate
3,6-Dioxaoctamethylene dimethacrylate
Biphenyl dimethacrylate
Glycerolphosphate dimethacrylate

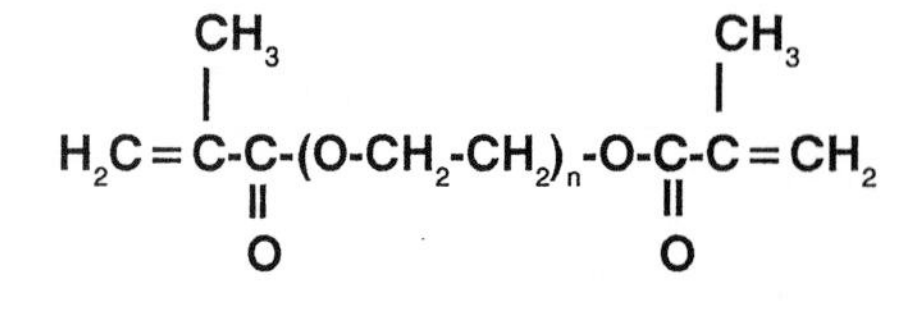

$$H_2C = \overset{\displaystyle CH_3}{\underset{\displaystyle \underset{\displaystyle O}{\|}}{C}} - C - (O-CH_2-CH_2)_n-O-\overset{\displaystyle CH_3}{\underset{\displaystyle \underset{\displaystyle O}{\|}}{C}} - C = CH_2$$

FIGURE 25–12 • Chemical formulas of *n*-ethyleneglycol dimethacrylates.

n = 1:   ETHYLENEGLYCOL DIMETHACRYLATE   (EGDMA)
n = 2:   DIETHYLENEGLYCOL DIMETHACRYLATE   (DEGDMA)
n = 3:   TRIETHYLENEGLYCOL DIMETHACRYLATE   (TREGDMA)

curable acrylates in inks and coatings has increased tremendously. In the can-coating industry, UV printing inks are used on beverage and beer cans as well as on crown caps and aerosol containers. UV-curable acrylate coatings are used as wood finishes, mat varnishes, parquet varnishes and sealers, and as varnishes and coatings in the manufacture of furniture.[1]

TMPTA and PETA can both be used in the production of polyfunctional aziridine added to paint primer and floor top coatings as self-curing cross-linker or hardener.[51–53] In the absence of oxygen and in the presence of metals, anaerobic acrylic sealants (e.g., Loctite, Treebond, and Sta-Lok) polymerize rapidly. Dimethacrylates are their principal components.[50, 54–56] Diethylene glycol dimethacrylate oligomer is most often used for screw-thread locking, whereas urethane dimethacrylate is used for retaining and locking flat metal surfaces.[1]

Prepolymers

Acrylate resins, based on the conventional thermoplastic resins, into which two or more reactive acrylate or methacrylate groups have been introduced, are called prepolymers. The most commonly used prepolymers are acrylated epoxy resins, acrylated polyurethanes, acrylated polyesters, and acrylated polyethers.

Epoxy Acrylates

Epoxy acrylates is another name for the beta-hydroxyester acrylates, because they are usually obtained by reacting epoxy resins or glycidyl derivatives with acrylic acid (Fig. 25–15). Both aromatic and aliphatic epoxy acrylates are available, as are acrylated epoxydized oils. Epoxy acrylates have found a wide range of useful applications in UV and electron beam curing.

The addition-reaction product between bisphenol A and glycidyl methacrylate or an epoxy resin and methacrylic acid is bis-GMA; 2,2-bis{4-(2-hydroxy-3-methacryloxypropoxy)phenyl}propane (see Fig. 25–15). Bis-GMA can thus be classified as a dimethacrylated epoxy, although it does not contain a reactive epoxy group. Bis-GMA is the prepolymer most commonly used in dental composite restoration materials. Several similar compounds have also appeared as substitutes for bis-GMA or in addition to bis-GMA in dental resins. Such dimethacrylates based on bisphenol A with various chain lengths are bis-MA; 2,2-bis(4-(methacryloxy)phenyl)-propane, bis-EMA; 2,2-bis(4-(2-methacryloxyethoxy)phenyl)-propane, and bis-PMA; 2,2-bis(4-(3-methacryloxypropoxy)phenyl)-propane (see Fig. 25–15).

The industrial applications of bis-GMA resins and the other similar derivatives are many. Acrylates based on bisphenol A or epoxy resin can be polymerized not only by exposure to electron

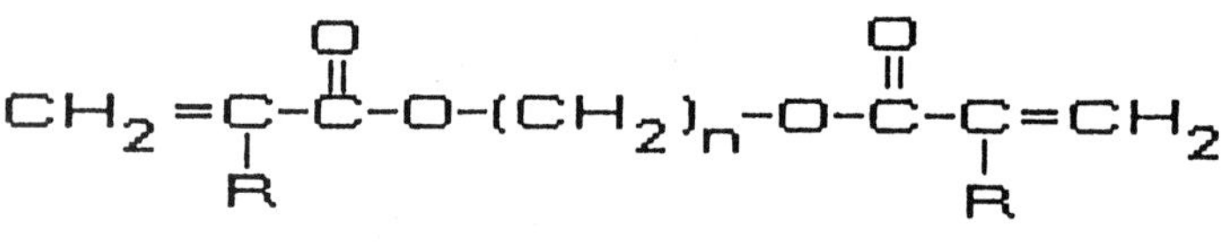

$$CH_2 = \overset{\displaystyle \underset{\displaystyle R}{|}}{C} - \overset{\displaystyle \overset{\displaystyle O}{\|}}{C} - O-(CH_2)_n-O-\overset{\displaystyle \overset{\displaystyle O}{\|}}{C} - \overset{\displaystyle \underset{\displaystyle R}{|}}{C} = CH_2$$

R = H & n = 6:   **1,6-Hexanediol diacrylate**   **(HDDA)**

R = CH$_3$ & n = 4:   **1,4-Butanediol dimethacrylate**   **(BUDMA)**

FIGURE 25–13 • Chemical formulas of 1,6-hexanediol diacrylate and 1,4-butanediol dimethacrylate.

FIGURE 25–14 • Chemical formulas of two common UV-curable multifunctional acrylates.

$$(H_2C = CH\text{-}C\text{-}O\text{-}CH_2)_3\text{-}C\text{-}CH_2\text{-}R$$
$$\overset{\|}{O}$$

R = OH: PENTAERYTHRITOL TRIACRYLATE   (PETA)

R = CH$_3$:   TRIMETHYLOLPROPANE TRIACRYLATE (TMPTA)

beams, UV light, or even visible light, but also can be chemically activated by various peroxides.

Urethane Acrylates

Many types of acrylated urethanes are on the market. While some are based on aromatic isocyanates, others are of the aliphatic types. Acrylated urethanes are used not only in prepolymers in UV-curable inks or coatings, as for instance vinyl floorings, but also as resins with dental applications. The acrylated urethanes used in dentistry are the methacrylate types.

Polyester Acrylates

There are various types of polyester acrylates on the market, and they are used mostly in UV-curable lacquers and printing inks for wood and paper coatings.[1]

Effects of Acrylate Esters on the Skin

The skin-irritating potential of various acrylic monomers has shown that the diacrylates are strong irritants to guinea pig skin, monoacrylates weak to moderate irritants, and monomethacrylates and

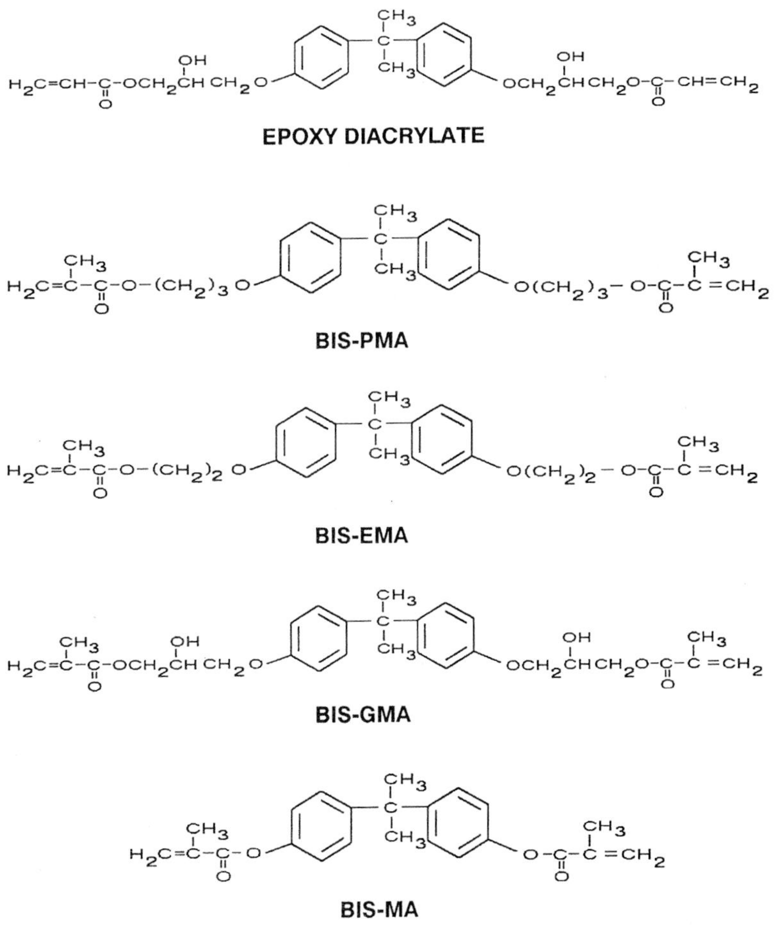

EPOXY DIACRYLATE

BIS-PMA

BIS-EMA

BIS-GMA

FIGURE 25–15 • Chemical formulas of di(meth)acrylates based on bisphenol A and epoxy resin.

BIS-MA

dimethacrylates weak irritants or innocuous.[57–65] Multifunctional acrylates as well as acrylated pre-polymers seem to be more skin irritating than the corresponding methacrylates. These effects have been seen when patchtesting both humans and guinea pigs.[65] Bullous irritant skin reactions have been reported in workers exposed to tetramethyl-ene glycol diacrylate.[66] A peculiar delayed irrita-tion from butanediol diacrylate and hexanediol diacrylate has been observed by Malten and asso-ciates.[67] Tetraethylene glycol diacrylate can cause delayed cutaneous irritant reactions as well as allergic contact dermatitis.[68] The irritant effect of various acrylate compounds has been reviewed by Kanerva and coworkers.[28, 29]

The sensitizing potential of many mono(meth)-acrylates, multifunctional (meth)acrylates, and ac-rylated resins has been thoroughly studied in guinea pigs by many authors.[57–65] Tests have shown that monoacrylates are strong sensitizers whereas mono(meth)acrylates have little to moder-ate sensitizing potential.[57, 59, 61, 65] Thus, the intro-duction of a methyl group reduces the sensitizing potential of monoacrylates. Of the multifunctional acrylates, the di- and triacrylic compounds should be regarded as potent sensitizers.[60, 62, 65] The meth-acrylated multifunctional acrylic compounds are weak sensitizers.[62, 65]

Among the various di(meth)acrylates based on bisphenol A or epoxy resin, the allergenicity seems to diminish when the acrylates have three or more methylene groups in the molecular chain.[60–65] It is more difficult to predict the sensi-tizing capacity of the various prepolymers. Epoxy acrylates are strong sensitizers and their sensitiz-ing capacity is due to the entire molecule. This excludes the possibility that the epoxide group is the sole sensitizing part of the compounds.[65] Free epoxy resin may be present in epoxy acrylates, which may sensitize separately or simultane-ously.[62]

The whole molecular structure of polyester ac-rylate probably acts as an allergen as well; how-ever, the reactive terminal acrylate and methacry-late groups seem to be very important for antigen formation and sensitization.[63] The carboxy ethyl side group seems to be important for antigenic-ity.[45]

The aliphatic urethane acrylates are more potent sensitizers than the aromatic ones, whereas the aliphatic urethane methacrylate commonly used in dental resins is a weak sensitizer.[64, 70]

There are many reports on contact allergy to mono(meth)acrylates in humans. Contact derma-titis due to 2-HPMA in printers exposed to print-ing plates and to UV-curing inks has been re-ported.[71, 72] Contact allergy to 2-HEMA, one of

the ingredients in a photo prepolymer mixture, has been described.[73] 2-HEMA is a water-soluble form of methacrylate resin and thus is commonly used as a dentine-bonding compound. The bonding sys-tems used contain a primer and an adhesive. The dentine is first treated by the primer, followed by the adhesive. This is polymerized with a visible light curing unit, and then a dental composite resin is applied to the tooth and cured chemically or with light. 2-HEMA is a common allergen for dental personnel. Fingertip dermatitis is common in dentists and dental assistants allergic to dentine-bonding acrylates.[49, 74–77]

Contact dermatitis from 2-EHA in an acrylic-based adhesive tape has been reported.[78] Orthope-dic surgeons, surgical technicians, nurses, and dental technicians are exposed to methyl methac-rylate monomer when preparing bone cement and dentures. Contact allergy to methyl methacrylate monomer is rare in patients undergoing hip sur-gery.[79]

In the last decades, many reports about contact allergy caused by various multifunctional acrylic compounds have been published.[1, 49, 50] At risk of developing contact allergy to multifunctional tri- and diacrylates are those who work with UV-curable inks or coatings, whereas contact allergy to dimethacrylates is more common in dentistry, in workers with anaerobic acrylic sealants, and in those exposed to acrylic fingernails.[49, 50, 65, 74–77] There are some reports of allergic contact derma-titis to dimethacrylates based on bisphenol A or epoxy resin in dental composite materials. At risk for developing contact dermatitis are dentists, den-tal technicians, and dental patients.[49, 50, 74–77] Pa-tients allergic to bis-GMA may also react to epoxy resin MW 340.[62, 80] It is not clear whether any residual epoxy resin monomer is left unreacted or whether it is formed in the synthesis of the bis-GMA monomer.[62] Methyl methacrylate and 2-HEMA can cause paresthesia of the fingertips for months after discontinuation of contact with the monomer.[81–83] Effects on the peripheral nervous system have also been described for acrylamide.[84]

Acrylonitrile

Acrylonitrile ($H_2C=CH-CN$) is used as a copoly-mer in approximately 25% of all synthetic fibers. It is also used for synthetic rubbers and for the production of acrylonitrile-butadiene-styrene plas-tics and styrene-acrylonitrile plastics. These ter- and copolymers are used in the automobile indus-try and in the production of housewares, electrical appliances, suitcases, food packaging, and dispos-able dishes. Acrylonitrile can also be a constituent of fabrics and paints.[1]

Skin Problems from Acrylonitrile

There are only a few reports of contact allergy to the acrylonitrile monomer.[85–88] In the guinea pig maximization test, however, acrylonitrile has shown strong allergenic potential.[88]

Acrylamide and Derivatives

Acrylamide ($H_2C=CH-CO-NH_2$) is an odorless, white, crystalline solid used as a monomer or as a raw material in the production of polyacrylamides and other compounds. Most of the acrylamide monomer is produced and used as an aqueous solution. The reactive acrylamide monomer is used in the production of other compounds, mostly polymers of acrylamide, and as a grouting agent in the construction or rehabilitation of dams, buildings, sewers, tunnels, and other structures. Acrylamide grouts are used predominantly as barriers against groundwater seepage into sewers. About 95% of the acrylamide produced is consumed in the production of other compounds and polyacrylamide products that are widely used as flocculents in potable water and wastewater treatment, mineral ore processing, sugar refining, water flow control agents in oil well operations, and adhesives in paper making and construction. The remaining 5% is used as a monomer. Acrylamide and its derivatives are also used in the production of photopolymer printing plates. Because acrylamide is produced by catalytic or sulfuric acid hydration of acrylonitrile, acrylamide production workers can also be exposed to acrylonitrile.

Health Effects

Polyacrylamide products are generally considered not hazardous. The monomer can be irritating and can cause contact allergy. Skin problems are seen among printers exposed to photopolymerizing printing plates. Acrylamide and their acrylamide compounds N,N'-methylene-bis-acrylamide and N-methylol acrylamide have been described as allergens.[89–94] N-methylol acrylamide sensitization has also been observed in workers making PVA-acrylic copolymers for paints. Acrylamide, N-hydroxymethyl acrylamide, and N,N'-methylene-bis-acrylamide are moderate sensitizers when tested in guinea pigs.[58]

Acrylamide monomer may be neurotoxic, carcinogenic, genotoxic, and hazardous to reproduction. Recent studies confirm that acrylamide exposure causes cancer and reproductive effects in animals, but epidemiological studies have not demonstrated these effects in humans. The neurotoxic effects from acrylamide exposure include peripheral nerve damage and central nervous system effects.[84, 92–94] Allergic contact dermatitis from

piperazine diacrylamide used as a reagent and as cross-linker for acrylamide gels in electrophoresis and column chromatography has been described by Wang and colleagues.[95]

Cyanoacrylates

Cyanoacrylates ($H_2C=C(CN)-COOR$) are also called *super glues*. The structure of the side chain (R) defines the different alkyl 2-cyanoacrylates and varies with the alcohol that has been used; for instance, methanol gives methyl 2-cyanoacrylate, ethanol gives ethyl 2-cyanoacrylate. Methyl 2-cyanoacrylate is mainly instant glue for household use. Ethyl 2-cyanoacrylate is the one used most commonly in industry, and most of the different adhesive products on the market are manufactured by Loctite. Commonly used as medical adhesives are n-butyl 2-cyanoacrylate and isobutyl 2-cyanoacrylate.

Glues based of cyanoacrylates are widely used as contact adhesives for metal, glass, rubber, plastics, and textiles and for biological materials, including binding tissues and sealing of wounds in surgery. The bonding action of cyanoacrylates is generally believed to be a result of an anionic polymerization that is highly exothermic and rapid, occurring within seconds or minutes, even at room temperature. Catalysts are not required for this reaction, since weak bases such as water and alcohols or nucleophilic groups on proteins (e.g., amine or hydroxyl groups) already present on the adherent surfaces initiate the polymerization. Vaporized cyanoacrylates are known to irritate the eyes and respiratory tract. Irritation and discomfort in the face and eyes may occur in workers owing to associated low humidity.[96, 97]

Contact sensitization to cyanoacrylates is considered extremely rare because of the immediate bonding of the cyanoacrylate to the surface keratin.[96] The adhesive was thus believed never to come into contact with immunocompetent cells farther down in the epidermis. For instance, Parker and Turk[59] were unable to sensitize guinea pigs with methyl or butyl 2-cyanoacrylate; although, in the last decade some case reports have been published that strongly indicate that cyanoacrylates are able to induce contact allergy.[98–105]

Patchtesting with cyanoacrylate glue might give false-negative reactions when it is dissolved in acetone using the Finn chamber (aluminum) technique. Patchtesting with petrolatum as a vehicle in a plastic chamber is recommended.[105] Cyanoacrylates, in addition to causing skin sensitization and irritation, have also been shown to cause occupational asthma and to be mutagenic. Furthermore, cyanoacrylates are suspected to be carcinogenic and to induce peripheral neuropathy.

Precautions for Handling Acrylic Resins

Gloves are recommended to protect the hands against various acrylic compounds. Methyl methacrylate as well as other acrylic monomers such as butylacrylate and acrylamide easily penetrate natural rubber latex gloves, however.[58, 106] Vinyl gloves are even more inferior in this regard.[107, 108] Polyethylene gloves protect best against methyl methacrylate diffusion.[58] Nitrile gloves give better protection than neoprene gloves against UV-curable acrylate resins.[1, 107] New multilayer glove material of the folio type, with ethylene-vinyl-alcohol copolymer laminated with the polyethylene on both sides, has especially good chemical resistance.[42] Because acrylics used in dentine-bonding systems are strong sensitizers and quickly penetrate most gloves, dentists and dental personnel should use no-touch techniques.[43, 49]

Most of the acrylic compounds used in UV-curable acrylic resins should be regarded as irritants and relatively potent sensitizers. Accordingly, care should be taken to minimize contact with skin. Measures that seem effective in preventing the dermatitis include use of impervious protective gloves and protective clothing. Face shields and goggles are recommended whenever there is risk of splatter. Contaminated skin should be washed with soap and water, and contaminated clothing should be removed promptly. It is necessary to keep clean and contaminated clothing separate. Thorough education of employees regarding skin hazards is also recommended.[1]

Patchtesting with Acrylic Compounds

In general, to avoid patchtest sensitization a patchtest concentration of 2% in petrolatum is recommended for the methacrylated monomers and 0.1% in petrolatum for the acrylated monomers.[109]

POLYURETHANE RESINS

Polyurethanes (PU) are plastics formed by the reaction between diisocyanates and polyhydroxy compounds (polyols). The polyurethanes are of the thermosetting type of plastic, and the polymerization is a polyaddition reaction. A *thermoplastic* material is produced when both components are only difunctional. When one or both components are more than difunctional, *thermosetting* end

products are produced. The polyhydroxy compounds used are mainly polyalcohols, polyesters, or polyethers, but isocyanates can also react with other molecules when they carry active hydroxyl groups. Isocyanates are low–molecular weight aromatic, aliphatic, or cycloaliphatic compounds characterized by a highly reactive −N=C=O group. Some isocyanates used in the production of polyurethane plastics are shown in Figure 25–16. The most commonly used difunctional isocyanates are toluene diisocyanate (TDI), often as mixtures of the isomers 2,4-TDI and 2,6-TDI. Diphenylmethane-4,4′-diisocyanate (MDI) is used industrially as crude MDI, which is a mixture of 4,4′-MDI with 2,4′-MDI and 2,2′-MDI. Crude MDI is also named *polymethylene polyphenyl isocyanate* (PAPI or PMPPI). Phenyl isocyanate is usually a contaminant in MDI. 1,6-Hexamethylene diisocyanate (HDI) is the most commonly used diisocyanate in lacquers, coatings, and paints. Examples of other diisocyanates include isophorone diisocyanate (IPDI), trimethyl hexamethylene diisocyanate (TMDI) (a mixture of the two isomers 2,2,4-TMDI and 2,4,4-TMDI), naphthalene diisocyanate (NDI), triphenylmethane triisocyanate (TPMTI), and dicyclohexylmethane diisocyanate (DMDI).[1, 89, 97, 110, 111]

Many auxiliary substances are also used in the manufacter of PU products. The hardening process can be modified by heat or with a catalyst (e.g., diaminodiphenylmethane or methylenedianiline [MDA]), triethylenediamine, triethylamine, cobalt naphthenate, or nickel salts.

Diisocyanates are used in a prepolymerized form. These prepolymers are synthesized by adding a small amount of the isocyanate to a polyol. The various prepolymers can be extended by adding water. When used as activators or hardeners, diisocyanates are often dissolved in aliphatic or aromatic hydrocarbon solvents or mixtures of different organic solvents (e.g., aliphatic hydrocarbon solvents, petroleum, and butylacetate). Adhesives, varnishes, and paints can also contain solvents. Polyurethanes have many uses—for coatings, paints, lacquers, adhesives (one- or two-component glue), binding agents, castings, elastomers, foams, fibers, and synthetic rubber. Flexible polyurethane foams are used for mattresses, cushions, dashboards, and packaging.[1, 111]

Skin Problems from Polyurethane Resins

The main occupational hazards caused by polyurethane chemicals are asthma and rhinitis, hypersensitive pneumonitis or alveolitis, conjunctivitis, and

FIGURE 25–16 • Chemical formulas of various isocyanates used in the production of polyurethane plastics.

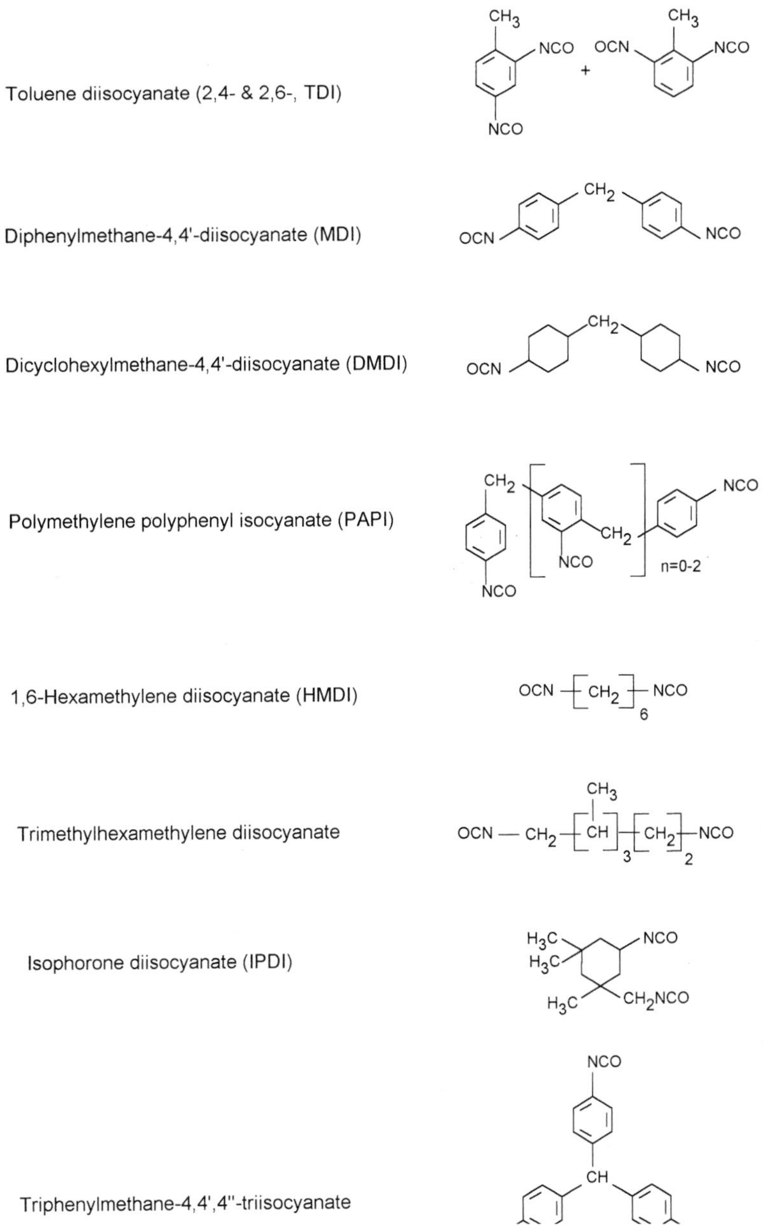

Toluene diisocyanate (2,4- & 2,6-, TDI)

Diphenylmethane-4,4'-diisocyanate (MDI)

Dicyclohexylmethane-4,4'-diisocyanate (DMDI)

Polymethylene polyphenyl isocyanate (PAPI)

1,6-Hexamethylene diisocyanate (HMDI)

Trimethylhexamethylene diisocyanate

Isophorone diisocyanate (IPDI)

Triphenylmethane-4,4',4''-triisocyanate

chronic obstructive lung disease.[112–114] Isocyanates are considered toxic chemicals.[113]

Exposure to isocyanates can produce both allergic and irritant contact dermatitis and urticaria.[97, 110, 111, 115–117] Diisocyanates are strong contact sensitizers, as has been shown from the results of animal studies[118]; however, in spite of this, the reports on allergic eczema are fewer in number, despite extensive use of these chemicals in manufacturing processes and other applications. Probably the rigorous rules that workers must follow when working with polyurethanes to minimize the hazard of isocyanates to the respiratory tract have also decreased the prevalences of all kind of skin hazards.

Isocyanates are described as mild to strong irritants, and irritant contact dermatitis seems to have been more common than allergic contact dermatitis.[28] Skin irritation can also be caused by amine accelerators (e.g., MDA, triethylenediamine, and triethylamine). Contact allergy to TDI, MDI, IPDI, HDI, TMDI, and DMDI has been reported.[97, 111, 116, 119–121] MDI-positive patients may also react to 4,4'-diaminodiphenylmethane, but it is not clear that MDI is the actual allergen, as MDI and water form 4,4'-diaminodiphenylmethane. 4,4'-Diaminodiphenylmethane may also represent cross-allergy to *p*-phenylenediamine.[115, 122]

Completely hardened polyurethane products usually do not cause skin problems. Unreacted isocyanate monomer may, however, remain in surplus inside polyurethane foams, even after curing. This can create isocyanate exposure when polyurethane dust is produced during machining or cutting.[117, 123, 124] When polyurethanes are heated above 250°C they decompose into isocyanates and nitrogen oxides and, again, could cause dermatitis. Animal experiments have been performed with guinea pigs and mice, and MDI, TDI, and HDI were found to be sensitizers.[118]

Patchtesting with Polyurethane Resins

Patchtesting of workers exposed to polyurethane chemicals should include MDI, TDI, HDI, MDA, and the actual chemicals to which they have been exposed.[111]

PHENOL-FORMALDEHYDE RESINS

Phenol-formaldehyde resins (phenolic resins) are polycondensation products of phenols and aldehydes, in particular phenol and formaldehyde. They are classified as resols and novolaks. When phenol reacts with an excess of formaldehyde under alkaline conditions, a resol resin is produced. As formaldehyde is in excess in the process, various low–molecular weight methylol phenol compounds are formed. These are 2-methylol phenol (2-MP), 4-methylol phenol (4-MP), 2,4-dimethylol phenol (2,4-MP), 2,6-dimethylol phenol (2,6-MP), 2,4,6-trimethylol phenol (2,4,6-MP) and, to a limited extent, 3-methylol phenol (3-MP; Fig. 25–17).[126] The polycondensation of the products has been stopped deliberately before completion. During processing, the polycondensation can be restarted by heating, which means that the resols are self–cross-linking and can be considered prepolymers.[1, 125, 126]

Novolak resins are formed when formaldehyde reacts with an excess of phenols under acidic conditions. Methylol phenols, mainly dihydroxydiphenyl methanes (HPM, bisphenol F isomers), are also present, but only in very low concentrations. These are 2,2'-HPM, 4,4'-HPM, and 2,4'-HPM. In the case of novolaks the polycondensation is brought to completion. The novolaks can be cross-linked by adding curing agents such as formaldehyde, paraformaldehyde, or hexamethylenetetramine in addition to heating, and give end products similar to resols.[1, 125, 126] The final cured polymer for both novolaks and resols is called *resite* or *C-stage resin*.

Commercially available phenol-formaldehyde resins are most often based on phenol itself, but other phenols such as cresols, xylenols, resorcinol (1,3-dihydroxybenzene), bisphenol A (diphenylolpropane), *p-tert*-butylphenol, 4-isooctylphenol, and 4-nonylphenol can be used. Besides formaldehyde, other aldehydes (e.g., acetaldehyde, glyoxal, furfural; 2-furancarboxaldehyde) can be used.[1, 125, 126] Phenolic resins are available as solids (broken pieces, flakes, pastilles, or granules) or as solutions or liquids.[125]

Phenol-formaldehyde and *p-tert*-butylphenol-formaldehyde resins have many industrial applications. Adhesives, glues, and glue films based on phenol-formaldehyde resins are used in the plywood industry. Because of their moisture resistance, the glues and laminates are used in the building industry and in boat and aircraft construction. The resins are also good insulators against electricity; they are thus used in many electronic and electrical appliances. In addition, they can be used to produce decorative laminates and coatings and to coat rigid constructions (e.g., pipelines and reaction vessels) because of their strong chemical resistance. They are also used as binders for glass and mineral fibers in the production of hearth-, noise-, and fire-insulating materials, in foundry moulding sand, and in abrasives such as sandpaper, abrasive cloth, and flexible sanding discs. Novolak resins can be used in the production of grinding wheels, brake linings, and clutch facings. They are also used as raw materials for polyfunctional epoxy resins.[1, 125–127]

The *p-tert*-butylphenol-formaldehyde resins are used in adhesives based on neoprene and other rubbers used in shoes, leather products, automobile interiors and upholstery, furniture, adhesive tapes and labels, and in the gluing of certain floor coverings.[1, 125, 126] The *p-tert*-butylphenol-formaldehyde resin is also used as adhesive for leather, artificial fingernails, and labels. The third large group is phenolic resins modified by natural resins. Rosin-modified phenolic resins are used as binders for book offset printing inks.[126]

Skin Hazards of Phenol-Formaldehyde Resins

Workers handling phenol-formaldehyde resins suffer mostly skin problems. Contact dermatitis is common and usually is caused by the contact allergy, but immediate contact reactions to the resins have also been reported.[128] Most of the reported cases of contact dermatitis are due to sensitization to *p-tert*-butylphenol-formaldehyde

2-methylolphenol

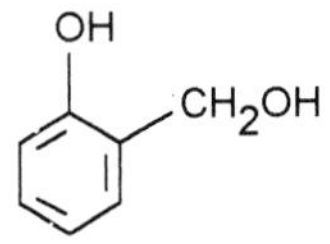

4-methylolphenol

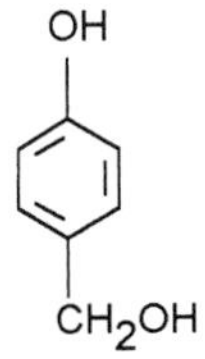

2,4-dimethylolphenol

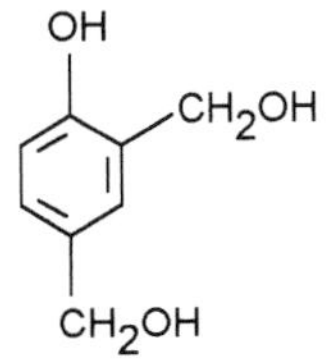

2,6-dimethylolphenol

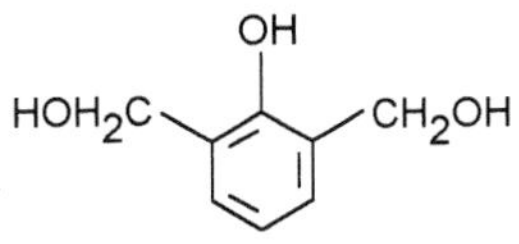

2,4,6-trimethylolphenol

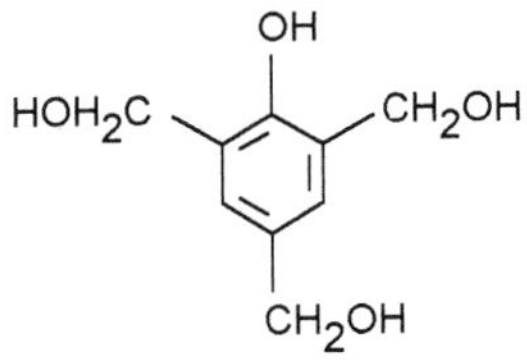

4,4'-dihydroxy-3,3'-dimethylol-
diphenylmethane

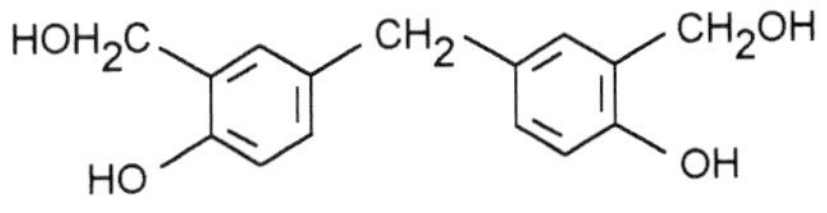

FIGURE 25–17 ● Chemical formulas of various methylolphenols.

resins. Reviews of *p-tert*-butylphenol-formaldehyde resin–induced occupational eczema have been published.[126, 129–131]

The *p-tert*-butylphenol-formaldehyde resins consist of hundreds of substances, the vast majority of which are not chemically defined. The major sensitizers in *p-tert*-butylphenol-formaldehyde resin are 2-methylol-*p-tert*-butylphenol (2-MPTBP) and 2,6-dimethylol *p-tert*-butylphenol (2,6-MBTBP).[132] Other allergens in *p-tert*-butylphenol-formaldehyde resin are *p-tert*-butylphenol (BTBP), some degradation product, and a few larger phenolic compounds. Guinea pigs sensitized to 2,6-MBTBP show cross-reactions to 2-MPTBP and to *p-tert*-butylcathecol (PTBC), but not to *p-tert*-butylphenol (BTBP).[132]

The *p-tert*-butylphenol-formaldehyde resin and resins based on other types of phenols and formaldehyde do not necessarily contain the same sensitizer.[126, 133] Bruze and Zimerson patchtested patients, with contact allergy to phenol-formaldehyde resin and at least one methylolphenol, with six additional methylolphenols and 13 chemically related compounds. They found probable cross-reacting substances to be *o*-cresol, *p*-cresol, salicylaldehyde, 2,4-dimethylolphenol, and 2,6-dimethylolphenol.[134] Formaldehyde is not the main sensitizer in phenol-formaldehyde resins, and the presence of at least 14 contact sensitizers—4,4′-dihydroxy(hydroxymethyl)-diphenyl methanes being the most potent allergens—has been demonstrated in resins and products based on phenol-formaldehyde resins. Simultaneous reactions to phenol-formaldehyde resins, colophony/hydroxyabietyl alcohol and balsam of Peru/perfume mixture can occur.[126, 127, 135–137]

Phenol-formaldehyde resins can also irritate the skin and cause chemical burns and depigmentation. Phenol and furfural are primary skin irritants and concentrated phenol can even cause corrosive chemical burns. Besides being a potent sensitizer, formaldehyde is a skin irritant.

Occupational irritant dermatitis has been reported in the manufacture of the electrical insulation material Bakelite, which is phenol-formaldehyde resin made of incompletely condensed resin powder in molds.[138] Irritant dermatitis was also common among workers in the manufacture of decorative laminates made of paper sheets impregnated with phenol-formaldehyde resins.[139, 140]

Patchtesting with Phenol-Formaldehyde Resins

In addition to *p-tert*-butylphenol-formaldehyde resin it is also necessary to patchtest with the actual resin to which the worker is exposed, as no single test substance reliably detects allergy to the wide variety of phenolic resin types. Bruze found 2.5 times more patients with contact allergy to phenol-formaldehyde resins when routinely patchtested with the resin based on phenol and formaldehyde (P-F-R-2) in addition to *p-tert*-butylphenol-formaldehyde resin.[141]

POLYESTER RESINS

Polyester resins are polycondensation thermosetting compounds of two different forms: saturated and unsaturated. The *saturated polyesters*, also termed *unmodified alkyd resins*, are produced from dicarboxylic acids, usually phthalic acid or its anhydride, and polyalcohols, usually glycerol, pentaerythritol, or trimethylolpropane. The saturated polyester synthesized in this way is a macromolecule commonly used as a plasticizer for other plastic materials. Alkyd resins are formed by a modification with oils containing fatty acids, which bind to free hydroxyl groups on the polyfunctional alcohol. In this form the resin is often used in modern water-based paints and other surface coatings (Fig. 25–18).

Unsaturated polyesters are produced through esterification of organic acids or their anhydrides (e.g., maleic anhydride, phthalic anhydride, or fumaric acid) and of diols (e.g., diethylene glycol or 1,2-propylene glycol). The unsaturated polyester is cured by cross-linking between parts of the linear macromolecule. Unsaturated monomers (e.g., styrene) are used as solvents and for copolymerization with unsaturated groups along the polyester chain. Vinyl toluene and methyl methacrylate can also be used for cross-linking. An initiator or catalyst is required to start the cross-linking process. The catalyst is usually a peroxide such as benzoyl peroxide or methyl ethyl ketone peroxide. Accelerators (e.g., cobalt naphthenate, or tertiary amines such as dimethyl aniline, diethyl aniline, and dimethyl-*p*-toluidine) are necessary for the curing of plastics at room temperature. In styrene there are usually inhibitors (e.g., *p-tert*-butylcatechol or hydroquinone). The peroxide-cured unsaturated polyesters have been used commercially for many years, but unsaturated polyesters cured by UV light have equivalent properties. The UV-curable polyester system is used as top coats in the furniture industry and for orthopedic casts. Casts curable by UV light usually consist of an unsaturated polyester with vinyl toluene as the cross-linking agent and a benzoin-ether molecule as photoinitiator. The resin is impregnated into woven glass fiber. Reactive (meth)acrylate groups can be attached to the molecular backbone of the

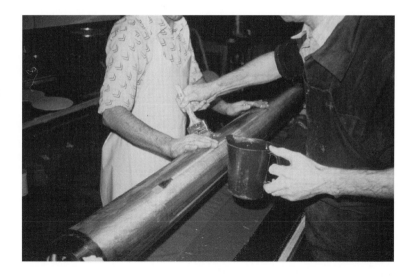

FIGURE 25–18 • Polyester resins are widely used in the manufacture of structural items; here, a mixture of resin and catalyst is applied with a paintbrush. Polyester resins, however, are not common allergic sensitizers.

unsaturated polyesters through functional group such as hydroxyl and anhydride, forming acrylated polyesters used in UV-curable inks or coatings for wood and paper.

Unsaturated polyesters have been used extensively in the reinforced plastics industry in the manufacturer of products for transportation, construction, and marine applications. They are also used for coatings, finishes, lacquers, cement, and glues.

Skin Problems from Polyester Resins

Contact dermatitis from *saturated polyesters* appears to be very rare. Allergic contact dermatitis has, however, been caused by a three-functional epoxy compound, triglycidyl isocyanurate (TGDI), used as cross-linker in heat-cured polyester paints.[142] Phthalic anhydrides have been reported to cause immediate IgE-mediated hypersensitivity, asthma, allergic rhinitis, and urticaria.[142] Alkyd resins are not sensitizing, but phthalic anhydrides used in the manufacturer of alkyd resins can cause irritation.

Unsaturated polyester resin is a rare sensitizer. Those at risk are workers employed in manufacturing, with few exceptions.[144–149] According to Malten, unsaturated polyester no longer appears to have sensitizing capacity, presumably because the formation of sensitizing free maleic acid esters is prevented by the avoidance of monoalcoholic impurities.[150] Should the diols contain monoalcohols like ethanol and butanol, then the ethyl maleate and dibutyl maleate can be formed, which are strong contact sensitizers. Diethylmaleate was reported to be a sensitizer in four men who worked with unsaturated polyester resins.[144] Allergic contact dermatitis from unsaturated polyester resins has more frequently been attributed to the auxiliary ingredients, catalysts,[144, 151] and cross-linking agents.[151–153]

The main irritants in unsaturated polyester resin system are styrene and organic peroxides. Unsaturated polyester resin may contain 30% to 60% styrene by weight. Styrene is classified as a mild skin irritant.[28, 154] Repeated skin contact with liquid styrene, however, causes drying of the skin and can cause irritant dermatitis.[151] In addition, workers in the reinforced plastics industry are exposed to many skin irritants, such as glass fiber, solvents, and other additives.

Peroxides are used in 3% to 10% by weight to catalyze hardening of unsaturated polyester resins. These reactive organic peroxides have been reported to cause stinging on uncovered skin areas during spray lamination.[154]

AMINO PLASTICS

Amino plastics is the common name for plastics formed by the reaction between an aldehyde and a compound of one or more amino groups. The most common aldehyde is formaldehyde, but sometimes hexamethylenetetramine, a formaldehyde releaser, can be used. Amino plastics always contain an excess of formaldehyde. The most common amino compounds are urea or carbamide ($H_2N-CO-NH_2$) and melamine (2,4,6-triamino-1,3,5-triazine). The reaction with formaldehyde produces thermosetting urea-formaldehyde and melamine-formaldehyde resins by a polycondensation-type reaction. The amino resins are cured by heat, usually with an inorganic acid as catalyst. Although both resins are quite similar in appearance, the melamine-formaldehyde resins have water resistance superior to that of cured urea-formaldehyde resins. Both amino plastics are relatively unaffected by common organic solvents, oils, and greases and are widely used as laminating and bonding materials in the wood and furniture industry. They are used as wood glues and surface coatings, and to improve the wet strength of paper and crease resistance of textiles. Powders from urea-formaldehyde resins can be molded to make containers for cosmetics products, electrical fittings, and bottle caps. Urea-formaldehyde foams have found application as insulation in refrigerators and the walls of houses. Other typical uses of urea-formaldehyde resins are clock cases, toilet seats, and buttons. Melamine-formaldehyde resin powders filled with cellulose are used to make plates and cups. High-quality decorative laminates are made of melamine-formaldehyde resins. Amino plastics are often used in conjunction with fillers and reinforcements such as glass mat and cloth, silica, cotton fabrics, and certain synthetic fibers.

Skin Problems from Amino Plastics

Usually, the finished product does not cause primary sensitization, but occasionally the uncured substance does. Textile dermatitis caused by urea- and melamine-formaldehyde resins is rare. Those with contact allergy to amino resins often also have formaldehyde allergy.[155, 156]

Urea and melamine do not cause contact allergy. Sensitization to amino plastics has developed from urea-formaldehyde resin used as textile finish[156] and melamine-formaldhyde resin in orthopedic casts,[157] gypson molds,[156] or the coating of plastic tubes intended for cosmetics.

The irritancy of amino plastic is due mainly to formaldehyde, which can be released from plastics. Nowadays, resins used in textiles release less free formaldehyde than they once did.[156] Occupational irritant contact dermatitis from fiberboard containing urea-formaldehyde resin has been reported.[158] Dust from urea-formaldehyde isulating foam has caused airborne irritation.[159]

POLYSTYRENE

Polystyrene is a hard, transparent plastic. It is manufactured by polyaddition polymerization of styrene ($CH_2=CH-C_6H_5$) using peroxide as an initiator. Polystyrene resin is one of the thermoplastics. As a foam, polystyrene plastic is an important packaging and isulation material. Modified polystyrene plastics with a co- or terpolymer structure (e.g., styrene-butadiene [SB], styrene-acrylonitrile [SAN], acrylonitrile-butadiene-styrene [ABS] are used in household utensils, toys, electrical appliances, handles, bags, and pipes. Polystyrene products are also widely used for food packaging and disposable tableware. Polystyrene products can usually be identified by the metallic sound they make when dropped on a hard surface. To increase the light stability of styrene-based plastics, stabilizers such as benzophenones, benzotriazoles, and organic nickel compounds are usually added.

Skin Problems from Polystyrene Resins

Contact allergy to styrene is extremely rare. One styrene-sensitive patient cross-reacted at patchtesting to 2-, 3- and 4-vinyltoluene (2-, 3- and 4-methylstyrene) and to the metabolites styrene epoxide and 4-vinylphenol (4-hydroxystyrene). It is assumed that styrene is a prohapten metabolized in the skin by aurylhydrocarbon hydroxylase to styrene epoxide, which acts as a true hapten. Styrene occurs both in nature and as a synthetic product, and vinyltoluenes (methylstyrenes) occur as synthetic products in plastics.[153] Cases of immediate allergy to styrene have been reported.[151, 153, 160, 161] Styrene defats the skin and can give rise to primary irritation, but it is nevertheless classified as a mild irritant.[28, 154] Styrene has been reported to cause chemical burns.[151, 162]

POLYVINYL RESINS

The chemical structure of a vinyl compound is $CH_2=CH-R$. ($CH_2=CH-$ is the vinyl group, and R is the symbol for different chemical groups used to synthesize various polyvinyl resins.) Some examples of vinyl compounds are vinyl chloride (R:Cl−), vinyl acetate (R:CH_3COOH-), vinyl acetal (R:$CH_3(CH_2)_n-O-$, $n=0, 1, 2 . . .$), vinyl alcohol (R:OH−), and vinylidene chloride (R:$CH_2=CCl_2$). The polyvinyl resins are polymerized through a polyaddition reaction and belong to the group of thermoplastics. Vinyl chloride ($CH_2=CH-Cl$) is a gaseous monomer, polymerized by suspension, emulsion, solution, and bulk processes. The repeating unit of PVC is as follows: −CH_2 −CHCl−.

There are various additives in PVC plastics, such as antioxidants, light stabilizers, initiators, plasticizers, flame retardents, and pigments, among others. As initiators, potassium persulfate, benzoyl peroxide, lauryl peroxide, percarbonate, and some azo-compounds can be used. The presence of chlorine in the hydrocarbon backbone gives rigidity and toughness to the polymer, but

PVC liberates hydrogen chloride when exposed to high temperatures. To prevent this, stabilizers are added to the polymer. There are several kinds of stabilizers on the market. The most important ones contain lead, tin, calcium, zinc, and barium. Plasticizers, mainly phthalates, are added to PVC to impart flexibility to the finished products and to improve processibility of the melt. In almost all PVC, plasticizers are added. Hard PVC contains approximately 10% plasticizers and soft PVC up to 60% to 70%. The plasticizers are mostly in the form of phthalic acid esters, most commonly diethylhexyl phthalate (DEHP), often termed *dioctyl phthalate* (DOP). More than one plasticizer is usually used when properties other than flexibility are also desired in the end product. Sometimes uncured epoxy resin is added to PVC as a plasticizer and stabilizer. Soft or plasticized PVC is very popular in applications such as artificial skin, wallpaper, laminated tablecloths, carpets, toys, garden hose, wire coatings for electrical cables, shower curtains, adhesive plasters, foils, bandages, casts, and protective gloves.

PVC is one of the most inexpensive thermoplastics and is the most frequently used plastic, after polyethylene. The toughness and rigidity of hard PVC give rise to applications in sewage systems, agricultural products, drinking water pipes, furniture, window frames, dishes, and packages of various shapes.

Skin Problem from Polyvinyl Resins

Workers processing PVC plastics can develop contact dermatitis.[163, 164] The vinyl chloride polymer (PVC) does not sensitize, and its additives seldom do. In the final PVC product there are always molecules of the monomer as well as a number of additives, which may cause contact dermatitis,[163, 167] irritant dermatitis,[164, 168] or contact urticaria.[169] Allergic contact reaction to epoxy resin in PVC plastic film and to the phenylthiourea and phenylisothiocyanate in PVC adhesive tape has been reported.[166, 170] Diphenylthiourea is a heat stabilizer in PCV and is partly decomposed to phenyl isothiocyanate.

The irritancy of polyvinyl resins is due to the plasticizers and stabilizers, dibutyl thiomaleate, dibutyl sebacate, or dioctyl phthalate.[28, 168] PVC powder may irritate in a special environment. An outbreak of acneiform eruptions in a PVC factory has been reported.[171] The cause was probably the combination of heat, high humidity, and the irritation of the PVC powder. Toxic PVC disease from the manufacture of PVC consists of Raynaud's phenomenon, lytic disease of bone, and scleroderma.

POLYOLEFINS

Polyolefins belong to a group of thermoplastics polymerized through polyaddition reaction of olefins (unsaturated hydrocarbons). The most important polyolefins are ethylene (ethene), $CH_2=CH_2$, which when polymerized yields polyethylene, and propylene (propene) $CH_2=CHCH_3$, which yields polypropylene.

Polyethylene, the most important in volume among the plastics, was already known more than half a century ago. The repeating unit of polyethylene is $-CH_2-CH_2-$. The polymerization is produced at high or low pressure, aided by catalysts and initiators. According to their density, polyethylenes are grouped into three main categories: low-density, linear low-density, and high-density polyethylenes.

All of these types are lighter than water and belong to the most inexpensive group of plastics. Films and sheets for packaging uses are the most widespread forms of polyethylene plastics. Because low-density polyethylene is soft and flexible, transparent, and nontoxic owing to the absence of plasticizers, it is used for food packaging. Shopping bags and sacks are the other most popular applications of low-density polyethylenes. Linear low-density polyethylene is the main plastic in the film-manufacturing industry, owing to its mechanical strength. Because low-density polyethylene has outstanding chemical and frost resistance, its main applications are for hoses, coatings of electric cables and wires, and many kinds of household utensils such as jars, containers, deep-freeze boxes, and cases. High-density polyethylenes are used mainly for bottles and containers but also for shopping bags and pipes.

Polypropylene has the repeating unit $-CH_2-CH(CH_3)-$. Polypropylene is similar to high-density polyethylene but is slightly harder and tougher. In addition to filament applications such as home furnishings, nonwoven products, and carpets, polypropylene is generally used as pipes and films.

Skin Problems from Polyolefins

Irritant or allergic contact dermatitis from polyethylene or polypropylene is rare. Incompletely cured resins can cause contact dermatitis. It is most likely to be caused by added ingredients such as catalysts and initiators. When sawing and grinding polyolefins the heat may cause depolymerization and release chemicals such as aldehydes, ketones, and acids, which might cause airborne contact dermatitis. Itching caused by the irritancy of heat-decomposed polyethylene plastics has been reported.[172]

POLYAMIDES

The polyamides are thermoplastics manufactured by condensation polymerization of adipic acid; $HOOC-(CH_2)_4-COOH$; and hexamethylene diamine; $H_2N-(CH_2)_6-NH_2$. The resulting polymer has a linear structure with the repeating unit $-OC-(CH_2)_4CONH-(CH_2)_6-NH-$. Other polyamides can be polymerized from caprolactam and water.

The polyamides are made into fibers known as nylon. The transparency of polyamide films makes them very useful for packaging. Hospital wares made of polyamide plastics have good stability at sterilization temperatures, and combined films of laminates are used, for example, in vacuum-sealed packages of meat.

Skin Problems from Polyamides

Irritant and allergic contact dermatitides from polyamides are rare.[1]

POLYCARBONATES

A polycarbonate plastic is characterized by the $-O-CO-O-$ group. It can be made from phosgene ($COCl_2$) and bisphenol A (4,4'-dihydroxydiphenyl-2,2-propane) and has the structure: $-O-(C_6H_4)-C(CH_3)_2-(C_6H_4)-O-CO-$. Bisphenols other than bisphenol A can also be used. Polycarbonate plastic is a very transparent, tough, and inert material that is extremely resistant to sunlight and weather. It is used, among other things, for safety helmets, bullet-proof windows, shields, doors, bottles, and lamp globes; however, the plastic is relatively expensive and thus has limited applications.

Skin Problems from Polycarbonates

Irritant and allergic contact dermatitis from polycarbonates are rare.[1]

OTHER PLASTICS

Plastics of less dermatological importance are coumarone-indene polymers, cellulose polymers, and cyclohexanone resins. It is not known for certain whether the monomers, additives, or impurities are the cause of the dermatitis in reported cases.[173, 174]

ADDITIVES IN SYNTHETIC POLYMERS

Additives are used to modify the properties of a plastic material. The major classes of additives to plastics are plasticizers, fillers and reinforcements, biocides, flame retardants, heat stabilizers, antioxidants, UV light absorbers, blowing agents, initiators, lubricants and flow control agents, antistatic agents, curing agents, colorants, solvents, and optical brighteners. Nearly 2,500 individual chemicals or mixtures are utilized in these major classes of additives. In the plastics industry the word *compound* denotes a chemical product of the plastic resin mixed with additives. Compounds are delivered to the plastics industry as powders or pellets. Masterbatch is a concentrated mixture of additives in the plastics.

Plasticizers

Plasticizers constitute a broad range of chemically and thermally stable products of a variety of chemical classes that are added to improve the flexibility, softness, and processibility of plastics. Their principal use is in thermoplastic resins, and 80 to 85% of the world's production of plasticizers is used in PVC manufacturing. Approximately 450 plasticizers are commercially available. Many are esters of carboxylic acids (e.g., phthalic, isophthalic, adipic, benzoic, abietic, trimellitic, oleic, and sebacic acids) or phosphoric acid. Other plasticizers are chlorinated paraffins, epoxidized vegetable oils, and adipate polymers.

Although about 100 phthalates have been employed as plasticizers, some 14 or 15 phthalates account for more than 90% of commercial phthalate production. The most commonly used phthalate is diethylhexyl phthalate (DEHP), which is often called *dioctyl phthalate* (DOP). Other plasticizers used are butyl benzyl phthalate (BBP), diisononyl phthalate (DINP), diisodecyl phthalate (DIDP), methyl-, ethyl-, butyl phthalate, dialkyl (C_6C_{11}) phthalate, and diethylhexyl adipate. Adipates and other aliphatic diesters are used in low-temperature applications, whereas trimellitics are used for high-temperature applications. Methyl-, ethyl-, and butyl phthalates are more often used as solvents than as plasticizers in the plastics industry.

Flame Retardants

Flame retardants are required for high-performance thermoplastic resins because they are used in electrical and high-temperature applications. Numerous chemicals are used as flame retardants. Chlorine- and bromine-containing aliphatic, cycloaliphatic, and aromatic compounds are used most widely. Others are antimony trioxide, aluminium hydrate, and chlorparaffins. A more fire-resistant epoxy resin can be produced by bromating bisphenol A in epoxy resins to tetrabromobisphenol A.

Heat Stabilizers

Plastics, particularly polymers containing chlorine, are susceptible to thermal decomposition when exposed to high temperatures or prolonged heating. Several kinds of stabilizers are on the market. The most important contain lead, tin, calcium and zinc or barium and zinc. Epoxidized oils and esters are also used. Diphenylthiourea is used as a heat stabilizer in PVC.

Antioxidants

Oxidative degradation of polymers during the manufacturing process or during their useful lifetime is a major industrial concern. Examples of antioxidants are alkylated phenols and polyphenols (e.g., butylated hydroxytoluenes [BHT] and 4-tert-butylcatechol), epoxidized soybean oil, propylphenolphosfit, thiobisphenol, organic phosphates, bisphenol A, benzophenone, hydroquinones, and triazoles.

Ultraviolet Light Absorbers

Radiation from the sun or fluorescent light is responsible for the rapid degradation of most plastics. The most widely used UV absorbers belong to seven distinct chemical classes: benzophenones, benzotriazoles, salicylates, acrylates, organonickel derivatives, hindered amines, and metal complexes with dialkyldithiocarbamate

The most widely used UV absorbers are 2-hydroxy-benzophenones, 2-hydroxy-phenyl-benzotriazoles, and 2-cyanodiphenyl-acrylate.

Initiators

Most commercial synthetic polymers are produced by a chain reaction polymerization process. Some of the many initiators used are various peroxides (e.g., benzoyl peroxide, di-tertiary-butyl peroxide, cyclohexanone peroxide, and methyl ethyl ketone peroxide). More than 65 organic peroxides are commercially available in more than 100 formulations.

Curing Agents

The usefulness of a number of plastics such as unsaturated polyester, epoxy, and phenolic resins is limited unless their linear polymer chains are cross-linked or cured. The various curing agents and compounds used as initiators (accelerators or catalysts) are discussed under the various plastics.

Biocides

Biostabilizers prevent the growth of microorganisms on the plastic's surface and in the pores of some plastics. Plastic materials easily attacked by microorganisms are PVC, polyurethane, silicon products, and fiber products based on polypropene and polyamide. Microorganisms usually cause discoloration but can also crack plastic materials. Biocides are usually added to plastic products used in environments of high temperature and humidity (e.g., saunas, showers, pools, and boats). The most used biocides are methyl- and octyl-isothiazolinones and oxybisphenoxarsin (OBPA).

Colorants (Dyes and Pigments)

Pigments are inert and, unlike dyes, insoluble in the medium in which they are incorporated. Both inorganic and organic pigments are used in plastics. Most colorants are inorganic pigments, titanium dioxide being the most commonly used one, and iron oxides the second most common.

Metals and Metal Salts

Many metals and metal salts and metallic compounds are used as additives in plastics. They are used as stabilizers, pigments, fillers, flame retardants, and antistatics. The most commonly used metals are aluminium, titanium, lead, zinc, antimony, tin, chromium, and molybdenum. Nickel, copper, and zirconium compounds are used to a lesser extent.

Skin Problem from Additives

Allergic and irritant contact dermatitis to various additives is mentioned briefly in connection with the various plastics. In spite of the fact that the phthalates are the most widely used additives, there are only a few reports in the literature. Allergic contact dermatitis from dibutyl phthalate has been reported when used in a plastic watch strap, in an antiperspirant spray, and in a steroid cream.[175–178] Contact dermatitis from diethyl phthalate has been reported from spectacle frames and hearing aids of cellulose ester plastics.[179, 180] Two cases of contact allergy to dimethyl phthalate in computer mice have been reported by Capon and associates.[181]

In an aircraft factory an outbreak of dermatitis was caused by o-diglycidyl phthalate, among other chemicals.[5] Burrows and Rycroft have reported contact allergy to tricresyl ethylphthalate in a plastic nail adhesive.[182] Phthalates can also appear in deodorant formulations, perfumes, emollients, and insect repellants.[183] Triphenylphosphate allergy from spectacle frames has been reported.[184, 185]

The International Contact Dermatitis Research

Group in 1976 examined the incidence of sensitization to the flame retardant tris(2,3-dibromopropyl)phosphate and found two cases among 1,103 subjects. One of the two cases was reported in detail by Andersen.[186] Contact allergy to UV light absorbers such as 2-hydroxybenzophenone, resorcinol monobenzoate, 2-(2-hydroxy-5-methylphenyl)benzotriazole (Tinuvin P) and bis-(2,2,6,6)-tetramethyl-4-piperidyl-sebacate has been encountered.[187, 188] Organic pigments, mostly the azotypes, are potentially sensitizing additives to plastics.[189, 190] Other additives of dermatological importance are hydroquinone, *p-tert*-butyl-catechol, cobalt naphthenate, benzoyl peroxide, dimethylaniline, methyl-4-toluene sulfonate, *p*-tolyldiethanolamine, and dimethyl-, diethyl-, and diphenylthiourea. These agents can cause both allergic and irritant contact dermatitis.[1, 28]

References

1. Björkner B. Plastic materials. In: Rycroft RJG, Menné T, Frosch PJ, eds. *Textbook of Contact Dermatitis*. Berlin: Springer-Verlag; 1995:539.
2. Muskopf JW, McCollister SB. Epoxy resins. In: Gerhartz W, Yamamoto YS, Kaudy L, Rounsavill JF, Schulx G, eds. *Ullmann's Encyclopedia of Industrial Chemistry*, 5th ed, Vol A9. Weinheim: VCH Verlagsgesellschaft; 1987:547.
3. Fregert S. *Manual of Contact Dermatitis*, 2nd ed. Copenhagen: Munksgaard; 1981.
4. Fregert S. Contact dermatitis from epoxy resin systems. In: Maibach HI, ed. *Occupational and Industrial Dermatology*, 2nd ed. Chicago: Year Book; 1987:341.
5. Burrows D, Fregert S, Campbell H, Trulsson L. Contact dermatitis from the epoxy resins tetraglycidyl-4,4′-methylene dianiline and o-diglycidyl phthalate in composite material. *Contact Dermatitis* 1984;11:80.
6. Thorgeirsson A, Fregert S, Magnusson B. Allergenicity of epoxy-reactive diluents in the guinea pig. *Derm Beruf Umwelt* 1975;23:178.
7. Jolanki R. Occupational skin diseases from epoxy compounds. Epoxy resin compounds, epoxy acrylates and 2,3-epoxypropyl trimethyl ammonium chloride [doctoral dissertation]. *Acta Derm Venereol (Stockh)* 1991[Suppl]: 159.
8. Jolanki R, Estlander T, Kanerva L. Occupational contact dermatitis and contact urticaria caused by epoxy resins. *Acta Derm Venereol (Stockh)* 1987[Suppl]: 134:90.
9. Birmingham DJ. Clinical observations on the cutaneous effects associated with curing epoxy resins. *Arch Ind Health* 1959;19:365.
10. Bourne LB, Milner FJM, Alberman KB. Health problems of epoxy resins and amine-curing agents. *Br J Ind Med* 1959;16:81.
11. Gaul LE. Sensitizing structure in epoxy resin. *J Invest Dermatol* 1957;29:311.
12. Gaul LE. Sensitivity to bisphenol A. *Arch Dermatol* 1960;82:1003.
13. Calnan CD. Epoxy resin dermatitis. *J Soc Occup Med* 1975;25:123.
14. Thorgeirsson A, Fregert S. Allergenicity of epoxy resins in the guinea pig. *Acta Derm Venereol* 1978;58:332.
15. Fregert S, Thorgeirsson A. Patch testing with low molecular oligomers of epoxy resins in humans. *Contact Dermatitis* 1977;3:301.
16. Jolanki R, Sysilampi M-L, Kanerva L, Estlander T. Contact allergy to cycloaliphatic epoxy resins. In: Frosch PJ, Dooms-Goossens A, Lachapelle J-M, Rycroft RJG, Scheper RJ, eds. *Current Topics in Contact Dermatitis*. Berlin: Springer-Verlag; 1989:360.
17. Dahlquist I, Fregert S. Allergic contact dermatitis from volatile epoxy hardeners and reactive diluents. *Contact Dermatitis* 1979;5:406.
18. Fregert S. Physiochemical methods for detection of contact allergens. *Dermatol Clin North Am* 1988;6:97.
19. Fregert S, Trulsson L. Simple methods for demonstration of epoxy resin of bisphenol A type. *Contact Dermatitis* 1978;4:69.
20. Lembo G, Balato N, Cusano F, Baldo A, Ayala F. Contact dermatitis to epoxy resins in composite material. In: Frosch PJ, Dooms-Goossens A, Lachapelle J-M, Rycroft RJG, Scheper RJ, eds. *Current Topics in Contact Dermatitis*. Berlin: Springer-Verlag; 1989:377.
21. Thorgeirsson A. Sensitizing capacity of epoxy resin hardeners in the guinea pig. *Acta Derm Venereol (Stockh)* 1978;58:332.
22. Mathias CGT. Allergic contact dermatitis from a nonbisphenol A epoxy in a graphite fiber reinforced epoxy laminate. *J Occup Med* 1987;29:754.
23. Lachapelle J-M, Tennstedt D, Dumont-Fruytier M. Occupational allergic contact dermatitis to isophorone diamine (IPD) used as an epoxy resin hardener. *Contact Dermatitis* 1978;4:109.
24. Dahlquist I, Fregert S. Contact allergy to the epoxy hardener isophorone diamine (IPD). *Contact Dermatitis* 1979;5:120.
25. Jolanki R, Estlander T, Kanerva L. Contact allergy to an epoxy reactive diluent: 1,4-butanediol diglycidyl ether. *Contact Dermatitis* 1987;16:87.
26. Jolanki R, Kanerva L, Estlander T, et al. Occupational dermatoses from epoxy resin compounds. *Contact Dermatitis* 1990;23:172.
27. Kanerva L, Estlander T, Jolanki R. Occupational allergic contact dermatitis caused by 2,4,6-tris-(dimethylaminomethyl)phenol, and review of sensitizing epoxy resin hardeners. *Int J Dermatol* 1996;35:852.
28. Kanerva L, Björkner B, Estlander T, et al. Plastic materials: occupational exposure, skin irritancy and its prevention. In: van der Valk PGM, Maibach HI, eds. *The Irritant Contact Dermatitis Syndrome*. New York: CRC Press; 1996:127.
29. Krajewska D, Rudzki E. Sensitivity to epoxy resins and triethylenetetramine. *Contact Dermatitis* 1976;2:135.
30. Fregert S, Rorsman H. Hypersensitivity to epoxy resins with reference to the role played by bisphenol A. *J Invest Dermatol* 1962;39:471.
31. Prens EP, de Jong G, van Joost T. Sensitization to epichlorohydrin and epoxy system components. *Contact Dermatitis* 1986;15:85.
32. van Joost T, Roesyanto ID, Satyawan I. Occupational sensitization to epichlorohydrin (ECH) and bisphenol A during the manufacture of epoxy resin. *Contact Dermatitis* 1990;22:125.
33. van Joost T. Occupational sensitization to epichlorohydrin and epoxy resin. *Contact Dermatitis* 1988;19:278.
34. Tarvainen K, Jolanki R, Estlander T, et al. Contact urticaria due to airborne methylhexahydrophthalic anhydride and methyltetrahydrophthalic anhydride. *Contact Dermatitis* 1995;32:204.
35. Kanerva L, Jolanki R, Tupasela O, et al. Immediate and delayed allergy from epoxy resins based on diglycidyl ether of bisphenol A. *Scand J Work Environ Health* 1991;17:208.
36. Allen H, Kaidbey K. Persistent photosensitivity following

occupational exposure to epoxy resin. *Arch Dermatol* 1979;115:1307.

37. Göransson K, Andersson R, Andersson G, et al. An outbreak of occupational photodermatosis of the face in a factory in northern Sweden. In: Berglund B, Lindvall T, Sundell J, eds. *Indoor Air*, Vol 3. Stockholm: Swedish Council for Building Research; 1984:367.

38. Maguire HC. Experimental photoallergic contact dermatitis to bisphenol A. *Acta Derm Venereol* 1988;68:408.

39. Pegum JS. Penetration of protective gloves by epoxy resin. *Contact Dermatitis* 1979;5:281.

40. Roed-Petersen J. A new glove material protective against epoxy and acrylate monomer. In: Frosch PJ, Dooms-Goossens A, Lachapelle J-M, Rycroft RJG, Scheper RJ, eds. *Current Topics in Contact Dermatitis*. Berlin: Springer-Verlag; 1989:603.

41. Blanken R, Nater JP, Veenhoff E. Protection against epoxy resins with glove materials. *Contact Dermatitis* 1987;16:46.

42. Blanken R, Nater JP, Veenhoff E. Protective effect of barrier creams and spray coatings against epoxy resins. *Contact Dermatitis* 1987;16:79.

43. Estlander T, Jolanki R. How to protect the hands. In: Taylor JS, ed. Occupational Dermatoses. *Dermatol Clin* 1988;6:105.

44. Freeman S, Lee M-S, Gudmundsen K. Adverse contact reactions to sculptured acrylic nails: 4 case reports and a literature review. *Contact Dermatitis* 1995;33:381.

45. Koppula SV, Feldman JH, Storms FJ. Screening allergens for acrylate dermatitis associated with artificial nails. *Am J Contact Derm* 1995;6(2):78.

46. Kanerva L, Lauerna A, Estlander T, et al. Occupational allergic contact dermatitis caused by photobonded sculptured nails and a review of (meth)acrylates in nail cosmetics. *Am J Contact Derm* 1996;7:109.

47. Henmer W, Focke M, Wantke F, et al. Allergic contact dermatitis to artificial fingernails prepared from UV light–cured acrylates. *J Am Acad Dermatol* 1996;35:377.

48. Fisher AA. Adverse nail reactions and paresthesia from "photobonded acrylate 'sculptured' nails." *Cutis* 1990;45:293.

49. Kanerva L, Estlander T, Jolanki R, Tarvainen K. Dermatitis from acrylates in dental personnel. In: Menne T, Maibach HI, eds. *Hand Eczema*. Boca Raton, FL: CRC Press, 1994:231.

50. Kanerva L, Estlander T, Jolanki R. Occupational allergic contact dermatitis from acrylates: observations concerning anaerobic acrylic sealants and dental composite resins. In: Frosch PJ, Dooms-Goossens A, Lachapelle J-M, et al, eds. *Current Topics in Contact Dermatitis*. Berlin: Springer-Verlag; 1989:352.

51. Dahlquist I, Fregert S, Trulsson L. Contact allergy to trimethylolpropane triacrylate (TMPTA) in an aziridine plastic hardener. *Contact Dermatitis* 1983;9:122.

52. Cofield BG, Storrs FJ, Strawn CB. Contact allergy to aziridine paint hardener. *Arch Dermatol* 1985;121:373.

53. Kanerva L, Estlander T, Jolanki R, et al. Occupational allergic contact dermatitis and contact urticaria caused by polyfunctional aziridine hardener. *Contact Dermatitis* 1995;33:304.

54. Dempsey KJ. Hypersensitivity to Sta-Lok and Loctite anaerobic sealants. *J Am Acad Dermatol* 962;7:779.

55. Ranchoff RE, Taylor JS. Contact dermatitis to anaerobic sealants. *J Am Acad Dermatol* 1985;13:1015.

56. Conde-Salazar L, Guimaraens D, Romero LV. Occupational allergic contact dermatitis from anaerobic acrylic sealants. *Contact Dermatitis* 1988;18:129.

57. van der Walle HB. *Sensitizing Potential of Acrylic Monomers in Guinea Pig*. Thesis, Katholieke Universiteit te Nijmegen, Holland, Kripps Repro Meppel, 1982.

58. Waegemaekers T. *Some Toxicological Aspects of Acrylic Monomers, Notably with Reference to the Skin*. Thesis, Katholieke Universiteit te Nijmegen, Holland, 1985.

59. Parker D, Turk JL. Contact sensitivity to acrylate compounds in guinea pigs. *Contact Dermatitis* 1983;9:55.

60. Björkner B. Sensitization capacity of acrylated prepolymers in ultraviolet curing inks tested in the guinea pig. *Acta Derm Venereol (Stockh)* 1981;61:7.

61. Cavelier C, Jelen G, Herve-Bazin B, et al. Irritation et allergique aux acrylates et methacrylates. Monoacrylates et monomethacrylates simples. *Ann Derm Venereol* 1981;108:549.

62. Björkner B, Niklasson B, Persson K. The sensitizing potential of di(meth)acrylates based on bisphenol A or epoxy resin in the guinea pig. *Contact Dermatitis* 1984;10:286.

63. Björkner B. Sensitization capacity of polyester methacrylate in ultraviolet curing inks tested in the guinea pig. *Acta Derm Venereol* 1982;62:153.

64. Björkner B. Sensitizing potential of urethane (meth)acrylates in the guinea pig. *Contact Dermatitis* 1984;11:115.

65. Björkner B. *Sensitizing Capacity of Ultraviolet Curable Acrylic Compounds*. Thesis, University of Lund, Lund, Sweden, 1984.

66. Beurey J, Mougeolle J-M, Weber M. Accidents cutanes des resines acryliques dans l'imprimerie. *Ann Dermatol Syphilol (Paris)* 1976;103:423.

67. Malten KE, den Arend JACJ, Wiggers RE. Delayed irritation: hexa: diol diacrylate and butanediol diacrylate. *Contact Dermatitis* 1979;5:178.

68. Nethercott JR, Gupta S, Rosen C, et al. Tetraethylene glycol diacrylate. A cause of delayed cutaneous irritant reaction and allergic contact dermatitis. *J Occup Med* 1984;26:513.

69. Finnish Advisory Board of Chemicals. *Acrylate Compounds, Uses and Evaluation of Health Effects*. Helsinki, Finland: Government Printing Office; 1992.

70. Nethercott JR, Jakubovic HR, Pilger C, et al. Allergic contact dermatitis due to urethane acrylate in ultraviolet cured inks. *Br J Ind Med* 1982;40:241.

71. Bang Pedersen N, Senning A, Otkjaer Nielsen A: Different sensitizing acrylic monomers in NAPP printing plate. *Contact Dermatitis* 1983;9:459.

72. Björkner B. Contact allergy to 2-hydroxypropyl methacrylate (2-HPMA) in an ultraviolet curable ink. *Acta Derm Venereol (Stockh)* 1984;64:264.

73. Malten KE, Bende WM. 2-Hydroxy-ethyl methacrylate and di- and tetraethylene glycol dimethacrylate: contact sensitizers in photoprepolymer printing plate procedure. *Contact Dermatitis* 1976;5:214.

74. Kanerva L, Estlander T, Jolanki R. Occupational skin allergy in dental profession. *Dermatol Clin* 1994;12:517.

75. Kanerva L, Henriks-Eckerman M-L, Estlander T, et al. Occupational allergic contact dermatitis and composition of acrylates in dental bonding systems. *J Eur Acad Dermatol Venereol* 1994;3:157.

76. Kanerva L, Estlander T, Jolanki R. Allergic contact dermatitis from dental composite resins due to aromatic epoxy acrylates and aliphatic acrylates. *Contact Dermatitis* 1989;20:201.

77. Kanerva L, Estlander T, Jolanki R. Dental problems. In: Guin JD, ed. *Practical Contact Dermatitis*. New York: McGraw-Hill; 1995:397.

78. Whittington CW. Dermatitis from UV acrylate in adhesive. *Contact Dermatitis* 1981;7:203.

79. Fregert S. Occupational hazards of acrylate bone cement in orthopedic surgery. *Acta Orthop Scand* 1983;54:787.

80. Kanerva L, Estlander T, Jolanki R. Allergic contact dermatitis from dental composite resins due to aromatic

epoxy acrylates and aliphatic acrylates. *Contact Dermatitis* 1989;20:201.

81. Bohling HG, Borchard U, Drouin H. Monomeric methylmethacrylate acts on desheathed myelinated nerve and on node of Ranvier. *Arch Toxicol* 1977;38:307.

82. Kanerva L, Verkkala E. Electron microscopy and immunohistochemistry of toxic and allergic effects of methylmethacrylate on the skin. *Arch Toxicol* 1986; 9[Suppl]:456.

83. Matthias CGT, Turner MC, Maibach H. Contact dermatitis and gastrointestinal symptoms from hydroxyethyl methacrylate. *Br J Dermatol* 1979;110:447.

84. Edwards PM. Neurotoxicity of acrylamide and its analogues and effects of these analogues and other agents on acrylamides neuropathy. *Br J Ind Med* 1975;32:31.

85. Balda BR. Allergic contact dermatitis due to acrylonitrile. *Contact Dermatitis Newslett* 1971;9:219.

86. Balda BR. Akrylonitril als Kontaktallergen. *Hautarzt* 1975;26:599.

87. Romaquera C, Grimalt F, Vilaplana J. Methyl methacrylate prosthesis dermatitis. *Contact Dermatitis* 1985; 12:172.

88. Bakker RJG, Jongen SM, van-Neer FC, et al. Occupational contact dermatitis due to acrylonitrile. *Contact Dermatitis* 1991;1:50.

89. Malten KE. Printing plate manufacturing processes. In: Maibach HI, ed. *Occupational and Industrial Dermatology*, 2nd ed. Chicago: Year Book; 1987;351.

90. Malten KE, van der Meer-Roosen CH, Seutter E. Nyloprint-sensitive patients react to NN'-methylene-bis-acrylamide. *Contact Dermatitis* 1978;4:214.

91. Pedersen NB, Chevallier M-A, Senning A. Secondary acrylamides in Nyloprint printing plate as a source of contact dermatitis. *Contact Dermatitis* 1982;8:256.

92. Dooms-Goossens A, Garmyn M, Degreff H. Contact allergy to acrylamide. *Contact Dermatitis* 1991;24:71.

93. Lambert J, Matthieu L, Dockx P. Contact dermatitis from acrylamide. *Contact Dermatitis* 1988;19:65.

94. Pye RJ, Peachey RD. Contact dermatitis due to Nyloprint. *Contact Dermatitis* 1976;2:44.

95. Wang M-T, Wenger K, Maibach HI. Piperazine diacrylamide allergic contact dermatitis. *Contact Dermatitis* 1997;37:300.

96. Calnan CD. Cyanoacrylate dermatitis. *Contact Dermatitis* 1979;5:165.

97. Malten KE. Old and new, mainly occupational dermatological problems in the production and processing of plastics. In: Maibach HI, Gellin GA, eds. *Occupational and Industrial Dermatology*. Chicago: Year Book; 1982:237.

98. Jacobs MC, Rycroft RJ. Allergic contact dermatitis from cyanoacrylate? *Contact Dermatitis* 1995;33:71.

99. Fitzgerald DA, Bhaggoe R, English JS. Contact sensitivity to cyanoacrylate nail adhesive with dermatitis at remote sites. *Contact Dermatitis* 1995;32:175.

100. Tomb RR, Lepoittevin J-P, Durepaire F, et al. Ectopic contact dermatitis from ethyl-cyanoacrylate instant adhesives. *Contact Dermatitis* 1993;28:206.

101. Belsito D. Contact dermatitis to ethyl cyanoacrylate containing glue. *Contact Dermatitis* 1987;17:234.

102. Pigatto PD, Giacchetta A, Altornare GF. Unusual sensitization to cyanoacrylate ester. *Contact Dermatitis* 1986;14:193.

103. Fisher AA. Reactions to cyanoacrylate adhesives: "instant glue." *Cutis* 1985;35:18.

104. Shelley ED, Shelley WB. Chronic dermatitis simulating small-plaque parapsoriasis due to cyanoacrylate adhesive used on finger nails. *JAMA* 1984;252:2455.

105. Bruze M, Björkner B, Lepoittevin J-P. Occupational allergic contact dermatitis from ethyl-cyanoacrylate. *Contact Dermatitis* 1995;32:156.

106. Pegum JC, Medhurst FA. Contact dermatitis from penetration of rubber gloves by acrylic monomer. *Br Med J* 1971;2:141.

107. Rietschel RL., Huggins R, Levy N, Pruitt PM. In vivo and in vitro testing of gloves for protection against UV-curable acrylate resin systems. *Contact Dermatitis* 1984;11:279.

108. Munksgaard EC. Permeability of protective gloves to (di)methacrylates in resinous dental materials. *Scand J Dent Res* 1992;100:189.

109. Kanerva L, Estlander T, Jolanki R. Sensitization to patch test acrylates. *Contact Dermatitis* 1988;18:10.

110. Malten KE. Occupational dermatoses in the processing of plastics. *Trans St. John's Hosp Dermatol Soc* 1964;59:78.

111. Estlander T, Keskinen H, Jolanki R, et al. Occupational dermatitis from exposure to polyurethane chemicals. *Contact Dermatitis* 1992;27:161.

112. Zeiss CR, Kanellakes TM, Bellone JD, et al. Immunoglobulin E–mediated asthma and hypersensitive pneumonitis with precipitating anti-hapten antibodies due to diphenylmethane diisocyanate (MDI exposure). *J Allerg Clin Immunol* 1980;60:346.

113. Mowe G. Health risks from isocyanates. *Contact Dermatitis* 1980;8:44.

114. Baur X. Isocyanates. *Clin Exp Allerg* 1991;21[suppl 1]:241.

115. Rothe A. Zur Frage arbeitsbedingter Hautschädigungen durch Polyurethanchemikalien. *Derm Beruf Umwelt* 1976;24:7.

116. Kanerva L, Lähteenmäki M-T, Estlander T, et al: Allergic contact dermatitis from isocyanates. In: Frosch PJ, Dooms-Goossens A, Lachapelle J-M, eds. *Current Topics in Contact Dermatitis*. Berlin: Springer-Verlag; 1989:366.

117. Kanerva L, Estlander T, Jolanki R, et al. Occupational urticaria from welding polyurethane. *J Am Acad Dermatol* 1991;24:825.

118. Tanaka K, Takeoka A, Nishimura F, Hanada S. Contact sensitivity induced in mice by methylene bisphenyl diisocyanate. *Contact Dermatitis* 1987;17:199.

119. White IR, Stewart JR, Rycroft RJG. Allergic contact dermatitis from an organic di-isocyanate. *Contact Dermatitis* 1983;9:300.

120. Malten KE. Dermatological problems with synthetic resins and plastics in glues. Part I. *Derm Beruf Umwelt* 1984;32:81.

121. Malten KE. Dermatological problems with synthetic resins and plastics in glues. Part II. *Derm Beruf Umwelt* 1984;32:118.

122. Van Joost Th, Heule F, De Boer J. Sensitization to methylenedianiline and para-structures. *Contact Dermatitis* 1987;16:246.

123. Emmett EA. Allergic contact dermatitis in polyurethane plastic moulders. *J Occup Med* 1976;18:802.

124. Wilkinson SM, Cartwright PH, Armitage J, et al. Allergic contact dermatitis from 1,6-diisocyanatohexane in an anti-pill finish. *Contact Dermatitis* 1991;25:94.

125. Elvers B, Hawkins S, Schulz G, eds. *Ullmans's Encyclopedia of Industrial Chemistry*, 5th ed, Vol A19. New York: VCH; 1991:371.

126. Bruze M. Contact sensitizers in resins based on phenol and formaldehyde. *Acta Derm Venereol (Stockh)* 1995;119[Suppl]:1.

127. Estlander T, Tarvainen K, Jolanki R, Kanerva L. Occupational sensitization to a resin binder used in rock wool. In: *Books of Abstracts, Third Congress of the European Academy of Dermatology and Venereology*. Copenhagen: 1993:283.

128. Kalimo K, Saarni H, Kyttä J. Immediate and delayed type reactions to formaldehyde resin in glass wool. *Contact Dermatitis* 1980;6:396.

129. Foussereau J, Cavelier C, Selig D: Occupational eczema from para-tertiary-butylphenol formaldehyde resins: a review of the sensitizing resins. *Contact Dermatitis* 1976;2:254.

130. Schubert H, Agatha G. Zur Allergennatur der para-tert. Butylphenol-formaldehydeharze. *Derm Beruf Umwelt* 1979;27:49.

131. White IR. Adhesives. In: Adams RM, ed. *Occupational Skin Disease*, 2nd ed. Philadelphia: WB Saunders; 1990:395.

132. Zimerson E, Bruze M. Contact allergy to the monomers of *p*-tert-butylphenol formaldehyde resin in the guinea pig. *Contact Dermatitis.* Submitted.

133. Bruze M. Patch testing with a mixture of 2 phenol-formaldehyde resins. *Contact Dermatitis* 1988;19:116.

134. Bruze M, Zimerson E. Cross-reaction patterns in patients with contact allergy to simple methylol phenols. *Contact Dermatitis* 1997;37:82.

135. Bruze M. Simultaneous reactions to phenol-formaldehyde resins colophony/hydroabietyl alcohol and balsam of Peru/parfume mixture. *Contact Dermatitis* 1986;14:119.

136. Bruze M, Zimerson E. Contact allergy to 3-methylol phenol, 2,4-dimethylol phenol and 2,6-dimethylol phenol. *Acta Derm Venereol (Stockh)* 1985;65:548.

137. Bruze M. Sensitizing capacity of 4,4-dihydroxy-(hydroxymethyl)-diphenyl methanes in the guinea pig. *Acta Derm Venereol (Stockh)* 1986;66:110.

138. Fregert S. Irritant dermatitis from phenol-formaldehyde resin powder. *Contact Dermatitis* 1980;6:493.

139. Bruze M, Fregert S, Zimerson E. Contact allergy to phenol-formaldehyde resins. *Contact Dermatitis* 1985;12:81.

140. Bruze M, Almgren G. Occupational dermatoses in workers exposed to resins based on phenol and formaldehyde. *Contact Dermatitis* 1988;19:272.

141. Bruze M. Patch testing with a mixture of 2 phenol-formaldehyde resins. *Contact Dermatitis* 1988;19:116.

142. Mathias CGT. Allergic contact dermatitis from triglycidyl isocyanurate in polyester paint pigments. *Contact Dermatitis* 1988;19:67.

143. Venables K. Low molecular weight chemicals, hypersensitivity, and direct toxity: the acid anhydrides. *Br J Ind Med* 1989;46:222.

144. Malten KE, Zielhuis RL. *Industrial Toxicology and Dermatology in the Production and Processing of Plastics.* Elsevier: New York; 1964.

145. Wehle V. Arbeitsbedingte Ekzeme durch Polyester. *Allergie Asthma* 1966;12:184.

146. Lidén C, Löfström A, Storgårds-Hatam K. Contact allergy to unsaturated polyester in a boatbuilder. *Contact Dermatitis* 1984;11:262.

147. Dooms-Goossens A, De Jong G. [Letter to the editor.] *Contact Dermatitis* 1985;12:238.

148. Mac Farlane AW, Curley RK, King CM. Contact sensitivity to unsaturated polyester resin in a limb prosthesis. *Contact Dermatitis* 1986;15:301.

149. Tarvainen K, Jolanki R, Estlander R. Occupational contact allergy to unsaturated polyester resin cements. *Contact Dermatitis* 1993;28:220.

150. Malten KE. Dermatological problems with synthetic resins and plastics in glue. Part I. *Derm Beruf Umwelt* 1984;32:81.

151. Bourne L, Milner F. Polyester resin hazards. *Br J Indust Med* 1963;20:100.

152. Meneghini CL, Rantuccio F, Riboldi A. Klinisch-allergologische Beobachtungen bei beruflichen ekzematösen Kontakt-Dermatosen. *Derm Beruf Umwelt* 1963;11:181.

153. Sjöborg S, Fregert S, Trulsson L. Contact allergy to styrene and related chemicals. *Contact Dermatitis* 1984;10:94.

154. Schmunes E. Solvents and plasticizers. In: Adams RM, ed. *Occupational Skin Diseases*, 2nd ed. Philadelphia: WB Saunders; 1990.

155. Fregert S. Formaldehyde dermatitis from a gypsum-melamine resin mixture. *Contact Dermatitis* 1981;7:56.

156. Belsito DV. Textile dermatitis. *Am J Contact Dermatitis* 1993;4:249.

157. Ross JS, Rycroft RJG, Cronin E. Melamine-formaldehyde contact dermatitis in orthopaedic practice. *Contact Dermatitis* 1992;26:203.

158. Vale PT, Rycroft RJG. Occupational irritant contact dermatitis from fibreboard containing urea formaldehyde resin. *Contact Dermatitis* 1988;19:62.

159. Dooms-Goossens AE, Debusschere KM, Gevers DM, et al. Contact dermatitis caused by airborne agents. *J Am Acad Dermatol* 1986;15:1.

160. Conde-Salazar L, Gonzales M, Guimaraens D, et al. Occupational contact dermatitis from styrene. *Contact Dermatitis* 1989;21:112.

161. Moscato G, Biscaldi G, Cottica D, et al. Occupational asthma due to styrene: two case reports. *J Occup Med* 1987;29:957.

162. Bruze M, Fregert S. Chemical skin burns. In: Menne T, Maibach HI, eds. *Hand Eczema.* Boca Raton, Fla: CRC; 1994:21.

163. Vidovic R, Kansky A. Contact dermatitis in workers processing polyvinyl chloride plastics. *Derm Beruf Umwelt* 1985;33:104.

164. Schulsinger C, Möllegaard K. Polyvinyl chloride dermatitis not caused by phthalates. *Contact Dermatitis* 1980;6:477.

165. Fregert S, Rorsman H. Hypersensitivity to epoxy resins used as plasticizers and stabilizers in polyvinyl chloride resins. *Acta Derm Venereol (Stockh)* 1963;43:10.

166. Fregert S, Trulsson L, Zimerson E. Contact allergic reaction to diphenylthiourea and phenylisothiocyanate in PVC adhesive tape. *Contact Dermatitis* 1982;8:38.

167. Hills RJ, Ive FA. Allergic contact dermatitis from diisodecyl phthalate in a polyvinyl chloride identification band. *Contact Dermatitis* 1993;29:94.

168. Di Lernia V, Cameli N, Patrizi A. Irritant contact dermatitis in a child caused by the plastic tube of infusion system. *Contact Dermatitis* 1989;21:339.

169. Osmundsen PE. Contact urticaria from nickel and plastic additives, butylhydroxytoluene, oleyamide. *Contact Dermatitis* 1980;6:452.

170. Fregert S, Meding B, Trulsson L. Demonstration of epoxy resin in stoma pouch plastic. *Contact Dermatitis* 1984;10:106.

171. Goh CL, Ho SF. An outbreak of acneiform eruption in a polyvinyl chloride manufacturing factory. *Derm Beruf Umwelt* 1988;36:53.

172. Thestrup-Pedersen K, Madsen JB, Rasmussen K. Cumulative skin irritance from heat-decomposed polyethylene plastic. In: Frosch PJ, Dooms-Goossens A, Lachapelle J-M, Rycroft RJG, Scheper RJ, eds. *Current Topics in Contact Dermatitis.* Berlin: Springer-Verlag; 1989:412.

173. Bruze M, Boman A, Bergqvist-Karlsson A, et al. Contact allergy to cyclohexanone resin in humans and guinea pigs. *Contact Dermatitis* 1988:18:46.

174. Heine A, Laubstein B. Contact dermatitis from cyclohexanone-formaldehyde resin (L2 resin) in a hair lacquer spray. *Contact Dermatitis* 1990;22:108.

175. Husain SL. Dibutylphthalate sensitivity. *Contact Dermatitis* 1975;1:6:395.

176. Calnan CD. Dibutylphthalate. *Contact Dermatitis* 1975;1:6:388.

177. Sneddon IB. Dermatitis from dibutylphthalate in an aerosol anti-perspirant and deodorant. *Contact Dermatitis Newslett* 1972;12:308.
178. Wilkinson SM, Beck MH. Allergic contact dermatitis from dibutyl phthalate, propylgallate and hydrocortisone in Timodine. *Contact Dermatitis* 1992;27:197.
179. Smith EL, Calnan CD. Studies in contact dermatitis XVII. Spectacle frames. *Trans St John Hosp Derm Soc* 1966;52:10.
180. Oliwiecki S, Beck MH, Chalmers RJG. Contact dermatitis from spectacle frames and hearing aid containing diethyl phthalate. *Contact Dermatitis* 1991;25:264.
181. Capon F, Cambie MP, Clinard F, et al. Occupational contact dermatitis caused by computer mice. *Contact Dermatitis* 1996;35:57.
182. Burrows D, Rycroft RJG. Contact dermatitis from PTBP resin and tricresylethylphthalate in a plastic nail adhesive. *Contact Dermatitis* 1981;7:336.
183. Hamanaka S, Hamanaka I, Otsuka F. Phthalic acid dermatitis caused by an organostanic compound, tributyltinphthalate. Dermatology 1992;184:210.
184. Carlsen L, Andersen KE, Egsgaard H. Triphenylphosphate allergy from spectacle frames. *Contact Dermatitis* 1986;15:274.
185. Camarasa JG, Serra-Baldrich E. Allergic contact dermatitis from triphenylphosphate. *Contact Dermatitis* 1992;26:264.
186. Andersen KE. Sensitivity to a flame retardant, tris(2,3-dibromopropyl)phosphate (Firemaster L VT 23 P). *Contact Dermatitis* 1977;3:297.
187. Niklasson B, Björkner B. Contact allergy to the UV-absorber Tinuvin P in plastics. *Contact Dermatitis* 1989;21:330.
188. Ikarashi Y, Tsuchiya T, Nakamura A. Contact sensitivity to Tinuvin P in mice. *Contact Dermatitis* 1994;30:225.
189. Kanerva L, Jolanki R, Estlander T. Organic pigment as a cause of plastic glove dermatitis. *Contact Dermatitis*, 1985;13:41.
190. Jolanki R, Kanerva L, Estlander T. Organic pigments in plastics can cause allergic contact dermatitis. *Acta Derm Venereol (Stockh)* 1987[Suppl]:134:95.

26

Semiconductor Industry

GARY R. FUJIMOTO, M.D.

Since its beginning in 1948, the microelectronics industry has shown a remarkably rapid growth. It is estimated that by the year 2000, it will be the fourth largest industry in the U.S. Currently, 213,000 workers are employed, producing a product with a market value in excess of 24 billion dollars per year. Formerly operating almost entirely in California and Massachusetts, the industry has expanded to many more parts of the U.S. and abroad. Numerous small companies, many of them less than a few years old, surround the several giants of the industry, which is characterized by intense competition and rapid change in processes and techniques.

The rapid proliferation of the use of computers across all aspects of society has driven the demand for silicon chips to record levels. Many of the components of the silicon wafer are highly toxic despite the appearance of a clean industry. Within the semiconductor industry, technology is constantly pushed by the ever elusive need for even faster processing. Such technology is continually involved in searching for and introducing new materials and processes to achieve this end.

The silicon chip or wafer is essentially a complex, three-dimensional circuit board created by overlaying various chemical substrates in a microscopic network. The patterns and materials create the equivalent electronic interface that previously required large transistors, capacitors, and other devices. The electronic components that previously filled the floors in a building have been reduced to the size of small notebooks.

The exceedingly small size of these complex matrices requires the avoidance of dust and fine particulate matter in the production process. Dust disrupts the microscopic interface on the silicon surface. The solution to this problem has been the development of a filtration system that provides highly purified air to the production process. This system requires that the technicians in this area wear containment suits. They prevent the release of skin dander and other particulate material from the body. These suits are not personal protection equipment for the production staff since much of the highly filtered air is recirculated through these rooms. This pattern of airflow in the semiconductor clean room poses a potential health hazard since inadvertently released gases may also be recirculated within the production area.

The wafer is generated by the introduction of a seed crystal of silicon into a crucible containing molten silicon within an argon atmosphere. This process results in a highly purified rod or ingot of silicon. When cooled, the ingot is sliced and prepared by machine to thin wafers. These wafers are then highly polished and cleaned.

Silicon wafers undergo a series of chemical treatments that apply various compounds containing electron-rich or electron-poor areas. These "n" or negative regions and "p" or positive regions form the bases for the microscopic array of connections. The n-type regions are composed of materials that release electrons such as nitrogen, phosphorus, and arsenic. The p-type regions accept electrons and are composed of materials such as boron.

Hundreds of different steps are required to complete the semiconductor wafer fabrication. The basic components of this process include application of protective layers to the wafer and further processes to make these areas more or less reactive to subsequent chemical application.

Etching is a process whereby surface layers on the silicon wafer are removed by chemical dissolution. Wet and dry etching are the two systems that are utilized for this process.

Wet etching includes a variety of concentrated acids to remove the unprotected areas on the wafer surface. One of these acids, hydrofluoric acid

(HF), poses special problems because of the highly electronegative fluoride ion and not the pH of the acid. HF burns can cause liquefaction necrosis of the underlying tissues. The fluoride ion disrupts tissue membranes and binds avidly to calcium and magnesium. Skin exposures require the specific treatment described in Chapter 1. Systemic poisonings usually follow large dermal exposures with concentrated HF and can cause hypocalcemia, hypomagnesemia, and death.

Dry etching involves ionized gas, usually chlorine, fluoride, or bromine compounds, in an electric field. This process leads to a chemical reaction that etches the wafer surface.

Chemical doping on the silicon wafer involves application of selected gases, liquids, or solid agents to the matrix using compounds such as antimony, arsine, phosphine, or diborane to create the n and p regions. High temperature diffusion allows some of these compounds to penetrate into the unmasked areas on the silicon matrix.

Arsine (AsH_3) is a colorless, odorless, and non-irritating gas. It is the most toxic form of arsenic. Arsine can cause massive intravascular hemolysis and oliguric renal failure. Toxic symptoms may be delayed up to 24 hours. They have been reported to occur at levels as low as 3 to 10 parts per million (the OSHA PEL is 0.05 parts per million). Treatment includes hydration to maintain renal function, exchange transfusion for severe hemolysis, and hemodialysis for renal failure.

Phosphine is another potent toxic gas that has a strong fishlike or garliclike odor. Exposure can cause acute pulmonary irritation and delayed pulmonary edema as well as cardiovascular, hepatic, and renal damage. No specific treatment exists for exposure except supportive care.

Ion implantation involves generating a charged beam of dopant ions into the wafer's substrate. The gases in this process include arsine, phosphine, and diborane. While the process usually occurs in a high vacuum environment, off-gassing of the product as well as accidental release makes it a more hazardous step in wafer fabrication.

Once a layer of silicon is doped, an additional layer of silicon can be applied to create another electronic template. This process, known as epitaxy, electronically separates these layers and increases the storage capacity on the wafer.

Metallization is a process whereby a layer of metal is applied in a highly directed pattern, linking areas on the wafer together. This process is essentially a wiring system to interconnect the wafer surface into a functional system. Metals such as aluminum, copper, gold, chromium, nickel, silver, and platinum are frequently em-ployed. The two systems that use this method of deposition are evaporation and sputtering.

Evaporation involves heating the metal in a vacuum, which layers the metal on the wafer. In sputtering, an electric field is applied to argon gas. This accelerates these ions toward a metal target. Metal ions are generated and deposited on the wafer's surface.

Gallium arsenide is replacing silicon as the wafer substrate of choice due to the more rapid conduction of electrons on a gallium arsenide wafer. The toxic properties of this material, however, are significantly higher than those of silicon.

Newer systems to apply metals include various chlorinated and fluorinated gases along with metal silicates. As increasingly more exotic compounds are used in the search for superconducting materials, more complex and unusual toxicities can be expected.

WORKERS

The semiconductor industry tends to be "top heavy" with professional staff. Production workers constitute only 31% of the workforce. The remainder consists of a highly educated professional cadre supervising and constantly seeking innovations and expanded markets. The production workers tend to be young, female,[1] and foreign born. In 1997, the U.S. Bureau of Labor Statistics reported that the U.S. semiconductor industry ranked sixth of the 223 durable good manufacturing industries included in the 1996 survey with respect to the lowest rate of injuries and illnesses. The annual incidence of work-related injuries and illnesses among semiconductor workers was 3.3 per 100 full-time workers, compared with an incidence rate of 11.6 for durable goods workers and 10.6 for all manufacturing workers.[2]

The greatest number of reported injuries and illnesses are reported by workers in fabrication of the chip ("fab" workers), in which ergonomic stresses and chemical and physical hazards are present. Chemical exposures include dopants based on phosphorus, arsenic and boron compounds, solvents, photoresists, acids, and a variety of organic compounds. Among the physical hazards are x-rays and low-frequency electromagnetic and magnetic fields.[3] It has been claimed that the process controls that maintain the extreme purity of materials and the environment, without even the tiniest speck of dust, contribute to worker safety. However, there is no firm data to substantiate this claim. Nevertheless, if controls are poorly designed or implemented, or if there is equipment failure, poor maintenance, and sloppy work practices with inadequate training, preventable diseases and accidents could and will occur not only to production workers, but also to those in research and development.[1]

DERMATITIS

In a survey of the health of semiconductor workers, McCurdy, et al.[4] found dermatitis to be the second most common disorder, after respiratory symptoms. In the semiconductor industry, skin irritants abound,[5] especially in wafer production procedures during wet etching, which uses highly irritating HF and ammonium fluoride in a variety of mixtures to remove the silicon dioxide layer of the chip. As mentioned, in the ion implantation processes, several arsenic, boron, and phosphorus compounds are utilized. Other irritants in the industry include hydrochloric, orthophosphoric, and HF acids, phosphine gas, zinc and ammonium chloride, various organic acids, methylene chloride, aniline hydrochloride, ethylenediamine, and mono- and trithanolamine, arsine gas, and various organic solvents.[6]

SOLVENTS

Huge amounts of solvents are used as degreasers, diluents, cleansers, and chemical reactants in this industry. The most important are tri- and tetrachlorethylene; toluene; *N*-butyl acetate; xylene; acetone; 1,1,-trichloroethane; Freon; methanol; methylene chloride; ethylene glycol; methylethyl ketone; and *N*-methylpyralidone. Solvents tend to dry and defat the skin. From prolonged exposure, they can induce a chronic, scaling, fissured dermatitis. When occluded by gloves or solvent-soaked clothing, bullae may result, as McBirney[7] described in 1954, from exposure to the vapors of trichloroethylene (TCE). The vapors of hot solvents, such as those arising from open degreasing tanks, may cause severe burns. Inhalation of even small amounts of TCE, followed within an hour or two by consumption of alcohol, may result in a curious facial and neck erythema termed "degreaser's flush,"[8] as well as irritation of the mucous membranes of the upper respiratory tract and eyes. Varying degrees of inebriation may also result.[9]

Stevens-Johnson syndrome was reported in five electronics workers who worked in a poorly ventilated area where there was a partially enclosed degreasing tank containing TCE. The workers not only employed the solvent to clean parts but also employed the too common practice of wiping off their hands and forearms with the solvent. All developed chemical hepatitis and one died.[10] Cold urticaria, developed from a spray of TCE used to clean electronic contacts between various parts, was described by Bjorkner in 1981.[11] The information on the Material Safety Data Sheet (MSDS) regarding toxicity of solvents may not always be adequate in regard to cutaneous effects.[12] To determine an excessive exposure to TCE, urine can be checked for trichloroacetic acid and the serum for TCE. Both may still be present up to 4 to 5 days following exposure.[9]

SOLDERING FLUX

Solder is a filler metal with a melting point of less than 600°F (315°C). Most solder is composed of a lead-tin, low-melting alloy. Soldering consists of joining metal surfaces without melting the base metal. All metals have a surface film from the surrounding atmosphere consisting of various oxides, sulfides, carbonates, and other corrosion products. To obtain a good mechanical bond between two surfaces, it is important for the flux to remove this film. Fluxes contain various inorganic and organic acids, salts, amines, amides, and so forth. Most of these are irritating and corrosive on the skin. Some are rosin-based (e.g., abietic acid), in which the rosin may be present in the core of the solder. During soldering, the fumes may be released into the atmosphere, causing an airborne-type dermatitis in the worker.

Soldering first involves cleaning the base metal, using solvent, solvent vapor ("vapor degreasing"), or ultrasonic degreasing.[13] Next, a flux is applied. Proprietary fluxes are available in solid, paste, and liquid forms, which are applied by brushing, spraying, or dipping, or as a paste. Most manual soldering operations use a soldering iron, or by dipping, use a solder pot. Variations of this pot have been employed in the semiconductor industry for soldering printed circuit boards (Fig. 26–1). Furnace soldering is also common.

Although hand soldering is still done in joining the electrical connections, the trend has been automation of this process. Hand soldering may especially be used for rejected or returned parts where minor faults are discovered during inspection. Hand soldering is a common source of dermatitis, especially when performed without gloves (Fig. 26–2).[14] Fluxes cause both irritant and allergic contact dermatitis. Hydroxyethyl ethylenediamine, an activator present in some fluxes, may induce contact sensitization.[15] The dermatitis usually begins in the periungual areas and spreads along the fingers to the wrists. A more frequent cause of

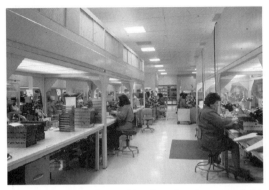

FIGURE 26–1 • Final assembly takes place in a remarkably clean environment. Soldering fluxes, adhesives, and various solvents used for cleaning, however, may cause dermatitis.

sensitization from soldering is colophony (rosin),[16, 16a] present as a core flux in many forms of solder.[17] Because the antigenic properties of the various rosin types may differ, Liden[18] and Mathias and Adams[19] have emphasized the importance of patch testing with the rosin actually used by the patient in its appropriate concentration.

During soldering, the flux is heated to a temperature of approximately 450°C, and fumes containing the allergen may induce an airborne der-

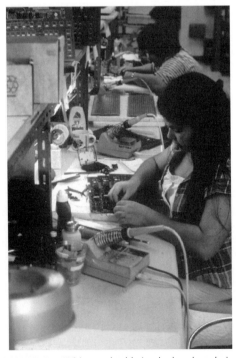

FIGURE 26–2 • Wiring and soldering by hand are being replaced by automation, eliminating a frequent cause of dermatitis in the semiconductor industry.

matitis of the face and neck, occasionally with asthmatic symptoms.[20] The latter occurrence helps to emphasize the importance of an effective exhaust system, especially during hand soldering.

For years, abietic acid was considered the chief allergen in rosin,[21] but it now appears that this acid acts as a prohapten.[16] The oxidation products of dehydroabietic acid are the allergens, especially 7-oxydehydroabietic acid and 15-hydroxydehydroabietic acid.

LATEX RUBBER GLOVES

Contact urticaria from latex rubber gloves has become an increasingly serious problem for the industry (see Chapter 6). The reaction develops within minutes of contact and can occasionally be very severe and even life-threatening. Contact allergic dermatitis results from the presence of antioxidants and accelerators in rubber and, rarely, from natural latex. The reaction is delayed, up to 48 hours following contact, and lasts for 7 to 10 days (see Chapter 29).

HYDROFLUORIC ACID

Without exception, the most important irritant in semiconductor work is HF acid, which is used in great quantities in the manufacturing process, especially in wet etching. Contact with HF acid in concentrations of from 15 to 20% may not cause symptoms initially, but as the acid penetrates into deeper layers of the skin and subcutaneous tissues, extensive tissue damage, including necrosis of bone may result, accompanied by excruciating pain (see Chapter 1).

The frequency of serious HF burns has been diminished, chiefly because of increased automation of the industry. Furthermore, worker education has played an important role, as has the provision of better protective clothing.

EPOXY RESIN

A fairly common cause of contact allergic sensitization in the semiconductor industry is epoxy resin. The usual source is a resin with a molecular weight of 340. These low-molecular-weight epoxies are usually cured with amine catalysts, making possible rapid polymerization and hardening. These epoxies have been utilized in chip manufacture less frequently, and today are almost always either premixed or mixed by an automated process, resulting in little or no skin contact. In countries where the electronics industry is the major industry, however, more than a third of all cases of epoxy-resin allergy originate from this industry.[22] Epoxy resins are very useful for die attach, device encapsulation, and ingot mounting prior to slicing into wafers. When allergic sensitization occurs, it may be severe, requiring transfer of the worker to an area that is completely epoxy free. The hardeners are less common causes of allergic contact dermatitis.

SILK-SCREENING

Silk-screening is an important process in the manufacture of printed circuit boards. The inks may be epoxy- or acrylate-based. A mesh-stencil process is used for coating the boards, which are exposed to ultraviolet light to complete the curing process. They are then placed in an oven to dry. In this process, workers may be exposed to highly sensitizing chemicals such as 4,4'-diaminodiphenylmethane, triglycidyl isocyanurate, and 2-hydroxyethyl methacrylate.[23]

ANAEROBIC SEALANTS

Anaerobic sealants are valuable in this industry not only because of their resistance to shock and vibration, but also because of their ability to polymerize almost instantly in the absence of air, immediately after being placed between two adjoining surfaces. The three most important commercial tradenames are Sta-Lok, Loctite, and Treebond (e.g., Crazy Glue and Super Glue). Because of their rapid action, it was thought that they induced only irritation;[24, 25] however, the first reported cases of contact allergy to these sealants was by Allardice[26] and later by Jansen.[27] In 1982, allergic contact dermatitis to Sta-Lok and Loctite was described by Dempsey[28] in three cases. Mathias and Maibach[19a] described three patients who assembled electronic parts and developed allergic contact dermatitis owing to the polyethylene glycol dimethacrylate (PEGMA) used as a sealant. In 1985, Ranchoff and Taylor[29] reported a case of sensitivity to three Loctite sealants in a machine assembler. Extensive patch testing revealed positive patch tests to polyethylene glycol dimethacrylate and to hydroxypropyl and hydroxyethyl methacrylate.

Patussi, et al.[30] described two cases of allergic dermatitis to Loctite 270 and 290 in which PEGMA also appeared to be the culprit. A study of six patients with allergic contact dermatitis to these sealants is by Conde-Salazar, et al.,[31] in which hydroxyethyl methacrylate gave the most positive responses. In most cases, because the application of these sealants requires manual dexterity, the dermatitis is predominantly on the distal part of the fingers and volar fingertips, especially the tips of the thumbs, index and middle fingers, with onycholysis in some cases.[31]

Various methacrylate resins are used in photoresists in which electron beams and x-rays are used for crosslinking. Because the processes take place in completely closed systems, skin contact is unlikely, except in those who charge and clean the reactors.

RUBBER

Allergic reactions to rubber are fairly common in this industry, especially from latex rubber finger gloves and cots. These articles are worn for many hours, and the opportunity for development of an allergic reaction is considerable. Allergic contact dermatitis from accelerators and antioxidants in rubber is not uncommon and may also develop from gloves worn to protect a preexisting irritant dermatitis. Contact urticaria from glove materials including powder also occurs (Chapter 6).

Certain photoresists are based upon polyisoprene or polybutadiene rubber, but because this stage of wafer processing is done under a completely closed system, skin contact is unlikely to occur, except in individuals cleaning and servicing the equipment.

PHYSICAL CAUSES

Clean rooms where fabrication takes place provide a remarkable "other-world" atmosphere—an environment almost totally lacking in common stimuli. The workers don special smocks, cloth head covers, masks, gloves, and booties, and enter the work area through a special passage resembling a wind tunnel that blows away contaminants from the clothing (Fig. 26–3). The workers are not permitted to use cosmetics, wear BandAids, or smoke for several hours prior to entering these rooms. The ambient air is continuously filtered and recirculated several times hourly to maintain an extremely low level of dust. The ambient temperature is ideally kept at approximately 50°F to 60°F, with a relative humidity between 30 and 35%, which may at times reach between 20 and 30%. This atmosphere is conducive to the development of dry skin. Atopic workers are especially likely to complain of itching and dermatitis. From friction from the masks, dermatitis of the neck and

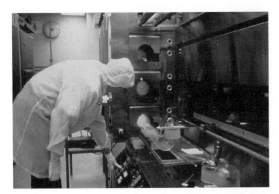

FIGURE 26–3 • Workers wear bunny-type suits in the fabrication areas, completely encasing their bodies, so that only a small portion of their faces is exposed.

face is common, aggravated by the low relative humidity and the drying of the skin.[32]

Fiberglass from printed circuit board workers can be a cause of an especially pruritic dermatitis.[33, 34]

Urticaria is also common in this type of environment, occurring more frequently in atopic workers and those with a tendency to dermographism. If a number of employees simultaneously develop similar symptoms, with itching, and if an unusual odor is also detected, the word may rapidly spread among the workers that a noxious substance has entered the enclosed, windowless workplace. Because a large portion of the air in clean rooms is recycled, solvent vapors and gases can become trapped in the system, either from "fugitive emissions" from production processes or through reentrainment from poorly placed ventilation intake and exhaust ducts.[1] When generalized itching is present, it is not difficult to understand how hysteria can disseminate among susceptible individuals.

Millions of dollars are spent each year investigating air pollution in the workplace. In some instances, the air circulation is indeed faulty and contributes to the complaints. If prompt environmental testing does not produce a satisfactory explanation for the workers' symptoms, however, mass psychogenic illness may result.[35, 36] This can result in temporary plant closings, extensive investigations, and much confusion and loss of worker confidence in the safety of the workplace.[37]

MISCELLANEOUS CAUSES

Numerous hazardous materials are used in the semiconductor industry. A distinct hazard is arsine gas, although the amounts involved are relatively small. Arsenic compounds are being used more and more frequently, however, replacing silicon as the wafer substrate. Arsine gas poisoning is unique in that rapid hemolysis results with relatively low exposure levels. Depending on the exposure, the symptoms vary and often are delayed 2 to 24 hours. They include abdominal pain, hematuria and jaundice, with laboratory findings consistent with Coombs-negative, hemolytic anemia. Treatment includes exchange transfusions, hemodialysis, and attention to arsine-induced, oliguric renal failure secondary to hemoglobinuria.

Although there have been no reports of arsenic-related carcinogenesis from this industry, a lag time of up to 30 to 35 years may be required before the characteristic arsenical keratoses and squamous cell carcinomas appear. Those who clean and repair reactors and diffusion furnaces appear to be at greatest risk.

Scleroderma and a scleroderma-like multisystem disease have been suggested to result from exposure to various solvents utilized in this industry, especially TCE.[38] The disorder seems to be limited to the skin of the hands and feet, where direct contact with solvent occurs.[39] A generalized morphea-like sclerosis has been described in association with exposure to various aliphatic hydrocarbons, including certain components of epoxy resins.[40, 41] Convincing proof of these claims has yet to be provided.

Nickel is found in hands tools and in many electronic assembly parts. It is unlikely that these contacts alone induce allergic sensitization to nickel, but in workers previously sensitized, especially from ear piercing, nickel dermatitis may result from contact with tools and nickel-plated parts. Electroplating with nickel also provides an occasional source of this allergy in sensitized persons.

A common etchant for stripping photoresist from wafers is ammonium persulfate, in combination with sulfuric acid. It is a potent oxidizing agent. As a bleach for hair it has been reported to cause contact urticaria, in which the reaction sometimes is very severe and widespread, with wheals, itching, and anaphylactoid responses that require the patient's hospitalization.[42, 43] Among workers who manufacture this chemical, irritant dermatitis is reported to be common.[44]

Other contact allergens that may occasionally be encountered in this industry are gold in electroplating and wiring, cobalt in manufacture of magnets, and platinum in electrical connections.

References

1. Wald PH, Jones JR. Semiconductor manufacturing: an introduction to processes and hazards. *Am J Indust Med* 1987; 11:203–221.

2. U.S. Bureau of Labor Statistics. Annual Survey, U.S. Semiconductor Industry, Durable Goods and All Manufacturing (1983–1996). Washington, D.C., 1997.

3. LaDou J. Health issues in the microelectronics industry. In: *Occupational Medicine: State of the Art Reviews*, Vol. 1. Philadelphia: Hanley & Belfus; 1986:1–11.

4. McCurdy SA, Pocekay D, Hammond SK, et al. A cross-sectional survey of respiratory and general health outcomes among semiconductor industry workers. *Am J Indust Med* 1995; 28:847–860.

5. Goh CL. Common industrial processes and occupational irritants and allergens—an update. *Ann Acad Med Singapore* 1994; 23:690–698.

6. Koh D. Electronics industry. *Clin Dermatol* 1997; 15:579–586.

7. McBirney RS. Trichloroethylene and dichloroethylene poisoning. *Arch Ind Hyg* 1954; 10:130–133.

8. Stewart RD, Hake CL, Peterson JE. Degreaser's flush. *Arch Environ Health* 1974; 29:1–5.

9. Bauer M, Rabens SF. Cutaneous manifestations of trichloroethylene toxicity. *Arch Dermatol* 1974; 110:886–890.

10. Phoon WH, Chan MOY, Rajan VS, et al. Stevens-Johnson syndrome associated with occupational exposure to trichloroethylene. *Contact Dermatitis* 1984; 10:270–276.

11. Bjorkner B. Occupational cold urticaria from contact spray. *Contact Dermatitis* 1981; 7:338–339.

12. Leira HL, Tiltnes A, Svendsen K, Vetlesen L. Irritant cutaneous reactions to *N*-methyl-2-pyrrolidone. *Contact Dermatitis* 1992; 27:148–150. (Solvent appeared very irritating, and more than reported on the MSDS.)

13. Burgess WA. Soldering in electronics. In: *Recognition of Health Hazards in Industry: A Review of Materials and Processes*, 2nd Ed. New York: John Wiley & Sons; 1995:375–382.

14. Koh D, Lee HS, Chia HP, et al. Skin disorders among hand solderers in the electronics industry. *Occup Med* 1994; 44:24–28.

15. Goh CL. Occupational dermatitis from soldering flux among workers in the electronics industry. *Contact Dermatitis* 1985; 13:85–90.

16. Karlberg A-T. Contact allergy to colophony. Chemical identifications of allergens, sensitization experiments and clinical experiences. *Kongl Carolinska Medico Chirurgiska Institutet*, 1988.

16a. Karlberg A-T, Bohlinder K, Boman A, et al. Identification of 15-hydroperoxyabietic acid as a contact allergen in Portuguese colophony. *J Pharm Pharmacol* 1988; 40:42–47.

17. Widstrom L. Contact allergy to colophony in soldering flux. *Contact Dermatitis* 1983; 9:205–207.

18. Liden C. Patch testing with soldering fluxes. *Contact Dermatitis* 1984; 10:119–120.

19. Mathias CGT, Adams RM. Allergic contact dermatitis from rosin used as soldering flux. *J Am Acad Dermatol* 1984; 10:454–456.

19a. Mathias CGT, Maibach HI. Allergic dermatitis from anaerobic acrylic sealants. *Arch Dermatol* 1984; 120:1202–1205.

20. Burge PS, Harries MG, O'Brien I, et al. Bronchial provocation studies in workers exposed to the fumes of electronic soldering fluxes. *Clin Allergy* 1980; 10:137–149.

21. Wahlberg JE. Abietic acid and colophony. *Contact Dermatitis* 1978; 4:55.

22. Leow YH, Ng SK, Wong WK, et al. Allergic contact dermatitis from epoxy resin in Singapore. *Contact Dermatitis* 1995; 33:355–356.

23. Jolanki R, Kanerva L, Estlander T, Tarvainene K. Concomitant sensitization to triglycidyl isocyanurate, diaminodiphenylmethane and 2-hydroxyethyl methacrylate from silk-screen printing coatings in the manufacture of circuit boards. *Contact Dermatitis* 1994; 30:12–15.

24. Fisher AA. *Contact Dermatitis*, 3rd ed. Philadelphia: Lea & Febiger; 1986:559.

25. Malten KE. Old and new, mainly occupational dermatologic problems in the production and processing of plastics. In: Maibach HI and Gellin GA, eds. *Occupational and Industrial Dermatology*. Chicago: Year–Book Medical Publishers; 1982:225.

26. Allardice JT. Dermatitis due to an acrylic resin sealer. *Trans St John's Hosp Dermatol Soc* 1967; 53:86–89.

27. Jansen K. Zur Haufigkeit und Prophylaxe allergischer Kontaktekzeme durch acrylat-Klebstoffe. *Berufs Dermaotsen* 1975; 23:183. (Frequency and prevention of allergic contact dermatitis from acrylic glue.)

28. Dempsey KJ. Hypersensitivity to Sta-Lok and Loctite anaerobic sealants. *J Am Acad Dermatol* 1982; 7:779–784.

29. Ranchoff RE, Taylor JS. Contact dermatitis to anaerobic sealants. *J Am Acad Dermatol* 1985; 13:1015–1020.

30. Patussi V, Kokelj F, Marcolina D. Dermatite da contatto alla Loctite. Serie 200. *G Ital Derm Ven* 1986; 121:117–119.

31. Conde-Salazar L, Guimaraens D, Romero LV. Occupational allergic contact dermatitis from anaerobic acrylic sealants. *Contact Dermatitis* 1988; 18:129–132.

32. Rycroft RJG, Smith WDL. Low humidity occupational dermatoses. *Contact Dermatitis* 1980; 6:488–492.

33. Koh D, Av TC, Foulds IS. Fiberglass dermatitis from printed circuit boards. *Am J Ind Med* 1992; 21:193–198.

34. Koh D, Khoo NY. Identification of a printed circuit board causing fiberglass skin irritation among electronics workers. *Contact Dermatitis* 1994; 30:46–47.

35. Boxer PA, Singal M, Hartle RW. An epidemic of psychogenic illness in an electronic plant. *J Occup Med* 1984; 26:381–385.

36. Colligan MJ, Urtes MA, Wiseman C, et al. An investigation of apparent mass pyschogenic illness in an electronics plant. *J Behav Med* 1979; 2:297–309.

37. Adams RM. Dermatitis in the microelectronics industry. In: LaDou J, ed. *Occupational Medicine: State of the Art Reviews*, Vol. 1. Philadelphia: Hanley & Belfus; 1986:156–161.

38. Walder BK. Do solvents cause scleroderma? *Int J Dermatol* 1983; 22:157–158.

39. Hautstein UF, Ziegler V. Environmentally induced systemic sclerosis-like disorders. *Int J Dermatol* 1985; 24:147–151.

40. Yamakage A, Ishikawa H. Generalized morphea-like scleroderma occurring in people exposed to organic solvents. *Dermatologica* 1982; 165:186–193.

41. Yamakage A, Ishikawa H, Saito Y, et al. Occupational scleroderma-like disorder occurring in men engaged in polymerization of epoxy resins. *Dermatologica* 1980; 161:33–44.

42. Brubaker MM. Urticarial reactions to ammonium persulfate. *Arch Dermatol* 1972; 106:413–414.

43. Calnan CD, Shuster S. Reactions to ammonium persulfate. *Arch Dermatol* 1963; 88:812–815.

44. White IR, Catchpole HE, Rycroft RJG. Rashes amongst persulfate workers. *Contact Dermatitis* 1982; 8:168–172.

Paints, Varnishes, and Lacquers

27

TORKEL FISCHER, M.D.
ROBERT M. ADAMS, M.D.

PAINTS

Paint has become much more complex than it was in the 1930s, when white or red lead with raw linseed oil were almost the only ingredients. Today, a paint may contain several synthetic resins, a carefully selected and balanced group of pigments, various solvents, driers, catalysts, extenders, plasticizers, mildew-proofing agents, and fire retardants. Even a soundproofing agent is incorporated in certain paints. The water-based latex paints, suitable for both interior and exterior applications, have captured the growing do-it-yourself market since their introduction in the 1950s.

As paint formulations have become more diverse and complex, the paint industry has moved steadily into the field of chemistry. For example, NASA has developed several completely inorganic paints for use on space vehicles. These paints contain a durable inorganic pigment such as titanium dioxide, a binder of alkali metals and silicate in combination with a phosphate wetting agent, an epoxy resin, and water and are able to withstand temperatures of more than 1800°F.

Paint may be defined as a liquid mixture that is applied to a surface to produce a dry, tough coating for protective and decorative purposes. Varnishes and lacquers, essentially paints without pigments, must be included in this definition. Printing inks have a similar composition but a different function. The protective function of paint is usually more important than the decorative one. Corrosion resistance is the chief consideration, though resistance to fire, fungi, and marine growth; electrical insulation; radiation protection; reduction of frictional resistance; and control of illumination are also essential.

Paint is composed of two parts, a solid pigment and a liquid vehicle. The vehicle contains a non-volatile component called a *binder* and a *solvent*, which can be either oil- or water-based. The most important ingredient is the binder, which leaves a tough, adherent skin as the paint dries. The skin forms with the evaporation of solvent and often also with polymerization of the binder. All the other ingredients are secondary, fulfilling special requirements as needed.

The composition of a particular paint is determined to a large extent by the service it must perform. Exterior house paint, for example, is required to withstand markedly varied climatic conditions. During the hot summer it must be sufficiently plastic to expand without cracking, and in winter it must contract. To achieve this ductility, much oil and little binder is usually required.

Interior paints, on the other hand, contain less oil and more binder to produce the characteristic, hard, glossy film that is easily cleaned. "Flat" paints for walls and ceilings contain little oil and almost 70% pigment. Other types of paint combine great strength and corrosion resistance with high gloss, colorfastness, and beauty. Water-based acrylic automotive paints are included in this class.

Pigments

Paint pigment serves two purposes: it imparts color, and it covers or hides a surface. Hiding power is very important and depends on the particle size of the pigment and what proportion it constitutes of the vehicle. Pigments having the greatest hiding properties include titanium dioxide, white lead, red lead, zinc oxide, and lithopone, to which small quantities of color are usually added for decorative purposes. Pigments may react with binders to increase the durability of the paint.

Today, most paint manufacturers supply retail stores with only three or four oil-based or emulsion-type paints. From these, approximately 2,000 different shades of color can be produced. The merchant simply consults a chart and selects a given "formula" of pigments from about 15 colors. These pigments are then measured exactly, added to the paint stock, and agitated to effect thorough mixing. With this simple procedure, the exact color desired by the purchaser can be obtained.

Most pigments used in paint making are inorganic metal oxides, but for special purposes various organic dyes may be used. The pigments discussed below are commonly used in the manufacture of paint but are sometimes also coloring agents for rubber goods, leather, plastics, ceramics, tiles, and other articles.

Inorganic Pigments

Titanium Dioxide. Obtained from the ores ilmenite and rutile, titanium dioxide was introduced as a paint pigment about 1924, supplanting white lead, which had held a preeminent position for centuries. Pure titanium dioxide is a fine white powder that has the greatest hiding power of all pigments. For this reason it is found in almost all paint, often in combination with other pigments such as zinc oxide. Titanium dioxide is biologically inert and does not cause dermatitis.

White Lead. Used since the fourth century B.C., white lead is basic lead carbonate (lead subcarbonate). It is an excellent pigment for exterior paint but tends to darken and yellow on exposure to sulfides in smoky or smoggy atmospheres. It also cracks when it weathers. White lead is still occasionally used as a paint pigment for certain outdoor coatings (although far less than it used to be), usually in combination with other pigments. At one time a white lead paint contained 65% white lead and about 35% zinc oxide, but many states have altogether prohibited lead in paint. Systemic poisoning is rarely seen today in workers manufacturing white lead paint.

Red Lead. Red lead, or lead oxide produced from the heating of litharge, is a bright red powder that reacts chemically with linseed oil to form tough, elastic films. It is markedly corrosion resistant and has wide application in the manufacture of metal primer paints, especially for steel.

Zinc Oxide. Zinc oxide came into use about 1840. Also called *zinc white* or *Chinese white*, zinc oxide imparts hardness to paint and has the greatest ultraviolet light absorption power of all commercial pigments. It is also a fairly effective fungus inhibitor and is frequently used in combination with other pigments.

Lithopone. Lithopone, a white powder, is a mixture of barium sulfate and zinc sulfide. The opacity of lithopone derives from zinc sulfide. It is widely found in white and tinted interior paints, often in combination with titanium dioxide.

Antimony Trioxide. Antimony trioxide is a brilliant white pigment obtained from antimony ore.

Zinc Chromate. Zinc chromate is a yellow powder of varying composition consisting principally of zinc oxide and chromic acid. It has excellent anticorrosion properties and is widely used as an undercoat. Primer paints of this type contain sufficient quantities of water-soluble chromates to cause dermatitis.[1]

Lead Chromate. Lead chromate pigments are the single most important class of yellow pigments, ranging in color from primrose to deep orange. Variations in color can be obtained by alternating the proportions of lead sulfate and lead chromate. As the amount of lead sulfate decreases, the color lightens to a chrome yellow that contains 93% to 98% lead chromate. Prepared by treating lead acetate with sodium dichromate, lead chromate pigments have good hiding power and excellent colorfastness, but they darken on exposure to light and air.

Carbon Black. Most black pigments are composed of a very pure form of carbon made by precipitating the carbon from cooled gases of a natural gas flame.

Cadmium Yellow. Cadmium yellow can be manufactured into a range of colors from light red to maroon. Cadmium pigments are resistant to light and heat but are decomposed by dilute acids.

Iron Oxides. Iron oxide pigments come in a variety of colors, from black-red and brown to yellow, and are commonly known as *ochers* or *burnt sienna*. Today, synthetics are commonly used in place of mineral types, chiefly in metal primer paints.

Iron Blue. Iron blue, also known as *Prussian blue*, is a generic name for blue pigments derived from ferric ferrocyanide. Sodium dichromate is used as an oxidizing agent in their manufacture. They are semipermanent pigments of good colorfastness. Their excellent resistance to light renders them useful for permanent industrial finishes and automobile paints.

Ultramarine Blue. Ultramarine blue, probably a double silicate of sodium and alumina with some sodium sulfide, is a light blue powder with a reddish tinge. It is found in nature as the semiprecious lapis lazuli. Incorporated into paint, it has poor hiding power. Lapis lazuli is no longer used in paints or coatings. The ultramarine colors green and blue are completely synthetic today and are made by grinding china clay with sulfur, sodium sulfate, and a resin.

Chromic Oxide. Chromic oxide, also known as *green cinnabar*, is prepared by heating dry ammonium dichromate. This pigment has excellent fade resistance and infrared reflectance. The chromium is in trivalent form.

Metallic Pigments. For metallic pigments, powdered or flaked aluminum is most frequently used, sometimes coated with stearic acid. Copper and copper alloys, nickel, silver, and zinc dust are also used.

Organic Pigments

Para-Red. Para-red, one of the oldest organic pigments used in the paint industry, is prepared by coupling diazotized *p*-nitroaniline with beta-naphthol. It is a red pigment of great brilliance.

Lithol Reds. Lithol reds are produced by combining 2-naphthylamine-1-sulfonic acid with beta-naphthol. These pigments have numerous color variations but relatively poor fade resistance.

Toluidine Toners. Toluidine toners are brilliant red azo- dyes with excellent colorfastness.

Alizarin. Alizarin (1,2-dihydroxyanthraquinone) is the parent form of many dyes and pigments. It is seldom used alone in paint today but is employed in the manufacture of other dyes and lakes.

Phthalocyanine Blue. Phthalocyanine blue, introduced in 1935, is a brilliant blue of complex structure. Pigments made from this substance are stable to light and chemicals and are used in many decorative enamels and automobile finishes. The phthalocyanine family (benzoporphyrins) produces various shades of blue and green. They are also used in printing inks, roofing granules, wallpaper, and rubber goods.

Rhodamine. Rhodamine is a basic red fluorescent dye structurally related to xanthene. It is used when brilliant fluorescence effects are desired. Others in this group include malachite green, methyl violet, and Victoria blue.

Thioflavin. Thioflavin is a yellow basic dye of the thiazole class. Under ultraviolet light it fluoresces to yellow or yellowish green and is thus used in fluorescent sign paints. The thioflavins are also used in textile dying.

Vehicles

A vehicle is a liquid in which the finely divided pigment particles are dispersed. It has two components: a nonvolatile or oleoresinous binder, consisting of one or more oils in combination with natural or synthetic resins, and a volatile part, which on evaporation leaves only the hardened oleoresinous binder containing the trapped pigment particles. The vehicle not only contributes to the framework for the resulting film but also affects the viscosity, brushability, drying time, gloss, durability, fade resistance, chemical resistance, and color retention of the paint.

Vegetable Oils

Linseed Oil. Linseed oil (flaxseed oil) was for years the most commonly used vehicle, especially for interior paints. It consists of a golden-yellow or amber oil obtained from the seeds of the flax plant. It has marked drying properties, probably because of the presence of unsaturated linoleic and linolenic groups that become oxidized. The highest grade of linseed oil is blown flaxseed oil, which dries to an exceptionally hard film, making it useful for enamels and interior paints. Linseed oil is a rare, and probably weak, contact allergic sensitizer.

Tung Oil. Tung oil is another fast-drying oil that produces a hard film and is waterproof and highly resistant to alkalies. First manufactured by the Chinese from seeds of native trees, tung oil has been produced in certain parts of the United States since 1905, though it is quite expensive. Reports of irritation and allergic sensitization were recorded by Mitchell and Rook.[2]

Perilla Oil. Perilla oil comes from the seeds of a mint plant grown in Japan and Korea. This light yellow oil is used as a substitute for linseed oil in varnishes and lacquers.

Pine Oil (Tall Oil). Pine oil is a byproduct in the manufacture of sulfate cellulose and in pure form is almost free of rosin.

Soybean Oil. Soybean oil is pressed or extracted from soybeans.

Ricinous Oil. Derived from the seeds of the ricinous bush or tree, ricinous oil itself is not drying but takes on drying properties after being dehydrated.

Natural Resins

Rosin. Rosin, also known as *colophony, pine rosin,* and *wood rosin,* is obtained from the oleoresin of the pine tree *Pinus polustris.* Rosin esters are used in paints and commonly in varnishes. Rosins are well-known allergic sensitizers (see Chapter 31).

Dammar. Consisting of natural resins obtained from several trees native to the East Indies and Malaya, dammar is more frequently a component of varnishes than of paints.

Copal. Copal is a class of fossil resins from the Philippines and Africa. Its principal use is in varnishes.

Synthetic Resins

Alkyd Resins. Alkyds are oil-modified polyester resins produced by heating a mixture of oil and rosin to 530°F. Alkyd resins are condensations of polybasic carboxylic acids, polyhydric alcohols, and monobasic acids. The polyalcohols and polyacids are usually derived from natural resins. Common polyacids are phthalic, adipic, and maleic acid; common polyalcohols include pentaerythritol, trimethyolyl propane, and glycerol. The monobasic fatty acids are derived from linseed oil, soybean oil, and pine oil, which contain oleic, linoleic, adipic, and sebacic acid. Linseed oil and similar drying oils, when combined with hard resins such as rosin, produce a paint that is resistant to climatic conditions and has good colorfastness and adhesiveness. The alkyds have been used extensively for years in house paints and in automotive and industrial finishes. The drawback of most alkyd paints is the need for a large proportion of organic solvent. Modern alkyd paints can also be prepared as water emulsions with little added solvent.

Latex Paints. Latex paint is a type of emulsion paint the binder of which consists of small plastic droplets, usually of polyvinyl acetate, acrylic resins or styrene-butadiene, about 1 μm in size, finely dispersed in water. Antirust additives such as sodium benzoate or sodium nitrite are commonly included in such water-based paints. Introduced by Glidden in 1948, the latex paints have made it possible for almost anyone to paint successfully.

Polyester Resins. Polyester resins, like alkyd resins, are formed by the interaction between polybasic acids or anhydrides and polyhydric alcohols. Styrene is used as the cross-linking agent and for faster drying. The usual dibasic acids and anhydrides are maleic or phthalic, which are linked with dibasic alcohols such as ethylene or propylene glycol. Organic peroxides are present as catalysts, and hydroquinone is used as the inhibitor. Polyester resins are remarkably resistant to corrosion, chemicals, solvents, weather, and smoggy atmospheres.

Phenol-Formaldehyde Resins. Phenol-formaldehyde resins are based on the reactions of formaldehyde with phenol, urea, or melamine. After the phenolic resins were discovered by Baekeland in 1907, they supplanted shellac, long used as the resin base of paint. Other aldehydes used include furfural and acetaldehyde. Phenol-formaldehyde resins are stable over wide temperature ranges and have excellent resistance to moisture, acids, and solvents. Paints containing such resins are sound deadening, because they inhibit transmission and amplification of sound waves.

Cellulose Resins. First introduced in 1870, cellulose resins are the products of cellulose nitrate and cellulose acetate; dibutyl phthalate or camphor is used as the plasticizer. Acrylic resins are often added to improve the properties, such as hardness, of these paints. Because they are fairly quick to dry, cellulose resins are particularly suitable for spray painting. They are extremely tough and have low water absorption. Their chief disadvantage is flammability. The name *pyroxylin* is often applied to solutions of nitrocellulose, which is frequently combined with melamine, formaldehyde, or acrylic resins in the manufacture of high-gloss enamels and lacquers.

Du Pont developed cellulose resins as automobile finishes, and General Motors introduced them in 1923 as the topcoat for the Oakland automobile. They held the preeminent position in automobile painting until after World War II, when melamine-formaldehyde resins were introduced.

Epoxy Resins. Epoxy resins—products of the reaction between epichlorohydrin and bisphenol A and cross-linked with curing agents such as organic peroxides or polyamides—improve the adhesion and toughness of paint. They are supplied as two-package systems and are used widely in asphalt, marine varnishes, floor coatings, as interior coatings of concrete pipe, and on airplane exteriors.

Polyurethane Resins. Made from polymerized isocyanate radicals in the presence of an amine or tin soap catalyst, polyurethane resins have great strength, heat resistance, and flexibility.

Acrylic Resins. Acrylic resins are based on one of a group of related compounds: acrylic acid, methacrylic acid, acrylamide, and acrylonitrile. Common monomers are methyl acrylate, butyl acrylate, ethyl acrylate, methyl methacrylate, butyl methacrylate, and 2-ethylhexyl acrylate. The catalyst for polymerization is usually benzoyl peroxide. Styrene and vinyl toluene may be cross-linking agents that add to the paint's toughness. An epoxy resin may be present. The polymethylacrylates are harder than the corresponding polyacrylates. They are often used as modifiers for vinyl and other resins and in preparing vehicles with solvent and wetting agents for emulsion-type paints. They have good shock resistance and high dielectric strength and are stable outdoors. They are highly resistant to the actions of water and of both acids and bases. As a result, they are widely used in many paints and lacquers, especially for household appliances, automobile bodies, and farm machinery. The development of water-soluble acrylic polymers has made possible water-based latex paints and enamels.

Polyvinyl Acetate Resins. Polyvinyl acetate is

produced by the polymerization of vinyl acetate with a peroxide catalyst. Because of their low cost and weather resistance, polyvinyl acetate resins are used chiefly in water-based latex paints.

Polystyrene. Polystyrene, made from polymerized styrene, is a very tough resin, having the highest insulating power of all the more commonly used synthetic resins.

Synthetic Rubber. Synthetic rubber, also known as *SBR* or *chlorinated rubber latex*, is frequently used in paint, especially for floor coverings and tank linings. Chlorinated biphenyls were used until recently as plasticizers.

Fluorocarbon Resins. Developed in the 1950s, fluorocarbon resins found industrial application in electrical devices, high-temperature equipment, and where resistance to ultraviolet radiation is required. Polyvinylidene fluoride is representative of this group.

Cyclohexanon Resin. Cyclohexanon resin may be added to increase the hardness and water resistance of the paint.

Miscellaneous Components

Solvents. The solvents are either water or a volatile organic fluid included to dissolve the binder and give proper viscosity to the paint. Organic solvents may be added to water-based paints to slow drying and thus aid in film formation. Solvents are described further in Chapter 28.

Hardeners. Hardeners, used to cure the system, include organic amines, organic peroxides, and polyamides.

Extenders. Extenders are noncovering pigments that are added to the paint to improve thickness, adhesion, durability, and gloss. They include barium sulfate (barates), calcium sulfate (gypsum, plaster of Paris), calcium carbonate (chalk), magnesium carbonate, silica (quartz, diatomaceous earth), magnesium silicates (talc, soapstone), kaolin, pumice, and mica.

Driers. Paints often contain more than one drier. Examples of driers are cobalt, lead, zinc, manganese, calcium, barium, zirconium, and tin naphthenates, oleates, octoates, and resinates.

Emulsifiers. Tetrasodium pyrophosphates, dioctyl sodium sulfosuccinate, sodium lauryl sulfate, and certain nonionic detergents are used as emulsifying agents.

Antifoaming Agents. To prevent foaming and blistering, nonionic detergents (used most commonly), pine oil, kerosene, castor oil soaps, dibutyl phthalate, and silicone derivatives are added.

Thixotropic Agents. Oil-based paints such as alkyd paints are made thixotropic by the addition of polyamides, whereas latex paints are made

more viscous by the addition of cellulose derivatives. Large amounts of cellulose affect the water resistance of latex paint.

Plasticizers. Dibutyl phthalate, adipic and sebacic acid and their esters, polyester resins, and sulfonamides are all used as plasticizers. Chlorinated diphenyls were used until recently but have been discontinued.

Stabilizers. Stabilizers include starch, dextrin, methylcellulose, sodium polyacrylate, casein, soya, and alginates.

Fungicides. Mercuric oxide, thymol, chlorothymol, organic mercurials, pentachloro-phenol derivatives, tetramethylthiuram disulfides, copper arsenates, and calcium-, zinc-, and aluminum-stearates are all used as fungicides. Water-based paints especially require a germicidal agent (Table 27–1).

Antifouling Agents. Antifouling agents are compounds of special toxicity added to marine paints to resist the growth of organisms under water. Arsenials, lead, and mercury were previously used. Today copper, organic tin, tetramethylthiuram disulfide, and zinc carbamates are the compounds most commonly used.

Antioxidants. Antioxidants include hydroquinone, phenols, and oximes.

pH Adjusters. Ammonia is the most commonly used pH adjuster.

Photoinitiators. Photoinitiators are a new group of chemicals now added to many paints to aid in curing. Benzophenones, which split by electromagnetic radiation into two energy-rich radicals, are the most common photoinitiators.

Manufacture

A four-story building is ideal for the manufacture of paint, because gravity can be used to pass raw materials and the manufactured products through the plant. The top floor is often used for raw materials, which are fed by chutes and pipes to mills and mixing machines on the third floor. After mixing, the paint passes through pipes to the second floor, where additional solvents and special pigments are added. Quality control is performed on this floor. The completed product is packaged and stored for shipment on the first floor. Since about 1950, many paint factories have been built entirely on one floor, using hydraulic pumps for moving the product through the plant. The most important aspect of paint manufacture is the fine dispersion and thorough mixing of all ingredients. To accomplish this, several types of mixing machines are employed. A roller mill (Fig. 27–1) equipped with three to five large, water-cooled steel rollers rotating in opposite directions

TABLE 27-1 • Some Germicidal Agents in Paints

Germicide	Trade Name	Manufacturer
Pentachlorophenol (PCP)	Dowicide 7	Dow
	Pentachlorophenol DP-2	Reichold
		Vulcan
Formaldehyde		
Sodium pentachlorophenoxide	Dowicide G-ST	Dow
2,4,5-Trichlorophenol	Dowicide 2	Dow
		Vertac
1,2-Phenylphenol	Dowicide I	Dow
Sodium 1-2-phenylphenoxide	Dowicide A	Dow
4-Tolyldiiodomethyl sulfone	Amical 48	Abbott
4-Chlorophenyldiiodomethyl sulfone	Amical 77	Abbott
1,2-Dibromo-2,4-dicyanobutane	Tektamer 38	Merck
Benzyl bromoacetate	Merbac 35	Merck
Phenylmercuric acetate	PMA-100	Cosan
	Troysan PMA	Troy
Di(phenylmercury)dodecenylsuccinate (PMDS)	Super-Ad-It	Tenneco
Tributyl tin oxide	Cotin 300	Cosan
	Keycide X-10	Ferro
Chloroacetamide	Intercide 340A	Interstab
Tributyl tin fluoride	Biomet 204	M&T
Barium metaborate	Busan 11-MI	Buckman Labs
2-(Hydroxymethyl)aminoethanol	Troysan 174	Troy
Hexahydro-1,3,5-triethyl-s-trazine	Vancide TH	Vanderbilt
Sodium dimethyldithiocarbamate (Sodam)	Thiostate, Thiostop N	Uniroyal
Trans-1,2-bis($\sim$propylsulfonyl)ethylene	Vancide PA	Vanderbilt
2,3,5,6-Tetrachloro-4-(methylsulfonyl)pyridine	Dowicil S-13	Dow
2,3,5-Trichloro-4-(propylsulfonyl)pyridine	Dowicil A-40	Dow
Tetrahydro-3,5-dimethyl-2H-1,3,5-thiadiazine-20-thione	Metasol D3T	Merck
(DMTT)	Biocide N-521	Stauffer
1,2-Benzisothiazoline-3-one (5)	Proxcel CRL	ICI America
2-N-Octyl-4-isothiazolin-3-one	Skane M-8	Rohm & Haas
	Kathon LP	
5-Chloro-2-methyl-4-isothiazolin-3-one	Kathon CG	
2-Methyl 4-isothiazolin-3-one		
2-(4-Thiazolyl)benzimidazole	Metalsol TK-100	Merck
N-(Trichloromethylthio)-4-cyclohexane-1,2-dicarboximide	Vancide 89RE	Vanderbilt
(Captan)	Orthocide	Chevron
N-(Trichloromethylthio)phthalamide (Folpet)	Cosan P	Cosan
	Phaltal	Chevron
	Fungitrol	Tenneco
Tetrachloroisophthalonitrile	Nopoocide N-96	Diamond Shamrock
1-(3-Chloroallyl)-3,5,7-triaza-1-azonia-adamantane	Dowicil 100	Dow
chloride		

Adapted from Kirk RE and Othmer DF: *Encyclopedia of Chemical Technology.* New York: John Wiley; 1979.

and at different speeds is very effective for blending. The clearance between the rolls is approximately 0.001 inch. A scraper blade removes the paint paste from the final roller. The bull, or pebble mill, is a horizontal drum about half full of pebbles or steel balls the size of golf balls. As the cylinder rotates, the cascading balls subject the mixture to thorough blending. This machine is the most common mixer today. A Morehouse mill is a large-capacity grinding machine used chiefly for water emulsions, finishes, and house paints. The oldest paint blenders in existence are stone mills, in which one circular stone revolves against a similar but stationary one. The pigment-vehicle mixture is fed through a hole in the revolving stone, and the grinding surfaces have grooves or channels for the passage of the paint as it is mixed. A Cowles dissolver is a large vertical steel tank with a round, serrated blade at the bottom that rotates at extremely high speeds. The principle of action is similar to that of a home food blender.

After the basic ingredients have been properly

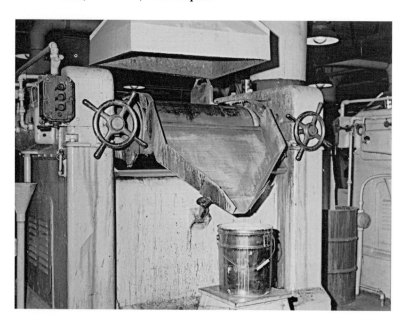

FIGURE 27–1 • A typical three-roller mill is used in many industries for thorough mixing of ingredients.

mixed, the paint flows into large vats with conventional paddle-type agitators that are kept in constant motion to prevent separation of the ingredients (Fig. 27–2). The completed paint may then be filtered through cheesecloth before quality control testing (Fig. 27–3).

Methods of Application

Brushing is still employed for small tasks and interior decoration. Large, flat surfaces are easily covered using a lamb's wool or nylon roller. For industrial painting, a variety of methods are employed, the most common being spray painting by hand or machine. Compressed air is driven across the opening of a small paint outlet on a gun, creating a fine mist of air and paint (Fig. 27–4).

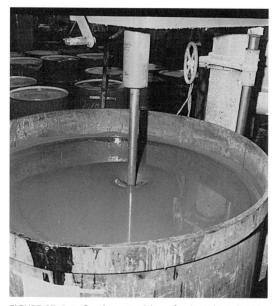

FIGURE 27–2 • Continuous mixing of paint takes place in large vats with agitators that keep the mixture in constant motion to prevent separation of ingredients.

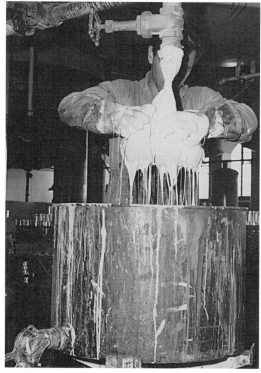

FIGURE 27–3 • It is important to filter the paint, in this case through cheesecloth, before quality-control testing.

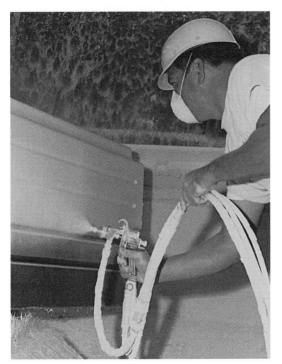

FIGURE 27–4 • Spray painting is a common method of paint application. Here the worker is applying a surface coating to a polyester shower stall.

Airless spraying uses direct pressure on the paint, breaking it up into fine droplets. A second method is the dipping process, which entails immersion of the object into the paint followed by drip drying. In roller coating, flat surfaces are coated mechanically by rolls that produce a film of paint in a line across the object. Tumbling is used for small objects, from buttons to hardware. Electrostatic spraying is accomplished by applying an electrostatic charge to a spray gun after grounding the object to be painted. Paint droplets take up a negative charge from the gun and are attracted to the positively charge object being painted. This method covers the object, especially any sharp corners and crevices, more efficiently than other methods.

Electrodeposition systems are used solely with water-based paint, which does not contain flammable solvents. The metal to be painted is immersed in a tank containing primer, where it acts as an anode. The charged resin particles are attracted to the metallic surface, resulting in uniform coverage even on interior surfaces and in corners and other inaccessible areas. Automobiles today are prime coated using this process. It is used increasingly for other objects, because it is fast, easily automated, and wastes little paint.

Methods of Curing

Baking in ovens and air curing are the methods most commonly used for curing. Polymerization initiated by an electric current, microwave heating, radiation, and electron beams have also been used more recently. Ultraviolet radiation, used for cans and other containers and for wood surface coating of furniture, is especially attractive because it eliminates solvent pollution.

VARNISHES

Varnishes are essentially unpigmented, oil-based paints consisting of a solvent and a binder. The latter is usually a drying oil, a natural or synthetic resin, rubber latex, or shellac. Japanese varnish contains asphalt, oils, and solvents. Varnishes produce clear, transparent coatings when dry and add to the natural beauty of wood surfaces.

Varnish is manufactured by cooking the drying oil and resin in a closed kettle at temperatures of 500° to 600°F. Powdered driers are added during cooking; on completion, the mixture is quickly cooled and thinned with a solvent. Liquid driers such as metallic naphthenates and oleates are then added, and the mixture is filtered, tested for quality control, and packaged. Drying oils include tung oil, linseed oil, and dehydrated castor oil. The primary varnish resins are copal, rosin, and dammar. Suitable synthetic resins include those of the phenol-formaldehyde class used as spar and other machine varnishes and for floors and porches as well as phenolic resins modified with other resins such as alkyds. The latter have become the most important resin class in the U.S. coatings industry.[3] The solvents are usually methanol, toluene, ketones, or naphtha.

LACQUERS

A lacquer is a protective coating containing a cellulose ester combined with a resin. To promote flexibility, plasticizers such as camphor, phthalates, rosin, and tricresyl phosphate are added. Nitrocellulose is the major binder used today and is often combined with an alkyd resin to improve durability. The finishing of wood products provides the largest market, lacquers being used in stains, sealers, toners, wood fillers, and topcoats. In addition to furniture of all kinds, these resins are used to coat wood paneling, flooring, automobile surfaces, and artificial leather. Nitrocellulose's compatibility with other resins has ensured its continued use in industry.

PAINT AND VARNISH REMOVERS

Paint and varnish removers are liquid or paste preparations intended to remove paints and varnishes in preparation for refinishing a surface. They are composed of volatile solvents such as methylene chloride, methyl alcohol, ethyl alcohol, benzene (rarely), or toluene. Paraffin is frequently used to retard the solvent action. Caustic agents such as sodium phosphate, sodium silicate, cresol, and caustic soda are frequently included in heavy-duty cleaners of this type.

Dermatitis from Paints, Varnishes, and Lacquers

Despite the myriad hazards of paint manufacturing, the incidence of occupational dermatitis is actually quite low. The majority of paints are now water based and less irritating than the solvent-based types were. Most cases of dermatitis among painters result from contact with water, soaps, detergents, and solvents.[4–6] A common source of irritation is clothing soaked with spilled solvents and paint that is allowed to remain against the skin too long. The incidence of dermatitis is higher among workers in the building trades than among workers in paint factories.

Screening the Danish national database on chemical products, including 2,713 paints and lacquers, 34 different allergens were found.[7] The most common ones were formaldehyde, epoxy resin, various amine hardeners, zinc chromate, urea- and phenolformaldehyde resins, and several preservatives.

Workers operating mixing machines must weigh and measure specified amounts of the dry ingredients by hand and then dump them into the containers. Liquids may be siphoned by a hand pump from barrels into measuring cans before being

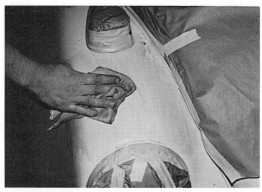

FIGURE 27–6 • Prior to spray painting, a surface must undergo careful preparation, including removal of grease and dirt with soap, water, lacquer thinners, and so forth.

added to the mix. Frequent spilling is almost unavoidable. After starting the mill and rotating valves to admit the steam that heats the mixture, the operators may test the substance between their fingers to determine the fineness of the grind. Mixing machine operators also clean the millstones, hoppers, and scrapers using a hot-water hose, solvents, and brushes.

Rollermill operators tend the machines that grind the ingredients to a paste. They must adjust the feed gate to let the mix flow from hopper to roll, and from time to time test the paste for fineness of grind, using a special gauge. They secure scraper blades to the takeoff rolls and bolt chutes to the scraper blades, allowing paste to flow from the roll into thinning and storage tanks. Using a spatula, they scrape the paste from the mill apron into the containers (Fig. 27–5). Mill operators must clean their equipment with solvents, blend specified extenders into the mix, and add thinners to the paint in the thinning tanks. Because of the continuous spilling and spattering that occur during the process, these operators are much exposed to paint and its ingredients.

Workers who tint and match colors for the preparation of small batches must add specified pigments and examine the result by dipping a wooden spatula into the mixture and comparing the color with a standard. They also send samples to the laboratory for colorimetric comparison. Since the work of tinters is done entirely by hand, considerable exposure to the ingredients is likely.

Varnish makers operate the equipment that melts, cooks, and mixes such ingredients as gums, oils, turpentine, resins, and solvents. They first weigh these ingredients, pouring them directly into the vat or agitator. The mixture is allowed to cook for a specified time, after which it is pumped into the reducing tank. The operator must periodi-

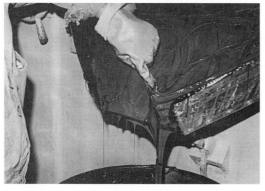

FIGURE 27–5 • Guiding the paint into the vats requires skin protection with suitable gloves.

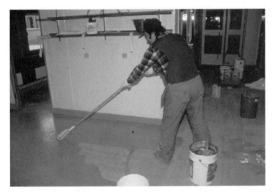

FIGURE 27–7 • There can be considerable clothing and skin contact during painting with brush and roller.

cally test samples for viscosity. Except for the mixing and testing procedures, little skin contact occurs in varnish manufacture. Fumes that escape when the lids of the varnish vats are lifted may be a source of airborne contact dermatitis.

Spray painters first must clean the product to be painted, removing grease and dirt with lacquer thinners, turpentine, and soap and water (Fig. 27–6). They also apply masking tape over areas to be left unpainted and fill cavities and dents with putty. In addition to operating spray guns, they may also use brushes to paint areas inaccessible to spraying.

Brush and roller painters (Fig. 27–7) may develop contact dermatitis from paint, paint removers, thinners, putty, plaster, or cement. They use large quantities of solvents, acids, soaps and detergents, steel wool, and sandpaper. They sometimes operate blowtorches and sandblasting equipment and have contact with masking tape, blueprints, inks, and stencils. Putty and plastic wood are also necessary articles of the trade. Painters working outdoors may develop dermatitis from contact with various plants, especially poison ivy or oak and English ivy, among others.

Solvent-based paints often irritate the skin, but allergic sensitization is less common. Sensitivity may occur occasionally to tung oil,[6] linseed oil, rosin, turpentine, synthetic resins,[8] and other substances (see section on Painters and Paperhangers). Modified colophony used in modern paints and lacquers may sensitize and does not always cross-react with natural colophony.[9, 10] Modern water-based paints contain several chemicals that may irritate the skin, alone or in combination, but these are rarely present in irritant concentrations.[11] The growing market for epoxy, acrylate, and phenol-formaldehyde resins in the construction and woodworking industries create problems; however, there are few reports of sensitivity to these compounds from painting and paint manufacture, probably because of low concentrations of monomers[5, 12–15] Allergy to constituents of ultraviolet (UV)-curing acrylate lacquers, such as 1,6-hexanedioldiacrylate, triethyleneglycol dimethacrylate, trimethylol-propanetriacrylate, tripropyleneglycol dimethacrylate, and amino-substituted diacrylate (BAPETG) have been reported.[16, 17] Contact allergy to polyester resins, increasingly used for surface coatings, is rare, and rarer still is sensitivity to the catalyst methyl ethyl ketone peroxide, which is used with an ultraviolet-curing polyester.[18]

Solvents recognized as both irritants and sensitizers include turpentine, oxidized limonene (dipentene),[19–21] and dimethylformamide.[22] Sensitivity to the solvent turpentine is still a frequent occurrence in some countries[23–28] and may even increase when interest in previously abandoned techniques is renewed. Glycols and glycol ethers function as solvents and film formers in both solvent- and water-based paints.[29–31] Except for sensitivity to propylene glycol and a few reports of sensitivity to hexylene glycol and phenoxyethanol, reports of allergy to glycols and their esters are rare.[5, 32, 33]

Pigments and dyes in paint are usually chemically stable, low-reactivity compounds that rarely sensitize. D&C yellow no. 11 and quinoline yellow used in spirit lacquers are exceptions, and have been reported to sensitize and to cross-react.[34]

Allergic and irritant contact dermatitis to germicidal agents (see Tables 27–1 and 27–2) is an increasing problem as water-based paints supplant those based on solvents.[35–39] Many different biocides, often as many as four simultaneously, are used to preserve water-based paints,[12, 40] among which are several known sensitizers (many also being irritants). These include benzyl alcohol mono(poly) hemiformal,[41] 1,2-dibromo-2,4-dicyanobutan (Tekamer 38AD, in Euxyl K 400)[42]; fomaldehyde and formaldehyde-releasing preservatives,[43] among them 2-bromo-2-nitro-1,3-propandiol (Bronopol)[44], N-methylolchloracetamide,[45] and chloracetamide[46–48], tetrachloroisophthalonitril[39, 49–51] and N-(trichloromethylthio)phthalimide.[5, 52] Chlorocresol is a weak sensitizer used to preserve wallpaper glue.[5, 53] For years, pentachlorphenol has been a common wood preservative. Long-term exposure has been reported to cause pemphigus.[54]

In 1980 Högberg and Wahlberg[55] conducted a field investigation of 2,239 Stockholm housepainters, and found 87 cases of occupational dermatitis, a prevalence of 3.9%. A common allergen was chloracetamide, which is used as a preservative

TABLE 27–2 • Painters' Test Series

Test Material	Concentration (%)	Vehicle
1,2-Benz-isothiazolin-3-one	0.1	Pet
Benzylalcohol-mono-(poly)-hemiformal	3.0	Aq
2-(2-Butoxyethoxy)-ethanol	20.0	Aq
n-Butylacrylate	0.1	Pet
Euxyl K400	0.1	Pet
Dibutylthiourea	1.0	Pet
Dichlorofluanid	0.1	Pet
d-Limonene	5.0	Pet
Di-iodomethyl-4-tolylsulphon	2.5	Pet
3-Iodo-propynylbutyl carbamate	0.5	Pet
2-Chloro acetamide	0.2	Pet
4-Chloro-3-cresol	1.0	Pet
2-Methyl-2,4-pentandiol	20.0	Aq
N-Methylol chloroacetamid	0.1	Pet
Nonylphenol ethoxylate	1.0	Pet
2-N-Octyl-3-isothiazolinon	0.1	Pet
Turpentine peroxides	0.3	Oo
N-(Trichloromethyltio)-phtalimide	0.1	Pet
2,2,4-Trimethyl-1,3-pentandiol diisobutyrate	5.0	Pet
Zirconium octoate	5.0	Pet
Propylene glycol	5.0	Pet
Methoxypropanol	10.0	Aq

Aq, deionized water; pet, white petrolatum; oo, olive oil.

many water-based paints.[47] On patch testing, five of 180 patients reacted positively to this preservative. Solvents used to clean the skin were also frequent causes of irritant dermatitis, especially among workers with a history of atopy (Fig. 27–8).[55]

During the last few years, isothiazolin-3-one derivatives, used as preservatives, have posed special problems, as they have assumed a significant place in the preservative market for both cosmetic and industrial products.[5, 35, 42, 48, 56–62] The isothiazolins are widely used as fungicides for latex paints under a variety of brand names.[63] A concentration of 30 ppm weight for weight (w/w) has been found to be sensitizing.[64] Despite its known toxicity, phenylmercuric acetate may still be used in indoor paint.[65]

Modern water-based paints are emulsions that may contain anionic, cationic, or nonionic surfactants, lecithin, zinc naphthenate, polyphosphates, polynonyl phenyl ethers, and dioctyl sodium sulfosuccinate. Most surfactants are irritants to some extent.[12] Dioxyl sodium sulfosuccinate may be a sensitizer.[66] Nonoxynols have also been reported to sensitize.[67–69] Accelerators and inhibitors of polymerization such as benzoyl peroxide, p-methoxy phenol, and hydroquinone may irritate the skin, but they are fairly innocuous.[12] Hydroquinone is rarely sensitizing. Triethylamine and other amines,

common ingredients in modern paints, may irritate and also sensitize.[70]

Plasticizers such as dibutyl phthalate rarely sensitize; however, the plasticizer and fire retardant triphenyl-phosphate is a low-grade sensitizer.[71] Primer paints containing chromate have been reported to cause allergic contact dermatitis in painters.[72, 73]

Antifouling organic tin compounds in paints, especially those used in marine paints, may be irritating. Because they are toxic to marine life, their use is currently decreasing.[37, 74] 2-Tert-butyl-amine-4-cyclopropylamine-6-methylthio-1,3,5-triazine, an antifouling agent used as a substitute for copper and tin compounds to prevent the growth of marine organisms, has recently been reported to sensitize.[75] Driers, especially cobalt salts (cobalt naphthenate and oleate), may sensitize.[76, 77]

Lacquer resin from the lacquer tree is used in making the famous handicraft lacquerware of Japan, China, Thailand, and Vietnam. The resin contains urushiol and is a common cause of allergic contact dermatitis when uncured.[78] Attempts have been made to reduce its allergenic potency by heat treatment,[79] but continuous contact with the lacquer is said to hyposensitize the workers.[80, 81]

Cyclohexanon resin, which is added to paint to increase hardness and enhance water resis-

have shown a significantly higher incidence of lung cancer than expected, spray painters appearing to be at greatest risk.[87] Cigarette smoking and inhalation of asbestos are additional predisposing factors to lung cancer. Paint guns can cause severe penetrating wounds of the hand. Released in a fine-jet stream of up to 7000 psi, the paint easily penetrates tissue deep below the skin.[88]

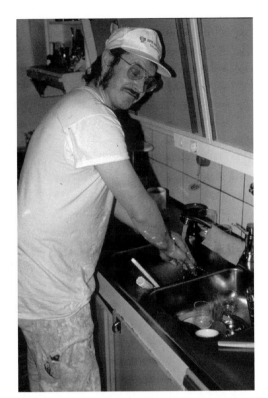

FIGURE 27–8 • Solvents used to clean the skin and brushes are common causes of irritant dermatitis, especially in workers with atopic backgrounds.

tance, has been reported to be a sensitizer.[82] The flame retardant, tri-(2,3-dibromopropyl)phosphate, which is also used as a plasticizer in lacquers, has caused several cases of contact dermatitis.[71, 83] Nickel- and chromium-sensitive workers may develop dermatitis when spray painting metal.[84]

Paint removers are usually very irritating and occasionally sensitize. Dibutyl-thiourea in a paint remover has been reported to cause contact dermatitis.[85]

Dermatologists should be aware of systemic symptoms that can result from inhalation of the fumes of oil-based paints and paint strippers. Painters who work long in poorly ventilated areas may experience dizziness, euphoria, headache, blurred vision, and slurred speech. Later, hallucinations, permanent disorientation, paralysis, and other nervous system disorders can result. Amateur home painters should consider wearing only masks approved by OSHA. Large paint stores and professional supply stores carry several brands of masks and also disposable-cartridge respirators, which are relatively inexpensive. In addition, long-sleeved shirts, long pants, and gloves are recommended.[86] Painters with exposure to zinc chromate primer paints for more than two decades

References

1. Adams RM, Fregert S, et al. Water solubility of zinc chromate primer paints used as antirust agents. *Contact Dermatitis* 1976; 2:357–358.
2. Mitchell J, Rook A. *Botanical Dermatology*. Vancouver: Greengrass; 1979.
3. American Chemical Society *Chemistry in the Economy*. Washington: National Science Foundation; 1973:158.
4. Moura C, Dias M, et al. Contact dermatitis in painters, polishers and varnishers. *Contact Dermatitis* 1994; 31:51–53.
5. Fischer T, Bohlin S, et al. Skin disease and contact sensitivity in house painters using water-based paints, glues and putties. *Contact Dermatitis* 1995; 32:39–45.
6. Schwartz L, Tulipan L, et al. *Occupational Diseases of the Skin*. Philadelphia: Lea & Febiger; 1957.
7. Flyvholm MA. Contact allergens in registered chemical products. *Contact Dermatitis* 1991; 25:49–56.
8. Piper R. Hazards of painting and varnishing. *Br J Industr Med* 1965; 22:247–260.
9. Karlberg AT, Gäfvert E, et al. Maleopimaric acid—a potent sensitizer in modified rosin. *Contact Dermatitis* 1990; 22:193–201.
10. Hausen BM, Loll M. Contact allergy due to colophony (VIII). The sensitizing potency of commercial products: an investigation of French and German modified-colophony derivatives. *Contact Dermatitis* 1993; 29:189–191.
11. Lovell CR, Rycroft RJ, et al. Contact dermatitis from the irritancy (immediate and delayed) and allergenicity of hydroxypropyl acrylate. *Contact Dermatitis* 1985; 12:117–118.
12. Hansen MK, Larsen M, et al. Waterborne paints. A review of their chemistry and toxicology and the results of determinations made during their use. *Scand J Work Environ Health* 1987; 13:473–485.
13. Kanerva L, Estlander T, et al. Sensitization to patch test acrylates. *Contact Dermatitis* 1988; 18:10–15.
14. Jolanki R, Kanerva L, et al. Occupational dermatoses from epoxy resin compounds. *Contact Dermatitis* 1990; 23:172–183.
15. Ortiz-Frutos FJ, Borrego L, et al. Occupational allergic contact dermatitis from epoxy varnishes. *Contact Dermatitis* 1993; 28:297–298.
16. Carmichael AJ, Foulds IS. Allergic contact dermatitis due to an amino-substituted diacrylate in a UV-cured lacquer. *Contact Dermatitis* 1993; 28:45–46.
17. Fischer T, Nylander-French L, et al. Dermatological risk to workers in the ultraviolet radiation wood surface curing industry. *Am J Contact Derm* 1994; 5:201–206.
18. Stewart L, Beck MH. Contact sensitivity to methyl ethyl ketone peroxide in a paint sprayer. *Contact Dermatitis* 1992; 26:52–53.
19. Calnan CD. Allergy to dipentene in paint thinner. *Contact Dermatitis* 1979; 5:123–124.
20. Falk A, Fischer T, et al. Purpuric rash caused by dermal exposure to *d*-limonene. *Contact Dermatitis* 1991; 25:198–199.
21. Karlberg A-T, Dooms-Goossens A. Contact allergy to oxi-

dized *d*-limonene among dermatitis patients. *Contact Dermatitis* 1997; 36:201–206.

22. Camarasa JG. Contact dermatitis from dimethylformamide. *Contact Dermatitis* 1987; 16:234.
23. Calnan CD. Turpentine in paint brush cleaner. *Contact Dermatitis* 1978; 4:57–58.
24. Foussereau J. Allergy to turpentine, lanolin and nickel in Strasbourg. *Contact Dermatitis* 1978; 4:300.
25. Calnan CD, Hill RN. Allergy to diphenyloxazole. *Contact Dermatitis* 1979; 5:269–270.
26. Cronin E. Oil of turpentine—a disappearing allergen. *Contact Dermatitis* 1979; 5:308–311.
27. Cachao P, Menezes Brandao F, et al. Allergy to oil of turpentine in Portugal. *Contact Dermatitis* 1986; 14:205–208.
28. Romaguera C, Alomar A, et al. Turpentine sensitization. *Contact Dermatitis* 1986; 14:197.
29. Sparer J, Welch LS, et al. Effects of exposure to ethylene glycol ethers on shipyard painters: evaluation of exposure. *Am J Indust Med* 1988; 14:497–507.
30. Ulfvarson U, Alexandersson R, et al. Temporary health effects from exposure to water based paints. *Scand J Work Environ Health* 1992; 18:376–387.
31. Wieslander G, Norrbäck D, et al. Occupational exposure to water based paint and symptoms from skin and eyes. *Occupational and Environmental Medicine* 1994; 51:181–186.
32. Dawson TA, Black RJ, et al. Delayed and immediate hypersensitivity to carbitols. *Contact Dermatitis* 1989; 21:52–53.
33. Kinnunen T, Hannuksela M. Skin reactions to hexylene glycol. *Contact Dermatitis* 1989; 21:154–158.
34. Björkner B, Niklasson B. Contact allergic reaction to D & C yellow No. 11 and quinoline yellow. *Contact Dermatitis* 1983; 9:263–268.
35. Pedersen NB. Occupational allergy from 1,2-benzisothiazolin-3-one and other preservatives in plastic emulsions. *Contact Dermatitis* 1976; 2:340–342.
36. Mathias CG, Andersen KE, et al. Allergic contact dermatitis from 2-*N*-octyl-4-isothiazolin-3-one, a paint mildewcide. *Contact Dermatitis* 1983; 9:507–509.
37. Goh CL. Irritant dermatitis from tri-*N*-butyl tin oxide in paint. *Contact Dermatitis* 1985; 12:161–163.
38. de Groot AC. Contact allergy to EDTA in a topical corticosteroid preparation. *Contact Dermatitis* 1986; 15:250–252.
39. Meding B. Contact dermatitis from tetrachloroisophthalonitrile in paint. *Contact Dermatitis* 1986; 15:187.
40. van Faassen A, Borm PJA. Composition and health hazards of waterbased construction paints: results from a survey in the Netherlands. *Environment Health Perspectives* 1991; 92:147–152.
41. Wurbach G, Schubert H, et al. Contact allergy to benzyl alcohol and benzyl paraben. *Contact Dermatitis* 1993; 28:187–188.
42. Mathias CG. Contact dermatitis to a new biocide (Tektamer 38) used in a paste glue formulation. *Contact Dermatitis* 1983; 9:418.
43. Dahlquist I, Fregert S. Formaldehyde releasers [Letter]. *Contact Dermatitis* 1978; 4:173.
44. Frosch PJ, White IR, et al. Contact allergy to Bronopol. *Contact Dermatitis* 1990; 22:24–26.
45. Farli M, Ginanneschi M, et al. Occupational contact dermatitis to *N*-methylol-chloracetamide. *Contact Dermatitis* 1987; 17:182–184.
46. Pedersen NB, Fregert S. Occupational allergic contact dermatitis from chloracetamide in glue. *Contact Dermatitis* 1976; 2:122–123.
47. Wahlberg JE. Högberg M, et al. Chloracetamide allergy in house painters. *Contact Dermatitis* 1978; 4:116–167.

48. Jones SK, Kennedy CT. Chloracetamide as an allergen in the paint industry. *Contact Dermatitis* 1988; 18:304–305.
49. Johnsson M, Buhagen M, et al. Fungicide-induced contact dermatitis. *Contact Dermatitis* 1983; 9:285–288.
50. Liden C. Facial dermatitis caused by chlorothalonil in a paint. *Contact Dermatitis* 1990; 22:206–211.
51. Jacobs MC, Rycroft RJ. Contact dermatitis and asthma from sodium metabisulfite in a photographic technician. *Contact Dermatitis* 1995; 33:65–66.
52. Lisi P, Caraffini S, et al. A test series for pesticide dermatitis. *Contact Dermatitis* 1986; 15:266–269.
53. Andersen KE. Contact allergy to chlorocresol, formaldehyde and other biocides. *Acta Derm Venereol* 1986; [Suppl 125]:1–21.
54. Lambert J, Schepens P, et al. Skin lesions as a sign of subacute pentachlorophenol intoxication. *Acta Derm Venereol* 1986; 66:170–172.
55. Högberg M, Wahlberg JE. Health screening for occupational dermatoses in house painters. *Contact Dermatitis* 1980; 6:100–106.
56. Thormann J. Contact dermatitis to a new fungicide, 2-*N*-octyl-4-isothiazolin-3-one. *Contact Dermatitis* 1982; 8:204.
57. Björkner B, Bruze M, et al. Contact allergy to the preservative Kathon CG. *Contact Dermatitis* 1986; 14:85–90.
58. Pilger C, Nethercott JR, et al. Allergic contact dermatitis due to a biocide containing 5-chloro-2-methyl-4-isothiazolin-3-one. *Contact Dermatitis* 1986; 14:201–204.
59. MacAulay JC. Orchid allergy. *Contact Dermatitis* 1987; 17:112–113.
60. Oleaga JM, Aguirre A, et al. Allergic contact dermatitis from Kathon 893. *Contact Dermatitis* 1992; 27:345–346.
61. Sanz-Gallen P, Planas J, et al. Allergic contact dermatitis due to 1,2–benzisothiazolin-3-one in paint manufacture. *Contact Dermatitis* 1992; 27:271–272.
62. Schubert H. Airborne contact dermatitis due to methylchloro- and methylisothiazolinone (MCI/MI). *Contact Dermatitis* 1997; 36:274.
63. Gruvberger B, Persson K, et al. Demonstration of Kathon CG in some commercial products. *Contact Dermatitis* 1986; 15:24–27.
64. de Groot AC, Bos JD, et al. Contact allergy to preservatives—II. *Contact Dermatitis* 1986; 15:218–222.
65. Agocs MM, Etzel R, et al. Mercury exposure from interior latex paint. *N Engl J Med* 1990; 323:1096–1101.
66. Fisher AA. *Contact Dermatitis*. Philadelphia: Lea & Febiger; 1986.
67. Nethercott JR, Lawrence MJ. Allergic contact dermatitis due to nonylphenol ethoxylate (nonoxynol-6). *Contact Dermatitis* 1984; 10:235–239.
68. Meding B. Occupational contact dermatitis from nonylphenolpolyglycolether. *Contact Dermatitis* 1985; 13:122–123.
69. Dooms-Goossens A, Deveylder H, et al. Contact allergy to nonoxynols as a cause of intolerance to antiseptic preparations. *J Am Acad Derm* 1989; 21:723–727.
70. Bittersohl C, Heberer H. Zur Toxicität von aliphatischen Aminen. *Z Gesamte Hyg Grenzgeb* 1978; 24:529–534.
71. Hjorth N. Contact dermatitis from cellulose acetate film. *Berufsdermatosen* 1964; 12:86–100.
72. Hall AF. Occupational contact dermatitis among aircraft workers. *JAMA* 1944; 125:179–185.
73. Engel HO, Calnan CD. Chromate dermatitis from paint. *Br J Ind Med* 1963; 20:192–198.
74. Lewis PG, Emmett EA. Irritant dermatitis from tri-butyl tin oxide and contact allergy from chlorocresol. *Contact Dermatitis* 1987; 17:129–132.
75. Anderson T. Occupational allergic contact dermatitis from 2-tert-butylamino-4-cyclopropylamino-6-methylthio-1,3,5-triazine. *Contact Dermatitis* 1997; 36:272.

76. Wehle U. Arbeitsbedingte Ekzeme durch Polyester. *Allerg Asthma* 1966; 12:184–186.

77. Pirilä V. On occupational disease of the skin among paint factory workers: painters, polishers, and varnishers in Finland. *Acta Derm Venereol* 1947; 27[**suppl 16**]:1–5.

78. Kullavanijaya P, Ophaswongse S. A study of dermatitis in the lacquerware industry. *Contact Dermatitis* 1997; 36:244–246.

79. Kawai K, Nakagawa M, et al. Heat treatment of Japanese lacquerware renders it hypoallergenic. *Contact Dermatitis* 1992; 27:244–249.

80. Kawai K, Nakagawa M, et al. Hyposensitization to urushiol among Japanese lacquer craftsmen. *Contact Dermatitis* 1991; 24:146–147.

81. Kawai K, Nakagawa M, et al. Hyposensitization to urushiol among Japanese lacquer craftsmen: results of patch tests on students learning the art of lacquerware [Comments]. *Contact Dermatitis* 1991; 25:290–295.

82. Bruze M, Boman A, et al. Contact allergy to a cyclohexa-none resin in humans and guinea pigs. *Contact Dermatitis* 1988; 18:46–49.

83. Andersen KE. Sensitivity to a flame retardant, tris(2,3-dibromopropyl)phosphate (Firemaster LVT 23 P). *Contact Dermatitis* 1977; 3:297–300.

84. Handfield-Jones S, Boyle J, et al. Contact allergy caused by metal sprays. *Contact Dermatitis* 1987; 16:44–45.

85. Kanerva L, Jolanki R, et al. Contact dermatitis from dibutylthiourea. Report of a case with fine structural observations of epicutaneous testing with dibutylthiourea. *Contact Dermatitis* 1984; 10:158–162.

86. Jepsen JR, Sparre Jörgensen A, et al. Hand protection for car-painters. *Contact Dermatitis* 1985; 13:317–320.

87. Dalager NA, Mason TJ, et al. Cancer mortality among workers exposed to zinc chromate paints. *J Occup Med* 1980; 22:25–29.

88. Mann RJ. Paint and grease gun injuries of the hand. *JAMA* 1975; 231:933.

89. Conde-Salazar L, Romero L, et al. Contact dermatitis in an oil painter. *Contact Dermatitis* 1982; 8:209–210.

28

Solvents

J.E. WAHLBERG, M.D.
ROBERT M. ADAMS, M.D.

A solvent is a substance capable of dissolving another substance to form a uniformly dispersed mixture at the molecular or ionic size level.[1] The use of hydrocarbon solvents began in 1823, when naphtha from crude coal tar was found to be an excellent solvent for rubber. Until recently solvents were employed almost exclusively to dissolve other substances or as diluents for adhesives and surface coatings. Today the chief uses are in the manufacture of other chemicals; as carriers for chemical reactions; as pressure transmitters for hydraulic systems; and in coatings, industrial cleaners, printing inks, and pharmaceuticals (Table 28–1). After water, the most common solvents are aliphatic and aromatic hydrocarbons, esters, ethers, ketones, amines, and nitrated and chlorinated hydrocarbons. Commonly used solvents are listed by chemical group in Table 28–2.

MANUFACTURE OF CHEMICALS

Solvents are most widely applied in the manufacture of other chemicals. Actually, solvents themselves are usually derived from other solvents—for example, methylethyl ketone from acetone, and formaldehyde from methanol. Exceptions are turpentine (from certain species of pine) and methyl or ethyl alcohol (from molasses, corn, and potatoes). But today most solvents are manufactured from petroleum, and synthetic turpentine has long been available.

Many solvents that were once leaders in their field are more important today as chemical intermediates. Benzene, until 1930 considered the outstanding solvent for greases and waxes, is now the starting material for phenol, aniline, styrene, and maleic anhydride. The majority of ethylene chloride produced today is used in the manufac-

ture of polyvinyl plastics; a much smaller percentage is used as a solvent. Carbon disulfide, up until 1930 the leading solvent for rubber, today is used almost exclusively in the making of viscose rayon.

Carriers for Chemical Reactions

Forty-five years ago it was estimated that more than 95% of all chemical reactions take place in a carrier solution.[2] Today that percentage is even greater. A carrier solution is a substance that dilutes another substance of primary importance, carrying it along through a complicated chemical process. The carrier does not react with the products or the catalysts, nor does it interfere with catalytic action. At the end of the reaction it should be possible to remove it from the solution.

TABLE 28–1 • Some End Uses of Solvents
Analytical chemistry
Carrier solutions for chemical reactions
Cleansing
Degreasing
Dry cleaning
Dyeing of fabrics, paper, plastics
Extraction processes
Floor laying
Froth flotation
Production of glass fiber polyesters
Graphics industries
Hydraulic systems
Painting and paint manufacture
Plastics manufacture
Printings
Rotogravure printing
Surface coating

TABLE 28–2 • **Common Solvents Classified by Chemical Group**

Solvent	Vapor Pressure (25°C, kPa)	Threshold Limit Value (ppm)	Skin Notation
Acetone	25	250	
Benzene	10	0.5	H
N-Butanol	0.6	15	H
Carbon disulfide	40	5	H
Carbon tetrachloride	12	2	H
Chloroform	21	2	
Dimethylformamide	0.4	10	H
Ethanol	6	500	
2-Ethoxyethanol	0.5	5	H
Ethyl acetate	10	150	
N-Hexane	16	25	
Isopropanol	4	150	
Methyl-N-butyl ketone	0.4	50	H
Methyl chloroform	13	50	
Methylene chloride	45	35	H
Methyl ethyl ketone	9	50	
Styrene	0.6	20	H
Tetrachloroethylene	1.9	10	
Toluene	2.9	50	H
Trichloroethylene	8	10	
White spirits distillates	<0.7		
Xylene	0.6–1.1	50	H

Solvents are ideal carriers and have numerous applications in the chemical industry for oxidation-reduction, esterification, hydrogenization, coupling, phosphorylation, and many other reactions.

Hydraulic Systems

Solvents are employed as pressure transmitters in hydraulic systems. For example, automobiles, lightweight trucks, and buses are all equipped with hydraulic brakes. The cylinders in each brake are constructed of aluminum, copper, brass, cast iron, or tin-plated steel and contain rubber seals. A hydraulic fluid must not corrode the metal or contribute to disintegration of the rubber. If too thin, the fluid will leak; if too viscous, unequal braking action results. Solvents such as lower alcohols, polyglycols of molecular weight 1,000 to 2,000 daltons, and glycol ethers are suitable for hydraulic systems and may be employed in combination with a castor oil derivative as a lubricant. Synthetic polymer mixtures of monobutyl ethers of oxyethylene and oxypropylene glycols are also used, along with mixtures of glycol ethers and additives for corrosion resistance, buffering, and so on. The composition and performance characteristics are specified by the Society of Automotive Engineers. Hydroquinone and bisphenol A are frequently added as antioxidants.

Froth-Flotation Processes

During the refining of many nonferrous metals (except aluminum), the froth-flotation process allows recovery of small quantities of minerals that would be lost were water alone used as solvent. First, the ore is thoroughly pulverized, treated with a surfactant and water, and mixed with a water-repellent solvent. Air is then forced into the mixture for agitation. Some of the ore particles are wetted by the surfactant and sink to the bottom. The minerals, however, remain unwetted, adhere to the air bubbles, and float to the surface, where they are skimmed off with the froth.

A *solvent-solvent* is a solvent for second-state extraction of difficult-to-extract metals such as gold, uranium, and thorium. An example is tributyl phosphine oxide, which is used in benzene or kerosene solution for the extraction of metal from the acids employed in mineral extraction.[3] The froth-flotation method, commonly used to concentrate copper, zinc, and lead from their ores, has become the most important and widely used concentration process in the mining industry. The method is also useful in recovering discarded minerals from industrial wastes, in purifying water, and in cleaning vegetables and fruits before commercial canning.

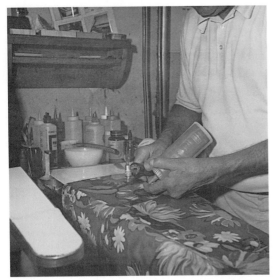

FIGURE 28–1 • Large quantities of solvents are used in dry cleaning, not only in tumblers but also in spotting soiled garments by hand.

DRY CLEANING

Solvents are indispensible in dry cleaning. First, spots are removed by gentle rubbing with a mixture of solvent and an aqueous detergent (Fig. 28–1). Then the cloth is treated by immersion–agitation and rinsed in nonaqueous solvents. Until 1925 petroleum naphtha was used for this purpose, but less hazardous solvents were soon employed. In 1928 *Stoddard solvent* was introduced, chiefly to replace the low–flash point, flammable naphtha.

Stoddard solvent is a petroleum distillate containing a mixture of straight and branched-chain paraffins, naphthenes, and alkyl derivatives of benzene, with a boiling range from 305° to 410°F. It is widely used in the industry, although chlorinated hydrocarbons have supplanted it to a large extent, especially perchloroethylene and trichloroethylene. Carbon tetrachloride was once the only chlorinated hydrocarbon used in the dry-cleaning industry but its use was discontinued because of its well-known hepatotoxicity. If the solvents used in dry cleaning, such as perchloroethylene, remain to some extent on clothing, skin irritation resembling a burn may result, especially on the legs, wrists, and neck.

ANTIKNOCK AGENTS

Antiknock agents have been added to gasoline since 1923 to prevent noisy spontaneous oxidation reactions in the cylinder head, a premature detona-

tion common to gasolines of certain octanes. Tetraethyl lead was the most effective and for years was the most common substance used for this purpose. Because of its significant role in air pollution, it has been removed from most gasolines, although it may still be present in trace amounts. Lead-free gasolines are now used in conjunction with catalytic converters, and the antiknock agents are methyl tert-butyl ether, or a mixture of methanol and tert-butyl alcohol.

METAL DEGREASERS

Solvent degreasing of metals is accomplished by several methods. Cold dipping is used for cleaning large objects such as engines; solvents for this method include Stoddard solvent, aromatic chlorinated hydrocarbons, ketones, Cellosolves, and others. Solvents may be applied to metal surfaces by brushing, wiping, or spraying, methods that require adequate ventilation at all times. In vapor degreasing, the part to be cleaned is lowered into a machine containing a solvent vapor. The part is lowered to approximately 2 feet above the boiling solvent. Solvent droplets condense on the cool metal surface and wash away grease and oil films. Coils containing cool water must be located at the level where parts are hung to decrease vapor contamination of the environment (Fig. 28–2). The metal objects being cleaned must remain long enough to reach the temperature of the vapor; otherwise, considerable solvent comes out of the tank with the dripping parts, contaminating the workers' skin and clothing.

Degreasing machines also operate by total immersion in boiling solvents or by pressure spraying with warm solvents. Ultrasonic degreasers are often valued for cleaning small objects. For years the solvent preferred for water-cooled degreasing machines was trichloroethylene; more than 90% of the total amount produced was used in degreasing machines and in dry cleaning.[4] Because of reports of hepatocellular carcinomas in mice given trichloroethylene by gastric intubation[5] and a subsequent ruling by OSHA, the solvent is now little used. Today perchloroethylene is used most widely as a dry-cleaning solvent, and fluorinated chlorohydrocarbons have nearly replaced trichloroethylene for degreasing. Ethylene dichloride and methyl chloroform are also used.

Inhibitors such as hydroquinone are often added to trichloroethylene to prevent its degradation. Epstein[6] reported dermatitis in two patients sensitive to trichloroethylene to which epichlorohydrin had been added as a stabilizer. Cleaning large degreasing machines creates a major hazard. Workers

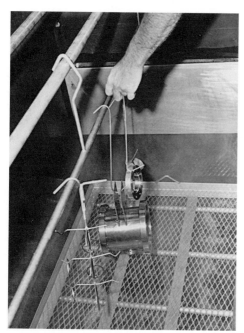

FIGURE 28–2 • Vapor degreasing is employed to clean small metal parts. The object to be cleaned is lowered into the hot vapor in a special vat. Care must be taken to avoid contact with the fumes.

TABLE 28–3 • Adverse Systemic Effects of Solvent Inhalation or Percutaneous Absorption
Carcinogenicity
Teratogenicity
Miscarriage
Nephrotoxicity
Hepatotoxicity
Neurotoxic and neuropsychiatric disorders
Hematopoietic effects
Cardiovascular effects
Respiratory effects
Gastrointestinal effects

must be supplied with respirators and a lifeline hose to the outside of the tank. A buddy system can prevent workers from being overcome with fumes, and gloves, sleeves, and aprons must be worn to avoid skin contact.

SOLVENT DERMATITIS

Occupational dermatitis from solvents is confined almost exclusively to people who use them in their work, since manufacturing processes for these substances take place in almost completely closed systems, allowing little or no skin contact. Almost all manufacturing plants use significant amounts of solvents. There are few occupations that do not use solvents in some manner.

Dermatologists should also be aware of systemic injury from inhalation or percutaneous absorption of solvents (Table 28–3), including narcosis, liver and kidney damage, pulmonary injury, hematopoietic effects, and peripheral neuritis. Some solvents have specific target organs—for example dimethyl formamide, the liver and benzene, bone marrow. Adverse effects are sometimes caused by the solvent itself; in other cases by its metabolite(s). In fact, the metabolites may be more toxic than the parent compound. In addition, the ever present hazards of fire and explosion must always be kept in mind.

In most studies of occupational dermatitis, solvents have been found to be responsible for as much as 20% of cases,[7, 8] the most frequent cause being the time-honored practice of washing the hands and arms in raw solvent (Fig. 28–3). The solvent varies with the occupation: plastics workers use acetone and methylethylketone; auto mechanics, gasoline and kerosene; printers, type wash; dry cleaners, perchloroethylene and Stoddard solvent; painters, paint thinners and turpentine; and so on. Additional damage may occur from prolonged immersion in water or repeated washing with soaps and detergents, particularly so-called waterless hand cleaners, which may themselves contain significant amounts of solvent.

Adverse skin effects of solvents are shown in Table 28–4. Almost all solvents are irritants, some more than others; only a few, such as turpentine, are also sensitizers (Table 28–5). In many instances of dermatitis caused by a solvent thought to be allergic, the disease is really due to irritation. Sensitization can be due to one or more of the additives, however.[9] Considering the extent of

TABLE 28–4 • Adverse Effects of Skin Exposure to Solvents
Subjective irritation
Irritation
Contact urticaria
Flushing (Stevens-Johnson syndrome)
Whitening
Irritant contact dermatitis
Chemical burns
Allergic contact dermatitis
Scleroderma
Dermatoses from higher boiling point distillates
Percutaneous absorption (systemic toxicity)
Enhanced skin penetration

TABLE 28–5 • Reports of Contact Allergy from Solvents

Turpentine/delta-3-carene[73, 74, 105]
d-Limonene[76–78, 106]
Dioxane[107]
Alcohols[21]
Styrene[104]

their use and the size of the exposed population, allergic contact dermatitis to solvents is rare. It should be remembered that, because of their strong potential for skin *irritancy*, it may be nearly impossible to demonstrate *allergenicity* by the conventional occlusive patch test technique.

In 1947 Klauder and Brill[10] demonstrated an inverse correlation between the boiling point of a solvent and its primary irritant effect. They demonstrated that the low–boiling range (below 450°F) petroleum solvents have the greatest defatting action and, thus, potential for causing dermatitis. Testing with petroleum solvents and oils of paraffin origin ranging from kerosene (initial boiling point 345°F) to light spindle oil (end boiling point 340°F) has shown that the irritant effects decrease as the boiling range increases. In general, the lower–boiling point naphthas, kerosene, and light oils are irritants, but petroleum distillates obtained at temperatures above 600°F, mainly heavier oils such as lubricating, spindle, transformer, machine, and cutting oils, have less defatting action but are more keratogenic. They cause comedos, acne, photosensitivity, melanosis, keratoses, and epitheliomas.[10] Workers, however, are

rarely exposed to only one solvent; more often they are exposed to mixtures of several. Mineral spirits, kerosene, gasoline, and various thinners are some widely used mixtures. Clinically, it is often difficult to demonstrate the relative importance of a single ingredient in mixtures.

The irritant action of solvents is based on dissolution of the surface lipids, the lipid material in the stratum corneum, and the fatty fraction of the cell membranes. This defatting action is responsible for the feeling of dryness and the whitening of the skin that follow contact with volatile solvents. Workers often report stinging, tingling, or burning from solvent contact, but the skin appears normal to visual inspection. This phenomenon has also been reported from skin exposure to lactic acid and in workers exposed to visual display units (VDUs).

Whitening of the skin has been observed when nine particular solvents are applied, as with a cotton applicator (Table 28–6). Using the Doppler flowmeter to study this phenomenon, no decrease in cutaneous blood flow was found, indicating that the whitening is not due to vasoconstriction. It was observed that most of the solvents that cause whitening also are able to extract lipids from the stratum corneum.[11] On the other hand, solvents that do not extract epidermal lipids, such as dimethylsulfoxide, propylene glycol, and water, also do not cause whitening.

Erythema, edema, and drying are the most common side effects from single or repeated exposures to solvents (Table 28–7). Solvents that rapidly evaporate from the skin are not as likely to induce damage unless there is also occlusion, as from

TABLE 28–6 • Effects on Skin Blood Flow from Solvent (Neat) Exposure as Expression of Irritancy as Recorded with Laser Doppler Flowmetry[12, 37]

| Solvent | Increase (+) or No Change (0) | | Duration (min) |
	0.1 mL Pipetted onto Skin	Whitening After Rubbing with Cotton	
Dimethylsulfoxide	+	0	1
Trichloroethane	0	+	1
N-Hexane	0	+	5
Carbon tetrachloride	0	+	5
Toluene	0	+	5
1,1,1-Trichloroethane	0	+	5
1,1,2-Trichloroethane	0	+	5
Dodecane	0	+	15
Methyl ethyl ketone	0	+	No increase
Propylene glycol	0	0	
Ethanol	0	+	
Water	0	0	

Exposure in excess of 1.5 mL/3.1 cm^2. Time in minutes to obtain an increase.

TABLE 28–7 • Ranking of Edema-Inducing Capacity of Skin Exposure to Solvents (Neat) in Experimental Animals[108, 109]

Solvent	Guinea Pig	Rabbit
Trichlorethylene	1	1
Toluene	2	1
1,1,2-Trichloroethane	3	1
Carbon tetrachloride	4	2
1,1,1-Trichloroethane	4	2
Dimethylsulfoxide	5	Not tested
N-Hexane	6	4
Methyl ethyl ketone	7	3
Ethanol	7	5

clothing. The resulting erythema and edema may be transient or may develop into irritant contact dermatitis, the course of which is related to the type of solvent, its concentration and dose, and the duration of exposure (see Tables 28–6, 28–7). Individual susceptibility factors are shown in Table 28–8. It is important to note that a history of atopic dermatitis or an existing lesion is important in increasing human susceptibility to irritants, and that those in predominantly "wet-work" occupations are also very likely to suffer relapses. The importance of preemployment examinations and vocational guidance cannot be overstated (see Table 29–8; see Chapters 12, 13, and 17).

The Doppler technique, a highly sensitive method of measuring skin blood flow, has found use in studying the erythema-inducing capacity of solvents.[12, 13, 37] The technique is three or four times more sensitive than the naked eye.[13] Table 28–7 illustrates the results of experiments with various solvents on the skin. In the first series of experiments 0.1-mL doses of the neat solvents were pipetted onto the skin; in the third series they were applied in excessive amounts.

Through defatting action, solvents increase the percutaneous absorption of water and other substances.[14] Vinson and colleagues,[15] using electron micrographs to show marked alterations in the

TABLE 28–8 • Susceptibility Factors for Dermatitis Due to Organic Solvents

History of atopic dermatitis
History of asthma/rhinitis*
History of previous, recurring dermatitis
Dry or aged skin[10]

*Relationship disputed.

nuclear and organelle membranes of cells, showed that mixtures of solvents such as chloroform-methanol actually damage the stratum corneum cells and the barrier. Methyl- and ethyl alcohol, hexane, and acetone alone, however, increase permeability more by removing skin lipids and less through action on the barrier structure.

Pathologic Changes

Guinea pigs were exposed to 13 solvents (neat), and skin biopsy specimens were taken at 15 minutes, and at 1, 4, and 16 hours.[16–18] Progressing nuclear pyknosis, perinuclear edema, pseudoeosinophilic infiltration, spongiosis, and junctional separation of varying degrees were observed. There was much variability among various solvents, and the exposure time also figured importantly. The only exception was n-butyl acetate, which was not observed to produce any histological changes. With percutaneous exposure some solvents caused only slight changes in skin morphology but pronounced systemic toxicity. The histologic changes observed may be interpreted as local defense reactions to toxic solvents.

A study by Lupulescu and Birmingham[19] also showed that the pathologic alterations vary among solvents. Using combined transmission and scanning electron microscopy, they studied the structural changes in the epidermis after application of acetone and kerosene. The changes varied considerably between the two irritants. Acetone produced large, paranuclear vacuoles, swollen mitochondria, and clumped tonofilaments. Application of kerosene resulted in cytolysis, widening of the intercellular spaces, and marked disruption of the epidermal architecture. A protective gel applied before contact with the two solvents to some extent reduced the intensity of the reactions.

Irritation of the skin, especially of the neck and face, may result from contact with solvent vapors, especially those of highly volatile solvents such as toluene,[20] trichloroethylene, and tetrachloroethane. Irritation of the face and neck may also be caused by hand contamination. Open degreasing machines are a common source of such dermatitis, but contact with solvent-soaked clothing and cleaning rags provides additional opportunities for development of dermatitis.

Contact urticaria is common from contact with certain solvents. Some solvents, such as alcohols, may cause immune-mediated and other types of contact urticaria.[21] Case reports have been published on trichloroethylene[22] (see below), methyl ethyl ketone,[23] naphtha,[24] and dimethyl sulfoxide, xylene, and polyethylene glycol. It is important, however, not to mistake macular erythema for contact urticaria.[27] Inhalation of trichloroethylene followed by drinking ethyl alcohol can within a few minutes elicit erythema on extensive areas of the face, neck, and shoulders. Reported by Stewart and coworkers,[22, 26] it has been termed *degreaser's flush*. To confirm the diagnosis, testing with gas chromatographically pure ethanol ("as is") is recommended.[21] When useful data for other solvents are lacking, testing should be done with graded concentrations, in addition to using a large number of controls. Exposure to trichloroethylene has been associated with generalized dermatitis[27, 28] and Stevens-Johnson syndrome.[29] Fatal toxic hepatitis has also been reported.[29] From these reports, it is difficult to know the main route of absorption, whether inhalation or through the skin.[28]

Because of the observed risks of systemic toxicity and carcinogenicity from inhalation of solvents, the Threshold Limit Values (TLVs) have been gradually reduced. As a result, the percutaneous route has assumed greater prominence. While it is true that skin absorption from exposure is negligible for most of the commonly used solvent vapors, certain solvents, especially those that contain both a lipophilic and a hydrophilic moiety (glycol ethers and dimethylformamide are examples), are readily absorbed, and skin exposure may contribute significantly to the total uptake. Glycol ethers have low volatility and high boiling points as compared with other organic solvents. Certain other solvents, especially 2-chloroethanol, 5-butoxyethanol, carbon tetrachloride, 1,1,2-trichloroethane, dimethylformamide, and dimethylsulfoxide have caused the death of guinea pigs exposed percutaneously,[30] and fatalities in humans have also been reported. The conclusion of these reports is that percutaneous absorption contributes to the total body burden and militate strongly for reducing percutaneous uptake and inhalation of solvents. In Sweden today solvents that are known to be readily absorbed through the skin are given a notation marked with *H* (*Hud*, or skin; see Table 28–2 and Fig. 28–3).[30a]

Any condition associated with defects in the skin barrier can facilitate percutaneous penetration; however, in guinea pigs it has been shown that skin damage (from stripping, needle and sandpaper abrasion, removal of the lipid layer) increases the absorption rate for *n*-butanol, but the absorption of toluene and 1,1,1-trichloroethane, which are lipophilic solvents, decreases.[31] Thus, skin damage does not automatically lead to increased percutaneous absorption. It appears, instead, that the lipophilic and hydrophilic properties of the solvent are more important and, perhaps, crucial. Certain common ingredients of many topical medications are said to facilitate penetration of other ingredients. Alcohols and propylene glycol are frequently cited as facilitators of percutaneous penetration; and, in fact, patients who use creams containing these solvents sometimes complain of burning and irritation.

Prolonged contact with solvent-soaked clothing may result in severe burns (Fig. 28–4) and even death. Walsh and colleagues[32] described the case of a 13-year-old boy trapped under an overturned tractor for 1 hour in clothing soaked with spilled gasoline. A scaldlike burn developed over 50% of his body and he died after 12 days, from renal failure.

Koilonychia in six cabinet makers was reported by Ancona-Alayon.[33] Each was cleaning metal accessories for finished furniture, using a solvent mixture of methanol, toluene, and xylene in varying concentrations.

Dermatitis from solvents is common and is estimated at up to 20% of cases of occupational dermatitis.[34] Most cases of dermatitis are relatively benign, with the exception being generalized dermatitis and the Stevens-Johnson syndrome from trichloroethylene. Covering the years 1984 to 1991, occupational eczematous diseases from solvent exposure in Denmark[35a] represented 991 re-

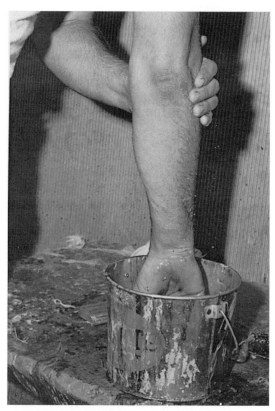

FIGURE 28–3 • Cleaning the skin with raw solvent is one of the most common causes of occupational dermatitis.

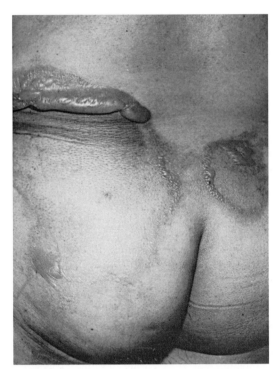

FIGURE 28–4 • This home gardener sprayed his clothing with pesticide. He was unable to remove his clothing for several hours. By that time, large bullae had formed, causing several weeks of disability, as well as permanent scarring.

ported cases (3.6%), fifth on the ranking list. Solvents were superseded by water (13.9%), detergents (11.6%), nickel (5.4%), and soaps and hand cleansers (3.9%).

Patch-testing Solvents

The irritant properties and volatility of some solvents make patch-testing very problematic. For example, in a comparative study with tetrachloroethylene, it was found that using the traditional patch-test technique and applying a 1% solution in olive oil produced, a reaction whereas open application (neat) was negative.[35] It was recommended, therefore, that to minimize evaporation, the solution should be applied immediately before application, using filter paper.

Since several solvents are potent skin irritants even after brief exposure (see Table 28–6), it is likely impossible to demonstrate allergenicity using conventional patch-test techniques. Information on suitable test concentrations and vehicles is rarely available to physicians, and testing with solvents is frequently a matter of trial and error. When a reaction is obtained, it is crucial to do serial dilution tests in the patient, using a sufficient

number of controls, preferably more than 25. Provocative use testing such as the repeated open application test (ROAT) has been used to clarify the relevance of a "positive" patch-test reaction to a solvent.[36]

Ethanol, methyl ethyl ketone, and acetone are recommended vehicles for patch-testing materials and products brought by patients, as it has been shown over many years that these solvents are only marginal irritants.[13] Under occlusion propylene glycol has irritant properties, and an optimal test concentration and vehicle have not yet been determined.[37]

CUTANEOUS EFFECTS AND COMMON USES OF SOLVENTS

Coal Tar–Based Solvents

Benzene

Discovered in 1825 by Michael Faraday from experiments with whale oil–based illuminating gas, benzene (benzol) was for many years one of the most widely used industrial solvents. It was relatively inexpensive and had superior solvent qualities. Today benzene has limited use as a general industrial solvent, but it is still used in analytical laboratories, as a specialty solvent, and in the synthesis of a number of important substances—ethyl benzene for production of styrene, and cyclohexane for nylon, among others. Exposure to benzene itself can still occur in rubber tire plants and in petrochemical plants and petroleum refineries, but usually it is used in closed systems that afford little opportunity for inhalation or skin contact.

The great potential hazard of benzene is damage to blood-forming organs, which often occurs from repeated exposure to comparatively small amounts. Before the hematopoietic hazards of benzene were realized and its use curtailed, the solvent was after lead the most important industrial poison. Individual susceptibility varies considerably: some workers show no toxicity even after heavy exposure. Purpura on the arms, legs, trunk, and mucous membranes may be one of the earliest manifestations of aplastic anemia from chronic benzene poisoning. Benzene has also been associated with all types of leukemia, but most frequently with the acute nonlymphocytic type.

Toluene (Methyl Benzene)

Toluene is today one of the most widely used industrial solvents, along with xylene. Produced mainly by the catalytic reforming of petroleum, it replaced benzene in many applications. High concentrations have a narcotic effect.[38] The local skin effect is drying, which may be caused by the vapor alone. It is used as blending stock in aviation and high-octane gasoline; as a solvent for paints and coatings; in gums, resins, many oils, rubber, and vinyl organosols; as a diluent and thinner for nitrocellulose lacquers; and in many other applications.

Xylene (Dimethylbenzene)

The mixture of the three isomers of xylene is known as *xylol*. Large amounts are used in gasoline, especially aviation gasoline. Approximately 10 to 15% is used in solvents.[39] It is also the starting material for acids in the manufacture of plastics, synthetic fabrics, paints, and pesticides and is a carrier in the manufacture of epoxy resins. Like other coal tar solvents, xylene exerts a defatting action on the skin and thus contributes to development of irritant dermatitis. Over the past decade environmental regulations have reduced its use.

Ethyl Benzene

Derived from benzene, ethyl benzene is a strong irritant, narcotic, and skin vesicant. It is considered the most severe irritant of the benzene series.[40] It is used as an intermediate in the production of styrene, as a paint and lacquer thinner, in motor and aviation fuels as a lead scavenger, and in other solvents, for the same reasons xylene is employed.

Cumene (Isopropyl Benzene)

Cumene is a high-volume solvent, produced in the United States chiefly for the production of phenol, acetone, and methyl styrene. It is used to improve the octane rating in aviation fuels and as a solvent for cellulose, paints, and lacquers.[41] Employed as a solvent for cellulose paints and lacquers, it is a skin and eye irritant that is slowly absorbed through intact skin, producing a narcotic effect.

Petroleum Solvents

Gasoline

Gasoline is the portion of petroleum distillate that vaporizes immediately before kerosene. Before the advent of the automobile, gasoline was discarded as a useless by-product. It contains hundreds of different hydrocarbons, including paraffins, cyclo-paraffins, and various aromatic hydrocarbons. To eliminate knocking and increase the octane number, methyl tert-butyl ether (MBTE) is added. This compound has replaced tetraethyl lead, which was used for decades before being abandoned because of serious environmental concerns about lead. Gasoline is irritating to the skin, especially through contact with gasoline-soaked clothing.[32] Vapors can have a narcotic effect. Contact allergy was suspected from a blue anthraquinone gasoline dye in a service station attendant, but allergic contact dermatitis to gasoline is very rare.[42] Service station attendants rarely develop dermatitis from the solvent action of gasoline, most likely because modern gasoline pumps rarely leak. Attendants still commonly use gasoline to clean their skin after repairing autos.

Kerosene

Also called *coal oil*, kerosene is a pale yellow, oily liquid containing approximately 10 hydrocarbons, including *n*-dodecane and derivatives of benzene and naphthalene. Until the manufacture of the automobile and the electric light, kerosene, because it was an illuminating fuel, was the major product of the petroleum industry. Today it is used as a cleaning solvent, as a fuel for jet, rocket and tractor engines, in domestic heating, as an illuminant, and as a carrier for insecticides, in which use it is a common cause of irritation.[43–45]

Stoddard Solvent

Also known as *Varnoline, Varsol,* and *white spirits*, Stoddard solvent is a petroleum distillate similar to gasoline that contains both aliphatic and aromatic hydrocarbons. It has been used as a dry-cleaning solvent especially for spot and stain removal, as a paint thinner and vehicle, as a carrier for herbicides and insecticides, in adhesives, and as a solvent in photocopier toners. Irritant dermatitis and chemical burns can occur.[46]

Hexane

Hexane is a widely used solvent derived from the fractional distillation of petroleum. It is a relatively inexpensive solvent for use in glues, varnishes, inks, rubber cements, and extraction of oils from seeds. It is readily absorbed by inhalation and to some extent through the skin. It causes respiratory and skin erythema and irritation, but the incidence of acute toxicity is rather low.[47] It also may cause anesthesia and neurobehavioral dysfunction. An isomer of hexane, *n*-hexane, causes peripheral neuropathy, especially in shoe- and sandalmakers, whose glues may contain *n*-hexane as solvent.[48] Paresthesias of the distal portions of the extremities, among the initial symptoms, lead to sensory loss and motor weakness of toes, arms, thighs, and forearms. Recovery usually follows removal of the source.

Chlorinated Hydrocarbon Solvents

Carbon Tetrachloride

Carbon tetrachloride is an excellent solvent that when absorbed or inhaled unfortunately produces severe liver and kidney damage. It also causes erythema, skin whitening (see Table 29–6), and dermatitis by its defatting action on the skin. In addition, it is a strong anesthetic. It has been used in metal degreasing and as a refrigerant, agricultural grain fumigant, and a solvent for fats, oils, rubber, and other products. It is still used (surreptitiously?) in commercial dry-cleaning establishments for spot-treating small soiled areas of clothing. It is not permitted in products intended for home use.

Trichloroethane

Because its solvent properties closely resemble those of carbon tetrachloride, trichloroethane (also known as *methyl chloroform*) has been widely and successfully used as a substitute. It is not as irritating to the skin and is less harmful to internal organs. It is considered one of the least toxic of the chlorinated hydrocarbon solvents, although it is a central nervous system depressant and administration to mice has induced neoplasms of the liver.[49] It is used as a solvent for natural and synthetic rubber, oils, waxes, tar, and alkyloids; as a degreaser; and in the synthesis of many organic compounds.

Tetrachloroethane

Produced by the chlorination of acetylene, tetrachloroethane (acetylene tetrachloride) was one of the first airplane "dopes" (adhesives) to be used, but because of its hepatotoxicity it was banned by the Germans shortly before World War I. It causes relatively mild skin irritation but is an extremely potent hepatic and kidney toxin and a powerful narcotic. It also causes chromosomal changes in leukocytes. Inhalation of the vapor is usually the main means of toxicity. Poisoning has occurred in the artificial silk and leather industries, and hepatitis was reported in a penicillin plant among almost 50 workers.[50] It is used in cleansing and degreasing metals, as a paint remover, in varnishes, lacquers, photographic films, resins and waxes, and as an intermediate in manufacture of other chlorinated hydrocarbons. It has also been used in dry cleaning for "spotting" and fabric cleaning.

Trichloroethylene

Trichloroethylene is a nonflammable solvent that until recently was used extensively in industry; however, laboratory studies have shown that it causes cancer in mice, and its use has been considerably curtailed.[51] It is not a strong irritant on the skin or mucous membranes, but owing to its defatting action it can cause dermatitis after repeated contacts. Contact with solvent-soaked clothing for long periods can result in severe blistering [52] Until recently, large amounts were used in degreasing and dry-cleaning machines.[4]

A curious cutaneous reaction that followed (1) ingestion of alcoholic beverages after (2) trichloroethylene inhalation was reported by Stewart and colleagues.[22] Termed *degreaser's flush*, it consists in erythema of extensive areas of the face, neck, and shoulders that develops within a few minutes after drinking alcohol. Nausea and vomiting also occurred in some persons. The reaction resembles the disulfiram reaction,[53] also called the *aldehyde syndrome*.[54] Further inhalation exposure induces intoxication, during which euphoria alternates with a narcotic effect. Liver toxicity has been reported.[55] Bauer and Rabens[27] reported four workers who exhibited generalized dermatitis and varying degrees of inebriation and one with toxic hepatitis after exposure. They described trichloroacetic acid in the urine to be a useful marker and test for exposure to this solvent. Chloroethanol may also be detected in the serum as long as 4 to 5 days after exposure. Breath analysis for trichloroethylene may be helpful as well.[26]

Rubber latex gloves are penetrated by trichloroethylene. Polyvinyl and butyl gloves appear to be more impermeable. It should be remembered that when trichloroethylene is used near a heat source such as a welding torch the vapor decomposes to phosgene gas and hydrochloric acid.

Trichloroethylene is widely used as a degreaser and in dry cleaning for textiles and furs. It is also used as a solvent for neoprene, and in the paint industry as a solvent for tar in paint for casks, vats, and so on. It is employed in extracting oils and fats from vegetable products, corn, olives, bones, leather, wool, and fish; and in recovering fat-free glue, the residues from tanneries, and wax and paraffin from refuse. At one time it was used to decaffeinate coffee; now methylene chloride is used. It is no longer used in the United States as a fumigant in agriculture.

Because trichloroethylene is somewhat unstable, stabilizers must be added. In the past these have included thymol and ammonium carbonate. More recently diisopropylamine with alkyl-*p*-hydroxyanisole are used.[56] The former is a mild skin irritant, and possibly a sensitizer.

Methylene Chloride

Methylene chloride (dichloromethane or carene) is a solvent used extensively in the electronics industry as a degreaser. Other major uses are as a paint remover, aerosol propellant, a substitute for fluorocarbons, blowing agent for polyurethane foams, and with other solvents for cleaning electric motors. It may also be used as a solvent for decaffeinating coffee beans and an extraction solvent for edible fats, cocoa, butter, beer flavoring in hops, perfumes, other flavorings, and drugs.

Methylene chloride is a mild skin irritant that is enhanced by occlusion with clothing such as shoes. It has a tendency to hydrolyze to form hydrochloric acid in small amounts, corroding containers and adding to its mild irritant properties.[57]

One of its metabolic products is carbon monoxide, and blood levels of carboxyhemoglobin can be used as a biological monitor. Persons with cardiac disease can be placed at increased risk by exposure to this substance,[58] but its principal toxic action affects the central nervous system, first as a narcotic and in higher concentrations as an anesthetic agent.

Ethylene Dichloride

A colorless liquid with an odor resembling chloroform, ethylene dichloride was one of the first anesthetic agents used by Sir James Simpson in 1848. It is a powerful narcotic and also is nephrotoxic and hepatotoxic. Contact dermatitis has been reported.[20] Ethylene dichloride is widely used in industry as a solvent for fats, turpentine, rubber, resins, and oils. It is also used as an insecticide and fumigant for furs, in fire extinguishers, household cleaning, and commercial dry cleaning fluids, and as a lead scavenger in antiknock gasoline.

Alcohol Solvents

Methyl Alcohol

Before 1906 the use of ethyl alcohol was illegal in U.S. industry, and methyl alcohol was the preferred solvent.[20] Many industrial poisonings were associated with inhalation, ingestion, or skin contact. When denatured ethyl alcohol was permitted by law in 1904, the prejudices against it were so strong that it gained acceptance only very slowly. It was not until Prohibition, in 1917, that the dangers of ingesting methyl alcohol were widely publicized, and only then did manufacturers renounce its use in industrial processes.

Until 1930, methyl alcohol was produced by the destructive distillation of wood; since then it has been made synthetically. It is used industrially in antifreeze, racing car and rocket fuels; as a solvent for paints, varnishes, shellacs, and paint removers; and in the manufacture of formaldehyde and formaldehyde resins. It is also used in small amounts in the manufacture of explosives, shoes, and linoleum.

Injury to the skin occurs by primary irritation, but more important are the dangers of blindness and death from ingestion or inhalation. Because it is eliminated slowly from the body, repeated exposure can result in increasing concentrations.[59] Ingestion of methyl alcohol (which often is done because it is mistaken for ethyl alcohol) can result in permanent blindness, and in severe cases, death, preceded by marked metabolic acidosis. Visual symptoms include eye pain, blurred vision, constriction of visual fields, and other vision complaints. Permanent blindness can develop after as little as 48 hours.[60]

Ethyl Alcohol

Ethyl alcohol, ethanol, is one of the most important solvents and intermediates in industry, being used in many products and processes. Approximately 85% is used in solvents, alone or as a derivative. Synthetic ethanol is made by the hydration of ethylene, a distillate of crude oil. Ethanol is also produced from the fermentation of corn.

Dermatitis from contact with ethanol is not common,[21] but irritation can occur from its mild solvent and drying action on the skin or, rarely, from substances used for denaturation. Numerous denaturants are used; all must be approved for use in the United States. Ethanol used for special purposes, such as hair tonics, may contain pine oil as a denaturant. Methyl alcohol has been used for years to denature ethanol, sometimes with disastrous results when it is taken internally. Other denaturants are tert-butyl alcohol, brucine (dimethoxystrychnine from nux vomica), quassin (from extract of quassia, bitterwood), sucrose octaacetate, and acetone oil. Denatured alcohol can be pink (amaranth) or blue (methylene blue).[61]

Ethanol has occasionally been reported to be a contact allergen.[62–64] Fregert's group[62] reported three patients with positive patch tests to methanol, ethanol, 1-propanol, 1-butanol, *and* 1-protenol. Two of the patients showed sensitivity to 2-protenol and one to 2-butanol. Testing with tertiary alcohols was negative. Two of the patients came in contact with the alcohols in their work. Van Ketel and Tan-Lim[64] reported severe dermatitis in a woman following gallbladder surgery during which ethanol was used on her skin. Patch testing with 60% ethanol was positive. Ethyl alcohol can also cause contact urticaria.[65, 66]

Isopropyl Alcohol

Isopropyl alcohol (dimethylcarbinol, isopropanol, 2-propanol) is made by treating propylene with sulfuric acid and hydrolizing the product. Isopropyl alcohol may be substituted for ethyl alcohol as a solvent for oils, alkyloids, gums, and resin. It is also used in electroplating drying baths; as a deicer for liquid fuels; in perfumes, cosmetics, and lacquers; and in medications.

As an irritant and drying agent, isopropyl alcohol is well-known, although it must be classified as a marginal irritant. Allergic sensitivity to it must be very rare, considering its wide use, particularly in alcohol "wipes"; however, some cases of sensitivity have been reported. In 1969 Fregert and coworkers[62] found two patients sensitive to this alcohol. Fisher[67] described erythema that developed within minutes after its application in a patch test, which suggested contact urticaria.

Jensen[68] reported two laboratory assistants who developed contact dermatitis from a commonly used disposable disinfectant swab containing 70% isopropyl alcohol and 1% propylene oxide. Both patients were positive on patch testing with propylene oxide, 0.1% in ethanol, and one also reacted to 70% isopropyl alcohol. Other instances of allergic contact dermatitis to isopropyl alcohol have been reported with positive patch-test reactions to dilutions as low as 5%.[69–71]

Other Solvents

Turpentine

Spirits of turpentine, also known as *turps*, is obtained by the distillation of an oleoresin exuded by pine wood, especially long-leafed and slash pine. It is a mixture of oils, mainly mono- and sesquiterpenes: alpha-pinene, beta-piinene, delta-3-carene, *d*-limonene, beta-phallandrene, sesquiterpene, longifolene, and others. The combination of ingredients varies depending on the tree and country of origin. After separation of the turpentine oils, the residue that remains is termed *rosin* or *colophony*. In addition to being used as a paint thinner and an ingredient of varnishes and lacquers, turpentine has also been employed as a rubber solvent and reclaiming agent, although it has been supplanted recently by less expensive solvents.

Pirila and coworkers[9, 72] determined that autooxidation products of delta-3-carene were the chief source of sensitization.[73, 74] In addition, there is evidence that turpentine left exposed to sunlight and air for a time is more likely than is fresh turpentine to cause irritation and allergic sensitization. Kirton[75] found that sunlight and air cause formation of hydroperoxides. Because of the trend in recent years toward using less toxic substances, organic solvents with less toxic properties have been recommended. Solvents containing high levels of *d*-limonene, for example, have found use

for metal degreasing, and may present a potent allergenic potential to workers in painting and cleaning assembly.[76–78]

Because the constituents of turpentine vary with its source, the allergenicity varies from country to country.[79] Swedish turpentine, for example, has much greater sensitizing potential than French turpentine.[80] Turpentine sensitivity in the United States is not common; however, the potential for sensitization was shown by Kligman,[81] who, using the human maximization test, sensitized 18 of 25 subjects. Magnusson and Kligman,[82] using the guinea pig maximization test, were also able to sensitize 16 of 25 animals.

Because of its allergic potential and its cost, turpentine is used much less frequently than it was in the past. It is still used to some extent by artists, and in Poland Rudzki[83] reported three house painters with turpentine allergy. He also found one cleaning woman who developed allergic dermatitis from contact with a floor polish containing turpentine. Porcelain painting has been a source of turpentine allergy.[84] Jordan[85] reported allergic contact dermatitis from eyeglass frames polished by tumbling in a mixture of beeswax and turpentine.

Although raw turpentine alone is hardly ever used in industry today, derivatives and the combination of turpentine with other substances have many valuable uses, especially as solvents and thinners. They are used in polishes for shoes, automobiles, and furniture, in printing inks, putty, and mastics, cutting oils and degreasing solutions. Terpex is the trademark for a polymerized turpentine modified with various additives and used as a component of coatings, especially aluminum paints. Terpex Extra is the trademark for a low–molecular weight liquid terpene resin used as a rubber tackifier and plasticizers, in adhesives, and as an oil extender. Terpinolene is a solvent for resins used in the manufacture of synthetic resins and is used in synthetic flavors and perfumes. Toxaphene is a commercial insecticide based on camphene from pinene.

At temperatures above 35°C turpentine releases a flammable vapor that can form explosive mixtures with air. In addition to its allergenic potential, turpentine is a skin irritant, producing bullous reactions, especially when occluded by clothing.

Ethyl Ether

Produced by the dehydration of ethyl alcohol, ethyl ether is not a strong skin irritant, although dryness and fissuring can result from prolonged contact. It is used as a solvent for waxes, oils, and resin; as a cleaning and spotting agent especially in the shoe industry; in the textile industry in the manufacture of cellulose acetate and rayon; in dyes; in the perfume industry; in the plastics industry mixed with ethanol; in the manufacture of photographic film; in the rubber industry; and as a surgical anesthetic.

Ketones

Ketone is a class of liquid organic compounds in which the carbonyl group, C—O, is attached to two alkyl groups. The simplest member of the series is acetone. They are used primarily as solvents, in lacquers, paints, explosives, and textile processing. Besides acetone, diethyl ketone and methyl ethyl ketone are chief members of this group. As a class they do not present serious acute health hazards, because irritation to the mucous membranes occurs long before central nervous system depression.

Acetone

In addition to being a valuable starting chemical for numerous other compounds, acetone is found in the paint, lacquer, and varnish industry, in rubber compounding, plastics, and dyeing. It is used as an active solvent in film casting, film formation, inks, cleaners, and thinners. It is also employed, as acetone oil, a denaturant for special alcohol formulas. It is very flammable and presents a serious fire hazard. Although acetone is a mild skin irritant that produces erythema and dryness, it is very volatile and when inhaled in large quantities can result in narcosis and collapse.

Methyl Ethyl Ketone

Methyl ethyl ketone (MEK, 2-butanone), is frequently combined with other solvents such as alcohol for use in cosmetics, fabric coatings, and pharmaceuticals. It is widely used as a constituent of dewaxing compounds and a solvent in the electronics industry. Fabricated plastics comprise approximately 30% of its end uses. It is also employed in the manufacture of methyl methacrylate and as a solvent for vinyl and acrylic resins. With exposure to the liquid and fumes it is a mild skin defatting agent, irritant, and contact urticant.[23] The metabolic pathways of this compound include methanol, and peripheral neuropathy has been observed after prolonged, heavy exposure.[86] Interaction between methyl ethyl ketone and 2-hexanone (methyl n-butyl ketone) appears to potentiate the neurotoxicity of 2-hexanone.[86]

Methyl Butyl Ketone

Also known as *2-hexanone*, methyl butyl ketone is an irritant to eyes and mucous membranes and narcotic in high concentrations. It is absorbed by the skin. It is used chiefly as a solvent in the lacquer industry. Toxic peripheral neuropathy has been reported.[88]

Carbon Disulfide

One of the most toxic solvents known, carbon disulfide is an extremely volatile liquid that has a sweet, ethereal odor and acrid taste. It was discovered in 1796 by Lampadius and was once used to treat a variety of diseases. It is one of the original, and most effective, rubber solvents and a solvent for sulfur, phosphorus, resins, and waxes. The first cases of poisoning from this chemical were observed a century ago in rubber vulcanization plants in France and Germany. It is also used in the manufacture of cellophane, explosives, and matches; in electroplating; and in the production of carbon tetrachloride. In viscose rayon plants it produces blisters resembling second- or third-degree burns on the fingertips of workers in reeling and spinning rooms.[89] Carbon disulfide is readily absorbed through the skin and is extremely irritating; in sufficient amounts it is a desiccant. It is also explosive, and when inhaled a potent narcotic and neurotoxin that sometimes produces permanent psychotic disturbances.[90] In the early days of rubber vulcanizing, many workers were affected with serious brain damage, and several were placed in mental institutions for long periods with the misdiagnosis of insanity.[89]

Ethylene Glycol Ether Solvents

Marketed under the trademark Cellosolve are a number of mono- and dialkyl ethers of ethylene glycol and their derivatives, which are widely used as industrial solvents. There are approximately 10 of these. They are strong solvents for paints, varnishes, plastics, and dyes. They also are used as anti-icing additives to fuels and brake fluids and as antistall agents in gasoline. Although they cause drying and defatting of the skin, the chief concern is ingestion—and to some extent absorption through the skin (Fig. 28–5).

Glycidyl Ethers

The glycidyl ethers are a group of complex organic compounds with at least one 2,3-epoxypropoxy radical. There are approximately 14 of these ethers incorporated into epoxy resin systems as reactive diluents to reduce the viscosity of the polymer. Exposure can occur in epoxy production and use, in electrical occupations, to other plastic products and rubber, and in communications occupations.

In addition to fire and explosion hazards, the toxicity of these compounds is related to primary skin and eye irritation and allergic sensitization.

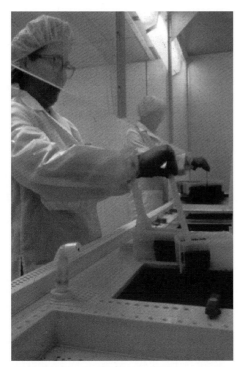

FIGURE 28–5 • The semiconductor industry uses great quantities of solvents. The protective measures are stringent in most plants, and dermatitis is rare. (Courtesy of Dr. Joseph LaDou.)

There have been no reports of carcinogenic, mutagenic, teratogenic, or reproductive effects of these ethers in humans.[91] The allergenicity of these ethers appears to be greatest with lower–molecular weight mono- and diglycidyl ethers, as opposed to the higher–molecular weight aliphatic polyglycidyl ether compounds.[92]

Ethyl Acetate

Ethyl acetate is a solvent for varnishes, lacquers, nitrocellulose and vinyl resins, and synthetic rubber, an ingredient of nail polish removers, and is used to make synthetic fruit essences. In 1971 Jordan and Dahl[85] reported contact dermatitis to ethyl acetate used as a plastic solvent to weld nose pads to eyeglass frames. The patient was also sensitive to ethylene glycol monomethyl ether acetate. Ethyl acetate is a mild irritant to the skin but less so than butyl and propyl acetate.

Amyl Acetate

n-Amyl acetate (pear oil) and isoamyl acetate (banana oil) are solvents for lacquers and paints; extraction of penicillins; in photographic film and leather polishes; as warning odors; in printing and finishing fabrics, and as a solvent for phosphors in fluorescent lamps. They are used as prespotting

agents in the dry-cleaning industry and as a stiffening agent in the manufacture of straw hats.[93] Like most other solvents, they are flammable, are mild defatting agents, and can cause irritant dermatitis.

Butyl Acetate

Butyl acetate is used as a solvent in nitrocellulose lacquers and other resins, leather and paper coatings, perfumes, flavoring extracts, and as a dehydrating agent. It is not especially irritating to the skin. Allergic contact dermatitis to butyl acetate was reported by Roed-Petersen[94] in a pharmaceutical factory worker employed in the purification of penicillin. Patch-testing to butyl acetate, 5% in olive oil, was positive, and control patch tests of 36 patients were negative. Protection with PVC gloves was not possible because PVC is soluble in butyl acetate.

Miscellaneous Solvents

Dimethylsulfoxide

Dimethylsulfoxide (DMSO) is an extremely powerful solvent that readily penetrates the skin, carrying along most substances dissolved in it.[95–98] It has been shown to release histamine from mast cells in the skin,[99] which may account for occasional contact urticaria reactions when it is used as an over-the-counter topical medication. Allergic contact sensitization has not been reported.

It is used as a solvent for polymerization reactions; as an analytical reagent; in manufacture of several synthetic fibers; in industrial cleaners, pesticides, paint strippers, and hydraulic fluids; and in veterinary medicine. After skin absorption, it is eliminated through the breath and the skin, giving the patients a characteristic garlicy odor. DMSO facilitates the penetration of other substances through the skin by increasing the permeability of the barrier layer.[100]

Dioxane

1,4-Dioxane (diethylene ether) is a widely used solvent that is very toxic when inhaled. It is also readily absorbed through the skin, to which it is not a particularly strong irritant, although it does defat it.[101] Dioxane is a solvent for cellulosics and for a wide range of organic products: lacquers, paints, varnishes; paint and varnish removers; wetting and dispersing agents in textile processing; cleaning and detergent preparations; and many others.

Fregert[107] described dermatitis in a man who cleaned metal parts by dipping his left hand into the solvent, which was used as a substitute for trichloroethylene. Patch-testing with 0.5% aqueous 1,4-dioxane was positive. Such prolonged and repeated exposure has been reported to result in irritation. Malignant liver tumors and other cancers have been demonstrated experimentally from exposure to dioxane.[102]

Styrene (Vinyl Benzene)

A natural component of the sap from styraceous trees, styrene is produced commercially by dehydrogenation of ethyl benzene. It is used in the plastics industry as a solvent for synthetic rubber and resins, particularly polystyrene plastics, as an odorant; as a solvent for polyester resins; as a starting material in the manufacture of emulsifying agents, as an intermediate in chemical synthesis; and in the manufacture of synthetic rubber. Hydroquinone, 3%, may be added to inhibit polymerization during storage.

Besides skin irritation, the chief problem with styrene is neurotoxicity (functional disorders of the nervous system) and hematopoietic changes such as leukopenia, and development of toxic hepatitis.[103] Contact allergy to styrene with cross-reaction to vinyltoluene has been reported.[104]

References

1. Hawley GG, ed. The Condensed Chemical Dictionary, 10th ed. New York: Van Nostrand Reinhold; 1981:958.
2. Doolittle AK. The Technology of Solvents and Plasticizers. New York: John Wiley; 1954.
3. Brady GS, Clauser HR. Materials Handbook, 11th ed. New York: McGraw-Hill, 1977:506, 728, 815–816.
4. Kirk-Othmer Encyclopedia of Chemical Technology, 2nd ed, Vol 5. New York: John Wiley; 1964:183.
5. Lloyd JW, Moore RM, Breslin P. Background information on trichloroethylene. J Occup Med 1975; 17:603–605.
6. Epstein E. Allergy to epichlorohydrin masquerading as trichloroethylene allergy. Contact Dermatitis Newslett 1974; 16:475.
7. Klauder JV, Gross BA. Actual causes of certain occupational dermatoses. III. Arch Dermatol 1951; 63:1–23.
8. Schwartz L, Tulipan L, Birmingham DJ. Occupational Disease of the Skin. Philadelphia: Lea & Febiger; 1957.
9. Pirilä V. On the primary irritant and sensitizing effects of organic solvents. In: Proceedings of the Twelfth International Congress of Dermatology, Vol 1. Amsterdam: Excerpta Medica; 1962:463.
10. Klauder JV, Brill FA. Correlation of boiling ranges of some petroleum solvents with irritant action on skin. Arch Dermatol 1947; 56:197–215.
11. Goldsmith LB, Friberg SE, Wahlberg JE. The effect of solvent extraction on the lipids of the stratum corneum in relation to observed immediate whitening of the skin. Contact Dermatitis 1988; 19:348–350.
12. Wahlberg JE. Erythema-inducing effects of solvents following epicutaneous administration to man: studied by laser Doppler flowmetry. Scand J Work Environ Health 1984; 10:159.
13. Wahlberg JE. Assessment of erythema: a comparison between the naked eye and laser Doppler flowmetry. In: Frosch PJ, et al, eds. Current Topics in Contact Dermatitis. Berlin: Springer-Verlag; 1989:549.
14. Rothman S. Physiology and Biochemistry of the Skin. Chicago: University of Chicago Press; 1954.
15. Vinson LJ, Singer EJ, Koehler WR, et al. The nature of the epidermal barrier and some factors influencing skin permeability. Toxicol Appl Pharmacol 1965; 7[Suppl 2]: 7–19.
16. Kronevi T, Wahlberg JE, Holmberg B. Morphological lesions in guinea pigs during skin exposure to 1,1,2-trichloroethane. Acta Pharmacol Toxicol 1977; 41:298.
17. Kronevi T, Wahlberg JE, Holmberg B. Histopathology of skin, liver, and kidney after epicutaneous administration of five industrial solvents to guinea pigs. Environ Res 1979; 19:56.
18. Kronevi T, Wahlberg JE, Holmberg B. Skin pathology following epicutaneous exposure to seven organic solvents. Int J Tissue Reac 1981; 3:21.
19. Lupulescu AP, Birmingham DJ. Effect of protective agents against lipid solvent–induced damaged skin. Arch Environ Health 1976; 31:33–36.
20. Browning E. Toxicity and Metabolism of Industrial Solvents. Amsterdam: Elsevier; 1965.
21. Ophaswongse S, Maibach HI. Alcohol dermatitis: allergic contact dermatitis and contact urticaria syndrome. Contact Dermatitis 1994; 30:1–6.
22. Stewart RD, Hake CL, Peterson JE. "Degreasers' flush." Dermal response to trichloroethylene and ethanol. Arch Environ Health 1974; 29:1–5.
23. Varigos GA, Nurse DS. Contact urticaria from methyl ethyl ketone. Contact Dermatitis 1986; 15:259–260.
24. Goodfield MJD, Saihan EM. Contact urticaria to naphtha present in a solvent. Contact Dermatitis 1988; 18:187.
25. Gollhausen R, Kligman AM. Human assay for identifying substances which induce non-allergic contact urticaria: the NICU test. Contact Dermatitis 1985; 13:98–106.
26. Stewart RD, Hake CL, Peterson JE. Use of breath analysis to monitor trichloroethylene exposures. Arch Environ Health 1974; 29:6–13.
27. Bauer M, Rabens SF. Cutaneous manifestations of trichloroethylene toxicity. Arch Dermatol 1974; 110:886–890.
28. Nakayama H, Kobayashi M, Takahashi M, et al. Generalized eruption with severe liver dysfunction associated with occupational exposure to trichloroethylene. Contact Dermatitis 1988; 19:48–51.
29. Phoon WH, Chan MOY, Rajah VS, et al. Stevens-Johnson syndrome associated with occupational exposure to trichloroethylene. Contact Dermatitis 1984; 10:270–276.
30. Wahlberg JE, Boman A. Comparative percutaneous toxicity of ten industrial solvents in the guinea pig. Scand J Work Environ Health 1979; 5:345.
30a. Occupational Exposure Limit Values. Statute Book of the Swedish National Board of Occupational Safety and Health. Ordinance 1996:2.
31. Boman A, Wahlberg JE. Percutaneous absorption of 3 organic solvents in the guinea pig. I. Effect of physical and chemical injuries to the skin. Contact Dermatitis 1989; 21:36–45.
32. Walsh WA, Scarpa FJ, Brown RS, et al. Gasoline immersion burn. N Engl J Med 1974; 291:830.
33. Ancona-Alayon A. Occupational koilonychia from organic solvents. Contact Dermatitis 1975; 1:367–369.
34. Anderson K. Solvent dermatitis. In: Riihimaki V, Ulfvarson U, eds. Symposium on Contact Dermatitis. Dermatol Clin 1984; 2:545–551.
35. Vail JT. False-negative reactions to patch testing with volatile compounds. Arch Dermatol 1974; 110:130.
35a. Halkier-Sørensen L. Occupational skin diseases. Contact Dermatitis 1996; 35(Suppl 1):11.
36. Wahlberg JE. Patch testing. In: Rycroft RJG, Menne T,

Frosch P J, eds. *Textbook of Contact Dermatitis*, 2nd ed. Berlin: Springer-Verlag; 1995:243.

37. Wahlberg JE. Propylene glycol: search for a proper and non-irritant patch test preparation. *Am J Contact Dermatitis* 1994; 5:156–159.

38. American Conference of Governmental Industrial Hygienists. *Documentation of the Threshold Limit Values for Chemical Substances in the Work Environment: Toluene.* Cincinnati: American Conference of Governmental Industrial Hygienists; 1986:578.

39. Ransley DL. Xylene and ethylbenzene. In: *Kirk-Othmer Encyclopedia of Chemical Technology*, 3rd ed, Vol 24. New York: John Wiley; 1982:709–741.

40. Oettel H. Einwirkung organisher Flussigkeiten auf die Haut. *Arch Exp Pathol Pharmakd* 1936; 183:641–696.

41. Kirk RE, Othmer DF. In: *Encyclopedia of Chemical Technology*, 3rd ed, Vol 7. New York: John Wiley; 1982:286–290.

42. Garcia-Perez A, Aparicio M. Dermatitis from a dye in petrol. *Contact Dermatitis* 1975; 1:265.

43. Tagami H, Ogino A. Kerosene dermatitis. *Dermatologica* 1973; 146:123–131.

44. Jee S-H, Wang J-D, Sun C-C, et al. Kerosene dermatoses among ballbearing factory workers. *Scand J Work Environ Health* 1985; 12:61–65.

45. Jarvholm B, Lavenius B, Bjorn A. Harmful health effect of exposure to kerosene and antirust oil. *Scand J Work Environ Health* 1986; 12:512.

46. Larsen LB, Shmunes E. Occupational health care report. No. 6—Stoddard solvent. *J Occup Med* 1974; 16:276.

47. Amdur MO, Doull J, Klaassen CD, eds. *Casarett and Doull's Toxicology, The Basic Science of Poisons*, 4th ed. New York: Pergamon; 1991.

48. Yamada S. An occurrence of polyneuritis by *N*-hexane in the polyethylene laminating plants. *Jpn J Ind Health* 1964; 6:192–194.

49. Bannasch P, Keppler D, Weber G, eds. *Liver Cell Carcinoma*. London: Kluwer Academic; 1989.

50. Elkins HB. Tetrachloroethane. In: *Encyclopedia of Occupational Health and Safety*. Geneva: International Labour Organization; 1983:2161–2163.

51. National Cancer Institute. *Carcinogenesis Bioassay of Trichloroethylene*, Publication 76-802. Carcinogenesis Technical Report Series, No. 2. Washington: US Dept of Health, Education and Welfare; 1976.

52. Schirren J M. Skin lesions caused by trichloroethylene in a metal working plant. *Berufsdermatosen* 1971; 19:240–254.

53. Stewart RD, Dodd HC. Absorption of carbon tetrachloride, trichloroethylene, tetrachloroethylene, methylene chloride, and 1,1,1-trichloroethane through the human skin. *Am Ind Hyg Assoc J* 1964; 25:439–446.

54. Fisher AA. *Contact Dermatitis*. Philadelphia: Lea & Febiger; 1986:541.

55. David A. Trichloroethylene. In: Parmeggiani L, ed. *Encyclopedia of Occupational Health and Safety*. Geneva: International Labour Organization; 1983:2214–2216.

56. Waters EM, Gerstner HB, Huff JE. Trichloroethylene I. An overview. *J Toxicol Environ Health* 1977; 2:671–707.

57. Methylene chloride passes early tests. *Chem Eng News* 1977; May 9:6.

58. Browning E. Dichloromethane. In: Parmeggiani L, ed. *Encyclopedia of Occupational Health and Safety*. Geneva: International Labour Organization; 1982:624–626.

59. Shmunes E. Methanol. In: Adams RM, ed. *Occupational Skin Disease*. Philadelphia: WB Saunders; 1990:448.

60. Andrews LS, Snyder R. Toxic effects of solvents and vapors. In: Amdur MO, Doull J, Klaassen CD, eds. *Casarett and Doull's Toxicology, The Basic Science of Poisons*, 4th ed. New York: Pergamon; 1991:701.

61. Fisher AA. *Contact Dermatitis*. Philadelphia: Lea & Febiger; 1973:79.

62. Fregert S, Groth O, Hjorth N, et al. Alcohol dermatitis. *Acta Derm Venereol* 1969; 49:493–497.

63. Haxthausen H. Allergic eczema caused by ethyl alcohol. *Acta Derm Venereol* 1944; 25:527–528.

64. van Ketel W, Tan-Lim KN. Contact dermatitis from ethanol. *Contact Dermatitis* 1975; 1:7–10.

65. Rilliet A, Hunziker N, Brun R. Alcohol contact urticaria syndrome (immediate-type hypersensitivity). *Dermatologica* 1980; 161:361.

66. Wilkin JK, Fortner G. Ethnic contact urticaria to alcohol. *Contact Dermatitis* 1985; 12:118–120.

67. Fisher AA. Contact dermatitis: the noneczematous variety. *Cutis* 1968; 4:567–571.

68. Jensen O. Contact allergy to propylene oxide and isopropyl alcohol in a skin disinfectant swab. *Contact Dermatitis* 1981; 7:148–150.

69. Wasilewski C. Allergen contact dermatitis from isopropyl alcohol. *Arch Dermatol* 1968; 98:502–504.

70. Kurwa AR. Contact dermatitis from isopropyl alcohol. *Contact Dermatitis Newslett* 1970; 8:168.

71. Fisher AA. *Contact Dermatitis*. Philadelphia: Lea & Febiger; 1986:353–354.

72. Pirilä V, Kilpio O, Olkkonin A, et al. On the chemical nature of the eczematogens in oil of turpentine. *Dermatologica* 1969; 139:183–194.

73. Hellerstrom S, Thyresson N, Widmark G. Chemical aspects of turpentine eczema. *Dermatologica* 1957; 115:277.

74. Rudzki E, Berova N, Czernielewski A, et al. Contact allergy to oil of turpentine: a 10-year retrospective view. *Contact Dermatitis* 1991; 24:317–318.

75. Kirton V. Reactions to ageing turpentine. *Contact Dermatitis* 1972; 11:302.

76. Karlberg A-T, Boman A, Melin B. Animal experiments on the allergenicity of *d*-limonene: the citrus solvent. *Ann Occup Hyg* 1991; 35:419.

77. Karlberg A-T, Magnusson K, Nilsson U. Air oxidation of *d*-limonene (the citrus solvent) creates potent allergens. *Contact Dermatitis* 1992; 26:332–340.

78. Karlberg A-T, Dooms-Goossens A. Contact allergy to *d*-limonene among dermatitis patients. *Contact Dermatitis* 1997; 36:201–206.

79. Preyss JA. Allergy to solvents, especially turpentine. *Berufsdermatosen* 1962; 10:214–217.

80. Cronin E. *Contact Dermatitis*. Edinburgh: Churchill-Livingstone; 1980:799.

81. Kligman AM. The identification of contact allergens by human assay. III. The maximization test: a procedure for screening and rating contact sensitizers. *J Invest Dermatol* 1966; 47:393–409.

82. Magnusson B, Kligman AM. Identification of contact allergens by animal assay. The guinea pig maximization test. *J Invest Dermatol* 1969; 52:268–276.

83. Rudzki E. Occupational contact dermatitis in 100 consecutive patients. *Berufsdermatosen* 1976; 24:100–104.

84. Foussereau J, Benezra C. *Les Eczemas Allergiques Professionelles*. Paris: Masson; 1970:377.

85. Jordan WP, Dahl MV. Contact dermatitis to a plastic solvent in eyeglasses. *Arch Dermatol* 1971; 104:524–528.

86. Parmeggiani L. Ketones. In: *Encyclopedia of Occupational Health and Safety*. Geneva: International Labour Organization; 1983;1171.

87. Couri E, Hetland LB, Abdel-Rahman MS, Weiss H. The influence of inhaled ketone solvent vapors on hepatic microsomal biotransformation activity. *Toxicol Appl Pharmacol* 1977; 41:285–289.

88. Allen N, Mendell JR, Billmaier DJ, et al. Toxic polyneu-

ropathy due to methyl *N*-butylketone. *Arch Neurol* 1975; 32:209–218.

89. Hunter D. *Diseases of Occupations.* London: Hodder and Stoughton; 1978.

90. Teisinger J. *Encyclopedia of Occupational Health and Safety.* Geneva: International Labour Organization; 1983:393–395.

91. Cook WA. Glycidyl ethers. In: Parmeggiani L, ed. *Encyclopedia of Occupational Health and Safety.* Geneva: International Labour Organization; 1982:787–789.

92. Thorgeirsson A, Fregert S. Allergenicity of epoxy resins in the guinea pig. *Acta Derm Venereol* 1978; 57:253–256.

93. Shmunes E. Amyl acetate. In: Adams RM, ed. *Occupational Skin Disease.* Philadelphia: WB Saunders; 1990:452.

94. Roed-Petersen J. Allergic contact dermatitis from butyl acetate. *Contact Dermatitis* 1980; 6:55.

95. Kligman AM. Topical pharmacology and toxicology of dimethyl sulfoxide. *JAMA* 1965; 193:796–804, 923–928.

96. Maibach HI, Feldman RJ. The effect of DMSO on percutaneous penetration of hydrocortisone and testosterone in man. *Ann NY Acad Sci* 1967; 141:423–427.

97. Stoughton RB, Fritsch W. Influence of dimethyl sulfoxide (DMSO) on human percutaneous absorption. *Arch Dermatol* 1964; 90:512–517.

98. Sulzberger MB, Cortese TA Jr, Fishman L, et al. Some effects of DMSO on human skin in vivo. *Ann NY Acad Sci* 1967; 141:437–450.

99. Leake C. Dimethyl sulfoxide. *Science* 1966; 152:1646–1649.

100. Klaassen CD, Rozman K. Absorption, distribution, and excretion of toxicants. In: *Casarett and Doull's Toxicology, The Basic Science of Poisons*, 4th ed. New York; Pergamon; 1991:61–62.

101. Patty FA. *Industrial Hygiene and Toxicology*, Vol 2. New York: Interscience; 1963:1500.

102. Woo Y-T, Argus MF, Arcos JC. Effect of mixed-function oxidase modifiers on metabolism and toxicity of the oncogene dioxane. *Cancer Res* 1978; 38:1621–1625.

103. Aldyreva MV. Styrene and ethyl benzene. In: *Encyclopedia of Occupational Health and Safety*, 3rd ed. Geneva: International Labour Office: 1983;2113–2115.

104. Sjoborg S, Dahlqvist I, Fregert S, et al. Contact allergy to styrene with cross-reaction to vinyltoluene. *Contact Dermatitis* 1982; 8:207–208.

105. Hellerstrom S, Thyresson N, Blohm S-G, et al. On the nature of the eczematogenic component of oxidized delta-3 carene. *J Invest Dermatol* 1955; 24:217.

106. Karlberg A-T, Magnusson K, Nilsson U. Influence of an anti-oxidant on the formation of allergenic compounds during auto-oxidation of *d*-limonene. *Ann Occup Hyg* 1994; 38:199.

107. Fregert S. Allergic contact dermatitis from dioxane in a solvent for cleaning metal parts. *Contact Dermatitis Newslett* 1974; 15:438.

108. Wahlberg JE. Edema-inducing effects of solvents following topical administration. *Derm Beruf Umwelt* 1984; 32:91.

109. Wahlberg JE: Measurement of skin-fold thickness in the guinea pig. *Contact Dermatitis* 1993; 28:141–145.

Natural and Synthetic Rubber

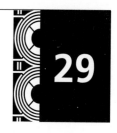

JERE D. GUIN, M.D.
CURT HAMANN, M.D.
KIM M. SULLIVAN

Rubber, natural or synthetic, has the ability to cause both allergic and irritant reactions in persons who, because of their personal health history, genetics, or occupational or recreational activities, are predisposed to sensitization. Irritation and delayed (type IV) reactions to rubber products have been recognized clinically for decades. More recently, natural rubber proteins have emerged as a cause of immediate (type I) hypersensitivity. Despite the fact that both medical and consumer natural rubber latex (NRL) products are safely used daily by millions of people throughout the world, many people can mount immune-mediated and nonimmune reactions to the intrinsic and extrinsic chemical and protein antigens that remain in these products.

Reports of irritation and delayed or immediate hypersensitivity have come from workers in various occupations (Table 29–1), health care workers, and certain patient populations (those with spina bifida) reporting the most type I reactions. Although there has been no formal update from the U.S. Food and Drug Administration (FDA) through the MedWatch Reporting Network on the frequency of NRL-related adverse events or product problems since 1992, there has been a dramatic rise in the number of type I cases reported in the medical literature during the past decade. In an attempt to prevent transmission of human immunodeficiency virus (HIV) and hepatitis viruses, many workers, particularly in health care fields, have either voluntarily chosen or been required to include routine use of personal protection devices and measures in their daily lives. The increase in frequency and duration of direct and indirect exposure to devices containing NRL—examination and surgical gloves, condoms, cathe-

ters, enema cuffs, and dental dams—is one explanation for the apparent rise in both occupational and nonoccupational cases, but questions remain: Why should surgeons or operating room nurses, who have worn NRL gloves for decades, suddenly emerge as a high-risk group for NRL hypersensitivity? Why now? What has changed? And how do we prevent the problem from escalating?

Although many theories attempt to explain the cause of this relatively new phenomenon of immediate allergy to NRL, the problem remains a matter of debate and is most likely a complex combination of various factors (Table 29–2). Understanding the chemical composition, manufacturing permutations, and how workers come in direct or indirect contact with rubber is the essence of determining diagnostic, preventive, and management strategies, and this is the focus of this chapter.

RUBBER

Rubber is made up of large molecules comprising thousands of carbon atoms arranged in repeating sequences in long, stringlike chains. Because of this molecular arrangement, rubber is classified as a polymer, from the Greek *poly* (many) and *meros* (parts).[1, 2] Typically, polymers are named after the raw material or the monomer that was used to make them. The most common rubber polymers used today are isoprene, butadiene, ethylene, styrene, chloroprene, and acrylonitrile (Fig. 29–1). It is the molecular weight, size, and structure of these basic polymers that determine the unusual physical properties and characteristics of rubbers, and what products are produced from them.[1] Rub-

TABLE 29–1 • Occupations Associated with Contact Allergy to Rubber

Agricultural worker (gloves, boots, milking machines)[37]	Groundskeeper (handle grips of power equipment)
Aircraft fitter	Hairdresser[311] (gloves)[37]
Aircraft repair and maintenance worker[26, 37]	Housework[37]
Automobile manufacture[350]	Health care provider[356]
Automobile salesperson	Hospital employee[192]
Automotive parts clerk	Housewife[356]
Automotive parts manufacture[351]	Machine operator
Bank teller[352]	Mechanic, body shop employee
Boiler maintenance worker	Metalworker (rubber chemicals)[37, 356]
Boilerman	Military radarscope operator[359]
Car factory[350]	Motorcycle rider
Car mechanic[353]	Painter
Car washer[72]	Papermaker[79]
Carpet worker[354]	Photographic film production[80]
Catering and food processing (gloves)[37]	Photographic processing (gloves)[37]
Cement tube worker[166]	Plant hire contractor[111]
Chemist[201]	Plumbing (gloves, hose packing)[37]
Church secretary[202]	Pneumatic drill operator[360]
Cleaning[37]	Policeman[196]
Coal miner[37]	Postal worker
Construction designer[355]	Postsorter[198]
Construction workers[356, 357]	Pottery[346]
Cushion manufacturer	Restaurant cashier[358]
Dairy farmer (milking machines)[76, 193, 194]	Rubber band factory worker[261]
Dentistry[37]	Salvage worker
Driver	Scuba diver (business or pleasure)[361]
"Elastic threads" worker[98]	Service station worker[72]
Electrical worker and cable repairmen (insulated wire)	Shoe and boot repairers
Electrician (insulation on electrical wiring)	Shoemaker[37]
Electronics worker[37, 358]	Stock clerk[211]
Embalmer[37]	Textile worker[218]
Engineer	Tire dealers, workers[72, 111, 112]
Factory worker[75]	Tire fitter
Farmers	Tire manufacture
Florist [Kanerva][211]	Tire retreader
Floristry, horticulture (gloves, boots)[37]	Tire salesmen
Footwear manufacturer[81]	Transportation industry[72]
Garage and parking attendant[111, 136]	Trucker
Greenhouse worker[77]	Veterinary medicine[37, 362]

ber can be extruded, shaped, dissolved, foamed, dipped, injected, and molded. Because of its electrical resistance, it is useful as insulation in protective gloves, shoes, and blankets and a variety of electrical instruments. Its relative impermeability to gases makes it useful for the manufacture of air hoses, balloons, balls, cushions, and medical devices. Rubber's resistance to various chemicals and water make it suitable for rainwear, diving gear, protective gloves, storage containers, equipment components, and tubing for chemical and medical applications. Abrasion resistance makes rubber valuable for tires, automotive parts, conveyor belts, handle grips, and housings, and its flexibility and elasticity make it ideal for use in the manufacture of a broad range of articles—hoses, toys, garments, sports equipment, and industrial/architectural shock absorbers.

Latex

The term *latex* (plural *latices*) originally referred to the agricultural source of natural rubber (NR), the milky white substance occurring in certain trees and plants. Rubber is also produced synthetically, and it can exist in a liquid latex form. Latex is therefore more accurately defined as "a stable dispersion of a polymeric substance in an essentially aqueous medium,"[1] which includes both naturally and synthetically derived rubber latices.

TABLE 29–2 • Possible Reasons for the Rise in NRL Allergy[5, 23, 363]

Natural Rubber Latex Harvesting
Changes in concentration or allergenicity of the proteins in NRL products
Changes in the *H. brasiliensis* or its harvesting
Change in the quality of the natural rubber
Changes in geographic locations of the source NRL
Rubber trees from new clones may produce an increase in quantity or quality of proteins in their latex

Manufacturing
Change in manufacturing practices in response to environmental and other health concerns
Changes in the location of manufacture causing a decrease in storage time
Augmentations to the amount and type of chemical additives in the NRL latex compounds
Manufacturing inexperience on the part of new NRL producers

Health Care
Increased NRL glove use in health care owing to compliance with Universal Precautions
Increased exposure to NRL-containing products
Increase in the duration of contact with NRL
Increased awareness among health care workers
Increased reporting to medical professional or regulatory agencies
Improved diagnostic awareness and acumen
Increased protein elution or dermal penetration due to the use of barrier creams, lotions, or topical creams for the treatment of dermal allergy or irritation
Increase in irritant dermatitis due to handcare regimen
Perspiration or high temperatures may promote the release of allergenic materials during repeated glove use
Misdiagnosis in earlier cases
Gamma irradiation does not provide the heat which may alter the NRL allergens as compared with earlier methods of steam autoclaving
Increase in airborne exposure to NRL protein allergens due to increasing levels of glove powder in the health care environment
Increased use of customized packs sterilized with ethylene oxide

General Environment
Increased exposure and duration of exposure to NRL-containing products
Increased reporting to medical professionals
Changes in the condition of NRL users skin due to preexisting dermatitis
Overall increase in allergies in the general population
The increased incidence of NRL allergen antibodies in asthmatics may be relevant to the high level of latex allergen in air pollution from tire dust
Changes in exposure to cross-reacting allergens
Changes in allergenicity of cross-reacting allergens due to ethylene (etephon) or ethylene oxide treatment (e.g., bananas, avocado, chestnuts, kiwis, drupes)
Changes in the spina bifida survival rates

With this in mind, it is clearly a misnomer to identify a person with a type I (Immediate) hypersensitivity to NRL protein as "latex allergic." Unfortunately, in the attempt to communicate the absence or presence of NRL proteins, many manufacturers of the synthetics (nitrile, neoprene, butyl, and styrene butadiene) label their synthetic rubber products as *latex free* or *non-latex*. Despite new regulations, many NRL manufacturers still omit material identification labeling on their packaging, adding to the confusion. To understand the nature of both delayed and immediate reactions to rubber it is essential to understand the differences and similarities among natural and synthetic rubbers, their uses, and the ways in which humans come in contact with them.[3]

Synthetic Rubber

Any artificially produced substance that resembles natural rubber in essential chemical and physical properties can be called a synthetic rubber. The basic units of synthetic rubber are monomers, which are compounds of relatively low molecular weight that are the building units of huge molecules called *polymers*. Synthetic rubber technology originated in 1860, when Charles Hanson Greville Williams, a British chemist, determined

Monomer and Polymer Structures

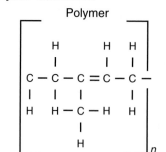

FIGURE 29–1 • Monomer and polymer structures.

Monomer

$C = C - C = C$

Isoprene

Polymer

$\left[\ C - C - C = C - C -\ \right]_n$

Polyisoprene (Natural Rubber)

Rubber Monomers

$C = C - C = C$

Butadiene

$C = C$

Styrene

$C = C - C = C$

Chloroprene

$C = C$

Acrylonitrile

$C = C$

Ethylene

that natural rubber was a polymer of the monomer isoprene. Although attempts were made to synthesize rubber in the laboratory by using isoprene as the monomer, it was not until 1927 to 1930 that an American chemist. Wallace Hume Carothers, and a German scientist, Hermann Staudinger, discovered that synthetic rubber can be prepared from monomers other than isoprene. He subsequently developed BUNA rubbers: BUNA-S (*bu*tadiene-*na*trium-*s*tyrene) and BUNA-A (*bu*tadiene-*na*trium-*a*crylonitrile), and chloroprene (neoprene). The name BUNA is derived from *bu*tadiene, one of the co-monomers, and *na*trium (sodium), which

was used as a catalyst. Produced from cyanide, acrylonitrile proved useful because of its resistance to oils and abrasion.

Efforts to develop synthetic rubbers were stepped up by the U.S. government during World War II, when the source of natural rubber was cut off owing to the occupation of the plantations in Southeast Asia. This shortage of natural rubber led to the development of another BUNA-type rubber called GR-S (government rubber-styrene). GR-S, a co-polymer of butadiene and styrene, was designated as a general-purpose rubber for the U.S. war effort and remains the basis of the modern synthetic rubber industry. The various grades of GR-S are classified in two categories, regular and cold, depending on the temperature of co-polymerization. Cold GR-S types, which exhibit superior properties, are used to make longer-wearing tires for automobiles and trucks. Although synthetic rubbers can be used in place of natural rubbers in many products because of their process-ability, design flexibility, cleanliness, biocompati-bility, and cost, they possess properties that are quite different from those of natural rubber. De-pending on the polymer, its composition, and its intended use, the features of elasticity, electrical insulating properties, chemical and fluid resis-tance, resistance to oxidative forces, and general durability vary. Unless the synthetic rubber is blended with NR, it does not contain the NRL proteins that are responsible for type I (immediate) hypersensitivity; however, many of the synthetics are cured by vulcanization and thus require many of the same sensitizing processing chemicals as NRL (Table 29–3).

Polyisoprene

Although it had been actively sought for nearly a century, polyisoprene (IR) was not successfully synthesized until 1950. The majority of the IR polymers produced today are of the high–cis-1,4 type, but synthetic *trans*-polyisoprene (similar to balata rubber) is also available. Both NR and IR exhibit good tack, high tensile strength (depending on the compounding), and good hot tear proper-ties. Although IR has a chemical structure similar to that of NR, the IR polymer tends to be easier to process, more consistent from lot to lot, and more compatible for blending with other polymers such as styrene-butadiene and ethylene propylene (see later). Additionally, like the other pure syn-thetic polymers, it does not contain the NRL pro-teins that have been implicated in type I hypersen-sitivity. IR, however, has poorer aging properties and less strength and requires longer cure time. IR may be found in shoes, tires, rubber bands, baby bottle nipples, cut threads, erasers, sponges, pharmaceutical supplies, sports equipment, and hoses. Carbon black–loaded compounds are found in tires, gaskets, and motor mounts.

Ethylene Propylene

Because of their physical properties and versatil-ity, ethylene propylene elastomers are one of the fastest-growing general-purpose rubbers in the world today. Like butyl rubber, they contain very few double bonds and require sulfur vulcanization and reinforcing pigments for strength.[1, 2] Ethylene propylene elastomers include the basic copoly-mers, as well as the terpolymers, which contain a small percentage of diene for unsaturation. Be-cause of their tensile properties and their resis-tance to temperature, water, oxidation, and heat, they are widely used for consumer, automotive, electrical, and construction products (e.g., wire and cable coverings, roofing materials, and sheet-ing, oil additives, tire sidewalls, and high-perfor-mance hoses and belts). Ethylene propylene and elastomers are often blended with polyethylene, polypropylene, or other thermoplastic resins to make thermoplastic elastomers. Depending on the blending of materials and the process utilized, these materials have varying degrees of heat and oil resistance and elasticity.[1, 2, 4]

Butyl Rubber

Butyl rubber, first produced in 1940, is used mainly for inner tubes in automobile tires. Pre-pared by co-polymerization of isobutylene with butadiene or isoprene, it can be compounded as natural rubbers but is difficult to vulcanize, thus requiring more active accelerators.[2] Thiuram sul-fides, dithiocarbamates, dioxime, dinitroso com-pounds, and polymethyl-phenol resins are also used to cross-link. Butyl rubber is not as resilient as natural rubber and other synthetics, but it is extremely resistant to oxidation, corrosive chemi-cals, or moisture, is impermeable to gases, and possesses enhanced thermal stability. Butyl rub-bers rank third in total consumption of synthetic rubbers and are used primarily in the tire industry but have found applications in adhesives, coatings, air cushions, conveyor belts, high-temperature hoses, inner tubes, pneumatic springs, and air bel-lows.

Nitrile Rubber

Nitrile rubber is a copolymer of two monomers, butadiene and acrylonitrile, and is a solvent-resis-tant rubber. It is most often used for fuel hoses, shoes, conveyor belts, and for waterproofing cloth, but owing to its good chemical, oil, and body fat resistance it is also used in the manufacture of medical grade and chemical-resistant gloves. These features vary with the acrylonitrile content. Nitrile products are typically less elastic than NR but offer good tensile and tear strength,[5] although reinforcing agents are required for high strength. Nitrile rubbers can be prepared by using similar compounding, dipping, and vulcanization used for natural rubber, typical compounds containing sul-fur accelerators and activators.[1]

Text continued on page 510

TABLE 29–3 • Selected Categories and Types of Rubber-Compounding Options*

Class or Chemical Name	Accelerators	Activators	Antidegradants Antioxidants	Antidegradants Antiozonants	Vulcanizing Agents	Retarders	Reinforcing Agents	Fillers	Pigments	Processing Aids	Blowing Agents
Acetaldehyde-ammonia	x										
Acetaldehyde-aniline	x		x								
Aldehyde-amines	x		x								
Aliphatic polysulfide polymers					x						
Alkyl phthalates										x	
Alkyl amines			x								
Alkyl sulfates										x	
Alkyl aryl sulfates										x	
Alkyl aryl-p-phenylenediamine			x								
Alkylated diphenylamines			x								
Alkylated phenols			x								
Alkylphenol disulfides					x						
Amines	x										
Aryl butylated reaction products			x								
Azobisfomamide											x
Benzoic acid						x					
Benzothiazoles	x				x						
Benzothiazole sulfenamides	x				x						
Benzothiazyl disulfide	x										
Bismuth salts	x										
Butylated hydroxytoluene (2,6-di-tert-butyl-p-cresol or BHT)			x								
Butylhydroxyanisole (BHA)			x								

	1	2	3	4	5	6	7	8	9	10	11
Calcium carbonate								x		x	
Calcium silicates								x			
Carbon black							x				
Chelating agents						x					
Cobalt naphthanate										x	
Dehydroabietic acid										x	
Diazo pigments									x		
Diethyldithiocarbamates	x										
Diethylthioureas	x										
Dihydroquinolones				x							
Diphenyl-p-phenylene diamines			x	x							
Diphenylamines										x	
Diphenylguanidines	x	x									
Diphenylthioureas	x										
Dithiocarbamates	x			x	x						
Dithiophosphates					x						
Esters										x	
Fatty acids		x			x						
Fine clays								x			
Formaldehyde	x										
Guanidines	x										
Heterocyclic amines	x										
Hydrazides											x
Hydroquinones	x										
Hydroxides										x	
Inorganic pigments									x		

Table continued on following page

TABLE 29-3 • Selected Categories and Types of Rubber-Compounding Options* Continued

Class or Chemical Name	Accelerators	Activators	Antidegradants		Vulcanizing Agents	Retarders	Reinforcing Agents	Fillers	Pigments	Processing Aids	Blowing Agents
			Antioxidants	Antiozonants							
Ketone-amines			x								
Lacquers									x		
Magnesium carbonate					x			x			
Magnesium oxide					x						
Metals	x										
Mineral oils										x	
Napthyl-p-phenylenediamines			x								
β-Naphthylamines (rarely used today)			x								
Nitrosobenzenes	x										
Organic peroxides					x						
Polyalkylaryl phosphites			x								
Potassium fatty acid complexes										x	
Salicylic acid						x					
Selenium	x				x						
Silicon dioxide							x				
Solvents										x	
Sulfenamides (50% of all accelerators)	x				x						
Sulfur and sulfur donors					x						
Tellurium	x				x					x	
Tetraalkylthiuram disulfides	x				x						
Tetraalkylthiuram monosulfides	x										

508

	1	2	3	4	5	6	7	8	9
Thiomorpholines	x				x				
Thiophosphates	x								x
Thioureas	x	x		x					
Thiuram sulfides	x				x				
Trimethylquinolines		x		x					
Trimethylthioureas	x								
Triphenylguanidines	x								
Urea				x					
Xanthates	x				x				
Zinc fatty acid derivatives		x							x
Zinc dithiocarbamates	x								
Zinc oxide	x	x			x				x
Zinc benzimidazole derivatives			x						

*More than 200 organic and inorganic chemicals are used today in various combinations to compose and stabilize the rubber compounds. It is estimated that five pounds of chemicals are incorporated into each 100 pounds of rubber during fabrication.

Neoprene

Neoprene, developed in 1931 by E.I. Du Pont de Nemours & Company, was one of the first successful synthetic rubbers. Today it is the generic name for polymers of the monomer chloroprene (2-chloro-1,3-butadiene) (see Fig. 29–1). The raw materials of chloroprene are acetylene and hydrochloric acid, and it is produced by two processes, one using acetylene, and the most common method, using butadiene. There are a wide range of neoprene vulcanizates with a broad spectrum of physical properties; However, no single compound provides all of the characteristic possibilities. Neoprene types include G type (amber colored), W type (white to gray), and the T types (cream to light amber).[2]

Neoprenes typically are vulcanized by heat; with zinc oxide and magnesium oxide are the preferred vulcanizing agents. Accelerators such as zinc salts of dialkyldithiocarbamates are often used to increase the sulfur vulcanization rate. Dipped products such as gloves may be produced on the same equipment as NRL products; however, neoprene requires a higher cure temperature and a longer cure time. Antioxidants are essential in neoprene latex compounds because, like NR, oxidation reduces the polymer chain length, which results in a softer and weaker material. Hindered bis-phenols, such as antioxidant 2246 and Wingstay L, have proved effective with limited staining. Because of their characteristic resistance to chemicals, atmospheric degradation, oils, and fats and their good elastomeric properties, neoprene latices may be blended with natural rubber to improve their resistance to oil, ozone, and weathering.[2, 4–6] Compounded neoprene latices are used to make a variety of products, including, but not limited to, foam; films; elasticized asphalt; fire, industrial, garden and automotive hoses; cable, cord and wire coverings; belts; appliance parts; bearings; seals; wet suits; coated fabrics; shoes; roof coatings; protective gloves; and adhesives for shoes, furniture, automotive products, and construction applications. Because of the broad range of physical properties imparted by each type of neoprene compound, no single vulcanizate provides all physical properties.

Polybutadiene

Polybutadiene (BR) is a newer polymer that was developed commercially only in the last 35 years. Most of the polybutadienes produced today are of the *cis*-1,4 type, but some may have a mixed-chain structure. It is most often manufactured by a solution process but can utilize an emulsion

method. Because of its superior abrasion resistance, resilience, and flexibility at low temperatures and its diminished cracking due to ozone resistance, it is useful in the production of tire treads and high-impact polystyrene (HIPS) found in golf ball cores and conveyor belts, among other things. Being an unsaturated elastomer, it is easily vulcanized with sulfenamide-type accelerators, thiurams, or guanidines. Because polybutadienes do not exhibit high gum tensile strength they are typically compounded with reinforcing fillers.[1]

Silicone

Silicone rubber (VMQ) has an entirely different polymer structure. It consists, not of a long chain of carbon atoms, but rather of a string of silicon and oxygen atoms. This structure is very flexible, having extremely weak interchain forces, and thus must be reinforced with a pigment such as silica powder. Silicone rubbers show little change when exposed to extreme temperatures and demonstrate excellent resistance to corrosion and solvents. Silicone rubber typically is vulcanized using peroxides and is used principally for adhesives, sealants, automotive and industrial products, and medical equipment.[1, 4]

Thiokol

Another specialty rubber is thiokol, produced by the co-polymerization of ethylene dichloride (CHCl:CHCl) and sodium tetrasulfide (Na_2S_4). This type, which can be compounded and vulcanized as natural rubber, is resistant to the action of oils and to organic solvents used for lacquers and is useful for electrical insulation because it does not deteriorate when exposed to electrical discharge and light.

Urethane Rubbers

Urethanes are produced through a specialized chain extension process that literally creates large macromolecules from smaller macromolecules rather than from monomers. This process has special advantages and allows for a wide range of variations in product features. Urethanes may be rigid or extremely elastic, depending on the type of short-chain polymer used (i.e., polyether, polyester) and the chain length.[1] Polyurethane elastomers typically are used for foams and surface coatings but are also useful in the manufacture of shoes, gaskets, and tires because of their tear and abrasion resistance, excellent load-bearing properties, and tolerance for abuse.[2]

Styrene-Butadiene Polymers

Styrene-butadiene rubbers (SBRs) are the most widely used general-purpose synthetic rubbers and are used principally in the manufacture of tires, mechanical goods, carpet backing, and thin-walled articles such as condoms and, surgical and examination gloves. Currently, it constitutes approximately 40% of all synthetic rubber utilized in the United States. SBR latices are prepared by emulsion polymerization of the desired ratios of butadiene and styrene monomers together with the required modifiers and catalysts. When the styrene content is less than 50%, the co-polymer is classed as a rubber latex. Some SBR latices utilize a dithiocarbamate as an antidegradant and stain in the presence of copper and other metals, although other SBRs are available that do not require chemical antioxidants.[1]

Thermoplastic elastomers (TPEs) are produced by creating an aqueous emulsion and dispersing a solvent-based (e.g., toluene) solution of the polymer in water and then removing the solvent. With an elastic block in the center and a thermoplastic block on the ends, TPEs typically have great tensile strength, high elongation, and low modulus, and are superior to natural rubber with their resistance to abrasion, cracking, and oxidative forces. SBRs' limitations are their poor resistance to heat, moderate tear strength, and poor tacking. Various physical properties and product features depend on what formulations and solvents are used. Kraton D and G (Shell Chemical Company) and Vector DPX (Dexco Polymers) thermoplastic elastomers are tri-block co-polymers. Kraton co-polymers are divided into three basic types: styrene-butadiene-styrene (SBS), styrene-isoprene-styrene (SIS), and styrene ethylene butylene styrene (SEBS). Vector DPX is available as SIS and SBS. Because these products are manufactured with solvents they are not resistant to similar solvents or chemicals that the end user may contact.[5] Compared with the numerous potentially allergenic chemicals that must be added to other rubbers, the manufacturing of TPEs is a relatively simple process that uses few ingredients. Whereas other polymers require vulcanization, TPEs develop their properties upon cooling or evaporation of solvent. Product applications include medical-grade gloves, condoms, catheters, and components for medical equipment.

Polyethylene

A large number of polymers exist as partially crystallized solids at normal temperatures. Polyethylene is an excellent example. This flexible plastic material is opaque owing to the presence of very fine crystallites, which refract and scatter light. These crystallites also tie together and restrict the motion of the polymer chains, so they lose their elasticity. Thus, the material retains its flexibility but loses some of its elasticity.[1]

Hypalon

Hypalon, developed by DuPont, is created by the simultaneous chlorination and chlorosulfonation of polyethylene in an inert solvent. Hypalon vulcanizates are widely used in the rubber industry because of their flexibility and resistance to abrasion, weathering, corrosive chemicals, oil, grease, fire, ozone, oxidation, and radiation. Additionally, they typically have excellent electrical properties, and their high tensile strength does not require the use of reinforcing fillers. They are used in cable coverings, insulation, nuclear power plants, industrial hoses, chemical containers, gaskets, and outdoor sports equipment.

Polyvinyl Chloride

Polyvinyl chloride (PVC) compounds may be extruded, calendered, injection molded, extrusion- or injection-blow molded, film blown, thermoformed, sheet molded, or dipped. This high–molecular weight polymer can be compounded to be rigid or extremely flexible. PVC is utilized in many diverse product applications, including blood bags, bottles, house siding, packaging, tubing, upholstery, pipes, coatings, toys, shoes, gloves, bumpers, and floor coverings (a quarter of all PVC dispersion resin consumption).[1] To achieve this processing range, the vinyl chloride monomer may be polymerized by adding any of a broad range of chemical additives such as plasticizers, thermal stabilizers, lubricants, modifiers, fillers, and pigments. Vinyl resins are classified by particle size and include general-purpose resins with an average particle size of 80 to 200 μm and dispersion resins (used to produce gloves) with an average particle size of 0.7 to 2.0 μm. The combination and selection of resin and plasticizer are important factors in controlling the physical properties of the desired finished product and may affect hardness, modulus, elongation, or surface friction.

Plasticizers in PVC are typically phthalate esters (i.e., butyl, butyl benzene, diisodecyl), but adipates and sebacates can also be used. Epoxidized soybean or linseed oil is often added as a secondary plasticizer and stabilizer with the esters. Because one of the limitations in PVC processing is its tendency to discolor and dehydrochlorinate at higher temperatures, thermostabilizers are often added—calcium stearate, lead stearate, epoxidized soybean oil, octyltin-thioglycolate, magnesium, calcium, and barium. Phosphates, antimony trioxide, aluminum, molybdenum, and zinc oxides may be added as smoke and flame retardants.[1] Although calcium carbonate is the most commonly used filler in PVC compounds, glass fibers, graphite, and other mineral microfibers are used in some products as reinforcing fillers, and nonreinforcing fillers such as calcium carbonate, clays (kaolin), silica, and silicates may be used in various combinations. Both organic and inorganic pigments may be added, depending on the product, whether inorganic—titanium dioxide, sulfates, sulfides, iron, lead, chromium, and cadmium, or organic—phthalocyanines and azo compounds.

Koroseal

A specialty rubber, koroseal is a polymer of vinyl chloride. Vinyl chloride polymers are resistant to heat, electricity, and corrosion and are not affected by exposure to light or by prolonged storage. Koroseal cannot be vulcanized and when not subjected to high temperatures is more resistant to abrasion than natural rubber or leather.

Natural Rubber

Pure crude natural rubber is a white or colorless hydrocarbon whose chemical name is *polyisoprene*. Because it consists of polymer chains with an almost perfect cis-1,4 structure (which means carbon atoms 1 and 4 are both on the same side as the double bond), the true name of this polymer is *cis-1,4-polyisoprene*.[1] Its structural formulation may be represented by the simple unit C_5H_8 multiplied many thousands of times (see Fig. 29–1).[1] Crude rubber is insoluble in water, alkalis, and weak acids but is soluble in benzene, gasoline, chlorinated hydrocarbons, and carbon disulfide. It is oxidized readily by chemical oxidizing agents and slowly by atmospheric oxygen.

MANUFACTURE OF NATURAL RUBBER LATEX

Historical Perspective

History does not record the use of natural rubber until 1496, when Christopher Columbus made his second voyage to the Americas and observed Haitian natives playing with bouncing balls made from the latex of the *cau-uchu,* or weeping wood tree. Archeological excavations, however, indicate that the first rubber articles were actually used by the native South Americans in religious ceremonies as early as 500 A.D.[1] Later, Spanish explorers brought back tales and examples of marvelous goods produced by the people of the New World, including such items as rubber balls, water bottles, shoes, and waterproof clothing.[1] Although impressed by the rubber articles, Europeans were unsuccessful at reproducing these unique waterresistant products, and interest in natural rubber quickly waned.

General scientific and manufacturing interest in the substance and its properties was finally revived in 1736, when on expedition to South America Charles Marie de la Condamine, a French geographer, brought back several rolls of crude rubber and a description of the many products that were being made by the people of the Amazon Valley. In 1770, the British chemist Joseph Priestley discovered that the material could erase pencil marks and subsequently coined the term *rubber.*[2] The first commercial application of rubber was initiated by Samuel Peal, who patented a method of waterproofing cloth by treating it with a solution of turpentine and rubber. He was followed by Charles Macintosh, a British inventor, who established a manufacturing facility in Glasgow to produce rainproof garments in 1823.

The widespread use of natural rubber remained limited owing to its inherent variability with temperature: it turned sticky and foul smelling in warm weather and rigid in colder temperatures. These problems were soon addressed when in 1820 Thomas Hancock discovered the means to soften, mix, and form rubber by the process now known as *mastication.* Charles Goodyear discovered the vulcanization process in 1839. These two important discoveries launched the development of numerous rubber products and the subsequent increased demand for the raw material. The wild rubber trees of South America continued to be the main source of crude rubber, and exports from Brazil of the raw material increased from approximately 400 metric tons in 1840 to 50,000 tons in 1910.[1, 2]

In the United States, rubberized goods had become popular by the 1830s, and rubber bottles and shoes made by the native South Americans were imported in substantial quantities. Other rubber articles were imported from England, and in 1832, at Roxbury, Massachusetts, John Haskins and Edward Chaffee organized the first rubber goods factory in the United States. Like the imported articles, however, the resulting products became brittle in cold weather and tacky and gummy in summer. In 1834 the German chemist Friedrich Ludersdorf and the American chemist

Nathaniel Hayward discovered that adding sulfur to gum rubber lessened or eliminated the stickiness of finished rubber goods. In 1839 the American inventor Charles Goodyear, using the findings of the two chemists, discovered that cooking rubber with sulfur, a process called *vulcanization,* removed the gum's unfavorable properties. Vulcanized rubber has greater strength, elasticity, and *greater* resistance to changes in temperature than unvulcanized rubber; it is impermeable to gases and resistant to abrasion, chemical action, heat, and electricity. Vulcanized rubber also exhibits high frictional resistance on dry surfaces and low frictional resistance on water-wet surfaces.

With the increased demand for this natural resource, it was apparent that additional sources for natural rubber would be essential. In 1876 Henry Wickham traveled to South America and collected 70,000 seeds from the *Hevea brasiliensis* tree and, despite a rigid embargo, smuggled them back to England in an attempt to cultivate rubber in other locations. Although only 3% of these seeds actually germinated, the majority of the seedlings were sent to Ceylon Sri Lanka (now) and Malaysia. Later, cultivation was expanded to include Indonesia, and by 1880 *Hevea* seedlings were distributed throughout much of Asia.[1] By 1890 rubber plantations began to make their appearance, and, thanks to the efforts of persons like Henry J. Ridley and John Perkins, the rubber industry began to make significant advances in latex production and harvesting.

With the development of the first pneumatic tire by John Dunlop in 1888 the tire industry was born, and the rubber industry accelerated its efforts in research and product development. The potential for new and innovative products manufactured from natural rubber seemed endless. In 1894, a surgeon at Johns Hopkins Hospital, W.S. Halsted, created the first pair of NRL surgical gloves, to protect the hands of his surgical assistant. His surgical nurse had developed severe hand dermatitis, most likely from using a chloride of lime solution to disinfect the hands.

By 1913 Southeast Asia's plantation rubber had surpassed the production of Brazilian wild rubber. Although attempts were made to establish rubber plantations in the Western Hemisphere during the early 1900s, these efforts failed owing to a fungal disease (*Microcyclus,* or leaf blight) that caused widespread tree loss and virtually destroyed the wild natural rubber industry in South America. Cultivation of natural rubber reached its peak in the years immediately before World War II. Approximately 4.5 million acres was under cultivation in India, Ceylon (now Sri Lanka), and Malaysia (then British possessions), and another 3.5 million acres of rubber plantations in Indonesia was held by the Netherlands. This combined 9 million acres produced the bulk of the world's natural rubber. Many of these plantations were destroyed or cut off from the world during the war, and the political and economic significance of natural rubber became evident. This acute natural rubber shortage forced the United States government to establish a program that cost more than $700 million to develop synthetic rubber–manufacturing plants. By 1952 annual plant capacity reached about 1 million metric tons of high-quality rubbers at prices comparable to that of natural rubber. Because of the high productivity achieved by the synthetic rubber industry, the natural rubber share of the elastomer market steadily decreased until 1980.[1] This decrease has been partially offset, however, by the increased consumption of the more expensive NRL-dipped goods, which utilize the higher priced liquid latex in their manufacture. Of the 15 million metric tons of the world's rubber production in 1990, only 5 million metric tons was natural rubber (Fig. 29–2). Although the use patterns of NRL vary among countries, it is estimated that 72% is used for tire products, 10% for latex products, 9% for industrial goods, 3.5% for engineering products, and the remaining 5.5% for footwear and adhesives (Fig. 29–3).[7]

Rubber Trees

Natural rubber exists as a colloidal suspension in the latex of more than 2,000 species of trees, shrubs, or vines (e.g., milkweed, poinsettia, dogbane, sapodilla, mulberry, poppy, chicory). Wounds exude this milky fluid, forming a protective layer, and in several plants it is bitter or poisonous, providing an excellent defense against bacteria, fungi, insects, and animals. Only the *Hevea* species and the guayule plant (*Parthenium argentatum*) of the sunflower family, however, are known to produce a high molecular weight linear polymer with a 100% *cis-* structure.[1, 2] Balata and gutta-percha occur in the *trans-* form. Because there are such structural similarities between guayule and *Hevea* rubber, efforts are constantly being made to develop guayule commercially, but it contains more impurities than does *Hevea* latex, including a sesquiterpene cinnamic acid ester that has been confirmed by guinea pig maximization testing to be a potent allergen.[8] It is the *H. brasiliensis* tree of the Euphorbiaceae family that is the source with the greatest commercial importance and that currently produces about 90% of all the natural rubber that is consumed today (Fig. 29–4).[9]

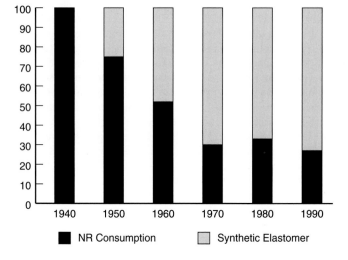

Year Consumption	NR (Tons per thousand)	% Total Elastomer
1940	1130	100
1950	1750	75
1960	2100	52
1970	3730	30
1980	3970	33
1990	5000	35

FIGURE 29–2 • World consumption of natural rubber.

■ NR Consumption   ☐ Synthetic Elastomer

Although China has succeeded in growing trees in colder climates, the *Hevea* tree grows best in tropical regions with average annual temperatures of 25° to 30°C and 2 m of annual rainfall.[1] Today, commercial cultivation of *H. brasiliensis* hybrids

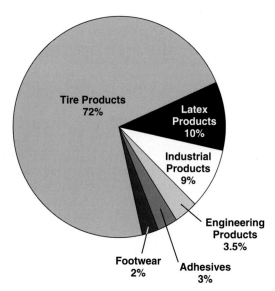

FIGURE 29–3 • Estimated division of the uses of natural rubber latex.

takes place predominantly in West Africa and Southeast Asia on small farms (less than 40 hectares or 100 acres) or larger plantations. The productive life of the tree is approximately 25 to 30 years, and at full maturity it reaches an approximate height of 20 m. Propagation is accomplished by vegetative reproduction utilizing selected seeds from high-yielding trees, bud grafting, or cloning (Fig. 29–5). All trees derived from a single "mother" tree are known as *clones,* each clone being cultivated to produce its own set of desired characteristics, such as rapid growth, high yield, or resistance to pests and disease. The characteristics of the NRL may likewise be engineered by cloning. These breeding programs, conducted principally in Malaysia and Indonesia, have increased the productivity of the trees, and high-yielding clones have now been transplanted throughout most of Malaysia and the rest of the NRL-producing regions of the world. Chemical yield stimulants such as 2-chloroethane phosphonic acid (Ethrel or Ethephon) and other methods such as secondary cloning and tapping augmentations are also being utilized to some extent.[1]

Natural Rubber Latex Protein

Fresh latex is in no way related to, or derived from, the tree's sap; rather, it is produced in the

FIGURE 29–4 • The *Hevea brasiliensis* tree of the family Euphorbiaceae.

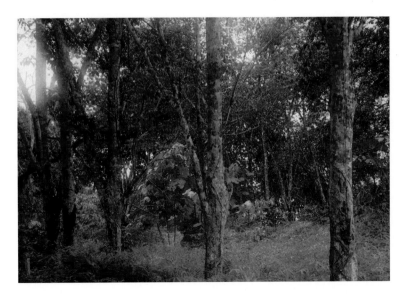

cytoplasm of the laticifer cells of the tree (Fig. 29–6). It contains approximately 60% water as a primary component, 35% natural polymeric rubber particles (0.1 to 2 μm in size) along with 5% non-rubber substances, which include, in varying proportions and combination, lipids, phospholipids, carbohydrates, resins, tannins, alkaloids, metals, sugars, and perhaps most important from an allergy perspective, a variety of proteins.[1, 2, 10] Some 40% of these proteins are dispersed in the aqueous serum, and 60% are bound to the rubber particles. Approximately 240 different polypeptides are contained in NRL, 57 of which have demonstrated the ability to bind immunoglobulin E (IgE) antibodies in sera from NRL-allergic persons.[11–13] Using both qualitative and semiquantitative methods, research efforts have focused on

understanding the character, identity, properties, and distribution of the relevant NRL allergens from various source materials and the IgE and IgG4 immunoreactivity of patients with various clinical symptoms.[14] Unfortunately, the lower–molecular weight peptides, which may be the relevant allergens, may escape detection by standard Western blotting.[10, 11, 13, 15–17]

Although little is currently known about the identity of these NRL allergens or their rates of elution from different products, it has been determined that the handling of the source material, chemical additives, and other processing variables have significant effects on the concentration of the extractable proteins (EP), and, thus, their allergenic potential.[11, 18] Fresh NRL contains approximately 30 to 50 mg/g of both water-soluble and

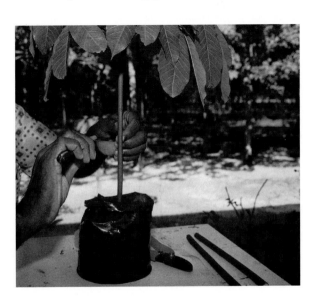

FIGURE 29–5 • Green budding and other breeding and cloning programs have increased the productivity of the trees.

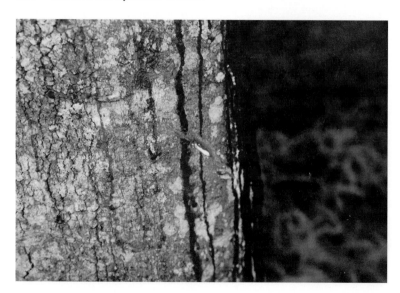

FIGURE 29–6 • Fresh latex is produced within the cytoplasm of the laticifer cells of the tree.

water-insoluble proteins.[19] During all processing stages, the level of EP is considerably lower than the total concentration of proteins (Table 29–4).

PROCESSING AND PREPARATION OF NRL

Tapping and Collecting

Natural *Hevea* latex is contained within specialized vessels arranged in channels that run up the length of the tree at 4-degree angles, forming a spiral. Natural latex is obtained, without damaging the trees, by tapping or cutting into the latex vessels at a 25- to 30-degree angle. This cut extends along a third to half the circumference of the trunk. Tapping is done before sunrise, when the turgor in the tree is at its maximum and the yield of NRL at its highest.[1] The latex is exuded from the cut through a spout and is collected in a small cup attached to the tree (Fig. 29–7). The amount of latex obtained on each tapping is about 30 mL (about 1 fl oz). Thereafter, to retap the tree, a thin strip of bark is shaved from the bottom of the original cut, usually every other day. When the cuts reach the ground, the bark is permitted to renew itself before a new tapping panel is started. About 250 trees are planted per hectare (100 per acre), and the annual yield for ordinary trees is about 450 kg/hectare (400 lb per acre) of dry crude rubber. For specially selected high-yield trees the annual yield may run as high as 2,225 kg/hectare (2,000 lb per acre), and experimental trees that yield 3,335 kg/hectare (3,000 lb per acre) have been developed. This raw natural latex has few uses because of its instability: it softens

when heated, hardens when cold, and deteriorates rapidly.

Preservation

Because NRL is very perishable and coagulates and spoils in a few hours a preservative—typically ammonia—is added in the field to prevent rapid coagulation and degradation by microorganisms.

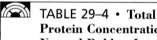

TABLE 29–4 • Total and Extractable Protein Concentrations During Natural Rubber Latex Processing

Processing Stage Protein (mg/g)	Protein (mg/g)	
	Total	Extractable
Raw latex	30–50	8–10
Preserved latex (ammoniated)	30–50	11–12
Enzyme-treated latex (alcalase)	6–10	0.10
Centrifuged HA latex (fresh)	16–20	0.50
Centrifuged HA latex (stored)	16–30	0.30–1.0
Double centrifuged latex	11–15	0.10–0.15
Compounded HA latex	16–20	>0.7
Prevulcanized latex	16–20	>1.5
Postvulcanized latex	16–20	2–4
Wet gel leaching (prevulcanization)	13–16	0.2–0.6
Dry gel leaching (postvulcanization)	13–16	0.2–0.4
Wet or dry gel leaching	13–16	0.2–0.4
Chlorination	13–16	0.02–0.05

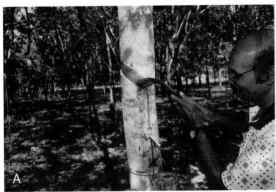

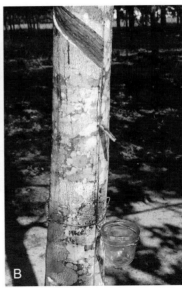

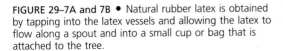

FIGURE 29–7A and 7B ● Natural rubber latex is obtained by tapping into the latex vessels and allowing the latex to flow along a spout and into a small cup or bag that is attached to the tree.

NO preserved by ammonia alone is known as *high-ammonia (HA) latex* (0.7%).[20] The trend since 1955 has been to use a reduced-ammonia or low-ammonia (LA) latex (0.2%) to obviate deammoniating it with formaldehyde down to 0.2% to 0.3%. If a low-ammonia latex is to be used, a secondary preservative such as sodium pentachlorophenate or zinc oxide, either tetramethylthiuram disulfide, sodium dimethyldithiocarbamate, or boric acid, is added.[20–22]

These chemicals act to preserve the latex, and over time they stabilize the rubber particles in preparation for transport. The mandatory holding period for the natural latex is 3 weeks, but it can extend for 4 to 8 weeks if the ammoniated liquid latex is to be exported. This incubation process causes several changes in the natural latex: It (1) kills bacteria; (2) inhibits regrowth; (3) prevents coagulation; (4) degrades proteins; (5) disrupts or hydrolyzes the protein coating of the rubber particles, releasing fatty acids that stabilize the latex; (6) allows for the reduction of trace metals through precipitation or sequestration; and (7) hydrolyzes and alters the electrophoretic profiles of the proteins and lipids, exposing a neoantigen or potentially significant epitope.[10, 13, 18, 19, 23–26] Upon the filming of nonammoniated, or green, latex, the EP content is approximately 8 mg per gram of rubber (see Table 29–4). Sodium dodecyl sulfate polyacrylamide gel electrophoresis (SDS-PAGE) confirms that the ammoniated latex (AL) contains fewer proteins than fresh latex, major proteins having partially decomposed to smaller molecular fragments and unidentified products, whereas the 24-kD polypeptide present on rubber particles in fresh latex has been demonstrated to disappear

completely.[10] Upon completion of the ammonification, the total protein content is 16 to 26 mg/g and the EP content 11 to 12 mg/g. Enzyme treatment of field latex has also been considered. Such deproteinized latex shows an EP content of 0.1 mg/g, and although it increases with compounding, it renders a final film lower in EP than ordinary latex concentrate.

Dry Rubber

At the plantation, most natural latex is reduced to solid sheets for export to processing plants and the manufacture of "dry rubber" products. The gathered latex is strained, diluted with water, and treated with acid to cause the suspended rubber particles in it to clump together. It is then placed in a treatment tank where the liquid begins to gel into a more solid form. After pressing between rollers (calendering) to consolidate the rubber into 0.6-cm (0.25-inch) slabs or thin sheets (crepe), the rubber is processed into conventional grades of rubber, air- or smoke dried, baled, and shipped to manufacturers.[2]

Centrifugation

Liquid preparations of rubber are used in waterproofing fabrics and manufacturing thin-walled articles such as medical and household gloves, condoms, diaphragms, and balloons. Because these articles are shaped by dipping a form into the solution, the rubber must be maintained in its liquid state. Before leaving the plantation, the liquid latex is centrifuged to reduce its water content, concentrate the rubber, and remove excess debris such as bark, dirt, and insects.[18] During centrifugation, the NRL is separated into three major fractions: *the rubber fraction* (27%), the upper most layer containing the rubber particles; *B fraction serum* (25%), the aqueous middle layer; and *C fraction serum* (48%), the bottom layer, which contains lutoids and other intracellular particles.[10, 27–29] The proteins associated with the rubber phase are predominantly water insoluble and attached to the polyisoprene matrix, but a few are water soluble and extractable in ammonia.[30, 31] The sera from the B and C fractions contain most of the water-soluble proteins. Many of these water-soluble proteins are extractable by the ammonia but a portion is lost during centrifugation owing to sedimentation and loss of some of the serum. Ion removal from the latex makes the remaining proteins less soluble.[10, 29, 32–34] At this point in the processing the EP content is approximately 0.5 mg/g, but it may be reduced by another 25% to 30% with a second or third run through the centrifuge.[10, 18, 28] Treatments with alcalase, papain, or endogenous proteolytic enzymes[22] may decrease EP content further, but the increased cure time and loss of important properties limit the usefulness of this approach. Surfactants used during centrifugation help to displace hydrophobic proteins from the polyisoprene particles and mobilize all proteins, facilitating their migration during processing.

Compounding

Before the raw NRL is suitable for use in anything other than crepe rubber or adhesives it must be blended with chemicals to produce the required durability, flexibility, and strength. The process of incorporating ingredients into either latex or dry rubber to modify its characteristics is called *compounding.*[1] In the rubber industry, the problem of selecting the basic raw materials for the preparation of a specific commercial product is assigned to the compounder, a trained chemist or chemical engineer. Such training is necessary because of the complex chemical reactions that must take place during production.[1] Water-soluble ingredients are added to the latex as aqueous solutions and water-insoluble in ones as emulsions. Dispersion is accomplished with ball, pebble, or colloid mills, or tanks equipped with disk agitators. When preparing dispersions it is essential that the particle size of the material be smaller than 5 mm. Particles that are too large produce imperfections on the surface of the product. It is also important that the chemicals be added to the latex in the proper order, to ensure a stable mixture.[20]

Many ingredients are used to prepare both natural and synthetic rubber products. Depending on the manufacturer and the desired characteristics of the finished product, as many as 200 different organic and inorganic chemicals are added to the latex in various combinations (see Tables 29–3 and 29–5).[32] It is estimated that 5 pounds of chemicals is added to every 100 pounds of rubber.[35] Although these chemicals are necessary to obtain optimal performance and cost effectiveness, some are potent sensitizers that produce irritant and type IV (delayed) skin responses. In general, these chemicals may be classified by their specific use; however, it is important to understand that many individual chemicals are capable of functioning in more than one capacity (e.g., zinc oxide may be added as an accelerator-activator, vulcanizing agent, filler, or pigment).[1]

Serum proteins clearly change during compounding. After compounding, the EP content may double and contain fewer high molecular weight proteins and proportionally less low molecular weight proteins.[10, 19] Because of the allergenic potential of these chemicals and their ability to affect the proteins in NRL, manufacturers must balance the barrier efficacy and performance requirements of the products against their potential allergenicity.

Although two functional classes (accelerators and antidegradants) make up 90% of the estimated consumption of rubber chemicals, the other chemical groups may also be of concern when attempting to determine the cause of contact dermatitis. The major categories are described next.[1, 7, 32, 35]

TABLE 29–5 • Effects of Natural Rubber Proteins

Property	Effects
Cure accelerators	Phospholipids and some proteins are natural.
Storage-hardening	Proteins and free amino acids react with abnormal groups in rubber.
Creep and stress	High contents of proteins and ash lead to moisture absorption, which results in high creep and stress relaxation in vulcanizates.
Modulus	Increased by proteins
Filler effect	Proteins act as fillers. One part protein equals high-abrasion-furnace (HAF) black.
Heat build-up	Increased by proteins
Tear strength	Increased by proteins
Dynamic crack growth	Resistance increased by proteins

Accelerators

For rubber to become useful its hydrocarbon chains must be permanently linked together. Vulcanization completes this task by creating sulfur linkages between the rubber chains. In combination with other vulcanizing agents, accelerators reduce the vulcanization time (cure time) by increasing the vulcanization rate. In most cases the physical properties of the product are improved.[1, 2] Although Goodyear's discovery of this process was a major breakthrough for the rubber industry, it still took hours, or even days, to vulcanize products. Accelerators were first discovered in 1906, with the introduction of anilines to the process. Efficiency of the process was again increased with the addition of newer accelerators in the 1920s. By 1930 the sulfenamides were incorporated, and today approximately 50% of all accelerators are sulfenamides, with benzothiazoles, dithiocarbamates, and thiurams making up the bulk of the remaining 50%.[35]

Accelerators are highly reactive chemicals. They function at normal curing temperatures except in latex, where they function at lower temperatures. Thanks to these new compounds, sulfur cross-linking of any unsaturated rubber can be accomplished in minutes. Different chemical accelerators work at different speeds. The *ultrafast accelerators* are thiurams, dithiocarbamates, xanthates, and thiophosphates. *Moderate accelerators* are sulfenamides, guanidines, and mercaptobenzothiazoles (MBTs), and *slow accelerators* are amines and thiourea derivatives.

Accelerator Activators

Primary accelerators are often combined with secondary accelerators that give a synergistic effect during processing. These ingredients form chemical complexes with the accelerators and help derive the maximum benefit from the accelerators.[1]

Antidegradants (Antiozonants and Antioxidants)

Rubber polymers are susceptible to deterioration in varying degrees. This deterioration occurs as a result of exposure to oxygen, ozone, light, heat, and radiation during natural and accelerated aging processes, and can dramatically affect the life of the product. The loss of physical properties associated with this aging process is usually caused by scission cracking, cross-linking, or some form of chemical alteration of the polymer chain.

Antidegradants are used to resist the formation of peroxides at points along the rubber polymer chain as a result of hydrogen atoms' being knocked off by some sort of energy (e.g., heat,

light, ozone). The loss of hydrogen creates a radical that reacts with oxygen to form the peroxide. Subsequently, the newly formed peroxide can remove another hydrogen atom from the same polymer chain or another one, which then produces another radical and a hydroperoxide. When two hydroperoxides react a rubber alkoxy radical and another rubber peroxide form. Both of these radicals then remove hydrogen from polymer chains, and polymer destruction accelerates.[35]

A major type of antidegradant was first developed more than 100 years ago, in response to fabricated rubber products' losing their flexibility, cracking, becoming sticky, and adhering to various surfaces, including skin. Before 1910, pitch, creosote, and naphthalene from coking coal were used. Later, organic chemicals were developed from purified coal tar or subsequent derivatives. Useful compounds today include aniline, various creosols, hydroquinone, phenol, and various simple amine and hydroxy derivatives of these compounds.[35]

Antioxidants

Oxidation occurs whenever rubber chains are broken and carbon radicals formed. Highly unsaturated polymers, such as NR, SBR, polybutadiene, and polyisoprene, oxidize more readily than saturated polymers such as ethylene propylene. These oxidative changes can cause rubber to either harden or soften, depending on the polymer. Natural and polyisoprene rubbers tend to soften as a result of chain breaking and depolymerization, while the remaining polymers tend to harden. Because of this weakness, compounders add chemicals called *antioxidants* to the rubber, which are compounds that competitively destroy oxy radicals before they have a chance to react with the rubber.[1]

Antioxidants work in one of two ways. In one, a hydrogen atom from the antioxidant reacting with the peroxide leaves a radical from the antioxidant that reacts with another peroxide, preventing it from removing another hydrogen atom from the polymer chain. The most common antioxidants that react with the peroxides are phenols, phosphites, and certain alkyl and aromatic amines. Antioxidants of the second type react with the hydroperoxides.

Antioxidants prolong the useful life of a large variety of finished products, from tires to gloves and tubing. Because phenolic antioxidants are not staining, they are frequently used in the manufacture of medical gloves and condoms.[2, 20] While NR usually requires antioxidants only, many synthetic polymers require both antioxidants and stabilizers, which protect polymers during storage.[36] The most widely used antioxidants are phenols, quinolones, alkylamines, and phosphites, with *p*-phenylenediamine being the most popular one.

Antiozonants

Ozone (O_3) is created in our atmosphere by photolysis, depending upon the amount and availability of sunlight or other ozone-generating source (e.g., electrical equipment). Ozone reacts directly with the polymer when it is stretched and cleaves the double bonds that solidify the rubber matrix. These broken bonds represent weakened areas of the material and are most prevalent in areas where the polymer is stretched, folded, or bent. Rubbers differ in their ozone resistance. Concentrations of 5 ppm or more crack most susceptible rubbers. Highly unsaturated rubbers such as NR, SBR, polybutadiene, and nitrile are readily cracked, whereas polyisobutylene and neoprene are moderately ozone resistant, and ethylene propylene elastomers are totally resistant.

Ozone cracking can be prevented in three ways. One is by the addition to the polymer of surface coatings (i.e., specialized waxes) that are intended to "bloom" to the surface, forming a protective barrier. Because the waxy surface coating is brittle, this application is feasible only when the finished product need not be flexible. Adding or blending with ozone-resistant polymers is another way to prevent ozone cracking. Finally, chemical antiozonants can be added. For products that must withstand continuous flexing, chemical antiozonants such as *p*-phenylenediamines, naphthylamines, 2,2,4-trimethyl-1,2-dihydroxyquinolone, and alkyl-aryl chemicals (typically in chloroprenes) are widely used. All are potent sensitizers.[35]

Like the phenylenediamines, napthylamines and quinolones can discolor rubber. Excessive exposure to hydroquinone has been reported to cause depigmentation of human skin.[23, 37, 38] Although these antiozonant chemicals are used in some household and medical gloves, they are more often used in the manufacture of darker-colored products such as tires, hoses, and industrial gloves. Styrenated or hindered phenols are thought to be nonstaining and thus are the antiozonants of choice for use in most gloves, condoms, catheters, and dental dams. Other antiozonants used today include urea- and thiourea derivatives and certain dithiocarbamates. These chemicals can also act as sensitizers.

Fillers

Fillers, or extenders, are used to reinforce or modify physical characteristics (i.e., tensile and tear strength), impart certain processing properties, or reduce the cost of the finished product. Reinforcing fillers that strengthen the finished product include carbon black, zinc oxide, magnesium carbonate, and various clays. Fillers that do not significantly increase the strength of the product include whiting, calcium carbonate, barite, and barium sulfate.[1, 2, 4]

Vulcanizing Agents

To obtain efficient vulcanization, vulcanizing agents are used, which donate a sulfur atom or other chemical cross-link during vulcanization. In addition to elemental sulfur, sulfur-containing accelerators can be used as well. Thiuram sulfides, thiomorpholines, and morpholinothiabenzolthiazoles are typical. Organic peroxides and metal oxides can also be used for sulfurless chemical cross-linking.

Retarders

Used principally in the tire industry, retarders act as antiscorching agents, prevulcanization inhibitors, and cure retardants, all actions that allow delays and afford flexibility during the production process overall. Benzoic acid and phenylamine derivatives may be used, but *N*-(cyclohexylthio) phthalimide is preferred because it is considered to be nonstaining and works well with many antidegradants.[35]

Pigments, Odorants, and Flavorants

Pigments color the finished rubber product. They include zinc oxide, lithopone, and a number of organic dyes (e.g., Irgalite orange F2G).[39, 40] Odorants are often required to hide the offensive smell associated with the compounding of various polymers, but they can also be added along with flavorants to products such as toys, dental gloves, baby nipples, and condoms. Some of these chemicals are known to cause irritation and contact sensitization.

Processing Aids

Materials added to rubber compounds as processing aids are diverse: some have extensive effects on the finished products; others do not. Plasticizers or peptizers (i.e., thiophenols) are often added during compounding to chemically retard repolymerization of the chains broken during mastication. Chemical softeners (petroleum products, oils, waxes, pine tar, fatty acids) are necessary when the mix is too stiff for proper incorporation of the various ingredients. They are used to aid mixing, promote greater elasticity, tack, viscosity, act as lubricants or dispersants, and extend or replace a portion of the rubber hydrocarbon without sacrifice of physical properties. Terpene softeners are synthesized by the *H. brasiliensis* tree, and, thus, many NRL manufacturers do not add other chemical softeners. Although their presence may be minimal in many finished products, they can cause both irritant and type IV reactions.

Blowing Agents

Blowing agents generate gas required for the production of blown sponge and microporous rubbers. Azo compounds and carbonates are typically used for their ability to release gas during vulcanization. *Foam rubber* is manufactured directly from latex by using emulsified compounding ingredients. The mixture is then whipped mechanically in a frothing machine into a foam containing millions of gas bubbles. The foam is poured into molds and vulcanized by heating to form such articles as mattresses and seat cushions, pillows, and cellular crepe rubber used in the shoe industry.

Dipping Technology

For the most part, thin-film devices (e.g., condoms, gloves, diaphragms, balloons, nipples, bathing caps, football bladders, toys, pacifiers) are manufactured on formers or molds made of porcelain, glass, metal, plastic, or plaster that are mounted on racks and then pulled through various processing steps along a continuously moving (hydraulic batch or chain-driven) production line (Fig. 29–8). A coating of the concentrated latex adheres to the form and is stripped from it after vulcanization. Although allergic reactions have been reported to other types of NRL manufactured products, dipped products are the most common cause of allergic reactions.[41–43] Since manufacturing methods have a significant impact on the even-

tual allergenicity of the product, the steps in dipping technology will be briefly reviewed.[21]

Straight Dipping

The former is immersed in the latex mix, withdrawn very slowly, and the latex that adheres to the former is dried and vulcanized. Greater thickness is achieved by reimmersing the former in the latex. The thickness of the rubber depends on the number of dips, the viscosity of the mix, and the total content of solids.[20]

Coagulant Dipping

Coagulant dipping is the most popular process for manufacturing many kinds of latex gloves. The former is initially immersed in a coagulant solution—consisting of calcium nitrate, magnesium, or zinc chloride in water, or methylated spirits—which acts to ensure uniform deposition of the latex emulsion on the former. Zinc coagulant complexes have demonstrated their ability to bind protein in the latex matrix more effectively and permanently than magnesium or calcium coagulant, helping to remove NRL proteins throughout the remaining processing. Environmental regulations in the mid-1980s limited their use and may have affected the quantity and quality of the residual NRL proteins in finished products.

Lubricants

Releasing agents (i.e., cornstarch powder, talc, *Lycopodium*, oatstarch, silicone oils) are used to reduce the surface drag and facilitate stripping or removing the product from the formers. Talc and *Lycopodium*, however, are no longer permitted in medical-grade glove production because of con-

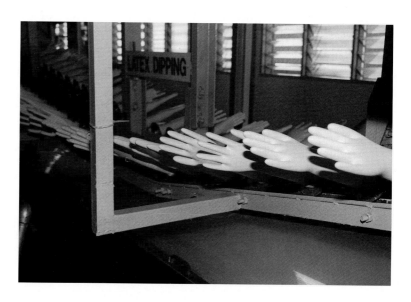

FIGURE 29–8 ● Thin-film devices such as gloves, condoms, and balloons are typically manufactured on formers made of porcelain or glass, which are immersed in the latex mix.

cerns about insolubility and promotion of postoperative adhesions. Current lubricants must meet the U.S.P. specifications for absorbable dusting powders. Powdered lubricants can also be combined with antimicrobials and wetting agents and are usually applied on line, where the formers are dipped into tanks of slurry powder lubricants in water or alcohol suspensions). Slurry dipping may take place either before or after drying. Water-based slurry solutions require the addition of preservatives, which can also be contact sensitizers.

Drying

After dipping, the formers are sequentially withdrawn and rotated into ovens for drying. This process has a profound effect on the migration of any unbound proteins, chemicals, salts, or fatty acids. Because of evaporation due to heat during drying or vulcanization, and pressure as the gelled latex matrix contracts, the water containing the unbound particles moves away from the surface of the formers. Because products such as gloves and condoms are inverted as they are removed from the formers, the inside—"skinside"—surface now contains the highest levels of chemical and protein allergens.[10] Methods such as water stripping, chlorination, enzyme treatments, surface coating, wet gel leaching, and postcure leaching are currently being utilized to remove the residual allergens effectively from both sides of the product.[10, 18, 44]

Latex Dip

The formers are dipped into tanks containing the compounded latex. In the NRL process the polymer is not dissolved but is an emulsion. The thickness of the product depends on the viscosity, dwell time, number of dips into the polymer, total solids content, and concentration and type of coagulant. The rotation and speed of the formers are crucial to the uniformity of the finished product.

Vulcanization

After rubber materials have been properly compounded, mixed, and shaped (molded, calendered, extruded, dipped, or fabricated into a composite item), they must be vulcanized so that the finished product will behave as a truly elastic material. The vulcanization process consists simply of introducing cross-links between the long-chain rubber molecules through reactions with vulcanizing agents and accelerators to form a continuous network of long, flexible three-dimensional structures, which transform the latex liquid into a strong elastic material. Vulcanization is accomplished by means of various chemical reactions, depending on the chemical structure of the macromolecule. The most common process involves sulfur and its compounds, which works very well with unsaturated elastomers such as NR, nitrile, neoprene, and some of the other synthetic polydienes.[1]

NRL can be *prevulcanized* or *postvulcanized*. Prevulcanization involves mixing the latex suspension with a dispersion of antioxidants and a fast accelerator, and both the compounded latex and the dipped film are heated to a temperature of 70°C for about 2 hours. Postvulcanization requires heating the dipped film alone. Vulcanization converts residual proteins to a water-soluble form, permitting more EPs to migrate to the surface. The EP content increases during prevulcanization, depending on the duration and temperature of the process. Postvulcanization shows a similar rise in EPs, but they are not extracted as easily from postvulcanized films, possibly owing to fusion of a less permeable sheet.[10]

Leaching

Dipped products are usually leached (washed) to remove water-soluble materials.[20] *On-line leaching* is carried out before drying; *off-line leaching*, on the dried, vulcanized film. Off-line extraction can take hours or days to complete, depending on the thickness of the product. It is always used when removal of all water-soluble substances is essential, as for electricians' gloves.[20] Leaching is particularly important for products like nipples and medical devices, to remove extractable NRL proteins and residual chemical in both natural and synthetic rubber products.[20] Leaching can reduce EP levels, but only under appropriate process conditions. For example, a nonleached, oven-dried film can still have less surface EP than a 5-minute–leached, oven-dried film. Short-term hydration swells the NRL matrix and facilitates protein migration to the surface, but is insufficient for protein removal. Factors such as soft or hard water, moving or standing water, duration of the leach, temperature, and rate of water exchange contribute to the efficacy of the residual removal.

Wet gel leaching involves soaking or rinsing the coagulated gel latex to remove the salts, residual chemicals, and water-soluble proteins from the product osmotically before drying or further vulcanization. Leaching is very effective and can remove as much as 85% of the EP from prevulcanized films and another 60% from postvulcanized films. Dual leaching of both pre- and postvulcanized films has also been proven effective in protein reduction and can remove as much as 90% of the extractable protein.[18]

Chlorination

Chlorination can also be an on-line or an off-line process. It reduces the surface drag of the product and removes powdered lubricants when a powder-free or reduced-powder product is required. An on-line process has cost and efficiency advantages but carries increased risk for workers and is extremely corrosive to production equipment. For these reasons, off-line chlorination is more common. The chlorine bath removes most of the powder, but also acts as a harsh surface treatment that undermines the physical properties of the product by accelerating oxidation. After chlorination, it is necessary to neutralize the chlorine with a dilute aqueous solution of ammonia or sodium bicarbonate followed by a water rinse. In addition to the effects of rewashing the product, the addition of chlorine renders the proteins insoluble—and perhaps forms a layer less permeable to protein migration,[20] bringing the EP level down to 0.02 mg/g or less. Chlorination does present significant challenges. The process is costly, potentially hazardous to the environment (wastewater), and can present challenges to maintaining a products' shelf life, integrity, and barrier efficacy.

Protein Identification and Quantification in Finished Products

To contain the growing problem of latex allergies, manufacturers have attempted to reduce or eliminate latex proteins from finished devices. The challenge of protein reduction is to maintain the physical properties necessary for adequate barrier protection and product viability. According to the U.S. Food and Drug Administration's 1996 Document, *Guidance for Medical Gloves: A Workshop Manual* (FDA 96-4257), anyone who intends to market a medical glove with a specified protein level must submit the proposed protein label and supporting test data to the FDA. At present the FDA's interim policy specifies 50 µg per gram to be the lowest acceptable protein value for medical-grade gloves. This value reflects the limited sensitivity of the Lowry protein assay, rather than any known safety threshold for NRL exposure.

Protein levels are to be determined by a standard test method that has been established by the American Society of Testing and Materials (ASTM). Currently, the standard test method for the analysis of total protein in NRL medical devices is the *Modified Lowry with Precipitation* (ASTM D5712).[10, 45, 46] The Lowry protein assay

was selected for its sensitivity to the complex mixture of polypeptides in NRL. Because all protein assays are susceptible to interference by chemical additives in the test sample, a precipitation technique that allows more than 85% protein recovery is utilized. Bovine serum albumin (BSA) or ovalbumin is used as the calibration protein.[10, 46, 47] Good correlation has been demonstrated between total protein measured by Lowry and skin prick testing ($R = 0.95$, $P > .001$).[48] The FDA recommends this method be used to help ensure uniformity in protein level determinations for medical devices. The labels for medical gloves that bear a claim for total water-extractable protein content must also bear the following cautionary statement:

> **Caution: Safe use of this glove by or on latex-sensitized individuals has not been established.**

In addition to the Lowry assay, the *Latex ELISA for Antigenic Protein (LEAP)* has been marketed to NRL manufacturers to determine antigenic protein levels in finished goods. This method employs an indirect ELISA technique, in which latex proteins are immobilized by absorption to plastic and reacted with rabbit antilatex antisera. The proteins eluted from NRL products are allowed to bind to microtiter wells, and the bound antigens are then detected by polyclonal rabbit IgE antibodies that have been raised against ammoniated latex. The primary advantages of this assay are its sensitivity and specificity for latex antigens; however, only a small portion of these are likely to elicit an allergic response relevant in type I allergy. This method remains controversial because the polystyrene surface allows for unpredictable attachment of mixtures of proteins so that the initial solid phase of the assay may be difficult to standardize. In addition, the LEAP assay has not been shown to correlate well against in vitro or in vivo methods that measure allergens such as the radioallergosorbent test (RAST) inhibition.[48] Reproducibility also presents challenges.[11, 21, 46, 49]

Although significant correlation has been reported in some studies between total protein content and symptom elicitation, the extent of the correlation may be too small to justify using total protein as a safe method for determining allergenicity of a product.[11, 30] While reducing total protein may theoretically prevent future sensitization, this has not yet been substantiated, and it is important to remember that minute concentrations are enough to elicit a response in sensitized persons.

Because not all latex proteins are allergens, total protein measurements are not always sufficient to monitor the allergenic properties of NRL products. The amount of protein eluted from product samples does not always correlate with its allergenicity. For example, a surgical glove with high total protein concentration demonstrated no allergenicity as determined by skin prick testing, whereas a household glove with a low total protein level demonstrated 95% skin prick test reactivity.[50] It is possible for an NRL product to test low in total protein but high in allergen.[30, 51]

Although total protein measurement is not perfect, allergen measurement presents its own set of challenges. The allergens that have been eluted from different NRL products in multiple studies vary much in type, range, potency. Differences in investigators, source materials, extraction and separation procedures, and testing techniques may account for this variability.[10, 11, 24, 52] In comparing various products, Makinen-Kiljunen, reports a 400-fold difference in NRL allergen activity in vitro, with condoms demonstrating levels similar to those in toy balloons and 20-fold variation between brands. Likewise, one brand of baby pacifier exhibited a 200-fold higher allergen level than another. Yunginger and coworkers also demonstrated this variability, with a reported 3,000-fold variation in the allergen levels in NRL medical gloves.[30] In addition, extract source materials (i.e., fresh latex, low-ammoniated latex, high-ammoniated latex, compounded latex, product extracts) have produced considerable differences in the IgE antibody responses of patients.[43, 53–55] For example, Alenius and associates found 10 allergens in fresh latex, nine in ammoniated latex concentrate, and none of these allergens in the product (glove) extract. In addition, two allergens were detected in the glove extract but not in either the fresh or ammoniated latex.[10, 11, 56]

Quantification and identification of the specific NRL allergens require human IgE-class antibodies (from a serum pool from sensitized persons) or experimentally produced monoclonal or polyclonal antibodies that recognize the dominant epitopes in the allergen. These dominant epitopes have not yet been characterized, but they are being sought aggressively by a variety of immunochemical methods.[11] With all methods, testing in vivo of sensitized persons is required to verify that the antigens measured are capable of eliciting allergic reactions. Serological variations in populations of sensitized subjects have also been demonstrated by Alenius' group[13] and indicate that no single antigen can be used to detect antibodies to NRL in all patients. Because NRL-allergic persons have been exposed to a variety of products, each con-

taining diverse proteins, unique antigenic epitopes, and different cross-reactive antigens, there are considerable differences in the IgE antibody responses of individual patients and among different patient groups (i.e., healthcare workers, spina bifida patients) to different antigen preparations. These variations in the immune responses between individuals and between patient groups may also be related to the manner of exposure, clinical sensitivity, and underlying disease.[10, 13, 43, 52, 54]

Although it is known that the amount of exposure necessary to cause an allergic reaction varies from person to person, little is known about the duration or level of exposure that is required to bring about sensitization to NRL. Thus, the more important challenge is to determine the level or threshold below which the NRL protein exposure may be regarded as "nonsensitizing."[57] A study of "low-allergen" gloves conducted with known NRL type I allergic persons by Gehring and colleagues was halted in 1997 when the test subjects reacted to the low-allergen test products.[58] Threshold labeling may be hindered by the fact that thresholds often depend on the route of sensitization and on the product source of the allergens. Because the research has not yet been completed that would establish a safe level for either total protein or allergen content, caution on the part of the consumer is prudent. When making product selections it is important that consumers understand their own personal requirements. Users who have type I (immediate) sensitivity to NRL protein should avoid NRL products. Those who have type IV (delayed) allergy will need specific details about the chemical composition from the manufacturer. Because the skin barrier can be compromised in type IV cases, subdermal NRL protein exposure may occur with subsequent sensitization and a progression to type I. Thus, timely and accurate diagnostic and management procedures are essential.

CLINICAL ASPECTS

Some cases of occupational contact dermatitis to rubber have been described as irritant and as allergic.[59] Although contact urticaria (Fig. 29–9) is more often caused by the proteins in the natural rubber latex than by an allergy to accelerators, allergic contact dermatitis (Fig. 29–10) is more often due to sensitivity to chemicals used as accelerators, antioxidants, and the like. The urticarial reaction presents within a few minutes and may cause rhinitis, respiratory problems, or even anaphylaxis, whereas allergic contact dermatitis is delayed and is largely limited to the skin. There

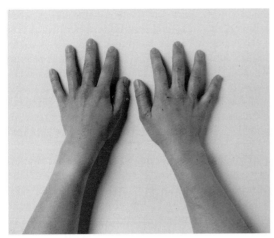

FIGURE 29–9 • Type I hypersensitivity to natural rubber latex.

are, however, patients whose eczematous eruptions are caused by type I allergic mechanisms. Hand eczema resembling dyshidrotic eczema can be caused by aromatic amines, and contact dermatitis to rubber can also have an atypical presentation.[60] Such manifestations include purpura,[61] pustulosis,[62, 63] depigmentation,[64] lichenification,[65, 66] erythema multiforme–like lesions,[67] depigmentation,[68] lichenoid lesions,[65, 69] and even a pellagrinoid appearance.[70]

While occupational contact reactions to rubber are often thought to occur principally in workers in rubber production, this presentation actually accounts for relatively few of the cases seen today. Because of improved technology in the rubber industry, the number of sensitized rubber workers is small compared with persons sensitized from using rubber products, especially latex gloves.[71, 72] For example, 34 of the 999 workers in a Yugosla-

vian tire factory had irritant reactions, but only three had allergic contact dermatitis and only two of those were reacting to chemicals in rubber.[73] In 1975 Fregert, reporting 20 years' experience in an occupational medicine clinic, found that only 20% of those who were rubber sensitive worked in the rubber industry and that most cases were caused by exposure to finished rubber products.[74]

Workers in many industries develop occupational sensitivity to both natural and synthetic rubbers or rubber-processing chemicals, including factory workers,[75] dairy farmers,[76] greenhouse workers,[77] metalworkers, potters,[78] paper manufacturing workers,[79] photographic film production personnel,[80] footwear manufacturers,[81] cleaners and janitors,[82, 83] construction workers,[84, 85] hospital cleaning personnel,[86] kitchen workers,[87] and those exposed during the manufacture or use of products such as rubber bands,[88] dolls,[89] and gloves themselves.[23, 90, 91] Workers at risk for occupational contact dermatitis from rubber sensitivity in Poland include metal industry workers (machine tool operators, electroplaters), healthcare workers, construction, footwear manufacture, stock breeders, and truck drivers. In a Canadian NRL glove factory, approximately 11% of the workers reported allergic symptoms in questionnaire data.[92] A list of published examples of related occupations is given in Table 29–1, but today rubber is so ubiquitous that exposure is possible in almost any occupation. The more common picture of rubber sensitivity is glove dermatitis. Both eczematous and urticarial lesions occur in a variety of workers who routinely wear gloves. Glove reactions can be irritant or allergic. They are most common in healthcare workers,[93, 94] but should be suspected when any worker who has a history of protective glove use develops an eruption on the hands.[90, 91, 95, 96] Problems from gloves are significantly more

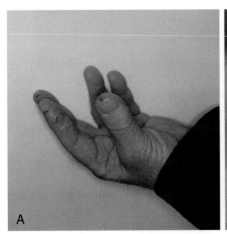

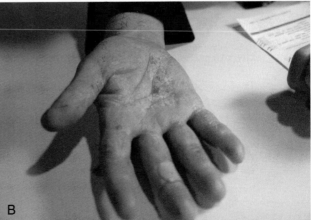

FIGURE 29–10A and B • Type IV hypersensitivity to MBT.

common in hospital workers who wear gloves more than 2 hours per day, and veterinarians may be at similar risk.[97]

Hairdressers may[98] or may not[98, 99] have increased risk of rubber allergy: observations vary. In two large groups of reactors, a few were allergic to carbamates or *p*-phenylenediamine mix, but this represented fewer than 3% of reactors in one group[100, 101] and only five of 143 (all to thiuram mix) in the other.[102] Unfortunately, classic patch testing may miss reactors with eczematous responses associated with type 1 allergy.[98] We have seen hairdressers with hand eczema develop contact dermatitis to gloves worn to protect their hands from chemicals, but this may be a regional problem, as in relatively large series several other investigators did not find hairdressers to react more often to thiuram mix[98, 99] or other rubber chemicals.

Rubber chemicals can also cause contact allergy in those who manufacture them,[103] and these workers will subsequently be allergic to rubber products that contain such compounds. Rubber sensitivity, relatively common in construction workers,[85] is, in fact, associated with chromate sensitivity, apparently from gloves worn to protect eczematous hands from chromate dermatitis.[74] This seems especially true in construction, where chromate allergy was found in 47 of 69 rubber-sensitive construction workers.[85] Related fungicides have also been associated with occupational allergy to rubber chemicals,[104] although this is not in the strictest sense an allergy to *rubber.*

Irritant Dermatitis from Rubber

Rubber workers frequently develop irritant dermatitis caused by chemical irritants such as solvents (i.e., naphtha, benzol,[105] petroleum ethers, heptane[60]) and exposure to antitackifiers or mechanical irritants such as dust, friction,[72] and "aggressive" hand cleaning.[60] Tire builders were singled out in one study as being at risk for (irritant) rubber dermatitis due to friction and cleansing solvents.[73] Schwartz and associates described irritation from soapstone, talc, and several amine antioxidants.[105] Mechanical irritation may occur from the shearing stress from tacky, uncured rubber or exposure to cut metal wire suspended in the rubber. Manufacture of the "bead" that holds a tire to a wheel (loops of rubber-coated wire wrapped in a fabric tape impregnated with a phenolic resin[60]) has been automated, but the "bead wrappers" must start the wrap and finish it. In doing so they can injure their fingertips. Production workers who experience irritant dermatitis at work may call the condition *rubber rash.*[60] It tends

to be more common in new workers or after holidays or during hot, humid weather.[60]

Nonallergic reactions are not limited to workers in the rubber industry. Occupations that require wearing gloves (i.e., maintenance works, computer processing, beautician, greenhouse work, and food service personnel) can all be affected. Healthcare professionals often wear gloves continuously throughout the workday and have reported "irritation" from both NRL and synthetic rubber gloves (with or without glove powder). Irritation associated with gloves may be a result of the processing chemicals in natural and synthetic rubber gloves, friction of the glove material against the skin, perspiration, heat, use of hand soaps or lotions, excessive hand washing, failure to dry the hands completely, permeation or penetration of other chemical irritants through the glove material, or of a disturbance in the natural barrier function of the skin.[106, 107]

Type IV Hypersensitivity to Rubber Chemicals

According to White,[108] of the hundreds of rubber chemicals in use, few are used in quantity and relatively few are important potential allergens. In one European patchtest clinic, 3.8% of those tested were rubber allergic, and about 55% of reactions to rubber chemicals were occupationally induced, 84% of them by rubber gloves.[109] In Europe, occupational exposure to tires[110] is a risk factor for sensitization to *N*-isopropyl-*N'*-phenyl-*p*-phenylenediamine (IPPD).[69, 111, 112] In a tire factory, antioxidants (particularly IPPD) were the dominant allergens, especially for assemblers, compounding room workers, equipment maintenance personnel, vulcanizers, atomizers, retreaders, tire balancers, and production workers. The *p*-phenylenediamine derivatives are followed by benzothiazole accelerators such as MBT.[26] This relationship, also seen in other countries,[113, 114] is probably related to opportunities for exposure. For example, MBT is certainly a relatively potent sensitizer in guinea pigs.[115] At one time it was, along with guanidines[116] and thiurams,[117] a prominent cause of rubber allergy. It still causes many cases of contact dermatitis to rubber, particularly to shoes[118–120] (including the insoles of even wooden shoes[121]), but despite the enormous amount of MBT used every year, tetramethylthiuram disulfide is a better screening antigen for rubber allergy.[122] In the United States the prevalence of MBT sensitivity in patients seen in patch test clinics is about 2.7%,[123] which is lower than that reported in previous years.[124, 125] Thiurams may be found in rubber-free materials such as soap,[126] and can cross-react or co-react with carbamates and chemically related fungicides such as maneb, zineb,[127] ziram,[128] benomyl, betanal, carbyne, carbofuran, carbaryl,[129] and mancozeb.[130, 131]

Lammintausta found that 4.7% of those tested in a contact dermatitis clinic were rubber allergic. Of these, almost half (73 of 158) tested positive to thiuram mix, followed by carba mix (51 of 158), p-phenylenediamine mix (40 of 158), and mercapto mix (19 of 158). Only three had immediate reactions to NRL.[132] Prevalence of contact sensitivity most likely depends on exposure more than on any inherent susceptibility.[133] Opportunity for exposure may also determine the prevalence of sensitivity to specific chemicals or categories, as there are scattered reports of epidemics from morpholines[134] (e.g., dithiodimorphiline or Sulfasan R), which may or may not be associated with sensitivity to other categories of rubber chemicals such as quinolines,[135] p-tert-butyl-catechol (used to inhibit polymerization of butadiene,[72, 105] and even dinitrochlorobenzene (as a contaminant[136]), but these are implicated less often, overall. Such rubber chemicals may affect not only rubber workers but also chemical workers who manufacture compounds for use in the rubber industry.[137]

RUBBER CHEMICAL ANTIGENS

Thiurams

Thiurams are rubber accelerators used in both natural rubbers and some synthetic ones. Thiurams contain a basic urea structure, except that a sulfur atom is substituted for oxygen, making the basic structure similar to that of a thiourea (Table 29–6). From patch test data in contact dermatitis clinics throughout the world, thiurams have been indicted as the most common cause of allergy to rubber chemicals. Approximately 5% of persons in the United States who have been patch tested have had relevant reactions to thiuram mix,[138] and this has changed little since 1974.[139] It has been theorized that this prevalence rate may be due to the increase in the widespread use of rubber products, especially NRL gloves, in many professions. This has become a major problem in healthcare, the majority of cases of contact dermatitis to gloves being caused by thiuram accelerators.[40]

Although glove dermatitis due to thiuram sensitivity is common in healthcare workers (i.e., surgeons, surgical scrub nurses,[141] dentists[142]), it also occurs frequently in other occupations (e.g., housekeeping employees,[143] beauticians, maintenance workers, computer assembly personnel, homemakers, and agricultural workers). Although the eruption itself may present in a glove-type distribution, it can also occur on the feet and other exposed areas. Thiuram allergies may be due to airborne exposure (e.g., agricultural chemical sprays of pesticides and fungicides,[144] or spray-on wound dressings[145]). Thiuram sensitivity may be associated with photodermatitis,[146] perhaps as part of the extended antigen syndrome. It may also be seen as systemic contact dermatitis, perhaps in several forms, including the pattern from administration of disulfiram (Antabuse[147]) with onset 5 hours after the first episode of diffuse itching, swelling of the feet, and a vesicular eruption of the face, arms, and feet (pompholyx), and acute nummular dermatitis of the extremities and dermatitis at an old scar site.[148] "Systemic disulfiram" can also cause flushing on exposure to alcohol, and exposure can be occupational.[149] Like sensitivity to other rubber accelerators, reactions are sometimes mounted to chemicals in "nonoccupational" items such as balloons, clothing, protective aprons, pillows, sponges, applicators, pesticides, putty, tires, rubber bands, adhesives, plastic-treated seeds, fungicides, neoprene (chloroprene), germicides, insecticides, soluble oils, paints, animal repellents, soaps, shampoos, fingercots, gaskets, and many, many others.

Exposure to thiurams may differ geographically, as allergies to tetramethylthiuram monosulfide and tetramethylthiuram disulfide are more common in Portugal,[150] Holland,[151] Finland,[93] and Poland.[152] In contrast, allergies to tetraethylthiuram disulfide and di-pentamethylenethiuram disulfide were at one time more common in England.[26] Two studies of thiuram reactivity in Europe in 1984 to 1987 and in 1989 showed response rates of 3.2% and 3%[154] in Belgium[153, 154] and 4.5% in a similar 10-year study.[155]

The test to thiuram mix is positive more often than those to other rubber mixes or mercaptobenzothiazole.[132] More than half of rubber-sensitive persons react to thiuram mix, so reactivity to this group is somewhat more common than that to the next most frequent screening antigen.[156] It is thus a much better antigen for screening rubber sensitivity than either MBT[122] or carba mix, which may not be as consistently positive.[157]

Mercaptobenzothiazole and the Mercapto Mix

Mercaptobenzothiazole (MBT) is used as an accelerator in the production of both natural and synthetic rubber products. It is also classified with other chemicals that are similar in structure, known as benzothiazoles. Although most rubber

Text continued on page 532

TABLE 29–6 • Structures of Representative Chemicals Used in the Manufacture of Rubber*

Chemical Name	Structure
Thiurams	
Tetramethylthiuram disulfide	
Tetramethylthiuram monosulfide	
Tetraethylthiuram disulfide	
Dipentamethylenethiuram disulfide	
Amine Compounds	
N-(1,3-dimethylbutyl)-N′-phenyl-p-phenylenediamine	
N,N′-bis(1,4-dimethyl pentyl)-p-phenylenediamine	
Phenyl-β-naphthylamine	
Phenyl-α-naphthylamine	
N-isopropyl-N′-phenyl-p-phenylenediamine	

TABLE 29–6 • Structures of Representative Chemicals Used in the Manufacture of Rubber* *Continued*

Chemical Name	Structure
N-cyclohexyl-N'-phenyl-p-phenylenediamine	
N,N'-diphenyl-p-phenylenediamine	
4,4'-diaminodiphenylmethane	
Hexamethylenetetramine	
N,N'-di-β-naphthyl-p-phenylenediamine	
Thiazoles 2-Mercaptobenzothiazole	
N-Cyclohexyl-2-benzothiazolesulfenamide	
2,2'-Dithiobisbenzothiazole	
N-tert-butyl-2-benzothiazolesulfenamide	
N-oxydiethylene-2-benzothiazolesulfenamide	

Table continued on following page

TABLE 29–6 • Structures of Representative Chemicals Used in the Manufacture of Rubber* *Continued*

Chemical Name	Structure
Thiourea Derivatives N,N'-Diphenylthiourea	
Diethylthiourea	
Dibutylthiourea	
Ethylenethiourea	
Guanidine Derivatives 1,3-Diphenylguanidine	
N,N'-di-ortho-tolylguanidine	
Quinoline Derivatives 1,2-Dihydro-2,2,4-trimethylquinoline	
6-Ethoxy-1,2-dihydro-2,2,4-trimethylquinoline	

TABLE 29–6 • Structures of Representative Chemicals Used in the Manufacture of Rubber* *Continued*

Chemical Name	Structure
Dithiocarbamates	
Zinc dibutyldithiocarbamate	$$\left[\begin{array}{c} C_4H_9 \\ N-C-S- \\ C_4H_9 \ \ \underset{S}{\overset{\parallel}{}} \end{array} \right]_2 Zn$$
Zinc diethyldithiocarbamate	$$\left[\begin{array}{c} C_2H_5 \\ N-C-S- \\ C_2H_5 \ \ \underset{S}{\overset{\parallel}{}} \end{array} \right]_2 Zn$$
Zinc dimethyldithiocarbamate	$$\left[\begin{array}{c} CH_3 \\ N-C-S- \\ CH_3 \ \ \underset{S}{\overset{\parallel}{}} \end{array} \right]_2 Zn$$
Zinc ethylphenyldithiocarbamate	$$\left[C_2H_3 - N - \overset{S}{\overset{\parallel}{C}} - S^- \right]_2 Zn^{++}$$
Sodium diethyldithiocarbamate	$$\begin{array}{c} C_2H_3 \\ \qquad \diagdown \\ \qquad N-\overset{S}{\overset{\parallel}{C}}-S^- \ Na^+ \\ \qquad \diagup \\ C_2H_3 \end{array}$$
Phenols	
Butyraldehyde-aniline reaction product	$C_2H_5 \quad (CH_2)_2CH_2$ ... C_2H_5
Butylated hydroxytoluene	$$(CH_3)_3C \overset{OH}{\diagup\diagdown} C(CH_3)_3$$ CH_3

Table continued on following page

TABLE 29–6 • Structures of Representative Chemicals Used in the Manufacture of Rubber* *Continued*

Chemical Name	Structure
Butylated hydroxyanisole	
p-benzyloxyphenol	
N-butyl-p-aminophenol	
(1,1′-biphenyl)diol	
2′,2′methylene bis 4-methyl-6-tert-butyl phenol	
4,4′-Thiobis (6-tert-butyl-m-cresol)	

*Note: Many of these chemicals have several synonyms. Alternative names can be found by searching the National Library of Medicine Databases (e.g., ChemID), which are accessible on line via Internet Grateful Med.

antigens in the standard tray are tested as mixes of three or four chemicals, in the United States, MBT is an exception. Formerly available as a component of the mercapto mix, it is now tested separately to provide optimal concentration. Because irritation is a problem when all of these (usually related) chemicals are used in optimal concentrations, the remaining three structurally similar chemicals used in routine testing now make up the mercapto mix. Each is now used in 0.33% concentration rather than 0.25%, which was necessary for four antigens when MBT was included. This permits screening with a higher concentration of all four benzothiazole antigens.

The mercapto mix comprises three benzothiazole-related rubber chemicals (see Table 29–6): N-cyclohexyl-2-benzothiazolesulfenamide (CBS), 2,2′-dithiobisbenzothiazole (MBTS), and 4-morpholinyl-2-benzothiazyl disulfide. In Europe, MBT is included as well, rather than being tested as a separate antigen. N-cyclohexyl-2-benzothiazolesulfenamide is an accelerator sometimes used in the manufacture of both natural and synthetic rubber tires, and as a substitute for MBTS/diphenylguanidine systems in other applications. The basic structure is that of MBT linked to the cyclohexyl structure through an amine linkage. The technical aspects are not important to the physician, but because a benzothiazole component is present in the structure one would expect it sometimes to cross-react with other benzothiazole accelerators. The structure of MBT closely resembles those of many other rubber chemicals, which again allows for significant cross-sensitivity. The morpholinyl derivatives may be even more sensitizing, according to Wang and Suskind,[158] but MBT probably picks up most of those sensitivities, as there is a prominent cross-reaction on challenge with MBT in morpholinyl derivative-allergic animals.[158]

Although MBT is a potential sensitizer in animal studies[122] and has been used in great quantities in the past, it causes fewer cases of contact sensitivity than the thiurams do. In the United States, the prevalence in a population tested for contact dermatitis is about 2.1%,[138] which is lower than figures for previous years collected by the same group.[124, 125] About 1.6% of persons younger than 40 reacted to MBT and 2.2% of those over 40 who were patch tested for suspected contact dermatitis. The prevalence is almost three times as great for occupational contact dermatitis,[159] but sensitivity is not limited to that group; it is also a common sensitizer in some pediatric populations.[160]

MBTS, also known as benzothiazole disulfide, is a dimer of mercaptobenzothiazole. It is used as an accelerator for both natural and synthetic rubber, and in the latter it may be combined with a secondary accelerator. It may be used in white and colored materials and in products intended to be in repeated contact with food (concentration limited to 1.5% by federal regulations). This is formed from 2-mercaptobenzothiazole by heat and oxidation and may be a sensitizer in some shoes. MBTS has been isolated, along with MBT, from athletic shoes that caused insole dermatitis but it is impossible to know whether it was used primarily or was formed chemically in the process from oxidative change. It may also be found in chloroprene rubber as a plasticizer. 4-Morpholinyl-2-benzothiazyl disulfide is used for thick treads or extrusions, in products that contain much furnace black, and in products that will be stored for long periods.

It was suggested that allergic reactions attributed to MBT might actually be caused by MBTS.[161] One group even postulated that MBTS is actually the allergen for MBT-allergic persons, as MBT is converted by oxidation to its dimer by heat and oxidation[161] and reduced back to MBT by glutathione.[162] Furthermore, there is cross-reactivity between members of the benzothiazole group such as those in the mercapto mix. Foussereau and associates[163] found that CBS, N-oxydi-

ethylene-2-benzothiazolesulfenamide, and other substituted benzothiazoles cross-react with MBT. Wang and Suskind ranked these agents in order of sensitization: 4,4′-dithiodimorpholine, N-oxydiethylene-2-benzothiazolesulfenamide, and MBT.[158] The reasons for differences have to do with absorption of and affinity for protein, but from the data of Foussereau's group and Wang and Suskind one would expect such mixtures to produce as many reactions as MBT or more. Allergy to mercapto mix has about the same prevalence as MBT sensitivity,[138] but Mitchell's data on mixes show that, of 171 persons allergic to MBT or mercapto mix or both, 48 reacted to MBT but not to the mix, whereas only 14 responded to the mix but not to MBT.[164]

Shoe dermatitis is a typical presentation of sensitivity to MBT, and some such cases are occupational. Insole dermatitis is typical. Severity varies enormously, probably with both the level of sensitivity and the degree of exposure. The leading source is shoes and boots, and especially the insoles,[119] where MBT is the most common allergen. It is used in many kinds of shoes, even safety shoes,[165] but the leading source is probably athletic shoes. In one case, when the antigen was extracted and examined the actual sensitizer was found to be MBTS, a dimer of MBT. One group believes that this is the predominant antigen in MBT sensitivity anyway,[162, 166] but this impression needs confirmation. Allergy to rubber chemicals in safety shoes (which is as often dye or chromate sensitivity as it is rubber allergy) is often due to MBT, but thiourea, IPPD, and phenyl-alpha-naphthylamine have also been implicated.[165]

A positive patch test to 2-MBT may be evidence of occupationally induced contact dermatitis when there is a relevant history of occupational exposure, such as reactions in "elastic thread" workers,[26] cement tube workers,[166] workers exposed to a conveyer belt,[167] postal clerks who use rubber bands (MBT was weaker than some other rubber allergens[168]), and persons who use rubber banknote counters,[26] and fingerstalls.[26] It is wise, however, to look everywhere for sensitizers, as reactions are often caused by nonoccupational exposure to a large variety of rubber products. Reported examples include brassiere cups,[169] rubber swim caps and face masks,[26] a Foley catheter,[170] medical prostheses,[171, 172] elastic bandages,[173] rubber stoppers in medical syringes,[174] shoes,[175] and baby bottle nipples,[176] to name a few. For a brief time MBT was found in some Spandex (polyurethane) elastomers,[177–179] but that has not been a problem for many years. It has also been found in sources other than rubber, such as an anticorrosive agent,[180] an antifreeze mixture,[26] and as a contaminant in digoxin injectable solution.[181] It occasionally causes allergy from condoms.[182, 183]

This chemical can be found in sources other than rubber, and exposure is more common among persons who present to a physician for occupational contact dermatitis. Products associated with MBT allergy include photographic film,[152] veterinary medications,[184] a "releasing" fluid,[185] antifreeze, soluble oils, clothing, tools, cements and adhesives, cleansers, detergents, paints, black tires, fungicides, slimicides, greases, insecticides,[186, 187] and even earrings.[188]

Black Rubber Mix

The black rubber mix contains certain chemicals used in rubber processing to make the product more resistant to breakdown, cracking, and crumbling in the air. Rubber would not weather well if it did not contain antidegradants protecting against damage from oxygen and ozone, from flex cracking and heat aging. The derivatives of *p*-phenylaminediamine comprise an excellent group of such chemicals. There are other (nonstaining) antioxidants, but the black rubber products provide good protection (at the cost of staining). Typical applications are tires, radiator hoses, etc. In the United States IPPD is seldom used today, but it is still present in some European products.[112] Most persons allergic to IPPD also react to 1,3-dimethylbutyl-phenyl-*p*-phenylenediamine, the chemical usually substituted for IPPD, so the test material used is still relevant. *p*-Phenylenediamine-related rubber chemicals are used in both natural and synthetic products, mostly in tires, but also in a wide variety of products that usually are recognizable by their black color.

Patients sensitive to these derivatives may or may not be sensitive to other rubber chemicals, and the percentage who are varies with the population studied. The *p*-phenylenediamine-related chemicals are often associated with occupational allergy.[189] In some series of industrial cases, *p*-phenylenediamine mix is the most common rubber sensitizer (reported prevalence 37 per 1000 subject).[189] Of 158 persons allergic to rubber, *p*-phenylenediamine mix produced a positive patch test in 40. It was third in order of frequency after thiurams and carbamates.[132] In countries where IPPD is still used, it may be the leading rubber allergen in tire manufacturing workers. In one European study 42 of 56 IPPD-allergic persons acquired the sensitivity through occupational exposure. Seventeen of them were in tire manufacture, nine automobile mechanics, and nine drivers, and seven had some other kind of industrial exposure.[190] Anyone who handles automotive parts like tires and hoses will probably be exposed. Mechanics and body shop employees, salvage workers, automobile salespersons, automotive parts clerks, tire fitters, and tire salesmen are all at risk. Service station, garage, and parking attendants, car washers, and drivers and truckers are also exposed. Persons who retread tires handle materials containing these chemicals. In one report, 38 of 51 reactors to black rubber were exposed at work, including drivers, motor mechanics, tire fitters, tire manufacturers, garage attendants, car washers, painters, engineers, machine operators, boilerman, farmers, aircraft fitters, and a plant hire contractor.[111] A tire worker might be expected to be sensitized by IPPD,[69] but some who are sensitive to that chemical do not react to products that contain it.[191]

Some occupational exposures are less obvious. Military personnel operating radarscopes, scuba divers (including recreational divers), motorcycle riders, policemen, hospital employees,[192] electrical workers who handle insulated wire and cable, and line repairmen. Bank tellers, postal workers, and florists all use elastic bands, which sometimes contain these chemicals. Dairy farmers may react to black rubber components of automatic milking machines.[193, 194]

Hand dermatitis is a common presentation of allergy to *p*-phenylenediamine derivatives, especially in workers exposed to automobile tires, radiator hoses, and the like. The eruption is often fissured dermatitis of the hands and lichenified dermatitis of the wrists and forearms,[65] as the antigen frequently contaminates the tires' surface.[195] The eruption can spread to other areas, such as the chest and axillas.[69] One reason for this may be the tendency for IPPD, *N*-cyclohexyl-*N'*-phenyl-*p*-phenylenediamine, and *N,N'*-diphenyl-*p*-phenylenediamine to concentrate on the surface of the black rubber objects, which predisposes workers to hand contact and transfer. In one large series, 47% of workers had hand involvement. Exposure often is caused by handling black rubber tires or hoses, but sometimes the sensitizing object is unusual: A policeman's rubber-covered billy club (truncheon or blackjack) produced a reaction that cleared on changing to leather.[196] Nonoccupational sensitization from holding the black rubber "wishbone" of a windsurfer was cured by changing to an aluminum component.[197] One report of dermatitis from rubber fingerstalls in postal sorters found IPPD in the product when the manufacturer ostensibly did not know it was there.[198] Perhaps another reason that we see surface transfer is that IPPD is a potent sensitizer, even at such low levels that it is tested at 0.1% concentration.[199]

IPPD can be transferred from the hands to the face, and the mechanism of this transfer may be difficult to identify. Some nonoccupational cases still illustrate the patterns of exposure and how it occurs. Shaw and Wilkinson reported on a patient who developed localized eczema on her leg after an injury. They found that she was aggravating the condition by rubbing it with the black rubber tip of her walking stick. She was, of course, allergic to black rubber mix. Other unusual presentations include purpuric contact dermatitis, erythema multiforme,[65] palmoplantar pustulosis,[62] and perhaps even photodermatitis.[200]

Identifying the cause of some occupational cases takes detective work. Dooms-Goossens reported the case of a chemist with a dermatitis of the hands and the perioral area who was allergic to black rubber mix. He was very cautious about sensitizers in his laboratory but experienced breakouts on attending monthly meetings of the European Economic Community in Brussels, where he regularly gave reports. The rash appeared on the day after the meetings and steadily improved until the next meeting. He so painstakingly avoided contact with black rubber that he even wore cotton gloves while searching diligently (but unsuccessfully) for the source. The investigators observed his behavior in the EEC building and discovered that he rode an escalator and grasped the handrail without realizing it was made of black rubber. Avoidance solved the problem.[201] Involvement of the face was apparently caused by hand transfer.

Another case of occupational contact with *p*-phenylenediamine derivatives followed *Candida* cheilitis.[202] The patient, a church secretary, had been given an ointment to treat the condition, and she soon developed circumoral contact dermatitis. On testing she was not allergic to the ointment but did react on patch testing to black rubber mix in the standard screening series. Apparently the oil-based ointment tended to degrade some rubber object that she touched, and she picked up the antigen and transferred it to her face. By carefully tracing her every step after flareups, she found the cause to be the black rubber pads on the undersurface of the stapler she used at work. Again, recognition and avoidance solved the problem.

p-Phenylenediamine

Another antigen in the standard tray that is structurally closely related to this group is *p*-phenylenediamine. This is sometimes confused with black rubber mix, which is a mixture of rubber antioxidants. While one might assume that patients would cross-react to both antigens owing to the similarity of structure, only about 37.5% of persons allergic

to black rubber mix also react to the *p*-phenylenediamine test.[86] Some amines are used in manufacturing both plastics and rubber (e.g., phenyl-α-naphthylamine, phenyl-β-naphthylamine, IPPD, and butylated hydroxytoluene.

Carba Mix

The carba mix comprises three rubber chemicals, two carbamate activators or accelerators and diphenylguanidine, each in a 1% concentration in petrolatum. Diphenylguanidine is a "medium" accelerator, used especially in curing the heavier, industrial types of rubber. The two carbamates are zinc diethyldithiocarbamate and zinc dibutyldithiocarbamate.

Carbamates are found in a wide variety of rubber products, both natural and synthetic. They are commonly present in latex gloves,[203] from which, in the presence of sweat, they can release as much antigen as patch test materials.[204] They are also used as agricultural chemicals and in antinematode preparations and soil fumigants,[205] any of which can produce sensitivity. The methyl carbamates have weak cholinesterase activity, whereas the phenyl carbamates are used as herbicides.[26]

The best-known of the former group are perhaps the fungicides maneb[206] and zineb. These chemicals are used on seeds and bulbs and are sometimes applied to plants. They are common sensitizers of agricultural workers,[129, 207] and can affect retail florists.[131] Some persons are sensitive to multiple agents of the same class,[208] although most reports do not show this.[209] Carbamate sensitivity occurred as an epidemic when in 1991 a train tanker car derailment in California caused a chemical spill of the soil fumigant sodium methyldithiocarbamate into the nearby Sacramento River. Many of the jail inmates and crew leaders who helped to remove dead fish developed dermatitis. Concentration of the chemical in the river water was measured at 20 to 40 ppb.[210]

Thiourea and Other Sources

Another hidden source of rubber sensitivity can be rubber or rubber chemicals in objects used after an occupational injury or dermatitis. Thiourea—in silver polish,[211] a knee brace, neoprene gloves—is an example. A large variety of other chemicals are used in rubber manufacture, and some cause sensitivity. Lowinox, an antioxidant related to butylated hydroxyanisole and butylated hydroxytoluene, proved to be the cause of latex glove sensitivity.[212, 213] Sometimes unexpected sensitivities can occur because of contaminants, chemical reaction by-products or both.[136] Sensitivity to some objects such as a wet suit[214, 215] may be either be occupational or recreational. Thiourea sensitivity is not necessarily caused by rubber exposure, as these chemicals are also used for other purposes, such as paint and glue remover,[216] corrosion inhibitor,[217] antioxidant, in diazo processes for textiles and paper,[218, 219] and in thermocoating plastic phonecards.[220] Chemicals related to the thioureas can also cause contact dermatitis and photodermatitis.[221]

PATCH TESTING METHODS

Often when contact dermatitis is suspected in a worker who responds on patch testing to one of the "rubber antigens," one should evaluate relevance, provide information on each positive antigen, and counsel the patient. The five rubber antigens—thiuram mix, MBT, mercapto mix, black rubber mix, and carba mix—were discussed earlier along with a bit of information on thioureas that can produce occupational problems. In the United States the standard series contains five patch test reagents associated with rubber sensitivity, one single chemical (MBT) and four mixes. In Europe IPPD is tested alone in place of the black rubber mix, and MBT is included in the mercapto mix. A series of individual rubber chemicals allows directed testing and can also be used as a screen. Such series are available from Chemotechnique and Trolab.

In addition to the standard test batteries, patients should be tested with personal-care products and occupational materials to which they have been exposed. Otherwise, many false-negative results will be reported. To confirm sensitivity to gloves by patch testing the gloves themselves as well as rubber chemicals (especially thiuram mix) should be tested. Rubber chemicals other than thiurams may be the allergens in work gloves,[222, 223] and some responses do not appear with the standard tray. Estlander's group[224] reported 108 cases of rubber dermatitis, 68 of which were caused by gloves. Of these, 38 reacted to both the patch test reagent and the gloves, 11 only to the patch test reagent, and 14 only to the gloves. Tested for glove material, 14 of 185 hospital workers with hand eczema reacted to glove material.[225] Such testing also helps to establish that the condition is occupational.[226] The chemical composition of these products is not nearly as simple as patch test data might suggest. Extraction and identification of antigens by high performance liquid chromatography (HPLC) and gas chromatography (GC) showed one pair of rubber work gloves to contain zinc ethylphenyldithiocarbamate, and surgical gloves may contain not only carbamates such as zinc dimethyldithiocarbamate, zinc diethyldithiocarbamate, and zinc dibutyldithiocarbamate, but also amines such as dimethylamine, diethylamine, and piperidine.[227]

Testing with mixes and with single chemicals are different in several ways, as Mitchell pointed out many years ago.[114] The concentration in mixes is usually weaker, which could lead to false-negative results, and this may be a problem with the mercapto mix. MBT has been separated and is now tested as a single antigen because the mix concentration was too weak. Mitchell worried about stability of all chemicals, and using four at once may increase the problem. One controversial form of interaction that he considered was quenching, which might occur in a mixture. This is the suppressive influence of one substance on the sensitizing ability of another (such as the effect of eugenol on sensitization by cinnamic aldehyde),[228] but this has not to our knowledge been shown for rubber chemicals. Another concern with mixes is false-positive reactions from irritation.[229] An additive effect from multiple weak responses is also theoretically possible, as, used together, weaker allergens might elicit a reaction in subthreshold concentrations.[230]

Patch testing to MBT is normally done at a 2% concentration in petrolatum; however, that vehicle may not be ideal, as both MBT and MBTS in high–molecular weight polyethylene glycol cause a more dramatic reaction than they do in the same concentration in petrolatum.[161] The concentration used (in a different vehicle) for the T.R.U.E. Test (Glaxo Wellcome Inc.) has been adjusted so that the result compares reliably with that to the 2% in petrolatum used as a control standard.[231] For this antigen, positive results are regularly confirmable with standard testing methods and on replicate testing.[98, 232] As with any allergen a positive test result may be related to previous allergy, to the present problem, or may be of unknown relevance.

In the United States the current composition of the mercapto mix is 0.33% each of CBS, MBTS, and 4-morpholinyl-2-benzothiazyl disulfide. According to Cronin,[26] the latter produces the most positive responses, followed by CBS and MBTS, in that order. All three are closely related in structure to 2-mercaptobenzothiazole, having the 2-thiol component necessary for cross-reactivity.[223] A positive response to the mix in a subject who does not react to MBT is uncommon.[234, 235] The reason may be that MBT is tested at 2% concentration whereas the total concentration in the mixes is less. With a mix comprising 0.25% of each of four antigens, only 14 of 169 allergic to either or both were "mix positive" and "MBT negative."[234] Even when the concentration was raised to 0.33% each, only eight of 73 allergic to MBT or the mix were MBT negative and mix positive.

Thiuram mix is a good screening agent for thiuram sensitivity, although mild reactions may be caused by an irritant effect or mild sensitivity.[151] The mix comprises four rubber chemicals of similar structure—tetramethylthiuram disulfide, tetraethylthiuram disulfide, dipentamethylenethiuram disulfide, and tetramethylthiuram monosulfide. In a group of masons who wore gloves to protect themselves and became allergic to the gloves, tetramethylthiuram disulfide was the most important sensitizer, the order of isolated reactions being: tetramethylthiuram monosulfide, tetramethylthiuram disulfide, tetraethylthiuram disulfide, and dipentamethylenethiuram disulfide.[150]

Black rubber mix contains three antioxidant chemicals: IPPD in a concentration of 0.1%; *N*-cyclohexyl-*N′*-phenyl-*p*-phenylenediamine; and *N,N′*-diphenyl-*p*-phenylenediamine, both in 0.25% concentrations. Black rubber mix is used in the United States and in the T.R.U.E. test, but in Europe the mix has been replaced with IPPD alone,[236] which detects 90% of reactors to black rubber mix.[237] Using the mix allows three or four chemicals to be tested at once, although usually in lower concentrations. In European centers about 0.6% to 0.7% of those tested react to the black rubber mix,[237] whereas in the United States screening examinations turn up a response in about 2.1%.[138] The prevalence may be much higher, however, in persons allergic to rubber from sources other than gloves, although it is not nearly as common as thiuram sensitivity, even in this group.[109] In the United States IPPD is tested at 0.1%, both in the mix and individually as part of a rubber tray. The other two compounds, when tested individually, are used at concentrations of 1%. These are commercial-grade chemicals, so there may be some contamination or cross-reactivity with other chemicals in the group. There is seldom any reason to go to great lengths to determine the specific *p*-phenylenediamine derivatives to which the patient is allergic, as the patient will not be able to determine which black rubber product contains which chemical anyway. The rank order for reactivity in the group is IPPD, *N*-cyclohexyl-*N′*-phenyl-*p*-phenylenediamine and *N,N′*-diphenyl-*p*-phenylenediamine.

Cross-reactions occur between IPPD and other *p*-phenylenediamine derivatives,[238] and are widespread throughout this group.[112, 239] Rubber chemicals have many uses, and sensitivity can occur in workers exposed to the chemical who were not exposed through contact with rubber itself.[112] Piperazine is sometimes used in rubber, but occupational reactions might more often be related to other uses, especially pharmaceuticals.[74, 240]

Carba mix contains two carbamates and diphenylguanidine. Recently, the need to test with this antigen has been questioned. Structurally, carbamates are closely related to the thiurams, and some have suggested that it is not necessary to test for both because of the overlapping results.[241] It is generally assumed that a positive result with carba mix together with a negative reaction to thiuram mix suggests sensitivity to diphenylguanidine, the unrelated component. Test results to the two mixes do not overlap completely, so we continue to use both. Carbamates in bleached clothing sometimes cause a reaction that is not detectable with the standard test agents,[242] but this is not usually occupational. Naphthyl mix, formerly a standard antigen in many areas, is still sometimes used in a series of rubber antigens, but it seldom produces a reaction.[26, 243]

Natural Rubber Latex Protein Antigens

NRL sensitivity is quite complex because natural rubber contains many immunogenic proteins, and these must be characterized before immunotherapy can be formulated or we can reliably recognize them all with test procedures. The suspected allergens in immediate reactions are proteins in natural rubber and can vary greatly in molecular weight.[21] Several immunoblot studies have identified IgE (and some IgG4)–binding proteins in NRL (or NRL products) that range from 2 kD to 110 kD in molecular weight.[27, 43, 244-248] Obviously, there are multiple bands of immunoreactive proteins that may appear to be the cause of NRL immediate sensitivity, depending on the source, the specific patient, or the method used to identify the underlying allergen. Antigens are probably different in different products, and are different in raw rubber and in finished products.[249] At least some are probably thermolabile.[250] Sensitivity to NRL is probably not based on a single reaction to one substance. Some of the causative allergens identified to date are hevein (Hev b 6.02), prohevein (Hev b 6.01), and rubber elongation factor (Hev b 1). Hevein, a 4.7-kD polypeptide involved in latex agglutination,[251] has been shown to contain the same antigenic epitopes as prohevein[252] (20-kD), and is considered to be a major source of IgE-mediated NRL immediate sensitivity particularly in healthcare workers.[253] Most latex-allergic patients are sensitive to this epitope common to both prohevein and hevein, which is a 43–

amino acid fragment.[254] Far less reactivity is found in prohevein's 14-kD C-domain.[27, 248, 255–257] Some 18% of NRL-allergic patients reacted to rubber elongation factor (Hev b 1);[258] this allergen may be more important in spina bifida patients.

Although urticarial reactions to rubber were not reported until 1978, such responses did exist. Since then, however, urticarial sensitivity in healthcare workers[259] and hospital employees[260] has become quite common, its prevalence perhaps being highest in operating room personnel.[261] Of American hospital-based physicians almost 10% were prick test positive to NRL (as compared with 3% of controls), and 24% of "atopic" physicians in the group were positive.[262] Twelve percent of dentistry workers were allergic to NRL in one setting,[263] and almost 14% of military dentists surveyed reported allergy.[264] About 8.7% of dental students are prick test positive, but the prevalence increased over time, from only 2% of those in their second semester to 10% by the 10th semester.[265]

On average, nurses in the operating room develop contact urticaria about 5 years after starting work there, and respiratory problems about 2 or 3 years later.[266] Asthma was found in 2.5% of hospital employees,[82] and anaphylactic or anaphylactoid reactions have been reported many times.[267–277] Furthermore, anaphylaxis may be recurrent if the cause is not recognized and eliminated.[270] This type of reaction is more common after mucosal exposure, but aerosolized exposure or cutaneous exposure can also provoke it.[95] Contact urticaria on exposure to glove powder may reflect sensitivity to the cornstarch itself[278, 279] or, more commonly, to the NRL allergens that were absorbed by, and subsequently, carried airborne in the powder.[246, 280, 281] Aerosolized powder can induce respiratory tract symptoms (especially from NRL contamination,[282, 283] and healthcare workers or their patients may contact NRL antigens left on inanimate objects by other healthcare workers who have donned or doffed powdered latex gloves. Contaminated glove powder may contain more than enough antigen to precipitate a prominent local skin, conjunctival,[281] respiratory tract,[280] or systemic response.[75, 246, 283] Even a syringe needle that punctures an NRL stopper in a medication vial bottle stopper on subsequent intravenous exposure can induce systemic reactions.[284] Allergy to cornstarch in gloves or condoms[278, 279, 285] may be more common than published reports might indicate. We have detected several cases in our clinic, especially in persons who exhibited a food allergy to corn on scratch or RAST testing.

The clinical presentation of immediate hypersensitivity to NRL in hospital workers is most often contact urticaria associated with gloves.[286] Within a few to 30 minutes the patient typically experiences erythema, pruritus, and wheal formation in the area of contact that disappears without treatment, usually in 1 to 2 hours.[91, 287] Where gloves are the cause, the dorsum of the hands is likely to be involved. Sensitive workers also may have allergic rhinitis[287–289] or occupational asthma from latex allergens.[87, 290–295] Furthermore, pulmonary function studies show these same workers to be hypersensitive to histamine, which suggests that they are likely to experience exacerbations from nonspecific stimuli. Turjanmaa rated the relative incidences of such manifestations in healthcare workers and those in other occupations with an immediate allergy to NRL: contact urticaria 79% and 72%, respectively; conjunctivitis, 28% and 16%; rhinitis, 16% and 13%; facial edema, 14% and 28%; asthma, 2% and 4%; generalized urticaria, 9% and 13%; and anaphylaxis, 7% and 10%. Another unexpected manifestation with type I hypersensitivity is hand eczema, 42% and 64%,[90, 91] with or without urticaria.

The prevalences vary: in one study[296] 10% of nurses demonstrated sensitivity to NRL; in another,[297] 17% of hospital workers did. In Japan, where latex sensitivity was once thought to be less prevalent than in some Western countries, more than 10% of hospital workers are affected. Approximately 8.5% of reportedly allergic[298] "medical workers" in one hospital in Japan, and 8.9% of nurses in another study had IgE antibodies to NRL that correlated to a history of penicillin allergy or atopy.[299] The prevalence among healthcare workers in Germany was between 4.5% and 10.7%,[300] and in hospital employees in Norway was 6.5% of 66 volunteers tested.[260] Immediate sensitivity to NRL is most frequently occupational, and Taylor and Praditsuwan[301] found that 38 of 44 persons with a documented type I NRL allergy had occupationally related sensitivity.

Contact urticaria from glove use is occasionally due to sensitivity to rubber accelerators rather than to NRL proteins.[244, 302–304] Such patients may also present with contact urticaria, rhinitis, conjunctivitis, hand eczema, or pruritus.[302] Scratch chamber testing[302] with the standard rubber antigens has been used to test for this, but it can produce false-positive responses.[305] We have successfully used patch test allergens in Finn chambers applied for 10 to 15 minutes to previously involved skin, usually the dorsum of the hand, in a manner similar to the method of Van Krogh and Maibach.[306]

Risk Factors

Workers in occupations where exposure to NRL is commonplace (e.g., healthcare and rubber factory workers) are at greater risk for type I hypersensitivity to NRL. Patients with spina bifida,[307, 308] urogenital anomalies, or paraplegia[302] are also at risk but these would not be considered occupationally related.[309] Persons with hand eczema who wear rubber gloves to protect their skin are also at risk for developing either type I or type IV sensitivity. Their eczema may be caused or exacerbated by underlying IgE sensitivity to NRL proteins or to rubber compounding chemicals.[138] The development of NRL type I and type IV sensitivities seems to parallel the opportunity for exposure. In addition, atopy is a significant risk factor for the development of NRL type I allergies. The prevalence in "atopic" children (16.7%) is higher than among "nonatopic" children (0.5%).[310] Work-related urticaria from NRL is also more common in atopic healthcare workers.[265, 270, 311–313]

Food Cross-Reactivity

Persons with contact urticaria to latex can experience cross-reactions with certain foods. These include banana, avocado, chestnut, kiwi, wheat germ agglutinin,[255] and others.[293, 314–318] The lack of in vitro competitive inhibition effects[319] and failure in many cases to see cross-reactivity[244, 320, 321] suggest that often the sensitizer is probably not the same protein, or perhaps not the same epitope. Food can also be contaminated by rubber during preparation.[322] Dental workers should avoid contact with gutta percha,[323] and persons allergic to unused glove powder should avoid corn and cornstarch.

DIAGNOSTIC TESTING

Diagnostic confirmation of contact urticaria to latex may involve skin prick tests (SPT), RAST, scratch chamber tests, or patch tests (for a few minutes). The RAST is positive in about 22% of those with contact urticaria and 66% of those with systemic symptoms. Sensitivity of one prominent commercial RAST test method is said to be between 40% and 70%[244, 324]; thus negative results are not reliable.

The SPT is currently the most convenient and accurate method for screening for type I allergy; however, no standardized eluants are commercially available in the United States today. Although work is progressing toward that end, variations in office-based antigen extraction methods and source materials have hindered direct comparisons in much of the current research. Unknown factors such as the relationship between sensitization and the amount of protein allergens in a given product as well as the concentration and availability of the extractable allergens in these products have further confounded the issue and made standardization difficult. NRL gloves have proven to be a good source of antigen,[325] but reproducibility is a concern. Although the antigen from nonammoniated latex (NAL) is more reliable on ELISA testing,[52] it is unlikely that many persons have been sensitized by contact with NAL. SPT is controversial, and concern has been expressed over the potential for producing sensitization or eliciting a severe reaction in an already sensitized individual.[326, 327] Because this potential exists, epinephrine and NRL-free resuscitation equipment should be immediately available where testing is done. The clinician's experience, the selection, preparation, and concentration of the allergen, and the type of lancet used are all significant factors in the safety and efficacy of the SPT.[23]

Generally, NRL skin prick testing uses glove eluate solutions prepared in sterile saline from commercially available medical grade gloves.[23, 90, 307] A drop of each eluate solution is placed on the volar surface of the forearm, and the skin is lightly pricked with separate sterile lancets. The "wheal" size reaction is compared with the response to positive (histamine) and negative (saline) controls administered in the same manner. NRL wheal size must be greater than half the size of the histamine wheal to be considered positive. The patient's score can range from negative (no reactions), to mildly positive or positive, to dermographic (all sites react, including the negative control).

Use Test and Provocation

Generally, when NRL gloves are implicated in occupational hand eczema, the patient is tested with a finger of the suspected glove (not the entire glove) for 15 to 30 minutes.[328, 329] If no response occurs in 15 to 30 minutes, a suspect glove can be applied to a wet hand for the same length of time, and a vinyl, polyethylene, or thermoplastic elastomer (TPE) glove to the other hand as a control.[21]

TREATMENT OF RUBBER SENSITIVITY

Avoidance of the offending substances is the first order of the day, but that may not be so easy for persons with anaphylactic reactions. Rubber objects are ubiquitous (Table 29–7), and the antigen is released into sweat[204] and carried by glove powder. Rarely are reactions due to the rubber

TABLE 29–7 • Products That Frequently Contain Natural Rubber Latex

Adhesives	Driveway sealants	Makeup
Amalgam carriers	Elastic bands	Markers
Ambu bag/mask	Elastic socks and stockings	Masks
Analgesia syringes	Elastic wrap	Mixing bowls
Anesthesia bag	Elastics in garments	Nasopharyngeal tubes
Anesthesia equipment	Electric cords	Needle counters
Anesthesia masks	Electrocardiographic straps	Neonatal incubator
Anesthetic carpule	Electrodes	Nipples
Art supplies	Emergency resuscitation masks	Orthodontic elastics
Autoinjectables	Endotracheal tube	Oximeter o-ring on percutaneous sheath
Automotive parts	Enema tips/cuffs supplies	Pacifiers
Baby bottle nipples	Epidural catheter injection adapters	Patient controlled peripheral nerve
Balloons	Erasers	stimulators
Balls	Esmarch bandages	Plasters
Bandages	Esophageal dilators	Polishing disks
Bed protectors	Esophageal protective cover	Portable suction apparatus
Bibs	ETO indicator/tape	Pressure-monitoring kit
Bicycle shorts	Evacuation tubing	Probe covers
Billy clubs	Examination gloves	Prophy cups
Bite blocks	Eyecup for binoculars	Pulmonary artery catheter
Blood pressure cuffs/tubing	Eyedropper bulbs	Raincoats
Blood warmer components	Eyeglass straps	Reservoir bag
Bonnets/caps/hoods	Eyelash curler	Retention suture
Bougies	Face mask fasteners	Rubber bands
Breathing bags	Feeding bag/tubes	Rubber pants
Breathing circuits	Feeding nipples	Rubber sheets/pillow/pad
Bungee cords	Finger cots	Rubber stamps
Burn bandages	Floor mats	Rubber stoppers on medicine
Camera eyepieces	Fluid circulating warming blankets	Sanitary belts
Carpet backing	Foam padding	Shoe covers
Catheter-dilating	Food handlers gloves	Shoes
Catheters-Malecot	Footwear	Shower caps
Catheters-external	Galoshes	Slipper socks
Catheters-Foley	Garments	Spinal trays
Catheters-suction	Gaskets	Sponges
Catheters-thoracic	Gastro supplies	Stethoscope/tubing
Catheters-urethral	Gloves	Stockinette
Cements	Goggles	Stretch textiles
Cervical dilator	Halloween masks	Stretcher mattress
Chux	Handgrips	Suction tips/tubing
Colostomy pouch	Handlebar grips	Surgical supplies
Compression bandages	Handles of sports equipment	Sutures
Condom catheters	Handles of tools	Swim fins
Condoms	Hemodialysis machine components	Swim suits
Connecting tubing/nitrous oxide	Heparin locks/T connection pieces	Syringe
Contraceptive sponges	Hoses	Tape
Converters sleeves	Hospital ID bands	Teeth protectors
Crib mattress pads	Hot water bottles	Telephone cords
Crutch padding	Ileostomy bags	Temperature probes
Crutch tips	Induction masks	Tires
Cuffs on tracheal tubes	Instrument mats	Tooth massagers
Cushions	Instrument pans in autoclave	Tourniquets
Cushions or padding	Insulation/electrical wiring	Toys
Dental dam	Intraaortic balloon	Tympanometer
Dentures	Intratracheal rubber cannula	Underwear
Diapers	Intubation tube	Urethral probe
Diaphragms	Irrigator tubing	Urethral stents
Diazosensitized photocopy paper	IV access/injection ports	Urinary drainage bag
Diving gear	Laser fiber	Urodynamics rectal press
Douche bulbs	Latex paints (craft)	Utility gloves
Drains	Liquid bandage	Ventilator bellows
Drapes	Liquid droppers	Wheelchair wheels, padding
Dressings		

molecule itself[330] or to glove powder.[331] The patient must be tested to determine the causative ingredient; it cannot be assumed. Even connubial contact dermatitis has been reported,[332] and physicians with contact urticaria to NRL may react to glove powder left on a patient's chart by other physicians. In extreme cases it may be necessary for physicians and nurses who sometimes work in a latex-free environment to use powder-free gloves even outside the area. Persons at risk for anaphylaxis and other severe reactions may need to use prophylactic measures and to prepare for a crisis. This may include having at hand latex-free resuscitation equipment. The treatment of urticaria is described elsewhere.[333]

Product Selection

Substitution of products—gloves, condoms, dental dams, catheters—that are free of the specific allergen requires some knowledge of the available materials and an accurate diagnosis of the patient's allergies. Although allergies can result from exposure to rubber chemicals from nonrubber sources such as disulfiram used as a medication[334] and fungicides, antigen substitution is usually effective.[335] For persons allergic to NRL protein, most investigators recommend substituting vinyl, TPE, nitrile, polyethylene (nonmedical uses), or chloroprene products (Table 29–8). For those suffering from irritation or a type IV allergy to the residual processing chemicals in certain products, it is possible to find another NRL or synthetic product that is manufactured without the offending chemical.[336] However, substitute gloves should be tested before they are used, as many people are sensitive to agents other than those found in standard test kits.[212, 330] One rubber worker became allergic to Hypalon, a chlorosulfonated rubber, apparently from the epoxy used as a stabilizer.[337]

Workers who wear gloves for protection can react to substances that permeate rubbers at different rates and at different breakthrough times. Surgical nurses and dental assistants frequently become allergic to glutaraldehyde. Healthcare workers frequently become allergic to glutaraldehyde (equipment cold sterilization solutions), acrylates (adhesives, bonding agents), and epoxy resins (restorative compounds) that can permeate gloves at different rates depending upon the glove material, chemical, concentration, and duration of exposure.[338–342] For example, acrylates permeate both NRL and TPE, but dissolve the latter nearly instantly. In contrast, glutaraldehyde permeates NRL more readily than SEBS, and this is time-, concentration-, and stress level–dependent.[341] In workers with occupationally based allergies, it is important to identify the chemical compatibility of all protective equipment.[338]

Long-term management for NRL protein–induced contact urticaria requires not only gloves that are free of NRL but also an environment that is free of significant amounts of glove powder contaminated with NRL protein.[307] Having non-allergic coworkers use gloves with a low NRL total EP content[343] or powder-free gloves seems to be beneficial.[343, 344] Avoidance of foods such as banana, kiwi, avocado, and chestnuts, is also wise. It is also prudent for physicians, dentists, and others who treat sensitized persons to ensure a "latex-safe" office and patient care environment. Patients also need counseling on what NRL products to avoid in the workplace and at home, including NRL toys, condoms, gloves, and so forth.[54, 345]

PROGNOSIS

Prognosis for latex sensitivity is guarded, as some persons change occupations to avoid contact and others change tasks the same profession. Cronin[26] found favorable outcomes in a large percentage of persons with contact dermatitis to rubber after the cause was identified and the sensitizer avoided. Most people with contact urticaria however, continue to experience problems, as exposure is difficult to avoid. With time, reactions can progress to contact urticaria, rhinitis, periorbital swelling and asthma in some.[42] Permanent symptoms were reported by 30% of men and 38% of women; periodic symptoms by 50% and 42%, respectively; and healing by 20% of both groups.[74] Many rubber reactions are to the carbamates commonly present in NRL gloves,[346] from which, in the presence of sweat, as much antigen can be released as patch testing materials contain.[347] Intercurrent reactions to chrome and rubber occur when rubber gloves are used to protect the hands from materials such as cement.[74]

Most healthcare workers who are allergic to NRL proteins continue to work but remain symptomatic.[300] Of 41 NRL-sensitive patients in one series, only one had to quit work, but eight others (20%) changed jobs to minimize exposure. Most patients eventually develop systemic symptoms, and anaphylaxis was reported in 13%. Often it is necessary not only for the patient to avoid NRL but for coworkers to use vinyl and other substitutes to minimize exposure in the workplace.[300] Many have switched to powder-free gloves because the powder carries NRL antigens in quantity sufficient to cause reactions, especially in more sensitive patients. When the workplace is free of

TABLE 29–8 • Surgical and Examination Gloves That Contain No Natural Rubber Latex

Type	Material	Brand Name*	Supplier	Phone
Surgical, powdered	TPE	ElastylLite	SmartCare	800 822 8956
	TPE	TactylLite	SmartCare	800 822 8956
	TPE	Allergard	Johnson & Johnson	800 526 3967
	TPE	Safeskin Tactylon	Safeskin	800 462 9989
	Nitrile	Pure Advantage	Tillotson HealthCare	800 445 6830
	Chloroprene	Neolon	Maxxim	800 727 7340
	Chloroprene	Dermaprene	Ansell	800 727 7340
	Chloroprene	Duraprene	Allegiance	800 422 9837
Surgical, powder-free	TPE	ElastylonPF	SmartCare	800 822 8956
	Polyurethane	Elite	Ansell	800 727 7340
	Nitrile	Pure Advantage PF	Tillotson HealthCare	800 445 6830
	Chloroprene	NeoTec	Regent	800 843 8497
	Chloroprene	Dermaprene PF	Ansell	800 727 7340
	Chloroprene	Neolon PF	Maxxim	800 727 7340
Examination, powdered	TPE	ElastylLite	SmartCare	800 822 8956
	TPE	TactylLite	SmartCare	800 822 8956
	Nitrile	N-Dex	Best Manufacturing	800 884 6413
	Nitrile	Nitrilite	Ansell	800 727 7340
	Nitrile	Pure Advantage	Tillotson HealthCare	800 445 6830
	Chloroprene	Dermaprene X-AM	Ansell	800 727 7340
	PVC	Royal Shield Vinyl	SmartCare	800 822 8956
	PVC	Vinylite	SmartPractice	800 522 0800
	PVC	SensiCare	Maxxim	800 727 7340
	PVC	Multi Care	Tillotson HealthCare	800 445 6830
	PVC	Tru-Touch	Maxxim	800 727 7340
	PVC	TriFlex	Allegiance	800 422 9837
Examination, powder free	TPE	ElastylonPF	SmartCare	800 822 8956
	Nitrile	N-Dex PF	Best Manufacturing	800 884 6413
	Nitrile	Nitra-Touch	Ansell	800 321 9752
	Nitrile	NitraPF	SmartCare	800 822 8956
	Nitrile	SmartPractice Nitrile PF	SmartPractice	800 522 0800
	Nitrile	Flexam Nitrile	Allegiance	800 422 9837
	Nitrile	Safeskin Nitrile	Safeskin	800 462 9989
	Nitrile	Dual Advantage	Tillotson HealthCare	800 445 6830
	Nitrile	Pure Advantage PF	Tillotson HealthCare	800 445 6830
	PVC	Royal Shield PF Vinyl	SmartCare	800 822 8956
	PVC	Vinylite PF	SmartPractice	800 522 0800
	PVC	SensiCare	Maxxim	800 727 7340
	PVC	Multi Care PF	Tillotson HealthCare	800 445 6830

*Brand names shown are either trademarked or registered.

NRL-contaminated glove powder and the allergic person has eliminated direct contact with NRL it is often possible for him or her to return to work.[348]

PREVENTION

Although the problem of type I hypersensitivity to the NRL proteins was not reported until 1979, the increase in reported reactions to NRL products has been met with a flurry of activity.[348a] While researchers struggle to understand the pathoimmunology and the molecular biology of such reactions, clinicians and healthcare facilities are working to develop better diagnostic, preventive and management strategies. Manufacturers are striving to ensure that products balance the need for barrier efficacy and nonsensitizing, and regulatory agencies are working to provide guidance for both manufacturers and consumers. Management of

NRL allergy also depends on understanding the major protein allergens. Standardized and well-characterized NRL extracts are essential for better diagnosis of allergic reactions. Furthermore, the ability to establish threshold limits for NRL products depends on this information.[349]

Effective September 30, 1997, the FDA mandated that the word *hypoallergenic* not be used in conjunction with NRL and established labeling requirements for both liquid and dry NRL products. Medical devices (e.g., gloves, catheters, tubing) must now be labeled as follows:

Caution: This product contains natural rubber latex, which may cause allergic reactions in some individuals.

The National Institute of Occupational Safety and Health (NIOSH) and the Occupational Safety and Health Administration (OSHA) have listed NRL allergies as a priority research topic and issued a position statement plus guidelines for NRL use. In addition, the Americans with Disabilities Act mandates that "reasonable accommodations" be made to enable disabled employees to continue their jobs. This could also affect NRL-allergic persons as they attempt to continue their careers. Hospital administrators and employee health personnel must view NRL hypersensitivity as a potential health risk for their patients and as an occupational hazard for employees that, if ignored could lead to poor morale, absenteeism, serious health problems, loss of career, worker's compensation claims, disability, litigation, and increased financial burdens. Although some institutions have developed NRL management policies and protocols, more widespread implementation is needed to prevent further symptom elicitation and sensitization. It is essential that hospital administrators and employee health personnel understand the importance of obtaining a complete and definitive diagnosis by a qualified professional. It is imperative to identify the specific cause or causes of a reaction before a comprehensive management strategy, including product selection or substitution, can be formulated. Until a complete diagnostic evaluation has been completed, the most conservative approach is to avoid contact and exposure to all NRL products.

Acknowledgements

We are grateful for the editorial assistance of Pamela Rodgers, Ph.D., and Kathy Wartner.

References

1. Morton M. *Rubber technology*, 3rd ed. New York: Van Nostrand Reinhold; 1987.
2. Subramaniam A. Commercial elastomers: natural rubber. In: *The Vanderbilt Rubber Handbook,* 13th ed. Norwalk, Conn: RT Vanderbilt; 1990:22–43.
3. Groce DF. The health care worker plague: latex allergy has stricken large numbers of workers in this decade and forced them to struggle daily to avoid latex proteins completely. *Occup Health Safety* 1996;October:170–180.
4. Adams RM. *Occupational skin disease,* 2nd ed. Philadelphia: WB Saunders; 1990.
5. Rubber Consultants. Latex protein allergy: the present position. London: Crain Communications; 1993.
6. Gelbert CH. *Basic Compounding of Neoprene Latex.* Technical Report. Wilmington, Del: Du Pont; 1986.
7. Kadir AASA. Natural rubber: current developments in product manufacture and applications. Kuala Lumpur, Malaysia: Rubber Research Institute of Malaysia; 1993.
8. Rodriguez E, Reynolds GW, Thompson JA. Potent contact allergen in the rubber plant guayule (*Parthenium argentatum*). *Science* 1981;21:1444–1445.
9. Pendle TD. Challenges for NR latex products in medical and food-related applications. In: Kadir AASA, Ed. Natural Rubber: Current Developments in Product Manufacture and Applications. Kuala Lumpur, Malaysia: Rubber Research Institute of Malaysia, 1993:3–18.
10. Audley BG. Protein allergies and latex products. In: Recent advances in latex technology, October 1993. Kuala Lumpur, Malaysia: Latex Technology Group; 1993:2–15.
11. Palosuo T. Immunological methods for determination of leachable proteins, antigens and allergens from medical gloves. 1994; CEN/TC 205 WG 3pt3: Washington, DC: US Government Printing Office.
12. Todt JC, Ownby DR. Amino acid analysis of allergenic proteins from raw non-ammoniated latex. *J Allerg Clin Immunol* 1994;93:283[Abstract].
13. Alenius H, Kurup V, Kelly K, et al. Latex allergy: frequent occurrence of IgE antibodies to a cluster of 11 latex proteins in patients with spina bifida and histories of anaphylaxis. *J Lab Clin Med* 1994;123:712–720.
14. Czuppon AB, Chen Z, Rennert S, et al. The rubber elongation factor of rubber trees (*Hevea brasiliensis*) is the major allergen in latex. *J Allergy Clin Immunol* 1993;92:690–697.
15. Makinen-Kiljunen S. Detection and characterization of atopic allergens. *Ann Intern Med* 1994;26:283–288.
16. Makinen-Kiljunen S. Banana allergy in patients with immediate-type hypersensitivity to natural rubber latex: characterization of cross-reacting antibodies and allergens. *J Allergy Clin Immunol* 1994;93:990–996.
17. Makinen-Kiljunen S, Turjanmaa K, Palosuo T, Reunala T. Characterization of latex antigens and allergens in surgical gloves and natural rubber by immunoelectrophoretic methods. *J Allergy Clin Immunol* 1992;90:230–235.
18. Subramaniam A. Reduction of extractable protein content in latex products. In: Food and Drug Administration. *Program and Proceedings. International Latex Conference: Sensitivity to Latex in Medical Devices.* Baltimore: 1992:63.
19. Hasma H. Proteins in natural rubber latex. Presented at Latex Protein Workshop (Paper no. 1), International Rubber Technology Conference, June 1993. Kuala Lumpur, Malaysia: Rubber Research Institute of Malaysia, 1993.
20. Mellstrom GA, Boman AS. Gloves: types, materials, and manufacturing. In: Mellstrom GA, Wahlberg JE, Maibach HI, ed. *Protective Gloves for Occupational Use.* Boca Raton, Fla: CRC Press; 1994:21–35.

21. Hamann CP. Natural rubber latex protein sensitivity in review. *Am J Contact Dermatitis* 1993;4:4–21.
22. Truscott W. Manufacturing methods sought to eliminate or reduce sensitivity to natural rubber products. In: Food and Drug Administration. *Program and Proceedings. International Latex Conference: Sensitivity to Latex in Medical Devices.* Baltimore: 1992:66.
23. Turjanmaa K, Makinen-Kiljunen S, Reunala T, Palosuo T. Natural rubber latex allergy: the European experience. *Immunol Allerg Clin North Am* Philadelphia: WB Saunders Company, 1995;15:71–88.
24. Tomaszic VJ, Withrow TJ, Fisher BR, Dillard SF. Latex-associated allergies and anaphylactic reactions. *Clin Immunol Immunopathol* 1992;64:89–97.
25. Hasma H. Proteins of natural rubber latex concentrate. *J Nat Rubber Res* 1992;102–112.
26. Cronin E. *Contact Dermatitis.* Edinburgh: Churchill-Livingstone, 1980.
27. Beezhold DH, Sussman GL, Kostyal DA, Chang NS. Identification of a 46-kD latex protein allergen in health care workers. *Clin Exp Immunol* 1994;98:408–413.
28. Pendle TD. The production, composition and chemistry of natural latex concentrates. In: FDA Center of Devices & Radiological Health, ed. *Program & Proceedings. International Latex Conference, Sensitivity to Latex in Medical Devices.* Baltimore: FDA, 1992:13.
29. Beezhold DH. Latex allergy. *Biomed Instrum Technol* 1992;26:238–240.
30. Yunginger JW, Jones RT, Fransway AF, et al. Extractable latex allergens and proteins in disposable medical gloves and other rubber products. *J Allergy Clin Immunol* 1994;93:836–842.
31. Aarons J, Fitzgerald N. The persisting hazards of surgical glove powder. *Surg Gynecol Obstet* 1974;174:4–6.
32. Hamann CP, Kick SA. Allergies associated with medical gloves: manufacturing issues. *Dermatol Clin* 1994; 12:547–559.
33. Dennis MS, Light DR. Rubber elongation factor from *Hevea brasiliensis.* Identification, characterization, and role in rubber biosynthesis. *J Biol Chem* 1989;264:18608–18617.
34. Dennis MS, Henzel WJ, Bell J, Kohr W, Light DR. Amino acid sequence of rubber elongation factor protein associated with rubber particles in *Hevea* latex. *J Biol Chem* 1989;264:18618–18626.
35. Greek BF. Rubber-processing chemicals. *Chem Eng News* 1987:29–49.
36. Fishbein L. Chemicals used in the rubber industry: an overview. *Scand J Work Environ Health* 1983;9[Suppl 2]:7–14.
37. Adams RM. *Occupational Skin Disease.* New York: Grune and Stratton; 1983.
38. Gellin GA. *Occupational and Industrial Dermatology.* Chicago: Year Book; 1982.
39. Kanerva L, Jolanki R, Estlander T. Organic pigment as a cause of plastic glove dermatitis. *Contact Dermatitis* 1985;13:41–43.
40. Axelsson IGK, Johansson SGO, Zetterstrom O. A new indoor allergen from a common non-flowering plant. *Allergy* 1987;42:604–611.
41. Wrangsjo K, Osterman K, van Hage-Hamsten M. Glove-related skin symptoms among operating theatre and dental care unit personnel. (II) Clinical examination, tests and laboratory findings indicating latex allergy. *Contact Dermatitis* 1994;30:139–143.
42. Wrangsjo K. Latex allergy in medical, dental, and laboratory personnel: a follow-up study. *Am J Contact Dermatitis* 1994;5:194–200.
43. Turjanmaa K, Laurila K, Makinen-Kiljunen S, Reunala T. Rubber contact urticaria: allergenic properties of 19 brands of latex gloves. *Contact Dermatitis* 1988;19:362–367.
44. Hashim MYA. Effect of leaching on extractable protein content. *Latex Protein Workshop (paper no. 4), Proceedings of International Rubber Technology Conference.* June 1993. Kuala Lumpur, Malaysia: Rubber Research Institute of Malaysia; 1993.
45. Alenius H, Kalkkinen N, Lukka M, et al. Prohevein from rubber tree is a major latex allergen. *J Allergy Clin Immunol* 1995;95:155.
46. Beezhold DH. Measurement of latex proteins by chemical and immunological methods. Amsterdam: *Proceedings of Latex Protein Allergy: The Present Position 1993.*
47. Yeang HY. The Lowry and Bradford assays for the quantitation of soluble latex glove proteins. Latex Protein Workshop (paper no. 2), International Rubber Technology Conference. June 1993. Kuala Lumpur, Malaysia: Rubber Research Institute of Malaysia, 1993.
48. Gehring LL. Support for healthcare workers with latex allergy. Source to Surgery 1994;2:1–4.
49. Beezhold DH. LEAP: latex ELISA for antigenic proteins: preliminary report. Guthrie J 1992;61:77–81.
50. Alenius H, Makinen-Kiljunen S, Turjanmaa K, Palosuo T, Reunala T. Allergen and protein content of latex gloves. *Ann Allergy* 1994;73:315–320.
51. Dreborg S. Skin tests used in type I allergy testing [Position paper]. *Allergy* 1989; 44[Suppl 10]:1–59.
52. Kurup VP, Kelly KJ, Turjanmaa K, et al. Immunoglobulin E reactivity to latex antigens in the sera of patients from Finland and the United States. *J Allergy Clin Immunol* 1993;91:1128–1134.
53. Wrangsjo K. *IgE-mediated Latex Allergy and Contact Allergy to Rubber in Clinical Occupational* Dermatology. Stockholm: National Institute of Occupational Health; 1993.
54. Turjanmaa K, Reunala T. Condoms as a source of latex allergen and cause of contact urticaria. *Contact Dermatitis* 1989;20:360–364.
55. Yunginger JW, Jones RT, Fransway AF, Kelso MA, Warner MA, Hunt LW. Extractable latex allergen contents of medical and consumer rubber products. In: Food and Drug Administration. *Program and Proceedings. International Latex Conference: Sensitivity to Latex in Medical Devices.* Baltimore: 1992.
56. Alenius H, Turjanmaa K, Palosuo T, Makinen-Kiljunen S, Reunala T. Surgical latex glove allergy: characterization of rubber protein allergens by immunoblotting. *Int Arch Allergy Appl Immunol* 1991;96:376–380.
57. Ansell Medical, Canadian Society of Allergy and Clinical Immunology, eds. Toronto: *Latex Allergy Symposium.* 1994.
58. Gehring LL, Fink JN, Kelly KJ. Evaluation of low allergenic latex gloves in latex sensitive patients. *J Allergy Clin Immunol* 1996.
59. Campion KM, Rycroft RJ. A study of attenders at an occupational dermatology clinic. *Contact Dermatitis* 1993;28:307.
60. White IR. Dermatitis in rubber manufacturing industries. *Dermatol Clin* 1988;6:53–59.
61. Roed-Petersen J. Purpuric contact dermatitis from black rubber chemicals. *Contact Dermatitis* 1988;18:166.
62. Schoel J, Frosch PJ. Allergic contact eczema caused by rubber containing substances simulating pustulosis palmaris. *Derm Beruf Umwelt* 1990;38:178–180.
63. Shmunes E, Darby T. Contact dermatitis due to endotoxin in irradiated latex gloves. *Contact Dermatitis* 1984; 10:240–244.
64. O'Malley MA, Mathias CG, Priddy M, et al. Occupa-

tional vitiligo due to unsuspected presence of phenolic antioxidant byproducts in commercial bulk rubber. *J Occup Med* 1988;30:512.

65. Calnan CD. Lichenoid dermatitis from isopropylaminodiphenylamine. *Contact Dermatitis Newslett* 1971;10:237.

66. Jordan WP. Contact dermatitis from *N*-isopropyl-*N*-phenylparaphenylenediamine. *Arch Dermatol* 1971;103:85–87.

67. Foussereau J, Cavelier C, Protois JC, Sanchez M, Heid E. A case of erythema multiforme with allergy to isopropyl-*p*-phenylenediamine of rubber. *Contact Dermatitis* 1988;18:183.

68. Zaitz ID, Proenca NG, Droste D, Grotti A. Achromatizing contact dermatitis caused by rubber sandals. *Med Cutan Ibero Lat Am* 1987;15:1–7.

69. Ancona A, Monroy F, Fernandez-Diez J. Occupational dermatitis from IPPD in tires. *Contact Dermatitis* 1982;8:91–94.

70. Lisi P, Caraffini S. Pellagroid dermatitis from mancozeb with vitiligo. *Contact Dermatitis* 1985;13:124–125.

71. Riboldi A, Lobaccaro M. Occupational contact dermatitis from rubber. *Clin Dermatol* 1992;10:149–155.

72. Brandao FM. Rubber. In: Adams RM, ed. *Occupational Skin Disease,* 2nd ed. Philadelphia: WB Saunders; 1990:462–485.

73. Varigos GA, Dunt DR. An epidemiological study in the rubber and cement industries. *Contact Dermatitis* 1981;7:105–110.

74. Fregert S. Occupational dermatitis in a 10-year material. *Contact Dermatitis* 1975;1:96–107.

75. Vandenplas O. Occupational asthma caused by natural rubber latex. *Eur Respiratory J* 1995;8:1957–1965.

76. Lintrum JC, Nater JP. Contact dermatitis caused by rubber chemicals in dairy workers. *Berufs Dermatosen* 1973;21:16–22.

77. Carrillo T, Blanco C, Quiralte J, Castillo R, Cuevas M, Rodriquez F. Prevalence of latex allergy among greenhouse workers. *J Allerg Clin Immunol* 1995;96:699–701.

78. Bajos N, Wadworth J, Ducot B, et al. Sexual behavior and HIV epidemiology: comparative analysis in France and Britain. *AIDS* 1995;9:735–743.

79. Meding B, Toren K, Karlberg AT, Hagberg S, Wass K. Evaluation of skin symptoms among workers at a Swedish paper mill. *Am J Ind Med* 1993;23:721–728.

80. Rudzki E, Napiorkowska T, Czerwinska-Dihm I. Dermatitis from 2-mercaptobenzothiazole in photographic films. *Contact Dermatitis* 1981;7:43.

81. Kiec-Swierczynska M. Occupational sensitivity to rubber. *Contact Dermatitis* 1995;32:171–172.

82. Vandenplas O, Delwiche J, Evrard G, et al. Prevalence of occupational asthma due to latex among hospital personnel. *Am J Respiratory Crit Care Med* 1995;151:54–60.

83. Sussman GL, Lem D, Liss G, Beezhold D. Latex allergy in housekeeping personnel. *Ann Allergy Asthma Immunol* 1995;74:415–418.

84. ASTM. Standard test for rubber—deterioration in an air oven. D 573-88. In: *Annual Book of ASTM Standards,* Vol 09.01. Philadelphia: ASTM; 1991:100–104.

85. Conde-Salazar L, Guimaraens D, Villegas C, Romero A, Gonzalez MA. Occupational allergic contact dermatitis in construction workers. *Contact Dermatitis* 1995; 33:226–230.

86. Singgih SI, Lantinga H, Nater JP, Woest TE, Kruyt Gaspersz JA. Occupational hand dermatoses in hospital cleaning personnel. *Contact Dermatitis* 1986;14:149.

87. Kanny G, Prestat F, Moneret-Vautrin DA. Allergic asthma to latex, proven by a bronchial provocation test. *Allergie Immunologie* 1992;24:329–332.

88. Rycroft RJ. Occupational dermatoses among office personnel. *Occup Med* 1986;1:32–38.

89. Orfan NA, Reed R, Dykewicz MS, Ganz M, Kolski GB. Occupational asthma in a latex doll manufacturing plant. *J Allerg Clin Immunol* 1994;94:826–830.

90. Turjanmaa K. Contact urticaria from latex gloves. In: Mellstrom GA, Wahlberg JE, Maibach HI, eds. *Protective Gloves for Occupational Use.* Boca Raton, Fla: CRC; 1994:241–254.

91. Turjanmaa K. Update on occupational natural rubber latex allergy. *Dermatol Clin* 1994;12:561–567.

92. Tarlo S, Wong L, Roos J, Booth N. Occupational asthma caused by latex in a surgical glove manufacturing plant. *J Allerg Clin Immunol* 1990;85:626–631.

93. Lammintausta K, Kalimo K, Aantaa S. Course of hand dermatitis in hospital workers. *Contact Dermatitis* 1982;8:327–332.

94. Nilsson E. Contact sensitivity and urticaria in "wet" work. *Contact Dermatitis* 1985;13:321–328.

95. Sussman GL, Tarlo S, Dolovich J. The spectrum of IgE-mediated responses to latex. *JAMA* 1991;265:2844–2847.

96. Kleinhans D. Contact urticaria to rubber gloves. *Contact Dermatitis* 1984;10:124–125.

97. Rudzki E, Rebandel P, Grzywa Z, Pomorski Z, Jakiminska B, Zawisza E. Occupational dermatitis in veterinarians. *Contact Dermatitis* 1982;8:723.

98. van der Walle HB, Brunsveld VM. Latex allergy among hairdressers. *Contact Dermatitis* 1995;32:17–78.

99. Conde-Salazar L, Baz M, Guimaraens D, Cannavo A. Contact dermatitis in hairdressers: patch test results in 379 hairdressers (1980–1993). *Am J Contact Dermatitis* 1995;6:19–23.

100. Guerra L, Tosti A, Bardazzi F, et al. Contact dermatitis in hairdressers: the Italian experience. *Contact Dermatitis* 1992;26:10–17.

101. Katsarou A, Koufou B, Takou K, Kalogeromitros D, Papanayiotou G, Varelzidis A. Patch test results in hairdressers with contact dermatitis in Greece (1985–1994). *Contact Dermatitis* 1995;33:34–78.

102. Suttipisal N, McFadden JP, Cronin E. Sensitization in atopic and nonatopic hairdressers with hand eczema. *Contact Dermatitis* 1993;29:20–69.

103. Hansson C. Allergic contact dermatitis from *N*(1,3dimethylbutyl)*N*′phenylphenylenediamine and from compounds in polymerized 2,2,4,trimethyl 1,2dihydroquinoline. *Contact Dermatitis* 1994;30:114–115.

104. Aguirre A, Manzano D, Zabala R, Raton JA, Diaz-Perez JL. Contact allergy to captan in a hairdresser. *Contact Dermatitis* 1994;31:46.

105. Schwartz L, Tulipan L, Birmingham DJ. Dermatoses in the manufacture of rubber. In: Schwartz L, ed. *Occupational Diseases of the Skin,* 3rd ed. Philadelphia: Lea & Febiger; 1957:574–595.

106. Burke FJT, Wilson NHF, Cheung SW. Factors associated with skin irritation of the hands experienced by general dental practitioners. *Contact Dermatitis* 1995;32:35–38.

107. Ramsing DW, Agner T. Effect of glove occlusion on human skin (II): long-term experimental exposure. *Contact Dermatitis* 1996;34:258–262.

108. White IR, Rubber. In: Maibach HI, ed. *Occupational and Industrial Dermatology,* 2nd ed. Chicago: Year Book; 1987:421–429.

109. von Hintzenstern J, Heese A, Koch HU, Peters K-P, Hornstein OP, Frequency, spectrum and occupational relevance of type IV allergies to rubber chemicals. *Contact Dermatitis* 1991;24:244–252.

110. Bieber P, Foussereau J. Role de deux amines aromatiques dans l'allergie au caoutchouc PBN et 4010 NA. *Bull Soc Franc Derm Syphlol* 1968;75:63–67.

111. Alfonzo C. Allergic contact dermatitis to isopropylaminodiphenylamine (IPPD). *Contact Dermatitis* 1979;5:145–147.

112. Herve-Bazin B, Gradiski D, Duprat P, et al. Occupational eczema from *N*-isopropyl-*N'*-phenylparaphenylenediamine (IPPD) and *N*-dimethy-1,3 butyl-*N'*-phenylparaphenylenediamine (DMPPD) in tyres. *Contact Dermatitis* 1977;3:1–15.

113. Fan X, Zhao B. Study on Chinese common allergens of contact dermatitis. *Derm Beruf Umwelt* 1990;38:158–161.

114. Hirano S, Yoshikawa K. Patch testing with European and American standard allergens in Japanese patients. *Contact Dermatitis* 1982;8:48–50.

115. Mosher WD, Bachrach CA. First premarital contraceptive use: United States, 1960–82. *Stud Fam Plann* 1987;18:83–95.

116. Bonnevie P, Marcussen PV. Rubber products as a widespread cause of eczema. *Acta Derm Venerol* 1945;25:163–178.

117. Hermann WP, Schultz KH. Hilfsstoffe der Gummials Ekzemnoxen. *Dermatologica* 1960;120:127–138.

118. Saha M, Srinivas CR, Shenoy SD, Balachandran C, Acharya S. Footwear dermatitis. *Contact Dermatitis* 1993;28:260–264.

119. Correia S, Brandao FM. Contact dermatitis of the feet. *Occup Environ Dermatoses* 1986;34:102–106.

120. Angelini G, Vena GA, Meneghini CL. Shoe contact dermatitis. *Contact Dermatitis* 1980;6:279–283.

121. Fogh A, Pock-Steen B. Contact sensitivity to thiram in wooden shoes. *Contact Dermatitis* 1992;27:348.

122. Ziegler V, Suss E. The allergenic effect of rubber accelerators tetramethyl thiuram disulfide (TMTD) and mercaptobenzothiazole (MBT). *Allergie Immunologie* 1974;20–21:281–285.

123. Nethercott JR, Holness DL, Adams RM, et al. Patch testing with a routine screening tray in North America. *Am J Contact Dermatitis* 1991;2:122–129.

124. Rudner E, Clendenning WE, Epstein E, et al. Epidemiology of contact dermatitis in North America. *Contact Dermatitis* 1980;6:309–315.

125. Storrs F, et al. Results of patch tests in North America. *J Am Acad Dermatol* 1989;20:1038–1044.

126. Dick DC, Adams RH. Allergic contact dermatitis from monosulfiram (Tetmosol) soap. *Contact Dermatitis* 1979;5:199.

127. Nater JP, Terpstra H, Bleumink E. Allergic contact sensitization to the fungicide Maneb. *Contact Dermatitis* 1979;5:24–26.

128. Manuzzi P, Borrello P, Misciali C, Guerra L. Contact dermatitis due to Ziram and Maneb. *Contact Dermatitis* 1988;22:77–80.

129. Sharma VK, Kaur S. Contact sensitization by pesticides in farmers. *Contact Dermatitis* 1990;23:77–80.

130. Kleibl K, Rackova M. Cutaneous allergic reactions to dithiocarbamates. *Contact Dermatitis* 1980;6:348–349.

131. Crippa M, Misquith L, Lonati A, Pasolini G. Dyshidrotic eczema and sensitization to dithiocarbamates in a florist. *Contact Dermatitis* 1990;23:203–204.

132. Lammintausta K, Kalimo K. Sensitivity to rubber. Study with rubber mixes and individual rubber chemicals. *Derm Beruf Umwelt* 1985;33:204–208.

133. Hegyi E, Buc M, Busova B. Frequency of HLA antigens in persons sensitive to *N*-isopropyl-*N'*-phenyl-*p*-phenylenediamine (IPPD). *Contact Dermatitis* 1993;28:194–195.

134. Heydenrich G, Ohlholm-Larsen P. 4–4'-Dithiodimorpholine, a new rubber sensitizer. *Contact Dermatitis* 1976;2:292–293.

135. Bjorkner B, Niklasson B. Contact allergy to AgeRite resin D. *Contact Dermatitis* 1986;14:122–123.

136. Zina AM, Bedello PG, Cane D, Bundino S, Benedetto A. Dermatitis in a rubber tyre factory. *Contact Dermatitis* 1987;17:17–20.

137. Romaguera C, Grimalt F. Occupational leukoderma and contact dermatitis from paratertiary butylphenol. *Contact Dermatitis* 1981;7:159–160.

138. Taylor JS, Melton A, Hamann CP. Selected highlights of the International Latex Conference: Sensitivity to latex in medical devices. *Am J Contact Dermatitis* 1993;4:101–105.

139. The frequency of contact sensitivity in North America 1972–1974. *Contact Dermatitis* 1975;1:277–280.

140. Guin JD. The doctor's surgical/examination gloves—problems with and without them. *Int J Dermatol* 1992;31:853–855.

141. Agathos M, Bernecker HA. Hand dermatitis in medical personnel. *Occup Environ Dermatoses* 1982;30:43–47.

142. Jokstad A. Contact dermatitis due to professional activity among dental health care personnel. *Norske Tannlaegeforenings Tidende* 1989;99:48–57.

143. Hansen KS. Occupational dermatoses in hospital cleaning women. *Contact Dermatitis* 1983;9:343–351.

144. Shelley WB. Golf course dermatitis due to thiuram fungicide. *JAMA* 1964;188:415.

145. Pock-Steen B. Contact allergy to Nobecutan. *Contact Dermatitis* 1988;18:52–53.

146. Hannuksela M, Suhonen R, Forstrom L. Delayed contact allergies in patients with photosensitivity dermatitis. *Acta Derm Venereol* 1981;61:303–306.

147. Webb PK, Gibbs SC, Mathias CT, Crain W, Maibach H. Disulfiram hypersensitivity and rubber contact dermatitis. *JAMA* 1979;241:2061.

148. van Hecke E, Vermander F. Allergic contact dermatitis by oral disulfiram. *Contact Dermatitis* 1984;10:254.

149. Mathelier-Fusade P, Leynadier F. Occupational allergic contact reaction to disulfiram. *Contact Dermatitis* 1994;31:121–122.

150. Themido R, Brandao FM. Contact allergy to thiurams. *Contact Dermatitis* 1984;10:251.

151. Van Ketel WG. Thiuram-mix. *Contact Dermatitis* 1976;2:232.

152. Rudzki E, Ostawszewski K, Grzya A. Sensitivity to some rubber additives. *Contact Dermatitis* 1976;2:24–27.

153. Sertoli A, Gola M, Martinelli M, et al. Epidemiology of contact dermatitis. *Semin Dermatol* 1989;8:120–126.

154. Sober AJ, Fitzpatrick TB. *Statistics of Interest to the Dermatologist.* St. Louis: Mosby–Year Book; 1990.

155. Sober AJ, Fitzpatrick TB. *Statistics of Interest to the Dermatologist.* St. Louis: Mosby–Year Book; 1989.

156. Song M, Degreef H, De Maubeuge J, Dooms-Goossens A, Oleffe J. Contact sensitivity to rubber additives in Belgium. *Dermatologica* 1979;158:163–167.

157. Van Ketel WG, Van Den Berg WHHW. The problem of the sensitization to dithiocarbamates in thiuram-allergic patients. *Dermatologica* 1984;169:70–75.

158. Wang XS, Suskind RR. Comparative studies of the sensitization potential of morpholine, 2-mercaptobenzothiazole and 2 of their derivatives in guinea pigs. *Contact Dermatitis* 1988;19:11–15.

159. Nethercott JR, Holness DL, Adams RM, et al. Patch testing with a routine screening tray in North America, 1987 through 1989: IV. Occupation and response. *Am J Contact Dermatitis* 1991;2:247–254.

160. de la Cuadra Oyanguren J, Marquina Vila A, Martorell Aragones A, Sanz Ortega J, Aliaga Boniche A. Contact allergic dermatitis in childhood: 1972–1987. *Anales Espanoles Pediatrio* 1989;30:363–366.

161. Jung JH, McLaughlin JL, Stannard J, Guin JD. Isolation, via activity-directed fractionation, of mercaptobenzothia-

zole and bibenzothiazyl disulfide as 2 allergens responsible for tennis shoe dermatitis. *Contact Dermatitis* 1988;19:254–259.

162. Hansson C, Agrup G. Stability of mercaptobenzothiazole compounds. *Contact Dermatitis* 1993;28:29–34.

163. Foussereau J, Menezes-Brandao F, Cavelier C, Herve-Bazin B. Allergy to MBT and its derivatives. *Contact Dermatitis* 1993;9:514–516.

164. Mitchell JC. Patch testing with mixes. Note on mercapto-benzothiazole mix. *Contact Dermatitis* 1981;7:98–104.

165. Foussereau J, Muslmani N, Cavelier C, Herve-Bazin B. Contact allergy to safety shoes. *Contact Dermatitis* 1986;14:233–236.

166. Fregert S. "Cement dermatitis" caused by rubber packing. *Contact Dermatitis Newslett* 1969;6:123.

167. Fregert S. Dermatitis due to a conveyer belt of Lycra. *Contact Dermatitis Newslett* 1972;12:325.

168. Kirton V, Williamson DS. Rubber band dermatitis in post office sorters. *Contact Dermatitis Newslett* 1972;11:257.

169. Verbov J. Rubber in brassiere cups. *Contact Dermatitis Newslett* 1969;5:98.

170. Petersen MC, Vine J, Ashley JJ, Nation RL. Leaching of 2-(2-hydroxyethyl-mercapto)benzothiazole into contents of disposable syringes. *J Pharm Sci* 1981;70:1139–1143.

171. Correcher BL, Perez AG. Dermatitis from shoes and an amputation prosthesis due to mercaptobenzothiazole and paratertiary butyl formaldehyde resin. *Contact Dermatitis* 1981;7:275.

172. Conde-Salazar L, Llinas Volpe MG, Guimaraens D, Romero L. Allergic contact dermatitis from a suction cup prosthesis. *Contact Dermatitis* 1977;3:217–218.

173. Malten KE. Sensitizers in leg bandages. *Contact Dermatitis* 1977;3:217–218.

174. Salmona G, Assaf A, Gayte-Sorbier A, Airaudo CB. Mass spectral identification of benzothiazole derivatives leached into injections by disposable syringes. *Biomed Mass Spectrom* 1984;11:450–454.

175. Bajaj AK, Gupta SC, Chatterjee AK, Singh KG. Shoe dermatitis in India: further observations. *Contact Dermatitis* 1991;24:149–151.

176. Blosczyk G, Doemling HJ. HPLC determination of 2-mercaptobenzothiazole in rubber baby bottle nipples. *Lebensmittelchem Gerichtl Chem* 1997;36:90[Abstract].

177. Joseph HL, Maibach HI. Contact dermatitis from spandex brassieres. *JAMA* 1967;201:880–882.

178. Tannenbaum MH. Spandex dermatitis. *JAMA* 1967; 200:899.

179. Allenby CF, Crow KD, Kirton V, Munro-Ashman D. Contact dermatitis from spandex yarn. *Br Med J* 1966;1:624.

180. Fregert S, Skog E. Allergic contact dermatitis from mercaptobenzothiazole in cutting oil. *Acta Derm Venereol* 1962;42:235–238.

181. Reepmeyer JC, Juhl YH. Contamination of injectable solutions with 2-mercaptobenzothiazole leached from rubber closures. *J Pharm Sci* 1983;72:1302–1305.

182. Wilson HTH. Rubber dermatitis. An investigation of 106 cases of contact dermatitis caused by rubber. *Br J Dermatol* 1969;81:175–179.

183. Fisher AA. Condom dermatitis in either partner. *Cutis* 1987;39:281–285.

184. Adams RM. Mercaptobenzothiazole in veterinary medications. *Contact Dermatitis Newslett* 1974;16:514.

185. Wilkinson SM, Cartwright PH, English JS. Allergic contact dermatitis from mercaptobenzothiazole in a releasing fluid. *Contact Dermatitis* 1990;23:370.

186. Taylor JS. Rubber. In: Fisher AA, ed. *Contact Dermatitis*, 3rd ed. Philadelphia: Lea & Febiger; 1986:606–643.

187. Guin JD. The MBT controversy. *Am J Contact Dermatitis* 1990;1:195–197.

188. Fowler JF, Adams RM. Earlobe contact allergy caused by rubber. *Am J Contact Dermatitis* 1992;3:111.

189. Kilpikari I. Occupational contact dermatitis among rubber workers. *Contact Dermatitis* 1982;8:359–362.

190. Foussereau J, Cavelier C. Has *N*-isopropyl-*N'*-phenyl-paraphenylenediamine a place among standard allergens? Importance of this allergen in rubber intolerance. *Dermatologica* 1977;155:164–167.

191. Herve-Bazin B, Foussereau J, Cavelier C. Contact allergy to *N*-isopropyl-*N'*-phenylparaphenylenediamine (IPPD) in different individual protective devices. *Derm Beruf Umwelt* 1980;28:82–88.

192. Carlsen L, Andersen KE, Egsgaard H. IPPD contact allergy from an orthopedic bandage. *Contact Dermatitis* 1987;17:119–121.

193. Nater JP. Hypersensitivity to rubber. *Berufs Dermatosen* 1975;23:161–168.

194. Lintrum JC, Nater JP. Allergic contact dermatitis caused by rubber chemicals in dairy workers. *Dermatologica* 1974;148:42–44.

195. Fregert S. Relapse of hand dermatitis after short contact with tires. *Contact Dermatitis Newslett* 1973;13:351.

196. Brandao FM. Occupational contact dermatitis from rubber antioxidants. *Contact Dermatitis* 1978;4:246.

197. Tennstedt D, Lachapelle JM. Windsurfer dermatitis from black rubber components. *Contact Dermatitis* 1981; 7:160–161.

198. Roed-Petersen J, Hjorth N, Jordan WP, Bourlas M. Postsorters' rubber fingerstall dermatitis. *Contact Dermatitis* 1977;3:143–147.

199. Wilkinson DS. Sensitivity to *N*-isopropyl-*N*-phenyl-*p*-phenylenediamine. *Contact Dermatitis Newslett* 1968; 3:37.

200. Levine MJ. Idiopathic photodermatitis with a positive para-phenylenediamine photo patch test. *Arch Dermatol* 1984;120:1488–1490.

201. Dooms-Goossens A, Degreef H, de Veylder H, Maselis T. Unusual sensitization to black rubber. *Contact Dermatitis* 1987;17:47–48.

202. Guin JD. Black rubber mix. In: Guin JD, ed. *Practical Contact Dermatitis*. New York: McGraw-Hill; 1995:243–252.

203. Heese A, Hintzenstern JV, Peters K-P, Koch HU, Hornstein OP. Allergic and irritant reactions to rubber gloves in medical health services. Spectrum, diagnostic approach, and therapy. *J Am Acad Dermatol* 1991; 25:831–839.

204. Egsgaard H, Knudsen B, Larsen E. Release of thiurams and carbamates from protective gloves to artificial sweat. *J Agri Food Chem* 1981;29:729–732.

205. Schubert H. Contact dermatitis to sodium *N*-methyldithi-ocarbamate. *Contact Dermatitis* 1978;4:370–371.

206. Piraccini BM, Cameli N, Peluso AM, Tardio M. A case of allergic contact dermatitis due to the pesticide maneb. *Contact Dermatitis* 1991;24:381–382.

207. Garcia-Perez A, Garcia-Bravo B, Beneit JV. Standard patch tests in agricultural workers. *Contact Dermatitis* 1984;10:151–153.

208. Peluso AM, Tardio M, Adamo F, Venturo N. Multiple sensitization due to bisdithiocarbamate and thiophthalimide pesticides. *Contact Dermatitis* 1991;25:327.

209. Guin JD. Carba mix (rubber). In: Guin JD, ed. *Practical Contact Dermatitis*. New York: McGraw-Hill, 1995:161–166.

210. Dermatitis among workers cleaning the Sacramento River after a chemical spill—California. *MMWR* 1991;40:825–837.

211. Dooms-Goossens A, Dedusschere K, Morren M, Roelandts R. Silver polish: another source of contact derma-

titis reactions to thiourea. *Contact Dermatitis* 1988; 19:133–135.

212. Rich P, Belozer ML, Norris P, Storrs FJ. Allergic contact dermatitis to two antioxidants in latex gloves: 4,4-thiobis (6-tert-butyl-meta-cresol) (Lowinox 44S36) and butylhydroxyanisole. *J Am Acad Dermatol* 1991;24:37–43.

213. Kanerva L, Estlander T, Jolanki R. Occupational allergic contact dermatitis caused by thiourea compounds. *Contact Dermatitis* 1994;31:228–242.

214. Reid CM, van Grutten M, Rycroft RJ. Allergic contact dermatitis from ethylbutylthiourea in neoprene. *Contact Dermatitis* 1993;28:193.

215. Sherertz EF, Medford KB. Patch testing may be important in chronic dyshidrotic eczema. *Am J Contact Dermatitis* 1994;5:180–181.

216. Kanerva L, Jolanki R, Plosila M, Estlander T. Contact dermatitis from dibutylthiourea. Report of a case with fine structural observations of epicutaneous testing with dibutylthiourea. Contact Dermatitis 1984;10:158–162.

217. Hawley CG. *The Condensed Chemical Dictionary,* 10th ed. New York: Van Norstrand Reinhold; 1981.

218. Dooms-Goossens A, Boyden B, Ceuterick A, Degreef H. Dimethylthiourea, an unexpected hazard for textile workers. *Contact Dermatitis* 1979;5:367–370.

219. Nurse DS. Sensitivity to thiourea in plain printing paper. *Contact Dermatitis* 1980;6:153–154.

220. Schmid-Grendelmeier P, Elsner P. Contact dermatitis due to occupational dibutylthiourea exposure: a case of phonecard dermatitis. *Contact Dermatitis* 1995;32:308–309.

221. Goh CL, Ng SK. Photoallergic contact dermatitis to carbimazole. *Contact Dermatitis* 1985;12:58–59.

222. Kaniwa MA, Nakamura A, Kantoh H, et al. Identification of causative chemicals of allergic contact dermatitis using a combination of patch testing in patients and chemical analysis. Application to cases for industrial rubber products. *Contact Dermatitis* 1994;30:20–25.

223. Camarasa JG, Romaguera C, Conde-Salazar L, et al. Thiourea reactivity in Spain. *Contact Dermatitis* 1985;12:220.

224. Estlander T, Jolanki R, Kanerva L. Dermatitis and urticaria from rubber and plastic gloves. *Contact Dermatitis* 1986;14:20–25.

225. Vaneckova J, Ettler K. Hypersensitivity to rubber surgical gloves in healthcare personnel. *Contact Dermatitis* 1994;31:266–268.

226. Daecke CM, Schaller J, Goos M. Value of patient's own test substances in epicutaneous testing. *Hautarzt* 1994;45:292–298.

227. Kaniwa MA, Nakamura A, Kantoh H, et al. Identification of causative chemicals of allergic contact dermatitis using a combination of patch testing in patients and chemical analysis. *Contact Dermatitis* 1994;31:65–71.

228. Opdyke DLJ. Inhibition of sensitization reactions induced by certain aldehydes. *Food Cosmetics Toxicol* 1976; 14:197–198.

229. Molinari JA. Dermatitis in dental professionals: causes, treatment, and prevention. *J. Pract Hyg* 1996;5:13–16.

230. McLelland J, Shuster S. Contact dermatitis with negative patch tests: the additive effect of allergens in combination. *Br J Dermatol* 1990;122:623–630.

231. Wilkinson JD, Bruynzeel DP, Ducombs G, et al. European multicenter study of Tru Test panel 2. *Contact Dermatitis* 1990;2:218–225.

232. Belsito DV, Storrs FJ, Taylor JS, et al. Reproducibility of patch tests: a United States multicenter study. *Am J Contact Dermatitis* 1992;3:193–200.

233. Fregert S. Cross sensitivity pattern of 2-mercaptobenzothiazole (MBT). *Acta Derm Venereol* 1962;49:45.

234. Lynde CW, Mitchell JC, Adams RM, et al. Patch testing with mercaptobenzothiazole and mercapto-mixes. *Contact Dermatitis* 1982;8:273–274.

235. Mitchell JC, Clendenning WE, Cronin E, et al. Patch testing with mercaptobenzothiazole and mercapto-mix. *Contact Dermatitis* 1976;2:123–124.

236. Bruynzeel DP, Andersen KE, Camarasa JG, Lachapelle JM, Menne T, White IR. The European standard series. European Environmental and Contact Dermatitis Research Group (EECDRG). *Contact Dermatitis* 1995; 33:145–148.

237. Menne T, White IR, Bruynzeel DP, Dooms-Goossens A. Patch test reactivity to the PPD-black rubber mix (industrial rubber chemicals) and individual ingredients. *Contact Dermatitis* 1992;26:354.

238. Rudzki E, Napiorkowska I. Active sensitisation to IPPD. *Contact Dermatitis* 1984;10:126–127.

239. Cavelier C, Herve-Bazin B, Foussereau J, Poitou P, Marignac B. Allergic properties of a series of *N*-phenyl*N'*-alcoyl paraphenylenediamines. *Derm Beruf Umwelt* 1980;28:45–47.

240. Rudzki E, Grzywa Z. Occupational piperazine dermatitis. *Contact Dermatitis* 1977;3:216.

241. Logan RA, White IR. Carbamix is redundant in the patch test series. *Contact Dermatitis* 1988;18:303–304.

242. Jordan WP, Bourlas MC. Allergic contact dermatitis to underwear elastic. Chemically transformed by laundry bleach. *Arch Dermatol* 1975;111:593–595.

243. Van Ketel WG. Low sensitization rate of naphthyl mix. *Contact Dermatitis* 1983;9:77.

244. Fuchs T, Wahl R. Immediate reactions to rubber products. *J Allergy Proc* 1992;13:61–66.

245. Alenius H, Reunala T, Turjanmaa K, Palosuo T. Detection of IgG4 and IgE antibodies to rubber proteins by immunoblotting in latex allergy. *J Allergy Proc* 1992;13:75–77.

246. Jaeger D, Kleinhans D, Czuppon A, Baur X. Latex-specific proteins causing immediate-type cutaneous, nasal, bronchial, and systemic reactions. *J Allergy Clin Immunol* 1992;89:759–768.

247. Akasawa A, Hsieh LS, Martin BM, Liu T, Lin Y. A novel acidic allergen, Hev b 5, in latex. Purification, cloning and characterization. *J Biol Chem* 1996; 271:25389–25393.

248. Akasawa A, Hsieh LS, Lin Y. Serum reactivities to latex proteins (*Hevea brasiliensis*). *J Allergy Clin Immunol* 1995;95:1196–1205.

249. Tomazic VJ, Withrow TJ, Hamilton RG. Characterization of latex allergen(s) in latex protein extracts. *J Allergy Clin Immunol* 1995;96:(5 Pt 1)635–642.

250. Rat JP. Latex allergy: is the allergen thermolabile? [French]. *Allergie Immunologie* 1994;26:219–220.

251. Gidrol X, Chrestin H, Tan HL, Kush A. Hevein, a lectin-like protein from *Hevea brasiliensis* (rubber tree) is involved in the coagulation of latex. *J Biol Chem* 1994;269:9278–9283.

252. Chen Z, Posch A, Lohaus C, et al. Isolation and identification of hevein as a major IgE-binding polypeptide in *Hevea* latex. *J Allergy Clin Immunol* 1997;99:402–409.

253. Alenius H, Kalkkinen N, Lukka M, Reunala T, Turjanmaa K, Makinen-Kiljunen S. Prohevein from the rubber tree (*Hevea brasiliensis*) is a major latex allergen. *Clin Exp Allergy* 1995;24:659–665.

254. Alenius H, Kalkkinen N, Reunala T, Turjanmaa K, Palosuo T. The main IgE-binding epitope of a major latex allergen, prohevein, is present in its N-terminal 43-amino acid fragment hevein. *J Immunol* 1996;156:1618–1625.

255. Beezhold DH, Kostyal DA, Sussman GL. IgE epitope analysis of the hevein preprotein as a major latex allergen. *Clin Exp Immunol* 1997;108:114–121.

256. Vallier P, Ballard S, Valentas R. Identification of profilin as an IgE-binding component in latex from *Heveas brasiliensis. Clin Exp Allergy* 1995;25:332–339.

257. Lu L, Kurup V, Hoffman D, Kelly K, Murali P, Fink J. Characterization of a major latex allergen associated with hypersensitivity in spina bifida patients. *J Immunol* 1995;155:2721–2728.

258. Alenius H, Kalkkinen N, Yip E, et al. Significance of rubber elongation factor as a latex allergen. *Int Arch Allergy Immunol* 1996;109:262–268.

259. Slater J. Latex allergy. *J Allergy Clin Immunol* 1992;68:203–211.

260. Holm JO, Wereide K, Halvorsen R, Thune P. Allergy to latex among hospital employees. *Contact Dermatitis* 1995;32:239–240.

261. Taylor J. Latex allergy. *Am J Contact Dermatitis* 1993;4:114–117.

262. Arellano R, Bradley J, Sussman G. Prevalence of latex sensitization among hospital physicians occupationally exposed to latex gloves. Anesthesiology 1992;77:905–908.

263. Safadi GS, Safadi TJ, Terezhalmy GT, Taylor JS, Battisto JR, Melton AL. Latex Hypersensitivity: its prevalence among dental professionals. *J Am Dent Assoc* 1996;127:83–88.

264. Berky ZT, Luciano WJ, James WD. Latex glove allergy: a survey of the US Army Dental Corps. *JAMA* 1992;268:2695–2697.

265. Heese A, Peters KP, Stahl J, Koch HU, Hornstein OP. Incidence and increase in Type I allergies to rubber gloves in dental medicine students [German]. *Hautarzt* 1995;46:15–21.

266. Allmers H, Kirchner B, Huber H, Chen Z, Walther JW, Baur X. Latenzzeit zwischen Exposition und Symptomen bei Allergie gegen Naturlatex. Vorschlage zur Prävention. *Dtsch Med Wochenschr* 1996;121:823–828.

267. Konrad C, Fieber T, Schupfer G. Anaphylactic reaction to latex in health care workers. *Anesth Analg* 1995;81:878–879.

268. Yoshino A, Nagashima S, Uchiyama M. Anaphylactoid reaction in a surgeon to surgical rubber gloves. *Anesth Analg* 1995;878–879.

269. Baykara N, Kati I, Arikan Z, Oz H. Intraoperative latex anaphylaxis observed in a farmer. *Anesthesiology* 1996;84:476–477.

270. Masood D, Brown JE, Patterson R, Greenberger PA, Berkowitz L. Recurrent anaphylaxis due to unrecognized latex hypersensitivity in two healthcare professionals. *Ann Allergy Asthma Immunol* 1995;74:311–313.

271. Laskin DM. Latex sensitivity: a potentially dangerous problem. *J Oral Maxillofac Surg* 1996;54:933.

272. Rosen A, Isaacson D, Brady M, Corey JP. Hypersensitivity to latex in health care workers: report of five cases. *Otolaryngol Head Neck Surg* 1993;109:731–734.

273. Hudgins LB, Hamdy RC, Miller MP. Anaphylaxis due to latex. *South Med J* 1993;86:948–949.

274. Chen MD, Greenspoon JS, Long TL. Latex anaphylaxis in an obstetrics and gynecology physician. *Am J Obstet Gynecol* 1992;166:968–969.

275. Ber DJ, Davidson AE, Klein DE, Settipane GA. Latex hypersensitivity: two case reports. *J Allergy Proc* 1992;13:71–73.

276. Marcos C, Lazaro M, Fraj J. Occupational asthma due to latex surgical gloves. *Ann Allergy* 1991;67:319–323.

277. Seifert HU, Seifert B, Wahl R, Vocks E, Borelli S, Maasch HJ. Immunoglobulin E–mediated contact urticaria and bronchial asthma caused by household rubber gloves containing latex: 3 case reports. *Derm Beruf Umwelt* 1987;35:(4)137–139.

278. Assalve D, Cicioni C, Perno P, Lisi P. Short communications: contact urticaria and anaphylactoid reaction from cornstarch surgical glove powder. *Contact Dermatitis* 1988;19:61.

279. Fisher AA. Contact urticaria due to cornstarch surgical glove powder. *Cutis* 1986;38:307–308.

280. Baur X, Ammon J, Chen Z, Beckmann U, Czuppon AB. Health risk in hospitals through airborne allergens for patients presensitised to latex. *Lancet* 1993;342:1148–1149.

281. Baur X, Jager D, Engelke T, Rennert S, Czuppon AB. Latex proteins as the trigger of respiratory and systemic allergies. *Dtsche Med Wochenschr* 1992;117:1269–1273.

282. Pisati G, Baruffini A, Bernabeo F, Stanizzi R. Bronchial provocation testing in the diagnosis of occupational asthma due to latex surgical gloves. *Eur Respir J* 1994;7:332–336.

283. Kujala VM, Reijula KE. Glove related rhinopathy among hospital personnel. *Am J Ind Med* 1996;30:164–170.

284. Schwartz HA, Zurowski D. Anaphylaxis to latex in intravenous fluids. *J Allergy Clin Immunol* 1993;92:358–359.

285. Fisher AA. Contact urticaria due to cornstarch powder. *J Dermatol Surg Oncol* 1987;13:224.

286. Molinari JA. Merging infection control issues: increasing incidence of latex. *Compend Contin Educ Dent* 1995;16:346–348.

287. Ahman M, Wrangsjo K. Nasal peak flow rate recording is useful in detecting allergic nasal reactions: a case report. *Allergy* 1994;49:785–787.

288. Fiser MP, Landwehr LP. Latex: a new occupational hazard for physicians. *J Ark Med Soc* 1993;90:636.

289. Kujala V, Pirila T, Niinimaki A, Reijula K. Latex induced allergic rhinitis in a laboratory nurse. *J Laryngol Otol* 1995;109:109–146.

290. Hopkins J. Rubber latex in the air: an occupational and environmental cause for asthma? *Food Chem Toxicol* 1995;33:895–899.

291. Nemery B. Latex induced occupational asthma [Letter; comment]. *Eur Respir J* 1994;7:172–174.

292. Voelker R. Latex-induced asthma among health care workers. *JAMA* 1995;273:764.

293. Brugnami G, Marabini A, Siracusa A, Abbritti G. Work-related late asthmatic response induced by latex allergy. *J Allergy Clin Immunol* 1995;96:457–464.

294. Konrad C, Schupfer G, Fieber T, Gerber H. Latex allergy not only a threatening danger to patients. A case report from an anesthesiological department. *Schweiz Rundschau Med Prax* 1996;85:482–485.

295. Vandenplas O, Delwiche JP, Sibille Y. Occupational asthma due to latex in a hospital administrative employee. *Thorax* 1996;51:452–453.

296. Marks D. Nearly 10 percent of nurses suffer from a latex allergy. *Am Nurse* 1996;28:7.

297. Yassin MS, Lierl MB, Fischer TJ, O'Brien K, Cross J, Steinmetz C. Latex allergy in hospital employees. *Ann Allergy* 1994;72:245–249.

298. Mizutari K, Kuriya N, Ono T. Immediate allergy to rubber gloves: a questionnaire study of hospital personnel. *J Dermatol* 1995;22:19–23.

299. Grzybowski M, Peyser PA, Schork MA. The prevalence of anti–latex IgE antibodies among registered nurses. *J Allergy Clin Immunol* 1996;98:535–544.

300. Rustemeyer T, Pilz B, Frosch PJ. Kontaktallergien in medizinschen Berufen. *Hautarzt* 1994;45:834–844.

301. Taylor JS, Praditsuwan P. Latex allergy. Review of 44 cases including outcome and frequent association with allergic hand eczema. *Arch Dermatol* 1996;132:265–271.

302. Belsito DV. Contact urticaria caused by rubber: analysis of seven cases. *Contact Dermatitis* 1990;8:61–66.

303. Helander I, Makela A. Contact urticaria to zinc diethyldithiocarbamate (ZDC). *Contact Dermatitis* 1983;9:327–328.

304. Van Ketel WG. Contact urticaria from rubber gloves after dermatitis from thiurams. *Contact Dermatitis* 1984; 11:323–324.

305. Turjanmaa K. Latex glove contact urticaria. *Acta Universitatis Tamperensis* 1988;254 Ser A:1–87.

306. Van Krogh G, Maibach HI. The contact urticaria syndrome—an updated review. *J Am Acad Dermatol* 1981;5:328–342.

307. Sussman GL, Beezhold DH. Allergy to latex rubber. *Ann Intern Med* 1995;122:43–46.

308. Moreno Ancillo A, Lopez Serrano MC, Barranco Sanz P, Dominguez Noche C, Ornia Fernandez N, Martinez Alzamora F. Latex sensitization in 28 patients. *Allergologia Immunopathologia* 1994;22:275–280.

309. Markey J. Latex allergy: implications for healthcare personnel and infusion therapy patients. *J Intravenous Nurs* 1994;17:359.

310. Akasawa A, Matsumoto K, Saito H, et al. Incidence of latex allergy in atopic children and hospital workers in Japan. *Int Arch Allergy Immunol* 1993;101:177–181.

311. Turjanmaa K, Reunala T. Contact urticaria from rubber gloves. *Dermatol Clin* 1988;6:47–51.

312. Beaudouin E, Pupil P, Jacson F, et al. Allergie professionelle au latex. Enquete prospective sur 907 sujets du milieu hospitalier. *Rev Fr Allergol* 1990;30:157–161.

313. Lagier F, Vervloet D, Lhermet I, Poyen D, Charpin D. Prevalence of latex allergy in operating room nurses. *J Allergy Clin Immunol* 1992;90:319–322.

314. Crisi G, Belsito DV. Contact urticaria from latex in a patient with immediate hypersensitivity to banana, avocado and peach. *Contact Dermatitis* 1993;28:24–25.

315. Dousson C, Ripault B, Leblanc MA, et al. Prevalence of latex allergy among personnel at a hospital. *Allergie Immunologie* 1994;26:367–373.

316. Randolph C, Fraser B. Latex hypersensitivity in a horse farmer. *Allergy Asthma* 1996;17:89–91.

317. Abeck D, Borries M, Kuwert C, Steinkraus V, Vieluf D, Ring J. Food-induced anaphylaxis in latex. *Hautarzt* 1994;45:364–367.

318. Dompmartin A, Szczurko C, Michel M, et al. Two cases of urticaria following fruit ingestion, with cross-sensitivity to latex. *Contact Dermatitis* 1994;30:250–252.

319. Caruso B, Caputo M, Senna G, Andri L. Immunoblotting study of specific antibody patterns against latex and banana. *Allergie Immunologie* 1993;25:187–190.

320. Safadi GS, Corey EC, Taylor JS, Wagner WO, Pien LC, Melton AL. Latex hypersensitivity in emergency medical service providers. *Ann Allergy Asthma Immunol* 1996; 77:39–42.

321. Fuchs T, Wahl R. Immediate allergic reaction to natural latex with special reference to surgical gloves. *Med Klin* 1992;87:355–363.

322. Schwartz HJ. Latex: a potential hidden "food" allergen in fast food restaurants. *J Allergy Clin Immunol* 1995;95:139–140.

323. Boxer MB, Grammer LC, Orfan N. Gutta-percha allergy in a health care worker with latex allergy. *J Allergy Clin Immunol* 1994;93:943–944.

324. Pecquet C, Leynadier F, Dry J. Contact urticaria and anaphylaxis to natural latex. *J Am Acad Dermatol* 1990;22:631–633.

325. Hamilton RG, Charous BL, Adkinson NF Jr, Yunginger JW. Serologic methods in the laboratory diagnosis of latex rubber allergy: study of nonammoniated, ammoniated latex, and glove (end-product) extracts as allergen reagent sources. *J Lab Clin Med* 1994;123:594–604.

326. Kelly KJ, Kurup V, Zacharisen M, Resnick A, Fink JN. Skin and serologic testing in the diagnosis of latex allergy. *J Allergy Clin Immunol* 1993;91:1140–1145.

327. Spaner D, Dolovich J, Tarlo S, Sussman G, Buttoo K. Hypersensitivity to natural latex. *J Allergy Clin Immunol* 1989;83:1135–1137.

328. Hjorth N. Diagnostic patch testing. In: Marzulli FN, Maibach HI, eds. *Dermatotoxicology*, 3rd ed. New York: Hemisphere; 1987:307–317.

329. Hamann CP, Kick SA. Diagnosis-driven management of natural rubber latex glove sensitivity. In: Mellstrom GA, Wahlberg JE, Maibach HI, eds. *Protective Gloves for Occupational Use*. Boca Raton, Fla: CRC; 1994;131–156.

330. Castelain M, Castelain PY. Allergic contact dermatitis from cetyl pyridinium chloride in latex gloves. *Contact Dermatitis* 1993;28:118.

331. Milkovic-Kraus S. Glove powder as a contact allergen. *Contact Dermatitis* 1992;26:198.

332. Karathanasis P, Cooper A, Zhou K, Mayer L, Kang BC. Indirect latex contact causes urticaria/anaphylaxis. *Ann Allergy* 1993;71:526–528.

333. Guin JD. Urticaria. In: Rakel RE, ed. *Conn's Current Therapy*. Philadelphia: WB Saunders; 1995;776–779.

334. Lachapelle JM. Allergic "contact" dermatitis from disulfiram implants. *Contact Dermatitis* 1975;1:218–220.

335. Adams RM. Possible substitution for mercaptobenzothiazole in rubber. *Contact Dermatitis* 1975;1:246.

336. Brehler R. Contact urticaria caused by latex-free nitrile gloves. *Contact Dermatitis* 1996;34:296.

337. Kilpikari I, Halme H. Contact allergy to Hypalon rubber. *Contact Dermatitis* 1983;9:529.

338. Fisher AA. Contact allergens that pass through ordinary rubber gloves. *Cutis* 1993;52:333–334.

339. Nethercott JR, Holness DL, Page E. Occupational contact dermatitis due to glutaraldehyde in health care workers. *Contact Dermatitis* 1988;19:219–220.

340. Di Prima T, DePasquale R, Nigro M. Contact dermatitis from glutaraldehyde. *Contact Dermatitis* 1988;19:219–220.

341. Lehman PA, Franz TJ, Guin JD. Penetration of glutaraldehyde through glove material: Tactylon versus natural rubber latex. *Contact Dermatitis* 1994;30:176.

342. Murer AJ, Poulsen OM, Roed-Petersen J, Tuchsen F. Skin problems among Danish dental technicians. A cross sectional study. *Contact Dermatitis* 1995;33:42–47.

343. Vandenplas O, Delwiche JP, Depelchin S, Sibille Y, Vande Weyer R, Delaunois L. Latex gloves with a lower protein content reduce bronchial reactions in subjects with occupational asthma caused by latex. *Am J Respir Crit Care Med* 1995;151:887–891.

344. Hunt LW, Boone-Orke JL, Fransway AF, et al. A medical-center–wide, multidisciplinary approach to problem of natural rubber latex allergy. *J Occup Environ Med* 1996;38:765–770.

345. Fisher AA. Condom advice in rubber urticaria [Letter]. *Contact Dermatitis* 1989;21:354.

346. Hesse A, Hinzenstern J, Peters KP, Koch HU, Hornstein OP. Allergic and irritant reactions to rubber glove in medical health services. *J Am Acad Dermatol* 1991; 25:831–839.

347. Knudsen BB, Larsen E, Egsgaard H, Menne T. Release of thiurams and carbamates from rubber gloves. *Contact Dermatitis* 1993;28:63–69.

348. Tarlo SM, Sussman GL, Contala A, Swanson MC. Control of airborne latex by use of powder-free latex gloves. *J Allergy Clin Immunol* 1994;983:985–989.

348a. Nutter AF. Contact urticaria to rubber. *Br J Dermatol* 1979;101:597–598.

349. Ownby DR. Is rubber elongation factor the major allergen of latex? *J Allergy Clin Immunol* 1993;92:633–635.

350. Eriksson G, Ostlund E. Rubber bank note counters as the cause of eczema among employees at the Swedish Post Giro Office. *Acta Derm Venereol* 1968;48:212–214.

351. Meding B, Barregard L, Marcus K. Hand eczema in car mechanics. *Contact Dermatitis* 1994;30:129–134.

352. Brandao FM. L'allergie de contact au PPD-mix. *Acta Dermatol Allerg II* 1980:113–120.

353. Raith L. Contact dermatitis from 4-isopropyl-amino-diphenylamine. *Contact Dermatitis* 1976;2:362.

354. White WG, Vickers HR. Diethylthiourea as a cause of dermatitis in a car factory. *Br J Ind Med* 1970;27:167–169.

355. Hamada T, Horiguchi S. Chronic melanodermatitis due to rubber peephole of a ship radarscope. *Contact Dermatitis* 1978;4:245–246.

356. Guin JD. 2-Mercaptobenzothiazole. In: Guin JD, ed. *Practical Contact Dermatitis*. New York: McGraw-Hill; 1995:179–193.

357. Ancona A, Suarez de la Torre R, Evia JR. Dermatitis from mercaptobenzothiazole in a Foley catheter. *Contact Dermatitis* 1985;13:339–340.

358. Rycroft RJG, Menne T, Frosch PJ. Occupational contact dermatitis. In: Rycroft RJG, ed. *Textbook of Contact Dermatitis*. 2nd ed. Berlin: Springer-Verlag; 1995:341–400.

359. Gola M, Sertoli A, Angelini G, et al. GIRDCA data bank for occupational and environmental contact dermatitis (1984–1988). *Am J Contact Dermatitis* 1992;3:179–188.

360. Geier J, Schnuch A. A comparison of contact allergies among construction and nonconstruction workers attending contact dermatitis clinics in Germany: results of the information network of Department of Dermatology from November 1989 to July 1993. *Am J Contact Dermatitis* 1995;6:86–94.

361. Torres V, Lopes C, Lobo L, Soares P. Occupational contact dermatitis to thiourea and dimethylthiourea from diazo copy paper. *Am J Contact Dermatitis* 1992;3:37–39.

362. Hjorth N, Roed-Petersen J. Allergic contact dermatitis in veterinary surgeons. *Contact Dermatitis* 1980;6:27–29.

363. Estlander T, Jolanki R, Kanerva L. Contact urticaria from rubber gloves: a detailed description of four cases. *Acta Derm Venereol* 1987; 134 [suppl]:98–102.

Petroleum and Petroleum Derivatives

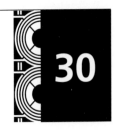

30

R. J. G. RYCROFT

PETROLEUM

Petroleum remains the major source of power for the engines of civilization and provides lubrication for virtually every piece of moving machinery. With most of the world's proven petroleum reserves in land areas having been developed, offshore developments have assumed ever increasing importance.[1] Petroleum supplies the starting materials for more than 3,000 petrochemicals that find their way into such diverse products as synthetic fibers, plastics, resins, synthetic rubber, soaps and detergents, solvents, medications, and surface coatings.[2] It provides the surfacing material for roads; the fuel for many households, small offices and factories, and hospitals; and, as a component in the manufacture of fertilizers and pesticides, it plays a major role in the expansion of the world's agriculture and food supply. Petroleum and petroleum gases are important sources of energy for jet engines and missiles.

Composition

Petroleum (crude oil) consists of the remains of incompletely decayed plants and animals buried under thick layers of rock during the past 600 million years. Crude oils are highly complex mixtures of hydrocarbons (including asphalt), with small quantities of sulfur-, nitrogen-, and oxygen-containing substances, and organo-metallic compounds of vanadium, nickel, and arsenic. Hydrocarbons constitute the largest fraction, the percentage varying with the field of origin. Alkanes (paraffins), isoalkanes, cycloalkanes (naphthenes), and aromatics constitute the bulk of these hydrocarbons.[3]

Recovery

Most of the world's crude oil occurs at depths of about 600 to 3,000 m and is normally recovered from there by rotary drilling.[4] Attached to the end of a revolving hollow pipe, a bit crushes the rock at the bottom of the borehole. While the bit is drilling, fluid (known as drilling mud) is pumped continuously down inside the rotating hollow pipe, emerging through holes in the drill bit and serving to cool and lubricate it, flush up the rock cuttings outside the drill pipe to ground level, and reduce friction between the drill pipe and the borehole. It also carries materials to treat and stabilize the borehole wall and protect it from penetration. To carry out all these functions, drilling muds, which originally consisted of muddy water, have become complex mixtures of chemicals based on either water or oil. Oil-based muds have been used increasingly in recent years. They consist of an oil phase, a brine phase, emulsifiers, filtration control agents, viscosifiers, wetting agents, and weighting agents. The base oil, which is the bulk of the fluid, was originally diesel fuel (gas oil), a relatively unrefined petroleum fraction, but now a deodorized kerosene or purified light mineral oil fraction, often called "clean oil," is frequently used instead. Viscosifiers (thickening agents) include blown asphalt and metallic soaps of tall oil or rosin acids.

The drilling process operates 24 hours a day, 7 days a week, until the flow of oil appears, interrupted only by hectic pauses to add another length of drill pipe or to pull out and replace a worn bit ("a round trip"). A typical drilling crew, working in shifts as long as 12 hours, consists of a driller, derrick operator, engine operator, and several helpers on the drill floor ("roughnecks"). The work has both physically and mentally demanding aspects, especially offshore, and roughnecks' overalls, gloves, and boots can become coated during a round trip with pungent, greasy drilling mud.[5]

When oil appears, if a well is able to produce its own flow by the force of underground pressure, it is "topped" by a system of pipes and valves known as a "Christmas tree," that carefully regulates the flow of oil and gas from the well. The network of tubing allows for tools for subsurface work to be introduced through the system. If the underground pressure is insufficient to produce spontaneous oil flow, a pump operated by a walking beam may be built at the site.

In nearly all crude oil wells, no more than one third of the oil can be recovered by the force of the reserves alone, called the *pressure decline method.* Some form of secondary recovery must be employed. Water flooding is one of the most widely used methods. Injection of gas, alcohol, liquid carbon dioxide, propane, and steam into the system, and even limited combustion *in situ,* are additional ways to recover the last drops of oil.

From the well, oil is sent by pipe to storage tanks, nearby or onshore, where gaugers and shippers check testtube samples for water and sand content and turn the valves to effect shipment by pipeline or tanker to refineries.

Oil can also be recovered from the ground in certain areas, including Scotland and the United States, by mining, crushing, and retorting oil-bearing rock known as *shale.*

Refining

The process of separating crude oil into its constituent parts is known as *refining,* the primary process of which is *fractional distillation.*[6] First the crude oil is heated in steel alloy tubes in a furnace to approximately 350°C (600°–800°F). The resulting mixture of vapor and oil passes from the furnace to fractionating columns, which rise vertically to 45 m (150 ft) or more. Each tower is supplied with approximately 50 perforated fractionating trays at intervals of about 2 feet all the way up. The vapor formed by heating rises up the tower and is cooled and condensed, and part of the condensed liquid is pumped back to the top of the tower (reflux). On each tray the hot vapor from the tray below preferentially evaporates some of the lower–boiling point material in the liquid on the tray, and some of the higher–boiling point material in the vapor is left behind in the liquid, which then falls to the tray below. In this way the "lower-boiling" material becomes concentrated toward the top of the column and the higher-boiling material toward the bottom. Liquid drawn off from an intermediate tray will have a boiling range intermediate between those of the top and bottom products. Lubricating oils come from the fraction withdrawn at the lowest level, gasoline from the highest level, and uncondensed hydrocarbon gases from the very top of the column.

Another important separation process is *solvent extraction* (or solvent refining), in which one liquid, the solvent, dissolves only certain molecules from another liquid containing many different hydrocarbons. The two liquids are then separated by gravity, and the solvent layer is removed. The first solvent to be used for this purpose was liquid sulfur dioxide, introduced in 1907. During the 1930s furfural began to be employed. Today diethylene glycol is especially important for the separation of the important benzene-toluene-xylene fractions from raw crude. Tetraethylene glycol and other glycols are also used in solvent extraction processes.

Adsorption is a third important method of petroleum refining. In this process, a stream of gaseous or liquid hydrocarbons is passed over or through an adsorbent compound, such as an aluminosilicate, called a *molecular sieve.* The very small pore diameters of these adsorbent compounds (approximately 10^{-8} cm) permit passage of only certain low–molecular weight hydrocarbons through their openings.

Crystallization is another refining process. The molecules to be separated are frozen and then filtered from the mixture. Hydrocarbons of great purity can be obtained by this process.

Conversion Processing or Cracking

After refining, the products are then converted to the desired compounds, usually by altering their molecular structure. The enormous demand for gasoline created by the automobile provided the impetus for the development of different conversion processes. Early in the 20th century it became apparent to petrol refiners that distillation of crude petroleum alone would never produce enough gasoline to satisfy the demand. The earliest method of converting hydrocarbons to gasoline and other products was *thermal cracking,* developed in 1913. This was the sole method until 1937, when *catalytic cracking,* using silica-aluminum compounds as catalysts, was introduced. The method of catalytic processing using a catalyst, heat, and pressure is called *hydrocracking.* Other methods include *polymerization, alkylation, catalytic reforming, dehydrogenation, isomerization,* and *coking and hydrotreating.*

PETROLEUM DERIVATIVES

Petroleum chemicals, also known as *petrochemicals,* are pure chemical substances produced from petroleum and natural gas.[2] The term usually refers to organic substances, but important inorganic compounds, such as ammonia and sulfur, are also included.

The petrochemical industry began about 1910 with the search for more and better gasoline, but it developed very slowly in the beginning, chiefly because of the inefficient cracking methods and primitive analytic techniques. Commercial production on a major scale began in 1920, and since the mid-1930s the industry has expanded tremendously, so that by the 1990s a very large percentage of the chemicals produced in the United States, western Europe, Russia, and Japan are in this class.

Each year more synthetic chemicals replace their natural counterparts. Notable examples are synthetic detergents, almost all of which are now derived from petroleum and have all but replaced conventional soaps for most industrial processes. Synthetic rubber products, the majority of which utilize butadiene as the starting material, are almost entirely derived from petrochemicals. Because the end products have little similarity to petroleum, we tend to forget the part petroleum plays in human life, from clothing to plastics, paints, insecticides, and photographic film, to name a few.

Gasoline

The nature of the crude oil determines how much gasoline can be refined from it. Gasoline is a complex mixture of hundreds of hydrocarbons, mostly saturated compounds with 4 to 12 carbon atoms per molecule.[2] Small amounts of highly volatile hydrocarbons are usually added to provide a readily combustible mixture for rapid engine starting. Tetraethyl lead was the main antiknock additive, but its use has progressively been restricted because of the hazards of lead air pollution.

Detergent additives such as polyolefin polyamine keep the carburetor and other combustion parts free of sludge and other deposits. Various glycols and surface-active agents (surfactants) function as de-icing agents. Antioxidants are usually derivatives of para-phenylenediamine. Various azo- and anthraquinone dyes are added for coloring. Combustion-control additives include tricresyl, cresyldiphenyl, and methyldiphenyl phosphates.

Diesel Fuels

Diesel fuels vary somewhat according to whether they are designed for high-speed diesel engines, for automotive purposes in trucks, buses, locomotives, and automobiles, or for stationary and ma-

rine diesel engines, which run at lower speeds. For high-speed diesel engines, gas oil is required, which overlaps to some extent with kerosene (also known as *paraffin* in the United Kingdom) in its boiling range. Gas oil is sometimes referred to in the United Kingdom as *derv* (*d*iesel *e*ngine *r*oad *v*ehicle). For lower-speed diesel engines, fuel quality is not so critical, and gas oil may be blended with some residual (asphaltic) material.

Lowering the sulfur content of high-speed diesel engine fuels has improved their general acceptability. For easier starting, amyl nitrate and other alkyl nitrates are added as cetane improvers. Detergents and dispersants, usually amines or sulfonates, are other important additives. Diesel fuels require several times more antioxidants than does gasoline. To combat the excessive smoke from diesel-fueled vehicles, barium compounds have been used.

Aviation Fuels

Ordinary aviation gasoline for piston-engined aircraft is the same as other motor gasolines, except that it usually has a very high octane rating. It is commonly known as *avgas*.

Jet fuels are commonly composed of a petroleum product similar to kerosene, often referred to in the United Kingdom as ATK or *avtur*. Commercial jets use kerosene-type fuels with varying freezing points, depending on the length of the flight: long-range flights require fuel with a lower freezing point than short- and medium-range flights. Military jets tend to mix kerosene with varying amounts of gasoline and other light petroleum distillates. Avtag (U.K.) or JP.4 (U.S.) is a wider–boiling range alternative aviation fuel.

Lubricating Oils

Lubricating oils contain paraffinic hydrocarbons (alkanes) from 17 carbons and up, with boiling ranges from 300° to 700°C. Hundreds of individual hydrocarbons are present, including those of the naphthenic (cycloalkane), aromatic, and polyaromatic series. Solvent extraction[6] with furfural is used to increase the viscosity of lubricating oil by removing low-viscosity aromatics. Further solvent extraction with mixtures of methyl ethyl ketone and toluene, or methylene chloride and dichloroethane, is then required to remove waxes so that the high-viscosity oil remains free flowing.

In addition to the basic materials, certain special chemical compounds are added to improve an existing property or to give the oil a new property.

Today hundreds of chemicals are employed as additives.

Greases

Greases are oils to which thickening agents have been added. Usually the concentration of thickening agents ranges from 3% to 30% by volume. The most common are fatty acid soaps of lithium, calcium, sodium, cobalt, aluminum, magnesium, and other metals, which add high-pressure strength to the final product. Inorganic clays, substituted ureas, lanolin, rosin, graphite, carbon black, talc, zinc oxide, waxes, and bitumens may also be employed as thickening agents.[7]

Automatic Transmission Fluids

General Motors introduced the first automatic transmission in the 1938 Oldsmobile, its key concept being a *fluid coupling*. The working principle of a fluid coupling is analogous to one fan setting the blades of another fan placed opposite it in motion: the transmission medium between the fans is air, whereas in a fluid coupling it is oil.

Transmission fluids must be mild, extreme-pressure lubricants, nonfoaming, resistant to oxidation and high temperatures, nonrusting, and noncorrosive, and must flow freely. Most transmission fluids contain mineral oil with detergents and oxidation inhibitors, various pour-point depressors, viscosity improvers, antiwear and antifoaming agents, sealants, and dyes.

Hydraulic Fluids

Hydraulic power is used for power transmission and machine movement of every conceivable description. Hydraulic systems have come to be widely used in aeronautical engineering (rudders, elevators, ailerons, flaps, retractable landing gear), because they can transmit and exert large forces without taking up much space. The majority of hydraulic systems employ fluids that are completely or primarily mineral oils. They also contain viscosity improvers, rust and corrosion inhibitors, and antiwear and other additives. Fire resistance in hydraulic fluids has also assumed increased significance and has led to the use of synthetic and water-based fluids in environments such as coal mines. Triaryl phosphate esters are used in fire-resistant hydraulic fluids.[7]

Asphalt

Asphalt is the heavy, solid to viscous fraction of crude petroleum consisting of natural bitumens. Bitumens are also found in lower grades of coal and tar sands and have been used for centuries as sealants and for waterproofing. In the United States about 80% of the asphalt used today is consumed in road-surfacing products, the remainder being employed in roofing materials, pipe coatings, cable laying, water engineering, and other uses. Like most other petroleum products, natural asphalt must be improved by various additives. Synthetic plastics and rubber are commonly added, as well as solvents, pigments, and various clays, gravels, and rocks. Rosin derivatives as well as epoxy compounds are frequently employed; epoxy compounds improve wheel grip at junctions and on inclines.

Cutting Fluids

When metal was first cut by machine it could be done only at low speeds because the heat generated at higher speeds destroyed the cutting edge of the steel tool. Early engineers found that higher speeds were possible when drilling gun barrels when a flow of cold water was used to reduce the temperature. However, water has the serious disadvantages of rusting ferrous metals, high surface tension, and poor lubricating action. Its high surface tension prevents it from adequately wetting the metal surface. Adding soap to water was found to improve both its wetting and lubricating power, and adding soda prevented rusting. This prototype of *water-based cutting fluids* was widely known as *suds* and remained in use until the 1920s.

One of the earliest alternatives to suds was the addition to water of triethanolamine (as a wetting agent) and nitrite (as a corrosion inhibitor). More sophisticated aqueous chemical solutions (synthetics; see Table 30–1), without the potential for nitrosamine formation, are widely used as cutting fluids in industry today, especially for metalworking operations that have an adverse effect on the stability of emulsions, such as the grinding of cast iron.

TABLE 30–1 • A Simple Classification of Cutting Fluids

Type of Cutting Fluid	Base
Neat oils	Mineral, fatty, and/or synthetic oils
Water-based fluids	Water
Soluble oils	Oil-in-water emulsion
Synthetics	Chemical solutions
Semisynthetics	Combinations

Type of Cutting Fluid	Composition
Mineral oils	Medium viscosity, solvent refined
Fatty oils	Animal or vegetable origin
Synthetic oils	Polyalkylene glycols
Emulsifiers	Petroleum sulfonates, fatty acid soaps, fatty amides, fatty alkanolamides, synthetic alcohol ethoxylates
Corrosion inhibitors	Alkanolamines, alkanolamine borates, sodium mercaptobenzothiazole
Extreme pressure additives	Free sulfur, sulfurized fats, chlorinated paraffinic oils, chlorinated paraffin waxes, triaryl phosphate esters, zinc dialkyldithiophosphates
Coupling agents	Aliphatic alcohols, glycols, and glycol ethers; xylenols, phenols, and cresols
Stabilizers	Copolymers of ethylene and propylene oxides, oleyl alcohol
Antifoaming agents	Silicones and waxes
Biocides	Chlorinated phenols and xylenols, formaldehyde releasers, isothiazolinones, orthophenyl phenol, sodium omadine, alkanolamine borates
Dyes	
Fragrances	

TABLE 30–2 • Composition of Water-Based Cutting Fluids

Lard was the earliest alternative to water as a cutting fluid. It was a better lubricant but a poorer coolant. Its major disadvantage was that it became rancid. When mineral oil became available in the mid-19th century, it was a natural substitute, though lard was still added to it initially to improve its machining properties. This was the prototype of present day neat (*insoluble*) oils.

By the end of the 19th century, these two lines of development had been combined to obtain the cooling property of water together with the lubricating property of oil. When lard was stirred rapidly into water containing soap and soda, an emulsion formed that was an effective cutting fluid. By the early 1900s the first emulsifiable mineral oils (*soluble oils*) came into use.

During the remainder of the 20th century, a complex technology has developed around attempts to combine as many desirable properties as

possible in single cutting fluids. Neat oils—and to a greater extent water-based fluids—have come to contain an increasing number of constituents. A simple working classification of cutting fluids is shown in Table 30–1, and examples of the possible constituents of water-based fluids are listed in Table 30–2.

The main functions and features of a satisfactory cutting fluid (Fig. 30–1) include these:

- Increased operating speed
- Improved dimensional accuracy of the workpiece
- Prolonged tool life
- Relatively cooler chip
- Removal of chips
- Improved surface finish
- Decreased energy requirement
- Long use life
- Anticorrosion properties
- Tolerable odor
- Ready disposability without pretreatment
- Economic viability

Neat (Insoluble) Oils

Neat oils are composed of naphthenic or paraffinic oils and certain additives that give them the qualities listed earlier. Fatty and synthetic oils and extreme pressure additives, similar to those listed for water-based fluids in Table 30–2, are commonly used. "Scavengers" such as epoxides may

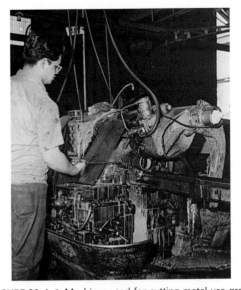

FIGURE 30–1 • Machines used for cutting metal use great quantities of cutting fluids (coolants), and some skin contact is inevitable. Automated cutting machines are widely used today, but smaller establishments still use cutting machines that involve close contact with the cutting fluids.

be added to "mop up" chlorine ions liberated from chlorinated paraffin extreme-pressure additives and thus prevent corrosion. Diluents, including kerosene, gas oil, white spirit, dipentene, and nonflammable chlorinated hydrocarbon solvents, are sometimes used to obtain lower viscosities.

Although the use of neat oils has decreased in the face of competition from water-based cutting fluids, they retain an advantage in certain machining operations and are still widely used. They are preferred, for example, when lubrication of a machining process is more important than cooling it, as in fine grinding and honing. They can be used in recycling systems in which metal fragments ("swarf") and other foreign matter are continuously removed. Biocides are not routinely required. The flammability of neat oils makes them a fire hazard.

Soluble Oils

Soluble oils are more properly called *emulsifiable* or *emulsified oils* and attract a variety of other names such as *suds, soup, slurry, mystic* (U.K.), or even *water.* They are almost always supplied to a plant or factory as concentrates, requiring emulsification in water before use, at dilutions usually between 1:10 and 1:100. This is most reliably done using purpose-made mixing valves. The emulsified micelles of mineral oil are large enough to reflect almost all incident light, and soluble oils are therefore easily recognizable by their opaque, or milky, appearance.

Soluble oils are better coolants than lubricants and, compared with neat oils, are more economical, cleaner, and safer because they do not present the same fire hazard. The addition of extreme-pressure additives improves their lubricating ability by increasing their adherence to metal surfaces. Because they contain water, corrosion inhibitors must be added to them in greater concentrations than to neat oils. Antifoaming agents, usually silicone derivatives, are also necessary because of the presence of the emulsifying agent, which tends to foam like a detergent. Various other additives are listed in Table 30–2, the most important of which from a dermatological standpoint are the biocides that have to be added to prevent microbial spoilage.[8]

Biocides are added to most soluble oil concentrates, at between 0.01% and 10%, to help control the growth of bacteria, yeasts, fungi, and algae, both before and after emulsification. Additional biocide may be added during the life of a soluble oil emulsion in use. The presence of microorganisms in soluble oils has several serious practical disadvantages, the most apparent of which are the generation of foul odors, corrosion and discolor-

ation of the workpiece, and eventually the breakdown of the emulsion ("mayonnaise effect").

Synthetics

Synthetic cutting fluids consist essentially of wetting agents and corrosion inhibitors in water. Their formulations now tend to include many more other additives than were originally used; these are similar to those employed in soluble oils, including biocides.

Synthetics have numerous advantages over both neat and soluble oils and, as a result, have been used increasingly in industry over the past 20 years. One major disadvantage, however, is their lack of lubricating ability, or oiliness, which may interfere with the smooth movement of the machine parts and the surface finish of the workpiece. Their large percentages of wetting agents are significant from a dermatological viewpoint.

Semisynthetics

Semisynthetic cutting fluids are a compromise between conventional soluble oils and chemical solutions. They can be described as emulsifiable oils containing less than 50% oily material in the concentrate. They tend to contain additives drawn from the formulations of both soluble oils and synthetics, including biocides.

Tramp Oil

Tramp oil is oil that leaks into a circulating cutting oil system from the metalworking machine's hydraulic and gearing systems. It may represent up to 2% of the cutting oil system, especially on older machines.[9]

DERMATITIS IN THE PETROLEUM INDUSTRY

Recovery

Oil folliculitis and photosensitivity can occur among oilfield workers, though contact dermatitis from crude petroleum is probably rare. Actinic keratoses and carcinomas on sun-exposed skin continue to be common cutaneous abnormalities found in oilfield workers, largely as a result of continuous and prolonged exposure to sunlight.[10] The incidence of skin cancer among Scottish shale oil workers appears to have been much reduced in the mid-20th century by the introduction of appropriate hygiene measures and workforce surveillance.[11]

Drillers are exposed to drilling muds, acids, detergents, and solvents, as well as to various insects, but their greatest hazard is injury from moving pipes and machinery. Drilling mud is subjected to temperatures of up to 200°C at the drill bit and returns to the surface commonly at 50° to 60°C, roughly the temperature of domestic hot water. Those working on the drill floor regularly become covered in drilling mud, and there is considerable opportunity for contact with unprotected skin. Irritant contact dermatitis occurs from oil-based muds, though the substitution of gas oils with "clean oils" is said to have reduced its incidence. Allergic contact dermatitis has also been reported from polyamines in the emulsifiers of oil-based muds.[11a]

Pumpers, in addition to operating the pumps and valves that control the flow of oil, collect and bottle samples of oil for laboratory analysis, examine the pipelines for leaks, and test and treat the oil to reduce its content of water and sediment. They experience little direct skin contact, however.

Acidizers and acidizer helpers operate the equipment designed to treat wells with acid to increase production. Acids (usually hydrochloric) and other chemicals are poured by hand into mixing devices and then pumped with the drilling mud into the well. The acidizers and helpers also use cement in their work for minor repair jobs at the well site. They must therefore run some risk of both irritant (acid and alkali) and allergic (chromate) contact dermatitis.

Gaugers measure oil levels in storage tanks before and immediately after the shipment of oil; they lower thermometers into tanks and pressure gauges at well sites, and they take samples of oil for analysis of water and mud content. Like pumpers, they usually experience little direct skin contact.

"Roustabouts" perform the routine duties of laborers on oil rigs and sometimes repair and maintain machinery. They may experience considerable exposure to oil and sunlight and to plants (including poison oak).

Crude oil pipelines, which connect the source of oil in the field with the distant refinery, are buried several feet beneath the ground. To protect the metal from underground corrosion, the pipe may be enveloped in a cover of asphalt, Fiberglas, and felt by a large wrapping machine, which moves along the pipe before it is placed in the ditch. The workers who operate these machines are exposed to large amounts of asphalt thrown from the whirling arms of the machine, and they uniformly exhibit marked hyperpigmentation of the skin, which is also exposed to sunlight (Fig. 30–2). They also frequently show folliculitis and contact dermatitis from contact with solvents, detergents, asphalt, and Fiberglas.

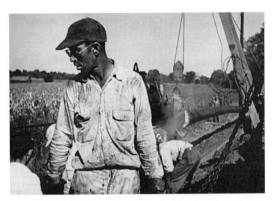

FIGURE 30–2 • Melanosis of exposed skin areas is almost inevitable in jobs such as this in which a worker is monitoring the laying of a pipeline coated with a hot petroleum-asphalt material.

Refining

In a modern refinery, much of the work is done by operators stationed at control panels, who may operate units that regulate the processing of thousands of different chemicals. In older refineries, total personnel numbered anywhere between 600 and 2,000, but because of automation, modern refineries typically operate with only 150 to 200 people. Refining and subsequent purification and blending are conducted in completely closed, complicated systems of towers, ovens, retorts, and vacuum flash units. Consequently, very little skin contact occurs during routine operations, but considerable and disastrous results may follow skin contact within these units during testing, inspection, and maintenance.

Most reports of dermatitis in today's refineries are from maintenance workers, such as electricians, carpenters, painters, welders, and boilermakers, who exhibit the dermatoses generally associated with these occupations. Contact dermatitis is occasionally reported among employees who monitor equipment and take samples for testing, and among chemists and laboratory technicians who work in research and development laboratories. It should always be remembered that considerably more skin contact occurs at the pilot plant stage of development than at the later stage of full production.

There is evidence of an excess Standardized Mortality Ratio (SMR) from malignant melanoma in several cohort studies of refinery workers.[12] The implications of this have not yet been determined.

Dermatitis from Petroleum Derivatives
Gasoline

Gasoline is a common mild irritant, especially when there is skin contact with gasoline-soaked clothing. Sufficient skin absorption can in fact be fatal.[13] Allergic contact dermatitis from gasoline is rare but has been reported, dyes or antioxidants being the causative agents.[14, 15]

Diesel Fuels

There are a number of cases of irritant contact dermatitis on record among those who have repeated contact with diesel fuel.[16] Such cases are particularly common among workers who calibrate fuel injection systems for diesel engines, and less irritating alternative fluids have been introduced as a result. Allergic contact dermatitis from isothiazolinones, used as preservatives in stored diesel fuel, has been described in a diesel mechanic.[17]

Aviation Fuels

Kerosene-type jet fuels undoubtedly have irritant potential and can cause or contribute to contact dermatitis among aircraft maintenance personnel. This can occur from working in wheel bays and other areas on aircraft that are heavily contaminated with jet fuel.

Lubricating Oils

Lubricating oils rarely seem to cause irritant contact dermatitis,[18] and reports of allergic contact dermatitis are few. In 1956, Hjorth and Brodthagen[19] reported dermatitis from a lubricating oil additive, with strong patch-test reactions. The additive was thought to be a phenolic antioxidant, but this was never confirmed by the manufacturers. The range of additives in lubricants, however, does make sensitization an occasional possibility. Burrows[20] reported chromium dermatitis in a tire fitter from chromate used as an anticorrosive in a tire-easing lubricant.

Greases

Greases rarely seem to cause contact dermatitis. If skin contact is sufficiently continuous and prolonged, the fatty acid soap content of certain greases may be capable of exerting a mild irritant effect. Again, their additives, particularly antioxidants, sometimes cause allergic contact dermatitis. Both phenyl-alpha-naphthylamine[21] and diphenylamine[22] have been reported to be contact allergens.

Automatic Transmission and Hydraulic Fluids

Automatic transmission and hydraulic fluids appear to be capable of both irritant contact dermatitis from their base oil content and allergic contact dermatitis from their additives, though published case reports are lacking.

Asphalt

Asphalt itself is a source of dermatitis, phototoxicity, and carcinogenicity, and additives such as rosin derivatives and epoxy resin can also sensitize.

Dermatitis from Cutting Fluids

The majority of metal machining is still carried out in the traditional manner, either by moving the workpiece and keeping the tool that cuts it still, as in a lathe, or by moving the tool while the workpiece is kept still, as in drilling machines. The success of these operations depends on the skills of machine tool operatives ("tool setters") in controlling and adjusting ("setting") the cutting tools. Even with an "automatic" lathe, tools have to be selected, set, and reset, or replaced during use by a tool setter. During machining operations, workpieces commonly have to be introduced and removed from the machine and checked for dimensions, while swarf routinely has to be cleared from the machining area. These duties are usually carried out by machine "operators" (distinct from setters). Since the great majority of such machine tools use high rates of flow of cutting fluid directed at the cutting tools, and splashing back tends to occur, the hands and forearms of both setters and operators can be heavily exposed to cutting oil throughout their shift, and gloves are often either unsafe or impractical to wear (Fig. 30–3).

The technology now exists to allow a workpiece to be fed to a computer-controlled machine (machining center) that orients the workpiece, selects the proper tools from storage, and carries out a series of machining operations, without the intervention of a human machine tool operative. The introduction of flexible manufacturing systems

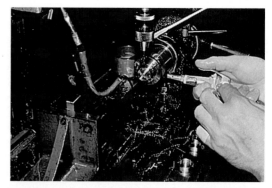

FIGURE 30–3 • During operation of cutting machines, bits of metal are blown away with an air hose, providing ample opportunity for skin contact with the cutting fluids as well as with sharp bits of metal.

(groups of computer-controlled machining centers linked by conveyors) is beginning to reduce the degree of skin contact with cutting fluids. Electronic plugboard–controlled lathes have already become more widely distributed, and they assist in reducing the degree of skin contact, though even flexible manufacturing systems tend to require swarf clearance and other periodic interventions that serve to maintain some degree of cutting fluid contact.

In the United States today there are approximately a half million machine tool operatives and, counting laborers, inspectors, assemblers, engineers, and others, a total of approximately 2 million workers who are exposed to some degree to cutting fluids. In regions of the country where engineering industries are concentrated, dermatitis caused by petroleum products may account for as many as 15% to 20% of reported cases of occupational skin disease. These figures are likely to be closely reflected in many other industrialized countries. Many of these operatives work in small factories where understanding of the dermatitis hazard of cutting fluids is generally poor.

One common factor in the causation of practically all forms of cutting oil dermatitis is likely to be mechanical trauma, not only visible lacerations but also scarcely perceptible friction and microtrauma.[23] The gradual buildup of such damage to the skin over many years is perhaps one of the reasons why dermatitis from water-based cutting fluids can occur for the first time in experienced workers *or* inexperienced ones.

Water-Based Cutting Fluids

Soluble oils, synthetics, and semisynthetics are similar in this respect: they all tend to cause an eczematous dermatitis, but not oil acne or folliculitis. The extent to which they cause contact dermatitis depends on many factors (Table 30–3), the most important of which is always likely to be the precise degree of skin contact. There is a world of difference, for example, between the exposure to soluble oil of a setter and that of a storeman on the same production line, the storeman being very unlikely to develop contact dermatitis from the cutting fluid and the setter being at high risk of doing so.

Irritation from water-based fluids is a major factor in the majority of cases of contact dermatitis. This irritation is caused principally by surfactants (emulsifiers or wetting agents) in their formulations. The damage that such surfactants inflict on the skin goes much deeper than the superficial "defatting" action that is frequently ascribed to them; damage to cell membranes deep in the epidermis and dermal disruption also occur. Such

TABLE 30–3 • Some Causative Factors of Water-Based Cutting Fluid Dermatitis

Man	Machine
Individual susceptibility	Machine type
Protective clothing	Control method
Barrier cream	Fixed features design
Conditioning cream	Alterable features design
Skin cleansers	Ease of cleaning sump
Systems of work and payment	**Water-Based Cutting Fluid**
Work habits	
Psychosocial	Chronic irritancy of surfactants
Unfamiliarity	Wetting and drying cycles
Other disability	Alkalinity
Other	Microtrauma from metal fragments
General factory environment	Cutting fluid type
Climate	Strength when made up
	Strength with use
	Deterioration with use
	Biocide addition in use
	Contact sensitizers

irritation is encouraged when concentrations are too strong—because they were improperly mixed or water was allowed to evaporate during use.[24]

There is no doubt, however, that the more scrupulously sensitization to additives in these fluids is sought, the more often it is found.[25] When such allergy is found by careful patch testing, it is usually impossible to know for sure how much *allergenicity* was responsible for the dermatitis and how much *irritancy* of the same cutting fluid, preceding, accompanying, or following the sensitization, was responsible. The prognosis for the more severe cases of dermatitis from water-based cutting fluids is often poor, sometimes even when an allergen is identified and an allergen-free cutting fluid is substituted for the original. In the absence of sensitization, however, the milder forms of irritant contact dermatitis can have a good prognosis, clearance often occurring without any loss of time from work.[26]

Additives known to be potential sensitizers in water-based cutting fluids are listed elsewhere in this text, the most frequent of which are the various biocides. The Grotan and Bioban ranges of biocides, mainly formaldehyde releasers, have featured most often in reports, along with the isothiazolinones, including also Proxels[27, 28] and Kathons. Patients allergic to formaldehyde releasers are often also allergic to formaldehyde,[29] but not always.[30]

The Grotan range includes these compounds:

- Grotan BK. Active ingredient: hexahydro-1,3,5-tris(2-hydroxyethyl)-*sym*-triazine.[31–38]
- Grotan HD. Active ingredient: *N*-methylol-chloroacetamide.[39]
- Grotan HD-2. Active ingredients: 2-chloro-*N*-(hydroxymethyl) acetamide; sodium tetraborate; potassium iodide.
- Grotan K and TK2. Active ingredients: 5-chloro-2-methyl-4-isothiazolin-3-one; 2-methyl-4-isothiazolin-3-one.

Eliminating all Grotans from coolant led to the clearance of dermatitis in patients who on patch testing reacted to formaldehyde but not to Grotans BK, OX, or TK2.[40]

The Bioban range includes the following compounds:

- Bioban P-1487. Active ingredients: 4-(2-nitrobutyl)morpholine; 4,4′-(2-ethyl-2-nitrotrimethylene)-dimorpholine.[41, 42]
- Bioban CS-1246. Active ingredient: 5-ethyl-1-aza-3,7-dioxabicyclo-3,3,0-octane.[29]
- Bioban CS-1248. Mixture of Bioban P-1487 and CS-1246.
- Bioban CS-1135. Active ingredients: 4,4-dimethyloxazolidine; 3,4,4-trimethyloxazolidine.

The active ingredient of Proxels is 1,2-benzisothiazolin-3-one. The active ingredients of Kathons are 5-chloro-2-methyl-4-isothiazolin-3-one and 2-methyl-4-isothiazolin-3-one together, or 2-*n*-octyl-4-isothiazolin-3-one alone. The Proxel isothiazolinone does not appear to cross-react with the Kathon isothiazolinones.

Other biocides reported during the past decade to be sensitizers include the formaldehyde releaser 2-hydroxy-methyl-amino-ethanol-tri-*N*-ethyl-hydroxy-2-amino-methylene (Forcide 78)[43]; 1-H benzotriazole[44]; *o*-phenylphenol (Dowicide 1)[45]; *p*-chloro-*m*-xylenol[46]; 2-(hydroxymethyl)-2-nitro-1,3-propanediol (Tris Nitro)[47]; and alkanolamine borates.[48]

Colophony sensitization is a particular problem for machine operatives because of the widespread use of fatty acids derived from wood rosin and tall oil in emulsifiers.[49] Sensitization to mercaptobenzothiazole (MBT)[50] is related to a much more limited range of water-based cutting fluids, particularly those used for metals containing copper. Oleyl alcohol (octadecanol), used to improve the solubility of other constituents in the finished product, has been reported to be a sensitizer.[51]

Machine operatives may also demonstrate allergy to nickel, chromium, and cobalt as a result of the leaching out of such metals by the cutting fluid during machining operations.[52–59] Ordinarily,

the levels of sensitizing metals in cutting fluids are too low to pose much of a threat of sensitization, though they are more likely to be causal in a previously sensitized person. The machining of alloys particularly high in the same metals can, however, release much higher levels.

There is no evidence that the microorganisms that proliferate in water-based cutting fluids themselves cause dermatitis by colonizing the skin,[60] though they might perhaps be capable of rendering the fluid more irritating because their metabolic activity lowers the pH or perhaps even because of release of bacterial exotoxins and endotoxins. When infected dermatitis does occur, the pathogenic organisms almost invariably are derived from the worker's own skin, nose, or throat. Opportunistic infections from cutting fluid microorganisms could, however, be a risk for immunodeficient or immunodepressed persons.

While there is no doubt that contact dermatitis from water-based cutting fluids may present in an enormous variety of clinical patterns, including even "dyshidrotic" eczema,[61] one particularly common presentation is patchy low-grade eczema of the backs of the hands, fronts of the wrists, and forearms, which can sometimes resemble discoid or nummular eczema and so escape diagnosis.[62]

Outbreaks of contact dermatitis from water-based cutting fluids occur in both large and small engineering factories, and the causes are often hard to identify.[63] Usually, however, such outbreaks arise against a background of an endemic lower prevalence of dermatitis that comes to be accepted as part of the job. Such background levels can involve as many as a third of the workforce with some degree of dermatitis during the course of a single year.[26]

Neat Oils

Although neat oils are used much less frequently than in the past, they are still responsible for numerous cases of dermatitis today. The most common skin abnormality seen from contact with these oils is folliculitis (oil acne), which results from chemical irritation of the follicular canal, provoking keratotic plugging (Fig. 30–4). Bacterial infection plays no primary role, though it may arise secondarily. Folliculitis develops in workers soon after initial exposure, usually appearing first on the extensor surfaces of the forearms and the dorsa of the hands and fingers in the form of open comedones or blackheads. The abdomen and anterior thighs are also commonly affected from contact with oil-soaked clothing. Comedones are present, in addition to numerous pruritic and erythematous perifollicular papules and pustules. Melanoderma may develop later. Persons with

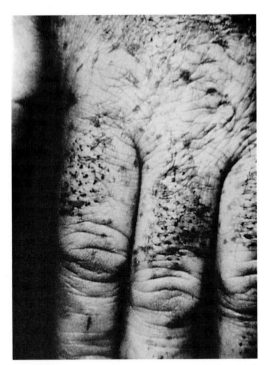

FIGURE 30–4 • Blackened comedones are a hallmark of oil exposure.

acne, large follicular openings, or heavy hair growth are more susceptible to folliculitis from neat oils. Machines with high cutting speeds and heavy oil flow, such as automatic lathes, increase the degree of exposure to cutting oil and thus pose the greatest risk.[64] Oil folliculitis can also occur from spraying the molds of prefabricated concrete with mineral oil.[65]

Although oil folliculitis can persist for months, time is rarely lost from work, and many workers frequently dismiss the condition as inconsequential. The main contributing factors to all cases of folliculitis are poor personal hygiene, failure to wear clean clothing daily, poor factory housekeeping, and substandard or nonfunctioning guarding of the machines. Inadequate supervision of workers and lack of adequate washing facilities nearby are also important.

Oil folliculitis must be differentiated from acne vulgaris, chloracne, drug eruptions, furunculosis, irritation from glass fiber, miliaria pustulosa, foreign body granulomas, and papulonecrotic syphilis.

Oil folliculitis can readily be distinguished from acne vulgaris because of the characteristic distribution of oil folliculitis, which localizes in body areas not commonly involved by acne, such as the abdomen and anterior thighs. Also, men over 30 years of age rarely develop widespread acne. Pru-

ritus sometimes is a clue to folliculitis. Chloracne develops more slowly, the lesions being deeper, more keratotic and hyperplastic. The "malar crescent," postauricular areas, and genitals are favored sites. Hepatic abnormalities sometimes are associated. Chloracne from cutting oils is almost never seen today,[65a] because chlorinated biphenyls are no longer used.[66] The melanosis resulting from contact with mineral oil (see Fig. 30–2) may be mistaken for hyperpigmentation after some nonoccupational dermatitis, melasma, a drug reaction, or Addison's disease.

Treatment of oil folliculitis is usually uncomplicated, as most cases clear rapidly and will not recur if proper cleaning methods are adopted. Some cases may require additional treatment of secondary bacterial infection. The work area should be inspected regularly to ensure that the machines are operated safely and that the operators wear proper protective clothing.

Neat oils also cause eczematous dermatitis, though much less often than water-based cutting fluids. The lesion is most often chronic irritant contact dermatitis, the irritancy of paraffinic oils being inversely related to their boiling range, and naphthenic and aromatic fractions having enhanced irritancy.[67] Sensitization to components of neat oils also (more rarely) occurs, sometimes to small amounts of additives such as epoxides.[68, 69] Dipentene has been reported to sensitize honing machinists.[70] The antioxidant tertiary-butylhydroquinone (TBHQ) has been identified as a cause of allergic contact dermatitis from a vegetable oil–based cutting fluid.[71]

Cutting oils, neat oils much more than soluble oils,[72] have also caused squamous cell carcinoma of the skin.[73] This was first recognized well before World War II,[74] but after the war became increasingly so.[75–77] Squamous cell carcinomas were produced on the skin of mice following repeated applications of cutting oils.[78] Polycyclic aromatic hydrocarbons have been shown to be carcinogenic.[79] The latent period before development of skin cancer may be as long as 20 to 25 years.[80] Thus, patients can still present from exposure at work before solvent-refined mineral oil was generally introduced in cutting fluids to diminish the levels of polycyclic aromatic hydrocarbons. When such cases occur in retired machine operatives, the fact that they were work related may be overlooked and go unreported.

Depigmentation of the hands of workers employed in a tappet assembly plant was caused by oils used to machine and test the tappets (valve lifters). Of the 270 workers in this plant, 60% had dermatitis, but only four showed depigmentation, some with widespread areas of involvement. The causative agent, confirmed by animal testing, was 4-*tert*-butylcatechol, used as an antioxidant in the oil.[81]

Prevention

The following general measures may help to prevent dermatitis caused by cutting fluids. Table 30–3 suggests further specific measures for water-based cutting fluids.

Substitution. If sensitization has occurred, ideally, the coolant responsible for the dermatitis should be replaced with one that does not contain the offending allergen (or is itself modified by allergen replacement). It will require several days to flush all traces of the coolant out of the system, and the worker should be cautioned not to return to the machine before this has been accomplished.

Maintenance of a Clean Environment. Splash guards, shields, and other machine parts that regularly come into contact with the skin should be kept free of oil and cleaned down regularly with disposable paper wipes, which should be discarded immediately and never kept in pockets.

Protection. Gloves, gauntlets, and aprons can provide protection if kept clean, but often they cannot safely be worn because of the danger of becoming caught in the machinery. Although the job may progress somewhat more slowly, workers willing to wear gloves for certain tasks, such as changing cutting tools, will decrease their chances of developing dermatitis.

Skin Cleansing. Barrier cream applied before work, appropriate skin cleansers, and conditioning cream applied after work together serve to promote effective skin cleansing while reducing associated skin damage. Waterless skin cleaners are preferable to organic solvents for removing oil from the skin.

Preplacement Recommendations. Workers with chronic hand eczema of any cause, and especially those with a history of atopic dermatitis, should not be trained as machinists in the engineering industry.

References

1. Schoonmaker GR. Oil and gas, offshore. In: *McGraw-Hill Encyclopedia of Science and Technology,* 7th ed. Vol. 12. New York: McGraw-Hill; 1992:308–310.
2. Speight JG. Petroleum products. In: *McGraw-Hill Encyclopedia of Science and Technology,* 7th ed. Vol 13. New York: McGraw-Hill; 1992:297–299.
3. Schmerling L. Petroleum: characteristics. In: *McGraw-Hill Encyclopedia of Science and Technology,* 7th ed. Vol.13. New York: McGraw-Hill; 1992:284–285.
4. Doscher TM. Oil and gas well completion, oil and gas well drilling. In: *McGraw-Hill Encyclopedia of Science and Technology,* 7th ed. Vol. 12. New York: McGraw-Hill; 1992:320–329.
5. Alvarez A. *Offshore: A North Sea Journey.* London: Hodder and Stoughton; 1986.
6. Speight JG. Petroleum processing. In: *McGraw-Hill Encyclopedia of Science and Technology,* 7th ed. Vol. 13. New York: McGraw-Hill; 1992:293–297.
7. *Concawe Report No. 5/87: Health Aspects of Lubricants.* The Hague: Concawe; 1987.
8. Rossmore HW. Antimicrobial agents for water-based metal working fluids. *J Occup Med* 1981; 23:247–254.
9. Welter ES. Manufacturing exposure to coolants and lubricants. *J Occup Med* 1978; 20:535–538.
10. Gusein-Zade KM. Characteristics of dermatoses morbidity in workers of Apsheron oilfields in relation to physicochemical properties of the petroleum produced. *Vestn Dermatol Venereol* 1982; 9:63–66.
11. Seaton A, Louw SJ, Cowie HA. Epidemiologic studies of Scottish oil shale workers: 1. Prevalence of skin disease and pneumoconiosis. *Am J Industr Med* 1986; 9:409–421.
11a. Ormerod AD, Wakeel RA, Mann TAN, et al. Polyamine sensitization in offshore workers handling drilling muds. *Contact Dermatitis* 1989; 21:326–329.
12. *Concawe Report No. 2/87: The Health Experience of Workers in the Petroleum Manufacturing and Distribution Industry.* The Hague: Concawe; 1987.
13. Walsh WA, Scarpa FJ, Brown RS, et al. Gasoline immersion burn. *N Engl J Med* 1974; 291:830.
14. Garcia-Perez A, Aparicio M. Dermatitis from dye in petrol. *Contact Dermatitis* 1975; 1:265.
15. Lamb JH, Lain ES. Occurrence of contact dermatitis from oil soluble gasoline dyes. *J Invest Dermatol* 1951; 17:141–146.
16. Fischer T, Bjarnason B. Sensitizing and irritant properties of 3 environmental classes of diesel oil and their indicator dyes. *Contact Dermatitis* 1996; 34:309–315.
17. Bruynzeel DP, Verbrugh CA. Occupational dermatitis from isothiazolinones in diesel oil. *Contact Dermatitis* 1996; 34:64–65.
18. Burrows D. Contact dermatitis to machine oil in hosiery workers. *Contact Dermatitis* 1980; 6:10.
19. Hjorth N, Brodthagen H. Contact dermatitis from lubricating oil additives. *Acta Dermatol Venereol* 1956; 36:146–149.
20. Burrows D. Chromium dermatitis in a tyre fitter. *Contact Dermatitis* 1981; 7:55–56.
21. Boman A, Hagelthorn G, Jeansson I, et al. Phenyl-alpha-naphthylamine—case report and guinea pig studies. *Contact Dermatitis* 1980; 6:299–300.
22. Herve-Bazin B, Foussereau J, Cavelier C. Allergy to diphenylamine in an industrial grease. *Contact Dermatitis* 1986; 14:116.
23. Kligman AM, Klemme JC, Susten AS, eds. The chronic effects of repeated mechanical trauma to the skin. *Am J Industr Med* 1985; 8:257–264.
24. Wigger-Alberti W, Hinnen U, Elsner P. Predictive testing of metalworking fluids: a comparison of 2 cumulative human irritation models and correlation to epidemiological data. *Contact Dermatitis* 1997; 36:14–20.
25. English JSC, Rycroft RJG. Cutting oil dermatitis: a review of 115 patients. In: Frosch PJ, Dooms-Goossens A, Lachapelle J-M, et al, eds. *Current Topics in Contact Dermatitis.* Berlin: Springer-Verlag; 1989:212–215.
26. Rycroft RJG. Soluble oil as major cause of occupational dermatitis. Cambridge: Cambridge University; 1982 [MD dissertation].
27. Brown R. Concomitant sensitization to additives in a coolant fluid. *Contact Dermatitis* 1979; 5:340–341.
28. Alomar A, Conde-Salazar L, Romaguera C. Occupational dermatoses from cutting oils. *Contact Dermatitis* 1985; 12:129–138.

29. Dahlquist I. Contact allergy to the cutting oil preservatives Bioban CS-1246 and P-1487. *Contact Dermatitis* 1984; 10:46.

30. Wrangsjö K, Martensson A, Widstrom L, et al. Contact dermatitis from Bioban P-1487. *Contact Dermatitis* 1986; 14:182–183.

31. Düngemann H, Borelli S, Reber E. Kontaktallergien gegen eine Gruppe neuer Desinfektionsmittel. *Medsche Klin* 1964; 59:170–175.

32. Rietschel E. Erfahrungen aus der werksärztlichen Praxis über Hautschaden bei Nasschleifern. *Berufsdermatosen* 1964; 12:284–291.

33. Schneider W, Huber M, Kwokzek JJ, et al. Weitere Untersuchungen zur Frage der Hautverträglichkeit hochverdünnter Kuhlmittel. *Berufsdermatosen* 1965; 13:65–85.

34. Keczkes K, Brown PM. Hexahydro, 1,3,5 tris(2-hydroxyethyl)triazine, a new bacteriocidal agent as a cause of allergic contact dermatitis. *Contact Dermatitis* 1976; 2:92–98.

35. Hesbert A, Darrigrand MC, Lemonnier M, et al. Study of bacterial contamination of cutting fluids: efficiency of preservatives on micro-organisms. *Arch Maladies Professionnelles* 1977; 38:569–579.

36. Poitou P, Marignac B. Sensitizing effect of Grotan BK in the guinea pig. *Contact Dermatitis* 1978; 4:116.

37. Rycroft RJG. Is Grotan BK a contact sensitizer? *Br J Dermatol* 1978; 99:346–347.

38. Dahl MGC. Patch test concentrations of Grotan BK. *Br J Dermatol* 1981; 104:607.

39. Hjorth N. *N*-methylol-chloracetamide, a sensitizer in coolant oils and cosmetics. *Contact Dermatitis* 1979; 5:330–331.

40. van Ketel WG, Kisch LS. The problem of the sensitizing capacity of some Grotans used as bacteriocides in cooling oils. *Dermatosen* 1983; 31:118–121.

41. Gruvberger B, Bruze M. Contact allergy to 4-(2-nitrobutyl)-morpholine and 4,4′-(2-ethyl-2-nitrotrimethylene)-dimorpholine as active ingredients of a preservative recommended for metalworking fluids in the guinea pig. *Dermatosen* 1995; 43:126–128.

42. Gruvberger B, Bruze M, Zimerson E. Contact allergy to the active ingredients of Bioban P 1487. *Contact Dermatitis* 1996; 35:141–145.

43. Hamann K. Forcide 78—another formaldehyde releaser in a coolant oil. *Contact Dermatitis* 1980; 6:446.

44. Ducombs G, Tamisier JM, Texier L. Contact dermatitis to 1-H benzotriazole. *Contact Dermatitis* 1980; 6:224–225.

45. Adams RM. Allergic contact dermatitis due to *o*-phenylphenol. *Contact Dermatitis* 1981; 7:332.

46. Adams RM. *p*-Chloro-*m*-xylenol in cutting fluids: two cases of allergic contact dermatitis in machinists. *Contact Dermatitis* 1981; 7:341–342.

47. Robertson MH, Storrs FJ. Allergic contact dermatitis in two machinists. *Arch Dermatol* 1982; 118:997–1002.

48. Bruze M, Hradile E, Eriksohn I-L, et al. Occupational allergic contact dermatitis from alkanolamine borates in metalworking fluids. *Contact Dermatitis* 1995; 32:24–27.

49. Fregert S. Colophony in cutting oil and soap water used as a cutting fluid. *Contact Dermatitis* 1979; 5:52.

50. Fregert S, Skog E. Allergic contact dermatitis from mercaptobenzothiazole in cutting oils. *Acta Dermatol Venereol* 1962; 42:235–238.

51. Koch P. Occupational allergic contact dermatitis from oleyl alcohol and monoethanolamine in a metalworking fluid. *Contact Dermatitis* 1995; 33:273.

52. Arndt KA. Cutting fluids and the skin. *Cutis* 1969; 5:143–146.

53. Gellin GA. Is a dermatitis-free cutting oil possible? *J Occup Med* 1969; 11:128–131.

54. Hodgson G. Cutaneous hazards of lubricants. *Industr Med* 1970; 39:68–73.

55. Samitz MH. Effects of metal working fluids on the skin. *Prog Dermatol* 1974; 8:11–15.

56. Einarsson Ö, Kylin B, Lindstedt G, et al. Chromium, cobalt and nickel in used cutting fluids. *Contact Dermatitis* 1975; 1:182–183.

57. Samitz MH, Katz SA. Skin hazards from nickel and chromium salts in association with cutting oil operations. *Contact Dermatitis* 1975; 1:158–160.

58. Fregert S, Gruvberger B. Chromate dermatitis from oil emulsion contaminated from zinc-galvanized iron plate. *Contact Dermatitis* 1976; 2:121.

59. Wahlberg JE, Lindstedt G, Einarsson Ö. Chromium, cobalt and nickel in Swedish cement, detergents, mould and cutting oils. *Berufsdermatosen* 1977; 25:220–228.

60. Rycroft RJG. Bacteria and soluble oil dermatitis. *Contact Dermatitis* 1980; 6:7–9.

61. de Boer EM, Bruynzeel DP, van Ketel WG. Dyshidrotic eczema as an occupational dermatitis in metalworkers. *Contact Dermatitis* 1988; 19:184–188.

62. Rycroft RJG. Soluble oil dermatitis. *Clin Exp Dermatol* 1981; 6:229–234.

63. Järvholm B, Ljungkvist G, Lavenius B, Rodin N, Peterson C. Acetic aldehyde and formaldehyde in cutting fluids and their relation to irritant symptoms. *Ann Occup Hyg* 1995; 39:591–601.

64. Finnie JS. Oil folliculitis: a study of 200 men employed in an engineering factory. *Br J Industr Med* 1960; 17:130–140.

65. Farkas I. Oil acne from mineral oil among workers making prefabricated concrete panels. *Contact Dermatitis* 1982; 8:141.

65a. Key MM, Ritter EJ, Arndt KA. Cutting and grinding fluids and their effects on the skin. *Am Industr Hyg Assoc J* 1966; 27:423–427.

66. Crow KD. The engineering and chemical aspects of soluble coolant oils. *Br J Dermatol* 1981; 105[suppl 21]:11–18.

67. Klauder JV, Brill FA. Correlation of boiling ranges of some petroleum solvents with irritant action on the skin. *Arch Dermatol Syph NY* 1947; 56:197–215.

68. English JSC, Foulds I, White IR, et al. Allergic contact sensitization to the glycidyl ester of hexahydrophthalic acid in a cutting oil. *Contact Dermatitis* 1986; 15:66–68.

69. Scerri L, Dalziel KL. Occupational contact sensitization to the stabilized chlorinated paraffin fraction in neat cutting oil. *Am J Contact Dermatitis* 1996; 7:35–37.

70. Rycroft RJG. Allergic contact dermatitis from dipentene in honing oil. *Contact Dermatitis* 1980; 6:325–329.

71. Meding B. Occupational contact dermatitis from tertiary-butylhydroquinone (TBHQ) in a cutting fluid. *Contact Dermatitis* 1996; 34:224.

72. Järvholm B, Lavenius B. Mortality and cancer morbidity in workers exposed to cutting fluids. *Arch Environ Health* 1987; 42:361–366.

73. Waldron HA. A brief history of scrotal cancer. *Br J Industr Med* 1983; 40:390–401.

74. Prosser-White R. *The Dermatergoses*, 4th ed. London: HK Lewis; 1934.

75. Cruikshank CND, Squire JR. Skin cancer in engineering industry from use of mineral oil. *Br J Industr Med* 1950; 7:1–11.

76. Cruikshank CND, Gourevitch A. Skin cancer of the hands and forearms. *Br J Industr Med* 1952; 9:74–79.

77. Mastromatteo E. Cutting oils and squamous cell carcinoma. Part I. Incidence in plant with report of six cases. *Br J Industr Med* 1955; 12:240–243.

78. Gilman JPW, Vesselinovitch SD. Cutting oil and squamous

cell carcinoma. Part II. Experimental study of carcinogenicity of two types of cutting oils. *Br J Industr Med* 1955; 12:244–248.

79. Fulk HL, Hotin P, Mehler A. Polycyclic hydrocarbons as carcinogens for man. *Arch Environ Health* 1964; 8:721–730.

80. Emmett EA. Occupational skin cancer: a review. *J Occup Med* 1975; 17:44–49.

81. Gellin GA, Possick PA, Davis IH. Occupational depigmentation due to 4-tertiarybutyl catechol (TBC). *J Occup Med* 1970; 12:386–389.

Plants and Woods

31

KATHRYN A. ZUG, M.D.
JAMES G. MARKS, JR, M.D.

Dermatitis as a consequence of occupational exposure to plants and woods is addressed in this chapter. We open with a brief review of taxonomy, followed by a discussion of several types of dermatoses caused by plants, epidemiology, occupations at risk, and general testing principles. The chapter focuses primarily on commonly reported plant and wood species and information about their role in occupational allergic contact dermatitis.

TAXONOMY

Plant taxonomy can be confusing if one is not a botanist. In 1735, the Swedish naturalist Carl Linnaeus developed the first systematic and widely applied classification of plants. His system grouped plants according to morphological similarities. Linnaeus' system of nomenclature was binomial: each plant was given two names, a generic (genus) name, followed by a specific (species) name. Present-day classifications consider plant biochemistry, genetics, cytology, and anatomy. Today, identification of a plant and its proper name are derived from the *International Code of Botanical Nomenclature*. Such a classification system allows plants to be aligned in groupings that in many cases have an evolutionary relationship, often sharing biochemical similarities.[1, 2]

Most plants relevant to a discussion of occupational dermatoses are in the major plant group Spermatophyta, which is divided into two parts, the Angiosperms, or flowering plants, and the Gymnosperms, among others the conifers. Angiosperms are divided into two classes based on the character of the first seed leaves. The Monocotyledons have one first leaf (cotyledon) on germination, and Dicotyledons have two. Most publications of relevance to this subject confine the discussion of plant taxonomy to family, genus, and species, in addition to the common (colloquial or vernacular) names of plants. Members of a plant family share some defining characteristic. The suffix *-aceae* (for example, Anacardiaceae), or sometimes *-ae*, is appended to most names of plant families. There may be one genus or several genera in a family. Since most laypersons use common, vernacular terms when referring to particular plants, it is often important to know both the scientific, binomial, and the vernacular names for a given plant. In binomial nomenclature, the genus of a plant is followed by the species name. By convention, the genus and species are italicized (e.g., the scientific name for the climbing type of poison ivy is *Toxicodendron radicans*). The family of the plant may also be cited. An initial or a surname often follows the scientific name and indicates the botanist who named the species, (e.g., in the scientific name for wild feverfew, *Parthenium hysterophorus* L., the L. is for Linnaeus). Specific cultivars are given varietal names by their cultivators.

To avoid confusion, appropriate identification of a particular plant should use the accepted scientific name. Most classification schemes are based on a plant's flowers, though the leaf shape, margination, venation, surface features, and leaves' relationship to one another and to the stem are also important for proper classification. The stem, fruit, and seed may also be useful in identifying a particular plant. Plants collected for identification should include these vital parts; they are best collected at the time of flowering. Professional or university botanists, master gardeners, and state or federal agricultural extensions can be helpful resources for proper plant identification.

Once collected, a plant specimen should be kept

moist and transported in an airtight container. Some experts advise freezing a plant for further study if the quantity is limited. Placing plant leaves and flowers onto absorbent paper and pressing them facilitates drying when immediate use or identification is not possible. Mitchell and Rook recommend dividing plant material into three parts which are then used, respectively, for identification, testing, and making plant extracts.[3]

WHEN TO SUSPECT PLANT DERMATITIS

Exposure history, and distribution and morphology of lesions may lead to a suspicion of plant-induced dermatitis. Exacerbations of dermatitis that correlate with workplace exposures, and clearing or improvement during periods away from work such as vacations suggest an occupational relationship. In many cases, exposure to certain plants is seasonal, and dermatitis may initially occur on a seasonal basis. However, with time and repeated episodes, a dermatitis can evolve into a chronic problem, and then a seasonal relationship may no longer be obvious. Occupationally related exposures to plants may be intentional and recognized or incidental and unrecognized. A florist working with *Alstroemeria* may be an example of the former, whereas a sawyer or woodsman who becomes sensitized to *Frullania* is an example of the latter.

A particular pattern of dermatitis may provide the strongest clue to the astute clinician. Linear streaks, large bullae, and weeping acute eczematous dermatitis on exposed skin is a well-known presentation of poison ivy dermatitis (Fig. 31–1). Other typical distributions of a plant-related dermatitis include the airborne distribution, characterized by dermatitis of the face, including eyelids, submental skin and exposed V of the neck, postauricular skin, including the postauricular triangle and posterior neck, and exposed hands and arms (Figs. 31–2). In some cases, a worker may present with a patchy facial and hand dermatitis. Another well-recognized pattern of plant dermatitis is tender, cracked, fissured, and erythematous fingertip dermatitis, a pattern described in tulip bulb and garlic handlers (Fig. 31–3). Any of these presentations plus known exposure should prompt suspicion of a plant dermatitis and further evaluation (Table 31–1).

WHO GETS IT? WHO IS AT RISK?

Many occupations involve exposure to plants, woods, and their products (Table 31–2). Forestry

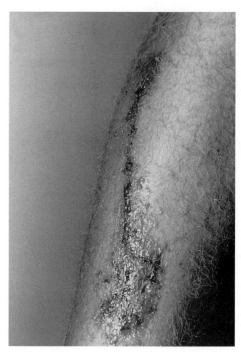

FIGURE 31–1 • Poison ivy dermatitis: typical linear vesicles and bullae.

workers, firefighters, landscapers, gardeners, florists, nursery workers, rural outdoor workers, food handlers, botanists, and horticulturists are among those most commonly reported at risk for plant-related dermatitis (phytodermatitis). The risk of developing dermatitis from occupational exposure to plants of any type is not accurately known. Studies are apt to underestimate the true incidence, as plant dermatitis may often go unsuspected by both the worker and the evaluating physician.[4] Additionally, dermatitis from a plant *known* to cause reactions often does not prompt a worker to seek medical treatment.

Agricultural Workers

Agriculture has consistently ranked highest among occupations that carry risk for skin disease. A study of California agricultural workers' time lost reported on compensation claims to the California Department of Industrial Relations between 1978 and 1983 demonstrated 2,722 claims for lost work time for skin disease among 2,355,802 agricultural workers. In the claims data studied for this period, more reported cases involved plants (52.1%) than chemical exposures (20.4%) or food products (12.5%). Forestry workers were the agricultural subdivision with the highest claims rate for skin disease related to plants (53.5 cases per 10,000 employed). Other agricultural jobs with elevated

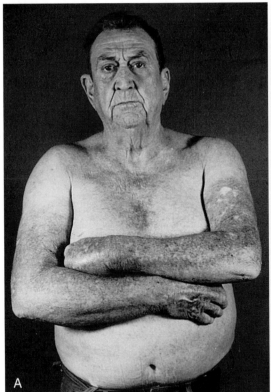
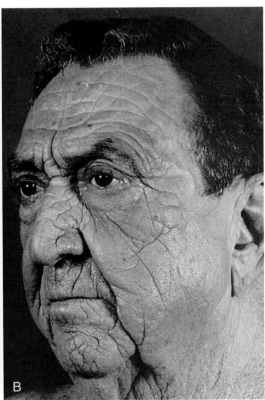

FIGURE 31–2A and B • Chronic, lichenified dermatitis on the face and exposed skin typical of an airborne distribution, presumably from dried, wind-borne particulate plant dust. This patient was allergic to Compositae plants and had concomitant photosensitivity.

claims rates for plant-related skin disease included landscaping services (35.9 per 10,000 workers), horticultural specialties (15.9), soil preparation services (9.9), general livestock farms (9.6), and animal specialties (7.6).[5] Including only reported cases involving at least 1 day lost from work and reported through claims data, this study provides some useful descriptive epidemiology. Such population-based data are difficult to obtain; however,

they too probably underrepresent the extent of occupational plant dermatoses. Pesticides are commonly used in agriculture and may confound the diagnosis of dermatitis in agricultural workers.[6]

The states of Oregon, Washington, and Ohio have been involved in a research program sponsored by the National Institute for Occupational Safety and Health (NIOSH) that is designed to reduce occupational dermatitis through a surveillance system and systematic collection of risk factor data. A retrospective analysis of 5 years (1988 to 1992) of Oregon Workers' Compensation Division's claims files found plant materials to be

FIGURE 31–3 • A dry, fissured dermatitis of the fingertips is classic for contact allergy to tulip bulbs.

TABLE 31–1 • Findings That Suggest Plant Dermatitis
Plant exposure through work or hobby
Distribution of lesions
Linear
Airborne
Patchy on hands and face
Fingertips
Seasonal lesions at first, then chronic ones

![icon] TABLE 31–2 • **Occupations Associated with Risk**	
Plant-Related Dermatitis	**Wood-Related Dermatitis**
Aromatherapist/ massage therapist	Cabinetmaker
	Boatbuilder
Bartender	Carpenter
Caterer	Instrument maker
Farmer	Flooring worker
Floral arranger/ florist	Framer
	Logger
Food cultivators, picker	Musician
Food handler	Sander
Forester	Sawyer
Greengrocer/market gardener	Turner
Landscaper	
Logger	
Nursery worker	

second only to chemicals as a source of claims for occupational dermatitis (44.1% versus 14.1% of 2,464 claims for lost work time due to dermatitis over 5 years). Farm workers and gardeners accounted for 75% of the accepted claims among agricultural workers. Contact with vegetation, including poisonous plants, accounted for 63% of cases among agricultural workers.[7] Similarly, the Sensor Dermatitis Project in Washington State has compared physician-reported data on work-related skin disorders with workers' compensation claims data from 1990 to 1997. Thus far, absent from the early sentinel event data supplied by physicians over a 2-year period of reporting are plants and vegetation, whereas the workers' compensation claims analysis done over a 7-year period has found vegetation to be the third most common source of dermatitis (8.1% of total). Chemicals and soaps and detergents accounted for 25.6% and 14.4% of the total number of cases, respectively.[8]

The prevalence of occupational contact allergy to plants has been studied, but estimates are likely low, given the referral bias of patients selected from large patch test clinic populations, and often the limited tests performed in screening patch test series. In 1994, 4.4% of occupational allergic contact dermatitis in Finland was caused by plants.[9]

During the period from 1990 to 1993, The Finnish Register of Occupational Diseases identified 22 cases of allergy to decorative plants, 1.4% of the 1,567 patients with occupational allergic contact dermatitis. From 1979 to 1993, the Finnish Institute of Occupational Health diagnosed 12 cases of occupational allergic contact dermatitis caused by decorative plants. Plant families implicated over this 14-year period included Composi-

tae (five patients with reactions to chrysanthemum, elecampane, gerbera, or feverfew), Alstroemeriaceae (five patients to *Alstroemeria*), Liliaceae (four patients to tulips and hyacinth), Amaryllidaceae (two patients to daffodil), and Caryophyllaceae (two patients to carnation or cauzeflower). Allergic patients were middle aged and had notably long average exposure time (13 years). Seven of 12 allergic patients could continue working, but five could not because of persistent, severe symptoms.

Florists and Nursery Workers

Hand dermatitis is a significant occupational problem for floral workers. Erythema and fissuring of the hands are often associated with the irritant effects of constant water exposure. The most frequent allergens for florists who design and arrange displays are *Alstroemeria* and chrysanthemums (*Dendranthema grandiflora*). One survey conducted among 20 floral shop workers in the United States yielded a dermatitis prevalence of 26% over 12 months.[10] A cross-sectional study of florists in Lisbon, Portugal found a similar prevalence of dermatitis, 29.8%.[11] The workers surveyed by questionnaire most frequently implicated cedar of florists, chrysanthemum, and *Dieffenbachia* as aggravating agents for hand dermatitis. Atopy has been identified as a risk factor for hand dermatitis in florists and shop assistants.

A mail survey of floral shops conducted by The Baltimore-Washington Allied Florists' Association found that one shop in three reported at least one worker affected by dermatitis, and most affected workers were floral designers.[12] In the United Kingdom reports of dermatitis in the floristry trade indicated a rate at least 10 times that expected for the number of workers in the field.[13] A Swedish study of the frequency of dermatitis among nursery workers who mainly handled tulips found 21.6% (11 of 51) to have work-related dermatitis; nine had allergic contact dermatitis (to either tulips or daffodils), and two were diagnosed with irritant contact dermatitis.[14] Allergy to pesticides may present an additional problem for these workers, although this is uncommon in the authors' experience. Santucci and Picardo evaluated workers exposed to chrysanthemums, poinsettias, geraniums, roses, and *Alstroemeria* and found about 20% of 200 to be affected by either mechanical or physical manifestations, 12% by a chemical irritant dermatitis, 8% by dermatoses due to pesticides, insecticides, or fungicides, and 5% to plant allergens.[15]

A survey of skin problems in retail floristry conducted in the United Kingdom identified a low level of formal training among many workers, and it correlated knowledge of hazards to the skin and better hygiene with formal training. Most of those interviewed did not feel that their rash was occupationally related, though 46% has reported a rash at some time in their employment. Few had ever consulted a physician about their rash.[16] Some experts note that occupational contact dermatitis in florists often requires a change of occupation.[17] Worker education early on about good skin care, especially hand care, may help decrease the number of workers in the floral industry who develop skin problems.

Food Handlers

Hand dermatitis is common among food handlers, preparers, and cooks.[18, 19] Tomatoes, carrots, garlic, onions, celery, lettuce, and potatoes are frequent causes.[20–22] Essential oils of citrus fruits such as lemon and orange have been implicated as a cause of chronic hand dermatitis in citrus pickers, bartenders, housewives, and food handlers.[23] Both contact urticaria and allergic contact dermatitis have been described. Consideration should be given early on to testing for type I hypersensitivity by immediate skin tests (prick and rub), and radioallergosorbent (RAST) tests for specific immunoglobulin E (IgE) antibodies in persons who develop symptoms of itching, redness, and swelling within minutes of handling food. Delayed-type patch testing to suspected foods can also be considered for patients with chronic eczema, though it is infrequently performed. Patch test challenges might include garlic or onion if exposure of the hands is identified (since they are the most common cause of food-related allergic contact dermatitis), limonene, a terpene of the essential oil from lemon and orange peel, and possibly its structural relatives geraniol and citral.[24]

TYPES OF PLANT DERMATITIS

Cutaneous reactions to plants are of several types: mechanical dermatitis, contact irritant dermatitis, contact allergic dermatitis, contact urticaria, phototoxic dermatitis, photoallergic dermatitis, and erythema multiforme–like reactions. So-called pseudophytodermatitis is a phenomenon in which the clinical appearance of a dermatitis mimics a plant dermatitis but the cause of the lesion is actually something else, possibly a pesticide, fungicide, insecticide, or even gloves worn by plant handlers.

Mechanical Dermatitis

Mechanically induced dermatitis can occur when thorns or spines of plants penetrate the skin. Hairy appendages such as trichromes and glochids from cacti can cause severe irritant reactions. Puncture injuries from plants can become secondarily infected with bacteria, mycobacteria, or fungi.[25] Pickers of the Mexican prickly pear, *Opuntia ficus indica* can develop "sabra dermatitis," a popular pruritic eruption resembling scabies but attributable to contact with the plant glochids.[26] Thorns that are not removed from the skin can cause foreign body granulomas.

Irritant Dermatitis

Irritant dermatitis, the most frequent type of plant-related dermatitis,[3] can manifest itself clinically as erythema, hyperkeratosis of the hands and fingers, papules, vesicles, necrosis, abrasions, or granulomas. Plant families most commonly implicated in irritant dermatitis are Cruciferae, Euphorbiaceae, Rutaceae, Ranunculaceae, Brassicaceae; less commonly implicated are the Dieffenbachia and Urticaceae.

A number of factors contribute to irritant dermatitis in plant handlers, among them frequent skin trauma and frequent exposure to water. Irritant reactions may be due to plant chemicals, mechanical factors or trauma, and follicular irritation. Repeated subthreshold irritation with mild plant irritants and repeated water exposure can lead to clinically evident cumulative irritant dermatitis. Plants contain a number of irritants such as acids, glycosides, proteolytic enzymes, phorbol esters, isothiocyanates, and calcium oxalate crystals.[27] Some plant families and their members with known irritant properties are listed in Table 31–3. The irritating capacity of certain plants is often known to experienced plant handlers; appropriate precautions when handling these plants can prevent dermatitis.

Phototoxic Dermatitis (Phytophotodermatitis)

Linear furocoumarins, commonly called *psoralens*, are implicated in phototoxic plant dermatitis. Bergapten, also known as 5-methoxypsoralen (5-MOP), and xanthotoxin, known as 8-methoxypsoralen (8-MOP) are the most common plant-derived phototoxic compounds. Phototoxic dermatitis is due to the reaction of these furocoumarins and ultraviolet light (UVA, wavelength 320 to 400 nm). Clinically it is initially recognized as large, usually nonpruritic bullae on exposed skin that

TABLE 31–3 • **Common Plant Irritants**

Common Name (Plant Part)	Family	Botanical Name	Irritant
Black mustard	Brassicaceae	*Brassica nigra*	Isothiocyanates (all)
Buttercup	Ranunculaceae	*Ranunculus* spp.	Protoanemonin (damaged plant parts)
California glory	Sterculiaceae	*Fremontodendron*	Sea urchin–like irritant hairs
Columbine	Ranunculaceae	*Aqualegia* spp.	Protoanemonin
Croton bush	Crotonoideae	*Croton tiglium*	Phorbol esters (stems, leaves)
Daffodil	Amaryllidaceae	*Narcissus* spp.	Calcium oxalate (stems, leaves, bulbs)
Dumbcane	Araceae	*Dieffenbachia* spp.	Calcium oxalate (leaves, fruit)
Hyacinth	Liliaceae	*Hyacinthus orientalis*	Calcium oxalate (bulbs)
Manchineel tree	Euphorbiaceae	*Hippomane mancinella*	Phorbol esters (stems, leaves, fruit)
May apple	Euphorbiaceae	*Podophyllum peltatum*	Podophyllin resin
Nettle	Urticaceae	*Urtica dioica* L.	Histamine, acetylcholine, 5-hydroxytryptamine
Pencil tree	Euphorbiaceae	*Euphorbia tirucalli*	Triterpene alcohols
Pepper	Solanaceae	*Capsicum annum*	Capsaicin
Poinsettia	Euphorbiaceae	*Euphorbia pulcherrima*	Phorbol esters
Pineapple	Bromeliaceae	*Ananas comosus*	Bromelin (stem, fruit)
Prickly pear	Cactaceae	*Opuntia vulgaris*	Spines
Spurge	Euphorbiaceae	*Euphorbia* spp.	Phorbol esters (stems, leaves, fruit)

Modified from Marks and DeLeo.

resolve in 7 to 10 days, leaving behind a characteristic, usually streaky, hyperpigmentation that can last months. The hyperpigmentation may be a result of decreased levels of glutathione leading to increased pigment production, since reduced glutathione is a known inhibitor of tyrosinase.[15]

Acute lesions may have a linear distribution (presumably from the worker having brushed by a plant). This eruption is nonselective and occurs in all exposed persons when specific conditions, such as exposure to a plant containing furocoumarin, dampness, and sunlight are present. Outdoor workers typically develop the characteristic phytophotodermatitis when exposed to these plants on a damp day when there is plenty of sunlight. The bullous eruption occurs within a few hours of exposure (up to 48 hours).[28] This form of dermatitis is also known as *meadow dermatitis* or *dermatitis bullosa striata et pratensis.*[29]

Table 31–4 provides a list of plants that contain phototoxic furocoumarins. Psoralens capable of causing phototoxic dermatitis are present in a number of plants, among them members of the Umbelliferae (Apiaceae) family, which include such common vegetables and herbs as garden parsley *(Petroselium sativum)*, celery *(Apium graveolans)*, and parsnip *(Pastinaca sativa)* and weeds like giant hogweed *(Heracleum mantegazzianum)*.[30] Umbelliferae have abundant furocoumarins in their roots and leaves. Members of the Rutaceae family that also have psoralens include

common rule *(Ruta graveolans)*, the burning bush or gas plant *(Dictamnus albus)*, and bergamot. The fig tree *(Ficus carica)*, a member of the family Moraceae, also contains psoralens. *Cneoridium dumosum*, a member of the Rutaceae family found in California and Mexico, was implicated in a severe phototoxic dermatitis in a biologist who walked through an area densely overgrown with this weed.[31]

"Weed whacker," or "strimmer," dermatitis is a pattern of photodermatitis that occurs on exposed skin and is induced by contact with newly cut plant fragments containing psoralens. Buckshotlike plant fragments are dispersed through the air by a string trimmer (strimmer) used to edge landscapes and cut weeds and grasses.[32] When such a machine is used to cut plants containing furocoumarins such as cow parsley *(Anthrisis sylvestris)* and hogweed *(Heracleum sphodylium)*, as in the cases reported by Reynolds and Burton, a widespread phytophotodermatitis can result.[33] Removing clothing on sunny days increases skin exposure. Initially the eruption is characterized by an acute, eczematous, and often bullous, dermatitis on exposed skin. On resolution, there are telltale hyperpigmented, often streaky macules.

Grocery workers and bartenders can also get this dermatosis, usually from celery or limes, respectively. A case report of a recurrent phototoxic eruption in celery harvesters makes the point that prevention can be achieved by using a broad-

TABLE 31–4 • Plants Implicated in Phototoxic Reactions

Family	Scientific Name	Common Name
Leguminosae	*Psoralea corylifolia*	Scurf pea
Moraceae	*Ficus carica*	Fig
Rutaceae	*Citrus aurantifolia*	Lime
	Citrus aurantium	Bitter orange
	Citrus bergamia	Bergamot orange
	Citrus limon	Lemon
	Dictamnus albus	Gas plant
	Ruta graveolans	Common rue
Umbelliferae	*Ammi majus*	False Bishop's weed
	Angelica archangelica	Angelica
	Anthriscus sylvestris	Wild Angelica
	Apium graveolans	Celery
	Daucus carota	Carrot
	Heracleum lanatum	Cow parsnip
	Heracleum mantegazzianum	Giant hogweed
	Heracleum sphondylium	Cow parsley
	Pastinaca sativa	Parsnip

spectrum sunblock, containing UVA-absorbing dimethoxydibenzoylmethane (Parsol 1789), octyl methoxycinnamate (Parsol MCX), and methyl benzylidene camphor (Eusolex 6300), applied several times a day.[34]

Photoallergy to plants containing psoralen is rare but has been reported.[35] It is said that in photoallergy the dermatitis is most severe earlier than is the expected maximum dermatitis of phototoxicity (48 to 72 hours). Ljunggren reported a case of photoallergy due to celery picking. Photopatchtesting with serial dilutions of 8-methoxypsoralen, 5-methoxypsoralen, and trimethylpsoralen was used to differentiate allergy from phototoxicity.

Contact Allergic Dermatitis

In different geographical regions the cause of plant contact allergy can vary markedly. Contact allergy to a given plant depends on several variables, including (1) the relative abundance of a plant or plant family containing related or similar allergens in a given region, (2) the frequency of individual exposure to potentially sensitizing plants, and (3) the sensitizing potential and concentration of a given compound or compounds in the plant.[36] Low–molecular weight compounds cause most cases of allergic contact dermatitis, though in some instances plant proteins are implicated in immediate or delayed contact reactions. Many plants are capable of causing allergic-type contact dermatitis; some do so more frequently

and are better known than others. Many of the plants most often implicated in occupational allergic contact dermatitis are reviewed in greater depth later in this chapter.

Contact Urticaria

Contact urticaria is sometimes an immune-mediated reaction and sometimes is not. Nonimmune contact urticaria (NICU) can be elicited nonspecifically in any (nonsensitized) person by contact. Plants or plant products containing cinnamic aldehyde, cinnamic acid, and balsam of Peru can cause NICU, probably through direct release of histamine from mast cells. Capsaicin, derived from chili peppers and cowhage can also cause this type of contact urticaria. Nettles *(Urticaria dioica)* have stinging hairs containing histamine, acetylcholine, and 5-hydroxytryptamine.

Immediate hypersensitivity, or type I hypersensitivity mediated by specific IgE, can be serious, presenting as angioedema and generalized urticaria or as dermatitis localized to areas of repeated contact, generally the hands. This type of reaction is also known as immunological contact urticaria (ICU). Atopic persons are prone to develop this form of hypersensitivity reaction. Preexisting irritant dermatitis may make a person more likely to develop type I reactions, perhaps by allowing better antigen penetration through damaged stratum corneum. Type I reactions are associated with a variety of proteins, many of which are contained in fruits and vegetables and others in plant pollens. Tulips and lilies can also cause contact urticaria.[37]

Preexisting hand eczema in food handlers can be exacerbated by contact urticaria.[38, 39] Apples, carrots, potatoes, beans, cucumbers and pickles, garlic, and strawberries are some fruits and vegetables implicated in this type of hypersensitivity reaction.[40] Table 31–5 contains plants, woods, and their products that can cause contact urticaria.

TESTING

Contact Urticaria

Testing for immediate-type contact urticaria to plants can be done in a number of ways. Testing must be conducted with caution: resuscitation equipment must be available as there is potential for induction of an anaphylactic reaction. The *skin application food test* is performed by applying a suspected food to the skin, and occluding with a Finn test chamber. The test site is examined for erythema and edema at 10-minute intervals over 30 minutes. *Prick testing* can also be performed; though more sensitive, it is also more likely to induce a systemic reaction. Prick testing is performed by placing a small piece of the plant material on the forearm then superficially pricking the skin with a blood lancet or hypodermic needle through the material. Some food allergens are available in standardized formulations for prick testing. A reading is taken immediately after pricking and after 15 minutes. A histamine and a

TABLE 31–5 • Plant and Wood-Related Allergens for Patch Testing

Commercial Allergen	Concentration (% in Petrolatum)	Source*	Plant Source; Allergen†
Achillea millefolium	1.0	C	Yarrow; SL: peroxyachifolid
Alantolactone	0.1	C	SL present in *Chrysanthemum* spp. (helenalin)
Alpha-methylene-gamma-butyrolactone	0.01	C	Plants containing SL
Arnica montana	0.5	C	Mountain tobacco; SLs: helenalin and helenalin acetate SLs; helenalin and its esters
Arnica	20.0 tincture	T	Mountain tobacco; SLs: helenalin and its esters
Atranorin	0.5	T	Lichens
Chamomilla romana (*Anthemis nobilis*)	1.0	C	Chamomile; SL: nobilin
Chrysanthemum cinerariaefolium (pyrethrum)	1.0	C	Chrysanthemum; SLs: parthenolide and santamarin
Colophony	20	C, T	Rosin, pine dust
Diallyl disulfide	1.0	C	Garlic
Feverfew flower extract	1.0	T	Feverfew; SLs: ambrosin, hymenin, hysterin, parthenin
Lichen acid mix Atranorin Usnic acid Evernic acid	0.3	C	Lichens
Primin	0.01	C, T	*Primula obconica*; primin
Propolis	10.0	C	
SL mix Alantolactone Dehydrocostuslactone Costunolide	0.1	C, T	Compositae and other plants containing SLs
Tanacetum vulgare	1.0	C	Tansy; SLs: arbusculin A and tanacetin
Taraxacum officinale	2.5	C	Dandelion; taraxinic acid glycoside
Usnic acid	0.1	T	Lichens

*Commercial sources, 1997 catalogs; C, Chemotechnique Diagnostics allergens. P.O. Box 80, Edvard Ols vag 2, s-230 42 Tygelsjo, Malmo, Sweden; T, Trolab patch test allergens., Omniderm Inc., Montreal, Quebec.
†Allergen is listed when different from commercial allergen.

normal saline (control) prick test are advised. A *scratch test* is performed by making a 5-mm scratch on the back of the forearm followed by application of the test material for 10 to 15 minutes. A reading is performed every 15 minutes for an hour. In the *scratch chamber test*, the skin is scratched and the test material is placed on the site and occluded with a Finn chamber for 15 minutes. Readings are performed when the material is removed and every 15 minutes, up to 1 hour.[25]

Contact Allergy

Specialized plant allergens are not included in the two contact allergy patch testing standard series currently widely available in the United States. A limited number of commercially prepared plant allergens are available through allergen manufacturers (Hermal or Chemotechnique). Table 31–6 contains a list of commercially available plant allergens in standardized dilution and vehicle. The

TABLE 31–6 • Some Causes of Occupational Contact Urticaria

Sensitizer	
Nonimmune-Mediated	Immune-Mediated
Plant Foods	
Cayenne pepper	Apple Mango
Mustard	Carrot Onion
Thyme	Corn Parsley
	Banana Potato
	Beans Runner bean
	Garlic Sesame, sunflower
	Kiwi seeds
	Lettuce Tomato
Plant and Tree Products	
Birch pollen	Colophony (rosin)
Nettles	Cornstarch
Seaweed	Limba (*Terminalia superba*)
	Obeche (*Triplochiton scleroxylon*)
	Ramin (*Gonystylus bancanus*)
	Dried (*Limonium tararicum*) flowers
	Henna
	Larch (*Larix decidua*)
	Latex rubber
	Teak (*Tectona grandis*)
	Tulips

Adapted from Amin S, Tanglertsampan C, Maibach HI. Contact urticaria syndrome. *Am J Contact Dermatitis* 1997;8:15–19.

lack of readily available testing materials and limited number of patients routinely tested with plant allergens probably lead to many missed diagnoses and a poor estimate of the number of cases of actual contact allergy caused by plants.

Guin has provided an excellent summary of procedures for patch testing to plants.[41] A suspect plant should be accurately identified before testing. If immediate use is not intended, plant materials should be properly stored by freezing or air drying. Mitchell and Rook recommend dividing plant material into three parts, one part for testing and one part for identification. The third part is frozen for possible future studies using a prepared plant extract.[3] Plants known to cause irritation either should not be tested or their extracts should be diluted to nonirritating concentrations. Flowering plants can be patch tested with parts of root, leaf, stem, and flower applied to Scanpor tape and then applied to the patient's back as a patch test. Guin recommends 1-hour exposure time for the testing of most Compositae plants to limit irritant reactions, although there is no widespread agreement on this. Many investigators perform these "as-is" plant part tests according to the standard exposure time of 48 hours. When testing bulbs, the outer scale should be removed and discarded; the fleshy outer layers are used for testing.[42]

Fresh plant material is generally advised for patch testing. At least 10 control subjects should be tested when using nonstandardized material. Another concern is the risk of sensitization when testing to plant parts or extracts. Plants known to be highly sensitizing, such as poison ivy and oak, should not be tested routinely. To limit the chance of testing to plants with known irritant properties or much sensitizing potential, consulting reference literature for testing recommendations is always wise before making an extract or testing a plant part. Testing with dilutions can be performed first to assess the possibility of irritation.

Variations of allergen concentrations in a plant lead to variations in extract; however, this is more easily standardized than testing as is with a fresh plant or its parts. Allergen concentration varies even in a single plant species; allergen content has been shown to vary according to seasonal factors, growing habitat, growth phase, and plant part used for allergen extraction.[43, 44]

Dr. Bjorn Hausen described a simple method for making plant extracts.[45] A short ether extract can be made by cutting fresh plant material into 20-cm-long pieces and "extracting" them for 90 seconds with peroxide-free ether at room temperature. The extract is dried over sodium sulfate for 1 hour, and the solvent is evaporated at 39° C under reduced pressure (waterpump vacuum). The extract is then incorporated into white petrolatum at the appropriate concentration. Before testing, irritancy threshold should be tested on 20 controls. A pharmacist, biochemist, or knowledgeable laboratory technician can be of assistance in preparing dilutions and extracts. Irritation and active sensitization are still possible using plant extracts.

Phototesting

Some plants cause phototoxicity or photoallergy. Testing for phototoxicity is not routinely considered necessary or appropriate. Testing for photoallergy is performed when indicated by the patient's clinical presentation. This testing is performed according to the standardized protocol for other photoallergens.[46] In the case of Compositae sensitivity, suspected actinic reticuloid, persistent light reactor, or an airborne or photo distribution of dermatitis, important parts of the evaluation are testing for light sensitivity by determining minimal erythema dose (MED) to UVB, minimal phototoxic dose (MPD) to UVA, and erythema threshold to visible light.

MAJOR AND REPORTED PLANT CAUSES

The following information reviews specific individual plants and plant groups that have been implicated in occupational contact dermatitis, principally the allergic type. Though it is not all inclusive, it focuses on important plants in terms of occupational exposure. Several of the less common but newly reported plants implicated in contact dermatitis are also included.

Alstroemeria

Native to Central and South America, *Alstroemeria*, otherwise known as *Peruvian*, or *Inca lily*, was imported to Europe early in the 20th century and has become a significant cause of allergic contact dermatitis in florists. Floral arrangers are particularly affected, many reported cases of dermatitis initially coming from Europe.[47, 48] *Alstroemeria* is a favorite cut flower for arrangements owing to its long-lasting bloom, year-round availability, and variety of colors. The flower resembles a lily, with a trumpet shape and streaked or dappled inner petals.[10, 49] *Alstroemeria* has been a popular cut flower with florists in the United States since its introduction in 1981. More than 50 species of *Alstroemeria* exist; *Alstroemeria ligtu L.* and *Alstroemeria aurantiaca* being most popular.

Alstroemeria cultivars are strong sensitizers. Dermatitis from *Alstroemeria* is most typically seen on the fingers and thumbs of both hands.[50, 51] A dry, cracked, and hyperkeratotic appearance of the distal fingertips, similar to the dermatitis known as *tulip fingers*, is characteristic (Fig. 31–4). Facial, forearm, and eyelid dermatitis may also be seen. Several reports detail delayed onset of the dermatitis after years of working with the flower.[51] Cross-reactivity is seen with tulip bulbs, since the allergen is alpha-methylene-gamma-butyrolactone (tulipalin A), which is also the allergen in tulip bulbs.[52] Contact urticaria to *Alstroemeria* has also been reported.[53]

Testing for allergy to *Alstroemeria* is done with tuliposide A, 0.01%, or one of its hydrolysis derivatives, tulipalin A (alpha-methylene-gamma-butyrolactone 0.01%) in petrolatum. Hausen recommends a methanol plant extract over an acetone extract, owing to the greater stability of allergen in the glycoside form. Such an extract can be stored at room temperature and diluted in petrolatum when needed. Patch testing can also be performed with the petal, leaf, or stem of the plant, though the amount of allergen is variable from species to species and from different plant parts, and Hausen notes that there is a high risk of sensitization and irritancy when testing is done to the plant itself.[44]

Penetration of this allergen through vinyl, but not nitrile, gloves was reported by Marks.[55] The liquid juice from the plants can also present a problem on scissors, work surface tabletops, and vases. DeHaan found polyvinylchloride and latex gloves to be inadequate in protection against dermatitis in tulipalin A–allergic handlers of *Alstroemeria*. Household-weight gloves, but not neoprene or nitrile ones, and the 4H glove provided 4 hours of protection.[56] High-performance liquid chromatography has been used to identify *Alstroemeria* species with lower allergen content.

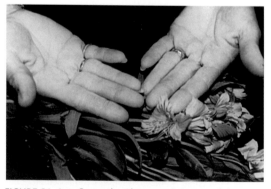

FIGURE 31–4 • Currently, *Alstroemeria* is one of the most common causes of contact allergy in florists.

Such systems are being used to develop less allergenic cultivars.[57] Some florists have chosen not to carry the flower, to avoid the hazards of disabling dermatitis.

Asparagus

Before automation in the 1920s and 1930s, hundreds of cases of allergic contact dermatitis were reported from the peeling of asparagus shoots in canning factories.[58] Hausen and Wolf identified 1,2,3-trithiane-5-carboxylic acid, an early-phase, sulfur-containing growth inhibitor seen in greater concentrations during the early growth of asparagus shoots, as a contact sensitizer. Though contact allergy to asparagus is now uncommon, cooks, food preparers, vegetable produce merchants, and specialty food cultivators may be at risk. The dermatitis' duration correlates strongly to the asparagus growing season.

Coleus

Several members of the *Coleus* genus are popular house plants. *Coleus* have multicolored leaves bearing fine hairs that may cause contact irritation. These plants are native to Africa and tropical Asia. Sensitization is rare, only a few cases having been reported. These cases involved airborne contact dermatitis manifested as facial and eyelid lesions in a gardener, a housewife, and a botanist doing thesis work on the plant.[59–61] A diterpene, coleon O, is one identified allergen with strong sensitizing potential.[62]

Compositae

Sesquiterpene lactones (SLs) are the main allergens in the Compositae, Jubulaceae *(Frullania)*, Lauraceae, and Magnoliaceae families.[63] Compositae dermatitis is often used as a synonym for SL dermatitis, though plants from the other families mentioned above also contain SLs. Some of the other names for dermatitis caused by SLs include *ragweed dermatitis, Australian bush dermatitis, Chrysanthemum dermatitis*, and *summer-exacerbated dermatitis*.

The Compositae family contains more than 25,000 species, about 200 of which reportedly cause allergic contact dermatitis.[64] Compositae species include common weeds, annual and perennial ornamental plants, and herbs. Compositae can be used for medicinal purposes, in aromatherapy, in so-called natural cosmetics and personal care products, naturopathy, massage therapy, and homeopathy. Compositae have worldwide distribution, which accounts for numerous series and reports of allergy from many countries. Workers at risk for dermatitis from Compositae or other SL–containing plants include florists, gardeners and horticulturists, floral arrangers, and perfumery, cosmetics, and food industry employees. Cases of allergy have been reported in herbalists and massage therapists.

SLs are the principal allergens implicated in allergic plant dermatitis caused by ragweed, feverfew, chrysanthemum, sneezeweed, sagebrush, wormwood, chamomile, burdock, artichoke, gaillardia, and lettuce, to name a few. SLs are not limited to the Compositae family; they occur in other unrelated plants, like the magnolia and bay trees, and in liverworts *(Frullania)*.[65] More than 600 SLs have been isolated and identified, and over 100 are allergenic. Unfortunately, cross-sensitivity cannot reliably be predicted in any individual patient.

The true incidence of both occupational and nonoccupational cases of dermatitis related to plants containing SLs, such as Compositae species, is unknown.[66] Rates reported from case series undoubtedly underestimate the problem. Many cases likely go unrecognized and are not referred for testing. In a British study of 114 cases of Compositae sensitivity diagnosed over a 4-year period, 15 were deemed occupational, owing to exposures in agriculture or floristry.[67] Menz and Winkelmann described 74 patients with Compositae sensitivity. The male-female ratio of affected patients was 1.4:1. Reported sources of exposure were the garden in 40%, outdoor work or recreational exposure in 17%, and farming in 15%.[64]

Perhaps the best-known epidemic of allergic contact dermatitis due to a plant source other than a *Toxicodendron* species is what has been called *the scourge of India*. The accidental introduction in 1956 of *Parthenium hysterophorus* (wild feverfew) seeds in imported grain in India resulted in widespread distribution of this fast-growing weed and in numerous cases of sensitization and dermatitis.[68]

The clinical presentation of plant dermatitis due to SLs often depends on the type of exposure. Floral shop workers, gardeners, arrangers, and sellers of these plants develop a dermatitis that is usually limited to the hands and concentrated on the fingertips, sometimes extending onto exposed forearm skin. If gloves are worn, the forearms alone may be affected. Additionally, these workers sometimes develop eyelid or facial dermatitis that can be due either to airborne particulate exposure or, probably more frequently, indirect transfer of allergenic material from contaminated hands. This distribution of dermatitis is more common in women than in men. An airborne contact dermatitis, a photodermatitis–like presentation or one of chronic actinic dermatitis, or persistent light reactivity has been described in outdoor workers, particularly middle-aged men employed in farming or forestry.[69–71] Initially, the dermatitis is seasonal, occurring from spring to late fall. Persistent exposure can lead to year-round dermatitis characterized by subacute or chronic eczematous lesions affecting the exposed skin of the face and neck, including the eyelids, postauricular skin, and submental areas, which often is so characteristic of an airborne dermatitis. The exposed face, forearms, and hands are also typically affected (Fig. 31–2). Sensitivity can be severe enough to result in erythroderma. Many patients have been described with Compositae sensitivity and multiple other positive patch tests. A high incidence of a history of atopy and concurrent allergies to balsam of Peru, wood tar, and colophony are most frequently described.[72]

Several studies have shown an association of light sensitivity in some patients with sensitivity to SLs.[73, 74] The degree of light sensitivity can be marked, reactivity occurring to such low-level light as 0.25 J/cm^2 UVA. The coexistence of SL sensitivity and light sensitivity varies; the larger studies show that 50% to 96% of patients have the combination.[75] Light testing in some of these patients has shown sensitivity to long-wavelength light (UVA) alone, short-wavelength light (UVB) alone, to light in the visible spectrum, and to a combination of UVA, UVB, and visible light. A small number of studies have shown photoaccentuation of SL patchtests.[76, 77] Photoaccentuation is defined as an increase in intensity of a patch test reaction that is brought about by the combination of UV light and the compound to which a patient is sensitized. Though coexisting photosensitivity is well-established, true photoallergy to Compositae allergens is rare.

Allergenicity is attributed to the alpha-methylene-butyrolactone moiety of the SL molecule. The SL mix generally has been used as a marker of allergy to Compositae and other plants containing sesquiterpene lactones.[78] The SL mix, 0.1% in petrolatum, is a mix of equal molar concentrations of three SLs: alantolactone, costunolide, and dehydrocostuslactone. Each of these compounds has a different sesquiterpene skeleton (eudesmanolide, germacranolide, and guaianolide, respectively). Routine screening in a standard series has uncovered many cases of otherwise unsuspected plant allergy, where reactive patients presented with hand or facial dermatitis, apparent photodermatitis, or generalized eczema.[79]

SL mix can serve as a screening test for Compositae plant and related SL-induced allergies but has been reported to be a test with limited sensitivity in identifying suspected cases of contact allergy to Compositae.[80–82] Green and Fergusen found that this test picked up only 35% of cases. Six patients reacted to both the SL mix and individual Compositae oleoresins, whereas 11 patients reacted to Compositae oleoresins but not to the mix.[80] A Compositae mix made of five Compositae plants (*Arnica montana* L., *Chamomilla recutita*, *Tanacetum parthenium*, *Tanacetum vulgare*, *Achillea millefolium*) reported by Hausen may offer a testing advantage by including other potential allergenic constituents—thiophenes and polyacetylenes—obtained through a short ether extract process.[79] The addition of these constituents may increase the sensitivity of this screening test, as thiophenes have also been identified as sensitizers in some Compositae species.[83]

Most authorities on the subject recommend aimed testing with individual dilutions of Compositae oleoresins to which a patient has been or may have been exposed so that allergens are not missed and advice on avoidance of specific plants can be given.[84] Although screening mixes are at times helpful, testing the specific plants either with plant parts or by making diluted extracts of specific oleoresins to which there is known exposure is an important way to identify allergy in an individual patient with a suspected plant dermatitis, since the mixes available may yield false-negative results (Fig. 31–5).[85, 86] Hausen described a technique for short ether extraction of SLs for use in testing. Basically, a whole plant is subjected to extraction for 30 seconds with highly purified peroxide-free diethyl ether. The ether extract is then dried over Na_2SO_4 for 8 hours (about 80 g/L) and then evaporated at room temperature using a waterpump vacuum. The dry weight of the extract is determined, and then tests can be made by diluting to appropriate concentration (often 1.0%, 0.1%, or 0.01%) in petrolatum.[87] For patients who present with an airborne-type dermatitis, phototesting is part of a complete evaluation and may prove useful in providing further information to the patient about what can trigger the dermatitis.

Treatment of Compositae dermatitis begins with avoidance of the allergens as much as possible. Some affected persons cannot completely avoid the allergen, despite removing the occupational exposure, as various Compositae are present in and around the patient's outdoor environment as indigenous plants and weeds. Successful treatment of patients whose dermatitis has evolved into a chronic and nonseasonal one is difficult. Immunosuppression with prednisone, azathioprine, or cyclosporine is potentially helpful, but adverse

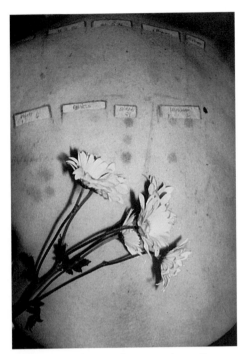

FIGURE 31–5 • Positive patch tests to chrysanthemum, a representative Compositae family member containing allergenic sesquiterpene lactones.

effects of these systemic medications require caution and close monitoring.[70, 88, 89] An outpatient, prednisone-assisted psoralen-plus-UVA (PUVA) protocol has been described as a useful treatment modality for these patients, many of whom are also light sensitive.[90]

Daffodils

Narcissus (common name daffodil) is a genus of the family Amaryllidaceae. *Narcissus* is naturally found throughout the Mediterranean, particularly on the Iberian Peninsula. The genus *Narcissus* contains more than 60 species, and there are multitudes of cultivars. Among the most popular species cultivated for cut flowers and the perfume industry include *Narcissus pseudonarcissus*, *Narcissus jonquilla*, and *Narcissus poeticus*.[91] Both allergic and irritant contact dermatitis from occupational exposure to daffodils have been reported.[92] *Narcissus* allergy and irritation have been described in flower cultivators during flowering, from March to May, and among perfumery workers.[93] Bulb handlers and those who cut the cultivated flower stems and sell the flowers in bulk are principally at risk. Irritation as a result of contact with the plant sap is much more common than allergy. The tulip bulb contains raphides of calcium oxalate, an irritant that can cause pruritus,

erythema, hyperkeratosis, and tender, dry fingertips in bulb handlers. Also implicated in irritant dermatitis are chelidonic acid and a number of alkaloids.[93]

Allergic dermatitis is most frequent in workers who pick and pack flowers. The dermatitis tends to occur on the sides of the fingers (especially the thumb and index finger), hands, forearms, neck, abdomen, and genitals. A hardening effect from repeated exposure has been reported.[93] The allergen is unknown but is present in both leaf and flower; two likely sensitizers are mansonin and homolycorin; mansonin is said to play the greater role. The bulbs may contain the greatest concentration of mansonin and homolycorin.[93] It is important to note that some *Narcissus* species or cultivars do not provoke contact dermatitis in patients sensitized to other species; they likely lack the specific sensitizing component or contain an insufficient amount to provoke dermatitis on testing.

The flower and leaf can be tested, as is. The corolla and calyx may yield the best results. Different allergens have been suspected in *Narcissus* allergy; testing should be considered to both alcohol and acetone extracts.

Garlic and Onion

Garlic (*Allium sativum* L.) is one of the most common food materials that cause allergic contact dermatitis in food handlers, caterers, farmers, and greengrocers. Raw uncooked garlic is responsible for the classic clinical appearance of dermatitis, which is characterized by scaling, erythema, and fissuring affecting the nondominant thumb, index, and middle fingers and the thumb of the dominant hand. It is the commonest cause of contact dermatitis in Asian Indian housewives.[20] Italian housewives with apparent irritant dermatitis of the hands had a high frequency of positive patch test reactions to garlic (8 of 62, 12.9%) in one study.[94] Widespread use of garlic in the local cuisine is felt to result in much exposure and frequent contact allergy. Patch testing can be performed with garlic extract, 2% to aqueous.[95] Diallyl disulfide, the implicated allergen, is tested at 2% in petrolatum.[96] Allylpropyldisulfide and allicin are additional allergens, which are also heat labile and eliminated by cooking.

Hydrangea

Hydrangea are flowering plants widely distributed in North, Central, and South America, China, Japan, and Europe. It is a cultivated decorative garden and potted plant and may also be used in floral arrangements. Contact dermatitis to hydrangea is rare, despite its relatively strong experimental sensitizing capacity.[97] This may be attributable to seasonal variation of the allergen hydrangenol, a chemical intermediate of lunularic acid, a plant-growth inhibitor. The allergen is present in the peripheral plant parts, roots, and in withered parts likely to be removed by deadheading or pruning. Hydrangenol (3,4-dihydro-8-hydroxy-3-(4-hydroxyphenyl)-isocoumarin) is the allergen in some, but not all hydrangeas.[98] Meijer and Hausen[97, 98] recommend a 0.1% concentration in petrolatum for patch testing and suggest that contact allergy may not be as rare as reported. Because florists have contact with so many plants, hydrangea could easily be overlooked and not often sought by testing.

Kiwi Fruit

Kiwi fruit, *Actinidia chinensis*, also known as *Chinese gooseberry*, is a major agricultural crop in New Zealand. Harvesting is still performed by hand, principally by transient workers hired for this autumn work. Immediate contact urticaria has been reported, as has contact dermatitis of the hands, in an orchard worker who handled kiwi fruit vines.[99, 100] The orchardist in that report was able to handle the fruit itself without developing dermatitis.

Lichens

Lichens are epiphytic plant forms resulting from a symbiotic relationship of an alga and a fungus. Among the thousands of lichen species, *Parmelia, Usnea, Evernia*, and *Cladonia* are the ones implicated in most cases of contact allergy. Lichen acids are strong sensitizers; however, allergy to lichens is not considered common. Foresters, woodcutters, and other outdoor workers are the main workers at risk for contact allergy to lichens, as lichens grow on the bark of tree trunks and branches. Salo and colleagues reported that 30 of 164 lichen pickers in Finland had dermatitis of the hands; at least 10% of them had delayed-type allergy.[103] Lichens are used in floral arrangements and for holiday decorations. Lichen extracts are used to produce perfumes and medicinals.

Allergy to lichens manifests as an eczematous dermatitis, typically in an airborne distribution, where exposed skin is affected. This distribution simulates the pattern of photodistribution. Airborne dispersal of allergen in dust particles during wet weather is one possible route of exposure, in addition to direct contact with exposed skin and possible inadvertent hand transfer of the allergen.

Allergy to lichens has also been called *woodcutter's* eczema. The waist, low back, genitals, ankles, thighs, and neck are other sites of involvement, presumed to be places where lichen particles are trapped by clothing.[102] Dermatitis can also progress to erythroderma. Immediate urticarial reactions have also been described.

The most common allergens in lichens are atranorin, *d*-usnic, and *l*-usnic acid.[103] Sandberg and Thune found atranorin to be the most frequent allergen but also reported other lichen acids, including *d*-usnic, evernic, fumarprotocetraric, lobaric, salazinic, diffractaic, and physodic/physodalic acid. Oak moss absolute, a fragrance extracted from lichens, contains atranorin, a weak to moderate sensitizer[104]; however, oak moss absolute more often causes allergy when used in cosmetics such as aftershave lotions and perfumes, than as an occupational hazard.

Several patients with persistent light reactivity and contact allergy to oak moss and purified lichen compounds have been described.[105, 106] In a selected Norwegian patient series of 18 elderly men with persistent light reactivity for 5 to 20 years, Thune and Eeg-Larsen found that allergy to lichen compounds was twice as common as allergy to Compositae oleoresins.[71] Solberg and Thune tested sensitized guinea pigs and failed to show clear-cut photoallergy or photoaugmentation of atranorin, evernic, usnic, or physodic acid. Others, however, have reported atranorin to evoke photoaugmentation (a stronger patch test with UV irradiation), whereas usnic acid is unlikely to do so.[76] Munos and de Corres reported photocontact allergy to oak moss[107]; however, true photocontact allergy to lichen acids is probably rare, and some cases of persistent light reactions may be due to other, concurrent photoallergens.[104] Testing for suspected allergy to lichens is with atranorin, 0.5% in petrolatum, and usnic acid 1% or 0.1%, both in petrolatum. Oak moss absolute may also be used for testing, as can oak moss extract, although it contains substances in addition to lichen compounds.[108]

Coexisting allergy to SLs has been reported, probably a result of cosensitization, since *Frullania* (liverwort) species and lichens often live on the same tree trunks.[109, 110] Testing to the SL mix and to alantolactone, each 0.1% in petrolatum, can be important in identifying the specific allergenic plant, as the two presentations can be indistinguishable. Because many patients have multiple allergies, it is recommended to test with a broad allergen screening tray, including balsam of Peru, lichen acids, fragrance mix, wood tars, and Compositae oleoresins or screening allergens, in addition to those mentioned above. A complete evaluation would include photopatchtesting to known photosensitizers (including sunscreens) on a screening tray, and phototesting to UVA and UVB for MED thresholds, as some cases reflect intercurrent photosensitivity or photocontact dermatitis.[111, 112]

Liverwort *(Frullania)*

Liverworts are small, reddish brown, primitive vascular plants belonging to the genus *Frullania*, a member of the Jubulaceae family. They are found worldwide growing on rocks and trees. Liverworts often grow on the bark of oak trees. They grow well in the Pacific Northwest, Coastal British Columbia, France, Spain, and other areas of Europe. Allergy to *Frullania* is most often described in country dwellers, farmers, sawmill workers, lumbermen, tree fellers, and carpenters.[113]

Frullania dermatitis is also known as *woodcutter's eczema, cedar poisoning*, and *oak wood dermatitis* because woodsmen, lumbermen, and those who fell timber are the occupational groups at risk for allergic contact dermatitis.[114] The clinical appearance of allergy is similar to that of Compositae dermatitis, often demonstrating chronic, lichenified dermatitis in a photodermatitis–like distribution. The hands, arms, neck, and face are commonly affected in lumbermen. Close, but not direct, contact with the plant can result in dermatitis, though it may not be recognized because presumably contact occurs via volatile airborne particles, especially during warm, humid weather.[115] Workers can be long exposed to liverworts before dermatitis appears: in Mitchell's series of 112 cases of contact allergy to *Frullania* onset of dermatitis varied after a few months to 15 years' occupational exposure.[119]

Two species are known: *Frullania dilatata* and *Frullania tamarisci*. The principal allergen is frullanolide, an SL, although other lactones can be sensitizers.[116] Cross-reactivity can be seen with plants of the Compositae family. *F. tamarisci* contains the levo (-) enantiomer, whereas *F. dilatata* contains the dextro (+) enantiomer.[117, 118] Testing is performed to both *F. dilatata* and *F. tamarisci*, or the *d*- and the *l*-enantiomers of frullanolide, since enantiomeric specificity can result in reactions only to the primary sensitizing *Frullania*. Patients may also react to alantolactone, 0.1% in petrolatum. Concurrent exposure to lichens in the forest environment may account for additional positive patch tests to *d*-usnic acid (1% in petrolatum), atranorin, or evernic or perlatolic acid.[119]

It is not recommended to test *Frullania* in routine screening allergen series, owing to the great potential for active sensitization.[120] Since the lactones of *Frullania* are chemically related to Compositae SLs, patch testing can be performed with the SL mix, 0.1% in petrolatum, though false-negative results can occur. The plant can also be tested as is: a small part is moistened before being tested.

Prevention of the dermatitis is difficult, and avoidance of the plant is usually necessary. Some less sensitive workers may continue to work and tolerate mild, persistent dermatitis. Usually a change of occupation is necessary for affected workers. Job changes often result in lower-paying work and substantial loss of income for the affected worker; however, some sensitized workers in Mitchell's series were able to continuing working in an interior, colder and drier province, where conditions are less optimal for growth of the liverwort.[119, 121]

Mayweed

Anthemis cotula, also known as *dog fennel* or *stinking daisy*, is a weed that grows on roadsides, pastures, and wastelands in the United States. *Anthemis* species, including *A. cotula*, have been reported to cause irritant contact dermatitis in field workers. In a case series of 14 affected field workers in California, the eruption consisted primarily of a burning, erythematous rash on exposed skin, with large blisters in many cases. Additionally, there were a few cases of an erythema multiforme–like rash.[122] The large number of affected workers and the clinical appearance of large bullae suggest a phototoxic reaction.

Peony

Peonies are decorative perennial shrubs that grow in temperate climates and are garden favorites. There are more than 33 species of the genus *Paeonia*, and many cultivars. Bruynzeel reported a case of a nursery worker who developed a vesicular hand dermatitis from exposure through his job, which entailed dividing peony roots.[123] Testing to the root, and leaf—as is, and as in 10% aqueous, ether, and acetone extracts—confirmed the contact allergy.

Perilla frutescens (Shiso)

P. frutescens (shiso) is a well-known contact allergen in Japan. The leaves from this plant, also known as the *beefsteak plant*, are a popular spice for sashimi, tempura, and Japanese apricot pickle. Owing to increased consumption over the last 20 years, the incidence of dermatitis among shiso farmers has risen.[124] L-Perillaldehyde, a strong sensitizer, is the implicated allergen.

Philodendron

Philodendron dermatitis can occur in nursery workers, tree trimmers in tropical and subtropical areas, and in housekeepers, as *Philodendron* species are popular houseplants. They are members of the Araceae family. Allergy to *Philodendron* is caused by resorcinols, which are antigenically similar to the catechols in members of the genus *Toxicodendron*. There are more than 275 members of the *Philodendron* genus; allergic contact dermatitis is most often reported to *Philodendron scandens scandens*, but allergy to other species has also been reported.[125] The six different resorcinols identified as allergens differ in the type and degree of saturation of the aliphatic side chains, which may be C15 (pentadecyl) or C17 (heptadecyl) resorcinols. The highly unsaturated triolefin resorcinol of *P. scandens* is 5-heptadecatrienylresorcinol, the principal allergen. It is wise first to identify the implicated species of *Philodendron* when allergy is suspected. In implicated species, the leaf's cuticle contains resorcinols, which can be extracted with alcohol or acetone and used for testing. The plant leaf and stem may also be used for testing.

Poison Ivy, Poison Oak, Poison Sumac

Poison ivy and poison oak are the most common agents of plant allergy and major causes of occupational contact dermatitis in the United States. Firefighters, foresters, woodsmen, farmers, and landscapers are frequently at risk. In California, Oregon, and Washington, one third of firefighters suffer disability from poison oak contact dermatitis through smoke containing oil droplets. In California, between 3,000 and 5,000 cases of occupational poison oak dermatitis are reported each year.[126] Poison oak dermatitis is a significant cause of lost time from work and of disability, accounting for nearly 1% of California's workers' compensation budget.

About half of the adult population are sensitive to poison ivy and develop dermatitis from contact with the plant. Perhaps another 35% who are subclinically sensitive develop a rash with heavy exposure.[126]

Though poison ivy has been transplanted to England and Europe, the spread of the plant has been slow and dermatitis from these plants is very rarely reported in Europe. Related plants containing cross-reacting compounds are found in Southeast Asia and Central and South America.

Poison ivy, poison oak, and poison sumac are members of the Anacardiaceae family and of the genus *Toxicodendron*. Other members of the Anacardiaceae family that can cause allergic contact dermatitis in poison ivy–sensitive persons include the mango tree *(Mangifera indica)*, cashew tree *(Anacardium occidentale)*, Ginkgo tree *(Ginkgo biloba)*, Japanese lacquer tree *(Rhus vernicifera)*, and the Indian marking nut tree *(Semecarpus anacardium)*.

There are five *Toxicodendron* species in the United States. Features common to the genus include (1) pinnate leaves with an odd number of leaflets, (2) a poisonous effluvium, (3) dark brown root hairs, (4) a tan, cream, or white outer layer of the ripe fruit, (5) white, fatty, and waxy mesocarp with black striations, (6) an axillary influorescence, (7) pendant fruit when clusters are large, (8) if present, fruit hairs that are not glandular, and (9) pollen grains less than 32 μm in length.[127] Poison ivy is usually recognized by its leaf characteristics; thus, the adage, *Leaves of three, let them be*. Leaf character, however, varies with locale and season. In summer leaves are green, and in fall change to deep red, and later yellow. Shiny black spots on the leaves at sites of damage may help in identification and often are found where sap has been released and has dried. *Toxicodendron* species differ in form, soil requirements, flowering, fruit maturation, and climatic requirements. Different forms of growth occur in different regions, in response to local habitat and climate, so recognition of the plant may require knowledge of its growth features in a specific region.

Two species of poison ivy exist, *Toxicodendron rydbergii*, a nonclimbing dwarf shrub, and *Toxicodendron radicans*, which grows either as a shrub or a climbing vine, typically up telephone poles or trees (Fig. 31–6). *T. rydbergii* is present in the northern and middle United States, and is the predominant form of poison ivy in Canada. It is typically found North of 44-degrees latitude and in some mountainous areas extending within 100 miles of Mexico. Poison ivy does not grow in Hawaii, but cross-reacting plants grow in Hawaii, Florida, the Caribbean, South America, and Asia. *T. radicans* (poison ivy) and *T. vernix* (poison sumac) are most common in the eastern United States. *T. radicans* is the most widespread plant of the genus and is the species with which most people are familiar. It is found on the Atlantic and Gulf coasts south of the 44th parallel, Bermuda, and the Bahamas; subspecies are found in China, Japan, and Mexico.[127]

There are two species of poison oak, commonly referred to as *eastern* and *western* poison oak.

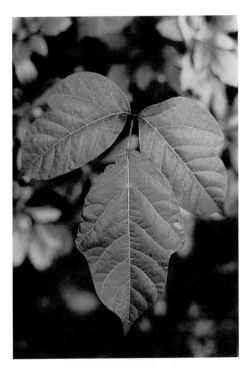

FIGURE 31–6 • Poison ivy.

Toxicodendron toxicarium (eastern poison oak) is found principally in the Southeast: *Toxicodendron diversilobum* (western poison oak) is found on the west coast. Poison oak does not grow well above 4,000 feet, in hot and humid climates, or in desert. The ideal environment is a temperate climate with a hot, wet summer. Exuberant growth is evident in the midwest, north, and southeast, and the eastern and western seacoasts. Poison oak tends to form a small shrub or tree.

Poison sumac *(T. vernix)* is found in moist areas such as peat bogs and swamps of the eastern United States and southeastern Canada. Poison sumac has an odd number (seven to 13) of smooth-edged, pointed leaves (Fig. 31–7).

Allergens

Urushiols are the allergenic chemicals in poison ivy, oak, and sumac. Urushiol (derived from the Japanese word for sap, *urushi*) is a colorless oil that runs in veins from the plant's roots to its leaves. Urushiol is also contained in the plant's berries. As the leaves dry in the fall, the oil content drops, but oil remains in the stems and root parts. Unsuspecting landscapers, woodcutters, and other outdoor workers can develop allergy through exposure to these plant parts during the winter. Urushiol content in these plants has been shown to vary seasonally and also among plants from different environments.[128] Gartner and colleagues showed the content of urushiol in poison oak to be significantly higher in plants from coastal areas, and in the late fall, when the leaves have begun to age.

Urushiols are catechols with long carbon side chains, ranging from C-13 (typical to poison sumac), C-15 (typical to poison ivy), and C-17 (typical to poison oak). The side chains are variably saturated; the more saturated the side chain, the less antigenic is the compound. Longer and more unsaturated side chains are more antigenic. Substitution on the catechol ring also reduces antigenicity.[129] The side chain position is also important: antigenicity is greater when the side chain is located at ring position 3. The carbons at positions 4, 5, and 6 determine protein binding. When carbons 4 and 5 are available for binding, they can bond with amino groups on proteins and sensitization occurs. Position 6 on the ring, if available, may bind to cysteine on proteins and result in nonreactivity or tolerance. In the presence of oxygen, urushiol is converted to a highly reactive *o*-quinone, which then is subject to nucleophilic attack at ring positions 4, 5, and 6. Binding via a sulfhydryl bond leads to reduced allergic contact dermatitis and tolerance via selective induction of suppressor cells, whereas binding with an amino carrier protein to form a complete hapten leads to selective activation of effector T cells and allergic contact dermatitis. Position C6 on the molecule reacts with thiol nucleophiles, while amino nucleophiles bind at the C5 ring position.[130]

Clinical Manifestations

In contrast to many other presentations of plant dermatitis, the dermatitis from poison ivy is often recognized for what it is. It begins any time from 6 to 72 hours after exposure, typically 24 to 48 hours. Exposed skin is affected with linear, streaky, often asymmetrical acute and subacute dermatitis. The reaction can be so strong as to

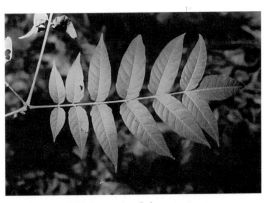

FIGURE 31–7 • Poison sumac.

produce variably sized bullae, which can become quite large and weep serous fluid. Severe sensitivity can lead to dramatic edema and erythema, which are often confused with secondary bacterial infection. Such edema typically occurs on the face or genitals, where the thin skin can become grossly swollen. When burned, poison ivy and oak resin can become airborne and be carried by wind in dust particles contained in smoke. About 10 to 15% of the population are extremely sensitive to poison ivy; such persons develop dermatitis of explosive onset whose swelling and bullae are extreme and dramatic. Untreated, resolution of the dermatitis typically takes 10 days to 2 weeks.

Crossreactions, Tolerance

Another important occupational exposure to urushiol is from the sap of the Japanese lacquer tree *(Rhus vernicifera).* Dermatitis from this tree has been recognized in Japan and China for more than 1,000 years. Decorative lacquerware is a traditional Japanese art and important industry. The raw lacquer contains 60% to 65% urushiol and can cause dermatitis even when dried on an ancient object.[131]

Hardening is a term coined by Jadassohn to describe the development of decreasing sensitivity to an allergen that previously provoked a greater allergic response. In most cases, repeated low-level allergen exposure is required for development of hardening (hyposensitization, or tolerance). The development of tolerance is generally regarded as uncommon; the mechanism is not yet established. An animal study has also shown that repeated cutaneous exposure to low concentrations of a sensitizing substance can result in hyposensitization.[132]

In questionnaire study, 232 lacquer craftsmen reported spontaneous improvement (hyposensitization) to urushiol in 158 of 189 craftsmen. Of these "hardened workers," 12.9% recovered from their dermatitis completely (described as *desensitization*), and 55.2% showed improvement (described as *hyposensitization*). The workers were not tested under experimental conditions, however. Three workers (1.3%) reported serious and continuous dermatitis.[133] The hardening phenomenon was documented experimentally in five of eight lacquer craftsmen who developed a positive patch test to urushiol 1 month after their first contact. Repeat testing after prolonged contact over 9 to 10 months resulted in negative or less markedly positive tests in all but one worker.[134] Clinically, these workers unexpectedly experienced improvement in their dermatitis after repeated exposure, despite a prolonged increase in contact with the lacquer.

A number of case series of cashew nut workers have described allergic dermatitis to cashew nutshell oil.[135, 136] The cashew tree *(Anacardium occidentale)* is cultivated principally in Brazil and India. Cashew shell oil, an irritant, contains the allergens cardol and anacardic acid, which are similar to the catechols of poison ivy and poison oak.[137] These allergens, as well as those of mango, are alk(en)yl resorcinols, which can cross-react with the substituted catechol allergens of poison ivy, oak, and sumac.[138] Heating the nuts before handling decreases the risk of contact dermatitis. Marks reported a series of workers in a factory that processed cashew nut oil into a solid material used to make auto brake linings. Workers who had a history of poison ivy dermatitis before going to work in the factory developed an eczematous eruption after beginning work. The eruption was short lived, lasting 3 weeks in 90% of affected workers. These workers developed decreased sensitivity, described as *tolerance* or *hardening*, which allowed them to continue working. About 10% of affected workers did not develop tolerance and had to change occupations.[139]

Of note, a hypersensitivity dermatitis known as an *internal-external* systemic eczematous reaction can occur from eating raw cashew nuts, since the cashew nut oil contains phenolic allergens that are antigenically similar to the catechols in toxicodendrons. This internal-external dermatitis is characterized by a pruritic, eczematous dermatitis, often on the buttocks (or bathing trunk area), flexural skin, and axillary folds.[140]

The mango tree *(Mangifera indica)* is another member of the Anacardiaceae family. Bark, leaves, stem, and the fruit's skin contain urushiol and other long-chain phenols such as cardol. Found in Florida, the Caribbean, and Central America, *Metopium toxiferum*, the poisonwood tree, contains similar allergenic catechols.[141] The rengas tree also contains a cross-reacting allergenic resin; exposure to furniture made from its wood can result in dermatitis.[142] Indian laundry workers exposed to the black juice of the Indian marking tree nut *(S. anacardium),* or bhilawa tree, may develop "dhobie mark dermatitis," due to the pentadecylcatechol in the black juice that is used to mark laundry in India and Malaysia.[143]

Prevention

The best protection against poison ivy and oak is recognizing the plant and avoiding it. Knowledge of where these plants are likely to be encountered, their identifying features, and basic information about how allergic contact dermatitis is contracted can be vital to preventing dermatitis in workers at risk. A mask can protect against windborne urushiol resins in particulate smoke dust. Extremely sensitive persons should avoid jobs where exposure to urushiol is likely. Urushiols can penetrate rubber gloves; heavy-duty vinyl gloves provide better hand protection.[144]

Destroying the plant is a difficult task, as herbicides are nonspecific and kill other plants. Ortho Poison Oak and Poison Ivy Killer Formula II contains triclopyr herbicide, which kills weeds and bushy plants, including poison ivy. As yet there is no effective biological method for eradicating these plants.

Washing exposed skin with soap and water has been shown to reduce the severity of the eruption, but only when it is done within 5 to 10 minutes of contact.[145] Protective clothing is often used as primary prevention against exposure to a variety of chemicals. Diverse clothing materials have been investigated, principally from the point of the fiber's binding urushiol; thus far they have limited practical application in the field because the binding efficacy of cloth alone is limited. Contaminated clothing of exposed workers could be removed in the field and decontaminated by immersion in a solvent system before being washed. Organic solvents readily solubilize urushiol and can effectively remove the urushiol resin from tools and animals. Use of such solvents to remove the resin from human skin is often limited by the 5- to 10-minute window of opportunity to remove the allergenic chemicals from the skin. Isopropyl alcohol is a readily available and inexpensive solvent that can be used in this way. It should be applied liberally and with caution to avoid redistributing the oil by vigorous or extensive rubbing of unaffected skin. Such an approach is effective only when used shortly after exposure.

Hyposensitization, Barrier Protection

Extracts of poison ivy and oak have been used to desensitize some patients. The procedure takes 2 to 4 months, requires cautious monitoring, and involves repeated low-level exposures. This approach has yielded anecdotal success and occasional severe flaring of dermatitis; controlled trials of desensitization have failed to show efficacy and safety,[146, 147] and extracts presently are not commercially available.

A variety of barrier creams have been investigated. A study of the barrier effect of ferric ammonium citrate found that it failed to diminish or protect from poison ivy.[148] Orchard and associates demonstrated that polyamine salts of linoleic acid dimer served as a skin protectant.[149] A polyamine linoleic acid dimer petrolatum-based product (Stokogard Outdoor Cream), a petrolatum-based ointment with vitamins A, D, and E (Hollister Moisture Barrier), and a silicone cream (Hydropel) were reported by Grevelink and colleagues to be effective in reducing the severity of experimentally induced dermatitis. Four of seven other barrier creams were not effective. These compounds likely limit or prevent dermatitis by inhibiting allergen penetration.[150]

Epstein tested an organoclay compound that was protective in experimental conditions up to 4 hours, and in some cases as long as 24 hours.[151] Five-percent quaternium-18 bentonite (bentoquatam) lotion, an organoclay material, applied 1 hour before patch testing was shown to prevent or limit poison ivy and poison oak dermatitis in a single-blind multicenter investigation. In the study by Marks and colleagues, 68% of 144 patients demonstrated to be allergic to a mixture of poison ivy and poison oak did not react after using the barrier lotion; the remaining 32% developed mild dermatitis as compared with that on control sites where no barrier lotion was applied.[152] This compound may work by interfering with absorption by acting as a physical block. It is now marketed in an over-the-counter lotion known as Ivy Block, manufactured by Enviroderm. It is the only FDA-approved topical poison ivy– and poison oak–preventive product.

Treatment

Acute poison ivy, oak, or sumac contact dermatitis is managed with corticosteroids. Wet compresses applied twice a day with dilute aluminum subacetate solutions (Domeboro) are soothing and help to remove crusts and to dry weeping lesions. They can be followed by topical corticosteroid creams such as triamcinolone, 0.1% cream. For generalized dermatitis, oatmeal baths are soothing, but treatment is usually best accomplished with oral corticosteroids. Prednisone, 40 to 60 mg daily, tapered slowly over 2 to 3 weeks can help avoid the flare-up seen when tapering is too rapid or treatment too brief. Oral antihistamines such as diphenhydramine or hydroxyzine can help provide relief from the unforgiving itch.

Primula

Primula obconica is a popular house plant in Europe and the most common cause of contact dermatitis to plants in European homemakers. *Primula* dermatitis is more often a consequence of caring for houseplants (primroses) than of occupational handling.[153] Cross-reactivity to some tropical woods, especially rosewood, has been reported. Facial dermatitis, at times combined with hand and arm dermatitis, is the most common distribution. The allergen is found on the plant surface in small glandular hairs.

The responsible allergen is primin (2-methoxy-6-pentyl-1,4-benzoquinone), a strong sensitizer, which should be tested at 0.01% concentration in petrolatum.[154] Primin is an allergen found on the standard European allergen tray. Krebs and Christensen extracted a related compound, miconidin, from *P. obconica*; primin may be another allergen in *P. obconica*.[155] Ethyl ether extraction removes most of the allergen.[156] The amount of allergen is greatest in the summer months and least in the winter. Avoidance of the plant prevents the dermatitis. A cultivar named *libra* is reported to be primin free and was cultivated especially to eliminate difficulty with this allergen.

Sabra

The vernacular name *Sabra*, or *Indian fig*, refers to a fruit-bearing prickly pear, *Opuntia ficus indica*. The plant is cultivated in warm climates for its sweet fruit, which is wrapped in a thick, bristly, glochid-covered skin. Described in fruit gatherers in Israel as a mimic of scabies, Sabra dermatitis is due to the fruit's glochids, or bristles, which break off and pierce the skin, producing irritant dermatitis.[157] These prickly pear pickers developed a pruritic, papular dermatitis on the fingers, wrists, genitals, trunk, and buttocks.

Trachelium caeruleum

This member of the Campanulaceae (bellflower) family bears a flower that is becoming increasingly popular in floral bouquets. It is indigenous to the Western Mediterranean region and to Portugal. Van Baar and Van der Valk recently reported a case of a male florist who was already allergic to *Chrysanthemum* species and who developed contact allergy to *T. caeruleum* after 1 year of handling and cultivation.[158] The allergen has not been determined but is not believed to cross-react with chrysanthemums, given the long latency before this florist previously sensitized to Compositae developed dermatitis.

Tobacco

Dermatitis from tobacco is generally considered rare. Work in the later stages of cultivation and processing are more often implicated in reported cases. Reports have involved cases from handling the cured leaves and in the manufacturing of cigars and cigarettes.[159–161] Allergy has also been reported in farm workers exposed to the green, uncured leaves.[162] The majority of reactions among tobacco workers are felt to be predominantly irritant in nature, from exposure to mechanical trauma, wet, alkaline leaves, and irritant effects of nicotine and other alkaloids.[163] A review of cases reported to the poison control center in Kentucky from 1990 to 1992 found one case of dermatitis reported each year, during the harvest seasons (August or September).[164] The reports of these three cases are nonspecific; they are described as erythema, pruritus, skin rash, and irritation occurring on the arms, face, legs, underarms, and sternum.

Tulips

Contact allergy from handling, packaging, sorting, and digging tulips was described many years ago and is well-known, especially in Europe.[165] Many reports come from the Netherlands, where bulb cultivation is a major industry. A Swedish survey of nursery workers involved mainly in the cultivation of tulips noted a 13.7% incidence of allergic contact dermatitis. Allergic contact dermatitis to tulips or daffodils was confirmed by patch testing in nine of 18 workers tested in this survey.[166] Eight of 12 patients with occupational contact allergy to decorative plants were allergic to tuliposide A; sensitivity was secondary to handling tulips and their bulbs or to handling *Alstroemeria*, which also contains this allergen. Other genera of the family Liliaceae also contain tuliposide A.

Tulip fingers is the classic description of allergy to tulip bulbs—a scaling, erythematous, and pruritic dermatitis, typically on the thumb and forefingers. The first and second fingers of the dominant hand are most often affected; however, as Bruze's group observed, dermatitis in nursery workers can be localized to the arms or the face, in addition to the hands.[14] This probably occurs principally through direct or incidental, unintentional transfer of allergen, although airborne contact dermatitis does occur in some cases.[167] Since the allergen is also found in the flowers, leaves, and stems of tulips, sensitivity can be acquired by handling the flowers or the bulbs.[168]

Gette and Marks[166] described five of nine (59%) of the workers in a bulb distribution business who sorted and packaged a variety of bulbs and developed a seasonal allergic contact hand dermatitis. The affected workers' dermatitis involved principally the dominant hand, mainly the fingertips, with erythematous, dry and scaling, painful and fissured lesions. In contrast to many presentations of contact allergy, pruritus and vesiculation were not part of the clinical picture. Nails were also sometimes dystrophic. Their investigation showed positive patch tests to tuliposide A, 0.1% pet in petrolatum, and to bulb epidermal pieces. Nitrile gloves were helpful in two of the workers and were recommended on the basis of prior testing, which was negative when tuliposide A was applied over a nitrile glove, but not over a vinyl glove.[14] Follow-up over several years has shown that nitrile gloves provide excellent worker protection.

Contact urticaria to tulips can manifest itself as irritation of the skin, mucous membranes, and eyes. Rhinitis, coughing, wheezing, and asthma attacks have been described, but rarely. Lahti reported a case of contact urticaria associated with exposure to a variety of tulip cultivars and "funeral lilies" (Lilium longiflorum) in an atopic floral shop worker. Patch tests to fresh tulip bulb, stem, and petal were negative, but prick and scratch chamber tests produced reactions within 30 minutes. The allergen was present in water, but not in acetone or ethanol extracts.[37]

The hydrolysis product of tuliposide A, alpha-methylene-gamma-butyrolactone, also known as tulipalin A, which has been identified as the allergen responsible for the characteristic fingertip allergic dermatitis seen in tulip workers, is commercially available for testing.[169] Testing is performed to tulipalin A, 0.01% in petrolatum, and to flower and bulb extracts, as described by Bruze and coworkers, or to the tulip flower, leaves, or stalk as is.[170] Tulipalin B has also been reported to be a sensitizer in tulips, but it is not commercially available. For this reason, testing to plant extracts may be more sensitive.[171] Limiting direct skin contact with the plant sap by changing work procedures and wearing protective gloves for handling the plants may help.

WOODS

Wood can cause folliculitis, allergic and irritant contact dermatitis, and contact urticaria. Erythema multiforme–like reactions have also been reported as a manifestation of contact allergy to woods. Alkaloids, saponines, anthraquinone, and phenols are compounds recognized to cause irritant contact dermatitis in woodworkers. Contact urticaria has been reported to woods such as ash, larch, limba, obeche, pine, spruce, and ramin.[172, 173] Many woods have been identified as causes of allergic contact dermatitis. The allergic form of dermatitis is frequently caused by quinones (benzo-, naphtho,- furano-, and phenanthrene quinones). Stilbenes, phenol compounds, and terpenes have also been implicated in reports of allergic contact dermatitis.[174]

Wood allergy can affect workers in a variety of woodworking occupations; reports detail affected carpenters, foresters, sawmill workers, shop teachers, cabinet builders, and boatbuilders, among others. Finished wood products infrequently produce contact allergy or irritation. Tiny dust fragments created by woodworking and sanding are most often the source of contact allergy to wood materials. Fine sanding jobs pose the greatest risk for both dermatitis and respiratory problems. In a study of furniture makers, 3.8% of 479 sanders had an occupational skin disease.[175] Pruritus (1.6%), irritant contact dermatitis (1.6%), and xerosis (1.4%) were the most common cutaneous diagnoses. Allergy to wood can also occur in musicians through prolonged and repeated direct contact with wooden instruments such as violins, recorders, and even (rarely) keyboard instruments.[176, 177] More comprehensive reviews of contact allergy to woods can be found in several reference texts.[26, 174]

Occupations at Risk

Some of the occupations that entail exposure to wood dust are woodworking instruction, forestry, carpentry, boatbuilding, cabinetry, and sawmill and papermill work. The incidence of occupational irritation and allergy to woods is small, though when it occurs, the consequences may have considerable financial impact for a skilled worker in a trade. Furniture makers and woodworkers are considered among those at highest risk. The 1-year prevalence of hand dermatitis in woodworking teachers in Sweden was 19%, whereas the baseline population's incidence was 9%. The dermatitis was generally mild, however, and minimal time was lost from work and medical consultation limited.[178] Allergic contact dermatitis to wood is infrequent but most often is reported to the so-called exotic woods from regions such as Asia, Africa, and Central and South America.

Clinical Manifestations

Wood dust from many conifers and hardwood trees can cause contact dermatitis of airborne distribution. The typical distribution of dermatitis from allergy to sawdust begins on the exposed hands and forearms and concurrently or subsequently appears on the face and neck, often involving the eyelids, submental skin, and postauricular area (which helps differentiate it from photoallergy). Wood dust can also be trapped by clothing and the reaction accentuated by sweating and friction in areas where clothing is snug, such as the waistline, boot tops, and periaxillary skinfolds.[179] The pruritic skin often becomes lichenified over time. An erythema multiforme–like reaction is an uncommon but occasional clinical manifestation of contact allergy to wood.[180]

Important Wood Contact Allergens

Several wood species implicated in allergic contact dermatitis are discussed next. A more extensive review of the topic can be found in the aforementioned texts by Mitchell and Rook, Benezra, and Hausen. The first step in the evaluation of a suspected wood allergic contact dermatitis is proper identification of the wood species. Testing methods are described at the chapter's end.

Apuleia leiocarpa Wood

Other names for *Apuleia leiocarpa* include *tatjuba*, *bagasse*, and *crebianco giono*; in Brazil it is known as *garapia* and *amarelao*. The International Technical Tropical Woods Association has proposed the common name *grapia*. A large tree of two varieties grown in Brazil, it is used for heavy construction purposes. A case of airborne contact allergy to the sawdust, accompanied by rhinitis and wheezing, has been reported.[181] The wood contains a number of flavones; the allergens are probably flavones, oxycyanin A, and oxycyanin B.

Australian Blackwood (Acacia melanoxylon R. Br.)

Also known as *Tasmanian blackwood*, the rich reddish brown wood of *A. melanoxylon* is used for furniture and cabinetry, paneling, billiard tables, and for decorations such as handles and inlays. It is one of the most commonly used woods in Australia and has been imported to Argentina, Sri Lanka, Chile, India, and Britain. According to experiments by Hausen, it has moderate to strong sensitizing capacity.[182] It has been reported to cause contact dermatitis in foresters and sawmillers in Tasmania.[183] Hausen has identified hydroxyflavan sensitizers (flavan-3,4-diols) to be primarily responsible for allergy. The primary sensitizer has been identified as melacacidin (2,3-cis-3,4-cis 3, 3′,4,4′7,8-hexahydroxyflavan). Hausen has pointed out the potential for cross-reactivity since melacacidin is also found in 125 Australian *Acacia* species and three African ones. Quinonoid components 2,6-dimethoxy-1,4-benzoquinone and acamelin have been identified as other weak sensitizing components.[114, 184] Correia and coworkers described a case of allergic contact dermatitis in a joiner exposed to airborne wood dust.[185] Testing can be performed with the sawdust incorporated into petrolatum in 1% and 5% concentrations.

Koa Wood *(Acacia koa)*

There are hundreds of *Acacia* species, most native to Africa or Australia. Koa wood is a hardwood of great economic importance to the Hawaiian islands. The Hawaiian koa tree (*Acacia koa* Gray) produces a reddish brown wood used in cabinetry, flooring, veneer, and furniture making. Knight and Hausen reported three cases of woodworkers' allergy to koa wood.[186] The sawdust was tested as is and as 1%, 3%, and 20% concentrations in petrolatum. Based on their results, 1% sawdust in petrolatum seems adequate for testing. Melacacidin was identified as the main sensitizer. More than 128 species of *Acacia* also contain this allergenic chemical.

Brazilian Box Tree Wood

The Brazilian box tree wood (*Aspidosperma* sp.) has both irritant and sensitizing capability. Jemec and Hausen reported a case of contact allergy in a beautician who used an "orange stick" made from the Brazilian box tree for manicuring, and in an organist with a fingertip, facial, and eyelid dermatitis associated with playing a keyboard made of the box tree wood. Testing can be performed with the wood scrapings in ethanol, or 10% and 1% ethanol extracts in petrolatum. Test results may be difficult to interpret given the known irritant potential of the wood.[176]

Cedar

A number of different woods are commonly referred to as cedar. *Cedar* is the common name given to four members of the genus *Cedrus*, family Pinaceae. The term *cedar poisoning* is a misnomer, since *Frullania*, and less often lichens, have been found to be the main causes of this dermatitis in foresters.[187] Western red cedar (*Thuja plicata*) is used in construction, boatbuilding, paneling, and shingling. Contact allergy to Western red cedar has been reported in a sawmill worker. Patch tests to an ethanol extract of the wood produced a reaction.[188] Further work demonstrated at least three allergens: gamma-thujaplicin, 7-hydroxy-4-isopropyltropolone, and carvacol.[189]

Cocobolo

Cocobolo (*Dalbergia retusa*), native to Nicaragua, Mexico, Panama, and Costa Rica, is a popular exotic wood because of its hardness, moisture resistance, and strength. Cocobolo is used to make cutlery, wooden jewelry, billiard cues, revolver stocks, and musical instruments. More than 100 cases of contact allergy to cocobolo have been reported.

Quinonoid compounds known as *dalbergiones* are the sensitizing allergens. There are a variety of quinones implicated in so-called exotic or tropical wood allergy; since many woodworkers use a variety of exotic woods, it is important to note that these chemically related moieties may show cross-reactivity.[190] Obtussaquinone and (R)-4-methoxy-dalbergione are the main sensitizers.[182] Some allergens that cross-react with the *Dalbergia* species may include the allergen primin, from primrose *(P. obconica)*, deoxylapachol from teak *(Tectona grandis)*, lapachenole from peroba *(Paratecoma peroba)*, and mansonone A from mansonia *(Mansonia altissima)*.[174]

Cordia

Boatbuilding, construction, and furniture making are a few of the uses for *Cordia* species grown in South America and Africa. Sensitization has been shown in animals, but there are no unequivocal cases reported in humans.[174]

Grevillea

A member of the Proteaceae family, the *Grevillea* genus has more than 170 species; dermatitis can result from exposure to the wood, flowers, and leaves. *Grevillea robusta* is also known as the Australian silky oak and the silver oak. The rapidly growing tree is used for shade and decoration and is indigenous to Australia, but it also grows in Hawaii, California, Arizona, and Florida. The light-colored heartwood is useful for decorative objects, plywood, and furniture. 5-Tridecylresorcinol (grevillol, 95%), 5-pentadecylresorcinol (5%), and 5-pentadecenylresorcinol (2%) are the three resorcinol compounds identified as sensitizers contained in the heartwood of *Grevillea*.[191, 192] The same resorcinol allergens are found in the botanically unrelated but phytochemically related *Philodendron* species, members of the family Araceae. The cashew nut tree, *A. occidentale* L., contains an identical allergen.

Case reports of allergic contact dermatitis to *Grevillea* wood have been described.[193–196] Telephone line and maintenance workers have used the term *Grevillol poisoning* to describe the reaction to this tree. Adams described a woodworker in a decorative box manufacturing plant who developed allergy to *Grevillea robusta* A. Cunn. 3 weeks after he began working with it. This case is typical of wood allergy, as this worker spent much of his time using a belt sander and was exposed to sawdust. Testing with the sawdust in 10% petrolatum yielded a reaction. In this case the worker had to give up his job.

Of note, cross-reaction has not been observed to another member of the Proteaceae family, the flowering shrub *Grevillea banksii* R. Br., also known as the *kahili flower*. The kahili flower is known to be a common cause of plant dermatitis in Hawaii. The main allergen in *G. banksii* is pentadecenyl resorcinols, which are unsaturated 15-carbon–side chain resorcinols with one double bond. A popular Australian *Grevillea* hybrid, "Robyn Gordon," from *G. banksii* and *Grevillea bipinnatifida* is the subject of case reports of contact allergy.[197] This flowering plant has been widely distributed in Australian gardens and parks since 1975 and has caused many cases of contact allergy in Australia. The testing challenges in this case were ether extracts of *Grevillea* Robyn Gordon, *G. banksii*, and *Grevillea hookerama* leaf and flower, diluted to 1% in petrolatum; all yielded positive results.

Iroko

Iroko is also known by the vernacular names *kambala, rokko, African teak, African oak, swamp mahogany, rock elm, West African mulberry,* and *bush oak*.[198] Iroko is used in the construction of heavy furniture and in general construction. It is among the more frequent tropical wood sources of occupational contact dermatitis.

Jelutong (Dyera costulata)

D. costulata grows in Southeast Asia and is a member of the family Apocynaceae. Its softness makes it easy to use in woodworking instruction, model workshops in car factories, carving, and for pencils. It has been used for woodwork teaching in Sweden; however, a study of 84 woodworking teachers in Stockholm investigated by questionnaire and patch testing showed (16 of 84) 19% to have patch-test reactions to dilutions of this wood's sawdust. Eight of the teachers had skin problems that could be related to working with this wood. Further testing and guinea pig sensitization experiments demonstrated strong sensitizing potential. As a result, the investigators recommended that other softwoods, such as alder and lime, be substituted for woodworking teaching in Swedish schools.[199]

Macassar Ebony

This expensive East Asian hardwood is used to manufacture furniture, cutlery handles, and musical instruments. The allergen is a macassar quinone, a moderately sensitizing naphthoquinone.[179]

Mahogany

Swietenia macrophylla is also called *American mahogany* and *Honduras mahogany*. This valuable hardwood was used so extensively in the past that demand outpaced supply and the resource was exhausted. African mahogany is used for furniture, boatbuilding, cabinetry, shelving, and other high-quality wood products. *Khaya* and *Entandrophragma*, genera of the family Meliaceae, are other hardwoods also called mahogany and today are used in place of American mahogany.[200] A West African mahogany, *Khaya anthoteca*, has been implicated in contact dermatitis in furniture makers, particularly in Great Britain.[201] Anthothecol and 2,6-dimethoxybenzoquinone are responsible for some allergic reactions to mahogany species, though there are probably other sensitizers.[174]

Oak

Dermatitis from oak wood is quite rare. A flavone from oak bark, quercetin, has mild sensitizing potential.[200]

Pao Ferro

Morado, caviuna vermelha, santos palisander, and *santos rosewood* are among the names used for pao ferro *(Macherium scleroxylum)*,[202] a less expensive and more readily available substitute for true rosewood *(Dalbergia)*. It is used to make furniture, knife handles, and decorative wood items. Pao ferro is both more sensitizing and more irritating than the *Dalbergia* species, though it is closely related to them. The main sensitizer is (R)-3,4-dimethoxydalbergione (R-3,4-DMD), the most sensitizing of the dalbergione compounds.[179] Cross-reactions can occur with other dalbergiones: (R)-methoxydalbergione, (S)-4,4'-dimethoxydalbergione, and (S)-4'-hydroxy-4-methoxydalbergione. Like some other wood dusts, pao ferro can also cause rhinitis and respiratory tract symptoms. Erythema multiforme–like reactions have also been reported.[203]

Pine

Pines are evergreen conifers commonly found in the northern temperate zones. Pine species (genus *Pinus*) are widely used timbers in construction, flooring, cabinetry, furniture making, and pulp and paper manufacturing. A dermatitis of airborne distribution with involvement of the face and hands is typical of allergic dermatitis to pine dust.[204] Handling pine and pine resins only occasionally leads to allergy.[205] Dermatitis in pine forest workers is also uncommon. Oil of turpentine and colophony account for most allergic dermatitis due to *Pinus* species.[3] A monoterpene, delta 3-carene, present in the turpentine oleoresin is responsible for sensitization to turpentine.

Mackey and Marks reported a case of a cabinetmaker who developed allergic contact dermatitis to Western white pine, *Pinus monticola*, 9 years after beginning work with it. The worker showed positive reactions to pine sawdust (10% petrola-

tum), and 2,6-dimethoxy-1,4-benzoquinone, in addition to several other allergens.[205] Interestingly, this worker also experienced a flare of his dermatitis while camping near pine trees.

Varying amounts of abietic acid and dehydroabietic acid, the main components of rosin (colophony), are present in pine and spruce. Oxidation products of these acids are felt to be the main contact allergens.[206] Pine, juniper, and spruce contain compounds also present in colophony. Colophony is present on the American and European standard trays and may identify allergy to pine dust. Persons with delayed-type contact allergy to colophony are likely also to be sensitive to pine and spruce dust, although it is not clear whether enough of these components are present in the wood dust itself to produce primary sensitization.

Poplar

Oliwiecki and coworkers reported a case of allergic contact dermatitis in a tree surgeon whose duties included tree climbing and sawing, clearing, and disposing of limbs. Rash occurred on his face, neck, finger webs, antecubital spaces, perineum, and waist.[207] Patch testing was positive to propolis, 10%, 3-methyl-2-butenyl caffeate, phenylethyl caffeate, and "LB-1," 1%, all as 0.1% extracts in petrolatum. Though poplar buds contain at least 15 different compounds, the primary sensitizers in poplar are thought to be "LB-1" (a mixture of three caffeic acid phentenyl esters typically found in poplar buds), phenylethyl caffeate, and benzyl salicylate. These are also felt to be the sensitizers in propolis, a poplar bud–derived bee glue.[208, 209] Cross-reactions have been reported to balsams of Tolu and of Peru.

Rosewood (Dalbergia)

So-called rosewoods are *Dalbergia* species. Brazilian rosewood *(Dalbergia nigra)* is a very durable wood used for furniture, cabinetry, musical instruments, jewelry, and decorative handles. Pao ferro resembles this wood and may be used as a substitute. More than 20 cases of contact allergy have been reported.[174] Allergy most often results from exposure to wood dust from sawdust and shavings.

The benzoquinone allergens in Brazilian rosewood and other *Dalbergia* species are called dalbergiones and are moderately strong sensitizers. Cross-reactions have been reported with deoxylapachol in teak.[174] East Indian rosewood *(Dalbergia latifolia* Roxb.) contains allergenic dalbergiones, (R)methoxy-dalbergione, and smaller amounts of (S)-4,4'-dimethoxydalbergione.[210] A case of airborne contact dermatitis in a knife handle maker was recently reported. This worker's symptoms included excessive tearing, coughing, and rhinorrhea. Symptoms of rhinitis and asthma have occasionally been reported in woodworkers.[171]

Teak

Native to India, Burma, and Thailand, teak *(Tectona grandis)* is an attractive, durable, and valuable wood typically used for furniture, boatbuilding, framing, flooring, and paneling. Teak was reported to be the most common wood allergen among dermatitis patients at St. John's Hospital in London in 1976.[114] Testing may result in false-positive irritant reactions. Hausen recommends patch testing with a 0.01% dilution of the sawdust in petrolatum.[200] Deoxylapachol is the primary sensitizer; lapachol is another allergen that can be tested as 1% in petrolatum.[211]

Patch Testing

The type of wood handled by a worker suspected to have allergic or irritant contact dermatitis should be accurately identified before testing is considered. If testing is indicated, wood can be tested by making an extract or using shavings or diluted sawdust. Again, cautious attention should be paid to testing and test interpretation, as some woods, particularly in the form of sawdust, can be irritating when used for patch testing and could produce false-positive reactions. Teak and pao ferro are known to be irritating, and if testing is

necessary it should be performed initially with caution and with dilute concentrations. Most non-irritant woods can be tested as sawdust diluted to a 10% concentration in petrolatum. Wet sawdust or wood shavings can be irritating. Some 10 to 20 control subjects must be tested to evaluate irritancy. Extracts can be formulated in alcohol vehicles, which are evaporated before patch testing. Extracts typically are tested at 10% concentration. Irritant reactions and active sensitization are possible. When wood dermatitis is suspected, specific, cautious patch testing should be performed. Careful consideration of patchtest-material concentration and vehicle, and similar testing of control subjects, are also important (Table 31–7).

Prevention

Preventing wood-related allergic dermatitis is difficult, as most cases are due to particulate wood dust exposure produced by wood-processing procedures, and small quantities of exposure can provoke severe flares of dermatitis. Irritant dermatitis often clears more easily with the help of dust control measures and protective clothing. Dust from processing, cutting, and sanding readily becomes airborne. Proper dust evacuation and ventilation are important for primary prevention and clearing of persistent dermatitis in allergic persons. Clothing may provide some protection; ideally, soiled clothing should be removed in the

TABLE 31–7 • Known Contact Allergens in Wood Species

Botanical Name	Contact Allergen and Suggested Patch-test Concentration
Khaya anthotheca	Anthothecol, 1% pet
Chlorophora excelsa	Chlorophorin, 1%–10% pet
Cordia and *Patagonula*	Cordiachromes, 0.1% pet
Tectona grandis L. and *Tabebuia*	Deoxylapachol, 0.01%–0.1% pet
Tectona grandis L. and Bignoniaceae	Lapachol, 1%–10% pet
Macherium	R-3,4-dimethoxydalbergione, 0.01% pet
Dalbergia	S-4,4′-dimethoxydalbergione, 1% pet
	S-4′-hydroxy-4-methoxydal, 1% pet
Different wood species	2,6-Dimethoxy-1,4-benzoquinone, 10%
Grevillea robusta A. Cunn.	Grevillol, 0.1%
Paratecoma peroba Fr. Al.	Lapachenole, 1%
Diospyros celebica Bakh.	Macassar quinone, 1%
Thuja plicata Donn ex D. Don	Thujaplicin, 0.1%–1%
Brya ebenus DC.	7,8-Dihydroxy-2′,4′,5′-trimethoxy-isoflavane, 1%
Mansonia altissima A. Chev	Mansonone A, 0.1% pet
Dalbergia retusa Hemsl.	Obtusaquinone, 1% pet
Distemonanthus benthamianus Baill.	Oxyayanin A and B, 1% pet
Calocedrus decurrens (Torr.) Florin	Thymoquinone, 0.1% pet
Acadia melanoxylon R. Br.	Acamelin, 1% pet
Thespesia populnea L. (milo wood)	7-Hydroxy-2,3,5,6-tetrahydro-3,6,9-trimethylnaphtho[1,8 bc] pyran-4,8-dione (Mansonone A)

work area, after which skin cleansing, preferably showering, is in order. Filtered masks can protect the face from particulate dust. Barrier creams have not yet shown efficacy. Although some persons may be at risk for hyposensitization from repeated exposures over time, this cannot be reliably predicted. Allergic persons whose problems persist despite education and preventive and protective measures may need to change occupations or avoid wood and plant products that have potential for cross-sensitivity.

References

1. Hansen M. Identification of plants. *Semin Dermatol* 1996;15:122–123.
2. Beamon JH. Plant taxonomy. *Clin Dermatol* 1986;4:23–30.
3. Mitchell J, Rook A. *Botanical Dermatology. Plant and Plant Products Injurious to the Skin.* Vancouver: Greengrass; 1979.
4. Roed-Petersen J, Hjorth N. Compositae sensitivity among patients with contact dermatitis. *Contact Dermatitis* 1976;2:271–281.
5. O'Malley MA, Mathias CG. Distribution of lost-work-time claims for skin disease in California Agriculture: 1978–1983. *Am J Ind Med* 1988;14:715–720.
6. O'Malley MA, Smith C, Krieger RI. Dermatitis among stone fruit harvesters in Tulare County, 1988. *Am J Contact Dermatitis* 1990;1:100–111.
7. CD Summary. Center for Disease Prevention and Epidemiology. Oregon Health Division. 1993;42:1–2.
8. Sensor Dermatitis Project in Washington State. *Safety & Health Assessment & Research for Prevention (SHARP).* Washington State Department of Labor & Industries; 1997.
9. Lamminpaa A, Estlander T, Jolank R, et al. Occupational allergic contact dermatitis caused by decorative plants. *Contact Dermatitis* 1996;34:330–335.
10. Thiboutot DM, Hamory BH, Marks JG. Dermatoses among floral shop workers. *J Am Acad Dermatol* 1990;22:54–58.
11. Pereira F. Hand dermatitis in florists. *Contact Dermatitis* 1996;34:144–145.
12. Hoogasian C. Dermatitis concerns spark industry study. *Florist* 1988;21:95–99.
13. Rycroft RJ. Dermatitis in florists. *Semin Dermatol* 1996;15:83–86.
14. Bruze M, Björkner B, Hellström AC. Occupational dermatoses in nursery workers. *Am J Contact Dermatitis* 1996;7:100–103.
15. Santucci B, Picardo M. Occupational contact dermatitis to plants. *Clin Dermatol* 1992;10:157–165.
16. Merrick C, Fenney J, Clarke EC, et al. A survey of skin problems in floristry. *Contact Dermatitis* 1991;24:306.
17. Bangha E, Elsner P. Occupational contact dermatitis toward sesquiterpene lactones in a florist. *Am J Contact Dermatitis* 1996;7:188–190.
18. Cronin E. Dermatitis of the hands in caterers. *Contact Dermatitis* 1987;17:265–269.
19. Hjorth N, Roed-Petersen J. Occupational protein contact dermatitis in food handlers. *Contact Dermatitis* 1976;2:28–42.
20. Sinha S, Pasricha J, Sharma R, et al. Vegetables responsible for contact dermatitis of the hands. *Arch Dermatol* 1977;113:776–779.
21. Alonso MD, Martin JA, Cueva M. Occupational protein

contact dermatitis from lettuce. *Contact Dermatitis* 1993;29:109–110.
22. Hausen BM, Andersen KE, Helander I, et al. Lettuce allergy: sensitizing potency of allergens. *Contact Dermatitis* 1986;15:246–249.
23. Audicana M, Bernaola G. Occupational contact dermatitis from citrus fruits: lemon essential oils. *Contact Dermatitis* 1994;31:183–185.
24. Cardullo AC, Ruszhowski AM, Deleo VA. Allergic contact dermatitis resulting from sensitivity to citrus peel, geraniol and citral. *J Am Acad Dermatol* 1989;21:395–397.
25. Lovell CR. Current topics in plant dermatitis. *Semin Dermatol* 1996;15:113–121.
26. Lovell CR. *Plants and the Skin.* Oxford: Blackwell Scientific; 1993.
27. Epstein WL. House and garden plants. In: Jackson EM, Goldner R, eds. *Irritant Contact Dermatitis.* New York: Marcel Dekker; 1990:127–165.
28. Aberer W. Occupational dermatitis from organically grown parsnip. *Contact Dermatitis* 1992;26:62.
29. Oppenheim M. Dermatite bulleuse striée consecutive aux bains de soleil dans les pres. *Ann Dermatol Syphilol* 1932;3:1–7.
30. Pathak MA, Daniels F, Fitzpatrick TB. The presently known distribution of furocoumarins (psoralens in plants). *J Invest Dermatol* 1962;39:225–239.
31. Tunget CL, Turchen SG, Manoguerra AS, et al. Sunlight and the plant: a toxic combination: severe phytophotodermatitis from *Cneoridium dumosum. Cutis* 1994;54:400–402.
32. Freeman K, Hubbard SHC, Warin AP. Strimmer rash. *Contact Dermatitis* 1984;10:117–118.
33. Reynolds NJ, Burton JL. Weed wacker dermatitis. *Arch Dermatol* 1991;127:1419–1420.
34. Vale PT. Prevention of phytodermatitis from celery. *Contact Dermatitis* 1993;29:108.
35. Ljunggren B. Psoralen photoallergy caused by plant contact. *Contact Dermatitis* 1977;3:85–90.
36. Nandakishore TH, Pasricha JS. Patterns of cross-sensitivity between 4 Compositae plants, *Parthenium hysterophorus, Xanthium strumarium, Helianthus annuus* and *Chrysanthemum coronarium,* in Indian patients. *Contact Dermatitis* 1994;30:162–167.
37. Lahti A. Contact urticaria and respiratory symptoms from tulips and lilies. *Contact Dermatitis* 1986;5:317–319.
38. Hjorth N, Roed-Petersen J. Occupational protein contact dermatitis in food handlers. *Contact Dermatitis* 1976; 2:28–29.
39. Orange AP, Van Gysel D, Mulder PGH, et al. Food-induced contact urticaria syndrome (CUS) in atopic dermatitis: reproducibility of repeated and duplicate testing with a skin provocation test, the skin application food test (SAFT). *Contact Dermatitis* 1994;31:314–318.
40. Hannuksela M, Lahti A. Immediate reaction to fruit and vegetables. *Contact Dermatitis* 1979;3:79–84.
41. Guin JD. Patch testing to plants: some practical aspects of what has become an esoteric area of contact dermatitis. *Am J Contact Dermatitis* 1995;6:232–235.
42. Mitchell JC. Patch testing to plants. *Clin Dermatol* 1986;4:77–82.
43. Gartner BL, Wasser C, Rodriguez E, et al. Seasonal variation of urushiol content in poison oak leaves. *Am J Contact Dermatitis* 1993;4:33–36.
44. Hausen BM, Pratter E, Schubert H. The sensitizing capacity of *Alstroemeria* cultivars in man and guinea pig. *Contact Dermatitis* 1983;9:46–54.
45. Hausen BM. A simple method for extracting crude sesquiterpene lactones from Compositae plants for skin tests,

chemical investigations and sensitizing experiments in guinea pigs. *Contact Dermatitis* 1977;3:58–60.

46. Marks JG, Deleo V. *Contact and Occupational Dermatology*, 2nd ed. St. Louis: Mosby–Year Book; 1997:204–207.

47. Cronin E. Sensitivity to tulip and *Alstroemeria*. *Contact Dermatitis Newslett* 1972;11:286.

48. Van Ketel WG, Verspyck Mijnssen GAW, Neering H. Contact eczema from *Alstroemeria*. *Contact Dermatitis* 1975;1:323.

49. Marks JG. Allergic contact dermatitis to *Alstroemeria*. *Arch Dermatol* 1988;124:914–915.

50. Rook A. Dermatitis from *Alstroemeria*. Altered clinical pattern and probable increasing incidence. *Contact Dermatitis* 1981;7:355–356.

51. Adams RM, Daily AD, Brancaccio RR, et al. *Alstroemeria*: a new and potent allergen for florists. *Dermatol Clin* 1990;8:73–76.

52. Rook A. *Alstroemeria* causing contact dermatitis in a florist also allergic to tulips. *Contact Dermatitis Newslett* 1970;7:166.

53. Piirila P, Keskinen H, Leino T, et al. Occupational asthma caused by decorative flowers: review and case reports. *Int Arch Occup Environ Health* 1994;6:131–136.

54. Christensen LP, Kristiansen K. A simple HPLC method for the isolation and quantification of the allergens tuliposide A and tulipalin A in *Alstroemeria*. *Contact Dermatitis* 1995;32:199–203.

55. Marks JG. Allergic contact dermatitis to *Alstroemeria*. *Arch Dermatol* 1988;84:446–448.

56. Rietschel RL. Selected highlights of the Second Congress of the European Society of Contact Dermatitis. *Am J Contact Dermatitis* 1995;6:128–129.

57. Christensen LP, Kristiansen K. Isolation and quantification of a new tuliposide (tuliposide D) by HPLC in *Alstroemeria*. *Contact Dermatitis* 1995;33:188–192.

58. Hausen BM, Wolf C. 1,2,3-Trithiane-5-carboxylic acid, a first contact allergen from *Asparagus officinalis* (Liliaceae). *Am J Contact Dermatitis* 1996;7:41–46.

59. Saihan EM, Harman RR. *Coleus* sensitivity in a gardener. *Contact Dermatitis* 1978;4:234–235.

60. Dooms Goossens A, Borghijs A, Degreef H, et al. Airborne contact dermatitis to *Coleus*. *Contact Dermatitis* 1987;17:109–110.

61. Byrld LE. Airborne contact dermatitis from *Coleus* plant. *Am J Contact Dermatitis* 1997;8:8–9.

62. Hausen BM, Devriese EG, Geun JMC. Sensitizing potency of coleon O in *Coleus* species. *Contact Dermatitis* 1988;19:217–218.

63. Mitchell JC, Dupuis G, Geissman TA. Allergic contact dermatitis from sesquiterpenoids of plants. Additional allergic sesquiterpene lactones and immunologic specificity of Compositae, liverwort and lichens. *Br J Dermatol* 1972;87:235–240.

64. Menz J, Winkelmann RK. Sensitivity to wild vegetation. *Contact Dermatitis* 1987;16:169–173.

65. Mitchell JC, Fritig B, Towers GHN. Allergic contact dermatitis from *Frullania* and Compositae. The role of sesquiterpene lactones. *J Invest Dermatol* 1970;54:233–239.

66. Paulsen E. Compositae dermatitis: a survey. *Contact Dermatitis* 1992;26:76–86.

67. Ross JS, du Peloux Menage H, Hawk JL, et al. Sesquiterpene lactone contact sensitivity: clinical patterns of Compositae dermatitis and relationship to chronic actinic dermatitis. *Contact Dermatitis* 1993;2:84–87.

68. Towers GHN, Mitchell JC. The current status of the weed *Parthenium hysterophorus* L. as a cause of allergic contact dermatitis. *Contact Dermatitis* 1983;9:465–469.

69. Quirce S, Tabar AI, Muro MD, et al. Airborne contact dermatitis from *Frullania*. *Contact Dermatitis* 1994; 2:73–76.

70. Menage H, Ross JS, Norris PG, et al. Contact and photocontact sensitization in chronic actinic dermatitis: sesquiterpene lactone mix is an important allergen. *Br J Dermatol* 1995;4:543–547.

71. Thune P, Eeg-Larsen T. Contact and photocontact allergy in persistent light reactivity. *Contact Dermatitis* 1984; 11:98–107.

72. Warshaw EM, Zug KA. Sesquiterpene lactone dermatitis. *Contact Dermatitis* 1996;7:1–23.

73. Frain-Bell W, Johnson BE. Contact allergic sensitivity to plants and the photosensitivity dermatitis and actinic reticuloid syndrome. *Br J Dermatol* 1979;101:503–512.

74. Addo HA, Johnson BE, Frain-Bell W. A study of the relationship between contact allergic sensitivity and persistent light reaction. *Br J Dermatol Suppl* 1980:103:20–21.

75. Addo HA, Sharma SC, Ferguson J, et al. A study of Compositae plant extract reactions in photosensitivity dermatitis. *Photodermatology* 1985;2;68–79.

76. Thune PO, Solberg YJ. Photosensitivity and allergy to aromatic lichen acids, Compositae oleoresins and other plant substances. *Contact Dermatitis* 1980;6:64–71.

77. Frain-Bell W, Hetherington A, Johnson BE. Contact allergic sensitivity to chrysanthemum and the photosensitivity dermatitis and actinic reticuloid syndrome. *Br J Dermatol* 1979;101:491–501.

78. Ducombs G, Benezra C, Talaga P, et al. Patch testing with the "sesquiterpene lactone mix": a marker for contact allergy to Compositae and other sequiterpene lactone–containing plants. *Contact Dermatitis* 1990;22:249–252.

79. Hausen BM. A 6-year experience with Compositae mix. *Am J Contact Dermatitis* 1996;7:94–99.

80. Green C, Fergusen J. Sesquiterpene lactone mix is not an adequate screen for Compositae allergy. *Contact Dermatitis* 1994;31:151–153.

81. Ducombs G, Benezra C, Andersen KE, et al. Patch testing with the "sesquiterpene lactone mix": a marker for contact allergy to Compositae and other sesquiterpene lactone–containing plants. *Contact Dermatitis* 1990;22:249–252.

82. Paulsen E, Andersen KE, Hausen BM. Compositae dermatitis in a Danish dermatology department in one year (I). Results of a routine patch testing with the sesquiterpene lactone mix supplemented with aimed patch testing with extracts and sesquiterpene lactones of Compositae plants. *Contact Dermatitis* 1993;29:6–10.

83. Hausen BM, Helmke B. Butenylbithiophene, *alpha*-terthienyl and hydroxytremetone as contact allergens in cultivars of marigold (*Tagetes* spp.). *Contact Dermatitis* 1995;33:33–37.

84. Dawe RS, Green CM, MacLeod TM, et al. Daisy, dandelion and thistle contact allergy in the photosensitivity dermatitis and actinic reticuloid syndrome. *Contact Dermatitis* 1996;35:109–110.

85. Gomez E, Garcia R, Galindo PA, et al. Occupational allergic contact dermatitis from sunflower. *Contact Dermatitis* 1996;35:189–190.

86. Lovell CR, Rowan M. Dandelion dermatitis. *Contact Dermatitis* 1991;25:185–188.

87. Hausen BM. A simple method for extracting crude sesquiterpene lactones from Compositae plants for skin tests, chemical investigations and sensitizing experiments in guinea pigs. *Contact Dermatitis* 1977;3:58–60.

88. Roed-Petersen J, Thomsen K. Azathioprine in the treatment of airborne contact dermatitis from Compositae

oleoresins and sensitivity to UVA. *Acta Derm Venereol (Stockh)* 1979;275–277.

89. Roelandts R. Chronic actinic dermatitis. *J Am Acad Dermatol* 1993;28:240–249.

90. Burke DA, Corey G, Storrs FJ. Psoralen plus UVA protocol for Compositae photosensitivity. *Am J Contact Dermatitis* 1996;7:171–176.

91. Gonçalo S, Freitas JD, Sousa I. Contact dermatitis and respiratory symptoms from *Narcissus pseudonarcissus*. *Contact Dermatitis* 1987;16:115–116.

92. Van der Werff PJ. Occupational diseases among workers in the bulb industries. *Acta Allergol* 1959;338–355.

93. Gude M, Hausen BM, Heitsch H, et al. An investigation of the irritant and allergenic properties of daffodils (*Narcissus pseudonarcissus* L. Amaryllidaceae). A review of daffodil dermatitis. *Contact Dermatitis* 1988;19:1–10.

94. Lembo G, Balato N, Patruno C. Allergic contact dermatitis due to garlic *(Allium sativum)*. *Contact Dermatitis* 1991;25:330–331.

95. Burden AD, Wilkinson SM, Beck MH, et al. Garlic-induced contact dermatitis. *Contact Dermatitis* 1994; 30:299–315.

96. Papageorgiou C, Corbet JP, Mendez Brandao F, et al. Allergic contact dermatitis to garlic (*Allium sativum* L.). Identification of the allergens: the role of mono-, di-, and trisulphides present in the garlic. *Arch Dermatol Res* 1983;275:229–234.

97. Meijer P, Coenraads PJ, Hausen BM. Allergic contact dermatitis from hydrangea. *Contact Dermatitis* 1990; 23:59–60.

98. Hausen BM. Hydrangenol, a strong contact sensitizer in hydrangea (*Hydrangea* sp.; Hydrangeaceae). *Contact Dermatitis* 1991;24:233–235.

99. Veraldi S, Schianchi-Veraldi R. Contact urticaria from kiwi fruit. *Contact Dermatitis* 1990;22:244.

100. Rademaker M. Allergic contact dermatitis from kiwi fruit vine *(Actinidia chinensis)*. *Contact Dermatitis* 1996; 34:221–222.

101. Champion RH. Atopic sensitivity to algae and lichens. *Br J Dermatol* 1971;85:551–557.

102. Tenchio F. Etiologie de l'eczema des bûherons. *Dermatologica* 1948;97:72–77.

103. Salo H, Hannuksela M, Hausen BM. Lichen picker's dermatitis. *Contact Dermatitis* 1981;7:9–13.

104. Sandberg M, Thune P. The sensitizing capacity of atranorin. *Contact Dermatitis* 1984;11:168–173.

105. Frain-Bell W, Johnsen BE. Contact allergic sensitivity to plants and the photosensitivity dermatitis and actinic reticuloid syndrome. *Br J Dermatol* 1979;101:503–512.

106. Addo HA, Ferguson J, Johnsen BE, et al. The relationship between exposure to fragrance materials and persistent light reaction in photosensitivity dermatitis with actinic reticuloid. *Br J Dermatol* 1982;107:261–274.

107. Fernandez de Corres L, Munos D, Leaniz-Berrutia J, et al. Photocontact dermatitis from oak moss. *Contact Dermatitis* 1983;9:528–529.

108. Dahlquist I, Fregert S. Atranorin and oak moss contact allergy. *Contact Dermatitis* 1981;3:168–169.

109. Mitchell JC, Fritig B, Singh B, et al. Allergenic contact dermatitis from *Frullania* and Compositae. *J Invest Dermatol* 1970;54:233–239.

110. Quirino AP, Barros MA. Occupational contact dermatitis from lichens and *Frullania*. *Contact Dermatitis* 1995;33:68.

111. Thune PO. Contact allergy due to lichens in patients with a history of photosensitivity. *Contact Dermatitis* 1977;3:267–272.

112. Thune PO, Solberg YJ. Photosensitivity and allergy to aromatic lichen acids, Compositae oleoresins and other plant substances. *Contact Dermatitis* 1980;6:81–87.

113. Foussereau J, Muller JC, Benezra C. Contact allergy to *Frullania* and *Laurus nobilis*: cross sensitization and chemical structure of the allergens. *Contact Dermatitis* 1975;1:223–230.

114. Woods B, Calnan C. Toxic woods. *Br J Dermatol* 1976; 95 [Suppl 13]:1–97.

115. Quirce S, Tabar AI, Muro MD, et al. Airborne contact dermatitis from *Frullania*. *Contact Dermatitis* 1994; 30:73–76.

116. Foussereau J, Muller JC, Benezra C. Contact allergy to *Frullania* and *Lauris nobilis*: cross sensitization and chemical structure of the allergens. *Contact Dermatitis* 1975;1:223–230.

117. Benezra C, Stampf JL, Barbier P, et al. Enantiospecificity in allergic contact dermatitis. *Contact Dermatitis* 1985; 13:110–114.

118. De Corres LF. Contact dermatitis from *Frullania*, Compositae and other plants. *Contact Dermatitis* 1984;11:74–79.

119. Mitchell JC. Industrial aspects of 112 cases of allergic contact dermatitis from *Frullania* in British Columbia during a 10-year period. *Contact Dermatitis* 1981;7:268–269.

120. Tomb RR. Patch testing with *Frullania* during a 10-year period: hazards and complications. *Contact Dermatitis* 1992;26:220–223.

121. Storrs FJ, Rasmussen JE, Mitchell JC. Contact hypersensitivity to liverwort and the Compositae family of plants. *Cutis* 1976;18:681–686.

122. O'Malley MA, Barba R. Bullous dermatitis in field workers associated with exposure to mayweed. *Am J Contact Dermatitis* 1990;1:34–42.

123. Bruynzeel DP. Contact dermatitis due to *Paeonia* (peony). *Contact Dermatitis* 1989;20:152–153.

124. Kanzaki T, Kimura S. Occupational allergic contact dermatitis from *Perilla frutescens* (shiso). *Contact Dermatitis* 1992;26:55–56.

125. Knight T. *Philodendron*-induced dermatitis: report of cases and review of the literature. *Cutis* 1991;48:375–378.

126. Epstein WL. Occupational poison ivy and oak dermatitis. *Dermatol Clin* 1994;12:511–516.

127. Guin JD, Gillis WT, Beaman JH. Recognizing the *Toxicodendrons* (poison ivy, poison oak, and poison sumac). *J Am Acad Dermatol* 1981;4:99–114.

128. Gartner BL, Wasser C, Rodriguez E, et al. Seasonal variation of urushiol content in poison oak leaves. *Am J Contact Dermatitis* 1993;4:33–36.

129. Marks JG. Poison ivy and poison oak allergic contact dermatitis: *Immunol Allergy Clin North Am* 1989;9:497–506.

130. Dunn IS, Leberato DJ, Castagnoli N, et al. Contact sensitivity to urushiol: role of covalent bond formation. *Cell Immunol* 1982;74:220–233.

131. Toyama I. *Rhus* dermatitis. *J Cutan Dis* 1918;36:157–165.

132. Boerringer GH, Scheper RJ. Local and systemic desensitization induced by repeated epicutaneous hapten application. *J Invest Dermatol* 1987;88:3–7.

133. Kawai K, Nakagawa M, Kawi K. Hyposensitization to urushiol among Japanese lacquer craftsmen. *Contact Dermatitis* 1991;24:146–147.

134. Kawai K, Nakagawa M, Kawi K, et al. Hyposensitization to urushiol among Japanese lacquer craftsmen: results of patch tests on students learning the art of lacquerware. *Contact Dermatitis* 1991;25:290–295.

135. Pasricha JS, Skiniwas CR, Shankar K. Contact dermatitis to cashew nut *(Anacardium occidentale)* shell oil, pericarps and kernel. *Indian J Dermatol Venereol Leprol* 1988;43:36–37.

136. Pasricha JS, Skiniwas CR, Krupashankar DS, et al. Occupational dermatoses among the cashew nut workers in Karnataka. *Indian J Dermatol Venereol Leprol* 1988;54:15–20.

137. Diogenes MJ, DeMorais SM, Carvalho FF. Contact dermatitis among cashew nut workers. *Contact Dermatitis* 1996;35:114–115.

138. Guin J. When is "poison ivy dermatitis" not poison ivy dermatitis? [Editorial]. *Am J Contact Dermatitis* 1993; 4:133–135.

139. Reginella RF, Fairfield JC, Marks JG. Hyposensitization to poison ivy after working in a cashew nut shell oil processing factory. *Contact Dermatitis* 1989;20:274–279.

140. Ratner JH, Spencer SK, Grainge JM. Cashew nut dermatitis. *Arch Dermatol* 1974;110:921–923.

141. Lampe KF. Dermatitis-producing Anacardiaceae of the Caribbean area. *Clin Dermatol* 1986;4:171–182.

142. Beaman JH. Allergenic Asian Anacardiaceae. *Clin Dermatol* 1986;4:191–203.

143. Livingood CS, Rogers AM, Fitz-hugh T. Dhobie mark dermatitis. *JAMA* 1943;123:23–26.

144. Fisher AA. Poison ivy/oak dermatitis. Part 1: Prevention—soap and water, topical barriers, hyposensitization. *Cutis* 1996;57:384–386.

145. Howell JB. Evaluation of measures for prevention of ivy dermatitis. *Arch Dermatol Syph* 1943;48:373–378.

146. Marks JG, Trautlein JJ, Epstein WL, et al. Oral hyposensitization to poison ivy and poison oak. *Arch Dermatol* 1987;123:476–478.

147. Epstein WL. Allergic contact dermatitis to poison oak and ivy. Feasibility of hyposensitization. *Dermatol Clin* 1984;2:613–617.

148. Del Savio B, Sherertz EF. Failure of ferric ammonium citrate to work as a barrier against poison ivy dermatitis. *Am J Contact Dermatitis* 1994;5:242–243.

149. Orchard S, Fellman JH, Storrs FJ. Poison ivy/oak dermatitis: use of polyamine salts of linoleic acid dimer for topical prophylaxis. *Arch Dermatol* 1986;122:783–789.

150. Grevelink SA, Murrell DF, Olsen EA: Effectiveness of various barrier preparations in preventing and/or ameliorating experimentally produced *Toxicodendron* dermatitis. *J Am Acad Dermatol* 1992;27:182–188.

151. Epstein WL. Topical prevention of poison ivy/oak dermatitis. *Arch Dermatol* 1989;125:499–501.

152. Marks JG, Fowler JF, Sherertz EF, et al. Prevention of poison ivy and poison oak allergic contact dermatitis by quaternium-18 bentonite. *J Am Acad Dermatol* 1995;33:212–216.

153. Tabar AI, Quirce S, Garcia BE, et al. *Primula* dermatitis: versatility in its clinical presentation and the advantages of patch tests with synthetic primin. *Contact Dermatitis* 1994;30:47–48.

154. Inger A, Menne T. Primin standard patch testing: 5 years experience. *Contact Dermatitis* 1990;23:15–19.

155. Krebs M, Christensen LP. 2-Methoxy-6-pentyl-1,4-dihydroxybenzene (miconidin) from *Primula obconica*: a possible allergen? *Contact Dermatitis* 1994;33:90–93.

156. Fregert S, Hjorth N. The *Primula* allergen primin. *Contact Dermatitis* 1977;3:172–173.

157. Shanon J, Sagher F. Sabra dermatitis. An occupational dermatitis due to prickly pear handling simulating scabies. *Arch Dermatol* 1956;74:269–275.

158. Van Baar HM, Van der Valk PM. Contact allergy due to *Trachelium caeruleum*. *Contact Dermatitis* 1994;21:118–119.

159. Pecegueiro M. Airborne contact dermatitis to tobacco. *Contact Dermatitis* 1987;17:50–51.

160. Rycroft RJG. Tobacco dermatitis. *Br J Dermatol* 1980; 103:225–229.

161. Rycroft RJG, Smith NP, Stok ET, et al. Investigation of suspected contact sensitivity to tobacco in cigarette and cigar factory employees. *Contact Dermatitis* 1981;7:32–38.

162. Nakamura T. Tobacco dermatitis in Japanese harvesters. *Contact Dermatitis* 1984;10:310.

163. Gonçalo M, Couto J, Gonçalo S. Allergic contact dermatitis from *Nicotiana tabacum*. *Contact Dermatitis* 1990;22:188–189.

164. McKnight RH, Rodgers GC. Occupational tobacco dermatitis reported to a regional poison center. *Contact Dermatitis* 1995;32:122.

165. Welker WH, Rappaport BZ. Dermatitis due to tulip bulbs. *J Allergy* 1932;3:317.

166. Gette MT, Marks JE Jr. Tulip fingers. *Arch Dermatol* 1990;126:203–205.

167. Hausen BM. Airborne contact dermatitis caused by tulip bulbs. *J Am Acad Dermatol* 1982;7:500–503.

168. Slob A, Jekel B, De Jong B. On the occurrence of tuliposides in the *Lilliflorae*. *Phytochemistry* 1975;14: 1997–2005.

169. Mijnssen GA. Pathogenesis and causative agent of "tulip finger." *Br J Dermatol* 1969;81:737–745.

170. Bruze M, Trulsson L, Bendsoe N. Patch testing with ultrasonic bath extracts. *Am J Contact Dermatitis* 1992;3:133–137.

171. Benezra C, Ducombs G, Sell Y, et al. *Plant Contact Dermatitis*. Toronto: BC Decker; 1985.

172. Beck MH, Hausen BM, Dane VK. Allergic contact dermatitis from *Machaerium scleroxylum* Tul. (Pao ferro) in a joinery shop. *Clin Exp Dermatol* 1984;9:159–166.

173. Schmidt H. Contact urticaria to teak with systemic effects. *Contact Dermatitis* 1978;4:176–177.

174. Hausen BM. *Woods Injurious to Human Health: A Manual.* Berlin: de Gruyter; 1981.

175. Gan SL, Goh CL, Lee CS, et al. Occupational dermatosis among sanders in the furniture industry. *Contact Dermatitis* 1987;17:237–240.

176. Jemec GB, Hausen BM. Contact dermatitis from Brazilian box tree wood (*Aspidosperma* sp.). *Contact Dermatitis* 1991;25:58–60.

177. Hausen BM. Chin rest allergy in a violinist. *Contact Dermatitis* 1985;12:178–180.

178. Meding B, Åhman M, Karlberg AT. Skin symptoms and contact allergy in woodwork teachers. *Contact Dermatitis* 1995;34:185–190.

179. Hausen BM. Contact allergy to woods. *Clin Dermatol* 1986;4:65–76.

180. Irvine C, Reynolds A, Finlay AY. Erythema multiforme–like reaction to "rosewood." *Contact Dermatitis* 1988; 29:224–225.

181. Dejobert Y, Martin P, Bergoend H. Airborne contact dermatitis from *Apuleia leiocarpa* wood. *Contact Dermatitis* 1995;32:242–243.

182. Hausen BM, Bruhn G, Tilsley DA. Contact allergy to Australian blackwood (*Acacia melanoxylon* R. Br.): isolation and identification of new hydroxyflavin sensitizers. *Contact Dermatitis* 1990;23:33–39.

183. Tilsley DA. Australian blackwood dermatitis. *Contact Dermatitis* 1990;23:40–41.

184. Hausen BM, Schmalle HW. Quinonoid constituents as contact sensitizers in Australian blackwood *Acacia melanoxylon* R. Br. *Br J Ind Med* 1981;38:105–109.

185. Correia O, Barros MA, Mesquita-Guimaraes J. Airborne contact dermatitis from the woods *Acacia melanoxylon* and *Entandophragma cylindricum*. *Contact Dermatitis* 1992;2:343–344.

186. Knight TE, Hausen BM. Koa wood (*Acacia koa*) dermatitis. *Am J Contact Dermatitis* 1992;3:30–32.

187. Storrs F, Mitchell JC, Rasmussen JE. Contact hypersensitivity to liverwort in the Compositae family of plants. *Cutis* 1976;18:681–686.

188. Bleumink E, Natar JP. Contact dermatitis from Western red cedar *(Thujaplicata)*. *Contact Dermatitis Newslett* 1972;12:339–342.

189. Bleumink E, Mitchell JC, Natar JP. Allergic contact dermatitis from cedar wood. *Br J Dermatol* 1973;88:499–504.

190. Rackett SC, Zug KA. Contact dermatitis to multiple exotic woods. *Am J Contact Dermatitis* 1997;8:114–117.

191. Ritchie E, Taylor WC, Vautin STK. Chemical studies of the Proteaceae. *Aust J Chem* 1965;18:2015–2020.

192. Ridley DD, Ritchie E, Taylor WC. Chemical studies of the Proteaceae II. *Aust J Chem* 1968;21:2979–2988.

193. Adams RM, Arnau J-MC. Allergic contact dermatitis caused by the sawdust of *Grevillea robusta* A. Cunn. *Am J Contact Dermatitis* 1991;2:192–193.

194. Knight TE, Whitesell CD. *Grevillea robusta* (silver oak) dermatitis. *Am J Contact Dermatitis* 1992;3:145–149.

195. Menz J. Contact dermatitis from plants of the *Grevillea* family. *Aust J Dermatol* 1985;26:74–76.

196. Lothian N. *Grevillea* species and hybrids causing contact dermatitis. *Australas J Dermatol* 1989;30:111–113.

197. Menz J, loc. cit.

198. Hinnen U, Willa-Craps C, Elsner P. Allergic contact dermatitis from iroko and pine wood dust. *Contact Dermatitis* 1995;33:251–252.

199. Meding B, Karlberg A-T, Åhman M. Wood dust from jelutong *(Dyera costulata)* causes contact allergy. *Contact Dermatitis* 1996;34:349–353.

200. Hausen BM, Adams RM. In: Adams RM, ed. *Occupational Skin Disease*, 2nd ed. Philadelphia: WB Saunders; 1990:524–536.

201. Wilkinson DS, Budden MG, Hambly EM. A 10-year review of an industrial dermatitis clinic. *Contact Dermatitis* 1980;6:11–17.

202. Chiergato C, Vincenzi C, Guerra L, et al. Occupational airborne contact dermatitis from *Machaerium scleroxylon*. *Contact Dermatitis* 1993;29:164–165.

203. Holst R, Kirby J, Magnusson B. Sensitization to tropical woods giving erythema multiforme–like eruptions. *Contact Dermatitis* 1976;2:295–296.

204. Watsky K. Airborne allergic contact dermatitis from pine dust. *Am J Contact Dermatitis* 1997;8:118–120.

205. Mackey SA, Marks JG. Allergic contact dermatitis to white pine sawdust [Letter]. *Arch Dermatol* 1992;128:1660.

206. Karlberg AT, Bohlinder K, Boman A, et al. Identification of 15-hydroperoxyabietic acid as a contact allergen in Portuguese colophony. *J Pharm Pharmacol* 198;40:42–47.

207. Oliwiecki S, Beck MH, Hausen BM. Occupational allergic contact dermatitis from caffeates in poplar bud resin in a tree surgeon. *Contact Dermatitis* 1992;27:127–128.

208. Hausen BM, Stuewe HI, Koenig WA, Wollenweber E. Propolis allergy (IV). Studies with further sensitizers from propolis and constituents common to propolis, poplar buds and balsam of Peru. *Contact Dermatitis* 1992;26:34–44.

209. Hausen BM, Wollenweber E, Senff H, Post B. Propolis allergy (I). Origin, properties, usage and literature review. *Contact Dermatitis* 1987;17:163–170.

210. Gallo R, Guarra M, Hausen BM. Airborne contact dermatitis from East Indian rosewood *(Dalbergia latifolia* Roxb.). *Contact Dermatitis* 1996;35:60–61.

211. Schmidt H. Contact urticaria to teak with systemic effects. *Contact Dermatitis* 1978;4:176–177.

Bibliography

Benezra C, Ducombs G, Sell Y, et al. *Plant Contact Dermatitis*. Toronto: BC Decker; 1985.

Hausen BM. *Woods Injurious to Human Health: A Manual*. Berlin: de Gruyter; 1981.

Lovell CR. *Plants and the Skin*. Oxford: Blackwell Scientific; 1993.

Mitchell J, Rook A. *Botanical Dermatology. Plant and Plant Products Injurious to the Skin*. Vancouver: Greengrass; 1979. http://bodd.cf.ac.uk. (Courtesy of RJ Schmidt.)

Pesticides and Other Agricultural Chemicals

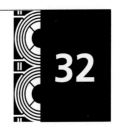

32

DANIEL J. HOGAN, M.D.
LEE H. GRAFTON, M.D.

Farmers and other agricultural workers are exposed to a wide variety of chemical, biological, and physical hazards at work.[1] It is estimated that farmers apply 60% of all domestic agricultural chemicals. In this chapter we review dermatological disorders due to pesticides and other agricultural chemicals.

A *pesticide* is any toxic chemical used to control insects, fungi, viruses, weeds, or rodents. Insecticides, herbicides, fungicides, bactericides, defoliants, miticides/acaricides, nematocides, silvicides (trees and shrubs), fumigants, and rodenticides are all pesticides. The use of herbicides in particular has increased in recent years. Other agricultural chemicals reviewed in this chapter are plant growth inhibitors and repellents against insects. The classification of pesticides used in this chapter is based on that of *Pesticides Studied in Man.*[2] The *Farm Chemical Handbook*[3] and the *Merck Index*[4] are used as the sources for the names, chemical structures, and uses of pesticides and agricultural chemicals.

More than 13,000 pesticide products are registered for use in California alone. These products contain more than 800 active ingredients and more than 1,000 inert ingredients. These products are formulated in many different ways—as liquids, wettable powders, dusts, and fumigants. About 600 million pounds of pesticides are sold annually in California alone.[5]

Large quantities of pesticides are used in nonagricultural settings. Institutional, industrial, and structural pest control uses accounted for an average of 34% of the pesticides employed in California. Some 15% of pesticides sold was used in homes and gardens. In California approximately a third of reported illnesses and injuries due to pesticides involve the skin.[5]

Adverse reactions to pesticides, especially fatal reactions, are more common in Third World countries,[6] but the majority of reports on adverse cutaneous reactions to pesticides originate in North America and Europe.

Lessenger and coworkers[7] reviewed the charts of 190 cases of patients who presented alleging pesticide illness. Important predictors of mild to moderate pesticide illness were found to be anxiety, nausea, vomiting, tearing, weakness, and vertigo. The presence of a rash was not predictive of pesticide exposure and was more often secondary to irritant contact dermatitis or scabies, according to these family physicians.

It has been stated that, considering the extent of their use,[8] contact dermatitis due to pesticides is rare, but it is possible that pesticides cause more contact dermatitis than is reported.[9, 10] Experimentally, certain pesticides are strong sensitizers.[11–12] Diluting pesticides before use in the field minimizes their capacity to sensitize exposed workers, as induction of sensitization requires a certain concentration of an allergen.[12] Once sensitized to a pesticide a person may react on patch testing to dilutions of the pesticide in acetone as weak as 1 in 1 million parts.[11, 13] Contact dermatitis may be the principal adverse health effect of certain pesticides in humans. In California where physicians are required by law to report all cases of illness or injury that might have resulted from exposure to pesticides, there have been reports of epidemics of pesticide contact dermatitis.[14] The agricultural sector was noted to have the highest rate of occupational skin disease of any industry in California.[15] The risk of occupational skin disease in agriculture was four times higher than the all-industry average risk, and twice as high as the rate in the manufacturing sector. Occupational skin diseases usually account for fewer than 40% of all occupational disease, but in California they accounted for approximately 70% of occupational disease in agriculture. The risk of occupational skin disease and the types vary with crops, livestock, farming practices, and climate. In California pesticides were second to poison oak as reported causes of occupational skin disease in agriculture.

Irritant contact dermatitis to pesticides is more frequent than allergic contact dermatitis. The chief cutaneous irritants among the pesticides are inorganic compounds such as copper sulfate. Fungicides such as carbamates, captan and similar chemicals, and benomyl have been the most frequently reported causes of allergic contact dermatitis due to pesticides.[16, 17]

CUTANEOUS EXPOSURE TO PESTICIDES

Under field conditions the skin is the organ most exposed to pesticides.[18] Farmers and agricultural workers are exposed while mixing, loading, and spraying pesticide formulations and while cleaning spray equipment and disposing of pesticide containers (Figs. 32–1 and 32–2).[19] Skin exposure to pesticides is maximal on the hands during mixing, loading, and spraying of pesticides from tractor-powered sprayers (Fig. 32–3). Protective gloves markedly reduce cutaneous exposure to pesticides. With knapsack-type spraying equipment the legs, especially the lower legs, are most exposed to pesticides (Fig. 32–4). Using a knapsack sprayer with a boom helps minimize exposure of the hands to pesticides.[20] Hand spraying (i.e., with a hand wand), which may be the most common application method, poses the highest risk for skin exposure.[21]

The distribution of pesticides on the skin after occupational exposure has been evaluated in the past using patch-test techniques. In 1990 Fenske published a report showing the distribution of pesticide exposure as demonstrated with a fluorescent tracer. He demonstrated that the proportion of skin surface in a specific body area that is exposed may be relatively small—and highly variable.[22]

All states in the United States regulate pesticide use under the Federal Insecticide, Fungicide, and Rodenticide Act (FIFRA). Each state has different requirements, including written tests and classes to ensure that persons who use pesticides are properly trained and educated to do so safely.

Earlier surveys in Saskatchewan found that only a minority of farmers always used skin protection while handling pesticides (data on file, Sections of Dermatology and Respirology, Department of Medicine, University of Saskatchewan, Saskatoon). Skin protection when using pesticides is most likely to be inadequate in hot weather and during very busy work periods. Field workers in California vineyards are most likely to develop skin rashes after thinning vines and on very hot days.[23] In this study pesticides in general, and propargite in particular, did not appear to be major causes of skin rashes, although outbreaks of rashes in grape field workers have been attributed to exposure to propargite or sulfur in California.

The year-to-year variability in reports on dermatitis due to agricultural use of pesticides has been found to be related to exposure to residues in the field. In the two California counties of Kern and Tulare, which reported more than half of all California cases of pesticide dermatitis, most episodes occurred in June and July, but some major ones in May and August. It was also found that table grapes are the most likely cause, as they are grown there and are tended intensively. The acaricide propargite was identified as the agent of several major outbreaks of dermatitis. Reentry intervals (the number of days that must elapse between pesticide application and unrestricted access to the treated field) for fields treated with propargite were subsequently extended, resulting in fewer reported cases.[24]

Adequate washing facilities frequently are not available in the fields where the pesticides are being applied, and some farmers cannot afford expensive safety equipment. Barrier creams have not been proven effective in protecting skin from pesticides. Pesticides are reported to persist long on the skin. Chlordane and dieldrin can persist on the skin as long as 2 years.[25] Ordinary laundering is not very effective in removing pesticide residues from clothing. Special laundering precautions are recommended. The degree of contamination of the worker's skin and clothing by pesticides also varies with the skill and attitude of the pesticide applicator, type of pesticide spray (low-volume concentrate, conventional spray), type of crop (orchard or row crop), wind, and quality of spray equipment.[19]

Certain highly toxic pesticides such as the organophosphate parathion are rapidly absorbed through the skin without producing dermatitis. Severe neurologic symptoms and death have been reported after percutaneous absorption of certain organophosphate pesticides.[26] Experimentally, percutaneous absorption is five times greater in some persons than in others and is greater through inflamed skin than through normal skin. Feldmann and Maibach[27] studied percutaneous absorption of 12 pesticides. The least absorbed was diquat and the most absorbed, carbaryl.

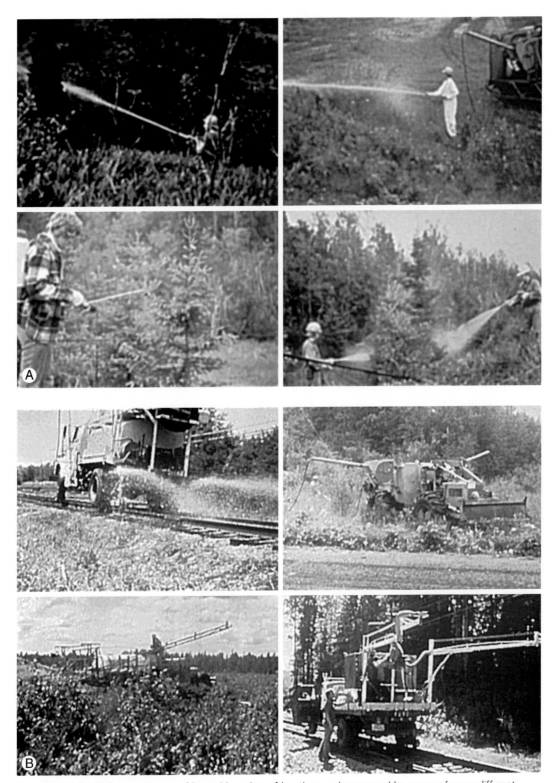

FIGURE 32–1 • Pesticide sprays are used in a wide variety of locations and are spread by means of many different application systems. (Courtesy of the Crop Protection Institute of Canada, W. Squires.)

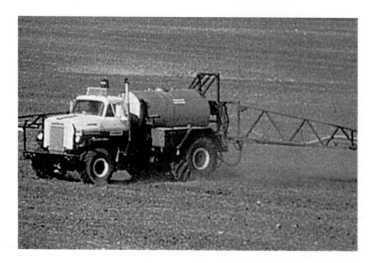

FIGURE 32-2 • Custom application of pesticides. (Courtesy of the Crop Protection Institute of Canada, W. Squires.)

The Environmental Protection Agency (EPA) in the United States recommended that workers not be allowed into fields treated with pesticides until an adequate interval has elapsed. For organophosphate and *N*-methyl carbamate pesticides, which cause acute dermal toxicity, a 48-hour interval was proposed. The EPA recommended rubber or chemical-resistant gloves for exposed workers and protective aprons to reduce exposure for mixers and loaders from splashes and spills from handling bulk pesticides. Other protective equipment for high-toxicity compounds includes headgear, face shields, and chemical-resistant footwear. Water, soap, and single-use towels should be available for decontamination near where the workers are. Workers who use organophosphate compounds for 3 consecutive days should have their serum cholinesterase level determined.

Pesticide sprays contain emulsifiers, adjuvants, carrier liquids, and surfactants. These ingredients may be considered proprietary information by manufacturers. Petroleum distillates are the most common solvents. Hydrocarbon-dissolved pesticides are usually diluted for application by adding measured amounts of water to form emulsions. Pesticide formulations with a pH of less than 5 or more than 8 are skin irritants. To prove that a case of allergic contact dermatitis is due to a particular pesticide it is necessary to perform patch testing to a nonirritating concentration of analytical-grade pesticide in an appropriate vehicle. Contaminants may be the main allergen in pesticide formulations. For example, diethyl fumarate was found to

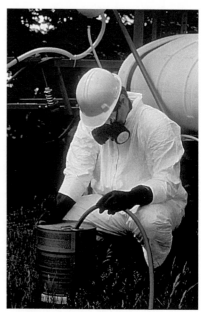

FIGURE 32-4 • Recommended protective equipment for the application of most pesticides. (Courtesy of A. J. Cessna, Ph.D., Agriculture Canada.)

FIGURE 32-3 • Tractor-mounted pesticide spraying. Spray nozzles may become blocked, and workers may be heavily exposed to pesticides when repairing malfunctioning nozzles in the field. (Courtesy of the Crop Protection Institute of Canada, W. Squires.)

be the sensitizer in technical-grade malathion.[13] Tests to assess a pesticides's capacity to induce allergic contact dermatitis are required before a pesticide can be registered for sale.[28]

STRESS IN FARMING

It was reported a decade ago that farming was ranked the 12th most stressful occupation in a field of 136.[29] The unpredictability of weather and the need for planting and harvesting crops during brief periods have always been stressful. Farmers work long hours to complete a task as quickly as possible and may not always remember to follow safety procedures.

PESTICIDES DERIVED FROM PLANTS

Pyrethrum

Pyrethrum is a powerful and degradable contact insecticide. It has a low order of systemic toxicity for humans and produces no harmful residues on food crops. The active principals of pyrethrum are obtained from the plant *Chrysanthemum cinerariaefolium*. The flowers are the source of the principles. The flowers and extracts are imported from Kenya and Ecuador into the United States. The active principals are pyrethrins I and II, cinerins I and II, and jasmolin I and II. The active principals are known collectively as *the pyrethrins*.

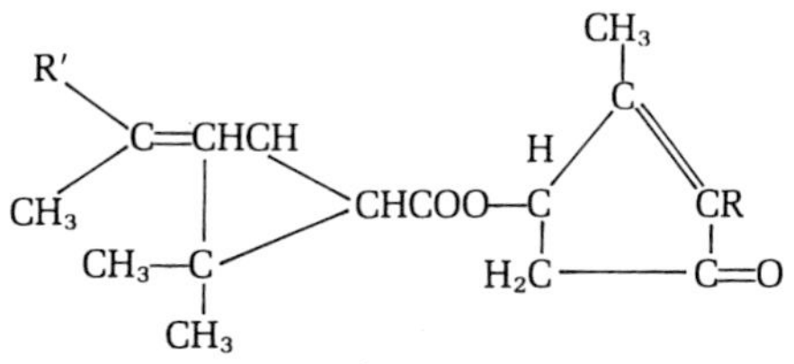

Pyrethrum

Pyrethrum extracts are used extensively in livestock sprays, pet sprays, household sprays, aerosols, and as food protection in warehouses. Pyrethrins are stable for long periods in water-based aerosols, where modern emulsifiers are used. Dermatitis from natural pyrethrin usually affects parts of the body exposed to the spray. The substance is a moderately potent allergic sensitizer. Cross-reactions occur among pyrethrum, chrysanthemum, shasta daisy, and ragweed oleoresin.[30, 31] Asthma and urticaria have also been reported as reactions to natural pyrethrin.[32, 33] In 1972 Mitchell and coworkers[31a] found that a sesquiterpene lactone, pyrethrosin, was the chief allergen in pyrethrin. Contact dermatitis due to pyrethrum is usu-

ally mild, but bullous reactions have been reported.[2] In Denmark positive patch-test reactions to pyrethrum were observed in 1% to 2% of dermatitis patients.[34]

Pyrethroids

Pyrethroids are synthetic compounds produced to duplicate the biological activity of the active principles of pyrethrum. Pyrethroids have a longer duration of activity against insects than pyrethrum and are neither teratogenic nor mutagenic. These compounds include allethrin, alphametrin, barthrin, bioresmethrin, biopermethrin, cismethrin, cyclethrin, cyfluthrin, cypermethrin, decamethrin, deltamethrin, dimethrin, fenothrin, fenpropanate, fenvalerate, flucythrinate, fluvalinate, furethrin, indothrin, permethrin, phthalthrin, resmethrin, and tetramethrin. Allergic contact dermatitis due to pyrethroids has not been reported. Temporary paresthesias, manifested by numbness, itching, burning, tingling, and warmth, have been reported after cutaneous exposure to the synthetic pyrethroid fenvalerate. Fenvalerate is produced in the United States. It produces more paresthesias after topical exposure than pyrethrin and other pyrethroids. It was reported that topical vitamin E acetate was highly effective in treating paresthesias induced by pyrethroids.[35]

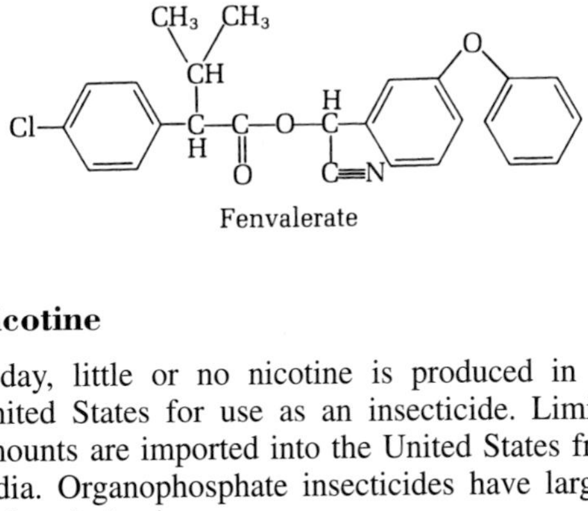

Fenvalerate

Nicotine

Today, little or no nicotine is produced in the United States for use as an insecticide. Limited amounts are imported into the United States from India. Organophosphate insecticides have largely replaced nicotine.

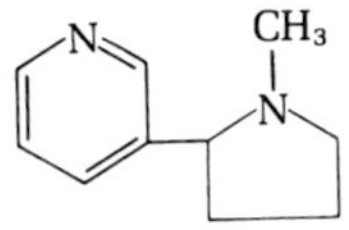

Nicotine

Allergic sensitization to nicotine was rare, as Sulzberger noted[36] in a study of patients with thromboangiitis obliterans, and Samitz and coworkers[37] in cigar makers. In a study of occupational dermatoses in Indonesia, Nasution's group[38] found that the dermatitis in tobacco workers was usually an irritant dermatitis of the hands that was caused either by the leaves that workers sorted and graded or the fertilizers and insecticides used on the plants. Vero and Genovese[39] patch tested a number of workers with dermatitis who made cigars from various tobacco leaves; no positive reactions were observed. Nicotine can be absorbed through the skin of tobacco harvesters. Exposed workers may develop nausea, vomiting, dizziness, prostration, and weakness. Skin abrasions sustained during tobacco leaf harvesting increase percutaneous absorption of nicotine. Wearing work gloves significantly decreases nicotine absorption in these workers.[40]

The transdermal nicotine patches that help people stop smoking have caused contact dermatitis.[41] Bircher described five cases of contact sensitization to nicotine and suggested that the optimal concentration for patch testing was an aqueous solution of 10% nicotine base.[42]

Rotenone

Rotenone is a selective contact insecticide with some acaricidal properties. In the United States cube is now the only commercial source of rotenone for insecticide production, although derris, timbo, and other related plants containing rotenone have been utilized. Peru is the main source of the cube root, which can be ground into a dust or extracted to provide concentrate. Rotenone has been used for a long time as dust for garden insects and for lice and ticks on animals. Rotenone emulsions are also used for eliminating or controlling fish populations to improve fishing in certain bodies of water. Rotenone can also be used in combination with pyrethrin and piperonyl butoxide (a synergist) for control of a wide variety of insects on food crops. Skin irritation from rotenone has been reported among workers in rotenone-processing plants in South America. Skin inflammation was most notable in intertriginous areas and where the powder was trapped by perspiration on the skin.[2] A similar outbreak was reported among workers in France, but improved ventilation and dust masks diminished the rate of dermatitis in these workers.[2]

Rotenone

Quassia

Quassia amara, or bitterwood, yields Surinam *Quassia*, an insecticide that was formerly used, particularly in Europe, to control horticultural insect pests. Mitchell and Rook[43] mentioned quassia wood dermatitis due to an extract of *Quassia* wood.

INORGANIC AND ORGANOMETAL PESTICIDES

Arsenic

The earliest insecticides against chewing insects were the arsenicals, chiefly copper acetoarsenite (Paris green), lead arsenate, and calcium arsenate. Sodium arsenite has been used as a sterilant herbicide and a potato-vine killer. Inorganic arsenic is both a cutaneous irritant and a sensitizer.[10] Hyperkeratosis, hyperhidrosis, and melanosis are all considered signs of chronic systemic exposure. The hyperpigmentation is most marked on surfaces exposed to light; it does not extend to mucous membranes. There may be speckled depigmentation of pigmented areas in a "raindrop" pattern. Compounds similar or identical to those used as pesticides have caused skin cancer in humans.[2] Agricultural workers are also exposed to much ultraviolet light, and Emmett believed that UV exposure was a more significant carcinogenic factor than their exposure to inorganic arsenic.[44]

Inorganic arsenicals have been superseded because of their hazards to humans and animals. Sodium arsenate was formerly the toxicant in many ant syrups for household use, but this application also has been discontinued. At present organic arsenicals are the most desirable pesticidal arsenicals because of their selective herbicidal activity.

Sulfur

Sulfur is a common fungicide. It is also an acaricide and is compatible with most other insecticides and fungicides. It is insoluble in water but soluble in organic solvents. Wettable sulfur is prepared by adding wetting and dispersing agents to finely ground sulfur. Micronized wettable sulfur is made by a special manufacturing process to ensure extremely fine particle size. Grapes and peanuts are examples of crops that require a fungicide such as sulfur. Many cases of contact dermatitis are attributed to sulfur in California,[5] but there are very few reports of sensitivity to it.[45]

Triphenyltin Hydroxide

Triphenyltin hydroxide is a fungicide used on a variety of crops. Irritant patch-test reactions are very common when patients are patch tested to 1% triphenyltin (phentin hydroxide).[16]

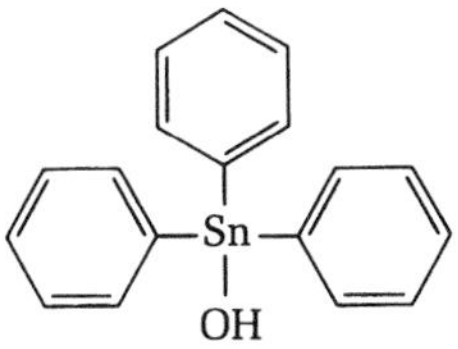

Triphenyltin Hydroxide

Tributyltin Oxide

Tributyltin oxide is a powerful skin irritant but not a sensitizer.[46]

Copper Sulfate

Copper sulfate is a fungicide and an algicide. Lisi and coworkers reported positive patch-test reactions to 1% copper sulfate solutions in agricultural workers.[16]

Phenylmercury Nitrate

Phenylmercuric salts were once widely used as herbicides and agricultural fungicides. Phenylmercury nitrate is still used for dressing tree wounds. Contact dermatitis to phenylmercury nitrate used as a herbicide has been reported.[47]

SOLVENTS

Kerosene

Kerosene was apparently the first petroleum oil to be used for insect control, back in 1877. Today it is widely used as a solvent for household and industrial pesticide sprays. The kerosene may be sulfonated to provide an odorless oil, or deodorants may be added. Kerosene is a cutaneous irritant. Barnes and Wilkinson[48] have described skin lesions similar to those of toxic epidermal necrolysis in a boy whose clothing was soaked with kerosene.

FUMIGANTS

A fumigant is a substance or a mixture of substances that produce gas, vapor, fume, or smoke intended to destroy insects, bacteria, or rodents. Fumigants can be volatile liquids or solids or naturally gaseous substances. They may be used to disinfect the interiors of buildings or objects and materials that can be enclosed so as to contain the fumigant or soil.[3]

Ethylene Oxide

Ethylene oxide, or epoxy ethane, is used as a fumigant and a sterilant. Severe irritant dermatitis and chemical burns have been reported from direct skin contact with ethylene oxide.[2] Ethylene oxide was first used as an agricultural fumigant in 1928.[49] It is effective against all microorganisms. It is a potent skin irritant and may produce immediate or delayed contact hypersensitivity. Epidemiological studies strongly indicate that ethylene oxide is carcinogenic in humans.[50]

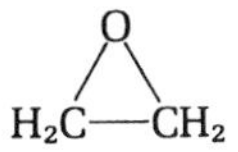

Ethylene Oxide

Methyl Bromide

Methyl bromide is a fumigant used for insect control in grain elevators, mills, ships, and greenhouses. The gas is a soil fumigant as well. It is also used for termite control, agricultural fumigation, and rodent control. Direct skin contact with methyl bromide produces chemical burns.

Acrylonitrile

Toxic epidermal necrolysis was reported by four patients 11 to 21 days after their homes were fumigated with a 2:1 mixture of acrylonitrile and carbon tetrachloride,[51] and three of the four died. This fumigant was subsequently discontinued.

Metam-Sodium

Metam-sodium (methylisothiocyanate, MITC) is a broad-spectrum soil fumigant. It is a fungicide, insecticide, nematocide, and herbicide. Richter[52] opined that allergic contact dermatitis to metam-sodium may be significant among exposed persons. He regarded it as a potent sensitizer. He also attributed hepatitis in one patient to metam-sodium.

In 1991 a train accident in California spilled 19,000 gallons of metam-sodium into the Sacramento River. Metam-sodium, when diluted in water, decomposes to MITC, a known skin irritant. Many workers cleaning up the spill suffered dermatitis of the lower extremities that was believed to be irritant contact dermatitis secondary to prolonged exposure to MITC or to methylamines produced by the decomposition of fish and other river life.[53]

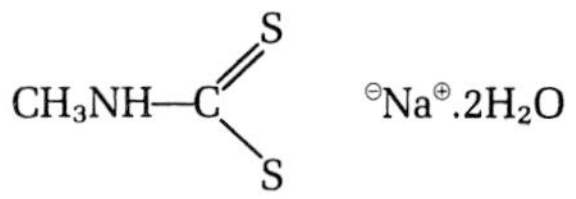

Metam sodium dihydrate

DD

DD is a very toxic mixture of 1,3-dichloropropene, 1,2-dichloropropane, epichlorhydrin, and related compounds. It is a cutaneous irritant and is used as a soil fumigant. Nater and Gooskens[54] obtained positive patch tests to 1% DD in acetone. They concluded that DD occasionally provoked allergic contact dermatitis.

Dazomet

Dazomet is used as a nematocide, soil fumigant, herbicide, and algicide. Dazomet hydrolyzes to formalin. Black described dazomet as a strong sensitizer, a primary irritant, and possibly a vesicant.[55]

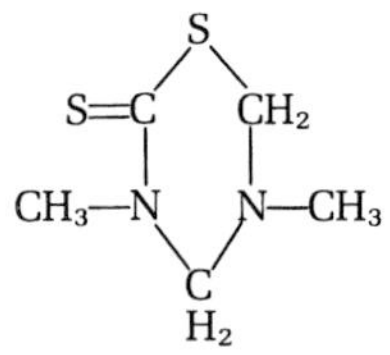

Dazomet

CHLORINATED HYDROCARBON INSECTICIDES

Dichlorodiphenyltrichloroethane DDT

Since January 1, 1973, DDT has been banned in the United States for any use except emergency public health measures. Allergic contact dermatitis due to DDT was never convincingly reported.[56–59] Positive patch-test reactions to 3% DDT were reported in cotton workers with dermatitis on exposed areas. No positive patch-test reactions to 1% DDT were observed among 665 routine eczema patients patch tested by the International Contact Dermatitis Research Group (I.C.D.R.G.).[10]

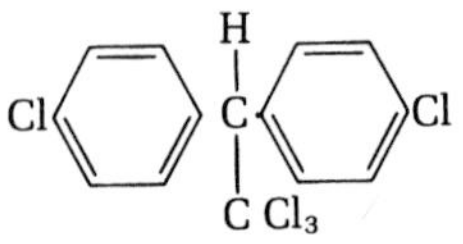

DDT

Lindane

Lindane is used for seed treatment to control wireworms and seedcorn maggots on various crops. It is also used to protect tobacco transplants from cutworms and wireworms and as soil treatment, a foliage treatment on fruit and nut trees, vegetables, ornamentals, and timber, and for wood protection.

It is a skin irritant, but allergic contact dermatitis is very rare. No positive patch-test reactions to 1% lindane were observed in 665 routine eczema patients patch tested by the I.C.D.R.G.[10]

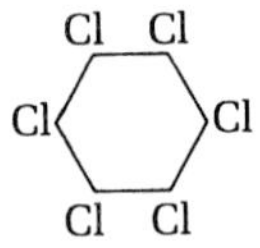

99 percent
γ-isomer
Lindane

Dieldrin

Dieldrin, an insecticide, is used only in the United States for termite control. Dieldrin probably caused dermatitis of the lower legs in 200 of 1,209 police recruits who sweated while wearing socks mothproofed with dieldrin.[60]

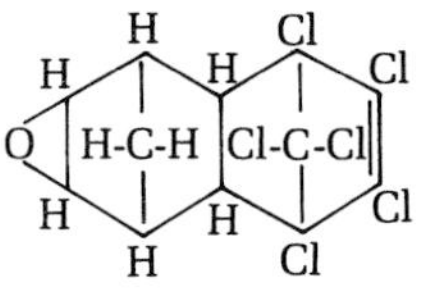

Principal constituent of Dieldrin

ORGANOPHOSPHATE PESTICIDES

Parathion and Methyl Parathion

Organophosphate pesticides came into wide use after DDT was banned. Parathion is an insecticide that is extremely toxic to humans and animals. It is a restricted-use pesticide in the United States, and workers must wear rubber gloves, protective clothing, goggles, and a respirator. The mask or respirator must be approved by the U.S. Bureau of Mines for parathion protection. Parathion was found on the skin of the hands of one worker 2 months after his last known contact with it.[25]

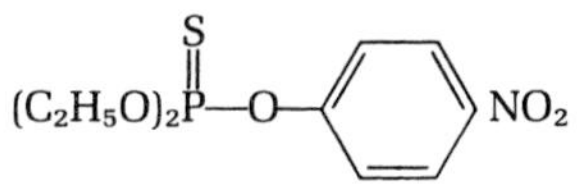

Parathion

Parathion is an experimental contact sensitizer.[16] Allergic contact dermatitis to parathion was reported in a German vintner.[61]

Elsewhere a gardener cut his finger and then used a very concentrated spray containing parathion and emulsifiers on begonias. The cut finger became swollen and bluish red a day later but was cool and painless. The author believed the patient had an unusual reaction to parathion.[62] Erythema multiforme has been reported in a woman who inhaled methyl parathion (Dalf).[63] Experimental reexposure reproduced her lesions.

Malathion

Malathion is used to control a large variety of insects. Milby and Epstein[13] found that nearly half of 87 volunteers developed contact sensitization after a single exposure to 10% malathion and that many of them reacted to dilutions as weak as 1 ppm. Kligman reported similar results.[12] However, it was found in the first study that only about 3% of people with occupational exposure to malathion had a positive patch-test reaction to 1% malathion, and no worker had to change work because of malathion allergy. Only one positive patch-test reaction to 0.5% malathion was observed in 455 routine eczema patients patch tested by the I.C.D.R.G.[10] The relevance of that one reaction was not known. In practice, malathion appears to be a rare allergic contact sensitizer. Kligman has suggested that the working concentration of malathion is too low to provoke sensitization. Milby and Epstein determined that the sensitizer in malathion is diethyl fumarate, which is used in its manufacture. Diethyl fumarate was present at 3% concentration in technical-grade malathion.[13] Diethyl fumarate can produce non–immune-mediated contact urticaria.[64]

$$(CH_3O)_2\overset{\overset{\displaystyle S}{\|}}{P}-S-CH-\overset{\overset{\displaystyle O}{\|}}{C}-OC_2H_5$$
$$CH_2-\overset{\overset{\displaystyle O}{\|}}{C}-OC_2H_5$$

Malathion

Dichlorvos (DDVP)

DDVP is an insecticide used in sprays, wettable powder, aerosols, resin strips (No Pest Strip insecticide), and flea collars. It is also formulated as an anthelminthic for swine, horses, and dogs. Strong reactions were reported in two humans whose dermatitis was attributed to contact with dogs wearing DDVP-impregnated flea collars.[65] Cronce and Alden[66] reported primary irritant contact dermatitis to DDVP flea collars in four patients. Patch testing produced bullous primary irritant reactions in four patients and five control subjects. Mathias[67]

noted negative patch tests to 1% and 0.1% DDVP in petrolatum in a truck driver who developed prolonged contact dermatitis to DDVP. This man also had systemic symptoms of organophosphate toxicity after being exposed to a DDVP spill in his truck. Mathias emphasized that those who develop dermatitis from skin contact with pesticides should be questioned carefully about general symptoms. This is particularly important for organophosphate insecticides.

$$(CH_3O)_2-\overset{\overset{\displaystyle O}{\uparrow}}{P}-O-CH{=}CCl_2$$

DDVP

Tetmosol

Tetmosol (tetraethylthiuram monosulfide) is used to treat parasitic infestations in dogs and cats. It is used as a scabicide and sometimes as a fungicide. Cronin[10] has reported a 58-year-old woman with chronic eczema whose dermatitis flared after she treated her cat with Tetmosol even though she wore rubber gloves. She had positive patch-test results to Tetmosol solution and to both 1% tetramethylthiuram disulfide and 1% tetramethylthiuram disulfide in petrolatum.

Naled

Naled is an insecticide-acaricide. It is intermediate in toxicity between malathion and parathion. Allergic contact dermatitis to naled has been reported in a few workers.[68]

Naled is broken down by hydrolysis within a few hours. Patients allergic to it may work with plants sprayed with naled once a suitable time interval has elapsed.

$$\overset{\displaystyle CH_3O}{\underset{\displaystyle CH_3O}{}}\overset{\overset{\displaystyle O}{\uparrow}}{P}-O-CH-\overset{\displaystyle C}{\underset{Br}{|}}-Cl_2$$

Naled

Thiometon

Thiometon is a systemic insecticide used to control aphids, thrips, and mites. A case of contact dermatitis was attributed to it.[2]

$$\overset{\displaystyle CH_3O}{\underset{\displaystyle CH_3O}{}}\overset{\overset{\displaystyle S}{\|}}{P}-S-CH_2-CH_2-S-C_2H_5$$

Thiometon

Rodannitrobenzene

Rodannitrobenzene has been used in insecticide sprays for home use. Fregert[69] has reported a case of severe contact dermatitis due to rodannitrobenzene.

Azamethiphos

Azamethiphos is an organophosphate compound that has been widely used as a pesticide in the last 10 years. Iliev reported a case of contact dermatitis from azamethiphos in a 34-year-old chemical worker who had been working on the packaging line for 2 weeks. Testing with a 2% aqueous dilution of azamethiphos yielded positive results. The worker also had a positive patch test to mancozeb, to which he had previously been exposed.[70]

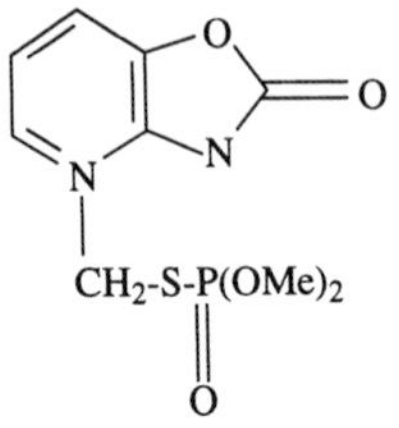

Azamethiphos

Dimethoate

Contact dermatitis to dimethoate is rare, but there are case reports. In 1992 Schena described a case of erythema multiforme–like contact dermatitis from dimethoate.[71]

$$S$$
$$(CH_3O)_2P–S–CH_2CONHCH_3$$

Dimethoate

Omethoate

Contact dermatitis has been reported with omethoate. In 1996 Haenen reported a case of contact dermatitis in a 38-year-old rose grower who was exposed to omethoate. Her patch test revealed reactivity to both omethoate and dimethoate, and Haenen proposed the possibility of cross-sensitivity between omethoate and dimethoate, as they are structurally very alike.[72]

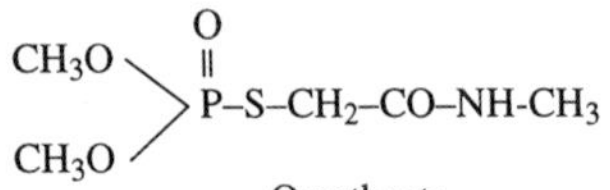

Omethoate

CARBAMATE INSECTICIDES

Promecarb

Promecarb is a contact insecticide. Contact dermatitis has been reported in two workers.[2]

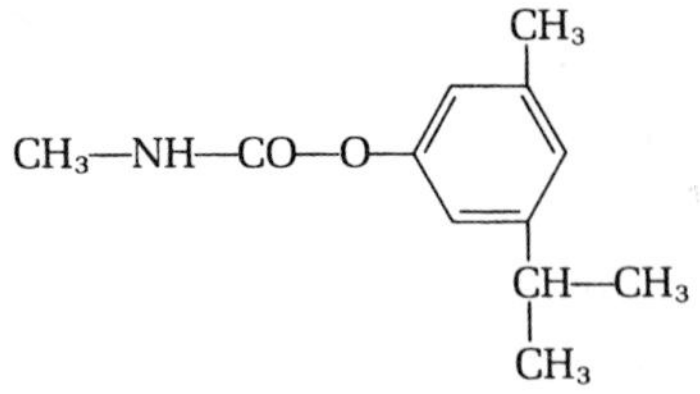

Promecarb

Carbaryl

Carbaryl, a broad-spectrum insecticide, is used on more then 120 different crops. A case of contact dermatitis to carbaryl spray was reported.[2]

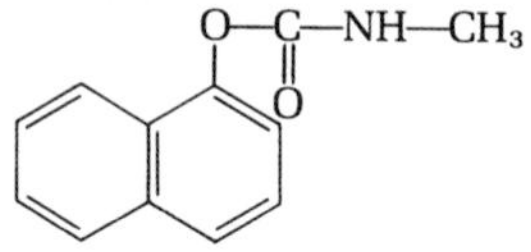

Carbaryl

NITRO COMPOUNDS AND RELATED PHENOLIC PESTICIDES

Chlorinated phenols are very effective fungicides, but owing to their toxicity are used only for fabrics and woods.

Pentachlorophenol (PCP)

PCP was first synthesized in 1841, but commercial production began only in 1936. It has been used as a molluscicide, insecticide, herbicide, fungicide, bactericide, antimildew agent, and preservative. It is used particularly as a wood preservative. Lumber impregnated with PCP is relatively resistant to bacteria, fungi, and termites, and the wood retains its natural appearance.[73]

Vaguely defined rashes and skin irritation, possible chloracne, and susceptibility to skin infections have been attributed to long-term exposure to PCP. Lambert and associates[73a] linked pemphigus vulgaris in a 41-year-old man and a 28-year-old woman and chronic urticaria in a 35-year-old man to long exposure to PCP.

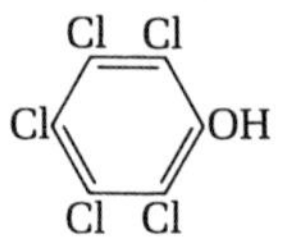

PCP

Pentachlorophenate

Kentor[74] reported a patient who developed urticaria and angioedema from contact with PCP. The condition was believed to be immune-mediated contact urticaria. He developed urticaria and angioedema at sites distant from his hands, which had come in contact with PCP.

Chlorocresol and Chloromethylphenoxyacetic Acid

A positive patch-test reaction to 0.1% chlorocresol in alcohol was reported by Fregert[75] in a man who developed dermatitis on two occasions after using chloromethylphenoxyacetic acid (MCPA) spray. Patch testing to 1% MCPA was negative. Chlorocresol is used in the manufacture of MCPA.

4,6,Dinitro-*o*-Cresol (DNOC)

DNOC is an insecticide, fungicide, herbicide, and defoliant. It is used in North America as a dormant spray for killing insect eggs and controlling apple scab. Nail dystrophy has been reported after fingernail contact with 5% DNOC.[76]

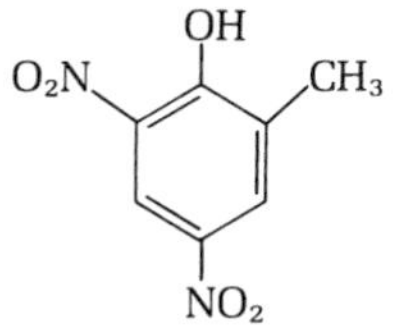

DNOC

Dinocap

Dinocap is a foliage fungicide and acaricide. One case of allergic contact dermatitis has been ascribed to dinocap.[22]

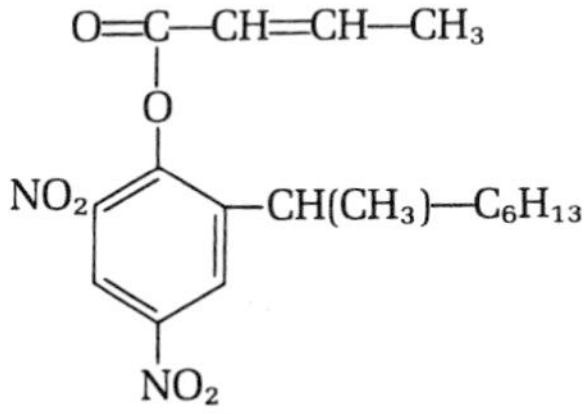

Dinocap

Tecnazene (Tetrachloronitrobenzene)

Tecnazene is a fungicide and growth regulator. Cotterill[77] reported on a farmer who developed acute dermatitis while throwing tecnazene granules onto a conveyor belt carrying potatoes. Patch testing to tecnazene was negative, but this farmer had a strong positive patch-test reaction to 0.01% DNCB. Cotterill attributed his patient's contact dermatitis to DNCB contaminating the tecnazene granules. DNCB could have been formed during production of tecnazene.

Phenothiazine

Phenothiazine (thiodiphenylamine) is an oral insecticide and anthelminthic. The earliest organic insecticide, it was introduced in 1925. It is provided in salt or mineral supplements to control fly larvae and certain internal parasites. Workers spraying apple orchards with phenothiazine in the state of Washington developed severe phototoxic reactions.[78] Phototoxic reactions also occurred in workers who prepared the raw materials. The reactions resemble sunburn, and the hair turns pinkish red and the fingernails brown.[79]

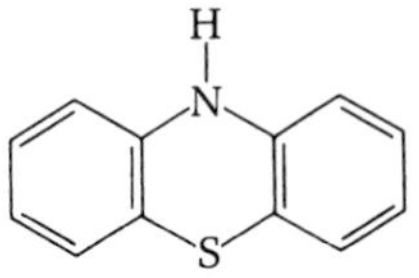

Phenothiazine

RODENTICIDES

Warfarin

Warfarin is a rodenticide that is highly effective in controlling Norway rats and house mice. A positive patch-test reaction to 0.05% warfarin in an agricultural worker was reported.[16]

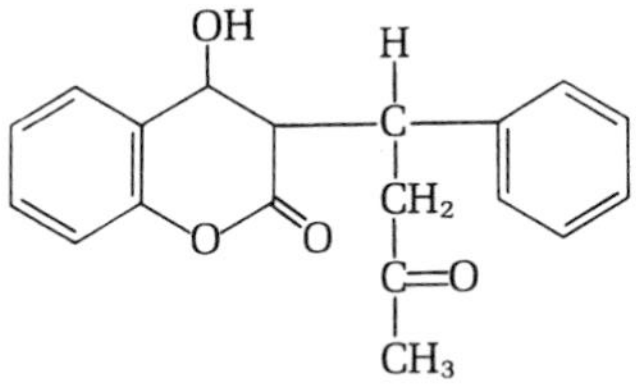

Warfarin

ANTU

ANTU is a rodenticide for adult Norway rats. A case of occupational contact dermatitis to ANTU was reported.[2]

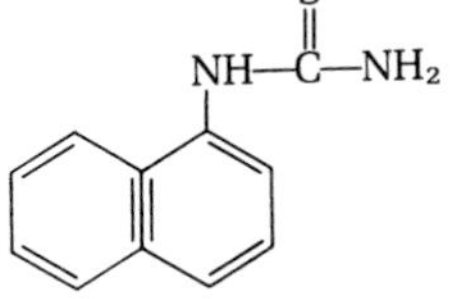

ANTU

HERBICIDES

Herbicides are frequently used in place of hand labor or machine cultivation to control unwanted plants.

Glyphosphate

Glyphosphate (Roundup) is a nonselective, post-emergent herbicide. In 1986, contact dermatitis attributed to glyphosphate was reported in 33 workers who mixed it or loaded it.[5] Maibach[80] investigated glyphosphate intensively and found it not to be a sensitizer and to be less irritating to the skin than baby shampoo. A phototoxic reaction to benzisothiazolone has been reported. Benziso-thiazolone is a preservative in commercial gly-phosphate spray. Phototoxicity to glyphosphate itself was not demonstrated.[81]

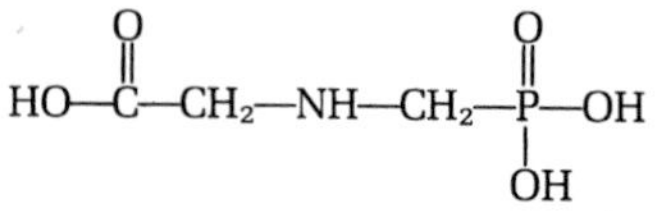

Glyphosphate

Paraquat

Paraquat is a contact herbicide and desiccant. Irritant contact dermatitis has been reported to para-quat. Workers in paraquat factories are at increased risk for occupational keratoses, Bowen's disease, and squamous cell carcinoma of the skin.[82, 83] Paraquat itself is probably not the agent of these premalignant and malignant skin lesions. Discoloration or deformity of fingernails, onychol-ysis, and loss of nails have been reported in workers whose nails came into contact with paraquat sprays and concentrates.[76, 84] A case of periungual eczematous dermatitis with striking nail lesions due to paraquat was reported by Botella and co-workers.[85] Patch testing to paraquat, 0.001% and 0.01% in water, was negative. A necrotic ulcer of the scrotum followed direct contact with paraquat solution.[86] A death was also reported to arise from percutaneous absorption of paraquat.[87]

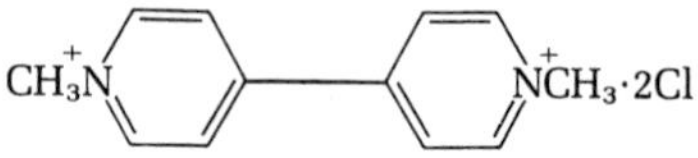

Paraquat

Nitralin

Allergic contact dermatitis to nitralin and its precursor 4-chloro-3,-5-dinitrophenylmethyl sulfone was reported in a man working in a factory that produced this herbicide. He also showed cross-sensitivity to DNCB.[88] Manufacture of nitralin in the United States has since been discontinued.

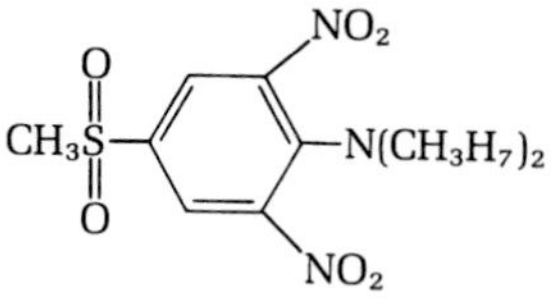

Nitralin

Amitrole

Amitrole (aminotriazole) is a systemic herbicide used to control nonselective grasses, broadleaf weeds, cattails, poison ivy, and certain aquatic weeds. One case of allergic contact dermatitis to aminotriazole was reported in a contract weed control operator.[89]

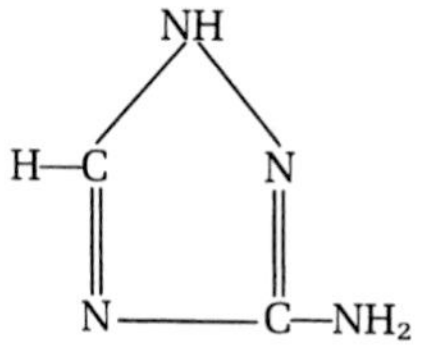

Amitrole

Chloridazon

Chloridazon (pyrazon), a herbicide used to protect beets, persists in the soil for several months. Allergic contact dermatitis to chloridazon spray was reported in a farmer by Bruze and Fregert.[90]

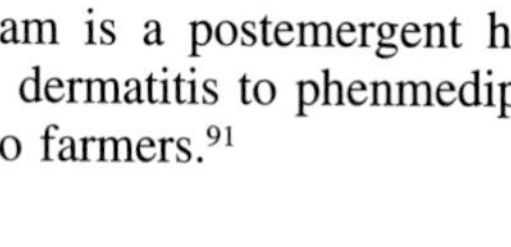

Chloridazon

Phenmedipham

Phenmedipham is a postemergent herbicide. Severe allergic dermatitis to phenmedipham was reported in two farmers.[91]

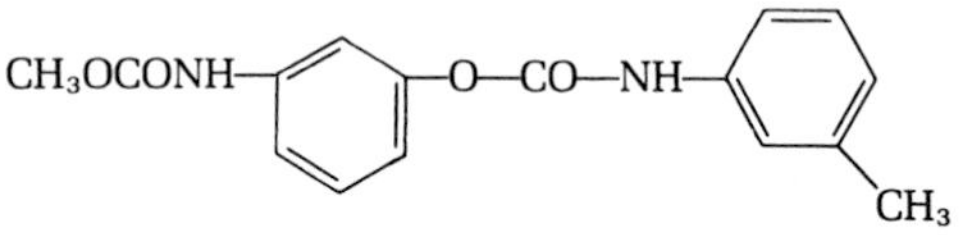

Phenmedipham

Dichlobenil

Dichlobenil is a herbicide. Six men engaged in mixing or bagging it developed dermatitis within 1 week to 5 months after first exposure. Although the lesions involved comedones and were described as chloracne, no cysts were observed, and, judging from the description and one photograph, the dermatitis was not severe. The possibility that this mild condition might have been associated with a contaminant does not seem to have been explored.[2]

Atrazine

Atrazine is a widely used selective herbicide. Severe contact dermatitis to atrazine was reported in a farmer with a history of dermatitis from propachlor. This patient had a patch-test reaction to a 1:1,000 dilution of a commercial atrazine formulation.[2]

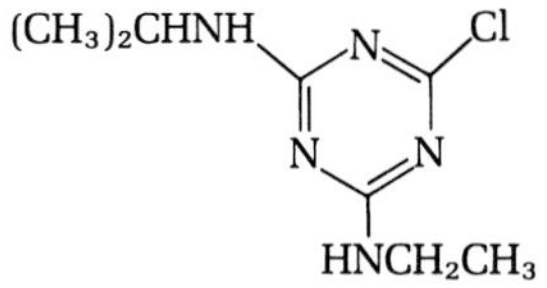

Atrazine

Propazine

Propazine and simazine are selective herbicides. Many cases of contact dermatitis have been reported among workers who manufacture them.[2]

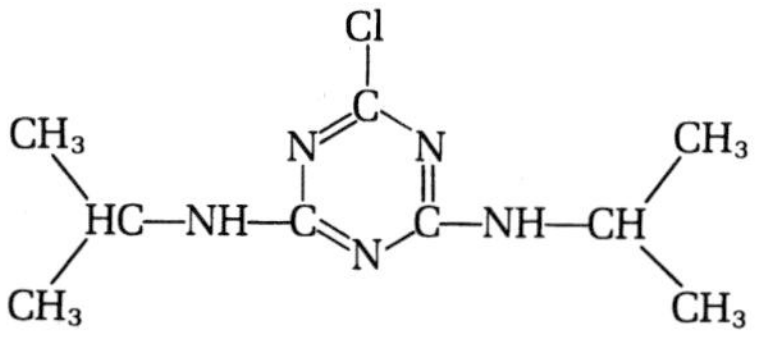

Propazine

Oxydiazol

Chloracne has been reported in workers who manufacture oxydiazol (methazole) 2-(3,4-dichlorophenyl)-4-methyl-1,2,4-oxadiazolidine-3,5-dione. This resulted from exposure to 3,4,3',4'-tetrachloroazoxybenzene (TCAB), an extraneous intermediate produced during the manufacture of the herbicide.[92]

Alachlor

Alachlor (Lasso) is a preemergent herbicide. Iden and Schroeter[93] have reported five persons who had allergic patch-test reactions to alachlor. They found that three of the 21 patients patchtested to alachlor reacted to both alachlor and propachlor (Ramrod).

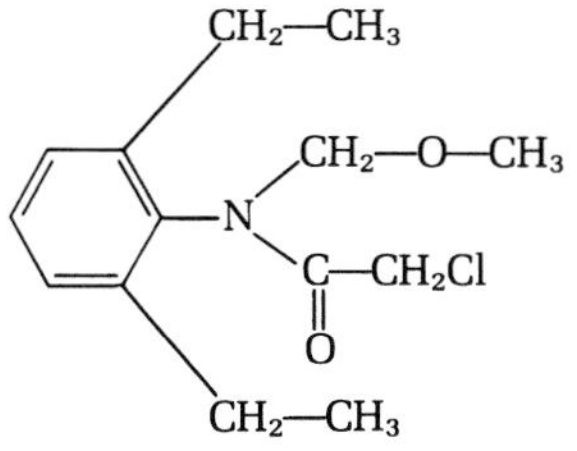

Alachlor

Allidochlor

Allidochlor (Randox) is a selective preemergent herbicide. Spencer[94] reported severe allergic contact dermatitis to allidochlor. The herbicide has since been banned in the United States.

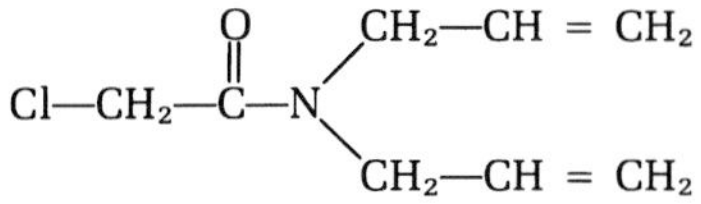

Allidochlor

Propachlor

Propachlor is a preemergent and early postemergent herbicide. Skin irritation to propachlor was reported in 1966.[94] It has been banned in the United States.

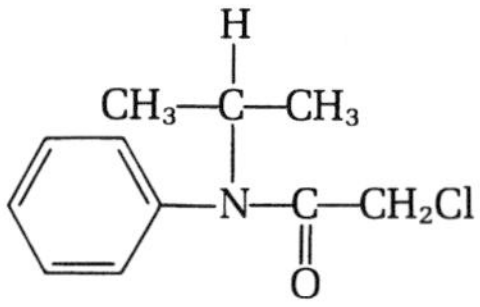

Propachlor

Trichlorobenzyl

Trichlorobenzyl chloride is a herbicide used in preemergence applications only in combination with allidochlor (Randox). Skin irritation to this chemical was also reported by Spencer.[94]

2,4-Dichlorophenoxyacetic Acid (2,4-D)

2,4-D, a selective herbicide, is used to control weeds, water hyacinths, and various other plants. A large number of companies manufacture 2,4-D. 2,4,5-Trichlorophenoxyacetic acid (2,4,5-T) salts and esters are used widely to control woody plants on industrial sites and rangeland. Amine formulations are used extensively to control weeds on rice. The actions and properties of these compounds are similar to those of 4,5-T preparations.

2,4-D–2,4,5-T-mixtures are used to destroy

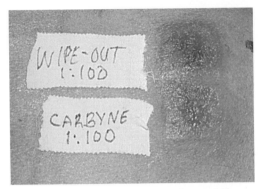

FIGURE 32–5 • Positive patch-test reactions at 48 hours from dilutions of commercial preparations of barban.

mixed-growth stands of woody and herbaceous plants. Severe contact dermatitis was reported in response to a mixture of 2,4-D and 2,4,5-T.[2] A major epidemiological study in Kansas found an association between the use of 2,4-D and non-Hodgkin's lymphoma. The greater the use of 2,4-D, the greater was the incidence of non-Hodgkin's lymphoma among exposed farmers.[95] This study did not confirm previously reported associations between use of 2,4-D and soft-tissue sarcoma or Hodgkin's disease.[96–102]

OCH₂COOH

2,4-D

Barban

Barban (barbamate, barbane, chlorinate) is a selective herbicide with low systemic toxicity. Allergic contact dermatitis to barban has been documented (Fig. 32–5).[11, 103] Marked sensitivity can develop — such that only minute concentrations of barban are sufficient to produce strong patch-test reactions. Hypopigmentation was noted after one case of allergic contact dermatitis (Fig. 32–6). Barban is a potent experimental sensitizer.[103]

Barban

Nitrofen

Nitrofen is a preemergent or postemergent herbicide used for broad-spectrum weed control in a variety of crops.

Nitrofen

Solomons[104] described a 50-year-old farmer with dermatitis of the forehead, face, neck, forearms, and hands and a patch-test reaction to 0.5% nitrofen. He had used nitrofen to spray a hedge. Because of the possibility of carcinogenesis, nitrofen has been withdrawn from the market.

A 0.5% concentration in water produced a reaction on patch testing, and a significant reaction also occurred 96 hours after testing.

Norflurazon

Norflurazon, a herbicide used to control broadleaf weeds and grasses, is a fluorinated phenol pyridasinone derivative. Leow and Maibach reported a case of contact dermatitis from this herbicide in a professional weed sprayer. His patch test was positive at 2 and 4 days in response to 1.0% and 0.1% aqueous challenges.[105]

Norflurazon

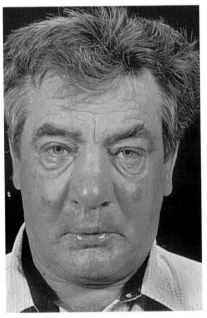

FIGURE 32–6 • Allergic contact dermatitis from the herbicide barban.

Trifluralin

Trifluralin is a soil-incorporated herbicide used to prevent the growth of certain grasses and weeds. It has been shown to cause skin and eye irritation. Allergic contact dermatitis was reported to occur in a laboratory supervisor in a chemical pesticide company. He tested positive to trifluralin and benefin (discussed below) at concentrations of 0.5% in petrolatum.[106]

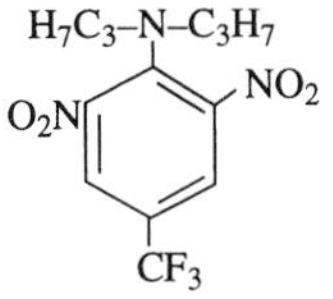

Trifluralin

Benefin

Benefin is a substitute dinitroaniline herbicide used to control grasses and weeds on food crops. It has also been shown to cause irritant dermatitis, and there is a report of contact dermatitis secondary to trifluralin (see Trifluralin).[106]

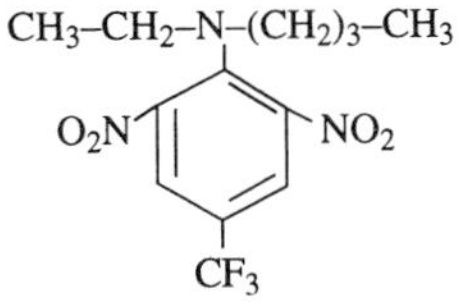

Benefin

FUNGICIDES

Benomyl

Benomyl is a systemic fungicide that is used widely for control of a broad range of diseases of fruits, nuts, vegetables, field crops, and ornamentals. Allergic contact dermatitis in exposed areas was reported in seven Japanese women who worked in a hot, humid greenhouse where benomyl was being sprayed on carnations. Ten Hispanic coworkers were not affected. Undiluted benomyl and benomyl diluted 1:5 in olive oil produced negative patch tests in three controls, but a Japanese medical assistant developed a 2+ reaction when these patch-test sites were exposed for 30 seconds to UV light. The seven Japanese workers had positive patch-test reactions to benomyl 1:10 in olive oil.[107] Fregert[108] reported one case of a positive patch-test reaction to benomyl 0.1% in water. He wondered whether most cases of dermatitis due to benomyl were transient. Van Ketel[109] reported a begonia grower with contact dermatitis due to this fungicide. The dermatitis was caused not by spraying but by picking the leaves. Patch testing with 1% in petrolatum was positive. Van Joost and coworkers[9] asserted that picking plants containing residues of benomyl is an important source of sensitization to the chemical.

Larsen studied 62 workers with a history of benomyl exposure and found only weak sensitization. He proposed that earlier case reports of contact dermatitis secondary to benomyl may have represented cross-reactions and that contact dermatitis in response to benomyl requires previous exposure to other chemically related pesticides.[110] A limited recall of batches of Benlate DF (benomyl) occurred in 1989 after farmers and nurseries blamed crop stunting deformities and plant death on this product. Claims were most frequent in Florida, Puerto Rico, and Hawaii. The manufacturer paid out more than $500 million in voluntary crop damage settlements, most of it to Florida growers, before refusing to settle hundreds of other lawsuits claiming adverse plant and human effects from Benlate DF.[111, 112]

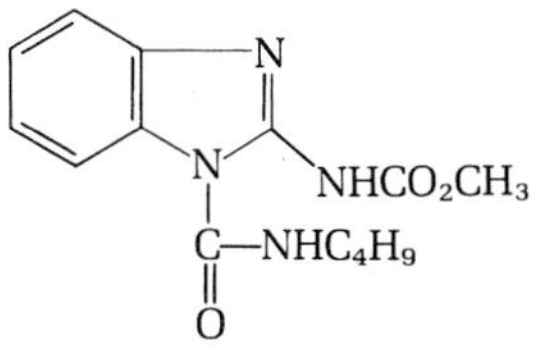

Benomyl

Hexachlorobenzene

Hexachlorobenzene is a seed protectant used on wheat. Contact may cause slight skin irritation. Hexachlorobenzene produced an epidemic of severe porphyria cutanea tarda in Turkey from 1955 to 1959. The disease occurred almost exclusively in persons who admitted eating wheat distributed for seed, not for food. The wheat had been treated with hexachlorobenzene. Many infants died from exposure to hexachlorobenzene in this epidemic.[113]

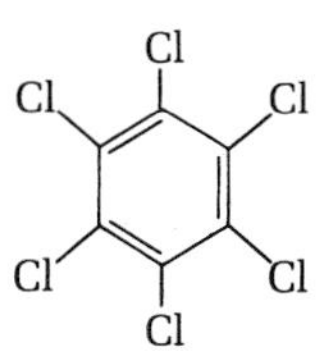

Hexachlorobenzene

Thiophanatemethyl

Thiophanatemethyl is a systemic fungicide that has a broad spectrum of activity for plant diseases. Many cases of apparent irritant contact dermatitis to thiophanatemethyl have been reported but few cases of allergic contact dermatitis.[2]

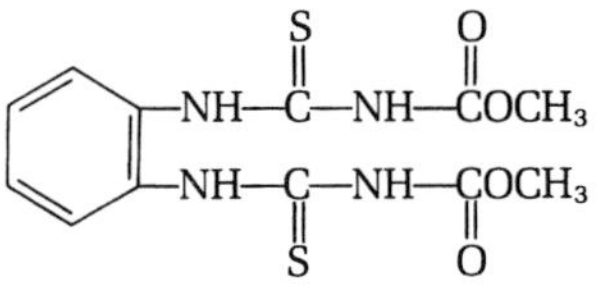

Thiophanatemethyl

Captafol

Captafol is used to prevent blight on potatoes and on fruit and farm crops. Camarasa[114] reported severe pruritus, morbilliform urticarial eruptions, and asthma among 7 of 41 workers in a company that packed captafol (difolatin). Four of these patients had strong patch-test reactions to captafol. The sudden appearance of vesiculation and edema on the face and hands of a welder associated with wheezing was attributed to contact with bags of captafol. Subsequent reexposure led to recurrences.[2] Irritant contact dermatitis has been associated with the use of captafol by Japanese tangerine orchardmen. Some 25% to 30% of workers were affected,[10] and some reactions were severe.[2] Captafol was the pesticide that accounted for the greatest number of cases of contact dermatitis in Japan from 1968 to 1970.[115] In 1996 a study was published on the skin sensitization associated with the use of pesticides in southern Taiwan. The authors used patch testing to determine that the Taiwanese fruit farmers were most often sensitive to captofol, folpet, and captan and that the dermatitis often presented on the volar aspects of the hands.[17]

Stoke[116] reported that at least one third of exposed workers develop dermatitis to captafol when adequate precautions were not taken. As many as 65% of exposed workers were reported to develop captafol dermatitis. The risk of dermatitis from captafol can be minimized by proper worker training and industrial hygiene. The manufacturers regard it as a potent sensitizer.[117] Cottel also reported two farmers with dermatitis on exposed areas who had positive patch tests to 0.1% captafol in water.

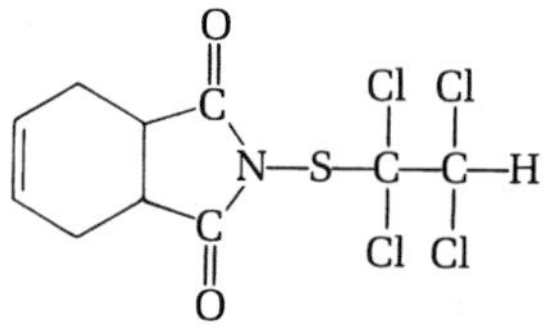

Captafol

Captan

Captan is a widely used protectant-eradicant fungicide. Agricultural workers may be much exposed during and after spraying operations. One California vineyard applied it 75 times in one season alone. The EPA reviewed the chemical because bacterial and rodent studies suggested that it is mutagenic and carcinogenic. Urticaria due to captan has been documented in a gardener who reacted to the chemical and to plants treated with it.[2] Fregert[118] reported a fruit farmer who developed dermatitis of the hands and face after 3 weeks' exposure to captan. Patch testing with captan and the related folpet (phaltan), 1% in petrolatum, gave positive reactions. Marzulli and Maibach[119] demonstrated that captan, in a concentration of 1%, is a significant contact allergic sensitizer. Out of 205 human test subjects, nine were sensitized. The International and North American Contact Dermatitis Groups later found captan in a 1% concentration to be irritant on patch testing; 0.25% in petrolatum is now preferred for patch testing. Relevant allergic reactions to captan appear to be rare.[10] It has been reported to be a successful topical treatment for tinea versicolor.[2, 120]

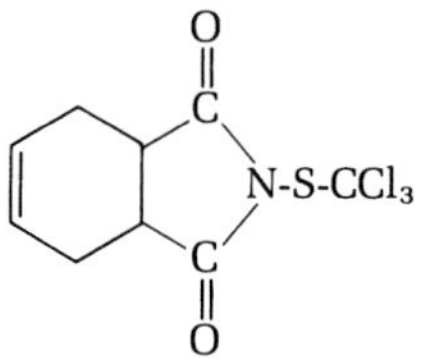

Captan

Folpet

Folpet is a protective fungicide used as a 50% wettable powder and in various dusts for fruits, berries, vegetables, flowers, and ornamentals. Six agricultural workers had patch-test reactions to 0.1% folpet, and irritant reactions were seen in some controls.[16] The I.C.D.R.G. patch tested 509 patients with suspected contact dermatitis to folpet. Fifty had patch-test reactions, but only one was relevant. When 107 patients were patch tested to 0.1% folpet, three had reactions, but none were deemed relevant.[10]

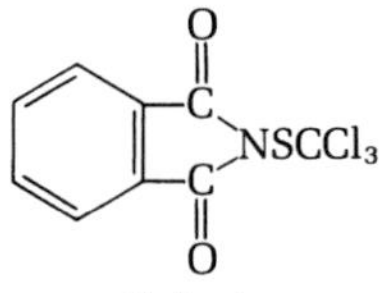

Folpet

DNCB

Occupational allergic contact dermatitis was reported when dinitrochlorobenzene (DNCB) was used as an algicide.[121, 122] Adams and coworkers[123] emphasized that this potent sensitizer should be used only in completely enclosed systems that do not allow skin contact with DNCB.

PCNB

Pentachloronitrobenzene (PCNB) is used as a soil fungicide and seed treatment. It is especially useful for Brussels sprouts, broccoli, and artichokes.

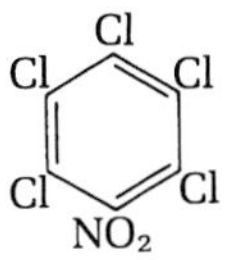

PCNB

Cronin[10] described a 46-year-old pesticide powder packer who developed eczema on his arms, legs, forehead, trunk, and scrotum. Patch testing to PCNB, 1% in petrolatum, was positive. The patient's shoes were heavily contaminated with PCNB dust. DCNA (2,6 dichloro-4-nitroaniline) is a related compound.

Ditalimfos is a contact fungicide used for the control of powdery mildews and scab on apples and pears. It is marketed only in Europe. Allergic contact dermatitis to ditalimfos used as a rose spray was reported by van Ketel.[124]

Dyrene (Anilazine)

Dyrene is a foliar fungicide and is a contact sensitizer.[125, 126] It has been reported to be a cause of allergic contact dermatitis among tomato field workers and in a lawn care worker.

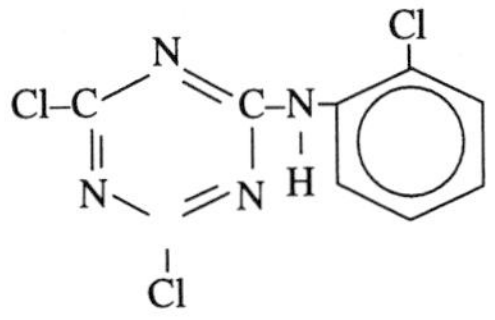

Anilazine

Plondrel

Plondrel is sprayed on roses to protect them from mildew. It is left on the roses, so both sprayers and florists are exposed. Four patients with occupational allergic contact dermatitis to plondrel were reported in 1975.[124] Cronin[10] also reported a case of occupational contact dermatitis due to plondrel in 1980.

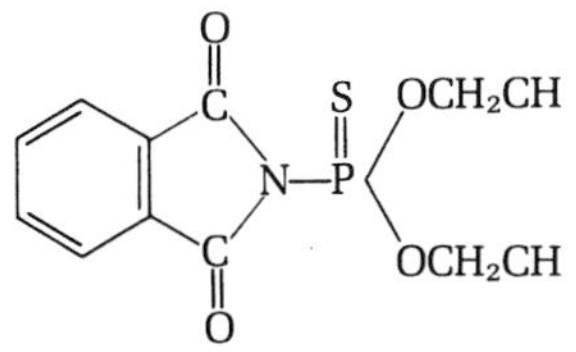

Ditalimfos

Maneb and Zineb

Maneb and zineb are used to treat many plant diseases. Maneb may be used in combination with other pesticides, including lindane, hexachlorobenzene, captan, and zineb. Zineb may be combined with other pesticides, including thiram and sulfur. Maneb and zineb are related to the carbamate class of rubber accelerators and have relatively little systemic toxicity. Nevertheless, they are important allergic sensitizers.

Matsushita and coworkers,[127] using the guinea pig maximization test, demonstrated the strong potential of maneb and zineb for allergic sensitization. Scepa and Ippolito reported six patients with dermatitis from zineb in 1959.[10] Cases of allergic contact dermatitis in workers spraying tobacco were reported by Laborie.[128] Nater and colleagues[129] described three cases of allergic contact sensitization due to maneb. Two of the patients worked in rooms decorated with many plants, and the third was a florist. Patch testing was done with 1%, 2%, and 5% concentrations, but no studies of cross-reactions to zineb and other dithiocarbamates were done. Cronin[10] has reported a rose gardener who had a strong patch-test reaction to maneb rose spray and zineb 1%.

Adams and Manchester[130] reported a case of allergic contact dermatitis to maneb in the wife of a residential gardener. Several severe episodes of dermatitis occurred before the cause was discovered: the patient's husband had stored a large bag of maneb next to the washing machine in the garage. Patch tests to both 1% maneb and 1% thiram in petrolatum produced strong reactions, whereas testing with zineb was negative.

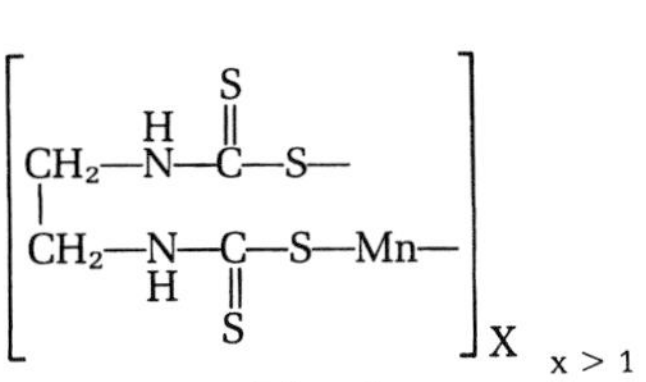

Maneb

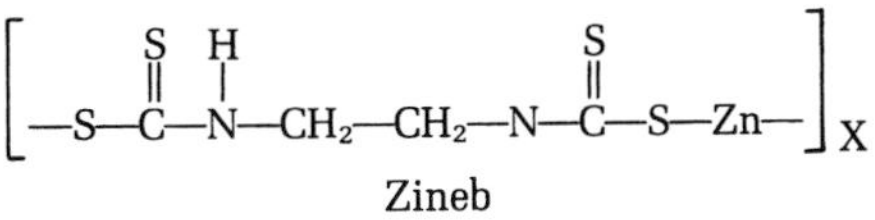

Zineb

Members of the I.C.D.R.G. tested 655 eczematous patients with zineb 1% and maneb 1% in petrolatum. Three patients had positive reactions to zineb, but none was thought relevant. Although 35 patients had reactions to maneb, only one was thought relevant. Allergic contact dermatitis to ethylenediamine used in the manufacture of zineb has been reported.[131]

Ziram

Ziram is a fungicide used extensively on almonds and peaches. It is the most stable of the metallic dithiocarbamates. A patch-test reaction to ziram in an agricultural worker was reported.[16]

Ziram

Mancozeb

Mancozeb (manzeb) is a fungicide related to both maneb and zineb. It combines the benefits of these two earlier fungicides into a distinctive chemical used on a wide range of crops. It has an acute dermal median lethal dose (LD_{50}) of more than 15,000 mg/kg in rats. Burry[132] reported allergic contact dermatitis from mancozeb in South Australia in a worker who treated barley and wheat seeds and in a farmer who planted the seeds. Patch testing was performed at 0.5% concentration; 10 controls were negative. Testing for cross-reactivity to thiram was not done. Allergic contact dermatitis due to mancozeb was also reported in an agricultural worker by Lisi and Carafinni.[133] This patient was also allergic to maneb. In 1996 Koch reported a case of contact dermatitis in a vineyard worker who tested positive to mancozeb at 0.5% and 1% concentrations in petrolatum.[134] This patient also reacted to metiram 1% in petrolatum and to four other chemicals that had not been used in the vineyard, suggesting the possibility of cross-reactivity. Iliev and Elsner reported allergy to mancozeb in a chemical worker.[70]

Thiram

The chemical name is bis(dimethylthiocarbamoyl) disulfide, or tetramethylthiuram disulfide. Thiram, thirame, and TMTD are common names for this fungicide, seed protectant, and animal repellent. Schultz and Herrmann[135] first reported TMTD dermatitis in five dockworkers who unloaded treated bananas. Shelley[136] described dermatitis associated

with TMTD fungicide on a golf course. Cronin[10] related dermatitis in a man who had applied thiram to his garden. TMTD was reported to cause allergic contact dermatitis in a Polish flower vendor. She was in contact with flowers treated with the Polish fungicide Sadoplon, which is 75% TMTD.[137] Fisher[138] published a list of fungicides and animal repellents that may contain thiram.

Thiram

Chlorothalonil

Chlorothalonil (tetrachloroisophthalonitril) is a broad-spectrum fungicide approved for use on vegetables, fruits, flowers, and trees. A 0.1% solution in acetone is a moderate cutaneous irritant. The same concentration in petrolatum is much less irritating and in saline is not irritating to the skin of New Zealand white rabbits.[35] It is stable in UV light. It has a half-life of about 2 months. Contact dermatitis has been reported in vegetable growers, woodworkers, and flower growers.[139] Patch testing is performed with 0.01% chlorothalonil in petrolatum, a marginally irritant concentration. Chlorothalonil is a strong cutaneous irritant in the concentrations used in spraying.

Chlorothalonil is used as a wood preservative in Northern Europe. Johnsson[140] reported an epidemic of contact dermatitis in a Norwegian woodenware factory in which 14 of the 20 workers had work-related skin complaints, seven of them contact dermatitis. Bach and Pedersen[141] reported contact dermatitis to tetrachloroisophthalonitril in a cabinet maker, and Spindeldreier and Deichmann[142] reported three other cases of contact dermatitis.

Fatal toxic epidermal necrolysis has been attributed to chlorothalonil. A 30-year-old Navy pilot had played 81 holes of golf in the week before he developed toxic epidermal necrolysis. The golf course had been sprayed with chlorothalonil. Special photographic techniques using UV light demonstrated chlorothalonil on the deceased's golf clubs, balls, and shoes.[143]

Chlorothalonil has been reported as a possible cause of pigmented dermatitis in 39 banana plantation workers.[144]

Photoallergic contact dermatitis was reported in a patient who used Daconil, whose main component is tetrachloroisophthalonitril, in his garden. Positive results were obtained with both patch- and photopatch testing with Daconil, 0.002% aqueous.[145] The latter produced the stronger result.

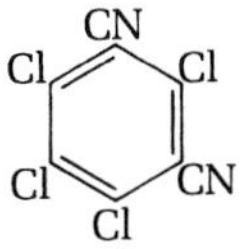

Chlorothalonil

Dithianon

Dithianon is a broad-spectrum fungicide. Calnan[146] reported dermatitis in a female horticulturist in a fruit orchard who became sensitive to dithianon. She came in contact with sprayed trees during pruning and while cleaning the spraying machines. Patch testing was positive with 1% dithianon in petrolatum.

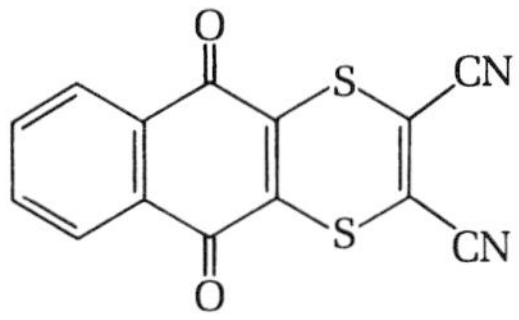

Dithianon

Dinobuton

Dinobuton is a fungicide and acaricide used to control the mites of deciduous fruit trees and citrus trees, cotton, and cucumbers and other vegetables. It is also valuable for controlling powdery mildew on apples, cucumbers, hops, and other crops.

In 1974 Wahlberg reported yellow staining of the hair and nails of workers who acquired contact allergic dermatitis while manufacturing dinobuton in a factory in northern Sweden. Dinobuton did not appear to be a strong primary irritant: patch testing with 40% dinobuton caused spontaneous flare reactions (sensitization) in two workers 9 to 10 days after application. The chemical relationship to picric acid was considered significant.[147]

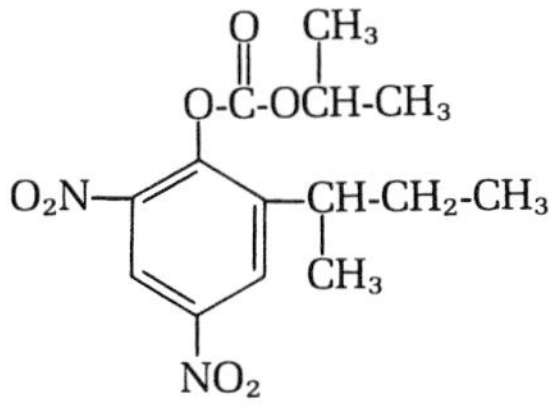

Dinobuton

Octhilinone

Octhilinone is a biocide used in industrial cooling water, cutting oils, cosmetics, and shampoos and as a leather preservative. Two cases of occupational allergic contact dermatitis to octhilinone

used as a fungicide for surface paint of sheet roofing were reported by Thormann.[148] Both workers had severe allergic contact dermatitis. Allergic reactions to other chemically related preservatives have been reported (1,2 benzisothiazolin-3-1 and 3-ethyl amino-1,2 benzisothiazol hydrochloride [Etisazol]).[149, 150] Etisazol is a veterinary antifungal agent.

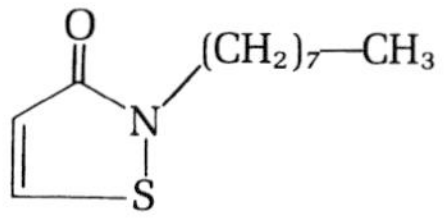

Octhilinone

Triforine

Triforine is a fungicide used to treat *Ascochyta* blight and is used by chrysanthemum growers. In 1994 Ueda and colleagues[151] performed mass examination of chrysanthemum growers, who commonly used triforine. The highest rate of positive patch testing was to triforine, and there was evidence of a cross-sensitization between triforine and dichlorvos (DDVP, a known sensitizer).

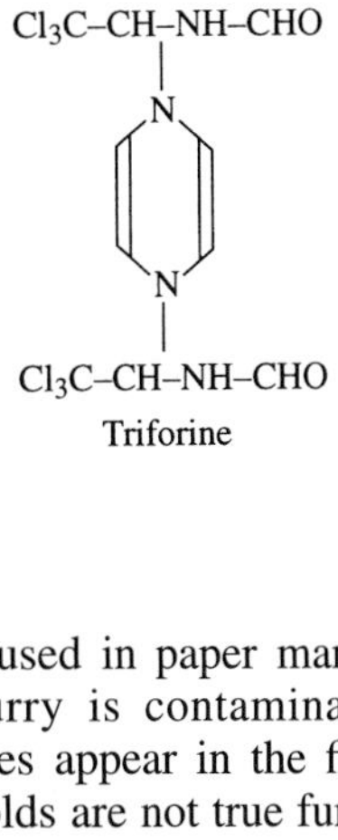

Triforine

Slimicides

Slimicides are used in paper manufacture. When wood pulp slurry is contaminated with slime molds, blemishes appear in the final paper products. (Slime molds are not true fungi, even though they possess like characteristics.) Slimicides are added to wood pulp slurry to prevent growth of slime molds. Rycroft and Calnan[152] reported irritant contact dermatitis to slimicides in a paper mill. The active constituents in the slimicides include bis-1,4-bromoacetoxy-2 butene and 2,3-dichloro-4-bromo-tetrahydrothiophene-1,1-dioxide.

ANTIBIOTICS

Streptomycin is used to control bacterial plant diseases such as fireblight, sometimes in combination with oxytetracycline or tetracycline. It has been reported to cause allergic contact dermatitis in agricultural workers.[153]

MITICIDES

Propargite

Irritant contact dermatitis to propargite has been reported.[10] The active ingredient in Omite-30W, a miticide widely used on California grapes, propargite is also the active ingredient of Omite-CR, used on citrus. An outbreak of dermatitis affected 114 of 198 orange pickers exposed to Omite-CR. The dermatitis appeared predominantly on exposed areas of the neck and chest. The prolonged residual action of propargite in Omite-CR was suggested to be the cause of this outbreak.[14] Dienchlor is a miticide of low toxicity that has been used for 20 years. The *Farm Chemical Handbook* states that it is neither a primary irritant nor a sensitizer, but a patch-test reaction to dienchlor was reported in a florist with hand dermatitis.[9]

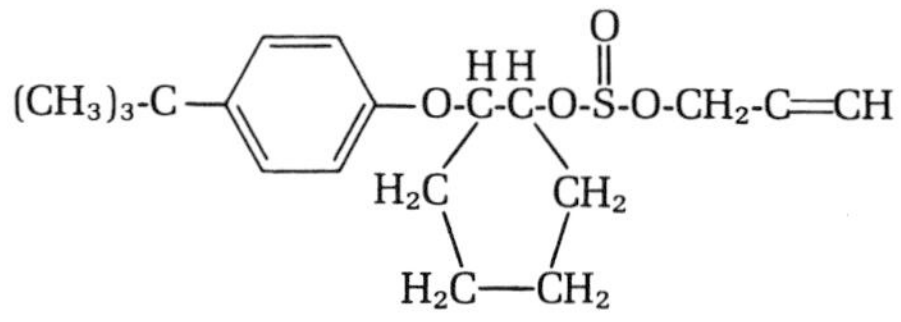

Propargite

PLANT GROWTH INHIBITORS

Choline Chloride

Choline chloride is a growth inhibitor used in agriculture. Fischer[154] reported a case of contact dermatitis related to choline chloride.

INSECT REPELLENTS

DEET

Diethyltoluamide (DEET) was first synthesized in 1954 and came into use as an insect repellent in 1957. It is relatively insoluble in water but is soluble in ethanol and propylene glycol. Diethyltoluamide is considered the best all-purpose insect repellent.[155] It is especially effective against mosquitoes. It remains effective for several hours after it is applied. Concentrations of DEET in sprays, liquids, or sticks formulated for application to skin or clothes vary from 1% to 70%.

Antecubital erythema progressing to hemorrhagic bullae was reported in 10 young soldiers.[155] The antecubital area was involved in two patients who had permanent scarring. Some American soldiers in Vietnam developed bullae, followed by scarring, from DEET.[156] DEET has been reported to exacerbate seborrhea and acne vulgaris and to produce contact dermatitis.[2] Maibach and Johnson[157] elegantly documented immune-mediated contact urticaria to DEET. Rarely, toxic encephalopathy and death have been reported in children who had skin contact with DEET.

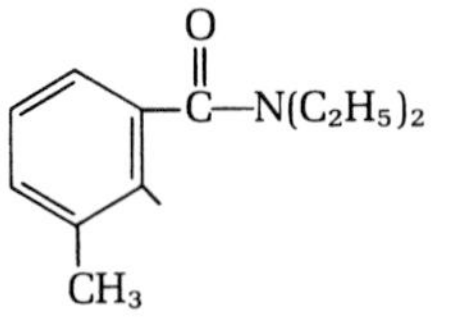

DEET

LIVESTOCK TREATMENTS

Disinfectants that can cause irritant or allergic contact dermatitis are often used to clean udders in preparation for milking.[153] Equipment is cleaned with sodium hydroxide and nitric acid. Dairy farmers are also exposed to hypochlorite, iodine, phenolic compounds, quaternary ammonium compounds, and hairs and secretions from cows.

Farmers can develop irritant contact dermatitis to animal feeds. Medicaments mixed in feeds can be primary irritants or sensitizers. Farmers sometimes neglect to wear protective gloves while mixing drugs to be administered to animals. Antimicrobial agents, including antibiotics, are used in feed both to treat disease and to promote growth. Contact dermatitis due to ethylenediaminedihydroiodide (as a source of iodine), furazolidone (a synthetic derivative of nitrofurazone), the antioxidant hydroquinone, and halquinol (as an antibacterial agent) have been reported from animal feed ingredients.[158, 159] Allergic contact dermatitis to the antioxidant ethoxyquin in animal feed has been reported in farmers and in feed mill workers. Also used to control scald in fruit, ethoxyquin was reported to cause allergic contact dermatitis in apple pickers.[158, 160]

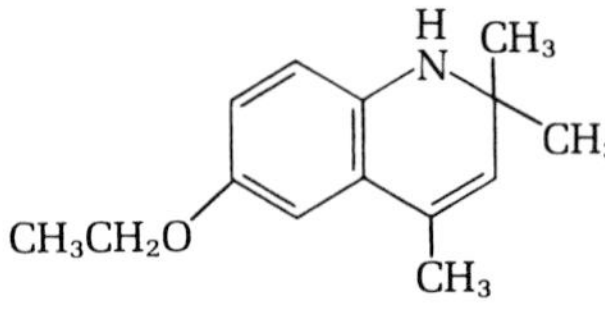

Ethoxyquin

Quindoxin once was used as a growth stimulant additive in animal feeds. Photocontact dermatitis has been attributed to quindoxin in animal feed. Quindoxin photosensitivity with a persistent light

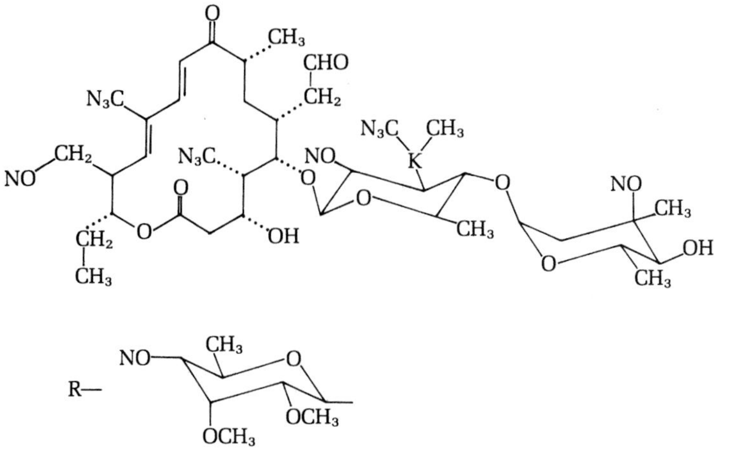

Tylosin

reaction was reported in pig farmers.[161] Quindoxin is not registered for use in the United States or Canada.

Dawson and Scott[162] reported severe contact eczema due to quinoxaline in animal feeds. It is also an acaricide. Olaquindox is a derivative of quinoxaline that is added to feed to prevent bacterial enteritis in pigs. Both allergic contact and photocontact dermatitis due to olaquindox have been reported in Italy.[163, 164]

Photocontact dermatitis with persistent photoallergy due to airborne olaquindox has been reported, and it is recommended that farmers minimize dust generation and contact with the skin.[165] Photoallergic contact dermatitis has been reported in farmers who used chlorpromazine to tranquilize pigs.[166]

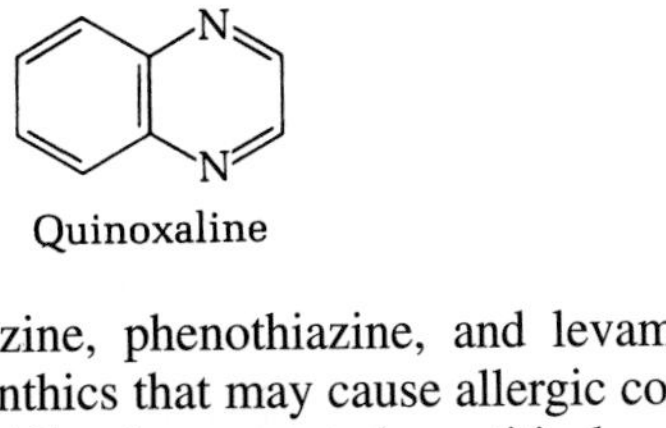

Olaquindox

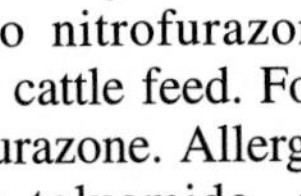

Quinoxaline

Piperazine, phenothiazine, and levamisole are anthelminthics that may cause allergic contact dermatitis. Allergic contact dermatitis has been reported to nitrofurazone. This anticoccidian is added to cattle feed. Formaldehyde is the allergen in nitrofurazone. Allergic contact dermatitis to 3,5 dinitro-*o*-toluamide, an anticoccidian used in chickenfeed, has been reported.[153]

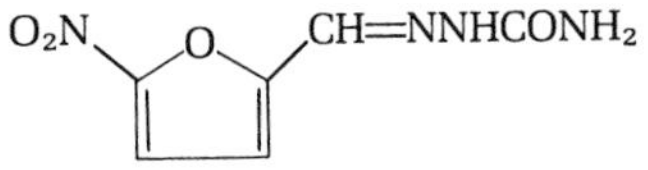

Nitrofurazone

Neomycin, ethylenediamine, and thiabendazole have also been used as feed additives. Sulfacetamide, sulfamethazine, chlortetracycline, oxytetracycline, and bacitracin have been used as growth promoters for livestock.[167] Farmers have become allergic to both nitrofurazone and tylosin in animal feed, particularly feed for hogs. Spiramycin and tylosin were the most common sensitizers among antibiotics used by farmers in Denmark.

Tylosin is a macrolide antibiotic used in the United Kingdom to combat swine dysentery in pigs and respiratory infections in poultry. Tylosin can produce both irritant and allergic contact dermatitis.[168] Cases of occupational allergic contact dermatitis due to the macrolide spiramycin and tylosin have been reported in hog farmers and veterinarians.[169, 170] Allergic contact dermatitis to virginiamycin, a food additive for pigs and poultry, has also been reported.[171]

Veien[172] patch tested 180 farmers to 5% virginiamycin in petrolatum but obtained no reactions. Approximately half of veterinarians surveyed in Scandinavia have occupational contact dermatitis, predominantly irritant contact dermatitis. Occupational dermatoses occasionally force veterinarians to abandon general veterinary practice.[173] Penethamate has been reported to be a common sensitizer of veterinarians. Penethamate is a powerfully sensitizing penicillin derivative used in Europe for local treatment of mastitis in cows.[170, 173]

MILK TESTERS

Chromate has been used as a preservative for milk samples to be analyzed for health and quality

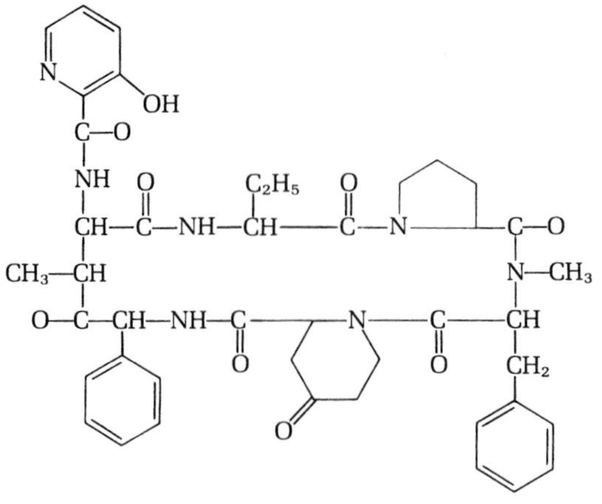

Virginiamycin S_1

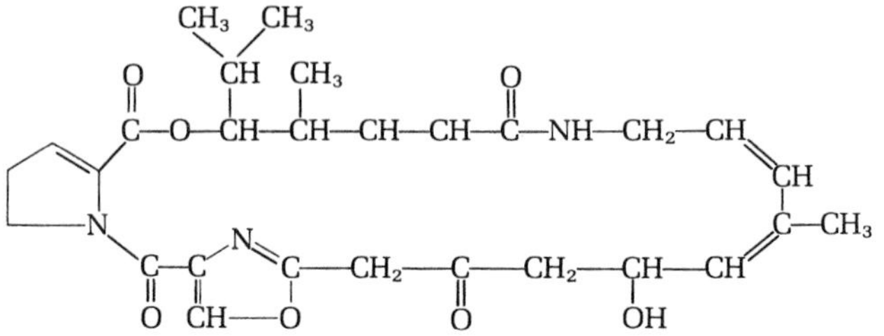

Virginiamycin N_1

control purposes. Several reports document chromate allergy in milk testers and in analysis laboratory workers.[174–176] Milk preservative solutions in the United Kingdom now contain 8% bronopol and 20% methylchloroisothiazolinone and methylisothiazoline (Kathon CG). Allergic contact dermatitis to bronopol and Kathon CG was reported in three milk recorders.[177] Bronopol has also been used in some countries as a seed treatment and foliar spray.

PATCH TESTING

After excluding nonoccupational causes of dermatitis, agricultural workers suspected of suffering from occupational allergic contact dermatitis should be patch tested to all plants and to the pesticides they are exposed to. Pesticides may be generally patch tested in 1% dilution.[9] A dilution of 0.1% is also suggested to avoid false-positive patch-test reactions. A minority of pesticides are commercially available in proper vehicles and concentrations for patch testing. Patch testing with insecticides[120] can be associated with false-negative reactions. Fear of systemic toxicity may deter physicians from patch testing with adequate concentrations of organophosphorus insecticides such as parathion. Pesticides that are dissolved in pri-

mary irritants must be extremely diluted for patch testing. The addresses of American pesticide manufacturers are listed in the *Farm Chemical Handbook*. A number of authors have suggested appropriate patch-test concentrations for pesticides (Appendix 32–1).[16, 138, 178, 179]

References

1. Hogan DJ, Lane PR. Dermatologic disorders in agriculture. *Occup Med* 1986; 1(2):285–300.
2. Hayes WJ. *Pesticides Studied in Man.* Baltimore: Williams & Wilkins; 1982.
3. *Farm Chemical Handbook.* Willoughby, OH: Meister; 1986.
4. Windholz M, ed. *Merck Index: An Encyclopedia of Chemicals, Drugs, and Biologicals.* Rahway: Merck & Co.; 1996.
5. Edmiston S, Maddy KT. Summary of illnesses and injuries reported in California by physicians in 1986 as potentially related to pesticides. *Vet Hum Toxicol* 1987; 29(5):391–397.
6. Jeyaratnam J, de Alwis Seneviratne RS, Copplestone JF. Survey of pesticide poisoning in Sri Lanka. *Bull WHO* 1982; 60:615–619.
7. Lessenger JE, Estock MD, Younglove T. An analysis of 190 cases of suspected pesticide illness. *J Am Board Fam Pract* 1995; 8:278–282.
8. Rycroft RJG, Wilkinson JD. The principal irritants and sensitizers. In: Rook A, Wilkinson DS, et al, eds. *Textbook of Dermatology.* Oxford: Blackwell; 1986:551.
9. van Joost TH, Naafs B, van Ketel WG. Sensitization to benomyl and related pesticides. *Contact Dermatitis* 1983; 9:153–154.

10. Cronin E. Pesticides. In: *Contact Dermatitis*. Edinburgh: Churchill Livingstone; 1980:393–413.

11. Hogan DJ, Lane PR. Allergic contact dermatitis due to a herbicide (barban). *Can Med Assoc J* 1985; 132:387–389.

12. Kligman AM. The identification of contact allergens by human assay. III. The maximization test: a procedure for screening and rating contact sensitizers. *J Invest Dermatol* 1966; 47:393–409.

13. Milby TH, Epstein WL. Allergic contact sensitivity to malathion. *Arch Environ Health* 1964; 9:434–437.

14. Saunders LD, Ames RG, Knaack JB, et al. Outbreak of Omite-CR–induced dermatitis among orange pickers in Tulare County, California. *J Occup Med* 1987; 29:409–413.

15. Mathias CGT: Epidemiological aspects of occupational skin disease in agriculture. In: Dosman JR, Cockroft D, eds. *Occupational Health and Safety in Agriculture*. Boca Raton, Fla.: CRC Press; 1989:285–287.

16. Lisi P, Carafinni S, Assalve D. Irritation and sensitization potential of pesticides. *Contact Dermatitis* 1987; 17:212–218.

17. Guo YL, Wang BJ, Lee CC, Wang JD. Prevalence of dermatoses and skin sensitisation associated with use of pesticides in fruit farmers of southern Taiwan. *Occup Environ Med* 1996;53(6):427–431.

18. Wolfe HR, Armstrong JF, et al. Pesticide exposure from concentrate spraying. *Arch Environ Health* 1966; 13:340–344.

19. Yoshida K. Cutaneous exposure of pesticide spray applicators. In: Dosman JA, Cockroft D, eds. *Occupational Health and Safety in Agriculture*. Boca Raton, Fla.: CRC Press; 1989:297–300.

20. Abbott IM, Bonsall JL, Chester G, Hart TB, Turnbull GJ. Worker exposure to a herbicide applied with ground sprayers in the United Kingdom. *Am Ind Hyg Assoc J* 1987; 48:167–175.

21. Rutz R, Krieger RI. Exposure to pesticide mixer/loaders and applicators in California. *Rev Environ Contam Toxicol* 1992; 129:1121–1139.

22. Fenske RA. Nonuniform dermal deposition patterns during occupational exposures to pesticides. *Arch Environ Contam Toxicol* 1990; 19:332–337.

23. Winter CK, Kurtz PH. Factors influencing grape worker susceptibility to skin rashes. *Bull Environ Contam Toxicol* 1985; 35(3):418–426.

24. Mehler LN, O'Malley MA, Krieger RI. Acute pesticide morbidity and mortality: California. *Rev Environ Contam Toxicol* 1992; 129:51–66.

25. Kazen C, Bloomer A, Welch R, Oudbier A, Price H. Persistence of pesticides on the hands of some occupationally exposed people. *Arch Environ Health* 1974; 29:315–319.

26. Upholt WM, Kearney PC. Pesticides. *N Engl J Med* 1966; 275:1419–1426.

27. Feldmann RJ, Maibach HI. Percutaneous penetration of some pesticides and herbicides in man. *Toxicol Appl Pharmacol* 1974; 28:126–132.

28. Ritter L. Assessment of pesticide toxicity: regulatory viewpoints. In: Dosman JA, Cockroft D, eds. *Occupational Health and Safety*. Boca Raton, Fla.: CRC Press; 1989:211–213.

29. Haverstock LM. Farm stress: research considerations. In: Dosman JA, Cockroft D, eds. *Occupational Health and Safety in Agriculture*. Boca Raton, Fla.: CRC Press, 1989:381–384.

30. Feinberg SM. Pyrethrum sensitization: its importance and relation to pollen allergy. *JAMA* 1934; 102:1557–1558.

31. Mitchell JC. Allergic contact dermatitis from Compositae. *Trans St Johns Hosp Derm Soc* 1969; 55:174–183.

31a. Mitchell JC, Dupuis G, Towers GHN. Allergic contact dermatitis from pyrethrum. *Br J Dermatol* 1972; 86:568–573.

32. Garratt JR, Bigger JW. Asthma due to insect powder. *Br Med J* 1923; 2:764.

33. Epstein E. Urticaria due to an insecticide (pyrethrum). *Urol Rev* 1938; 48:829.

34. Magnusson B, Blohm S-V, Fregert S, et al. Routine patch testing IV. *Acta Derm Venereol* 1968; 48:110–116.

35. Flannigan SA, Tucker SB, Key MM, et al. Synthetic pyrethroid insecticides: a dermatological evaluation. *Br J Indust Med* 1985; 42:363–372.

36. Sulzberger MB. Studies in tobacco hypersensitivity. I. A comparison between reactions to nicotine and to denicotinized tobacco extract. *J Immunol* 1933; 24:85–91.

37. Samitz MH, Mori P, Long CF. Dermatological hazards in the cigar industry. *Ind Med Surg* 1949; 18:434–439.

38. Nasution D, Klokke AH, Nater JP. A survey of occupational dermatoses in Indonesia. *Berufsdermatosen* 1973; 21:215–222.

39. Vero F, Genovese S. Occupational dermatitis in cigar makers due to contact with tobacco leaves. *Arch Dermatol* 1941; 43:257–263.

40. Ghosh SK, Gokani VN, Parikh JR, Doctor PB, Kashyap SK, Chatterjee BB. Protection against "green symptoms" from tobacco in Indian harvesters: a preliminary intervention study. *Arch Environ Health* 1987; 42:141–144.

41. Vincenzi C, Tosti A, Cirone M, Guarrera M, Cusano F. Allergic contact dermatitis from transdermal nicotine systems. *Contact Dermatitis* 1993; 29(2):104–105.

42. Bircher AJ, Howald H, Rufli T. Adverse skin reactions to nicotine in a transdermal therapeutic system. *Contact Dermatitis* 1991; 25(4):230–236.

43. Mitchell J, Rook A. *Quassia Amara in Botanical Dermatology*. Vancouver: Greengrass; 1979:646–647.

44. Emmett EA. Occupational skin cancer. A review. *J Occup Med* 1976; 17:44–49.

45. Wilkinson DS: Sulphur sensitivity. *Contact Dermatitis* 1975; 1:58.

46. Gammeltoft M. Tributyltin oxide is not allergenic. *Contact Dermatitis* 1978;4:238.

47. Morris GE. Dermatoses from phenylmercuric salts. *Arch Environ Health* 1960;1:53–55.

48. Barnes RL, Wilkinson DS. Epidermal necrolysis from clothing impregnated with paraffin. *Br Med J* 1973; 4:466–467.

49. Taylor JS. Dermatologic hazards from ethylene oxide. *Cutis* 1977; 19:189–191.

50. Becker CE. Recognizing the health hazards of ethylene oxide. *West J Med* 1988; 148:75.

51. Radimer GF, David JH, Ackerman AB. Fumigant-induced toxic epidermal necrolysis. *Arch Dermatol* 1974; 110:103–104.

52. Richter G. Allergic contact dermatitis from methylisothiocyanate in soil disinfectants. *Contact Dermatitis* 1980; 6:183–186.

53. Koo D, Goldman L, Baron R. Irritant dermatitis among workers cleaning up a pesticide spill: California 1991. *Am J Ind Med* 1995; 27:545–553.

54. Nater JP, Gooskens VH. Occupational dermatosis due to a soil fumigant. *Contact Dermatitis* 1976; 2:227–229.

55. Black H. Dazomet and chloropicrin. *Contact Dermatitis Newslett* 1973; 14:410–411.

56. Dunn JE, Dunn RC, Smith BS. Skin-sensitizing properties of DDT for the guinea pig. *Public Health Rep* 1946; 61:1614.

57. Leider M. Allergic eczematous contact-type dermatitis caused by DDT. *J Invest Dermatol* 1947; 8:125–126.

58. Niedelman ML. Contact dermatitis due to DDT. *Occup Med* 1946; 1:391–395.

59. Stryker GV, Godfrey B. Dermatitis resulting from exposure to DDT. *J Missouri Med Assoc* 1946; 43:384.

60. Ross CM. Sock dermatitis from dieldrin. *Br J Dermatol* 1964; 76:494–495.

61. Pevny I. Pesticide allergy—allergic contact eczema of a vintner. *Derm Beruf Umwelt* 1980; 28:186–189.

62. Svindland HB. Subacute parathion poisoning with erysipeloid-like lesion. *Contact Dermatitis* 1981; 7:177–179.

63. Bhargava RK, Singh V, Soni V. Erythema multiforme resulting from insecticide spray. *Arch Dermatol* 1977; 113:686–687.

64. Lahti A, Maibach HI. Contact urticaria from diethyl fumarate. *Contact Dermatitis* 1985; 12:139–140.

65. Farber GA, Burks JW. Flea-collar dermatitis. *Cutis* 1972; 9:809–812.

66. Cronce PC, Alden HS. Flea collar dermatitis. *JAMA* 1968; 206:1563–1564.

67. Mathias CGT. Persistent contact dermatitis from the insecticide dichlorvos. *Contact Dermatitis* 1983; 9:217–218.

68. Edmundson WF, Davies JE. Occupational dermatitis from naled. A clinical report. *Arch Environ Health* 1967; 15:89.

69. Fregert S. Allergic contact dermatitis from the pesticide rodannitrobenzene. *Contact Dermatitis Newslett* 1967; 2:4.

70. Iliev D, Elsner P. Allergic contact dermatitis from the fungicide Rondo-M and the insecticide Alfacron. *Contact Dermatitis* 1997; 36(1):51.

71. Schena D, Barba A. Erythema–multiforme-like contact dermatitis from dimethoate. *Contact Dermatitis* 1992; 27(2):116–117.

72. Haenen C, deMoor A, Dooms-Goossens A. Contact dermatitis caused by the insecticides omethoate and dimethoate. *Contact Dermatitis* 1996; 35:54–55.

73. Wood S, Rom WN, White GL, Logan DC. Pentachlorophenol poisoning. *J Occup Med* 1983; 25:527–529.

73a. Lambert J, Schepens P, Janssens J, Dockx P. Skin lesions as a sign of subacute pentachlorophenol intoxication. *Acta Derm Venereol* 1986; 66:170–172.

74. Kentor PM. Urticaria from contact with pentachlorphenate. *JAMA* 1986; 256:3350.

75. Fregert S. Allergic contact dermatitis from *p*-chloro-*o*-cresol in a pesticide. *Contact Dermatitis Newslett* 1968; 3:46.

76. Baran RL. Nail damage caused by weed killers and insecticides. *Arch Dermatol* 1974; 110:467.

77. Cotterill JA. Contact dermatitis following exposure to tetrachloronitrobenzene. *Contact Dermatitis* 1981; 7:353.

78. De Eds F, Wilson RH, Thomas JO. Photosensitization by phenothiazine. *JAMA* 1940; 114:2095–2097.

79. Pennsylvania Dept of Health, Division of Occupational Health. *Occupational Health News and Views*. Winter, 1969.

80. Maibach HI. Irritation, sensitization, photoirritation and photosensitization assays with a glyphosphate herbicide. *Contact Dermatitis* 1986; 15:152–155.

81. Hindson PC, Diffey BL. Phototoxicity of a weed killer: a correction. *Contact Dermatitis* 1984; 11:260.

82. Bowra GT, Duffield DP, Osborn AJ, Purchase FH. Premalignant and neoplastic skin lesions associated with occupational exposure to "tarry" byproducts during manufacture of 4,4'-bipyridyl. *Br J Ind Med* 1982; 39:76–81.

83. Wang JD, Li WE, Hu FC, Hu KH. Occupational risk and the development of premalignant skin lesions among Paraquat manufacturers. *Br J Ind Med* 1987; 44:196–200.

84. Hearn CED, Keir W. Nail damage in spray operators exposed to Paraquat. *Br J Ind Med* 1971; 28:399–403.

85. Botella R, Sastre A, Castells A. Contact dermatitis to Paraquat. *Contact Dermatitis* 1985; 13:123–124.

86. Sharvill DE. Reaction to paraquat. *Contact Dermatitis Newslett* 1971; 9:210.

87. Newhouse M, McEvoy D, Rosenthal D. Percutaneous Paraquat absorption. *Arch Dermatol* 1978; 114:1516–1519.

88. Nishioka K, Asagami C, Kurata M, Fujita H. Sensitivity to the weed killer DNA-nitralin and cross-sensitivity to Dinitrochlorobenzene. *Arch Dermatol* 1983; 119:304–306.

89. English JSC, Rycroft RJG, Calnan CD. Allergic contact dermatitis from aminotriazole. *Contact Dermatitis* 1986; 14:255–256.

90. Bruze M, Fregert S. Allergic contact dermatitis to chloridazon. *Contact Dermatitis* 1982; 8:427.

91. Nater JP, Grosfeld JCM. Allergic contact dermatitis from Betanol (phenmedipham). *Contact Dermatitis* 1979; 5:59–60.

92. Taylor JS, Wuthrich RC, Lloyd KM, Poland A. Chloracne from manufacture of a new herbicide. *Arch Dermatol* 1977; 113:616–619.

93. Iden DL, Schroeter AL. Allergic contact dermatitis to herbicides. *Arch Dermatol* 1977; 113:983.

94. Spencer MC. Herbicide dermatitis. *JAMA* 1966; 198:169–170.

95. Hoar SK, Blair A, Holmes FF, Boysen C, et al. Agricultural herbicide use and risk of lymphoma and soft-tissue sarcoma. *JAMA* 1986; 256:1141–1147.

96. Honchar PA, Halperin WA. 2,4,5-T, trichlorophenol, and soft-tissue sarcoma. *Lancet* 1981; 1:268–269.

97. Cook RR. Dioxin, chloracne, and soft-tissue sarcoma. *Lancet* 1981; 1:618–619.

98. Moses M, Selikoff IJ. Soft-tissue sarcomas, phenoxy herbicides, and chlorinated phenols. *Lancet* 1981; 1:1370.

99. Johnson FE, Kugler MA, Brown SM. Soft-tissue sarcomas and chlorinated phenols. *Lancet* 1981; 2:40.

100. Cantor KP. Farming and mortality from non-Hodgkin's lymphoma: A case-control study. *Int J Cancer* 1982; 29:239–247.

101. Burmeister LF, Everett GD, Van Lier SF, et al. Selected cancer mortality and farm practices in Iowa. *Am J Epidemiol* 1983; 118:72–77.

102. Buesching DP, Wollstadt L. Cancer mortality among farmers. *Int J Natl Cancer Inst* 1984; 72:503.

103. Brancaccio RR, Chamales MH. Contact dermatitis and depigmentation produced by the herbicide Carbyne. *Contact Dermatitis* 1977; 3:108–109.

104. Solomons B. Sensitization to Nitrofen. *Contact Dermatitis Newslett* 1972; 12:336.

105. Leow Y, Maibach HI. Allergic contact dermatitis from norflurason (Predict). *Contact Dermatitis* 1996; 35:369–370.

106. Pentel MT, Andreozzi RJ, Marks JG. Allergic contact dermatitis from the herbicides trifluralin and benefin. *J Am Acad Dermatol* 1994; 31:1057–1058.

107. Savitt LE. Contact dermatitis due to benomyl insecticide. *Arch Dermatol* 1972; 105:926–927.

108. Fregert S. Allergic contact dermatitis from two pesticides. *Contact Dermatitis Newslett* 1973; 13:367.

109. van Ketel WG. Sensitivity to the pesticide benomyl. *Contact Dermatitis* 1976; 2:290–291.

110. Larsen AI, Larsen A, Jepsen JR, Jorgensen R. Contact allergy to the fungicide benomyl. *Contact Dermatitis* 1990; 22(5):278–281.

111. Winter JM, Teaf CM: Benlate. A medical and scientific controversy. *J Florida Med Assoc* 1993; 80(6):400–402.

112. *Tampa Tribune*, 1996.

113. Cripps DJ, Gocmen A, Peter HA. Porphyria turica. Twenty years after hexachlorobenzene intoxication. *Arch Dermatol* 1980; 116:46–50.

114. Camarasa G. Difolatan dermatitis. *Contact Dermatitis* 1975; 1:127.

115. Matsushita T, Nomura S, Wakatsuki T. Epidemiology of contact dermatitis from pesticides in Japan. *Contact Dermatitis* 1980; 6:255–259.

116. Stoke JCJ. Captafol dermatitis in the timber industry. *Contact Dermatitis* 1979; 5:284–292.

117. Cottel WI. Difolatan. *Contact Dermatitis Newslett* 1972; 11:252.

118. Fregert S. Allergic contact dermatitis from the pesticides captan and phaltan. *Contact Dermatitis Newslett* 1967; 2:28.

119. Marzulli FN, Maibach HI. Antimicrobials: Experimental contact sensitization in man. *J Soc Cosmet Chemists* 1973; 24:399–421.

120. Hjorth N, Wilkinson DS. Contact dermatitis. II. Sensitization to pesticides. *Br J Dermatol* 1968; 80:272–274.

121. Zimmerman MC. Dinitrochlorobenzene in water systems. *Contact Dermatitis Newslett* 1970; 7:165.

122. Malten KE. DNCB in cooling water. *Contact Dermatitis Newslett* 1974; 15:466.

123. Adams RM, Zimmerman MC, Bartlett JB, Preston JR. 1-Chloro-2,4-dinitrobenzene as an algicide: report of four cases of contact dermatitis. *Arch Dermatol* 1971; 103:191–193.

124. van Ketel WG. Allergic dermatitis from a new pesticide. *Contact Dermatitis* 1975; 1:297–300.

125. Schuman SH, Dobson RL, Fingar JR. Dyrene dermatitis. *Lancet* 1980; 2:1252.

126. Mathias CGT. Allergic contact dermatitis from a lawn care fungicide containing Dyrene. *Am J Contact Dermatitis* 1997; 8:47–48.

127. Matsushita T, Arimatsu Y, Nomura S. Experimental study on contact dermatitis caused by dithiocarbamates maneb, mancozeb, zineb, and their related compounds. *Int Arch Occup Environ Health* 1976; 37:169–178.

128. Laborie F, Laborie R, Dedieu EH. Allergie aux fongicides de la gamme du menebe et du zinebe. *Arch Mal Prof Med Travail Securite Soc* 1964; 25:419–424.

129. Nater JP, Terpsta H, Bleumink E. Allergic contact sensitization to the fungicide maneb. *Contact Dermatitis* 1979; 5:24–26.

130. Adams RM, Manchester RD. Allergic contact dermatitis to maneb in a housewife. *Contact Dermatitis* 1982; 8:271.

131. Tsyrkunov LP. Toksiko-allergicheskii dermatit ot vozdeistviia etilendiamina v proizvodstve gerbitsida tsineba. *Gig Tr Prof Zabol* 1987; 8:45–46.

132. Burry JN. Contact dermatitis from agricultural fungicide in South Australia. *Contact Dermatitis* 1976; 2:288–296.

133. Lisi P, Carafinni S. Pellagroid dermatitis from mancozeb with vitiligo. *Contact Dermatitis* 1985; 13:124–125.

134. Koch P. Occupational allergic contact dermatitis and airborne contact dermatitis from 5 fungicides in a vineyard worker. Cross-reactions between fungicides of the dithiocarbamate group. *Contact Dermatitis* 1996; 34(5):324–329.

135. Schultz KH, Hermann WP. Tetramethylthiuramdisulphide, ein Thioharnstoffderivat also Ekzemnoxe bei Hafenarbeiten. *Berufsdermatosen* 1958; 6:130–135.

136. Shelley WD. Golf course dermatitis due to thiram fungicide. *JAMA* 1964; 188:415–417.

137. Rudzki E, Napiorkowska T. Dermatitis caused by the Polish fungicide Sadoplon 75. *Contact Dermatitis* 1980; 6:300–301.

138. Fisher AA. *Contact Dermatitis*. Philadelphia: Lea & Febiger; 1986.

139. Bruynzeel DP, van Ketel WG. Contact dermatitis due to chlorothalonil in floriculture. *Contact Dermatitis* 1986; 14:67–68.

140. Johnsson M, Buhagen M, Leira HL, Solvang S. Fungicide-induced contact dermatitis. *Contact Dermatitis* 1983; 9:285–288.

141. Bach B, Pedersen NB. Contact dermatitis from a wood preservative containing tetrachlorisophthalonitrile. *Contact Dermatitis* 1980; 6:142.

142. Spindeldreier A, Deichmann B. Contact dermatitis against a wood preservative with a new fungicidal agent. *Derm Beruf Umwelt* 1980; 28(3):88–90.

143. Lord JT, Moats R, Jones J. Too much golf. *J Forensic Sci Soc* 1984; 24:359.

144. Penagos H, Jimenez V, Fallas V, et al. Chlorothalonil, a possible cause of erythema dyschronicum perstans (ashy dermatitis). *Contact Dermatitis* 1996; 35:214–218.

145. Matsushita S, Kanekura T, Saruwatari K, et al. Photoallergic contact dermatitis due to Daconil. *Contact Dermatitis* 1996; 35:115–116.

146. Calnan CD. Dithianone sensitivity. *Contact Dermatitis Newslett* 1969; 6:119.

147. Wahlberg JE. Yellow staining of hair and nails and contact sensitivity to dinobuton. *Contact Dermatitis Newslett* 1974; 16:481.

148. Thormann J. Contact dermatitis to a new fungicide, 2-*n*-octyl-4-isothiazolin-3-one. *Contact Dermatitis* 1982; 8:204–221.

149. Bang Pedersen N. Occupational allergy from 1,2-benzisothiazolin-3-one and other preservatives in plastic emulsions. *Contact Dermatitis* 1976; 2:340–342.

150. Dahlquist I. Contact allergy to 3-ethylamino-1,2-benzisothiazole hydrochloride, a veterinary fungicide. *Contact Dermatitis* 1977; 3:277.

151. Ueda A, Aoyama K, Fumi M, et al. Delayed-type allergenicity of triforine (Saprol). *Contact Dermatitis* 1994; 31:140–145.

152. Rycroft RJG, Calnan CD. Dermatitis from slimicides in a paper mill. *Contact Dermatitis* 1980; 6:435–439.

153. Foussereau J, Benezra C, Maibach HI, Hjorth N. Agricultural occupations. In: *Occupational Contact Dermatitis*. Copenhagen: Munksgaard; 1982:90–107.

154. Fischer T. Contact allergy to choline chloride. *Contact Dermatitis* 1984; 10:316–317.

155. Reuveni H, Yagupsky P. Diethyltoluamide-containing insect repellent: adverse effects in worldwide use. *Arch Dermatol* 1982; 118(8):582–583.

156. Lamberg SI, Mulrennan JA Jr: Bullous reaction to diethyl toluamide (DEET) resembling a blistering insect eruption. *Arch Dermatol* 1969; 100:582–586.

157. Maibach HI, Johnson HI. Contact urticaria syndrome. *Arch Dermatol* 1975; 111:726–730.

158. Burrows D. Contact dermatitis in animal feed mill workers. *Br J Dermatol* 1975; 92:167–170.

159. Peachey RDG. Skin hazards in farming. *Br J Dermatol* 1981; 105[Suppl 21]:45–50.

160. Wood WS, Fulton R. Allergic contact dermatitis from ethoxyquin in apple packers. *Contact Dermatitis Newslett* 1972; 11:295–296.

161. Johnson BE, Zaynoun S, Gardiner JM, Frain-Bell W. A study of persistent light reaction in quindoxin and quinine photosensitivity. *Br J Dermatol* 1975; 93[suppl 11]:21–22.

162. Dawson TJA, Scott KW. Contact eczema in agricultural workers. *Br Med J* 1972; 3:469–470.

163. Bedello PG, Goitre M, Cane D, Roncarolo G. Allergic contact dermatitis to Bayo-N-OX-1. *Contact Dermatitis* 1985; 12:284.

164. Francalanci S, Giola M, Georgini S, Muccinelli A, Sertoli A. Occupational photocontact dermatitis from Olaquindox. *Contact Dermatitis* 1986; 15:112–114.

165. Schauder S, Werner S, Geier J. Olaquindox-induced air-

borne photoallergic contact dermatitis followed by transient or persistent light reactions in 15 pig breeders. *Contact Dermatitis* 1996; 35:344–354.

166. Klein HM, Schwanitz HJ. Photocontact allergy to chlorpromazine in farmers. In: CMD-Scientific Secretariat, ed. *Volume of Abstracts 17th World Congress of Dermatology Part II.* Karlsruhe, Germany: G Braun Druckerei und Verlage; 1987:346.

167. Neldner KH. Contact dermatitis from animal feed additives. *Arch Dermatol* 1972; 106:722–723.

168. Verbov J. Tylosin dermatitis. *Contact Dermatitis* 1983; 9:325–326.

169. Veien NK, Hattel T, Justesen O, Norholm A. Occupational contact dermatitis due to spiramycin and/or tylosin among farmers. *Contact Dermatitis* 1980; 6:410–413.

170. Hjorth N, Weismann K. Occupational dermatitis among veterinary surgeons caused by Spiramycin, Tylosin, and Penethamate. *Acta Derm Venereol* 1973; 53:229–232.

171. Tennstedt D, Dumont-Fruytier M, Lachapelle JM. Occupational allergic contact dermatitis to virginiamycin, an antibiotic used as a food additive for pigs and poultry. *Contact Dermatitis* 1978; 4:133–134.

172. Veien NK. Occupational dermatoses in farmers. In: Maibach HI, ed. *Occupational and Industrial Dermatology.* Chicago: Year Book Medical; 1987:436–446.

173. Falk ES, Hektoen H, Thune PO. Skin and respiratory tract symptoms in veterinary surgeons. *Contact Dermatitis* 1985; 12:274–278.

174. Rudski E, Czerwinska-Dihnz I. Sensitivity to dichromate in milk testers. *Contact Dermatitis* 1977; 3:107–108.

175. Huriez C, Martin P, Lefebre M. Sensitivity to dichromate in a milk analysis laboratory. *Contact Dermatitis* 1975; 1:247.

176. Rogers S, Burrows D. Contact dermatitis to chrome in milk testers. *Contact Dermatitis* 1975; 1:387.

177. Grattan CEH, Harman RRM, Tan RSH. Milk recorder dermatitis. *Contact Dermatitis* 1986; 14:217–220.

178. Jung HD, Rothe A, Heise H. Zur Epikutantestung mit Pflanzenschutz. *Dermatosen* 1987; 35:43–51.

179. Fisher AA. Occupational dermatitis from pesticides: patch testing procedures. *Cutis* 1983, 31:483–492.

Bibliography

Atsushi U, Kohji A, Fumi M, Tadako U, Yoshihiro K: Delayed-type allergenicity of triforine (Saprol). *Contact Dermatitis* 1994; 31:140–145.

Benlate: Buried Secrets. http://www.tampatrib.com/reports/benlate/benissu.htm

Bruecker G, Hofs W. Kobalthaliges Futtermittel fur Wiederkauer als berufliches Ekzematogen. *Derm Wochenschr* 1966; 152:528–530.

Bruynzeel DP, de Boer EM, Brouwer EJ. Dermatitis in bulb growers. *Contact Dermatitis* 1993; 29:11–15.

Cohen ML, Moll MB, Maley PW, Linn HI. Statistical description of agricultural injuries in the United States. In: Dosman JA, Cockroft D, eds. *Occupational Health and Safety in Agriculture.* Boca Raton, Fla.: CRC Press; 1989.

Dimiter I, Elsner P. Allergic contact dermatitis from the fungicide Rondo-M and the insecticide Alfacron. *Contact Dermatitis* 1997; 36:51–55.

Flannigan SA, Tucker SB: Influence of the vehicle on irritant contact dermatitis. *Contact Dermatitis* 1985; 3:177.

Garcia-Perez A, Garcia-Bravo B, Beneit SV. Standard patch tests in agricultural workers. *Contact Dermatitis* 1984; 10:151–156.

Hoffman MS. Farms—number and acreage by States. In: Hoffman MS, ed. *The World Almanac Book of Facts 1988.* New York; Pharos Books; 1988:119.

Kleibl K, Rackova M. Cutaneous allergic reactions to dithiocarbamates. *Contact Dermatitis* 1980; 6:348–349.

Lane HU. Hired farmworkers—workers and earnings 1970 to 1983. In: Lane HU, ed. *The World Almanac Book of Facts 1986.* New York: Scripps Howard; 1985:162.

Lisi P, Carafinni S, Assalve D. A test series for pesticide dermatitis. *Contact Dermatitis* 1986; 15:266–269.

Nater JP. A survey of occupational dermatoses in Indonesia. *Berufsdermatosen* 1973; 21:215–222.

O'Malley MO, Mathias CGT, Coye MJ. Skin injury associated with pesticide exposure in California 1974 to 1983. In: Dosman JA, Cockroft D, eds. *Occupational Health and Safety in Agriculture.* Boca Raton, Fla.: CRC Press; 1989:301–304.

Samman PD, Johnston ENM. Nail damage associated with handling of Paraquat and Diquat. *Br Med J* 1969; 1:818–819.

Scott KW, Dawson TAJ. Photo-contact dermatitis arising from the presence of quindoxin in animal feeding stuffs. *Br J Dermatol* 1974; 90:543–546.

Yueliang LG, Wang B, Lee CC, Wang J. Prevalence of dermatoses and skin sensitization associated with the use of pesticides in fruit farmers of southern Taiwan. *Occup Environ Med* 1996; 53:427–431.

Zaynoun S, Johnson BE, Frain-Bell W. The investigation of quindoxin photosensitivity. *Contact Dermatitis* 1976; 2:343–352.

Appendix 32–1. Patch-test Concentrations for Pesticides and Agricultural Chemicals

ANIMAL REPELLENTS

Citronella oil 1%
Diethylphthalate 2%
Eucalyptus oil 1%
Nicotine sulfate 5% aqueous
Oil of lemon grass 1%
Paradichlorobenzene 1% in alcohol
Pine tar 1%
Synthetic oil of mustard 0.1%
Thiram 1%

FUMIGANTS, NEMATOCIDES

Anthraquinone 2%
Carbon tetrachloride 10% in olive oil
Chloropicren (?) 0.25% aqueous
1,4 Dichlorobenzene 1 1%
*†Dichlorpropene 1
Ethylene oxide 0.01% aqueous
Fumarontile (Do not test)
Metam sodium
Methylisothiocyanate 0.03%
Naphthalene 2% in alcohol
†Propylene dichloride 1% in acetone

FUNGICIDES

Anilazine 0.1%
Antisapstain 1%
Benomyl 0.1%
Benzisothiazoline 1%
o-Benzyl p-chlorophenol 1% aqueous
Calcium chloride 2% aqueous
Captafol 0.1%
Captan 0.25%
Chloranil 1%
Chloro-2-phenylphenol 1%
Chlorothalonil (tetrachloroisophthalonitril) 0.01%
  in acetone
Chloromethylphenoxyacetic acid 1%
p-Chloro-o-cresol 0.1% in alcohol
Copper sulfate 1%
Creosote 10% (olive oil)

Cuprobam 1%
Dazomet 0.025% aqueous
Dichlone 1%
Dichlorophen 0.5%
Difolatan 0.1%
4,6-Dinitro-o-cresol 0.5%
Dinobuton 1%
Dinocap 0.5%
†Ditalimfos 0.01%
Dithianone 1%
DNCB 0.1% aqueous
Dowicide B 1%
Dowicide E 1%
Dowicide F 1%
Dowicide 1 1%
Dowicide 3 1%
Dowicide 61 1%
Dowicide 7 1%
Dyrene 0.1%
Fentichlor 1%
Ferbam 1%
Folpet 0.05%
Mancozeb 1%
Maneb 0.5%
Manzeb 0.5%
Mercaptobenzothiazole 1%
Metiram 1%
Nitrofen 0.5%
o-Phenylphenol 1% aqueous
p-Chloro-o-cresol 0.1%
Pentachloronitrobenzene 0.5%
Pentachlorophenol 1% aqueous
Paraformaldehyde (formaldehyde) 2% aqueous
Phaltan 0.01%
Phenylmercuric acetate nitrates 0.01%
Propineb 1%
Tetrachlorodihydroxydiphenyl 1% aqueous
Thiram (thiuram) 1%
Tributyltin hydroxide 0.01% aqueous
Zineb 1%
Ziram 1%

GROWTH INHIBITOR

Chlorphenesin 1%

HERBICIDES

Alachlor 1%
Allidochlor 0.1%

---

*Marginal irritant concentration.
†Manufacture has been discontinued in the United States.

Amitrole 1%
†Aminoguanidine 5%
Atrazine 0.1% aqueous
Barban 0.1% (acetone)
†Chloridazon 0.1%
Chlorpropham 1% aqueous
Cyanamide 1% aqueous
2,4-D 1% aqueous
Dazomet 0.25%
DEET 5% in alcohol
Desmetryn 1%
†Dichlorobenzene 5% in chloroform
Diquat 0.1%
DNCB 0.1% in acetone
Ethylene thiourea 1%
*MCPA/2.4-D 1% aqueous
Molinate 1%
Nitrofen 0.5%
*Paraquat 0.1% aqueous
Pentachlorophenol 1%
Phenmedipham 2% aqueous
*Propachlor 1 1% aqueous
Propanil 1%
Simazine 1%
†Trichlorobenzylchloride 1%

INSECT REPELLENTS

DEET 5% alcohol (open)
1,3-Ethylhexanediol 5% in olive oil

INSECTICIDES

Aldrin 1%
Arsenic 1%
Arsenic trioxide 5% (starch powder)
Arsenate sodium 1% aqueous
Azinphos methyl 1%
Benzyl benzoate 5%
Carbamates (methyl) 1%
Carbaryl 1%
Chlordane 5% acetone
Chorobenzene 5% in olive oil
Chlorothion 1% in alcohol
Dazomet 0.25% aqueous
DD 1% in alcohol
DDD 1% in acetone
DDT 1% in petrolatum
Diazinon 1%
Diazonium 1% in alcohol (open)
*Dichlorophen 1%
Dichlorodiphenyl 5% in acetone
Dichlorvos (DDVP) 0.05% aqueous

Dieldrin 1%
Difluorodiphenyltrichloroethane 5% in acetone
†Dilan 5% in acetone
Dimethoate 1%
Dinobuton 1%
Endosulfan 1%
Fentichlor 1%
Flit 25% in olive oil
Flusides 1%
Kerosene
Lead arsenate 20%
Lindane 1%
Malathion 0.5%
Metacide 1% alcohol (open)
Metaldehyde 1%
Naled 1%
Nicotine 5% aqueous
Ovex 5% acetone
†Paraoxon 1% in alcohol (open)
Parathion ethyl 1%
Parathion methyl 1% in alcohol
†Paris green 2% in acetone
Petroleum 20% in olive oil
Phenothiazine 1% aqueous
Phorate 1%
†Potasan 1%
Propargite 1%
Pyrethrum 2%
Rodannitrobenzene 1%
Rotenone powder 5% in talcum
Sodium sulfide 2% aqueous
Streptomycin 1% (bactericide)
Sulfur 5%
†TDE 1 5% acetone
Tetmosol 1%
Topocide R (as is)
Xylene 50% in olive oil

BACTERICIDES

Bronopol 0.25%

PLANT GROWTH REGULATORS

Choline chloride 1%

RODENTICIDES

ANTU 1%
Thallium 1% aqueous
Warfarin 0.05%

VETERINARY MEDICATIONS AND FEED ADDITIVES

Benzalkonium chloride 0.01% aqueous
Chlorpromazine 1%
Cinnamon oil 0.5%
Cobalt 1%
3,5-Dinitro-*o*-toluamide 1%
Ethoxyquin 0.5%
Furadantin 5%
Furazolidone 3%
Furfuraldehyde 3%

Laurylgallate 2%
Neomycin 2%
Nitrofurazone 3%
Olaquindox 0.5% (photopatch)
Olaquindox 10%
Penethamate 25% in olive oil
Penicillin 1%
Piperazine 5% aqueous
Phenothiazine 2.5%
Quindoxin 0.01%
Spiramycin 10%
Tylosin 1%

Appendix: Job Descriptions with Their Irritants and Allergens

ROBERT M. ADAMS, M.D.

ABATTOIR WORKERS

This group of workers includes occupations concerned with killing animals for food or byproducts, cutting up carcasses, and preserving and flavoring food and related products by salting or smoking.

The *sticker* severs the jugular vein of a previously stunned animal. The animal is then suspended from an overhead rail or shackled on a table. The head is severed, and, after the blood has drained, the skin is removed with a large knife. A *skinner* skins sections of the animal, or the whole animal, and trims meat or fat from the skin, pulling, cutting, and forcing his hands between the hide and carcass to break connective tissue and separate it from neck, sides, shoulders, flanks, back, and tail. He then breaks and severs the legs, removing tails and genital organs and so forth. The hide is removed from the carcass either by hand or with pinchers. The skin may be pulled off with a winch, and bone may be sawed. The *offal separator* separates edible portions of the viscera from the offal by cutting, skinning, and washing parts, cutting off ends of oxtails, and trimming loose tissue using either a knife or a rotary brush. The intestines and bladder, are flushed with a water hose, and the worker then squeezes them to remove slime and foreign matter. Casings of intestines may be bleached by soaking in solutions. The plant's identification number is then stamped on edible organs with a rubber stamp. The worker may brand tails and tongues with an electric iron. The carcasses are then washed *(washer)* and wrapped in muslin cloth *(shrouder)* to protect the meat and enhance its appearance.

In this work there is the constant hazard of lacerations and abrasions. The work is wet, and the animal parts are greasy and often irritating. Protein contact urticaria frequently occurs, not only from raw meat but also from blood and amniotic fluid.[271, 487] In a study of 144 slaughterhouse workers by Hansen and Petersen,[532] a prevalence of protein contact dermatitis of 22% was found, with the highest in workers who eviscerated and cleaned gut. Type I reactions are more common in atopics.[1338] Eczematous dermatitis in slaughterhouse workers accounted for 3.2% of all notified occupational eczematous disease in a Danish study covering the years 1984 to 1991.[517] Contact urticaria caused by raw pork may be more common than previously suspected, according to Kanerva.[674] Cow hair and dander,[695, 1009] as well as natural rubber latex in gloves, are frequent causes of this condition.[680] Occupational rhinitis and asthma[1245] may also occur. Cow dander has been considered the most common cause of occupational contact urticaria in Finland.[695] The classic report of protein contact dermatitis was by Hjorth and Roed-Petersen[602] in 1976.

Patch test to standard and vehicle preservative allergens, with special attention to the following.

Standard Allergens

Nickel sulfate, 2.5% pet; 0.2 mg/cm² (knife handles)
Wool alcohols, 30% pet; 1.00 mg/cm² (sheep carcasses)
Neomycin sulfate, 20% pet; 0.23 mg/cm² (medications for cuts, abrasions)
Caine mix, 3%; 0.63 mg/cm² (medications)
Fragrance mix, 8% pet; 0.43 mg/cm² (deodorizers, medications, barrier creams)
Colophony, 20% pet; 0.85 mg/cm² (adhesive tapes)
Quinoline mix, 6% pet; 0.19 mg/cm² (medications, veterinary products)
Balsam of Peru, 25% pet; 0.80 mg/cm² (protective creams)
p-tert-Butylphenol–formaldehyde resin, 1% pet; 0.04 mg/cm² (leather gloves)
Paraben mix, 16% pet; 1 mg/cm² (barrier creams, cosmetics)
Carba mix, 3% pet; 0.25 mg/cm² (rubber gloves)
Black rubber mix, 0.6% pet; 0.075 mg/cm² (rubber)
Cl + Me-isothiazolinone, 0.01% pet; 0.0040 mg/cm² (Kathon CG) (barrier creams)
Quaternium 15, 1% pet; 0.1 mg/cm² (preservative in cosmetics, creams)
Mercaptobenzothiazole, 2% pet; 0.075 mg/cm² (rubber)
Formaldehyde, 1% aq; 0.18 mg/cm² (released by quaternium 15, disinfectants, preservatives)
Mercapto mix, 1% pet; 0.075 mg/cm² (rubber)
Thiuram mix, 1% pet; 0.025 mg/cm² (rubber gloves)

AGRICULTURAL WORKERS

The pattern of farming in general has changed markedly over the last several decades, from the small family establishment, operating with one or two family members and occasional hired helpers, to large properties with hundreds of full-time employees. However, because of mechanization and shared use of farm machines, persons farming smaller plots of land often can still operate with relatively few full-time employees. In general, the work of farmers ranges from clearing and tilling the soil to planting, fertilizing, cultivating, and harvesting crops. Large quantities of pesticides are used throughout the year, varying with the desired result and the season. Farmers who raise livestock must feed and care for the animals and repair and clean barns, pens, milking sheds, and other farm areas. They also repair machinery, erect and paint fences and sheds, mix and spread agricultural chemicals, medicate sick animals, and, when professional help is unavailable, perform minor surgical procedures, vaccinate cattle and poultry, and assist at the birth of animals. They may also mix livestock feed and additives and pack, store, and transport crops.

Agriculture in the United States employs approximately 1% of the work force. Sharp et al.[1118] have reviewed long-term health problems such as reproductive hazards, carcinogenesis, and neurological disorders of agricultural workers. An epidemiological study of dermatitis among California farm workers showed a prevalence of contact dermatitis of 2%.[455] Agriculture, along with manufacturing, has consistently reported the highest rate of disease, with skin disease accounting for nearly two-thirds of all occupational illness.[868] Besides dermatitis from various irritants and allergens, including pesticides, skin damage due to excessive sunlight exposure and skin cancers are increasingly reported by agricultural workers. Sunlight exposure, especially in sun-sensitive individuals, is an important cause of the increasing incidence of malignant melanoma in agricultural workers.[705] Photoallergic contact dermatitis has been reported from the broad-spectrum fungicide Daconil (tetrachloroisophthalonitrile).[872] Phototoxic dermatitis may occur from numerous plants, such as celery infected by *Sclerotinia sclerotiorum*,[45, 82] and also from contact with healthy, uninfected celery.[79] Vale[1224] has recommended application of a water-resistant sunblock cream containing octyl methoxycinnamate (Parsol MCX), butyl methoxydibenzoylmethane (Parsol 1789), and methyl benzylidene camphor (Eusolex 6300) applied several times daily to prevent phototoxic dermatitis from celery. Even sunscreens, though not common causes of dermatitis, should be considered as potential causes of photoallergic dermatitis, especially sunscreens with *p*-aminobenzoic acid (PABA) and its derivatives and oxybenzone.[285] Photoallergic contact dermatitis may also result from several growth promoters, such as quindoxin, quinoxaline, and olaquindox, used in pig farming.[420, 741]

Phytophotodermatitis is especially likely to occur when grass and brush containing psoralens (such as hogweed, wild parsnip, and cow parsley) are cut, as with a strimmer—a hand-held, powered rotary cutter.[422, 641] Culprits may be *Heracleum spondylium*, *Pastinaca sativa* (both related to wild parsnip), and *Dictamnus albus* (gas plant), among others (Fig. AP–1).

Scleroderma-like changes have been reported, but not

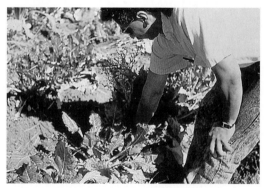

FIGURE AP–1 • Hand and arm contact with plants is repeated and heavy in most agricultural work, often when the plants are damp from irritation or rain.

entirely proved, in workers handling certain pesticides, such as chlodane, malathion, parathion, DDT, hepachlor, sodium dinitro-orthocresolate, 7-chlorocyclohexane,[230, 757] and paraquate.[946] Nail damage has also been reported from the herbicide paraquat.[58, 574, 1079]

Chlorothalonil, a commonly used fungicide, has been reported as a cause of contact urticaria and anaphylaxis in an employee of a redwood plant nursery[261] and also has been suspected as a possible cause of erythema dyschromicum perstans (ashy dermatitis) among Central American banana harvesters.[993]

Methyl parathion, a powerful restricted-use anticholinesterase-type pesticide, is approved only for outdoor agricultural use on cotton, soybeans and other crops, where it rapidly breaks down from exposure to ultraviolet light; indoors, it may persist for many months or even years.[208] It is a potential cause of serious field worker poisoning in the United States.

Sulfur dioxide gas, used as a fumigant, grape preserver, and fungicide, is a strong irritant to mucous membranes and poses an increased health risk for asthmatics, for example.

Until recently, the so-called inert ingredients of pesticide products have been declared trade secrets. As a result of a lawsuit brought by two environmental groups in Oregon, the EPA is now required to release the common names and Chemical Abstracts Service Registry Numbers of the inert ingredients from each pesticide's Confidential Statement of Formula.[533] Although most companies are committed to the safety of inert ingredients, the possibility always exists of contact allergy even to those ingredients generally considered "safe."

Attempts have been made to develop herbicide-resistant crops using genetic engineering. Bioengineered cotton varieties have been treated with bromoxynil, a broad-lead herbicide made by Rhone-Poulenc and sold as Buctril. The cotton seeds are modified by a bacterial gene that detoxifies bromoxynil; its use was approved in 1994 by the U.S. Department of Agriculture. Herbicide-resistant soybeans have also been treated with a nonselective herbicide known as Roundup (glyphosate). Other genetically altered plants will likely be available in the future.

Work-related contact urticaria is common in agricultural workers, especially in farmers and forestry workers. Cow hair and dander,[1009] grains and feed, as well as natural rubber latex in gloves and agricultural appliances are frequent causes of this condition.[680] Occupational rhinitis and asthma[1245] may also occur. Cow dander has been considered the most common cause of occupational contact urticaria in Finland.[695] The very effective insect repellent diethyltoluamide (DEET) against mosquitoes, biting fleas, gnats, and chiggers[116] may also induce contact urticaria and, rarely, serious allergic, neurological, and cardiovascular toxic reactions, especially in children.

Among polychlorinated biphenyls, trichlorophenol, 2,4,5-T (TCP), also known as Dowicide 2 and Dowicide 2S, was widely used as a fungicide, systemic herbicide, and defoliant until 1983, when the EPA cancelled registration of pesticides containing TCP, of which 2,3,7,8-tetrachlorodiabenzo-*p*-dioxin (TCDD, dioxin) has been a contaminant. It should be recalled that EPA jurisdiction is for the United States only and chiefly banned the spraying of 2,4,5-T on forests, pastures, and rights of way. These chemicals are extremely persistent in the environment and have been shown to be carcinogenic in rodents. An association between exposure to these compounds and the development of soft tissue sarcomas and lymphomas in humans has been a subject of debate.[215] Chloracne, a definitive marker for exposure to TCDD, has been reported in humans following exposure to TCP, while TCDD-contaminated materials have long been suspected to be responsible for the development of human cancers as well,[955] but the evidence is less convincing. Suskind and Hertzberg[1175] could find no increase in the risk for cardiovascular diseases, liver disease, kidney damage, or central nervous system problems from an accidental workplace exposure to herbicide contaminants, including dioxin.

Dermatitis from common plants occurs frequently, especially from plants of the Compositae family. Sesquiterpene lactones are a diverse group of chemicals found in this family and are responsible for almost all cases of dermatitis, some of which are phototoxic. Common wild-growing plants of this family are listed at the end of this section. Many of these plants cause irritant dermatitis, sometimes with severe bullous reactions, especially on exposure to sunlight (Fig. AP–1).[962] Patients with photosensitivity dermatitis and actinic reticuloid are especially susceptible to allergic contact dermatitis with such plants as daisy, dandelion, and thistle.[267] In India, the common weed *Parthenium hysterophorus* has been responsible for a large number of cases of contact dermatitis.[799, 823] Another weed, *Xanthium strumarium*, has more recently also been found to cause allergic dermatitis in agricultural workers.[823]

Agricultural workers are exposed to a wide variety of microorganisms and parasites. Cattle farmers commonly develop dermatophytoses from *Trichophyton verrucosum*, the reactions to which can be inflammatory. Milker's nodules, ecthyma contagiosum (orf), erysipeloid, and reactions to the bites of ticks are common (see Chapter 5). Lyme disease, caused by the tick-borne strains of the spirochete *Borrelia burgdorferi*, is manifested by erythema migrans, which begins at the site of a tick bite. Untreated, the condition may persist for weeks or months.[363] The most effective repellent for ticks is said to be permethrin, which can also be sprayed on clothing; it is said to be less likely to cause dermatitis than other and older repellents such as DEET.[116]

Atopic allergy to animals is common not only in farmers but also in veterinarians and in the biomedical laboratory workers who have done much of the research on occupational animal allergy.[1194]

Irritants

Soaps and detergents (barns, milking areas, and machines)
Scouring agents
Germicidal agents (especially those to sterilize milking machines and clean and "sterilize" cows' teats)
Grain dusts[613]
Plants, plant parts (thorns, hairs, weeds, seeds) (Fig. AP–2)
Animal hair, saliva, and secretions[170, 192, 1174, 1231]
Pesticides and insect repellents and their carriers, diluents, and so forth (contact urticaria, especially diethyl fumarate in malathion[1295] and diethyltoluamide in insect repellents)[1024]
Emulsifiers and surfactants in pesticide formulations[2]
Fertilizers
Gasoline and diesel fuel
Solvents
Oils and greases
Paints
Cement
Heat and humidity
Wet work

Patch test to standard and vehicle preservative allergens, with special attention to the following.

Standard Allergens

Potassium dichromate, 0.25% pet; 0.023 mg/cm^2 (cement, leather, preservative in milk testing)[492, 632]
Wool alcohols (lanolin), 30% pet; 1.00/cm^2
2-Mercaptobenzothiazole, 1% pet; 0.075 mg/% (rubber boots, milking machines)

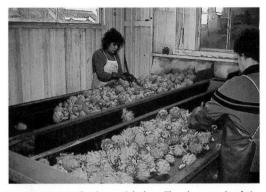

FIGURE AP–2 • Sorting artichokes. The sharp ends of the leaves are a source of irritation.

Neomycin sulfate, 20% pet; 0.23 mg/% (medications, animal feed additives)[159]

Balsam of Peru, 25% pet; 0.80 mg/cm² (medications)

Carba mix, 3% pet; 0.25 mg/cm² (pesticides,[2] rubber)

Nickel sulfate, 2.5% pet; 0.2 mg/cm²; (hand tools, possible contaminant in fertilizers)[980]

Cobalt chloride, 1% pet; 0.02 mg/cm² (feed additive, fertilizers)[935, 1215]

Kathon CG, 0.02% aq; 0.0040 m/cm² (germicidal agent, preservative for milk testing)[492, 586]

Mercapto mix, 1% pet; 0.075 mg/cm² (rubber)

Ethylenediamine dihydrochloride, 1% pet; 0.05 mg/cm² (medications)

Fragrance mix, 8% pet; 0.43 mg/cm² (masking fragrances in pesticides[424])

PPD mix (Black rubber mix), 0.6% pet; 0.075 mg/cm² (rubber boots,[957] milking machine rubber)

Quinoline mix, 6% pet; 0.19 mg/cm² (topical veterinary medications)

Thiuram mix, 1% pet; 0.025 mg/cm² (fungicides, rubber gloves and boots, animal repellents)

Formaldehyde, 2% aq; 0.18 mg/cm² (disinfectants, treatment of animal horns)

Nickel sulfate, 2.5% pet; 0.2 mg/cm² (hand tools)

Rosin (colophony), 20% pet; 0.85 mg/cm² (animal repellents)

Thimerosal, 0.1% pet; 0.0080 mg/cm² (medications)

p-tert-Butylphenol–formaldehyde resin, 1% pet; 0.04 mg/cm² (leather finishes, harnesses, gloves)

Additional Allergens

Ammoniated mercury, 1% pet (mercury in pesticides and medications)

Arnica tincture, 20% pet (Compositae plants, medications)

Barley dust, as is (?)[241]

Benzalkonium chloride, 0.01% aq (cleaning solutions)

Benzocaine, 5% pet (medications)

Bronopol, 0.25% pet (preservative in milk)[492]

p-Aminoazobenzene, 0.25% pet (gasoline additives)

BHA, 2% pet (feed additives)

BHT, 2% pet (feed additives)

Bronopol, 05.% (germicidal agent, milk preservative in test laboratories)

Chlorocresol, 1% pet (topical medications)

Chlorothymol, 1% pet (topical medications)

Chlorpromazine, 1% pet (feed additives for poultry)

Coal tar, 5% pet (wood preservatives)

Daconil (fungicide, tetrachloroisophthalonitrile), 0.002% aq[872]

Dibutyl phthalate, 5% pet (animal repellents)

Dichlorophene, 1% pet (topical medications)

p-Dimethylaminoazobenzene, 1% pet (gasoline dye)[408, 754]

Fluazinam, 0.5% pet (fungicide, 3-chloro-*N*-[3-chloro-5-trifluoromethyl-2-pyridyl]-a,a,a-2,6-dinitro-*p*-toluidine)[130]

Hexylresorcinol, 1% pet (medications)

N-isopropyl-*N'*-phenyl-*p*-phenylenediamine (IPPD), 0.1% pet (rubber milking machines and hoses)[792]

Metam-sodium, 0.1% pet (pesticide)[1100]

Methyl salicylate, 2% pet (disinfectants, medications)

Paraquat, 0.1% pet (pesticide)[1264]

Phenylmercuric nitrate, 0.5% pet (fungicides)

Pine oil, 10% olive oil (disinfectants, cleaning compounds)

Procaine, 1% pet (medications)

Propolis (bee glue), as is[566, 567]

Propylene glycol, 4% aq (medications)

Pyrethrins, 1% pet (insecticides)

Pyrethrum powder, 2% pet (insecticides)

Resorcinol, 2% pet (disinfectants, medications)

Sesquiterpene lactone mix, 0.1% pet (Compositae plants)

Streptomycin, 2% pet (antibiotic for cattle)[460]

Triclosan, 2% pet (medications)

Tylosin, 10% aq (bacteriostatic antibiotic)[1215]

Wood tars, 5% pet (preservatives)

The allergens in poison oak/ivy are not usually used for routine testing.

Infections

Fungal infections (*Trichophyton verrucosum, Microsporum canis, Trichophyton mentagrophytes, Candida imitis*)

Bacterial infections (anthrax [rare], pyodermas [common])

Viral infections (milkers' nodules,[766] cowpox, papular stomatitis[100])

Parasites (grain, straw, barley "itch" due to *Pyemotes vetricosus*)

Harvest mites (*Trombicula autumnalis*), chicken mites (*Dermanyssus galinae*)

Veterinary Medications

Penicillin

Streptomycin[460]

Sulfonamides

Formaldehyde releasers

Imidazole derivatives[301, 555]

Phenothiazines

Plants

Compositae

Ragweed (short)

Feverfew (*Parthenium hysterophorus* L.[1211])

Pyrethrum

Sneezeweed

Chamomile

Goldenrod

Dahlia

Burweed

Sunflower[564]

Chrysanthemum

Chicory

Endive

Lichens on trees, rocks, and soil[554, 905, 1199, 1200]

Mayweed (*Anthemis cotula*)[962]

Miscellaneous

Lettuce
Artichoke
Bulbs
Primula
Algerian and English ivy
Geranium
Carrots
Poison oak/ivy and other urushiol-containing plants are
    extremely common causes of allergic contact
    dermatitis[459]
Common ivy (*Hedera helix* L.)

Pesticides

Most allergic reactions due to pesticides are due to
fungicides. Insectides, herbicides, and fumigants less
commonly cause allergic contact dermatitis.

Parathion and related organophosphate pesticides
should *not* be used in patch testing because of the
rapidity with which they are absorbed by the skin and
their rapid systemic poisonous effects.

Aminotriazole, 1% pet (herbicide)[339]
Barban (Carbyne), 0.1% pet[103, 614]
Benomyl (Benlate),* 1% pet[242, 1241]
Bromophos, 0.1% pet[671]
Captafol, 1% pet
Captan, 0.5% pet[856]
p-Chloronitrobenzene, 1% pet[242]
Chlorothalonil, 0.001% acetone (Daconil)[126, 993]
Choline chloride, 1% aq (growth inhibitor)[373]
Copper sulfate, 1% pet[795]
Daconil (tetrachloroisophthalonitrile, TPN), 0.002%
    aq[872]
Diazinon, 1% pet[795]
1,3-Dichloropropene (D-D 92) 0.05% pet (nematocide,
    soil fumigant)
Difolatan (Captafol), 0.1% pet[118, 873]
Dimethoate, 1% pet[795] (1% alc[515])
4,6-Dinitro-*o*-cresol, 1% pet[795]
Dinocap, 0.5% pet[795]
Dyrene, 0.1% pet[1101]
Fluazinam, 0.5% pet (fungicide, a dinitro-*p*-toludine
    compound)[130]
Ferbam, 0.5% pet[1100]
Folpet, 0.1% pet[795]
Glyphosate (Roundup, Monsanto), 10% aq[826]
Lindane, 1% pet
Malathion (diethyl fumarate—contact urticaria,
    nonimmunological) 0.5% pet[795]
Mancozeb, 0.5%[167, 635, 728, 873]
Maneb, 0.5% pet[10, 728, 873, 932]
Metam-sodium, 0.1% pet[1100]
Omethoate, 1% aq[515]
Paraquat, 0.1% pet[795, 1264]
Propachlor (Ramrod), 0.05% aq[1098]

Propanil, 1% pet[795]
Propargite (Omite), 0.05% pet[242]
Pyrethrum, 2% pet[397, 795]
Sulfur (sublimed), 5% pet[1090, 1307]
Tetrachloroisophthalonitrile (fungicide), 0.001%
    acetone[51, 398, 659]
Thiuram, 2% pet[1123]
Zineb[728, 873]
Ziram, 1% pet[408]

Fumigants

Carbon tetrachloride (with acrylonitrile)
1,3-Dichloropropene (D-D 92), 0.05% pet
    (nematocide, soil fumigant)[931]
Formaldehyde
Sulfur dioxide
Metam-sodium, 0.1% pet[1100]
Methyl bromide[71]
Hydrogen cyanide
Ethylene oxide

Feed Additives

Ethoxyquin, 0.5% alc[108, 159]
Quinoxaline (1,4-benzodiazine)
Cobalt
Olaquindox, 1% pet[741]
Nitrofuran
p-Phenetidine
Penicillin
Nitrofurazone[935]
Streptomycin
Bacitracin
Chlortetracycline
Erythromycin
Griseofulvin
Imidazoles (e.g., miconazole, econazole,
    tioconazole)[313, 555]
Novobiocin
Nystatin
Olaquindox (food additive in pig feed,
    photoallergen)[318]
Oleandomycin
Oxytetracycline
Quindoxine (antibiotic and growth-promoting factor in
    pig feed, no longer marketed)
Spiramycin[1255]
Sulfadimethoxine
Sulfaethoxypyridazine
Sulfamerazine
Tylosin[605, 937, 1255, 1259]
Virginiamycin, 5% pet[1193]
Vitamin K_3 sodium bisulfite (menadione), 0.1%
    pet[194, 297, 1043]
Vitamin B_{12}, 10% pet[1036]
Lincomycin

Animal Repellents

Dogs and Cats

Synthetic oil of mustard
Lemon grass oil

---

*Because of suspected problems with the fungicide Benlate,
including plant damage and possible health problems in humans, the manufacturer, DuPont, has released it for sale only
to agricultural dealers solely as a wettable powder.

Eucalyptus oil
Citronella oil
Pine tar
Nicotine
Diethylphthalate

Rabbits, Deer, and Meadow Mice

Thiuram (up to 20%)

Squirrels

p-Dichlorobenzene
Lemon grass oil
Synthetic oil of mustard

Birds

Anthraquinone

Causes of Phytophotodermatoses

Umbilliferae (*Pastinaca sativa* L.: parsnip; *Heracleum mantegazzianum*, Somm. and Lev.: parsnip tree; *Ammi majus* L.; carrot, celery, dill, fennel, parsley, parsnip)
Rutaceae (citrus genus: limes, lemons, tangerines, gas plant; rue)
Moraceae (*Ficus carica* L.: fig trees)
Leguminosae (*Psoralea corylifolia*: Coronilla glauca)

Causes of Contact Urticaria

See Chapter 6.
Latex rubber
Flour
Pesticides such as lindane and diethyltoluamide
Arthropods
Moths
Caterpillars
Nettles
Animal hair
Cow dander[695]
Saliva
Serum
Placenta
Numerous decorative plants
Storage mites
Fruits
Vegetables such as lettuce, endive, and chicory[738]

Common Wild-Growing Plants of the Compositae Family[1283]

Vernacular Name	Scientific Name
Feverfew	*Tanacetum parthenium* (L.) Schul-Big
	Chrysanthemum parthenium (L.) Bernh.
Wild feverfew	*Parthenium hysterophorus* (L.)
Pyrethrum	*Tanacetum cinerariaefolium* (Trev.) Vis.
	Chrysanthemum cinerariaefolium (Trev.) Vis. *Pyrethrum cinerariaefolium* Trev.
Elecampane	*Inula helnuim* L.
Marsh elder	*Iva angustifolia*
	Iva xanthifolia
Costus root	*Saussurea lappa* (Decne) C.B. Clar
Sneezeweed	*Helenium autumnale* L.
Ordinary milfoil/ yarrow	*Achillea millefolium* L.
Tansy	*Tanacetum vulgare* L.
Mugwort	*Artemisia vulgaris* L.
American ragweed	*Ambrosia* species
Arnica/mountain tobacco	*Arnica montana* L.
German chamomile	*Matricaria chamomilla* L.
Field chamomile	*Anthemis arvensis* L.
Dandelion	*Taraxacu officinale* Weber

AIR HAMMER OPERATORS

The term *air hammer* includes hammers, drills, saws, tempers, paving breakers, and vibrators. These tools utilize compressed air and are powered by gasoline or electricity. Operators must wear safety goggles and hard hats. They often work on scaffolding around concrete structures.

The worker attaches an air hose to the hammer and inserts the proper tool, such as a chisel, bull point, pile driving shoe, steel drill bit, or spade, into the chunk. Then the operator starts the hammer and guides it into the material, lifting and moving it about as the material is broken up. The handles of the air hammers often have rubber grips (Black rubber).

Besides reacting to the irritants and allergens listed below, air hammer operators may develop Raynaud's vibration syndrome (see Chapter 3). Cutaneous reactions to sunlight are common.

Irritants

Dust
Heat
Friction and pressure (calluses)
Flying rocks, gravel, and other eye and skin irritants
Ultraviolet (solar) radiation
Moisture
Compressed air

Patch test to standard and vehicle preservative allergens, with special attention to the following.

Standard Allergens

Potassium dichromate, 0.25% pet; 0.023 mg/cm^2 (leather gloves, shoes, wet cement, concrete)

2-Mercaptobenzothiazole, 1% pet; 0.075 mg/cm² (rubber grips, hoses, safety goggles)
Carba mix, 3% pet; 0.25 mg/cm² (rubber, as above)
Mercapto mix, 1% pet; 0.075 mg/cm² (rubber, as above)
PPD mix (Black rubber mix), 0.6% pet; 0.075 mg/cm² (hard black rubber, grips, handles)
Thiuram mix, 1% pet; 0.025 mg/cm² (rubber, especially gloves)
Nickel sulfate 2.5% pet; 0.2 mg/cm² (tools, handles)

Additional Allergens

Diethylthiourea, 1% pet (safety shoes)[410]
Poison ivy, oak, sumac, other plants
Sunscreen photoallergens (see Chapter 10)

AIRCRAFT WORKERS

This occupational group comprises those concerned with manufacturing and repairing aerospace and aircraft vehicles (which include guided missiles, spacecraft, fixed and rotary wing aircraft, gliders, helicopters, airships, balloons, and surface-effect vehicles) and the manufacturing of parts (such as engines, propulsion units, hydraulic and mechanical equipment, and landing gear).

Because this industry has become extensively automated, and also because of its strong emphasis on preventive medicine, the incidence of occupational skin disease has fallen considerably in the last two to three decades. Nevertheless, some studies have shown the incidence of skin disease in some establishments to still be unacceptably high.[140] Most of the skin problems are irritant contact dermatitis, while allergic contact dermatitis occurs less frequently.[202] Machinists, assemblers, hydraulic workers, painters and electricians are most commonly affected with dermatitis.

Sealants are used to repair leaks and breaks in such areas as the wings. The resin, usually an anaerobic acrylic compound, may be injected onto rivets prior to insertion into the section of the plane. The dermatitis commonly affects the distal parts of the first three fingers of the dominant hand,[1311] with subungual inflammation, hyperkeratosis, and onycholysis.[202, 867] A polysulfide-polymer resin is also frequently used.[1311] Accelerators for certain epoxy sealants may contain hexavalent chromium.[523] Adhesives and sealants, including polysulfide types with chromium, appear to be among the most common contact allergens.[137]

Irritants

Abrasives
Degreasing agents
Paints
Solvents
Coolants and cutting oils[41]
Metal chips
Greases
Soaps and detergents[466]
Heat
Sealants

Patch test to standard and vehicle preservative allergens, with special attention to the following.

Standard Allergens

Potassium dichromate, 0.25% pet; 0.023 mg/cm² (coolants, rarely)[177, 520]
2-Mercaptobenzothiazole, 1% pet; 0.075 mg/cm² (rubber aprons, coolants)[444]
Carba mix, 3% pet; 0.25 mg/cm² (rubber)
Balsam of Peru, 25% pet; 0.80 mg/cm²[973]
Cobalt chloride, 1% pet; 0.02 mg/cm² (metal parts, especially hand grinding, polishing, and etching)[375, 1072]
Epoxy resin, 1% pet; 0.05 mg/cm²
Mercapto mix, 1% pet; 0.075 mg/cm² (rubber)
Ethylenediamine dihydrochloride, 1% pet; 0.05 mg/cm² (coolants)[193, 249]
Quaternium 15, 1% pet; 0.1 mg/cm² (preservative in barrier and hand creams)
PPD mix (Black rubber mix), 0.6% pet; 0.075 mg/cm² (black rubber, gaskets, seals, and so forth)
Thiuram mix, 1% pet; 0.025 mg/cm² (rubber gloves, aprons)
Formaldehyde, 2% aq; 0.18 mg/cm² (formaldehyde-releasing agents in soluble coolants)
Kathon CG, 0.01% pet; 0.0040 mg/cm² (preservative; hand cleaners)[281]
Nickel sulfate, 2.5% pet; 0.2 mg/cm² (small tools; leaching from machined metals)[323, 1078]
Rosin (colophony), 20% pet; 0.85 mg/cm² (cutting fluids)

Additional Allergens

Bioban CS 1246, 1% pet (preservative in coolants)[143, 811]
Bioban P 1487, 1% pet (preservative in coolants)[254, 498, 1328]
Bioban CS 1135, 1% pet (preservative in coolants)[811]
Bronopol, 0.25% pet (preservative; coolants and soaps)[202]
Chloroacetamide, 0.2% pet (coolants) (tested at 2% pet[754])
n-Methylol chloroacetamide, 0.1% pet (Parmetol K 50)[601]
p-Chloro-m-xylenol, 1% pet (coolants, protective creams)
Chlorocresol, 1% pet (germicidal agents)[32]
Dichlorophene, 0.5% pet (germicidal agent)
Diethylthiourea, 1% pet (safety shoes)[410]
Euxyl K 400, 0.5% pet (hand creams, germicidal agent)
Fluorescein sodium, 1% pet[607]
Grotan BK, 1% aq (germicidal agent)[1055, 1248]
Hydrazine sulfate, 1% pet (coolants)
N-isopropyl-N'-phenyl-p-phenylenediamine (IPPD), 0.1% pet (rubber)

Loctite, polyethylene glycol dimethacrylate (PEG), 1% pet[867]
Monoethanolamine (2-amino ethanol), 1% aq[727]
Oleyl alcohol, 6% aq (cutting fluids)[727]
o-Phenylphenol, 1% pet (germicidal agents, coolants)[4]
Pine oil, 10% olive oil (cutting fluids)[384]
Phenylmercuric nitrate, 0.05% pet (cutting fluids)
Polysulfide sealants, 1% pet (Thiokol)[1311]
Propylene glycol, 10% aq
Proxcel (1,2-benzisothiazolin-3-one), 0.05% alc[18, 19]
Tribromosalicylanilide, 1% pet (germicidal agents)
Triethanolamine, 1% pet (cutting fluids)[384]

ANODIZERS

Anodizing, also called *conversion coating*, is the process of applying an oxide coating to aluminum or magnesium, and sometimes other metals, by passing a high-voltage electric current through a bath in which the metal is suspended as an anode. The bath contains sulfuric, chromic, and oxalic acids.

The worker selects a holding rack appropriate to the size, shape, and number of the objects to be anodized, then wires or clips the objects to the anodizing rack, and immerses the rack in a series of baths, either by hand or with automatic equipment, usually in the following sequence:

1. Cleaning solutions (containing degreasers, soaps, detergents, water, heat, and usually caustics)
2. Etching bath (nitric, sulfuric, and hydrofluoric acids)
3. Rinsing bath (water)
4. Treatment bath (sulfuric, chromic, and oxalic acids; sodium dichromate; sodium carbonate)
5. Sealing bath (5% sodium dichromate)
6. Rinsing bath (water)

The objects are then oven or air dried.

The objects may be immersed in a dye bath to color them for decorative or identification purposes. A corrosion-resistant material may be anodized onto the article, usually using automated equipment that automatically cleans, rinses, and coats.

Hydrogen bubbles emitted during this process may contain corrosive mists, and proper ventilation is extremely important.

Because anodized aluminum is extremely porous, the surface can be sealed by a method termed *cold impregnation* using nickel fluoride. The method was introduced about 15 years ago and may be an unsuspected source of contact allergic dermatitis due to nickel.[786]

Protective clothing is very important in anodizing and should include appropriate goggles, aprons, gloves, and boots.

Irritants

Sulfuric acid
Hydrofluoric acid
Nickel fluoride

Nitric acid
Sodium chromate and dichromate
Chromium trioxide
Oxalic acid
Solvents
Caustics
Soaps and detergents
Hot water

Patch test to standard and vehicle preservative allergens, with special attention to the following

Standard Allergens

Potassium dichromate, 0.25%; 0.023 mg/cm^2 (anodizing solutions)
2-Mercaptobenzothiazole, 1% pet; 0.075 mg/cm^2 (rubber articles)
Carba mix, 3% pet; 0.25 mg/cm^2 (rubber)
Mercapto mix, 1% pet; 0.075 mg/cm^2 (rubber, as above)
Black rubber mix, 0.6% pet; 0.075 mg/cm^2 (rubber gaskets, hoses)
Thiuram mix, 1% pet; 0.025 mg/cm^2 (rubber, especially gloves)
Nickel sulfate, 2.5% pet; 0.2 mg/cm^2 (hand tools, dips, "cold-impregnated" aluminum)[786]

ARTISTS

The term *artist* covers a wide range of occupations—commercial artists, designers, illustrators, painters, sculptors, and those who work with wood, ceramics, and metal, to name but a few. The irritants and allergens found in art work are so numerous and varied that only the most important can be listed.

Irritants

Solvents used for cleaning and degreasing
Soaps and detergents
Paint removers
Clay
Wire brushes
Scraping tools
Soldering flux
Sandpaper
Turpentine
Rust removers (hydrofluoric acid)
Metal preservatives
Plaster of paris
Varnishes
Welding fluxes

Patch test to standard and vehicle preservative allergens, with special attention to the following.

Standard Allergens

Potassium dichromate, 0.25% pet; 0.023 mg/cm^2 (welding fumes; fixative in image-transferring processes for fabrics)[804]

2-Mercaptobenzothiazole, 1% pet; 0.075 mg/cm² (rubber, erasers)

Carba mix, 3% pet; 0.25 mg/cm² (rubber, erasers)

Cobalt chloride, 1% pet; 0.02 mg/cm² (colorants, especially blue)

p-Phenylenediamine, 1% pet; 0.090 mg/cm² (dyes)

Epoxy resin, 1% pet; 0.05 mg/cm² (adhesives, plastics, silk screening)

Mercapto mix, 1% pet; 0.075 mg/cm² (rubber erasers)

Black rubber mix, 0.6% pet; 0.075 mg/cm² (rubber)

Thiuram mix, 1% pet; 0.025 mg/cm² (rubber gloves and erasers)

Formaldehyde, 2% pet; 0.18 mg/cm² (preservatives)

Nickel sulfate, 2.5% pet; 0.2 mg/cm² (hand tools, pigments)

Rosin (colophony), 20% pet; 0.85 mg/cm² (soldering flux; in graphic art)[701]

Additional Allergens

p-Aminoazobenzene, 0.25% pet (dyes)

p-Aminophenol, 1% pet (dyes)

Ammoniated mercury, 1% pet (mercury pigments)

Beeswax (propolis), 30% pet (models)

Benzoyl peroxide, 1% pet (catalyst for plastics, especially polyesters)

Camphor, 10% pet (plasticizer in plastics)

N-isopropyl-N'-phenyl-p-phenylenediamine (IPPD) (in Black rubber mix, above), 0.1% pet (rubber)

MEK peroxide, 1% pet (catalyst, especially for polyester resins)

Methyl methacrylate, 2% pet

Turpentine, 10% olive oil

Exotic woods, such as cocobolo, rosewood, and teak (see Chapter 31)

Toluene diisocyanate (TDI), 0.1% pet

ASPHALT WORKERS

Asphalt is a cement-like material, black or dark brown in color, solid or semisolid in texture, containing bitumens from the residue of petroleum refining. It contains paraffinic and aromatic hydrocarbons and heterocyclic compounds. It is used in paving, roofing, and waterproofing materials; paints; oil-based drilling muds; dielectrics; diluents and fungicides; as a softener for rubber; and as a coating for carpentry nails. It has been used for years as a wood preservative. In *road paving*, three types of workers are primarily involved: paving machine operators, asphalt rakers, and asphalt mixers.

A *paving machine operator* drives the machine that spreads and levels the hot-mix bituminous paving material. He or she bolts extensions to the screed to adjust width. Burners are lighted to heat the mixture. The operator then guides the dump truck driver into dumping position at the hopper. The engine is started and controlled to push the dump truck and maintain a constant flow of asphalt into the hopper. As the machine moves along the roadway, the operator watches the distribution of the paving material, controls its direction to eliminate voids at curbs and joints, and adjusts the temperature so that the material flows evenly and does not harden on the screed. A deep gauge is punched through the paving material from time to time to determine its thickness. Operators usually work in pairs, one worker driving and the other riding on the back of the machine controlling the depth of the paving material.

Asphalt rakers rake asphalt paving materials evenly over road surfaces to the thickness desired. They follow the hot-mix paving machine or spreader, distributing the cold-mix paving over the surface and raking the paving material into seams to eliminate any voids at seams and ensure smooth surfaces. They also smooth the surface after it has been compacted by a truck or a pneumatic-tired roller.

Asphalt mixers tend the machines that weigh the ingredients and mix asphalt in the mechanism that automatically weighs sand, stone, and asphalt. The contents are discharged into the truck by levers.

Heaters tend the portable or stationary heating unit, heating asphalt for application on road surfaces. They light the burners and regulate the fuel supply, screw hose connections to the heater unit to connect the circulating system between tank and unit, start the pump to circulate the asphalt through the heating unit, and adjust the blower and damper controls to maintain the required temperature.

Irritants

Asphalt

Ultraviolet (the combination of asphalt and ultraviolet enhances development of actinic keratoses, keratoacanthomas, squamous cell and basal cell carcinomas, and melanosis)

Solvents

Sand

Gravel (= aggregates)

Crushed rock

Wood chips

Glass particles

Sulfur (40% of asphalt is sulfur)

Phosphoric anhydride (added to increase resistance to weathering)

Heat (burns from hot asphalt)

Patch test to standard and vehicle preservative allergens, with special attention to the following.

Standard Allergens

Potassium dichromate, 0.25% in pet; 0.023 mg/cm² (leather gloves)

2-Mercaptobenzothiazole, 1% in pet; 0.075 mg/cm² (rubber)

Carba mix, 3% in pet; 0.25 mg/cm² (rubber)

Cobalt chloride, 1% in pet; 0.02 mg/cm² (driers)

Epoxy resin, 1% in pet; 0.05 mg/cm² (additive to asphalt to increase strength)

Mercapto mix, 1% in pet; 0.075 mg/cm² (rubber)

Black rubber mix, 0.6% in pet; 0.075 mg/cm² (rubber gaskets)

Thiuram mix, 1% in pet; 0.025 mg/cm² (rubber gloves)

Nickel sulfate, 2.5% in pet; 0.2 mg/cm^2 (hand tools)
Rosin (colophony), 20% in pet; 0.85 mg/cm^2 (additive in asphalt)
p-tert-Butylphenol–formaldehyde resin, 1% in pet; 0.04 mg/cm^2 (leather gloves)

Additional Allergens

Coal tar, 5% in pet (asphalt)
N-isopropyl-*N'*-phenyl-*p*-phenylenediamine (IPPD) (rubber), 0.1% in pet (in Black rubber mix, above) (e.g., rubber gaskets)
Diethylthiourea, 1% pet (insoles of safety shoes)[410]

ATHLETES

Physical trauma, friction blisters, "joggers' nipples," calluses, subungual hematomas and subungual hyperkeratoses, "black heel," piezogenic papules, sunburn and other photosensitivity reactions, and cold-induced injury[468] are among the health problems of athletes. Subungual hematomas and other traumatic nail disorders are especially common in joggers, tennis and soccer players, as well as bowlers[1045] and other athletes. Splinter hemorrhages are seen in cricket players and other athletes. Acne mechanica may result from the friction of athletic equipment such as football helmets and shoulder pads. Insect bites, stings, reactions from contact with aquatic creatures such as catfish and jellyfish, and trauma from coral are common.[383] Tinea pedis is most frequently seen in basketball, tennis, and football players and track runners, while yeast infections due to *Candida albicans* are common in running sports and swimming. In wrestlers, herpes simplex[67] and molluscum contagiosum are frequent infections. An epidemic of tinea corporis due to *Trichophyton tonsurans* occurred among 14 wrestlers in Sweden.[627] Infection with the immunodeficiency virus (AIDS) can result from transfer of blood between boxers.

Athletes use a variety of liniments, rub downs, grip enhancers, foot sprays, and adhesives, all of which may cause irritation and/or allergic contact dermatitis. Among hunters, long distance runners, and joggers, plant dermatitis (especially poison ivy/oak/sumac dermatitis) may occur. An occasional contact allergic sensitizer in athletes is compound tincture of benzoin, which may produce a generalized exanthem in addition to contact dermatitis.[1157] The insoles of athletic shoes[1033] and adhesive tapes were common sources of contact allergy in the past, and today topical antibiotics, especially neomycin and bacitracin, are frequent sources of contact allergy. A raccoon-like periorbital leukoderma has been observed from contact with swim goggles containing hypopigmenting chemicals such as derivatives of hydroquinone.[470] Allergic contact dermatitis can result from the thioureas in black sponge rubber in certain swim goggles.[21, 1187] Maibach[824] reported facial dermatitis in a scuba diver from *N*-isopropyl-*N'*-phenyl-*p*-phenylenediamine in a rubber face mask. A severe dermatitis may occur in divers from rubber diving suits containing thiourea accelerators.[5, 713] Additional athletic

articles containing these substituted thiourea rubber accelerators are diving gloves, leg warmers, and eyeglass bands, all of which may be manufactured of neoprene containing ethylbutylthiourea.[1023] Dermatitis from dry ice caused by a ruptured cold pack and abrasions from "astro turf" have also been included among the numerous dermatological problems of athletes.[77]

Irritants

Soaps and detergents
Solvents, especially chloroform (in liniments)
Adhesive tape
Fibrous glass (hockey sticks)[454]
Canvas mats (wrestlers)
Iodine (and povidone iodine)

Patch test to standard and vehicle preservative allergens, with special attention to the following.

Standard Allergens

Caine mix, 8% pet; 0.63 mg/cm^2 (topical anesthetics)
p-tert-Butylphenol–formaldehyde resin, 1% pet; 0.04 mg/cm^2 (leather, plastic finishes on footwear and gloves)
Wool alcohols (lanolin), 30% pet; 1.00 mg/cm^2 (lotions, creams)
2-Mercaptobenzothiazole, 1% pet; 0.075 mg/cm^2 (rubber)
Paraben mix, 12% pet; 1 mg/cm^2 (lotions, creams)
Neomycin sulfate, 20% pet; 0.23 mg/cm^2 (topical medications)
Balsam of Peru, 25% pet; 0.80 mg/cm^2 (lotions, liniments, creams)
Carba mix, 3% pet; 0.25 mg/cm^2 (rubber)
Mercapto mix, 1% pet; 0.075 mg/cm^2 (rubber)
Ethylenediamine dihydrochloride, 1% pet; 0.05 mg/cm^2 (medications)
Kathon CG, 0.01% pet; 0.0040 mg/cm^2 (medications and cosmetics)
PPD mix (Black rubber mix), 0.6% pet; 0.075 mg/cm^2 (Black rubber)
Paraben mix, 15% pet; 1 mg/cm^2 (creams, lotions, cosmetics)
Thiuram mix, 1% pet; 0.025 mg/cm^2 (rubber)
Formaldehyde, 2% aq; 0.18 mg/cm^2 (medications, shampoos)
Quaternium 15, 2% pet; 0.1 mg/cm^2 (creams, cosmetics)
Nickel sulfate, 2.5% pet; 0.2 mg/cm^2 (buttons, metal clips)
Rosin (colophony), 20% pet; 0.85 mg/cm^2 (grip aids)
Thimerosal, 0.1% pet; 0.0080 mg/cm^2 (medications, especially ear and eye drops)

Additional Allergens

Sunscreens
Benzocaine, 5% pet (topical anesthetics)
Benzoin tincture, 10% alc (liniments, adhesives)
Benzophenone 3 (oxybenzone), 1% pet

Benzophenone 4 (sulisobenzone), 1% pet
Benzophenone 8 (dioxybenzone), 1% pet
Octyl-dimethyl PABA (padimate O), 1% pet
Amyl-dimethyl PABA (padimate A), 1% pet
Glycerol PABA 1% pet
p-Amino-benzoic acid (PABA) 5% pet
Parsol 1789 (butyl methoxydibenzoylmethane), 1% pet
Bronopol, 0.25% pet (cosmetics, lotions, creams)
Butylate hydroxyanisole, 2% pet (preservative in lotions and creams)
Butylated hydroxytoluene, 2% pet (preservative in lotions and creams)
Camphor, 10% pet (liniments)
Chlorocresol, 1% pet (medications)
p-Chloro-*m*-xylenol, 1% pet (medications)
Imidazolidinyl urea, 2% pet (cosmetics)
Cinnamic aldehyde, 1% pet (axillary deodorants)
Dichlorophene, 1% pet (medications)
Disperse dyes, 1% pet (clothing, especially tights)
DMDM hydantoin, 1% pet (preservative in creams, lotions)
Ethylbutylthiourea, 1% pet (rubber, especially insoles, swim goggles, wetsuits)[5, 713, 1033]
Glutaraldehyde, 0.5% pet (preservatives)
8-Hydroxyquinoline, 5% pet (topical antiseptics)
Menthol, 1% pet (medications, liniments)
Methyl salicylate, 2% pet (liniments)
Nitrofurazone, 1% pet (medications)
Pine oil, 10% olive oil (liniments)
Propylene glycol, 4% aq (liniments)
Turpentine, 10% olive oil (liniments)

AUTOMOBILE MECHANICS

Mechanics repair engines, power suspension systems, and other mechanical units for cars, buses, tractors, trackless streetcars, graders, bulldozers, cranes, power shovels, portable air compressors, and other gasoline- or diesel-powered engineering equipment. Today an auto mechanic usually specializes in one area and is designated according to the type of work performed: brake and front-end work specialists, carburetor mechanic, wheel alignment mechanic, tune-up person, radiator mechanic, transmission specialist, and so on (see related occupational profiles, such as Body and Fender Workers).

The *generalist* examines vehicles to determine the nature and extent of malfunction or damage and plans the work. With hydraulic hoists and jacks, the vehicle is raised to gain access to mechanical units bolted to the underside. Engine, transmission, or differential are removed using wrenches and hoist. The units are disassembled and inspected using micrometers, calipers, and thickness gauges. Various parts such as pistons, rods, gears, valves, and bearings are repaired or replaced using hand tools. The carburetor may be overhauled and replaced, as may blowers, generators, distributors, starters, and pumps. The mechanic may rebuild parts such as crankshafts or cylinder blocks using lathes, shapers, drill presses, and welding equipment. The ignition system, lights, and instrument panel may be re-wired. A brake repair person may reline and adjust the brakes, align the front end, repair or replace shock absorbers, and solder leaks in the radiator. Damaged areas of the body are mended by hammering out or filling in dents with polyester resin impregnated with fibrous glass (Fig. AP–3); broken parts may also be welded. A mechanic also replaces and adjusts headlights and installs or repairs accessories such as radios, heaters, mirrors, and windshield wipers.

An automobile *radiator mechanic* repairs cooling systems and fuel tanks. Water or compressed air is pumped through the radiator to test it for leaks or obstructions. The radiator is flushed with a cleaning compound to remove rust and mineral deposits. The radiator core is removed and cleaned using rods or boiling water and solvent. These workers solder leaks in core or tanks using either a soldering iron or acetylene torch. They also disassemble, repair, and replace defective water pumps; replace faulty thermostats and leaky head gaskets; and install new cores, hoses, and pumps. They also clean, test, and repair fuel tanks.

When disassembling radiators by melting the solder joints using a hand-held acetylene torch, as well as when cleaning radiator parts with pressurized air in an abrasive bead-blaster filtration cabinet, lead exposure may occur. Because of the likelihood of lead contamination of the atmosphere, cleaning these cabinets with a wire brush should be discouraged.

Dry sweeping the floor also creates a risk of lead exposure; a high-efficiency particulate vacuum should be used instead. Solder may contain as much as 60% lead, and inhalation of fumes may lead to lead poisoning, especially when there is inadequate ventilation and exposure to lead dust. A comprehensive lead standard was enacted by OSHA in 1978, but unfortunately compliance with this standard is still often inadequate.[799]

Auto mechanics are exposed to a large number of irritants and potential sensitizers. These include gasoline, oils, greases, carburetor and brake cleaners, silicone lubricants, rust penetrants, throttle and air intake cleaners, fuel injector flushes, rust penetrants, and numerous others. Many of these are packaged as sprays. Rubber gloves, tires, tubing, black rubber insulation, and shock absorbers are important sources of contact allergy, especially to thiurams, mercaptobenzothiazole, and *N*-phenyl-*N'*-isopropyl-phenylenediamine.[1027] Oil folliculitis and chronic irritant hand eczema and nail dystrophies are common.[947] Diesel oil may also cause oil folliculitis.[263] Koilonychia is also fairly common, thought to be due to contact with motor oils.[266]

Solvents and other irritants are the most common causes of dermatitis in auto mechanics, especially in atopics and those with a personal or family atopic background. Atopics in general do very poorly as auto mechanics. Wearing of gloves is not possible for much of the work, particularly when applying small screws to parts and making fine adjustments.

Episodic flushing of the face, upper chest, and arms may result from the combination of alcohol ingestion and exposure to such workplace solvents as trichoroethylene,[62] carbon disulfide, and dimethylformamide.[231, 807]

Leukoderma may result from contact with certain

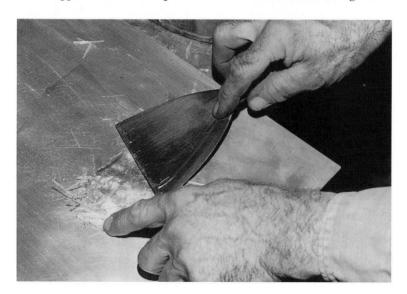

FIGURE AP–3 • Damaged areas of the car body are often repaired by filling in dents with polyester resin impregnated with fibrous glass.

phenolic compounds such as tertiary butylcatechol, which may be found as antioxidants in motor oils.[916]

Irritants

Solvents
Greases
Motor oils (koilonychia[266])
Metal-working fluids
Transmission fluids
Hydraulic oils
Carburetor cleaners
Brake fluids
Fibrous glass
Rust penetrants (e.g., toluene, methylene chloride)
Gasoline and other fuels[529]
Adhesives (especially cyanoacrylates)
Skin cleaners (especially those with abrasives) and strong detergents
Sharp metallic surfaces
Adhesives

Patch test to standard and vehicle preservative allergens, with special attention to the following.

Standard Allergens

Potassium dichromate, 0.25% pet; 0.023 mg/cm² (cooling system and carburetor cleaners, antifreezes, "yellow chromation" in primer paints for protection of zinc-plated components in assembly[596]; welding fumes)
Wool alcohols, 30% pet; 1.00 mg/cm² (creams, soaps)
2-Mercaptobenzothiazole, 1% pet; 0.075 mg/cm² (rubber gloves, gaskets, hoses, antifreeze)
Paraben mix, 12% pet; 1 mg/cm² (creams, especially "protective" creams)
Carba mix, 3% pet; 0.25 mg/cm² (rubber)
Cobalt dichloride 2% pet; 0.02 mg/cm² (lubricating oils, exhaust control devices, cobalt naphthenate; polyester resins)

p-Phenylenediamine, 1% pet; 0.090 mg/cm² (may crossreact with gasoline dyes and diesel fuel ingredients)
Epoxy resin, 1% pet; 0.05 mg/cm² (adhesives, sealants, undercoatings)
Mercapto mix, 1% pet; 0.075 mg/cm² (e.g., rubber gaskets)
PPD mix (Black rubber mix), 0.6% pet; 0.075 mg/cm² (e.g., rubber gaskets, weatherstripping)
Thiuram mix, 1% pet; 0.025 mg/cm² (rubber, especially gloves and aprons)
Formaldehyde, 2% aq; 0.18 mg/cm² (metal cleaners, radiator sealers, tire cleaners)
Nickel sulfate, 2.5% pet; 0.2 mg/cm² (hand tools, parts)
Quaternium 15, 2% pet (soaps and protective creams)
Kathon CG, 0.1% aq; 0.0040 mg/cm² (protective creams; diesel oil)[132]
Rosin (colophony), 20% pet; 0.85 mg/cm² (soldering cores, caulks, greases, waxes, polishes, gaskets)
p-tert-Butylphenol–formaldehyde resin, 1% pet; 0.04 mg/cm² (leather adhesives, neoprene adhesives for weather stripping)

Additional Allergens

Bronopol, 0.25% pet ("barrier" creams)
Chlorocresol, 1% pet (creams and hand lotions)
p-Chloro-m-xylenol, 1% pet (creams and hand lotions)
Imidazolidinyl urea, 2% pet (cosmetics)
Dichlorophene, 1% pet (fungicide in felt gaskets, lubricants)
DMDM hydantoin, 1% pet (preservative in creams, lotions)
Diethylthiourea, 1% pet (weather stripping)[1300]
Ethylbutyl thiourea, 1% pet (rubber, gaskets)
Glutaraldehyde, 0.5% pet (hand creams and lotions)
Methyl, ethyl, and butyl methacrylates, each 2% pet (rubber gaskets)[242]
p-Aminoazobenzene, 0.25% pet (gasoline and diesel fuel additives)

p-Aminophenol, 1% pet (gasoline and diesel fuel additives)

Benzoyl peroxide, 1% pet (polyester resin catalyst)

o-Benzyl-p-chlorophenol, 1% pet (auto cleaner, general cleaning compounds)

BHT, 2% pet (gasoline antioxidant, automatic transmission fluid, hydraulic fluids)

p-tert-Butylphenol, 2% pet (antioxidants in oils and greases, gasoline)

N,N'-di-sec-butyl-p-phenylenediamine, 1% pet (antioxidant for gasoline)

Diethylthiourea, 1% pet (rubber gaskets)

Dipentene, 2% pet (inactive form of limonene; auto waxes)[855]

Diphenylamine, 1% pet[583]

Hydrazine sulfate, 1% pet (soldering)

Hydroquinone, 1% pet (greases, oils, automatic transmission fluids)

N-isopropyl-N'-phenyl-p-phenylenediamine (IPPD), 0.1% pet (rubber door and window seals, tires, gaskets)[26, 172, 1027, 1306]

MEK peroxide, 1% pet (polyester resin catalyst)

Phenol-formaldehyde resin, 10% pet (brake linings, clutch facings)

Phenothiazine, 2.5% pet (antioxidant in oils and greases)

o-Phenylphenol, 1% pet (germicidal agent in oils and greases)

Pine oil, 10% olive oil (cleaning agents)

Polyester resin monomer, 10% pet (body repairs)[305]

Unsaturated polyester resin, 0.5% to 10% pet[1185]

Polyethyleneglycol (PEG) dimethyacrylate, 10% in pet (in certain anaerobic acrylic sealants of the Loctite type)[292, 734, 867]

Propylene glycol, 4% aq (antifreezes, deicers)

Resorcinol monobenzoate, 1% pet (steering wheel plastics)[665]

Tricresyl phosphate, 2% pet (oils, greases)

Triethylenetetramine, 0.5% pet (epoxy catalyst)

Zinc diethylbis(dithiocarbamate) (ZDC), 1% pet (greases)

BAKERS

The job description of a baker includes baker's helpers, batter mixers, cookie and cracker machine operators, dough feeders, doughnut machine operators, dough weighers, dusters, icers, oven operators, pan greasers, rack pullers, pie dough rollers, and others.

In general, using scales and graduated containers, bakers mix flour, sugar, shortening, and other ingredients to prepare batters, doughs, fillings, and icings. The ingredients are dumped into a mixing machine bowl or steam kettle to mix or cook according to specifications. Spices may be rolled into the dough by hand. The dough is rolled, cut, and shaped to form sweet rolls, piecrusts, tarts, cookies, and related products. The material is then placed in pans or bowls or on sheets and baked in ovens or on grills. After removal from the oven, a glaze, icing, or other topping may be applied to baked goods with a spatula or brush. In large bakeries,

workers may specialize in one type of product, such as bread, rolls, pies, or cakes.

Flour may cause contact urticaria,[584, 1254, 1336] and rye flour has been reported to cause asthma. Although contact allergy from flour rarely occurs,[1336] Calnan[174] reported dermatitis from malt flour. Veien and coworkers[1254] reported four bakers with dermatitis due to wheat and rye flour. Small amounts of chromium were found in flour in Germany, which Heine and Fox[576] reported as inducing eczema in bakers. FDA-approved food dyes rarely cause sensitization. The antioxidant sodium metabisulfite may cause allergic reactions, both immediate and delayed, including anaphylactic reactions,[393] and patch testing for delayed reactions should be done with concentrations of 1% or less to avoid irritant reactions.[38]

Contact and systemic contact-type dermatitis have been reported from nutmeg and mace, cardamom, turmeric, coriander, curry, cinnamon, and Laurus nobilis.[307, 836] Patch testing with these spices "as is" may result in confusing irritant reactions. Dilution in white petrolatum to 5% to 10% or less is preferable. A carefully drafted case history is also important in diagnosis.[307]

Additives are added to flour to speed up baking, reduce costs, and hopefully improve the product. These include α-amylase, proteases, and lipoxygenases. The amylases accelerate the rising of dough, improve browning, and appear to lengthen bread life. α-Amylase may cause urticaria, rhinitis, and asthma, as well as contact dermatitis.[917] The authors suggest routinely testing for α-amylase sensitivity those bakers in whom immediate or delayed allergy is suspected.

Most cases of dermatitis in bakers, however, are due to irritation. The wet, sticky dough is the most common cause, followed by the soaps and detergents used for cleaning. Atopics fare poorly in this occupation not only because of recurring skin complaints but also respiratory atopy, which is an important risk factor for the development of dermatitis in atopics.[1181] Monilial paronychia and interdigital monilial infections are very common. Rarely the food mites of flour and sugar induce a scabies-like dermatitis in persons mixing flour and other ingredients.

Bakers and confectioners increasingly add sugar artistry to their work. The sugar is warmed to about 50°C to liquify it and make it maleable. It is then worked into a variety of decorative objects. The mixture consists of granulated sugar, water, glucose, tartaric acid, and various food colorings. Because of firm manual contact with the hot material, there is increased sweating and erythema, often with blistering. Gloves should be worn to prevent burns.[56]

The persulfate flour improvers are banned in many countries; at one time they were the cause of contact allergy among bakers and their helpers. Combined with benzoyl peroxide, sodium or potassium persulfates were used to inhibit proteolytic enzymes and make the bread lighter.[1294]

Irritants

Acids (acetic, ascorbic, lactic)
Flour (especially wet dough)

Sugar
Spices[307, 836]
Soaps and detergents (especially those to remove dried flour on surfaces)
Oven cleaners
Persulfate bleaches[1294]
Fruit juices, especially citrus[243]
Essential oils (flavors)
Enzymes
Wet yeast

Patch test to standard and vehicle preservative allergens, with special attention to the following.

Standard Allergens

Wool alcohols, 30% pet; 1.00 mg/cm^2 (hand creams)
2-Mercaptobenzothiazole, 1% pet; 0.075 mg/cm^2 (rubber)
Paraben mix, 12% pet; 1 mg/cm^2 (candies, jellies, syrups)
Fragrance mix, 8% pet; 0.43 mg/cm^2
Balsam of Peru, 25% pet; 0.80 mg/cm^2 (flavors and spices)
Carba mix, 3% pet; 0.25 mg/cm^2 (rubber gloves)
Mercapto mix, 1% pet; 0.075 mg/cm^2 (rubber)
PPD mix (Black rubber mix), 0.6% pet; 0.075 mg/cm^2 (rubber gaskets)
Thiuram mix, 1% pet; 0.025 mg/cm^2 (rubber gloves)
Formaldehyde, 2% aq; 0.18 mg/cm^2 (cleaners, disinfectants)
Nickel sulfate, 2.5%; 0.2 mg/cm^2 (hand tools)
Potassium dichromate, 0.5% pet; 0.023 mg/cm^2 (flour,[576] Javel solution)

Additional Allergens

Ammonium persulfate, 2.5% pet (flour "improvers," bleaches)
α-Amylase, prick test 1:250 to 1:2,500 (contact urticaria)[917]
Beeswax, 30% pet (artificial flowers)
Benzoyl peroxide, 1% pet (flour-bleaching agents)[388]
BHA, 2% pet (antioxidants for lards and greases)[1039]
BHT, 2% pet (antioxidants for lards and greases)[1039]
Certified food dyes, 1% pet
Eugenol, 2% pet (crossreacts with flavors)
Karaya gum, as is[388]
Lauryl gallate, 0.2% alc (antioxidant in margarines, preservative)
Propyl and lauryl gallate, 0.5% pet (preservatives)
Sorbic acid, 2% pet (preservative)[388]
Sodium metabisulfite, 1% aq[38, 393, 917]
DL-α-tocopherol, 10% pet (antioxidant for fats)

Flavoring Agents[378, 836]

Vanilla extract, 10% acetone
Cinnamic aldehyde, 1% pet[1110]
Cinnamon oil, 0.5% pet (flavorings)[388, 597]
Cardamom seed (ground), 10%
Citronella oil, 1% pet

Coconut oil, as is
Eugenol, 2% pet
Anise oil, 25% pet
Ginger oil, 25% pet
Limonene oil, 1% alc
Methyl salicylate, 2% pet
Mustard oil, 05% pet
Nutmeg oil, 1% alc
Laurel oil, 2% pet
Clove oil, 1% pet
Peppermint oil, 1% pet
Cardamom oil, 2% pet[242]
Lemon oil, 1% pet
Lemon juice, as is

The above concentrations are not likely to be irritating, but caution should be used in interpretation of the results. In some instances, a lesser concentration should be employed.

BARBERS

Barbers cut, trim, and taper hair using scissors, combs, and clippers. They apply lather and shave beards or shape hair. They may apply hair dressings, lotions, dyes, tints, sprays and shampoos; style hair; and massage the face, neck, and scalp, often using a rubber vibrator that may induce dermatitis in barbers who are rubber sensitive. They may give permanent waves and color, straighten, or otherwise alter the hair style.

Allergic contact dermatitis is not as common in barbers as in cosmetologists who work with women. Granulomas may occur from hair cuttings that become embedded in the skin, especially the chest and abdomen.[226, 669] Fragments of hair may also be implanted under fingernails.[612] From standing for long periods, barbers with venous insufficiency in the legs are especially prone to development of stasis dermatitis and complications of varicose veins. Callosities and onychodystrophies are common.[526]

Glyceryl monothioglycolate in so-called acid permanent wave solutions causes disabling allergic contact dermatitis in barbers and hairdressers.[1170] It is important to remember that the allergen remains on hair for as long as 3 months after application (and perhaps longer), providing repeated opportunities for recurrent dermatitis in hairdressers allergic to the chemical.[918] Furthermore, the allergen readily passes through rubber gloves. A job change is frequently the only solution for barbers and hairdressers allergic to this potent sensitizer.

Irritants

Soaps and shampoos
Hair tonics
Hair tints and bleaches
Heat from blowers
Hair straighteners (ammonium thiosulfate, ammonium thioglycolate)
Wave solutions
Germicidal agents

Ammonium persulfate (urticarial reactions)
Depilatories

Patch test to standard and vehicle preservative allergens, with special attention to the following.

Standard Allergens

Wool alcohols, 30% pet; 1.00 mg/cm² (creams)
2-Mercaptobenzothiazole, 1% pet; 0.075 mg/cm² (rubber)
Balsam of Peru, 25% pet; 0.80 mg/cm² (cosmetics)
Carba mix, 3% pet; 0.63 mg/cm² (rubber)
Cobalt chloride, 1% pet; 0.02 mg/cm² (metallic hair dyes)
Mercapto mix, 1% pet; 0.075 mg/cm² (rubber)
PPD mix (Black rubber mix), 0.6% pet; 0.075 mg/cm² (rubber)
Thiuram mix, 1% pet; 0.025 mg/cm² (rubber) (Fig. AP–4)
Formaldehyde, 2% aq; 0.18 mg/cm² (germicidal agents, shampoos)[1096]
Fragrance mix, 8% pet; 0.43 mg/cm² (aftershaves, lotions)
Paraben mix, 12% pet; 1 mg/cm² (creams, lotions)
p-Phenylenediamine, 1% pet; 0.090 mg/cm² (permanent hair dyes)
Quaternium 15, 2% pet (cosmetics)
Nickel sulfate, 2.5% pet; 0.2 mg/cm² (scissors, hair clips, coins, metallic hair dyes)[1099]
Rosin (colophony), 20% pet; 0.85 mg/cm² (mustache wax)
Thimerosal, 0.1% pet; 0.0080 mg/cm² (preservatives)
p-tert-Butylphenol–formaldehyde resin, 1% pet; 0.04 mg/cm² (leather strap for sharpening straight razors)

Additional Allergens

p-Chloro-*m*-xylenol, 1% pet (preservatives in hair "tonics" and creams)
p-Aminodiphenylamine, 0.25% pet (hair dyes)
p-Aminophenol, 1% pet (hair dyes)

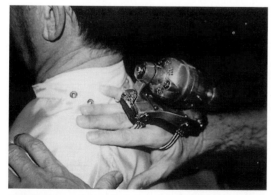

FIGURE AP–4 • Massaging the back following a haircut is common practice for barbers. The rubber on the massager may induce contact allergy. Tetramethylthiuram disulfide is often the allergen.

o-Aminophenol, 1% pet (hair dyes)
Beeswax, 30% pet (cosmetics, mustache wax)
Camphor, 10% pet (tonics)
Captan, 0.25% pet (shampoos)
Cetyl alcohol, 30% pet (tonics, creams)
Chlorocresol, 1% pet (tonics, creams)
Chlorothymol, 1% pet (tonics)
Dichlorophene, 1% pet (germicidal agents)
Eugenol, 2% pet (tonics)
Euxyl K 400, 0.5% pet[144, 551]
Glutaraldehyde, 0.25% aq (sterilizing solutions)
Glyceryl monothioglycolate, 1% pet ("acid" permanent wave preparations)[1170]
Hydroquinone, 1% pet (skin bleaches, hair dye developers)
Imidazolidinyl urea, 2% pet
Menthol, 1% pet (tonics)
Methyl heptidine carbonate, 0.5% pet (aftershaves)[1243]
Methyl salicylate, 2% pet (tonics)
Musk ambrette, 2% pet (aftershaves; photosensitizer)[763]
o-Nitro-*p*-phenylenediamine, 1% pet (semipermanent hair dyes)
PABA, 5% pet (sunscreens in creams)
m-Phenylenediamine, 2% pet (permanent hair dyes)
o-Phenylenediamine, 2% pet (permanent hair dyes)
o-Phenylphenol, 1% pet (germicidal agents for cleaning floors and walls)
Propylene glycol, 4% aq (creams, lotions)
Pyrogallol, 1% pet (hair dyes)
Resorcinol, 2% pet (hair dyes, tonics)
Sorbic acid, 2% pet (creams, lotions)
Stearyl alcohol, 30% pet (creams, lotions)
p-Toluenediamine, 1% pet (hair dyes)
p-Toluene-sulfonamide-formaldehyde resin, 10% pet (nail polish)
Triclosan, 2% pet (preservatives in soaps)

BARTENDERS

Bartenders mix and serve alcoholic and nonalcoholic drinks to patrons, following various recipes. They mix ingredients such as liquor, soda, water, sugar, and bitters in preparing cocktails and other drinks and serve wine and draft or bottled beer. They collect payment, make change, order supplies, and arrange bottled goods and glasses to make attractive displays. They also slice and pit fruit for garnishing drinks and prepare appetizers such as pickles, cheese, and cold meats. They also wash and rinse glasses and utensils in detergents, which may contain germicidal agents.

Irritant dermatitis is common among bartenders, especially atopics. Monilial paronychia, however, is also frequent because of the almost constant moisture. Allergic sensitization is uncommon.

Irritants

Water (wet work)
Soaps and detergents
Fruit juices
Alcohol

Bitters
Germicidal agents

Patch test to standard and vehicle preservative allergens, with special attention to the following.

Standard Allergens

Nickel sulfate, 2.5% pet; 0.2 mg/cm² (nickel measuring cups)[677]
Balsam of Peru, 25%; 0.80 mg/cm² (crossreacts with flavorings)[597]
Formaldehyde, 2% aq; 0.18 mg/cm² (disinfectants)
Fragrance mix, 8% pet; 0.43 mg/cm² (flavors, disinfectants)
Thiuram mix, 1% pet; 0.025 mg/cm² (rubber gloves)

Additional Allergens

Chlorhexidine digluconate, 0.5% (germicidal agents)
Cinnamon oil, 0.5% pet (flavorings, citrus rinds, vermouth, bitters)[597]
Sodium N-chloro-p-toluenesulfonamide, 1% pet (germicidal agents)
o-Benzyl-p-chlorophenol, 1% pet (germicidal agent for glasses)[1151]

BATH ATTENDANTS

This group of workers includes people who work at public baths, beauty establishments, reducing salons, health clubs, and so forth. They apply alcohol, lubricants, rubbing compounds, and cosmetics to patrons. They give massages using techniques such as kneading, pounding, and stroking the flesh with their hands, rubber, or vibrating equipment. They may also administer steam, dry heat, ultraviolet, infrared, or water treatments. They also sell and demonstrate cosmetics.

Irritants

Soaps and detergents
Water (especially steam) (wet work)
Alcohol
Dry heat
Ultraviolet light
Infrared
Stiff brushes
Leaves and twigs (birch and bay leaves)
Cleaning solutions

Patch test to standard and vehicle preservative allergens, with special attention to the following.

Standard Allergens

Wool (lanolin) alcohols, 30% pet; 1.00 mg/cm² (creams, lotions)
2-Mercaptobenzothiazole, 1% pet; 0.075 mg/cm² (rubber)

Paraben mix, 12% pet; 1 mg/cm² (creams, lotions)
Balsam of Peru, 25% pet; 0.80 mg/cm² (perfumes, rubbing compounds)
Carba mix, 3% pet; 0.25 mg/cm² (rubber)
Caine mix, 8% pet; 0.63 mg/cm² (local anesthetics)
Mercapto mix, 1% pet; 0.075 mg/cm² (rubber)
PPD mix (Black rubber mix), 0.6% pet (rubber, vibrators)
Thiuram mix, 1% pet; 0.025 mg/cm² (rubber gloves)
Formaldehyde, 2% aq; 0.18 mg/cm² (lotions, shampoos, disinfectants)
Quaternium 15, 2% pet; 0.1 mg/cm² (creams, lotions)
Kathon CG, 0.01% aq; 0.0040 mg/cm² (body creams, lotions)
Nickel sulfate, 2.5% pet; 0.2 mg/cm² (hand tools)

Additional Allergens

Arnica Tr., 20% pet
Beeswax, 30% pet (waxes, creams)
Benzocaine, 5% pet (topical anesthetics)
BHA, 2% pet (creams, lotions)
Bronopol, 0.25% pet (creams, lotions)
Cinnamic aldehyde, 1% pet (lotions, liniments, fragrances)
Camphor, 10% pet (creams, lotions)
Chlorocresol, 1% pet (creams, lotions)
Diazolidinyl urea, 1% pet
Dichlorophene, 1% pet (cleaning compounds)
Eugenol, 2% pet (fragrances)
Euxyl K400, 0.5% pet
Glutaraldehyde, 0.25% aq (sterilizing solutions)
Imidazolidinyl urea, 2% pet (creams, lotions)
Isoeugenol, 1% pet (cosmetics, rubbing compounds)
N-isopropyl-N'-phenyl-p-phenylenediamine (IPPD), 0.1% pet (rubber)
Lauryl oil, 0.2% pet[907]
Menthol, 1% pet (tonics, fresheners)
Methyl salicylate, 2% pet (fresheners, body rubs)
o-Phenylphenol, 1% pet (cleaning solutions for tables, floors, and walls; occasionally also in cosmetics)
Propylene glycol, 4% aq (lotions, creams)
DL-α-tocopherol acetate, 4% pet (vitamin E preparations)
Triclosan, 2% pet (preservatives in cosmetics and soaps)

BATTERY MAKERS

Because molten lead is used in the manufacture of lead storage batteries, the chief hazard of this work is lead poisoning (plumbism) from inhalation and ingestion of dust and fumes. In addition, exposure to mercuric oxide, which is used in the manufacture of the dry-cell battery, can cause mercury poisoning. Sulfuric acid is the chief electrolyte in the lead storage battery; splashes onto the eyes or skin can result in serious injury. The worker who fills the storage battery cells with sulfuric acid solutions preparatory to forming and charging the batteries is at the greatest risk of burns and irritant dermatitis. The battery casings are often constructed of fibrous glass.

Because spot welding with oxyacetylene torches is used at various steps in the manufacture, exposure to lead can be considerable during this activity. Medical evaluation of these workers should include blood tests for lead, as well as testing for free erythrocyte protoporphyrins and red blood cell protoporphyrins. Disposal of used batteries may also lead to considerable exposure to lead if precautions are not taken.

Cadmium is an integral component of nickel-cadmium storage batteries. Workers are at risk for kidney dysfunction, which increases with the number of years of work in this industry. Periodic examination for blood levels of cadmium has been recommended.[648] Epidemiological and toxicological data also suggest an association between cadmium exposure and cancer, especially prostatic cancer.[955]

Antimony is also widely used in storage batteries. Exposure to the fumes of melting antimony and antimony-containing dust may lead to follicular papules and pustules, especially if the skin is moist from perspiration. Epistaxis is also common, as well as obstructive lung disease, hematological disorders, and lung cancer after prolonged exposure.[1292]

Irritants

Sulfuric acid (electrolyte in lead storage batteries)
Zinc chloride (electrolyte solutions)
Potassium hydroxide (electrolyte solutions)
Sodium hydroxide (electrolyte solutions)
Phosphoric acid
Asphalt (sealants)
Oils and greases
Soaps and detergents
Solvents
Fibrous glass
Soldering flux

Patch test to standard and vehicle preservative allergens, with special attention to the following.

Standard Allergens

p-tert-Butylphenol–formaldehyde resin, 1% pet; 0.04 mg/cm² (leather and some plastic gloves)
2-Mercaptobenzothiazole, 1% pet; 0.075 mg/cm² (rubber)
Ammoniated mercury, 1% pet (mercury in dry cells)
Carba mix, 3% pet (rubber)
Cobalt chloride, 1% pet; 0.02 mg/cm²
Epoxy resin, 1% pet (adhesives, sealants)
Mercapto mix, 1% pet (rubber)
PPD mix (Black rubber mix), 0.6% pet (rubber)
Thiuram mix, 1% pet (rubber)
Nickel sulfate, 2.5% pet (battery parts, small hand tools; nickel-cadmium storage batteries)
Rosin (colophony), 20% pet (solder cores)

Additional Allergens

Cadmium chloride, 1% aq (nickel-cadmium storage batteries)

Hydrazine sulfate, 1% pet (solder flux)
Mercury (elemental), 0.5% pet

BEEKEEPERS

Also known as *apiculturists*, beekeepers cultivate bees for the production of honey and pollination of crops. They manually insert honeycombs into beehives, or they lead wild, swarming bees into hives of prepared honeycomb frames. The hives are then placed in orchards, clover fields, or near some other source of pollen and nectar. To force bees out of hives, a smoke pot may be used pads may be placed over hives. This makes it possible to inspect the hives and harvest the honeycombs. Parasites such as moth larvae must be removed, as well as vermin, birds, and mice. Royal jelly from queen bee cells is used for sale as a base for cosmetics and as a health food. Cyanide gas may be used to destroy diseased colonies. The hives are cleaned using various caustic solutions.

Propolis, a potent allergic sensitizer, is the resinous substance found in beehives. It contains approximately 10% cinnamic alcohol among dozens of other constituents. It is a common cause of allergic contact dermatitis in beekeepers. Because bees take the resinous material from the buds of various plants, the composition of propolis varies with the type of vegetation in the area. Studies have not confirmed, as previously believed, that cinnamic alcohol or cinnamic acid is the principal allergen of propolis.[892] Hausen and colleagues have shown that 1,1-dimethylallyl caffeic acid ester from poplar tree buds is the main contact allergen.[567]

Although propolis is a reported allergen in parts of Europe, there have been few reports of dermatitis from propolis in the United States. Most of the cases have occurred in persons using cosmetics containing propolis or when using it for self-treatment of various diseases, which is popular among users of folk remedies. Approximately 25% of the cases have occurred in beekeepers, however.[566]

Irritants

Honey and honeycombs
Caustics (to clean hives)
Pollen

Patch test to standard and vehicle preservative allergens, with special attention to the following.

Standard Allergens

Mercaptobenzothiazole, 1% pet; 0.075 mg/cm² (rubber protective clothing)
Rosin (colophony), 20% pet; 0.85 mg/cm²
Carba mix, 3% pet; 0.25 mg/cm² (rubber)
Thiuram mix, 1%; 0.025 mg/cm² (rubber gloves)
Formaldehyde, 1% aq; 0.18 mg/cm² (disinfectants)
p-tert-Butylphenol–formaldehyde resin, 1% pet; 0.04 mg/cm² (leather gloves)
Mercapto mix, 1% pet; 0.075 mg/cm² (rubber)

Black rubber mix (PPD mix, 0.6% pet; 0.075 mg/cm^2) (black rubber)
Balsam of Peru, 25% pet; 0.80 mg/cm^2 (pollen)
Nickel sulfate, 2.5% pet; 0.2 mg/cm^2 (tools)

Additional Allergens

Cinnamic alcohol, 5% pet (pollen)
Propolis, 20% pet

BLUEPRINT MAKERS

The techniques for copying engineering drawings include blueprinting and whiteprinting. In the older blueprint, or Prussian blue, method, introduced at the end of the nineteenth century, the drawing to be copied was made on translucent cloth or paper and laid on paper sensitized with a coating of ferric ammonium citrate and potassium ferricyanide. Today the making of blueprints is performed by either a diazo or a white printing machine. The operator selects sensitized paper according to the color of the line specified and then positions the original over paper. The light intensity is then regulated, as well as the exposure time (Fig. AP–5). Ammonia may be supplied to the machine automatically or by the operator pouring it by hand into the printer. After exposure and developing, the finished print is examined for color, intensity, and sharpness of the lines.

In the whiteprinting method, which was introduced in the 1920s, paper is sensitized with a diazonium salt, a coupler, and an acid to prevent coupling before use. Exposure to ultraviolet light destroys the diazonium salt. Treatment with ammonia gas neutralizes the acid, causing the coupling reaction to occur, making the lines of the drawing appear in color (usually blue) against a white background. The diazonium salt is either *p*-diethylaminobenzene diazonium chloride or a derivative such as *p*-diazodimethylaniline zinc chloride double salt, which is a rapid diazotype coupler. Whiteprinting,

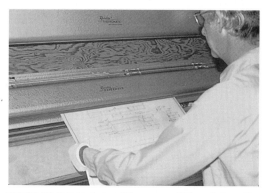

FIGURE AP–5 • In the ozalid process of blueprinting, the operator selects sensitized paper according to the color of the line specified and then positions the original over paper. The light intensity is then regulated, as well as the exposure time.

also known as the Ozalid or Radex method, is the common method used today.[226, 232, 536, 1260, 1261]

Most blueprint workers initially believe that ammonia is the cause of their dermatitis. While this may occasionally be true because of its irritant properties, allergic sensitization may also occur from contact with the diazonium dye on the paper. The paper must be kept in light-proof containers and patch testing done in a darkened room, the test patches covered with black, light-impermeable tape. Once the diazonium salt has been reduced by exposure to light, it loses allergenic properties.

Irritants

Ammonia
Ultraviolet light
Paper (especially "no carbon" paper)

Patch test to standard and vehicle preservative allergens, with special attention to the following.

Standard Allergens

Potassium dichromate, 0.25% pet; 0.023 mg/cm^2 (reducer in the ferric ammonium citrate process; rarely used today)
p-Phenylenediamine, 1% pet; 0.090 mg/cm^2 (may crossreact with azo dyes)
Thiuram mix, 1% pet; 0.025 mg/cm^2 (rubber gloves)

Additional Allergens

p-Aminoazobenzene, 0.25% (may crossreact with diazonium dyes)
p-Diethylaminobenzene diazonium chloride, 1% pet (a diazonium dye used on paper)
Diazodiethylaniline, 2% pet[226]
4-Diazo-2-methyl-pyrrolidinobenzene ZnCl$_2$, 1% aq[232]
Disperse orange 3, 1% pet (may crossreact with the paper dyes)
Disperse yellow 3, 1% pet (may crossreact with paper dyes)
Resorincol, 2% pet (developer)

BODY AND FENDER WORKERS

Body and fender workers repair damaged body parts of automobiles and light trucks. They examine the vehicle and estimate the damage and cost and then remove the upholstery, accessories, windows, and trim to gain access to the body and fenders. They chain or clamp the frame sections to alignment machines, which use hydraulic pressure to align the damaged metal, or they may place a dolly block against the surface of the dented area and beat the opposite surface with a hammer to remove the dents. They fill depressions with solder or plastic materials, especially fibrous glass impregnated with polyester resins. The resin and catalyst

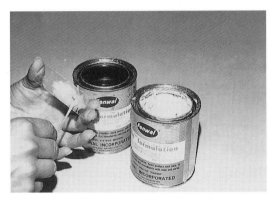

FIGURE AP–6 • To repair small areas, the resin and catalyst may be mixed by hand, often being squeezed from tubes and mixed with a spatula.

are usually mixed by hand (Fig. AP–6), often being squeezed from tubes and mixed with a spatula. Automatic mixers and dispensers are also employed. When testing for epoxy allergy, it is important to test with the resin actually used by the worker, appropriately diluted.

Excessively damaged parts such as fenders, panels, and grills are removed with wrenches and cutting torches; replacements are attached by bolting or welding them into position. Sealants containing polyethylene glycol dimethacrylate (Loctite 221) are commonly used and may be a source of contact allergic dermatitis.[292, 734, 867] Body and fender workers straighten bent frames using hydraulic jacks and pulling devices and file, grind, and sand surfaces using power and hand tools. They apply primer paint with a spray gun (Fig. AP–7), after which the surface is sanded. They also align headlights and wheels and bleed hydraulic brake systems. They may paint the surface after performing the repairs, but this is usually done by another worker. These workers often work in awkward or cramped positions; the workplace is often open to the weather, and the environment is usually dusty and dirty. Exposure to the fumes of paints and solvents is common. Atopics fare poorly in this work.

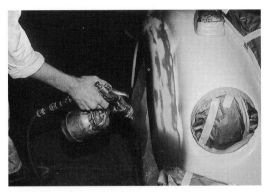

FIGURE AP–7 • A body and fender worker applying paint with a spray gun.

Irritants

Abrasives (abrasive wheels, sandpaper, abrasive skin cleaners)
Adhesives (plastics, especially cyanoacrylates)[867]
Metal cleaners
Soaps and detergents
Solvents
Plastics and catalysts
Hydraulic and brake fluids
Paints
Soldering flux
Heat torch
Fibrous glass
Metal parts

Patch test to standard and vehicle preservative allergens, with special attention to the following.

Standard Allergens

Potassium dichromate, 0.25% pet; 0.023 mg/cm^2 (primer paints)
2-Mercaptobenzothiazole, 1% pet; 0.075 mg/cm^2 (rubber)
Carba mix, 3% pet; 0.25 mg/cm^2 (rubber)
Cobalt chloride, 1% pet; 0.02 mg/cm^2 (drier in adhesives and polyester resins)
Epoxy resin, 1% pet; 0.05 mg/cm^2 (adhesives)
Mercapto mix, 1% pet; 0.075 mg/cm^2 (rubber)
PPD mix (Black rubber mix), 0.6%; 0.075 mg/cm^2 (rubber)
Thiuram mix, 1% pet; 0.025 mg/cm^2 (rubber, especially gloves)
Formaldehyde, 2% aq; 0.18 mg/cm^2 (metal cleaners)
Nickel sulfate, 2.5% pet; 0.2 mg/cm^2 (hand tools)
Rosin (colophony), 20% pet; 0.85 mg/cm^2 (solder)

Additional Allergens

Benzoyl peroxide, 1% pet (polyester resin catalyst)
p-tert-Butylphenol, 2% pet (oils, greases)
Dibutyl phthalate, 5% pet (plasticizer in resin systems)
Diethylenetriamine, 1% pet (epoxy catalyst)
Dibutyl and diethylthiourea, each 1% pet (safety shoes)[410]
Hydrazine sulfate, 1% pet (soldering flux)
Hydroquinone, 1% pet (oils, greases)
N-isopropyl-N'-phenyl-p-phenylenediamine (IPPD), 0.1% pet (gaskets, door seals)
MEK peroxide, 1% pet (catalyst in polyester resins)
Polyester resin monomer, 10% pet (repair resin)
Polyethylene glycol dimethacrylate (PEGMA), 10% in pet (anaerobic sealants)[867]
Triethylenetetramine, 0.5% pet (epoxy catalyst)

BOOKBINDERS

To bind books, the components must be cut, assembled, glued, and sewn according to specifications. Manually operated or automatic machines are used, as well as hand tools. The papers are sewn together by machine and glued together with a brush or machine. With a handpress or by machine, the book is compressed to the required thickness. The edges are trimmed by machine, and the back and cover are glued manually with a brush or by machine. The bound book is placed in a press that exerts pressure on the cover until the glue dries. Coloring is brushed on or applied by brush, pad, or atomizer. The cover material is usually leather, cloth, plastic, or paper. Lettering may be imprinted and embossed with designs or numbers on the cover in gold, silver, or colored foil with a stamping machine. Book binders often repair and rebind damaged or worn books for resale.

Irritants

Solvents
Glues
Paper (sharp edges)

Patch test to standard and vehicle preservative allergens, with special attention to the following.

Standard Allergens

2-Mercaptobenzothiazole, 1% pet; 0.075 mg/cm^2 (rubber aprons, adhesives)
Carba mix, 3% pet; 0.25 mg/cm^2 (rubber)
Mercapto mix, 1% pet; 0.075 mg/cm^2 (rubber)
Thiuram mix, 1% pet; 0.025 mg/cm^2 (rubber gloves, aprons)
Nickel sulfate, 2.5% pet; 0.2 mg/cm^2 (small hand tools)
Cobalt chloride, 1% pet; 0.02 mg/cm^2 (drier in polyester resins)
Epoxy resin, 1% pet; 0.05 mg/cm^2 (adhesives)
Formaldehyde, 2% aq; 0.18 mg/cm^2
Rosin (colophony), 20% pet; 0.85 mg/cm^2 (adhesives)

Additional Allergens

Dibutyl maleate, 5% pet (plasticizer in glues)[338]

BRAKE LINING WORKERS

A brake lining is usually made by twisting asbestos yarn with fine wire strands, treating this with a silicate solution, and then applying a binder, which may be rubber or derived from cashew nutshell oil or another type of phenolic resin, all under heat and pressure. (The cashew nutshell oil derivative used in brake linings is rarely allergenic.) The workers load vacuum tanks with rolls of asbestos lining stock using a hoist. They turn the valves to admit the required quantities of binder, often an asphalt solution, and adjust steam valves to heat the tanks. After the rolls of asbestos have been thoroughly impregnated, they are transferred to an oven, also with a hoist. The rolls are then heated for a specified time to cure the resin. Afterward, the rolls are

blown dry and the fumes removed by exhaust. A brake testing machine is used to be certain that the impregnated linings conform to specifications. The brake linings are cut into strips with a saw, the edges trimmed by machine, and the lining treated with resins using brush or spray gun. Because of the very considerable risk of pulmonary carcinoma in workers exposed to asbestos fibers, its use in brake linings has greatly diminished in recent years, being replaced with plastics of various types.

Irritants

Heat
Asphalt
Asbestos
Steam
Plastics
Solvents
Brake fluids

Patch test to standard and vehicle preservative allergens, with special attention to the following.

Standard Allergens

2-Mercaptobenzothiazole, 1% pet; 0.075 mg/cm^2 (rubber adhesives)
Carba mix, 3% pet; 0.25 mg/cm^2 (rubber)
Epoxy resin, 1% pet; 0.05 mg/cm^2
Mercapto mix, 1% pet; 0.075 mg/cm^2 (rubber)
PPD mix (Black rubber mix), 0.6% pet; 0.075 mg/cm^2 (rubber)
Thiuram mix, 1% pet; 0.025 mg/cm^2 (rubber gloves, adhesives)
Formaldehyde, 2% aq; 0.18 mg/cm^2 (phenolic resins)
Nickel sulfate, 2.5% pet; 0.2 mg/cm^2 (hand tools)

Additional Allergens

Cashew nutshell oil, 1% pet (rare sensitizer)
Diethylthiourea, 1% pet (safety shoes)[410]
Hexamethylenetetramine, 1% pet (in phenolic resins, rubber to textile adhesives)
Phenol-formaldehyde resin, acid catalyzed, 5% pet (binders)
Phenol-formaldehyde resin, alkaline catalyzed, 5% pet (binders)

BUTCHERS AND POULTRY PROCESSORS

Butchers cut, trim, and bone meats to prepare them for cooking using knives, saws, and cleavers. They chop or grind meats using meat grinders, shape and tie roasts, and portion steaks and chops for individual servings, determining size and portion according to the price of the meat to be served. They weigh meats to ensure that portions are uniform and store them in a refrigerator. They also handle fowl, fish, crabs, and other seafood.

The skin of a butcher is damp most of the time, and *Candida* infections and warts are frequent occurrences. Butchers often wear rubber boots at work, which may be a source of allergic contact dermatitis.[606] Other causes of allergic contact dermatitis are wooden knife handles,[245, 357] residues of penicillin,[95, 269] and povidone-iodine used for cleaning the skin.[744] Because of the need to walk in and out of refrigerators, sudden temperature changes may induce itching and, in atopics, a flare of dermatitis, which is also aggravated by frequent hand washing. Atopics generally do poorly in this work.[1269] Injuries among butchers and poultry processors are common from sharp tools, broken chicken bones, and so forth.[216, 1077] Friction calluses are universal among these workers, such as knuckle callosites in live-chicken hangers in poultry processing plants.[1026] Although bacterial infections are less common than in the past, they are still a professional hazard, and the term *chicken poison disease* is often used by poultry workers referring to skin eruptions caused by their work.[851] Erysipeloid is seen primarily among fish handlers, and pyodermas with lymphangitis are common.[96, 1282] Virus warts are extremely common,[998, 1339] especially in pork and beef butchers, in contrast to those who work only as packagers.[1339] Meat handlers may be unaware of the presence of flat warts especially.[1282] Four human papillomaviruses have been identified[966]; the most common is human papillomavirus type 7.[1285]

Contact urticaria may occur from contact with meat,[370, 381, 390, 602] poultry,[64, 1190] and fish[488] (see Chapter 6).

Irritants

Meat, fowl, fish (flesh, entrails, excrement)[602]
Water (wet work)
Soaps and detergents
Cleaning solutions for floors and walls
Spices (for making sausages and meatloaf)

Patch test to standard and vehicle preservative allergens, with special attention to the following.

Standard Allergens

2-Mercaptobenzothiazole, 1% pet; 0.075 mg/cm² (rubber gloves)
Carba mix, 3% pet; 0.25 mg/cm² (rubber gloves)
Mercapto mix, 1% pet; 0.075 mg/cm² (rubber gloves)
Thiuram mix, 1% pet; 0.025 mg/cm² (rubber gloves)
Formaldehyde, 2% aq; 0.18 mg/cm² (cleaning solutions)
Nickel sulfate, 2.5% pet; 0.2 mg/cm² (e.g., hand tools, saw handles)

Additional Allergens

Povidone-iodine (Betadine), 0.5% in ethanol (hand disinfectant)[744]
Spices, 1% pet (including onion and garlic)[604]
Oil of juniper berry, 2% pet
Teak, East Indian rosewood, *Dalbergia latifolia*,[357] and cocobolo woods used for knife handles; various sawdusts sprinkled on the floor (see Chapter 31)

CABINET MAKERS

Cabinet makers construct and repair wooden articles such as cabinets, store fixtures, office equipment, and furniture using woodworking tools and machines. They first study blueprints or drawings of the articles, mark the outlines or dimensions of the parts on paper or lumber stock according to the blueprint specifications, and match materials for color, grain, and texture. They then set up and operate woodworking machines such as power saws, jointers, mortisers, molders, and shapers to cut and shape parts from stock. (Workers who do only woodworking are known as millworkers.) Cabinet makers may trim the parts of joints to make them snug using planes, chisels, or wood files. They drill holes, either by hand or with a boring machine, for insertion of screws or dowels. They glue, fit, and clamp parts and subassemblies together to form complete units using clamps or clamping machines. They drive nails or other fasteners into joints and designated places to reinforce them; they sand and scrape surfaces and joints of articles to prepare them for finishing; they repair or refashion high-grade articles of furniture; and they coat assembled articles with stain, varnish, or paint by dipping, brushing, or spraying. Cabinet makers also install hardware, such as hinges, catches, and drawer pulls. A silk-screen processor may also be used for decorating certain types of furniture (see Silk-Screening Workers). Microwave radiation is used to cure adhesives in some establishments.

Contact dermatitis in cabinet makers usually results from contact with sawdust during sanding and sawing (Fig. AP–8). Irritation of the skin, eyes, and respiratory passages is common, and contact allergy can develop from the sawdust of a number of woods (see Chapter 31). Among the most common offenders is the rosewood substitute Pao ferro (*Machaerium scleroxylum* Tul), used especially for making high-quality, expensive furniture. The sawdust is a potent irritant and allergic sensitizer containing R-3,4-dimethoxydalbergione.[212, 226, 915, 1042] The dermatitis usually affects exposed site flex-

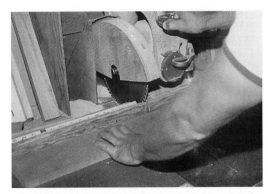

FIGURE AP–8 • In cabinet making there is heavy exposure to sawdust, sometimes sawdust of exotic woods, which can contain potent contact allergens.

ures and genitals. Oropharyngeal and pulmonary symptoms also occur,[212] as well as erythema multiforme.[642] Testing should be done at a concentration of 0.1% to avoid false-positive irritant reactions and sensitization of nonallergic persons.[65] It has been suggested that the incidence of rosewood (Pao ferro) dermatitis will likely increase because Brazilian Dalbergia rosewood has become difficult to obtain.[1325]

Allergic contact dermatitis to the sawdust of *Grevillea robusta* A Cunn (also known as Australian silky oak) has been reported in cabinet makers and other woodworkers.[7, 726] The allergen is a resorcinol compound related to the allergens of poison ivy and poison oak. The wood of *G. robusta* is also used for plywood, barrel and cask staves, and decorative articles such as bracelets, the latter reported to cause allergic contact dermatitis.[611] The allergen, present in the heartwood, is related to poison ivy and oak. Although less common, allergic contact dermatitis from coniferous woods such as pine, spruce, and juniper may also occur. Patch test sensitivity to rosin (colophony) may be an indicator of this, especially to pine.[888] Contact urticaria has been reported from teak.[1087]

In a study of 479 furniture sanders in Singapore, the prevalence of occupational skin disease was 3.8%. No cases of allergic contact dermatitis from wood dust were found, and the authors concluded that the woods used in furniture making were rather weak sensitizers.[456]

Fowler[412] has reported dermatitis in a woodworker from the sawdust of Honduran mahogany (*Swietenia* sp.), developing after the worker moved into a very dusty work area.

The resin from Thai and Japanese lacquer trees is used for cabinets, other furniture, trays, vases, jewelry boxes, and so forth. The trees are members of the Anacardiaceae family, and the allergen is related to poison ivy/oak/sumac. Craftsmen working in factories using these lacquers and exposed to the sawdust of these trees frequently develop dermatitis on their hands and uncovered body areas, especially at the beginning of their employment.[740]

Koa wood (*Acacia koa* Gray), closely related to the Australian acacia tree and used in furniture, flooring, veneer, cabinetry, and bowl-turning, was reported to cause dermatitis in several woodworkers in Hawaii. Each showed positive patch reactions to melacacidin, a hexahydroxyflavan. The sawdust was patch tested at 20% in petrolatum.[724]

Rengas wood resin is similar to that in poison ivy/oak and has been reported to cause dermatitis in a furniture factory worker.[476] Wood dust from jelutong (*Dyera costulata*), a tree growing in southeast Asia, causes contact allergy, as it does in model workshops in car factories and among woodwork teachers in schools.[888]

Western (Canadian) Red Cedar *(Thuja plicata)* has been known to cause asthma, and skin contact with the sawdust may cause a pruritic, vesicular, oozing dermatitis.[91] When the oil is used as a topical treatment for hemorrhoids, a severe contact dermatitis/erythema multiforme–like reaction may result.[1013]

Persons exposed for years to fine sawdust are also at risk for development of nasopharyngeal and sinonasal cancer.[291, 514, 638, 1223, 1316, 1321] Machine sanding of hardwoods may entail an especially high risk of development of cancers within the sinonasal area. Workers should be provided with respiratory protection and the workplace kept clean with a functioning exhaust apparatus. In workers exposed to wood dust, the risk of multiple myeloma also appears to be increased.[291]

Because of their frequent contact with organic solvents, koilonychia is common among cabinet makers.[29]

Irritants

Sawdust and other nuisance dusts
Abrasives
Glues
Wood bleaches
Compressed air (for cleaning)
Shellacs
Lacquers
Solvents
Stains (mostly from solvents)
Varnishes
Soaps and detergents
Fungicides

Patch test to standard and vehicle preservative allergens, with special attention to the following.

Standard Allergens

Potassium dichromate, 0.25% pet; 0.023 mg/cm^2 (wood preservatives)
2-Mercaptobenzothiazole, 1% pet; 0.075 mg/cm^2 (rubber)
Balsam of Peru, 25% pet; 0.80 mg/cm^2 (wood gums)
Carba mix, 3% pet; 0.25 mg/cm^2 (rubber)
Cobalt chloride, 1% pet; 0.02 mg/cm^2 (driers in stains and varnishes)
Epoxy resin, 1% pet; 0.05 mg/cm^2 (adhesives)
Mercapto mix, 1% pet; 0.075 mg/cm^2 (rubber)
PPD mix (Black rubber mix), 0.6% pet; 0.075 mg/cm^2 (rubber)
Thiuram mix, 1% pet; 0.025 mg/cm^2 (rubber)
Formaldehyde, 2% aq; 0.18 mg/cm^2 (solvents, adhesives, preservatives)
Rosin (colophony), 20% pet; 0.85 mg/cm^2 (varnishes, adhesives)
p-tert-Butylphenol–formaldehyde resin, 1% pet; 0.04 mg/cm^2 (adhesives)

Additional Allergens

Ammoniated mercury, 1% pet (wood preservatives)
Beeswax, 30% pet (adhesives and waxes)
p-tert-Butylphenol, 2% pet (glues, preservatives)
Phenol-formaldehyde resin, 10% pet (adhesives)
o-Phenylphenol, 1% pet (preservative in adhesives)
Pentachlorophenol, 1% pet (wood preservatives)
Resorcinol, 2% pet (adhesives and glues)
Propylene glycol, 4% aq (varnishes)
Polyurethane resins and catalysts (see Chapter 25)
Wood sawdust, 5% or 10% pet

Solvent Blue 36 (1,4-bis[isopropylamino]
  anthraquinone), 5% olive oil (dye used in wood
  stains and varnishes, as well as in felt-tipped
  pens)[899]
Tetrachloroisophthalonitrile (Daconil, Chlorothalonil),
  0.01% acetone (wood preservative and fungicide)[51]
Tricresyl phosphate, 2% pet (plasticizer in adhesives)
Triethylenetetramine, 0.5% pet (epoxy catalyst)
Turpentine, 10% olive oil (furniture polishes)
Urea-formaldehyde resin, 10% pet (fiberboard
  adhesives)
Various wood dusts, 1% to 10% pet (see Chapter
  31)[412, 547, 915, 1154]

CANDLE MAKERS

Candles are made by hand as well as with a machine. When they are made by hand the operator places a wick over the center of one section of a mold, presses the mold halves together, and fastens them with a rubber band. Wax is then poured through the opening, and the mold is placed in cold water to harden the wax, after which the mold is separated from the candle. Excess wax is then scraped away from the surface with a knife, and the candle is then examined for defects and color uniformity.

Candle-molding machines were developed during the nineteenth century and consist of rows of molds in a metal tank. The raw materials are first melted in steam-heated vats and the molten wax poured by a machine operator by one of two methods: (1) positioning metal pins in the center of molten wax to form holes for candle wicks and then pouring a specified quantity of wax into the molds; (2) pouring the molten wax into a large vat over which wicks are positioned on an automatic taper-candle-dipping machine resembling a large chandelier, onto which many candles can be made simultaneously. The assembly is dipped into the liquid wax several times, then intermittently immersed in cool water to harden the wax; the final wax layers are completed by hand-dipping. These popular hand-operated casting machines can produce up to 3,000 candles a day.

In addition to dyes, more than 120 fragrances are incorporated into the wax during molding, including jasmine, pine, lemon, and rose.

Household candles are usually composed of a mixture of spermaceti from the head cavity of the sperm whale and paraffin wax from petroleum. The basic candle stock is a composite of stearic and palmitic acids in paraffin. Ceresin, a wax distilled from ozocerite, or earth wax, is also sometimes used. Church candles are composed of a mixture of beeswax and spermaceti in paraffin; some today are still hand-molded. Of the vegetable waxes, carnauba, candella, and Japan wax are the most common. Mineral waxes such as ozokerite, paraffin wax, ceresin, and montan wax have been widely used, as well as refined waxes such as stearic or palmitic acid and even the so-called candle grease.

Wicks are made from braided cotton impregnated with ammonium chloride, ammonium phosphate, ammonium sulfate, borax, boric acid, and potassium nitrate.

Japan wax, also called sumac wax or Japan tallow, is sometimes added as an extender for beeswax in candles. Japan wax contains japonic acid obtained from the fruit of a species of *Toxicodendron* after boiling the fruit in water. Inorganic and organic dyes are used to tint the candles, and small amounts of perfumes are often added. So-called insect-repellent candles usually contain oil of citronella.

Burns from hot wax are an ever-present hazard, although there is less hazard if the wax is maintained at temperatures below 70°C. Because of the great quantity of molten wax present, there is inevitable spillage and the hazard of slippery floors.

Irritants

Hot wax
Water (wet work)
Solvents
Soaps and detergents

Patch test to standard and vehicle preservative allergens, with special attention to the following.

Standard Allergens

2-Mercaptobenzothiazole, 1% pet; 0.075 mg/cm² (gloves, rubber bands)
Balsam of Peru, 25% pet; 0.80 mg/cm² (crossreacts with some fragrances)
Carba mix, 3% pet; 0.25 mg/cm² (gloves, rubber bands)
Cobalt chloride, 1% pet; 0.02 mg/cm² (dyes)
Fragrance mix, 8% pet; 0.43 mg/cm² (scents)
Mercapto mix, 1% pet; 0.075 mg/cm² (gloves, rubber bands)
Thiuram mix, 1% pet; 0.025 mg/cm² (gloves, rubber bands)
Nickel sulfate, 2.5% pet; 0.2 mg/cm² (handles, tools, molds)

Additional Allergens

Beeswax, 30% pet
Bayberry wax, 30% pet(?)
Citronella oil, 2% pet (insect-repellent candles)

CANNERY WORKERS

Cannery workers (washers, dumpers, sorters, peelers, trimmers, and machine maintenance personnel) perform all sorts of tasks in canning, freezing, preserving, and packing foods. The food products are first dumped onto a conveyor belt, hopper, or sorting table. The workers sort and grade them according to size, color, and quality. The products are then fed into processing equipment such as washers, refrigerators, peelers, corers, pitters, trimmers, grinders, cookers, and slicing machines. Often the workers trim, peel, and slice the products by hand, using knives and paring tools. Sometimes the cans or packages are hand-filled using a scoop or a filling form, but they are usually filled by machine. The processed items are counted, weighed, and tallied according to specifications. The containers are then loaded onto trays or racks or into boxes and moved by hand or hand truck into a storage area prior to shipment. Finally, the containers are cleaned of dust and other debris with an air hose.

In addition to the time-honored method of preserving foods by heating and storing in glass containers and tins, ionizing radiation sterilization has recently been used, using gamma-emitting radioisotopes such as cobalt 60. Microwave sterilization is also commonly employed today. Sun drying is still used, as well as freeze drying.

Burns and scalding are fairly common occurrences in cannery work; they sometimes occur from the steam cleaning of equipment. Contamination of floors with oils, fats, and water can lead to injuries.

In addition to irritation from alkalis, acids, and cleaning compounds, a common dermatosis in these workers is moniliasis in the fingerwebs and periungual regions from the continual wetness. There is occasional dermatitis from the fruit or vegetables and the sugar used in canning; rarely, allergic contact dermatitis occurs, from sodium metabisulfite, for example, which may be used to keep produce such as cauliflower white, although this is less likely today. Food handlers may be subject to skin infections such as erysipeloid and atypical tuberculosis infections, warts due to a virus in fish, as well as anthrax and actinomycosis. However, in modern canneries there is little direct skin contact with raw ingredients. Noise is often a serious health hazard in many modern canneries.

Irritants

Soaps and detergents
Fruits and fruit juices
Vegetables and vegetable juices
Brines and syrups
Water (wet work)
Fish
Meat
Heat, high humidity, and cold

Patch test to standard and vehicle preservative allergens, with special attention to the following.

Standard Allergens

Potassium dichromate, 0.25% pet; 0.023 mg/cm^2
    (preservative once used in milk laboratories*)[587]
2-Mercaptobenzothiazole, 1% pet; 0.75 mg/cm^2
    (rubber in gloves, gaskets, and conveyor belts)
Carba mix, 3% pet; 0.25 mg/cm^2 (rubber)
Mercapto mix, 1% pet; 0.075 mg/cm^2 (rubber)
PPD mix (Black rubber mix), 0.6% pet; 0.075 mg/cm^2
    (Black rubber)

---

*Potassium dichromate is a recognized carcinogen. It is not used in milk laboratories in the United States today.

Thiuram mix, 1% pet; 0.025 mg/cm^2 (rubber gloves)
Formaldehyde, 2% aq; 0.18 mg/cm^2 (germicidal agent for floors and walls)
Nickel sulfate, 2.5% pet; 0.2 mg/cm^2 (small tools and instruments)

Additional Allergens

BHA, 2% pet (food preservative)
BHT, 2% pet (food preservative)
Ethoxyquin, 0.5% pet (apple packers)[1324]
Gallate esters (propyl and lauryl gallate), 1% pet (antioxidants)[121, 673]
Propylene glycol, 4% aq[382]
Sorbic acid, 2% pet (germicidal agent for yeast and bacteria)
Wooden knife handles (e.g., cocobolo), sawdust at 10% pet
Sodium metabisulfite, 1% aq ("whitener")

CARPENTERS

Carpentry is commonly divided into two categories—rough and finish. Rough carpentry includes building house frameworks, scaffolds, and wooden forms for concrete, as well as erecting docks, bridges, and supports for tunnels and sewers. Finish carpentry involves building stairs; installing doors, cabinets, wood paneling, and molding; and putting up acoustical tiles. Some carpenters do both rough and finish work; however, others limit themselves to laying hardwood floors, building wall frames, installing insulation or paneling, or even painting and varnishing (see related occupational profiles, such as Cabinet Makers).

Carpenters usually work from blueprints to plan or help plan the layout and measure the area and materials. They cut the woods or other materials and shape them with hand and power tools such as saws and drills. They join the materials with nails, screws, or adhesives, and they check the accuracy of their work with levels, rulers, and framing squares. All carpenters use hand tools, such as hammers, saws, chisels, and planes, and power tools such as power saws, drills, and rivet guns.

Dermatitis among carpenters is not common. When it occurs it is usually due to irritation from dusts, dirt, solvents, detergents, glues, wood preservatives, fibrous glass, and so forth. Carpenters are at a definite risk of injury from slips and falls, from contact with sharp or rough materials, and from the use of hazardous tools and power equipment. Many carpenters work outdoors and develop considerable actinic damage to exposed skin. Contact allergic sensitization, which is uncommon, may occur from the sawdust of allergenic woods such as Honduran mahogany (*Swietenia* spp.),[412] Pao ferro (*Machaerium scleroxylum* Tul),[65, 212] koa wood (*Acacia koa* Gray),[724] and *Grevillea robusta* A. Cunn[7, 726] (see Cabinet Makers) or plants such as poison ivy/oak, *Frullania,* and others. Although uncommon, coniferous woods such as pine, spruce, and juniper may cause allergic contact dermatitis, and sensitivity to rosin (colophony) may be an indicator of this, especially pine.[888]

Rosin (colophony) has been used to coat nails, and epoxy and other resins are used to some extent as adhesives.[1252] Hexavalent chromium in leather, cement, and wood preservatives[51] is occasionally responsible for sensitization. Chipboard is a composite consisting of wood particles bonded together with urea-formaldehyde resins. It may be covered with a thin epoxy resin surface coating to increase strength for processing. Allergic contact dermatitis to epoxy may occur from sawing this material in the preparation of wall board.[490]

Chloracne has been reported from contact with penta-chlorophenol-preserved wood containing considerable quantities of a dioxin.[219] A wood preservative containing tetrachloroisophthalonitrile (Daconil, Chlorothalonil) has been reported to cause contact dermatitis in a cabinet maker.[51]

Plywood may be treated with copper-chromium arsenate as a preservative, and, when the plywood is burned, workers (and family) can be exposed to fumes containing sufficient arsenic to develop poisoning. Arsenic can be detected in urine even 5 to 8 weeks after exposure; hair and/or nail levels may also show elevated levels.[622]

Rock wool and fibrous glass, used for thermal and acoustic insulation and fire protection, are notorious irritants,[195, 225] and, when impregnated with an epoxy resin, allergic sensitization may also occur.[251] Rock wool, on direct contact with the skin, may induce a dermatitis similar to that caused by fibrous glass and is also associated with severe itching.[391] The dermatitis is usually transient and chiefly caused by fibers with a diameter exceeding 4.5 μm. Fibers with the smallest diameter are the least irritating, while those with the largest are the most.[1160] Fibrous glass and rock wool dust may contain trace amounts of contaminants such as mercury, lead, arsenic, or cadmium. The mastics used in insulation may sometimes contain rosin acids.

Irritants

Sawdust and other dusts
Wood preservatives (especially those with bromine- or iodine-containing additives)
Wet cement
Fibrous glass
Rock wool
Resins and glues
Solvents and oils
Soaps and detergents

Patch test to standard and vehicle preservative allergens, with special attention to the following.

Standard Allergens

Potassium dichromate, 0.25% pet; 0.023 mg/cm^2 (cement, leather gloves, leather tool belts, wood preservatives)
2-Mercaptobenzothiazole, 1% pet; 0.075 mg/cm^2 (rubber gloves and tool handles)
Carba mix, 3% pet; 0.25 mg/cm^2 (rubber, as above)
Cobalt chloride, 2% pet; 0.02 mg/cm^2 (driers in varnishes)

Tetramethyl thiuram disulfide, 1% pet; 0.025 mg/cm^2 (rubber gloves)
Mercapto mix, 1% pet; 0.075 mg/cm^2 (rubber gaskets, hoses)
Formaldehyde, 2% aq; 0.18 mg/cm^2 (resins, cleaning agents)
Nickel sulfate, 2.5% pet; 0.2 mg/cm^2 (tools)
Epoxy resin, 1% pet; 0.05 mg/cm^2 resin (binder in fibrous glass and rock wool; surface coatings)[490]
Rosin (colophony), 20% pet; 0.85 mg/cm^2 (coating on nails, binder for rock wool and fibrous glass; pine dusts)
p-tert-Butylphenol–formaldehyde resin, 1% pet; 0.04 mg/cm^2 (adhesives)

Additional Allergens

Methyl methacrylate, 2% pet (adhesives)
Diethylthiourea, 1% pet (safety shoes)[410]
Pentachlorophenol, 1% aq (wood preservatives)
Phenol-formaldehyde resin, 10% pet (resins, glues, plywood)
Plants (e.g., *Toxicodendron, Frullania*)
Turpentine, 10% olive oil (solvents)
Wood sawdusts (especially teak, rosewood, mahogany and others), 10% pet (see Chapter 31)

CASHIERS

Cashiers are those employed in supermarkets, movie theaters, restaurants, and banks to handle money. They receive money, make change, fill out charge forms, and give receipts. Among the several types of machines they operate are cash registers that print the amount of the sale on paper tape and, more recently, electronic registers, computerized point-of-sale registers, and computerized scanning systems. Depending on complexity, a computerized system may automatically calculate the necessary taxes and record inventory numbers and other information. Cashiers also often operate adding and change-dispensing machines.

The skin problems of cashiers are not many, and most are due to nickel sensitivity from contact with coins.[204] Although it is unlikely that sensitization can be initiated by such contact, individuals previously sensitized to nickel from ear piercing, for example, may occasionally develop dermatitis on the fingers from prolonged and intensive handling of coins, especially if hyperhidrosis is present. Paper money may be coated with formaldehyde resins and minute amounts of phenolic germicides; however, allergic sensitivity to paper money is extremely rare. The computerized scanning machines in supermarkets emit small amounts of long-wave-length ultraviolet light. When the opening is large, the ultraviolet light exposure can be sufficient to induce photosensitivity in certain predisposed persons as, for example, when also in contact with psoralen-containing celery.

Irritants

Paper and paper tape

Patch test to standard and vehicle preservative allergens, with special attention to the following.

Standard Allergens

2-Mercaptobenzothiazole, 1% pet; 0.075 mg/cm^2 (rubber bands, rubber finger guards)

Carba mix, 3% pet; 0.25 mg/cm^2 (rubber, as above)

Mercapto mix, 1% pet; 0.075 mg/cm^2 (rubber, as above)

Thiuram mix, 1% pet; 0.025 mg/cm^2 (rubber, as above)

Formaldehyde, 2% aq; 0.18 mg/cm^2 (preservatives)

Nickel sulfate, 2.5% pet; 0.2 mg/cm^2 (coins)

CAULKERS

Caulkers apply caulking compounds (sealants) to seal crevices in parts of structures, such as stone coping, partition walls, and window frames, using a caulking gun. They load the gun by inserting the magazine of the gun with the caulking compound and pulling the plunger. They guide the nozzle along the joint or crevice while pressing the lever of the gun to discharge the compound into the crevice. They may apply the compound with a knife or trowel and very often smooth the surface with their fingers. They may mix the compound together, and they sometimes also brush the sealer into joints and crevices to prepare them for sealing.

The oldest caulking compound is putty, a mixture of calcium carbonate and linseed oil, to which white lead is occasionally added. Perhaps the best-known sealants are those composed of linseed oil, asphalt, and various waxes. Putty is most commonly used to cement window glass in place. (Putty should not be confused with "putty powder," a mixture of lead and tin oxides or tin oxide with oxalic acid, used rather as a polishing compound for stone, glass, and dental appliances.) Today most caulking compounds are composed of various synthetics, particularly rubber compounds, sometimes with lead peroxide (lead dioxide) used as the curing agent for polysulfide rubber. Polyester resins, in which benzoyl peroxide may be the catalyst, are also used. Other polymers are silicones, urethanes, acrylics, and polychloroprene. Linseed oil (in some putty), asphalt, and various waxes are also used. Cobalt oleate and naphthenate driers are often used to hasten curing. Rosin, 2-mercaptobenzothiazole, and thiuram are found in some caulks. Phenolic preservatives such as o-phenylphenol (Dowicide 1) and others may be used as preservatives.

Irritants

Solvents

Soaps and detergents

Asphalt

Dusts

Plastics

Resins

Patch test to standard and vehicle preservative allergens, with special attention to the following.

Standard Allergens

Potassium dichromate, 0.25% pet; 0.023 mg/cm^2 (cement caulks)

2-Mercaptobenzothiazole, 1% pet; 0.075 mg/cm^2 (rubber caulks)

Carba mix, 3% pet; 0.25 mg/cm^2 (rubber caulks)

Cobalt dichloride, 1% pet; 0.02 mg/cm^2 (drier for caulks)

Epoxy resin, 1% pet; 0.05 mg/cm^2 (adhesives)

Mercapto mix, 1% pet; 0.075 mg/cm^2 (rubber caulks)

PPD mix (Black rubber mix), 0.6% pet; 0.075 mg/cm^2 (rubber caulks)

Thiuram mix, 1% pet; 0.025 mg/cm^2 (rubber caulks)

Formaldehyde, 2% aq; 0.18 mg/cm^2 (preservatives)

Nickel sulfate, 2.5% pet; 0.2 mg/cm^2 (hand tools)

Rosin (colophony), 20% pet; 0.85 mg/cm^2 (adhesives)

Thimerosal, 0.1% pet; 0.0080 mg/cm^2 (preservatives)

Additional Allergens

Benzoyl peroxide, 1% pet (polyester and acrylic resin catalysts)

Coal tar, 5% pet (asphalt caulks)

Dichlorophene, 1% pet (preservatives)

Linseed oil, as is (putty)

MEK peroxide, 1% pet (polyester catalysts)

Methyl methacrylate, 2% pet (adhesives)

Phenylmercuric nitrate, 0.05% pet (preservatives)

o-Phenylphenol (Dowicide 1), 1% pet (preservatives)

Polyester resin monomer, 10% pet (caulks)

CEMENT WORKERS

Cement workers (including cement masons, cement finishers, cement pavers, concrete finishers, and concrete floaters) smooth and finish surfaces of poured concrete for floors, walls, sidewalks, and curbs using hand tools including floats, trowels, and screeds. Concrete today is frequently premixed at a nearby site with "aggregate" (usually sand or crushed stone) and water and delivered by large trucks with a large drum that rotates to avoid separation of the premixed ingredients. For small jobs it is usually mixed at the work site from bags of powdered cement and aggregate by a cement mason's helper using a hoe, trowel, or machine. The workers spread the concrete to the proper depth and consistency using a float to bring water to the surface and produce a soft topping. They level, smooth, and shape the surfaces of the freshly poured concrete using a straight-edged float (Fig. AP–9). Colored stone, powdered shell, or coloring powder may be sprinkled over the finished wet surface. They finish vertical surfaces by wetting the concrete and rubbing with abrasive stone and remove rough or

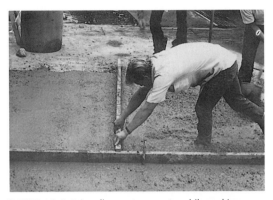

FIGURE AP–9 • Leveling wet concrete while making a driveway. The heavy, moist mixture can easily slide into the boots, resulting in a severe burn if not immediately recognized.

defective spots from the surfaces using a chisel or hammer. Old concrete is broken up using pneumatic and hand tools.

Mortar is a mixture of Portland cement, sand, water, and lime. Latex solids may be added to concrete to improve strength and adhesion. Curing may be retarded by adding methylcellulose and/or hydroxyethyl cellulose.

The most widely used construction cement is *Portland cement,* so named because in 1824 it reminded its inventor, Joseph Aspdin, of Portland stone, a limestone frequently used for building in England. It is a fine gray powder composed of limestone, chalk, cement, rock, clay, and slag. The basic ingredients are alumina, silica, iron oxide, di- and tricalcium silicates, and small amounts of magnesia, sodium, potassium, and sulfur. The gray color is due to the iron oxide. An additional raw material may be blast furnace slag (the source of dichromate?). The powder is rather soft and not particularly abrasive, causing skin irritation mostly when wet or moist from perspiration. Calcium hydroxide is formed on addition of water and is the chief irritant because of its high alkalinity. But the addition of sand and gravel also increases the irritant properties for other cement additives). Cement is very hygroscopic, causing drying and fissuring of the skin. The skin of cement workers is usually dry, hard, and thickened, often fissured, and occasionally ulcerated; their nails are often brittle, dry, and cracked.[164] Acute ulceration of the skin from kneeling on wet cement or from spills into the shoes is well recognized. Severe burns with scarring can result.[148, 386, 1056, 1210] During the period immediately following contact only burning and redness of the skin may be present; approximately 8 to 12 hours later blistering and later ulceration appear, which may develop into deep ulcers.[528] Healing may require many weeks.[1056] Amateur users of cement are the frequent victims and should be informed of its considerable hazards before use.[882]

Allergic contact dermatitis from cement almost always arises from the hexavalent chromium.[163, 169, 465, 626, 646] The chromium is thought to come either from the refractory bricks of the furnaces where the cement is made or from the raw materials (clay) themselves. Fregert[434] has noted that chromate did not appear in cement until the introduction of the modern horizontal kiln.

Although a small but significant number of workers may show positive patch-test reactions to hexavalent chromium and still be able to continue working without dermatitis,[47, 516, 626] the majority of cement workers who have chromate dermatitis continue to experience dermatitis[260] and disability even after changing occupations. The longer the dermatitis continues with the sensitivity undiagnosed, the more likely the dermatitis will continue despite avoidance (presumed) and treatment.[516] Early recognition, a job change into an industry where there is no contact with cement or hexavalent chromium salts, adequate financial support during job training, and a job that pays approximately the same as the previous job will greatly reduce the likelihood of persistent dermatitis.[793]

The total amount of chromium in Portland cement ranges between 20 and 100 ppm or between 0.002% and 0.1% chromium. Fresh U.S. concrete contains relatively high levels of hexavalent chromium, averaging 1.27 mg/kg.[1220] In 1983, legislation in Denmark required that the content of water-soluble chromate in dry cement not exceed 2 mg/kg (2 ppm).[451] To achieve this, since 1993 ferrous sulfate has been added to Danish cement, reducing the hexavalent chromium to the water-soluable trivalent form, which does not produce contact allergy. As a result, the level of hexavalent chromium in Danish cement today is very low, less than 0.01 mg/kg.[1220] This has markedly reduced the incidence of allergic cement eczema due to hexavalent chromium in Denmark.[1337] However, it should be emphasized that the addition of ferrous sulfate does not decrease the irritant properties of cement,[48] and home-users may still use cement containing allergenic levels of chromium.[1337] Elimination of the source of the chromium can be effective in reducing the incidence of chrome-caused allergic dermatitis in these workers. In Australia, to achieve this, changing magnesium-chrome refractories to those constructed of magnesium aluminate (spinel) has begun.[1184]

Dermatitis often also results from rubber chemicals, especially the thiurams, in gloves worn to protect the skin.[516, 1196] Cobalt sensitivity, although reported from European cement,[436] rarely results from U.S. cement.[995] Two cases of isolated cobalt sensitivity in Cuban cement workers have been reported.[458] For prevention of chrome dermatitis using the ferrous sulfate method, see Chapter 17.

Besides Portland cement, other types of cement include (1) *slag cements,* a granulated slag made by rapid chilling of molten slags from blast furnaces producing pig iron (a variety of this type is a supersulfated cement with 10% to 15% hard-burned gypsum and a small percentage of Portland cement); (2) *high alumina cement,* a fast-hardening cement from bauxite and limestone fused in an electric furnace; and (3) *expanding and nonshrinking cements,* which expand slightly on hydration, thus offsetting the small contraction that occurs when new concrete hardens for the first time. This type is a mixture of Portland cement and an expansive agent made by clinkering a mix of chalk, bauxite, and gypsum.

A comprehensive review of cement eczema is given by Avnstorp.[48, 49]

Irritants

Wet cement (cement burns)[1263]
Water (wet work)
Dust
Accelerators (calcium chloride)
Fiberglass
Concrete and brick cleaners (phosphoric acid, sulfamic acid, solvents)
Cement "parting agents" (solvents)
Zinc stearate
Plasticizers (alkyl aryl sulfonates, melamine-formaldehyde condensates)
Damp-proofing agents (soaps, soap derivatives)
Rock wool

Patch test to standard and vehicle preservative allergens, with special attention to the following.

Standard Allergens

Potassium dichromate, 0.25% pet; 0.023 mg/cm^2 (cement, leather in gloves)
2-Mercaptobenzothiazole, 1% pet; 0.075 mg/cm^2 (rubber)
Carba mix, 3% pet; 0.25 mg/cm^2 (rubber)
Epoxy resin, 1% pet; 0.05 mg/cm^2 (plastic additives; repairing cracks)[435]; cement additive[805]
Mercapto mix, 1% pet; 0.075 mg/cm^2 (rubber)
PPD mix (Black rubber mix), 0.6% pet; 0.075 mg/cm^2 (rubber)
p-tert-Butylphenol–formaldehyde resin, 1% pet; 0.04 mg/cm^3 (leather gloves)
Thiuram mix, 1% pet; 0.025 mg/cm^2 (rubber gloves)
Formaldehyde, 2% aq; 0.18 mg/cm^2 (phenolic resins)
Nickel sulfate, 2.5% pet; 0.2 mg/cm^2 (instruments, hand tools)
Cobalt chloride, 1% pet; 0.02 mg/cm^2 (cement, especially European)[458, 478, 480, 1007]

Additional Allergens

Methyl methacrylate, 2% pet
Phenylmercuric nitrate, 0.05% pet (mold retardants)
o-Phenylphenol, 1% pet (germicidal agent)
Melamine formaldehyde resin (Kaurit M-70), 10% pet

CERAMIC WORKERS

Ceramic materials are manufactured by firing certain materials, such as silicon and its oxides, and compounds at very high temperatures. Ceramic floor and wall tiles are composed of different clays that contain such compounds as hydrated aluminum silicates, and various quantities of the oxides of calcium, magnesium, sodium, potassium, iron, titanium, manganese, carbon, and phosphorus. Besides floor and wall tiles, they have numerous industrial applications, including electrical and chemical ceramics, dinnerware, and structural clay products such as bricks. Ceramics have great value because of their mechanical strength, chemical durability, and resistance to acids, bases, and other chemicals, as well as their ability to be decorated in a variety of colors and designs. Silk-screen printing is utilized prior to glazing the decorated piece.

Ceramics have been very important in the electronics industry as parts of microelectronic circuits, such as rectifiers, photocells, transistors, detectors, and modulators. They have been used for many decades as electrical insulators.

Freeze-drying is a valuable method of making ceramics that have a near-perfect microstructure. A water solution of salts with the desired cations is sprayed as a fine mist into a hydrocarbon (such as hexane) or a fluorocarbon (such as Freon) at very low temperatures. The mist freezes and is collected and dried by sublimation. The beads are then calcined (oxidized) in a furnace.

Workers who tend to machines that cook and coat metal objects with ceramic materials perform this job under closed conditions, observing the process by mirror reflection through a thick window. After removing the coated parts from the ovens, they may blow away the excess material with an air hose, but there should be almost no skin contact.

Dental ceramists, however, perform their work without special protection. They make and repair porcelain teeth according to a dentist's prescription, mixing the porcelain to the color of natural teeth. They first apply the mixture over a metal model of teeth using a spatula. They then brush excess porcelain from the teeth and place them in an electric furnace to harden. After removal, they brush on additional layers of porcelain and shape it with a spatula to the contour of a tooth. Repeated application followed by baking is performed until the denture reaches the specifications, and the surface has the desired glaze.

In a study of 139 workers from three ceramics factories in Italy,[1106] irritant dermatitis was predominant, with few cases of relevant contact allergy, which most likely can be explained because of automation in this industry. The classic papers on ceramic contact allergy describe cobalt as the predominant allergen.[1005, 1006] Turpentine allergy is a continuing problem and may be more common than allergy to the metals used in coloration; however, a more frequent allergen is α-pinene from Indonesian turpentine, which is reported to be more allergenic than the Portuguese variety.[765]

Irritants

Heat
Glazes
Clay dust
Wet clay
Acids
Alkalis

Soaps and detergents
Solvents
Turpentine

Patch test to standard and vehicle preservative allergens, with special attention to the following.

Standard Allergens

Potassium dichromate, 0.25% pet; 0.023 mg/cm²
Cobalt dichloride, 1% pet; 0.02 mg/cm² (black and blue pigments)[1005]
Epoxy resin, 1% pet; 0.05 mg/cm² (to repair defects)[1147]
Nickel sulfate, 2.5% pet; 0.2 mg/cm² (hand tools)
Kathon CG, 0.01% pet; 0.0040 mg/cm² (in ceramic paints)[493, 1032]

Additional Allergens

Chromium oxide, 1% (for green and pink colors)
Turpentine, 10% olive oil[407, 765]
Proxel (1,2-benzisothiazolin-3-one), 0.1% pet (biocide for releasing agents in molds[1147])

CHEMISTS

The term *chemist* embraces individuals who perform chemical tests, qualitative and quantitative analyses, and experiments for quality or process control and who develop new products and/or new basic knowledge. Nearly every industry employs chemists, and the irritants and allergens are countless and varied. Chemists are exposed to a large number of raw materials as well as finished products, and many of these may be toxic, flammable, and explosive. Personal and environmental protective measures are especially important in this work. Some of the chemicals that have been reported as contact irritants, allergens, and urticants in the last several decades are listed.

Some Allergens

4-Nitrophenyl-*N*-(2-chloroethyl)carbamate, 0.01% pet; 4-nitrophenyl-*N*-(2-chloroethyl)-*N*-nitrosocarbamate, 0.01% pet[951]
5-[(2-Aminoethyl)thiomethyl]-*N,N*-dimethyl-2-furanmethanamine (intermediate in H$_2$ antagonist synthesis), 1% aq[1060]
Benzisothiazolone (intermediate for isothiazolone germicides), 0.1% pet[1143]
Benzyl-1-amino-3-chloro-2-hydroxypropane (agricultural chemical intermediate), 0.1% ethanol[1246]
4-Bromomethyl-6,8-dimethyl-2(IH)-quinolone (intermediate in pharmaceutical industry), 1% pet[1059]
tert-Butyl catechol (polymerization of polyvinyl chloride), 0.1% pet[764]
2(*p*-Carboxyphenol)-4,5-diphenylimidzole (photo-processing agent), 1% pet[311]

bis-(4-Chlorophenyl)-methyl chloride (organic synthesis), 1% chloroform[988]
5-Chloro-1-methyl-4-nitroimidazole, 0.01% pet[661]
Cytosine arabinoside intermediates (synthesis of Ara-C) 1%, 0.5%, 0.1% aq[223]
N,N'-dicyclohexyldiimide (protein synthesis), 0.1% pet[265, 610, 1135, 1297, 1341]
2,6-Dichloropurine (intermediate in pharmaceutical industry), 1% pet[1058]
Diethyl-B-chloroethylamine (intermediate in pharmaceutical industry), concentration for patch testing not given[295]
Diethylfumarate (intermediate, cause of contact urticaria[1295]
Diisocyanoatodicyclohexyl methane (Hylene W) (chemical intermediate), 1% alc[835]
Dimethyl acetylenedicarboxylate (chemical synthesis)[1144]
Dinitrochlorobenzene[803]
4-Chloro-7-nitrobenzofurazan[115]
Diphenyloxazole (scintillator in radioimmunoassays), 2% MEK[189]
Hexylresorcinol (analysis of acrolein), 0.1% pet[166]
Hydrazine sulfate (intermediate in manufacture of aminoguanidine), 0.5% pet[1177]
N-Hydroxyphthalimide (peptide intermediate), 0.0001% in ethanol[441]
Methylenedianiline (epoxy and polyurethane resins), 0.05% pet[1240]
Methyl mercury (dimethyl mercury) (Potent systemic poison, one drop of which may result in mercury poisoning and death. Methyl mercury from ingestion of fish contaminated with methyl mercury was responsible for an epidemic of mercury intoxication in the Minamata district of Japan in the 1970s.)[1325a]
Palladium (Na$_2$PDCl$_3$)[920]
2-Phenyl tetralone tosylhydrazone (intermediate), 0.5% in chloroform[250]
Quinidine sulfate (pharmaceuticals), 1% aq[1274]
3,4,6-Trichloropyridazine (drug intermediate) (strong irritant)[303]
Winged bean (*Psophocarpus tetragonolobus*) (extracted oil is used in foods), causes contact urticaria[800]
4-Vinyl pyridine (organic solvent), 1.0% isopropyl alcohol[1082]

CIGARETTE AND CIGAR MAKERS

In the category of cigarette and cigar makers are included those who operate the machines that make the product: catcher, hopper feeder, making machine operator, inspector, and examiner, among others. Cigarette making is more automated than cigar making, and in the former there is less contact with tobacco. Besides cigarette and cigar making, the category includes making pipe and chewing tobacco and snuff.

The tobacco is received at the factory in bales and must first be conditioned and mixed with a variety of chemicals to make the type of tobacco desired. Before the bales are opened, they are moistened with water, usually by placing them into steam chambers. The wet bales are then opened and the stems removed by machine. A uniform and consistent quality of a particular type of tobacco is achieved by mixing on a conveyor belt or in a revolving drum or by shaking on a continuous belt. Then a variety of chemicals and vegetable substances, called *casings,* are added to improve the quality and/or to give some special characteristic or aroma. Adhesives are used to bind together the tobacco particles, which are mostly natural substances or polysaccharides such as carboxymethyl cellulose, hydroxyethyl cellulose, and others. Glyoxal may be used as a cross-linking agent. Humectants and plasticizers such as glycerol, proylene glycol, and 1,3-buylene glycol may be used. Nicotine is said to be removed by electrolysis or a current of ammoniated steam. To prevent fermentation, the moisture content must be reduced, initially by warming in roasters or in drying drums or by "panning," followed by cooling in a current of air. The tobacco is then machine-wrapped in paper to form a continuous cigarette or rod that is then cut to size at definite intervals. The cut cigarettes are then packaged for sale.

There is considerable hazard to exposure to tobacco dust, especially when it is moist or heated. Physical contact with the dust and the chemical substances used in the manufacture may result in conjunctivitis, dryness and irritation of the respiratory tract, dermatitis, and nail fragility. Adequate ventilation, a high degree of personal cleanliness, and good housekeeping are important preventive measures.

Rycroft et al.[1070] give a description of the cigar-making process in which there may be considerable contact with the leaf, especially between the thumbs and index fingers, as the desired shape of the tobacco leaf is being cut by machine. In cigarette assembly there is less contact with the plant because the filling and wrapping are done entirely by machine. Nevertheless, there can be contact with the tobacco leaves, especially during storage and loading them into hoppers. Urticarial reactions, erythema, and mild eczema are not uncommon among these workers,[1070] and bronchial asthma and rhinoconjunctivitis may also occur.[1209] Airborne contact dermatitis from dust has been reported.[978] Simple mechanical irritation from the leaf may also occur.[925] A report of skin hazards in the cigar industry is given by Samitz et al.[1078a] Allergic contact dermatitis from the natural, untreated tobacco leaf is very unusual.

Irritants

Tobacco dust
Tobacco leaves and stems (onycholysis)[1080]
Water and steam

Patch test to standard and vehicle preservative allergens, with special attention to the following.

Standard Allergens

Wool alcohols, 30% pet; 1.00 mg/cm² (hand creams)
2-Mercaptobenzothiazole, 1% pet; 0.075 mg/cm²
    (rubber gloves)
Balsam of Peru, 25% pet; 0.80 mg/cm² (flavorings)
Carba mix, 3% pet; 0.25 mg/cm² (rubber gloves)
Mercapto mix, 1% pet; 0.075 mg/cm² (rubber gloves)
Thiuram mix, 1% pet; 0.025 mg/cm² (rubber gloves)
Formaldehyde, 2% pet; 0.18 mg/cm² (cleaners, disinfectants)
Nickel sulfate, 2.5% pet; 0.2 mg/cm² (hand tools)

Additional Allergens

Camphor, 10% pet
Menthol, 1% pet
Propylene glycol, 2% aq
Glycerol, 1% aq

CONSTRUCTION WORKERS

Construction workers perform a variety of duties concerned with building, repairing, and wrecking buildings, bridges, dams, roads, railways, and so forth. The title includes engineer, equipment mechanic, inspector, estimator, and laborer. The work may involve mixing, pouring, and spreading concrete, asphalt, gravel, and other materials; digging ditches and excavating for foundations; and using pick and shovel or heavy equipment. These workers load and unload equipment, sort and stack lumber, paint, apply sealants to pipe, level earth, clean tools and equipment, and perform many other duties. Despite increasing mechanization and the more frequent use of precast concrete sections, contact with wet cement still occurs, particularly in spreading concrete and smoothing surfaces and during small jobs such as laying short distances of sidewalk. Although most construction workers are well aware of the hazards, contact with wet cement may cause severe burns, in addition to allergic skin sensitization. The method of spreading concrete by walking through it as it is being poured is a source of dermatitis and severe burns from spills over the tops of boots. The symptoms of wet cement burns develop rather slowly, and often not until 10 to 12 hours later are the burns noted.[1263] A major hazard of construction workers is working in confined, poorly ventilated spaces in which there may be exposure to potentially lethal substances such as nitropropane and other solvents.[539]

In a 1995 study of 205 workers in the construction industry (e.g., cement workers, bricklayers, and tile setters) the most common allergens were potassium dichromate, cobalt chloride, thiuram mix, *p*-phenylenediamine, and epoxy resin.[464] Dichromate allergy from cement continues to be a persistent cause of dermatitis in construction workers. At greatest risk are those who mix cement from bags at the worksite.[516] Those who develop contact dermatitis have a significantly worse prognosis than do workers in other industries,[1048] the dermatitis persisting even long after contact with cement has ceased.

Addition of ferrous sulfate during mixing has been found to reduce the incidence of chromate dermatitis in Denmark (see Chapters 17 and 24).

Epoxy resins are widely used in this industry as

binding agents. In the stone and marble industry, for example, epoxies are employed not only in creation of patterns, friezes, Greek frets, and decorative cornices but also in sealing the natural fissures in marble. Angelini et al.[36] reported that 10 out of 22 marble workers had contact and airborne dermatitis within a few weeks following initial exposure. The reactive diluent *o*-cresyl-glycidyl ether and the basic epoxy resin were responsible for most of the cases.

An association between operation of compressed-air and pneumatic tools and development of systemic scleroderma, especially if there is exposure to silica, has been claimed.[990] The validity of this finding awaits further study.

Irritants

Dirt
Acids (hydrochloric, hydrofluoric)
Fibrous glass and rock wool
Wet concrete
Gasoline
Solvents
Hand cleaners
Wood preservatives

Patch test to standard and vehicle preservative allergens, with special attention to the following.

Standard Allergens

Mercaptobenzothiazole, 1% pet; 0.075 mg/cm^2 (rubber gaskets, gloves)
Wool (lanolin) alcohols, 30% pet; 1.00 mg/cm^2 (protective creams)
Carba mix, 3% pet; 0.25 mg/cm^2 (rubber gaskets, gloves)
Cobalt chloride, 1% pet; 0.02 mg/cm^2
Thiuram mix, 1% pet; 0.025 mg/cm^2 (rubber gaskets, gloves)
Epoxy resin, 1% pet; 0.05 mg/cm^2 (adhesives)
p-tert-Butylphenol–formaldehyde resin, 1% pet; 0.04 mg/cm^2 (adhesives)
Kathon CG (Cl + Me-isothiazolinone), 0.01% pet; 0.0040 mg/cm^2 (preservatives, hand creams)
Mercapto mix, 1% pet; 0.075 mg/cm^2 (rubber)
Black rubber mix (PPD mix), 0.6% pet; 0.075 mg/cm^2 (rubber, gaskets, weatherseals)
Paraben mix, 12% pet; 1 mg/cm^2 (hand creams)
Potassium dichromate, 0.25% pet; 0.023 mg/cm^2 (wet cement and concrete, leather gloves)
Nickel sulfate, 2.5% pet; 0.2 mg/cm^2 (hand tools)

Additional Allergens

p-Chloro-*m*-cresol, 1% pet (protective creams)
o-Cresyl-glycidyl ether (epoxy reactive diluent), 0.25% pet[36]
Dichlorophene, 1% pet (preservatives)
Euxyl K 400, 1% pet (preservatives)
o-Phenylphenol, 1% pet (cleaners)
p-Chloro-*m*-xylenol, 1% pet (preservatives)

Chloroacetamide, 0.2% pet (preservatives, hand creams)
Diethylthiourea, 1% pet (safety shoes)[410]
Phenol-formaldehyde resin, acid catalyzed, 5% pet (adhesives)
Phenol-formaldehyde resin, alkali catalyzed, 5% pet (adhesives)
Urea-formaldehyde resin, 10% pet (fiberboard glue)
Various wood dusts, 1% to 10% pet (see Chapter 31)[412, 562, 915, 1154]

COOKS

See Food Preparation Workers.

COSMETOLOGISTS

The term *cosmetologist* includes beauty operators, hair stylists, beauticians, and manicurists. Hairdressers or hair stylists apply bleaches, dyes, and tints to hair using an applicator or brush. Prior to applying tints, a patch test is suggested to determine if the customer is allergic to the solution. Unfortunately, this is rarely done, and, if so, the patch often remains on the skin for only 12 hours or less, too short a time to determine allergy in most instances. Currently there are approximately 70 substances used to color hair, but allergic reactions are not common and occur from only a few, most frequently from *p*-phenylenediamine and its relatives.[640] Para-type azo and anthraquinone dyes have been found to be the most likely contact sensitizers. *p*-Phenylenediamine and its derivatives continue to lead the list of the most common contact allergens for hairdressers' hands,[220] as well as clients'. In hairdressers with hand dermatitis, contact sensitization to Disperse Orange 3 and *p*-aminoazobenzene is also reported to be common.[1107]

Cosmetologists also shampoo and rinse hair with water that may contain vinegar and lemon juice. Allergic contact dermatitis is rare from shampoos, even in those who are formaldehyde sensitive.[808] Cosmetologists also massage and condition the scalp. They style the hair by blowing, cutting, trimming, and tapering using clippers, scissors, razors, and blow driers. They apply wave or straightening solutions, wind the hair around rollers or pin curls, or "fingerwave" hair (Fig. AP–10). The tips of the second and third fingers are often primarily affected by dermatitis from contact with wave solutions.[1170] Cosmetologists set the hair by blowing it dry under a hot air drier, by natural setting, or by pressing the hair with a straightening comb. They may apply lotions and creams to the client's face and neck to soften and lubricate the skin. They also perform other beauty services, such as massaging the face or neck, coloring eyebrows or eyelashes, and removing unwanted hair with depilatories (Fig. AP–11).

Hairdressers intermittently wear gloves, usually latex. Contact urticaria from natural latex is fairly common among hairdressers (see Chapter 6). Also common is contact dermatitis from the allergenic, heat-activated

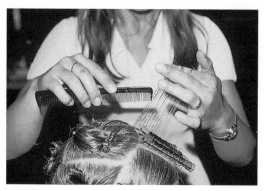

FIGURE AP–10 • Hairdressers apply wave or straightening solutions, wind the hair around rollers or pin curls, or "fingerwave" hair. The two major skin hazards are *p*-phenylenediamine and glyceryl monothioglycolate.

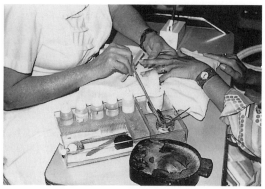

FIGURE AP–12 • The resins used to build artificial fingernails are complex acrylics, which can induce contact allergy in both operator and client.

permanent wave chemical glyceryl monothioglycolate, which readily passes through the operator's rubber gloves[1170] and remains on clients' hair for up to 3 months after application.[918] The contamination of the salon with this allergen is a significant factor in recurrence of dermatitis among hairdressers and is a major cause of disability, causing most affected operators to leave work entirely.[1234] Thiolactic acid (2-mercaptopropionic acid), which has also been reported to cause allergic contact dermatitis, has recently been recommended as a substitute for glyceryl monothioglycolate.[1173]

Antibacterials, necessary in personal care products, are found in numerous soaps and leave-on products such as hand creams. Chlorhexidine is widely used, and Ciba has recently patented a formulation that uses 10% triclosan.[719] Euxyl K 400 is a new, important allergen.

Common allergens among organic sunscreens are octyl methoxycinnamate and benzophenone-3. A new preservative is iodopropynyl butylcarbamate, which, because of its chemical structure, may prove to be a significant contact allergen and irritant.

Manicurists

Manicurists clean, shape, and polish customers' fingernails and toenails (Fig. AP–12). First, they remove any

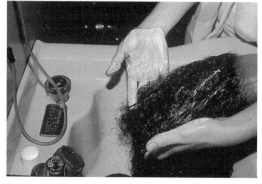

FIGURE AP–11 • Hair conditioner generously applied to lubricate the scalp and hair.

previously applied polish using an acetone-containing solvent on a swab. They shape and smooth the ends of the nails using scissors, files, and emery boards. They clean the customers' nails in soapy water using swabs, files, and orange sticks; soften the nail cuticle with water and oil; push back cuticles using a cuticle knife; and trim the cuticles using scissors and nippers. They may whiten the undersides of nails with white paste or pencil, buff the nails using powdered polish or buffer, and apply liquid polish and nail hardeners.

Toluenesulfonamide-formaldehyde resin, introduced in 1939, was until recently the most widely used resin for nail polish. Its monomers and dimers, however, are rather weak allergens when wet.[561] Liden et al.[787] and Tosti et al.[1207] have shown that even when dried the resin can cause clinical symptoms, usually dermatitis of the eyelids and neck from casual movements of the hand. Also, periungual dermatitis occurs more frequently than was previously recognized.[787] The currently popular substitute for toluenesulfonamide-formaldehyde resin is methyl acrylate, which Kanerva et al.[693, 694] have also reported as an allergic sensitizer.

Artificial nails are constructed by first applying fine linen or silk to the previously buffed nail plate, followed by an acrylic glue (often a cyanoacrylate). Additional glue is added, which rapidly hardens, and an artificial nail can then be "sculptured" by filing. The desired polish is then applied. The process is termed *nail wrapping* and is often used to strengthen the nails and repair splits. The resin Krazy Glue consists of 99.95% ethyl cyanoacrylate and is used to repair broken nails and attach preformed plastic nails. Although the resin dries and hardens almost immediately, it may cause allergic contact dermatitis not only in the clients but also in the manicurists.[72, 137, 427, 645] The dermatitis sometimes resembles small-plaque parapsoriasis.[1121] The resin has also been reported to cause periorbital dermatitis in a hair stylist attaching false hair to balding scalps.[1204]

While various methacrylate monomers have been recommended for artificial nails,[1049] in 1974 the FDA banned all artificial nail products containing methyl methacrylate monomer. Instead, longer chain methacrylate esters were used, such as ethyl methacrylate, and, although their sensitizing capacity may perhaps be somewhat less, they also have been found to be contact allergens.[686, 693] Koppula et al.[735] have suggested that a carboxy ethyl side group may be the prerequisite for development of allergic contact dermatitis to acrylates in artificial nails.

Dermatitis is especially frequent among young cosmetology trainees aged 16 to 21 years.[151, 830] Hairdressing is a poor career choice for individuals with a strong personal or family history of atopy, and young persons with this background should be counseled against choosing a career in cosmetology.[1310] Rystedt[1071] and Matsunaga et al.[870] have also reported a higher incidence of disabling dermatitis among hairdressers with atopic backgrounds. On the other hand, despite the fact that this work is very "stressful" to the skin and the high frequency of hand eczema among hairdressers, Majoie and Brunyzeel[830] failed to find a relationship to atopy or to prior nickel sensitivity.

The results of a multicenter study from Germany[997] in which 191 hairdressers were evaluated revealed contact allergy to nickel in 36.1%. Glyceryl monothioglycolate resulted in 34% positive reactions, heading the list of occupational allergens for hairdressers, with 10% of all patients tested and 20.7% of those with occupational contact allergy displaying sensitization solely to this common permanent wave chemical. The next most common allergens were the bleaching agent booster ammonium persulfate followed by the hair dyes *p*-phenylenediamine and *p*-toluenediamine. A coupling agent for the latter, pyrogallol, was demonstrated to be an allergen in 6.3% of cases.

In another large multicenter study of European hairdressers, glyceryl monothioglycolate was also the leading cause of contact allergy (19%), followed by *p*-phenylenediamine (15%) and the hair bleach ammonium persulfate and *p*-toluenediamine sulfate (each 8%) (see below).[446] In Spain, however, Conde-Salazar et al.[220] found positive patch test reactions to glyceryl monothioglycolate in only 3 of 111 hairdressers tested; *p*-phenylenediamine base and nickel accounted for the greatest number of allergic reactions.

For initial screening of hairdressers with suspected work-related allergic contact dermatitis, testing with *p*-phenylenediamine, glyceryl monothioglycolate, and formaldehyde has been suggested.[621]

Fragrance continues to be the most common cause of allergic contact dermatitis in cosmetics. The fragrance mix on the standard tray has been reported to detect between 50% and 80% of fragrance allergy.[277, 656, 762] Larsen et al.[761] reported that the fragrance mix co-reacts with 85.6% of positive responses to the fragrance ingredients on the U.S. standard tray. When Larsen et al.[761] added ylang ylang oil, narcissus oil, and sandalwood oil to the mix, the yield was increased to 94.2%; adding balsam of Peru increased it to 96%. In a study by Johansen et al.[656] the three most common allergens in the fragrance mix were geraniol, hydroxycitronella, and eugenol. Larsen et al.[761] and Johansen et al.[656] emphasize the importance of testing with the perfume actually used by the patient. It is also important to keep in mind that a fragrance may be composed of up to 300 separate chemicals, and, as yet, an ideal screening mixture for testing is not available. Artificial musks are

used in many fragrance formulations. Most of these are polycyclic musks, and new musk-like fragrances are currently being developed.[719] A review of fragrance reactions is given by de Groot and Frosch.[277]

Nickel allergy is also common among hairdressers.[706, 1271] Wahlberg[1272] believes that irritants in this work weaken the skin's barrier function and enhance penetration of various allergens, including and especially nickel, which is present in, for example, scissors, clips, pins, rollers, rods, and grips. Dahlquist et al.[256] and Brandao[107] have shown that permanent wave solutions release nickel from hair clips. Schubert and Prater[1099] have advised physicians to discourage young women with nickel allergy from becoming hairdressers. On the other hand, a recent study has found no correlation between nickel sensitivity and hand eczema in this occupation.[830]

In Europe, shampooing is done almost entirely by apprentices. Most Canadian and many American hairdressers shampoo throughout their careers, and hairdressers who experience repeated, even mild, episodes of irritant dermatitis, appear more readily to develop allergic contact dermatitis.[943] A strong sensitizer found in many shampoos is 3-dimethylaminopropylamine (3-DMAPA).[681] Cosmetologists may also be exposed to this allergen in hand cleansers. It should be kept in mind that hairdressers usually wash their clients' hair without gloves.

For more than 15 years minoxidil has been claimed to retard baldness in both men and women, and to treat alopecia areata. It is applied mostly by the clients themselves, but also by hairdressers. Although not common, allergic contact dermatitis has been reported.[20, 273, 1010] Veraldi et al.[1257] described a hairdresser with dermatitis localized to the fingers following application of minoxidil to the scalp of a customer with androgenic alopecia. Patch testing was positive with a 2% aqueous solution of minoxidil.

Ammonium persulfate is used as a "booster" or accelerator in hair bleaches, allowing less peroxide to be used and making lighter shades possible (e.g., "platinum blondes"). The use concentration ranges between 10% and 20% and is added separately from the tints. Anaphylactic reactions have occurred in some persons.[119, 190, 395, 1294] The mechanism appears to be histamine release in some patients, while in others it may be contact allergic urticaria. Scratch testing with ammonium persulfate should be done with caution, as it can lead to a severe asthmatic attack, syncope, and even death in highly sensitive persons.[125] However, in spite of such potentially serious consequences, reactions appear to be rare.[501]

Bleaching creams containing hydroquinone and its derivatives are commonly used to eradicate hyperpigmented areas, especially on the face. Although not common, allergic contact dermatitis may result from their use. Less well-known bleaching agents are bisulfites, used to fade dark blotches on skin and to bleach eyebrows.[970]

Henna, a red vegetable dye obtained from the leaves and stems of the henna plant *(Lawsonia inermis)*, is used worldwide for tinting hair and skin. The active ingredient is 2-hydroxy-1,4-naphthoquinone. Henna is sometimes mixed with indigo, beet, lemon, or walnut husk juice to give varying shades.[933] Immediate hypersensitivity reactions have been reported, consisting of angioedema, generalized urticaria, and wheezing.[240, 829, 1161] Whether the sensitivity is due entirely to the naphthoquinone or to other ingredients is unclear.[829] Occasionally henna is mixed with p-phenylenediamine, which in sensitive individuals can result in more severe, even fatal reactions.[511] In some Moslem cultures henna is also used for decorating the feet and other areas of skin. Considering its widespread use in this manner, contact allergic reactions are rarely reported.[975] Many young persons request hair colors that are considered "shocking," such as pink, bright yellow, and red. Some of these newer dyes have molecular weights around 200, which could have a greater tendency to sensitize; however, the molecular structure is patented. Although they may be more reactive than the common dyes, which have molecular weights from 800 to 1,000, lower concentrations are used.[719]

Studies have suggested that multiple myeloma is more common in female cosmetologists.[504, 573, 1156] Stasis dermatitis and varicose veins are common problems for cosmetologists, aggravated by the prolonged standing associated with this work.[573]

Over the last couple of decades there has been a trend toward use of "natural products" in cosmetics. There is a widespread belief that products labeled "natural" contain fewer harmful chemicals. In fact, most so-called natural products contain a large number of potential irritants and allergic sensitizers. For example, tree tea oil, from the leaves of *Melanleuca alternifolia* Cheel, a native of Australia, has been reported to cause contact dermatitis in patients using the oil for treating foot fungal infections, dog scratches, leg rashes, insect bites, and so forth.[725] The allergen appears to be D-limonene and can be patch tested at 1% in ethyl alcohol. The oil is found in a great many products, including cosmetics, lotions, suntan oils, deodorants, acne preparations, soaps, and household and laundry products.

Because of concerns over bovine spongiform encephalopathy (BSE), also known as "mad cow disease," the European Union in 1997 adopted a directive to ban cosmetic products containing tissues and ingredients derived from the encephalon, spinal cord, and eyes of cows, sheep, and goats. Specific regulations are planned for late June 1997. In the United States congressional committees are also considering measures to prevent an outbreak of BSE in the United States.[719]

A review of cosmetic preservatives is given by Fransway.[421]

Irritants[526]

Soaps, detergents, and shampoos
Wave solutions
Bleaches
Cuticle removers (potassium hydroxide and sodium hydroxide)
Organic solvents
Water (wet work)

Patch test to standard and vehicle preservative allergens, with special attention to the following.

Standard Allergens

Wool alcohols, 30% pet; 1.00 mg/cm² (creams and lotions, lanolin)
Balsam of Peru, 25% pet; 0.80 mg/cm² (cosmetics)[507]
Paraben mix, 12% pet; 1 mg/cm² (preservatives, weak sensitizers)
2-Mercaptobenzothiazole, 1% pet; 0.075 mg/cm² (rubber gloves)
Carba mix, 3% pet; 0.25 mg/cm² (rubber gloves)
p-Phenylenediamine, 1% pet; 0.090 mg/cm² (permanent hair dyes)[1095]
Mercapto mix, 1% pet; 0.075 mg/cm² (rubber gloves)
Thiuram mix, 1% pet; 0.025 mg/cm² (rubber gloves)
Formaldehyde, 2% aq; 0.18 mg/cm² (shampoos, germicidal agents, nail hardeners)
Fragrance mix, 8% pet; 0.43 mg/cm²
Kathon CG, 0.01% pet; 0.0040 mg/cm² (germicide in numerous skin care products and hair shampoos)[275, 405, 525, 949]
Quaternium 15, 2% pet; 0.1 mg/cm² (preservatives)
Nickel sulfate, 2.5% pet; 0.2 mg/cm² (tools)
Rosin (colophony), 20% pet; 0.85 mg/cm² (depilatory wax)

Additional Allergens

p-Aminoazobenzene, 0.25% pet[1107]
p-Aminodiphenylamine, 0.25% pet (hair dyes)[229, 501]
p-Aminophenol, 1% pet (hair dyes)[229]
Ammonium persulfate, 2.5% pet
Ammonium thioglycolate, 2.5% pet
Benzoyl peroxide, 1% pet
Bronopol, 0.5% pet
p-Chlorocresol, 1% pet (creams, lotions)
p-Chloro-m-xylenol, 1% pet
Chlorhexidine digluconate, 0.5% aq
Chloracetamide, 0.2%
Cinnamic alcohol, 2% pet
Cinnamic aldehyde, 1% pet
Cocamide diethanolamide (Cocamide DEA), 0.5% pet[1003]
Cocamidopropyl betaine, 1% aq (shampoos, shower gels)[279, 416]
Diazolidinyl urea (Germall II), 2% pet
Dimethylaminopropylamine (3-DMAPA) (surfactants and emulsifiers), 1% pet[681]
Disperse Orange 3, 1% pet[1107]
DMDM hydantoin, 2% aq
Euxyl K 400 (methyldibromoglutaronitrile), 0.5% pet[278] (preservative in numerous cosmetics)[449, 551]
Imidazolidinyl urea (Germall 115), 2% pet (preservatives)
Methyl, ethyl,[686] and butyl methacrylates, 5% pet (artificial nails)
Benzalkonium chloride, 0.01% aq (germicidal solutions)
BHA, 2% pet (antioxidant)[1206]
Bisphenol A, 1% pet

Bisphenol A dimethacrylate, 2%

Bronopol, 0.25% pet (preservatives)

Camphor, 10% pet (nail polish)

Captan, 0.25% pet (shampoos)[1265]

Chlorhexidine digluconate, 0.5% aq (cosmetic preservative)

Diazolidinyl urea, 1% pet (shampoos, hair preparations)[698]

Dimethyl-p-toluidine, 2% pet

DMDM hydantoin, 1% aq[275]

Ethyl cyanoacrylate resin, as is (allow to dry for approximately 15 to 20 minutes)[72]

Ethylene glycol dimethacrylate, 2% pet

Butyl methacrylate, 2% pet

Trimethylolpropane trimethacrylate, 0.1% pet

Diethlene glycol dimethacrylate, 0.1% pet

Tetraethylene glycol dimethacrylate, 2% pet

Triethylene glycol dimethacrylate, 2% pet[693]

Tripropylene glycol diacrylate, 0.1% pet[693]

Glyceryl monothioglycolate, 1% pet ("acid" permanent wave solutions)[918, 997, 1170]

Thiolactic acid, 1% pet (substitute for glyceryl monothioglycolate)[1173]

Hydroquinone, 1% pet (bleaches)

Sodium bisulfite, 1% aq (bleaches)[970]

Monotertiary butyl hydroquinone, 1% pet (antioxidant, lipstick)[183]

N-isopropyl-N'-phenyl-p-phenylenediamine (IPPD), 0.1% pet (rubber)

Lavender oil, 1% ethanol[109] (may induce hyperpigmentation[927])

L-limonene, 1% in ethyl alcohol[725]

D-limonene hydroperoxide, 0.5% pet[702]

Methyl heptine carbonate, 0.5% pet[1243]

Methyl methacrylate, 2% pet

Minoxidil, 2% aq[1257]

Monotertiary butyl hydroquinone, 1% pet (antioxidant in lipstick)[183]

o-Nitro-p-phenylenediamine, 2% pet (semipermanent hair dyes)

Oleyl alcohol, 30% pet (emulsifier)[503]

Orange oil, 2% pet (as in orange wood, as used by manicurists)[123]

m-Phenylenediamine, 2% pet (semipermanent hair dyes)

o-Phenylphenol, 1% pet (disinfectants, especially for counters, equipment, and so forth)

Propylene glycol, 10% aq (e.g., creams, lotions, nail polish)

Pyrogallaol, 1% pet (dyes)

Resorcinol, 2% pet (dyes)

Sorbic acid, 2% pet

Sudan III (Solvent Red 23), 1% pet (may crossreact with PPD)[871]

D-L-α-tocopherol (vitamin E), 10% pet[996]

p-Toluenediamine, 1% pet (permanent hair dyes)

Triclosan, 2% pet (widely used in soaps and cosmetics)

Tricresyl phosphate, 2% pet (nail polishes)

Ylang ylang oil, 2% pet (fragrances)[679]

Vitamin A acetate, 1% pet[92, 575]

DAIRY WORKERS

Dairy workers (including dairy field hands, dairy hands, and dairy helpers) feed cows and aid in calving, dehorning, and vaccination. They milk cows by hand or by milking machine and keep the barn, stalls, containers, and dairy equipment clean and sanitary. They may mix and blend feed for cows and keep dairy records. They frequently treat cows for various diseases such as mastitis and foot rot and for injuries such as cuts and bruises. They administer medications in pill and topical forms. They may spray the cows with insect repellents and drive the cows into baths of insecticides. Prior to milking they wash the udders of the cows. They clean the stalls and barns with disinfectants, which are often irritating and sometimes sensitizing. They may also perform other tasks such as maintaining gardens; painting barns, sheds, and fences; and plowing, cultivating, and so on.

Dairy workers may show skin reactions to the various irritants and allergens listed below. Bacterial and viral disease, fungal infections, and mite infestations are also commonly seen (see Chapter 5).

Irritants

Soaps and detergents

Disinfectants and germicidal agents

Medications (especially insecticides and dehorning compounds)

Water (wet work)

Ultraviolet light

Patch test to standard and vehicle preservative allergens, with special attention to the following.

Standard Allergens

Potassium dichromate, 0.25% pet; 0.023 mg/cm^2 (milk testing solutions[586, 632])

2-Mercaptobenzothiazole, 1% pet; 0.075 mg/cm^2 (rubber gloves, milking machines)[792]

Carba mix, 3% pet (0.25 mg/cm^2 (rubber)

Cobalt chloride, 1% pet; 0.02 mg/cm^2 (feed additives)

Wool wax alcohols, 30% pet; 1.00 mg/cm^2 (lanolin [anhydrous], creams, lotions)

Mercapto mix, 1% pet; 0.075 mg/cm^2 (rubber gloves, rubber on milking machines)

Black rubber PPD mix, 0.6% pet; 0.075 mg/cm^2 (rubber on milking machines)

Neomycin sulfate, 20% pet; 0.23 mg/cm^2 (feed additives, medications)

Thiuram mix, 1% pet; 0.025 mg/cm^2 (rubber gloves, rubber on milking machines)

Formaldehyde, 2% aq; 0.18 mg/cm^2 (disinfectants)

Nickel sulfate, 2.5% pet; 0.2 mg/cm^2 (tools)

Rosin (colophony), 20% pet; 0.85 mg/cm^2 (medications)

Additional Allergens

Ammoniated mercury, 1% pet (medications)

Animal feed additives (see section on Agricultural Workers)

Bacitracin, 20% pet

Benzalkonium chloride, 0.01% aq (disinfectants)

Chlorpromazine, 1% pet (medications)

Cinnamon oil, 0.5% pet (medications)

Coal tar, 5% pet (dust control oils)

Dichlorophene, 1% pet (disinfectants)

Euxyl K 400 (dibromodicyanobutane + phenoxyethanol), 1% pet (biocide, creams)

Menthol, 1% pet (medications)

o-Phenylphenol, 1% pet (disinfectants for floors, equipment)

Plant extracts (e.g., ragweed, poison ivy/oak, wild feverfew)

Tribromosalicylanilide, 1% pet (cleaning solutions)

Triclosan, 2% pet (soaps, detergents)

DENTAL PERSONNEL

Dentists

In addition to examining patients, dentists fill, extract, and replace teeth using rotary and hand instruments, dental appliances, medications, and surgical implements. They also design and fit bands and other orthodontic devices to straighten teeth. Rarely today do dentists clean teeth. Gloves, usually latex, are worn throughout the day by all chair dentists, with many changes.

Dental Hygienists

Dental hygienists remove calcareous deposits, accretions, and stains from teeth by scaling the accumulation of tartar from teeth and beneath the margins of the gums using a dental pick, rotating brush, rubber cup, and cleaning compounds. They apply medications to aid in arresting dental decay, and they also chart conditions of decay and disease for diagnosis and treatment by the dentist. They may expose and develop x-ray film, make impressions for casts, remove sutures and dressings, and administer topical anesthetic agents. They may place and remove rubber dams, matrices, and temporary restorations. They may place, carve, and finish amalgam restorations, as well as remove excess cement from surfaces of teeth. Gloves, usually latex, are worn during contact with patients.

Dental Laboratory Technicians

These technicians fabricate and repair full and partial dentures using hand tools, molding equipment, and bench fabricating machines. They position the teeth in a wax model and a specified plane of occlusal harmony, mold the wax around the base of the teeth, and verify the accuracy of occlusion using an articulator. They mold wax over the denture to form contours of gums using knives and spatulae and remove particles of plastic from the surface of the dentures using a bench lathe equipped with grinding and buffing wheels. They then cast plaster models of dentures using acrylics and molding equipment (Fig. AP–13). They fill cracks and separations with plastics, which are cured in pressure ports or ovens. The technicians then polish the metal, plastic, and porcelain surfaces to a specified finish using grinding and buffing wheels. They may solder gold and platinum wire to construct wire frames for dentures.

Acrylic dentures may be cured by heat or chemicals. (In the latter method the acrylic mixture is not always completely cured, and there can be residual monomer remaining on the surface that may persist up to 2 or 3 weeks, causing dermatitis in the denture wearer.) Almost all dentures are made of a mixture of acrylic monomer (methyl methacrylate) with a powder of polymethyl methacrylate. Acrylic denture materials have been recognized since 1954 as a cause of allergic sensitization.[377] It must be remembered that the acrylic monomer readily penetrates rubber and vinyl gloves. Technicians working with acrylates are especially likely to develop skin problems during the first months of work.[922] The so-called 4-H gloves, with three layers of fabric, are protective against acrylates for approximately 4 hours, but are cumbersome to wear and for many tasks impair dexterity.

Light-cured acrylic restoratives pose a potential hazard of allergic contact dermatitis for dental personnel.[1037] The most frequently used composite (mixture of filler and resin binder) materials are based on dimethacrylates such as BIS-GMA (2,2-bis[4-2-hydroxy-3-methacryloxypropoxyphenyl] propane) as the primary monomer and ethyleneglycol dimethacrylate (EGDMA), triethyleneglycol dimethacrylate (TEGMA), bisphenol-A-dimethacrylate, 2-hydroxyethyl methacrylate (2-HEMA), and methacrylic acid as diluents. This type can be polymerized by a peroxide/amine method or by UV light. When polymerization is accomplished chemically, benzoyl peroxide is usually the catalyst with dihydroxyethyl-p-toluidine as accelerator. Inhibitors such as p-methoxyphenol are added to prolong shelf life. UV stabilizers are phenyl-salicylate-glycidyl methacrylate and 1-hydroxy-4-dodecylbenzophenone. Dyes and pigments, usually inorganic metal oxides or sulfides, are added to color-match the restoration. Fillers such as lithium-aluminum silicate, barium glass, quartz, and barium-aluminum-silicate glass are also added.

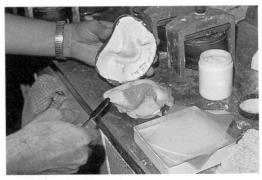

FIGURE AP–13 ● Dental technicians may cast plaster models of dentures using acrylics and molding equipment. The acrylics fill cracks and separations and the prosthesis is cured in pressure ports or ovens.

Acrylate allergy in dental personnel is becoming increasingly common.[1054] When allergic sensitivity develops, the prognosis for continued work is poor as relapses are difficult to avoid, and most workers must change occupations. A no-touch technique and adequate protective gloves are mandatory for all dental personnel, and careful and detailed instructions should be given to those new to the work.

The catalyst in the photo-polymerized systems is usually an ultraviolet-sensitive benzoin derivative such as benzoin-methyl-ether. The light is in the 320 to 365 nm UVA range. Shielding is accomplished with filters to eliminate radiation below 320 nm and stray, unfiltered radiation. A dental hygienist who was being treated for weeks for a chronic bladder infection with trimethoprim (a sulfa derivative) developed a widespread phototoxic facial eruption behind the ears and especially the submental area.[629] The dermatitis was associated with using BondWand for dental bonding, which emits UV at 400 to 500 nm. BondWand apparently was designed only for laboratory use, not for patients. Visible light is increasingly being used today for polymerization, having nearly replaced the original UV light curing systems. This is possible when a camphor quinone/amine catalyst is substituted for the benzoin-methyl-ether. Using visible light, the depth of polymerization is increased and is more complete.[23] Dental technicians and those who clean the work area are more likely to develop dermatitis from these materials than are dentists.

Epoxy resins are also used as sealants. The most durable of these are currently made of bisphenol A–glycidyl methacrylate (bis-GMA). Recent research has shown that when bisphenol A was fed to pregnant mice, the prostate glands of adult male offspring became 30% heavier than controls. Recently the National Institute of Dental Research and the American Dental Association have funded research to determine whether bisphenol A leaches from dental sealants and composites.[590]

For years, dental workers were at risk of exposure to significant levels of ionizing radiation,[1080] but radiodermatitis is today much less common than in previous years because the practice of holding the x-ray plate in the patient's mouth by the technician has been largely discontinued, and other protective measures are in place.

Because mercury has been used as a dental restorative material for more than 150 years, dental personnel have been at risk for poisoning from inorganic mercury. If amalgam mixing is not performed under strictly closed conditions, the office may be contaminated with significant amounts of mercury vapor (Fig. AP–14). Some dentists are said to still knead the amalgam mass in a mortar or even in their palms, squeezing the material by hand to rid it of excess mercury.[27] In the process mercury droplets fall to the floor, where they vaporize, particularly if they roll behind radiators.[496, 668] Mercury vapor is considered more toxic than inorganic and organic mercury compounds, except for methyl and ethyl compounds. Smoking cigarettes with mercury-contaminated hands may also be a source of exposure.[1178] Today the use of prepacked amalgam capsules has substantially reduced the hazard. Mercury is no longer a frequent contact allergen for dental personnel,[898] although

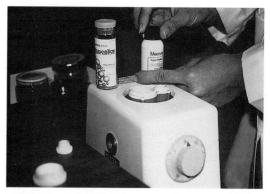

FIGURE AP–14 • Mixing mercury amalgam must be performed under strictly closed conditions, as shown in this illustration.

dentistry is still one of the largest users of mercury, including redistilled mercury.

Dentists are also exposed to a variety of infectious agents, especially the herpes simplex virus ("herpetic whitlow"),[664] but also streptococci, and hepatitis B and (probably) hepatitis C viruses. Acquired immunodeficiency syndrome (AIDS) is today a major hazard for dentists, dental hygienists, and their assistants, and measures must be taken to prevent its transmission.[1132] These include simple techniques such as using gloves, masks, and eye protection, as well as steam autoclave sterilization of dental instruments and strict attention to clean-up measures.[649] Three features of exposure to HIV seem to increase the likelihood of seroconversion: (1) deep injuries during exposure, as from instruments and needles; (2) the presence of blood on the penetrating device; and (3) exposure to a needle that had been in a patient's vein or artery. Seroconversion appears to be more likely when the source patient dies within 2 months after the exposure. Prophylaxis with a suitable medication following high-risk exposure is advisable.[908]

The wearing of latex rubber gloves, changing after each patient, has resulted in an increased incidence of acute contact urticaria due to latex, which can lead to life-threatening anaphylactic reactions[521, 1188, 1189, 1217, 1327] (see Chapter 6). The cornstarch powder in gloves appears to be a vehicle for the latex allergens, and it has been suggested that the complex antigen formed by the combination of latex and cornstarch may be more antigenic than the rubber alone and induce more serious reactions, including mucosal. Prepowdered gloves should not be used in dental offices.[69] In patients with latex reactions, the immunosorbent assay for serum latex-specific IgE is positive only in 20% to 30% of patients. However, skin prick and scratch testing is positive in most patients, but the risk of anaphylactic reaction is too great with this procedure, especially scratch testing, so that it should be performed only in offices with appropriate resuscitation facilities and trained personnel capable of handling such emergencies.[860]

Delayed-type contact allergy has been reported to natural rubber latex in the absence of sensitivity to the usual rubber accelerators and antioxidants.[1312]

Irritant dermatitis is common in dental personnel, as they wash their hands frequently and are in contact with potent contact irritants. Allergic contact dermatitis is also very common, which may develop from contact with the impression materials Impregum and Scutan, which are used for temporary crowns, bridges, and impressions.[1236] Kulenkamp et al.[739] found that the catalysts methyl dichlorobenzene sulfonate (for Impregum) and methyl-*p*-toluene sulfonate (for Scutan) are irritants as well as allergic sensitizers. The Impregum catalyst appears to be the more potent sensitizer.

Hindson[594] reported a dentist who developed dermatitis from contact with *o*-nitro-*p*-phenylenediamine from the dye of a patient's hair. Glutaraldehyde (Cidex-R and other brands) used for sterilizing the surfaces of counters, trays, instruments, and so forth is a very common sensitizer. It is also used for cold sterilization of instruments,[666] and it readily penetrates rubber gloves.[531] In a study of dental personnel from 1989 to 1994, glutaraldehyde was the second most common allergen.[1092] Patch testing at the usually recommended concentration of 1% (in petrolatum) may produce irritant reactions; a concentration of 0.5% is preferred.

Besides nickel allergy, sensitivity to palladium may occur[1249, 1251] and has been linked to oral lichen planus.[926] Sensitivity is uncommon, however, and often is found concomitantly with sensitivity to nickel and/or cobalt.[513] Titanium is a rare sensitizer, if at all.

Eugenol is also a fairly frequent allergen for dental personnel, as well as tetracaine, especially if the dentist applies the topical anesthetic to the gum with an ungloved finger,[453] which is almost unheard-of today (Fig. AP–15).

Toothpastes also may contain contact allergens,[1074] especially flavoring agents (e.g., cinnamic aldehyde, cinnamon oil, and peppermint). Preservatives include parabens and the isothiazolones.

Dentists often do not wear gloves when preparing temporary crowns, mixing resins, and so forth, donning them only for patient contact. Johnson and Mathias[657] suggested that the occlusive effects of gloves enhance

percutaneous absorption of methacrylate monomer, and so forth, thus more readily inducing allergic sensitization.

Irritants

Soaps and detergents
Wet work
Abrasives in polishing materials (pumice, plaster, silica, calcium carbonate)
Etching compounds (e.g., phosphoric acid)
Orthodontic plasters
Adhesives (epoxy and cyanoacrylates)
Coumarone-indene resins
Germicidal solutions
Resins and catalysts
Essential oils
Amalgam mixtures
Sodium hypochlorite
o-Phosphoric acid
Thymol-iodide (root canal sealer)
Solvents (alcohol, chloroform, methyl cellusolve)
Mechanical friction
Heat
X-rays

Patch test to standard and vehicle preservative allergens, with special attention to the following.

Standard Allergens

Potassium dichromate, 0.25% pet; 0.023 mg/cm² (fillings)
Wool alcohols, 30% pet; 1.00/cm² (lanolin, medications)
2-Mercaptobenzothiazole, 1% pet; 0.075 mg/cm² (rubber gloves, rubber bands, and rubber dams)
Balsam of Peru, 25% pet; 0.80 mg/cm² (medications, dental cement)
Caine mix, 3.5%² (topical anesthetics)
Cobalt chloride, 1% pet; 0.02 mg/cm² (metals)
Neomycin sulfate, 20% pet; 0.23 mg/cm² (medications, especially for root canal work)
Carba mix, 3% pet; 0.25 mg/cm² (rubber gloves, rubber bands, and dams)
Colophony, 20% pet; 0.85 mg/cm² (impression materials)
p-Phenylenediamine, 1% pet (clients' recently dyed hair)
Epoxy resin, 1% pet; 0.05 mg/cm² (bonding adhesives)
Fragrance mix, 8% pet; 0.43 mg/cm²
Mercapto mix, 1% pet; 0.075 mg/cm² (rubber gloves, rubber bands, and dams)
Ethylenediamine dihydrochloride, 1% pet; 0.05 mg/cm² (medications)
PPD mix (Black rubber mix), 0.6% pet; 0.075 mg/cm² (rubber gloves, rubber bands, and dams)
Thiuram mix, 1% pet; 0.025 mg/cm² (rubber gloves, rubber bands, and dams)
Formaldehyde, 2% aq; 0.18 mg/cm² (germicidal solutions and medications such as Formo-cresol)
Paraben mix, 12% pet; 1 mg/cm² (medications, toothpaste)

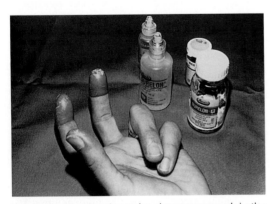

FIGURE AP–15 • Dentists today almost never work in the patient's mouth without wearing gloves. However, not long ago dentists who applied allergenic topical anesthetics to the gums without glove protection not infrequently developed a persistent, chronic allergic contact dermatitis of the fingertips.

Nickel sulfate, 2.5%; 0.2 mg/cm^2 pet (tools)

Rosin (colophony), 20% pet; 0.85 mg/cm^2 (impression materials, paste for gums, and soldering flux)

Thimerosal, 0.1% pet; 0.0080 mg/cm^2 (disinfectants)

Additional Allergens

Amethocaine (tetracaine), 5% pet (local anesthetics)[453, 1080]

Ammoniated mercury, 1% pet (amalgams)[27]

Benzocaine, 5% pet (often in gel at 20%)

Bisphenol A (in dental composite resin), 1% pet[662]

Cadmium chloride, 1% aq[1092]

Chlorhexidine digluconate, 1% aq (antiseptics)

p-Chloro-m-xylenol, 1% pet (antiseptics)

Methyl methacrylate monomer, 1% pet (dental materials)[377]

Cyclomethycaine, 5% pet (topical anesthetics; may crossreact with amethocaine)

Beeswax, 30% pet (impression materials)

Benzalkonium chloride, 0.01% pet (disinfectants)

Benzophenone, 1% pet (light absorber in plastic materials)

Benzoyl peroxide, 1% pet (caution: irritant[461])

Bronopol, 0.25% pet (medications)

Butanediol dimethacrylate, 2% pet

Cadmium chloride, 1% pet (caution: irritant[461])

Carnauba wax, as is

Chlorothymol, 1% pet (medications)

Cinnamic alcohol, 1% pet (toothpaste)

Cinnamic aldehyde, 1% pet (toothpaste)

Cinnamon oil, 1% pet (flavoring agent, antiseptic, medications, toothpastes)

Clove oil, 1% pet

Cresol, 1% pet (antiseptics)

N,N-dimethyl-p-toluidine 5% pet (catalyst)

Butyl acrylate, 0.1%

Ethyl acrylate, 0.1%

Eugenol, 1% pet (various dental materials)[816]

Eucalyptus oil, 1% pet

Glutaraldehyde, 0.25% to 0.5% pet (disinfectants, especially Cidex)

Gold sodium thiosulfate, 0.5% pet

Hexylresorcinol, 1% pet (medications)

Hydroquinone, 1% pet (photographic developer and fixer [Kodak]; inhibitor for acrylic resin systems)

2-Hydroxyethyl acrylate, 0.1%

2-Hydroxypropyl acrylate, 0.1%

N-isopropyl-N'-phenyl-p-phenylenediamine (IPPD), 0.1% pet (rubber)

Latex, ammoniated 1:10[1312]

MEK peroxide, 1% pet (catalyst for acrylic resin systems)

Menthol, 1% pet (medications, flavoring)

Mercury (metallic), 0.5% pet[27]

Methyl dichlorobenzene sulfonate, 0.5% pet (impression materials, Impregum catalyst)[239, 1236]

Methyl salicylate, 2% pet (toothpastes)

Penicillin, 1% pet

Procaine, 1% pet (anesthetics)

Methyl methacrylate, 2% pet[1054]

Ethyl methacrylate, 2% pet

N-butyl methacrylate, 2% pet

Ethyleneglycol dimethacrylate (EGDMA), 2% pet[1054]

1,4-Butanediol dimethacrylate, 2% pet

2-Hydroxyethyl methacrylate (2-HEMA), 2% pet (bonding agent)[697, 1054]

2-Hydroxypropyl methacrylate, 2% pet

Triethyleneglycol dimethacrylate (TEGMA), 2% pet

Trimethylolpropane triacrylate (TMPTA), 0.1% pet

Pentaerythritol triacrylate (PETA), 0.1%

Ethylene glycol dimethacrylate, 2% pet[657]

BIS-GMA (2,2-bis[4-2-(hydroxy-3-methacryloxypropoxy) phenyl] propane), 2% pet (acrylate restorative)[14, 689]

BIS-MA 2% pet (2,2-bis[4-(methacryloxy)phenyl]propane), 2% pet

BIS-EMA (2,2-bis[4-(2-ethacryloxyethoxy)phenyl]propane), 1% pet

1,4-Butanediol diacrylate (BUDA), 0.1% pet

1,6-Hexanediol diacrylate (HDDA), 0.1%

Urethane dimethyacrylate, 2% pet

N,N-dimethyl-4-toluidine, 2% pet

2-Hydroxy-4-methoxy-benzophenone, 2% (UV inhibitor)

Methyl dichlorobenzene sulfonate, 0.1% alc

Phenylmercuric acetate, 0.01% aq

Sodium thiosulfatoaurate, 0.5% (gold)

Thymol, 2% pet (antiseptics)

4 Tolyldiethanolamine, 2% alc

Urethane diemethyl methacrylate, 2% pet

Ammonium tetrachloroplatinate, 0.25% pet

Palladium chloride, 1% pet

DRY CLEANERS

Dry cleaners (including spot cleaners and spotters) operate dry-cleaning machines to clean garments, drapes, and other materials that cannot be washed in water without shrinkage or damage to the fabric. The following sequence of operations is used in the normal dry-cleaning procedure:

1. Soiled garments are marked and sorted.

2. Prespotting is performed when required.

3. Garments are rotated in a tumble-type centrifuge-type washer containing a dry-cleaning solvent.

4. The solvent is drained from the tumbler and most of the residue solvent removed by centrifugal extraction.

5. The small amount of remaining solvent is removed in heated driers.

6. Dirty solvent from the wash cycle is continuously passed through diatomaceous earth and activated carbon, or disposable cartridge filters, to remove as much of the dye and insoluble soil as possible and is recovered for future use.

7. The dry solvent–free garments are inspected and, if necessary, spot-cleaned a second time by hand.

8. The garment may be wet-cleaned at this point, but this step is usually omitted.

9. Clean garments are finished on suitable presses, puff irons, steam tunnels, or adjustable forms.

The *spotter* uses steam and air hoses, soap and water, various cleaning fluids, and brushes. Spots are removed from garments by treating the soiled area with a sponge or cloth saturated with a cleaning fluid or soap and water. The excess fluid and soap are then removed from the garment using a damp cloth, after which the garment is spread on a bench or table to dry. In another method the garment is placed on a padded table and steam forced through the padding and into the soiled area. Hot air is then circulated through the padding to dry the garment and prevent formation of cleaning rings. Special chemicals may be sprayed on or applied by hand to remove such substances as rust, blood, and wine stains.

The most common dry-cleaning solvent is perchloroethylene. Carbon tetrachloride, used for many years, has now been replaced by perchloroethylene. However, bottles of carbon tetrachloride and even benzene may be used surreptitiously and should be asked about. There have been claims that perchloroethylene may induce systemic scleroderma, as has been reported from vinyl chloride and certain other organic solvents.[1179] The greatest exposure to perchloroethylene, as measured by monitors, occurs when the operators load and unload the machines, when levels up to 2,000 ppm may be present. Stoddard solvent is also used, usually a fast-drying type with a narrow boiling range. Because Stoddard solvent is flammable, its use is restricted in some areas. A petroleum distillate similar to Stoddard solvent, called 140-Solvent because its flash point is 140°F, is available, but requires special equipment. A small amount of 1,1,1-trichloroethane is often used as a spotter, usually in closed systems. Note that hydrofluoric acid is widely employed to remove certain difficult stains, such as rust (as an "erusticator").[1163]

Many dry-cleaning establishments provide special services, such as repair of garments, dyeing, and water- and moth-proofing treatments. (Moth repellents include dichlorvos [DDVP], naphthalene, *p*-dichlorobenzene, and oil of cedarwood.) Many operators add optical brighteners and antistatic and sizing agents to improve the brightness and "feel" of a garment.

There are two major hazards in dry-cleaning work: flammability and toxicity. Although substitution of solvents with a higher flash point has reduced flammability during washing and extraction, they are less effective during tumbler drying when temperatures can be high. Stringent rules must be in place to minimize the possibility of explosion and fire. Adequate exhaust also must be present to prevent acute and chronic poisoning from retained vapors. Phosgene, a very toxic and corrosive gas, is produced when trichloroethylene or perchloroethylene vapors under certain conditions are exposed to high temperatures. The carcinogenicity of trichloroethylene and tetrachloroethylene has been shown in laboratory animals; in humans the exposure to dry-cleaning fluids may increase the risk of leukemia and liver cancer.[86]

Irritants

Cleaning substances of all kinds, especially grease removers and erusticators (especially hydrofluoric acid)[812]

Acids
Solvents (perchloroethylene)
Soaps and detergents
Steam

Patch test to standard and vehicle preservative allergens, with special attention to the following.

Standard Allergens

2-Mercaptobenzothiazole, 1% pet; 0.075 mg/cm^2 (rubber)
Carba mix, 3% pet 0.25 mg/cm^2 (rubber)
Mercapto mix, 1% pet; 0.075 mg/cm^2 (rubber)
PPD mix (Black rubber mix), 0.6% pet; 0.075 mg/cm^2 (rubber)
Thiuram mix, 1% pet; 0.025 mg/cm^2 (rubber gloves)
Formaldehyde, 2% aq; 0.18 mg/cm^2 (spotting agents)
Nickel sulfate, 2.5% pet; 0.2 mg/cm^2 (tools)
Rosin (colophony), 20% pet; 0.85 mg/cm^2 (certain soaps)

Additional Allergens

p-Aminoazobenzene, 0.215% pet (textile dyes)
Beeswax, 30% pet (rubbing compounds)
Disperse Blue 124, 1% pet[1107]
Disperse Orange 3, 1% pet (textile dyes, especially synthetics)
Disperse Yellow 3, 1% pet (textile dyes, especially synthetics)[1107]
Glyceryl ricinoleate, 20% pet (dry-cleaning soaps)[308]

See Textile Workers for additional dyes.

ELECTRICIANS

Electricians wire electrical fixtures, apparatus, and control equipment. They usually specialize in either construction or maintenance work. Construction electricians perform electrical work required in the building and remodeling of structures. They may plan new or modified installations. They measure, cut, thread, assemble, and install electrical conduits using hacksaws, pipe threaders, and conduit benders. They splice wires by stripping insulation from terminal leads with knives or pliers and twist or solder wires together, applying tape or terminal caps. They connect wiring to lighting fixtures and power equipment. They also install switches, relays, and circuit breaker panels, fastening them in place with screws or bolts using drills, masonry chisels, hammers, anchor bolts, and wrenches. After installing grounding leads they test the continuity of the circuits. They may occasionally pot materials using epoxy resin, and they often solder or weld.

Copper is increasingly being replaced by aluminum as a conductor. Aluminum is of poorer quality than copper; it requires a larger diameter of wire and shrinks to some extent with high voltages. It is difficult to join aluminum by soldering. The flux that is commonly used in soldering contains aminoethylethanolamine (hydroxyethyl ethylenediamine and fluorobate), which has reportedly caused dermatitis in cable joiners.[246] In Britain this chemical was later replaced by one less irritating and allergenic.

Epoxy resin sensitivity occurs with some frequency in electricians, especially in inexperienced workers, which emphasizes the need for detailed instructions on its safe use. Patch testing should be done with the resin actually used by the workers, in recommended and nonirritating dilution.

Because polychlorinated biphenyls (PCBs) were previously widely used in transformers, there has been concern that their toxic effects may pose a hazard for repair persons. A study of 55 transformer workers showed no classic PCB poisoning among those exposed, no neurobehavioral or irritant symptoms, and no chloracne.[331]

Irritants

Organic solvents
Epoxy resins and catalysts[950]
Hydrofluoric acid
Solvents
Antistatic agents[75]
Fiberglass
Soldering flux
Metal cleaners
Passivation of galvanized steel (after treatment with strong oxidizing agents)[128]

Patch test to standard and vehicle preservative allergens, with special attention to the following.

Standard Allergens

Potassium dichromate, 0.25% pet; 0.023 mg/cm² (welding fumes)
2-Mercaptobenzothiazole, 1% pet; 0.075 mg/cm² (rubber insulation and tape adhesive)
Carba mix, 3% pet; 0.25 mg/cm² (rubber insulation and tape adhesive)
Cobalt chloride, 1% pet; 0.02 mg/cm²
Epoxy resin, 1% pet; 0.05 mg/cm²
Mercapto mix, 1% pet; 0.075 mg/cm² (rubber insulation and tape adhesive)
PPD mix (Black rubber mix), 0.6% pet; 0.075 mg/cm² (rubber insulation and tape adhesive)
Thiuram mix, 1% pet; 0.025 mg/cm² (rubber insulation and tape adhesive)
Formaldehyde, 2% aq; 0.18 mg/cm² (phenolic resins, metal cleaners)
Nickel sulfate, 2.5% pet; 0.2 mg/cm² (hand tools)
Rosin (colophony), 20% pet; 0.85 mg/cm² (electrical insulating tape, soldering fluxes)
p-tert-Butylphenol–formaldehyde resin, 1% pet; 0.04 mg/cm² (leather in gloves, bonding agents)

Additional Allergens

Aminoethylethanolamine, 1% pet (soldering flux, especially for aluminum)[246]

Hydrazine sulfate, 1% pet (soldering flux)[1290]
N-isopropyl-N'-phenyl-p-phenylenediamine (IPPD), 0.1% pet (rubber)
Mercury, 0.5% pet (switches)
Phenol-formaldehyde resin, 10% pet
Polyethylene glycol dimethacrylate, 1% pet (anaerobic sealants)[224, 292, 867]
Triethylenetetramine, 0.5% pet (epoxy resin hardener)

ELECTRON MICROSCOPY WORKERS

These medical technicians are usually also histology technicians. They prepare tissues for examination and study, using a process similar to that used by the latter, but the imbedding material is often an epoxy resin. During the process, the technicians are exposed to a number of irritants and allergens,[655] especially epoxy resins and catalysts.[259]

Irritants

Acids (oxalic and chromic)
Solvents (xylene and others)
Propylene oxide (dehydrator and diluent for epoxy resin)[1244]
Glutaraldehyde
Formaldehyde
Osmium tetroxide (osmic acid)
Sodium citrate
Hydrochloric acid
Picric acid
Acrolein
Mercuric chloride
Freon 12 and 22
Acetone
Propylene oxide
Chloroform
Tetrahydrofuran
Dioxane
Potassium ferricyanide

Patch test to standard and vehicle preservative allergens, with special attention to the following.

Standard Allergens

Potassium dichromate, 0.25% pet; 0.023 mg/cm²
Epoxy resin, 1% pet; 0.05 mg/cm²
Ethylenediamine dihydrochloride, 1% pet; 0.05 mg/cm² (epoxy catalyst)
Formaldehyde, 2% aq; 0.18 mg/cm²

Additional Allergens

Diethylenetriamine, 0.5% pet (epoxy catalyst)
Triethylenetetramine, 0.5% pet (epoxy catalyst)
Dodecyl succinic anhydride, 0.5% acetone (epoxy catalyst)[486]
Glutaraldehyde, 0.25% pet (fixative)
Hydroquinone, 1% pet (photodeveloper)

Metol, 1% pet (photodeveloper)
Propylene oxide, 1% in ethanol[1244]
2,4,6-Tri(dimethylaminomethyl)phenol (DMP-30),
    0.1% pet (antioxidant)
Picric acid, 1% pet (fixative)
Mercuric chloride, 0.05% aq
Benzoyl peroxide, 1% pet
Beeswax, as is (embedding material)
Phenidone, 1% pet (photodeveloper)
Benzotriazole, 1% pet (photodeveloper)
Methyl methacrylate, 5% pet (embedding resin)
Butyl methacrylate, 5% pet (embedding resin)
Vinyl cyclohexene diepoxide, 0.25% pet(?)
    (embedding resin)[259]
Ethylene glycol diglycidyl ether, 0.25% pet
    (embedding resin)[259]

ELECTRONICS WORKERS

See Semiconductor Workers.

ELECTROPLATERS

Electroplating gives metal or plastic articles a protective surface and/or an attractive appearance. Plating metals include brass, bronze, cadmium, copper, chromium, gold, nickel (Fig. AP–16), silver, and tin. The object being plated is connected to one end of an electric circuit and placed in an appropriate solution; the other end of the circuit is connected to the plating material. By controlling the amount of electricity that flows from the plating material through the solution to the object being plated, electroplaters control the amount of metal applied to the final product. The process involves cleaning, pickling, rinsing, drying, inspection, and packaging in addition to electrolytic deposition. Sometimes dyes are used, especially in anodizing. The power sources depend on the operation and range from dry cell or storage batteries to disc rectifiers and large motor generators.

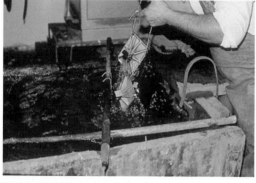

FIGURE AP–16 • During electroplating there is contact with the solutions from splashes and dripping from the parts. Here, the operator is removing plated objects from a nickel plating bath.

It is very important to clean the part first. Grease and dirt are removed by emulsion in organic solvents, in water with a wetting agent and alkali, or in aqueous alkaline solutions. Trichloroethylene and vapor degreasers or mixtures of water, kerosene, and soap are also used. The alkaline cleaners may be sodium hydroxide, sodium carbonate, sodium phosphate, and sodium silicate, and the solutions are usually very hot. Sometimes an electric current is applied to assist in the cleaning.

Pickling is usually required after cleaning to remove metal oxide from the surface. For this, acids such as sulfuric and hydrochloric acids are used. Certain mixtures give very bright finishes on metals and are termed *bright dips*.

Production platers tend the automatic equipment that conveys the metal objects through the cleaning, rinsing, and electrolytic plating solutions. They regulate the flow of electricity through the plating solution and control the immersion time of objects in the solutions, usually following written specifications. After adding water and other substances to maintain the mixture and level of the cleaning, rinsing, and plating solutions, the workers turn steam valves to maintain specific temperatures. They also maintain the plating conveyor parts, which includes lubricating them from time to time. They also may clean the plating and rinsing tanks, test the plating solution using a hydrometer or litmus paper, and take random samples for laboratory analysis. Fastening the metallic objects to hooks or racks or placing them in containers offers risk of skin and clothing contamination with the plating solutions.

A computer-controlled electroplating system that saves energy, boosts output, cuts pollution, and reduces the use of raw materials was developed by Bell Telephone Laboratories and Western Electric. The system is completely self-contained, carrying out all electrical and chemical processes in small, totally enclosed cells. The system permits almost no chemicals to evaporate into the plant or the air, greatly decreasing the risk of dermatitis and other injuries.

An electroplating technique that uses a laser to increase metal deposition over small areas was developed by IBM scientists. This technique makes it possible to produce small metal patterns in electronic circuitry, eliminating the need for the "masks" that are used in fabricating conventional photolithographic circuits. The cathodes used are tungsten molybdenum or nickel in layers approximately 0.1 μm thick, predeposited on glass substrates. The lasers are continuous-wave argon or krypton lasers. This techique is allegedly able to electroplate areas as small as 4 μm in diameter.[633]

Since its beginning in about 1920, chromium electroplating has utilized electrolysis of chromic acid with deposition of chromium on the plated components, which are usually steel- or zinc-based die casting, presurfaced with nickel and sometimes with a copper undercoat. A drawback to the use of hexavalent chromium electrolyte is that it must be heated to 40° to 50°C, generating an acid spray that is highly corrosive to the nose and throat, producing classic chrome ulcerations of the skin and mucous membranes called *chrome holes*. An exhaust system is absolutely necessary to protect workers from the fumes in these work areas. A chromium plating process based on trivalent chromium became available a number of years ago. Its advantages include the virtual elimination of the toxic, dermatitis-producing mist, creating more uniform metal deposition and automatically producing microcracked and microporous finishes.[806] The process is also said to be more economical and to permit easier disposal of the spent electrolytes. Widely used, it could eliminate many of the dermatological hazards of chromium plating.[165] However, the trivalent chromium is mildly corrosive at a pH of 2.5 to 3.4. The "purification reagent" contains 1% hydrazine.[165]

Most dermatitis among platers is due to irritants; airborne-type contact dermatitis from mists and steam is frequent. Atopics appear to be especially at risk of irritation, as from cyanide salts used in plating solutions.[861] Workers who develop chrome ulcers or nasal perforations are not necessarily allergic to chromate; in fact, most of them are not.[768] Burns due to chromic acid tend to be very chronic with persistent necrosis and to heal very slowly. The potentially lethal danger of percutaneous absorption must also be considered.[595] Mists from cadmium-containing electroplating baths have been considered possible sources of prostatic cancer in some workers.[956]

Gold sodium and potassium cyanide are especially irritating and probably should not be used for patch testing. Testing for gold sensitivity with potassium dicyanoaurate may result in negative results at the recommended test concentration of 0.002% pet and irritant reactions at higher concentration. Also, patch testing with gold chloride at 1% may also cause irritant reactions, and the reaction may persist for several months.[913, 1124] Goh[475] has recommended testing gold chloride at 0.5% aq. A reliable and now generally accepted nonirritating test preparation is gold sodium thiosulfate, used at a concentration of 0.5% in petrolatum.[414] There has been some doubt expressed about the reality of many reported gold sensitivity reactions, and it is likely that many reactions reported in the past were not allergic but irritative.[1017]

Irritants

Metal cleansers (alkaline soaks and alkalies such as sodium hydroxide, potassium hydroxide, sodium carbonate, trisodium phosphate; various solvents)
Heat
Pickling solutions (acids and dichromate)
Plating solutions (acids and alkalies)
Chromic acid (also fumes)[218, 595]
Cyanide plating solutions[861]
Heat
Abrasives
Solvents
Detergents
Dust from sandblasting prior to plating
Soaps and detergents

Patch test to standard and vehicle preservative allergens, with special attention to the following.

Standard Allergens

Potassium dichromate, 0.25% pet; 0.023 mg/cm² (plating solutions)
2-Mercaptobenzothiazole, 1% pet; 0.075 mg/cm² (rubber protective clothing)
Carba mix, 3% pet; 0.25 mgg/cm² (rubber)
Cobalt dichloride, 1% pet; 0.02 mg/cm²
Mercapto mix, 1% pet; 0.075 mg/cm² (rubber)
Ethylenediamine dihydrochloride, 1% pet; 0.05 mg/cm² (stabilizer, especially in copper plating)
PPD mix (Black rubber mix), 0.6% pet; 0.075 mg/cm² (rubber)
Thiuram mix, 1% pet; 0.025 mg/cm² (rubber gloves)
Formaldehyde, 2% aq; 0.18 mg/cm² (cleaning agent)
Nickel sulfate, 2.5% pet; 0.2 mg/cm² (nickel plating;[895] the first patch test with nickel was performed by Schittenhelm & Stockinger[1086])

Additional Allergens

Ammoniated mercury, 1% pet (mercury)
Coumarin, 5% pet (deodorant in plating baths)
Dioxane, 1% aq[430]
Gold sodium thiomalate, 0.1% pet (electroplating baths)[861]
Gold sodium thiosulfate, 0.5% pet[414]
Hydrazine sulfate, 1% pet ("purification reagent" in trivalent chromium plating solutions)
Platinum chloride, 1% aq
Sodium lauryl sulfate, 0.1% aq (cleaning baths)
Diethylthiourea, 1% pet (safety shoes)[410]
Triethanolamine, 1% pet

EMBALMERS

This category also includes funeral service workers. Embalmers prepare bodies for interment according to legal specifications. They wash and dry the body using germicidal soaps and towels or hot air driers. They insert convex celluloid or cotton between eyeball and eyelid to prevent slipping and sinking of the lid; depress the diaphragm to evacuate air from the lungs; join the lips using needle and thread or wire; and pack the body orifices with cotton saturated with embalming fluid to prevent escape of gases or waste matter. After making an incision in the arm or thigh using a scalpel, they insert pump tubes into the artery and drain blood from the circulatory system, replacing it with embalming fluid. They incise the stomach and abdominal walls and probe the internal organs, such as the bladder and liver, using a trocar to withdraw blood and waste matter and then attach the trocar to the pump tube, start the pump, and repeat probing to force embalming fluid into organs. Formaldehyde levels in the embalming room from the embalming fluid may show a level of 1 ppm or less.[572] Statistically significant excesses of malignancies of the lymphatic and hematopoietic system, including myeloid leukemia, and leukemia of other and unspecified cell types have been found in these workers. However, the excess malignancies of the lymphatic and hematopoietic systems could not be directly related to jobs held in the funeral industry.[572]

After closing the incisions using needle and suture, they reshape or reconstruct disfigured or maimed bodies using materials such as clay, cotton, plaster of paris, and wax. Embalmers dress the body, apply cosmetics, and place the body in a casket. They may also arrange funeral details, such as the type of casket or burial dress and place of interment, and keep records, such as itemized lists of clothing or valuables delivered with the body. The duties of embalmer and funeral director often overlap.

In recent years embalmers have been greatly concerned about infection with the AIDS virus and have instituted protective measures to guard against this and other infections. Because of the necessity to wear protective rubber gloves at all times during embalming procedures, contact urticaria to natural latex rubber gloves[959, 1188, 1189] may occur in this occupation, as may allergic contact dermatitis to the accelerators and antioxidants in rubber.

Erythema multiforme-like reactions have been reported from formaldehyde in a dissection-room worker.[53]

Irritants

Soaps and detergents
Water (wet work)
Hot air (driers)
Blood
Excreta (urine and feces)
Exudates
Embalming fluids
Formaldehyde
Plaster of paris
Waxes
Cleaning compounds for floors and walls
Phenol
Methyl alcohol
Radiation implants

Patch test to standard and additional allergens, with special attention to the following.

Standard Allergens

2-Mercaptobenzothiazole, 1% pet; 0.75 mg/cm² (rubber apparel and tubings)
Balsam of Peru, 25% pet; 0.80 mg/cm² (fragrances, cosmetics, deodorants)
Carba mix, 3% pet; 0.25 mg/cm² (rubber gloves)
p-Phenylenediamine, 1% pet; 0.090 mg/cm² (hair dyes)
Mercapto mix, 1% pet; 0.075 mg/cm² (rubber, as above)
Paraben mix, 15% pet; 1 mg/cm² (cosmetics)
Fragrance mix, 16% pet; 0.43 mg/cm² (cosmetics, deodorants, flowers)
PPD mix (Black rubber mix), 0.6% pet; 0.075 mg/cm² (rubber tubing)
Thiuram mix, 1% pet; 0.025 mg/cm² (rubber gloves)

Formaldehyde, 2% aq; 0.18 mg/cm² (embalming solutions)[619]
Quaternium 15, 2% pet; 0.1 mg/cm² (cosmetics)
Kathon CG (Cl + Me-isothiazolinone), 100 ppm aq; 0.0040 mg/cm² (cosmetics)
Nickel sulfate, 2.5% pet; 0.2 mg/cm² (tools)
Rosin (colophony), 20% pet; 0.85 mg/cm² (adhesives)
Wool (lanolin) alcohols, 30% pet; 1.00 mg/cm²

Additional Allergens

Ammoniated mercury, 1% pet (embalming fluids)
Methyl methacrylate monomer, 5% pet (reconstructive materials)
p-Aminophenol, 1% pet (hair dyes)
Benzalkonium chloride, 0.01% aq (germicidal solutions)
Beeswax, 30% pet (restorative waxes)
Bronopol, 0.25% pet (cosmetics)
Imidazolidinyl urea, 2% pet (cosmetics)
Camphor, 10% pet (deodorants)
Captan, 0.25% pet (cosmetics)
Chlorocresol, 1% pet (germicidal solutions)
Chlorothymol, 1% pet (deodorizers)
Cinnamic alcohol, 5% pet (cosmetics)
Dichlorophene, 1% pet (germicidal agents)
Eugenol, 2% pet (fragrances)
Flowers and other decorations, particularly chrysanthemums and ferns (see Chapter 31)
Glutaraldehyde, 0.5% pet (tissue fixative)
Euxyl K 400, 0.5% pet (preservative in cosmetics)
N-isopropyl-N-phenyl-p-phenylenediamine (IPPD), 0.1% pet (rubber, especially tubing)
Menthol, 1% pet (deodorants)
Methyl salicylate, 2% pet (deodorants)
Nitrophenylenediamine, 2% pet (hair dyes)
Phenylmercuric nitrate, 0.05% pet (germicidal agents)
o-Phenylphenol, 1% pet (deodorants)
Propylene glycol, 4% aq (cosmetics, embalming solutions)
p-Toluenediamine, 1% pet (hair dyes)
Triclosan, 2% pet (soaps, detergents)

ENGRAVERS

Engraving may be done by hand or machine on either hard or soft metals. Most engraving is done from copper plates, but iron, pewter, zinc, or silver may also be used. Hand engravers for soft metals do letter and ornamental designs on such items as silverware, trophies, aluminum or plastic eyeglass frames, and jewelry using engravers' hand tools. After brushing a chalk-like powder or solution on the object, they sketch the design in the powder; they sometimes use an inked rubber stamp. Then, after mounting the piece in a clamp-like device called a *chuck*, they fix the chuck in a jeweler's ball, a sort of rotating vice. The design is then cut using a chisel-like engraving tool. Punches, files, hammers, and shaping chisels are employed on hard metals. An anticorrosion agent may then be brushed over the surface of the metal.

Irritants

Anticorrosion paints
Etching acids
Paint removers
Solvents
Detergents
Adhesives (cyanoacrylates)[867]

Patch test to standard and vehicle preservative allergens, with special attention to the following.

Standard Allergens

Potassium dichromate, 0.25% pet; 0.023 mg/cm^2
  (etching compounds and anticorrosion agents)
Epoxy resin, 1% pet; 0.05 mg/cm^2 (adhesives)
Nickel sulfate, 2.5% pet; 0.2 mg/cm^2 (nickel-plated
  articles; "cold impregnation" of aluminum)[786]
Cobalt dichloride, 1% pet; 0.02 mg/cm^2

Additional Allergens

Gold sodium thiosulfate, 0.5% pet[414]
Ammonium tetrachloroplatinate, 0.25% pet (platinum
  jewelry)
Palladium chloride, 1% pet ("white gold" in jewelry)
Diethylenetriamine, 0.5% pet (epoxy catalyst)
Triethylenetetramine, 0.5% pet (epoxy catalyst)

FIREFIGHTERS

In addition to putting out fires, firefighters maintain the fire trucks and other emergency vehicles, operate engine pumping equipment, operate resuscitators, administer first aid, and maintain a clean and orderly environment in and about the firehouse. Frequently they prepare elaborate meals for themselves, rotating the duties of chef and kitchen help among their colleagues.

The greatest risk to firefighters in forestry is the dermatitis caused by poison ivy, poison oak, and poison sumac plants (see Chapter 31).

Irritants

Water (wet work)
Heat
Gasoline
Soaps and detergents
Polishes
Paints and solvents

Patch test to standard and vehicle preservative allergens, with special attention to the following.

Standard Allergens

2-Mercaptobenzothiazole, 1% pet; 0.075 mg/cm^2
  (rubber boots, hoses)
Carba mix, 3% pet; 0.25 mg/cm^2 (rubber)

Mercapto mix, 1% pet; 0.075 mg/cm^2 (rubber)
PPD mix (Black rubber mix), 0.6% pet; 0.075 mg/cm^2
  (rubber)
Thiuram mix, 1% pet; 0.025 mg/cm^2 (rubber gloves)

FLOOR LAYERS

Floor layers (including floor coverers and block layers) apply square strips or sheets of floor covering to floors, walls, and cabinets. They first disconnect and remove obstacles, such as radiators and light fixtures. After sweeping, scraping, sanding, or chipping dirt and irregularities from the surface and filling cracks with putty, plaster, or cement to form a smooth, clean foundation, they measure and cut the covering materials (which may be made of linoleum, vinyl, cork, or rubber) and also the foundation material (which may be made of felt or sponge rubber). They then spread adhesive cement over the floor and lay out the center lines, guidelines, and border lines on the foundation with chalk lines and dividers. They spread cement on the foundation material with trowels and lay the covering on the cement. Finally, the floor is rolled smooth to press the cement into the base and covering (Fig. AP–17).

When using solvent-based adhesives, protective clothing, including gloves and masks, should be worn. Even water-based adhesives are potentially harmful,[685] causing both allergic contact dermatitis and contact urticaria. Appropriate protective clothing should be worn and, as well, a "no-touch" technique used.

In patch testing with epoxy resins and hardeners it is important to test with the same product used by the patient in nonirritating concentrations.

Irritants

Dirt and dust
Putty, plastic, and cement
Adhesive cement
Solvents
Soaps and detergents

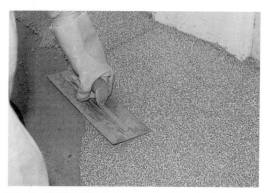

FIGURE AP–17 • The flooring material is mixed with an epoxy resin to create a hard surface. Here the floor is made smooth and even.

Floor strippers (sodium and ammonium hydroxides, monoethanolamine)

Patch test to standard and vehicle preservative allergens, with special attention to the following.

Standard Allergens

Potassium dichromate, 0.25% pet; 0.23 mg/cm^2 (cement, grout)

2-Mercaptobenzothiazole, 1% pet; 0.075 mg/cm^2 (rubber clothing, rubber knee pads)

Carba mix, 3% pet; 0.25 mg/cm^2 (rubber, as above)

Cobalt chloride, 1% pet; 0.02 mg/cm^2 (adhesive driers)

Epoxy resin, 1% pet; 0.05 mg/cm^2 (adhesives)

Mercapto mix, 1% pet; 0.075 mg/cm^2 (rubber, as above)

PPD mix (Black rubber mix), 0.6% pet; 0.075 mg/cm^2 (rubber, as above)

Thiuram mix, 1% pet; 0.025 mg/cm^2 (rubber gloves)

Formaldehyde, 2% aq; 0.18 mg/cm^2 (preservatives, synthetic resins)

Nickel sulfate, 2.5% pet; 0.2 mg/cm^2 (hand tools)

Rosin (colophony), 20% pet; 0.85 mg/cm^2 (adhesives)

p-tert-Butylphenol–formaldehyde resin, 1% pet; 0.04 mg/cm^2 (leather gloves, adhesives)

Additional Allergens

Methyl methacrylate monomer, 5% pet (adhesives)

Benzalkonium chloride, 0.01% aq (antistatic agent for carpets)

Dichlorophene, 1% pet (germicidal agent in carpet backing)

Disperse Orange 3, 1% pet (common colorant for carpeting; primary dye for nylon carpeting)

Disperse Yellow 3, 1% pet (common colorant for carpeting; primary dye for nylon carpeting today)

N-isopropyl-N'-phenyl-p-phenylenediamine (IPPD), 0.1% pet (rubber)

Isophorone diamine, 0.5% pet (catalyst in epoxy resin systems)[796]

Phenylmercuric nitrate, 0.05% pet (preservative)

Phenol formaldehyde resins, 5% pet

o-Phenylphenol, 1% pet (preservative)

Pine oil, 10% olive oil (wax strippers)

Polyfunctional aziridine (PFA) hardener, 0.5% pet[685]

Trimethylolpropane triacrylate (TMPTA), 0.1% acetone (hard plastic floor covering)[257] and aziridine hardener, Neocryl CX 100, 0.5% pet[535]

Urea formaldehyde resin, 10% pet

FLORISTS

Florists plan flower arrangements, select and trim the appropriate flowers and foliage, and prepare arrangements using wire, pins, floral tape, foam, trimmers, cutters, shapers, and so on. Not infrequently they pinch leaves and divide and break other plant parts by hand. They may decorate buildings, halls, churches, and other facilities. They pack and wrap completed arrangements

and estimate costs and prices. Contact hand dermatitis is common in this occupation, with the highest prevalence among designers and arrangers.[1197]

Over 95% of all cases of patch test–proven dermatitis reported have been caused by plants in a small number of families.[906] Dermatitis due to contact with chrysanthemums and other sesquiterpene lactone plants in the families Compositae and Magnoliaceae (Asteraceae) is very common.[55] The Compositae (Asteraceae) family is the second largest family and represents approximately 10% of the world's flowering plants.[1283] When patch testing is performed "as is" with sections of the plant of an unidentified culitivar, false-positive (irritant) and false-negative results are common. Depending on the species and season, using fresh plants in testing may sometimes result in severe bullous reactions, and plants collected in the spring may give greater skin reactions than do plants collected in the fall.[367] Patch testing has been recommended with sesquiterpene lactone and a Compositae mix (containing five Compositae plant extracts). Although this test material is probably adequate for routine screening, it is important to remember that as yet there is no completely reliable single screening mix.[976]

Schmidt and Kingston[1088] showed that all patients react to an extract of feverfew (*Tanacetum parthenium* Schulz-Bip) prepared by a relatively simple method described by Hausen.[546] This standardized test could be a useful and reliable method of diagnosing chrysanthemum allergy.

A plant commonly used for decoration in bouquets by florists is *Alstroemeria auranitiaca* Don (also *Alstroemeria ligtu* L.), commonly called "Inca lily" or "Peruvian lily." It is widely used on restaurant tables in the United States. The allergen tuliposide A (α-methylene-γ-butyrolactone) is identical to that in tulips[136] and hydrangeas.[126] Higher concentrations of tuliposide A are found in the flowers, leaves, and stalks of tulips than in the bulbs.[1142] On hydrolysis tuliposide A yields tulipalin A,[1142] which is patch tested at 0.01% pet.[136] Direct testing with the plant material may result in irritant reactions and active sensitization. Bruze et al.,[136] on the other hand, recommend patch testing with plant parts. Florists with allergic dermatitis due to tulips or the attractive, showy *Alstroemeria* may have considerable difficulty avoiding contact and usually must change occupations even when patch testing uncovers the culprit because in the workplace it is nearly impossible to avoid contact with the juice.[8, 74, 238, 848, 849, 901, 1046, 1047, 1065]

Contact urticaria with respiratory symptoms has also been reported from contact with tulips and lilies.[750]

The "English primrose" *Primula obconica* in the last decade has regained its past popularity in the United States and Europe. The dermatitis occurs more often at the end of the growing season, when the fading and dying leaves are plucked, resulting in dermatitis on the tips and sides of the fingers. Bedding the young, juicy plants in the spring is also a source of contact. Testing with the fresh leaves may result in irritant reactions or sometimes false-negative reactions (because of variation in amount of allergen in different parts of the plant). According to Hjorth,[598] false-negative reactions are potentially more serious because florists then believe they are not sensitive and continue to handle the plant. Hjorth[598] suggested that patients who are sensitized, even by patch testing, are fortunate because they can then avoid the plant. To avoid confusing irritant reactions it is probably safer to test only with synthetic primin available from commercial sources (Trolab or Chemotechnique Diagnostics).

Although contact allergy to orchids is uncommon, cultivation of these spectacular flowers is a frequent hobby of private fanciers. The allergen appears to be 2,6-dimethyl-1,4-benzoquinone[563] found in the stem juice of *Cymbidium* sp. Dermatitis has also been reported from *Cypripedium paphiodelium* in a commercial grower who pollinated the flower with bare hands, using a small brush to release pollen into the air.[809]

Workers sorting and trimming tulip, daffodil, hyacinth, and narcissus bulbs may develop irritant as well as allergic contact dermatitis.[127] Testing with α-methylene-γ-butyrolactone 0.01% in petrolatum is a reliable test material to confirm sensitivity.[136] Even the dust from hyacinth bulbs is a common cause of pruritus in these workers, especially atopics. The fungicide fluazinam used as a fungicide on bulbs may also cause allergic sensitization in workers handling the treated bulbs.[130] Chlorothalonil (also commonly known as Daconil and Bravo) is used as a plant fungicide and has been reported to cause contact urticaria in a plant nursery worker.[261]

Because of the frequent difficulty obtaining commercially prepared extracts of plants, Mitchell and Maibach[906] have recommended patch testing with the plants to which the patient was exposed. However, dried herbarium specimens cannot be used for this purpose. In testing with parts of a plant, the patient applies a lightly crushed piece of the plant 1 cm square to the forearm flexure, covering the site with a strip of paper tape. If irritation develops, the patch should be removed; otherwise it should remain for 24 hours, although Mitchell and Maibach[906] believe that even 4 hours may be sufficient for a reliable result to develop. It is important to remember, however, that patch testing with plants and plant extracts, especially in potentially irritant concentrations, can induce primary sensitization.[687] The "angry back" phenomenon is also common, especially when testing with multiple plants.[906] Furthermore, it is important not to test when any dermatitis is acute and actively spreading.

A review of allergic contact dermatitis caused by decorative plants, with suggested patch test concentrations, is given by Lamminpaa et al.,[755] who recommend testing with plant extract series available from companies manufacturing plant extract patch test allergens. For information on how to prepare plant extracts and how to test with plant materials themselves, consult Guin.[508]

Irritants

Soaps and detergents
Water (wet work)
Friction (twisting wires around stems)
Fertilizers

Herbicides and pesticides
Parasites
Irritating plants, plant parts, and juice

Patch testing to standard and vehicle preservative allergens, with special attention to the following.

Standard Allergens

2-Mercaptobenzothiazole, 1% pet; 0.075 mg/cm² (rubber)
Carba mix, 3% pet; 0.25 mg/cm² (rubber gloves)
Mercapto mix, 1% pet; 0.075 mg/cm² (rubber)
PPD mix (Black rubber mix), 0.6% pet; 0.075 mg/cm² (rubber)
Thiuram mix, 1% pet; 0.025 mg/cm² (rubber gloves)
Formaldehyde, 2% aq; 0.18 mg/cm² (disinfectants)
Nickel sulfate, 2.5% pet; 0.2 mg/cm² (hand tools)

Additional Allergens

Alantolactone (sneezeweed), 0.1% pet
α-Methylene-γ-butyrolactone, 0.01% aq (tulipalin A,[130, 132] tulips, narcissus, *Alstroemeria*)
2,6-Di-*tert*-p-cresol, 0.02% aq (stabilizer for tulipalin A)[132]
Phloroglucinol, 1% pet (preservative for cut flowers)
Bulbs (especially tulips, hyacinths, and narcissis)
English and Algerian ivy[553]
Ferns
Flowers (chiefly members of the Compositae family, such as chrysanthemums, marigold, pyrethrum, daisies, and others; also primrose *(Primula obconica), Alstroemeria,* hyacinths, tulips, nasturtiums[294, 296] and others (see Chapter 31)
Fluazinam, 0.5% pet (fungicide, a dinitro-*p*-toluidine compound)[132]
Laurus nobilis, 2% pet (laurel oil)
Parthenolide (feverfew), 0.1% pet
Philodendron *(Philodendron scandens)*, 0.1% to 0.005%, acetone extract[723]
Frullania (liverwort), piece of plant
Sesquiterpene lactone mix, 0.1% (useful for many Compositae plants)[55]
Compositae mix, 6.0% pet[552]
Primin, 0.01% pet (primrose, *Primula obconica*)

FOOD PREPARATION WORKERS

Food preparation embraces a number of occupations—fry cook, pastry cook, larder cook, kettle cook, railroad and ranch cook, short-order cook, and specialty cook. In addition to cooking, the occupation includes ordering food and other supplies and trimming, weighing, and washing meats, poultry, fish, and vegetables. Cleaning and a certain amount of paperwork are also required.

Dermatitis in the food industry has been studied extensively.[556] Hand dermatitis from immediate hypersensitivity among food handlers is frequent and commonly is misdiagnosed.[825] Persons with a history of eczema, asthma, and/or hay fever ("atopics") do very poorly in kitchen work, and it is advisable that they be counseled against this work when deciding on lifelong careers. They are more likely to experience immediate reactions (contact urticaria) to certain foods, such as seafoods, fruits, and vegetables.[527] A report of 50 caterers[243] revealed fish to be the most common cause of contact urticaria, while for allergic contact dermatitis garlic was most frequent and the only dermatitis exhibiting a recognizable diagnostic cutaneous pattern (on the tips of the first three fingers holding the garlic). Irritants are more common than sensitizers. In an Australian study,[428] seafood was found responsible for contact urticaria in 10 of 14 patients. In a classic study in 1976, Hjorth and Roed-Petersen[602] also found the major type I food allergens to be fish and shellfish, while the chief type IV allergens were commonly onion, garlic, and nickel from the metal tools used in preparation. Employing scratch tests with different fish products (fish juice from fillets, meat, skin, slime, juice from fish boxes and the hold of the fishing boats, and entrails), Halkier-Sorensen[519] found that all fish parts can cause irritant skin reactions, and the greater the postmortem age of the fish, the greater the irritation. Only the high-molecular-weight polypeptide fraction of fish juice seemed to produce symptoms.[518]

Peltonen et al.[991] reported more frequent occupational eczema in workers handling fish, meat, and vegetables than those making confectionery. Atopy again was a common background condition in many of these cases. Another important study was a retrospective analysis of 180 food handlers in Denmark,[1254] which emphasized that patients with type I protein dermatitis complained more often of a burning sensation than itching, appearing within minutes following contact.

Type I sensitivity to banana, chestnut, kiwi, papaya, peach, and avocado may be associated with immediate-type latex allergy.[88, 233] The presence of these sensitivities should alert physicians to the possibility of simultaneous latex rubber sensitivity and vice versa. Lahti and Hannuksela[751] recommend that when testing persons suspected of type I allergy, only the most fresh fruits and vegetables should be used. Anaphylactic antibodies have also been found in a patient with contact urticaria and anaphylactoid reactions to raw apples.[1001] White and Calnan[1293] also reported a nonatopic woman who experienced episodic swelling of the lips and tongue after eating apples. Raw potato may also be a cause of contact urticaria, first manifested with pruritus of the hands and fingers,[286] occurring in food preparation workers, especially atopics.[760] Atopy and exposure to latex are synergistic risk factors to latex sensitivity.[911] Coexistence of both types I and IV sensitization has been reported in occupational coffee allergy.[1212]

Cashew nut workers are susceptible to irritation and to the sensitizing ingredient cardol related to poison ivy/oak allergens.[846] The sensitizing potency of cardol is greatly reduced on heating.[298] Immediate hypersensitivity reactions to mustard and rape have been described in a cook,[885] and an anaphylactic reaction from the ingestion of mustard on a pizza was described by Panconesi et al.[972] A salad maker who had experienced recurrent hand dermatitis showed delayed hypersensitivity with a positive patch test to mustard; the dermatitis persisted for 2 years from contact with mustard contained in a salad cream and coleslaw.[262] Ingestion of peanuts has long been recognized as cause of immediate hypersensitive reactions, at times resulting in fatal anaphylactic reactions.

Garlic and onion are fairly common contact allergens.[1138] According to van den Akker et al.,[1229] the spices most commonly causing contact allergy are nutmeg, paprika, and cloves. Kanerva et al.[682] found the most frequent to be garlic, cinnamon, ginger, allspice, and clove. Goh and Ng[483] and Hata et al.[539] also reported allergic contact dermatitis from turmeric. Possible indicators of spice allergy are positive patch test reactions to colophony (rosin), balsam of Peru, fragrance mix, and/or wood tars.[1229]

In patch testing with spices, irritant reactions may occur if the concentration is too high. On the other hand, patch testing with spices is not performed often enough and should always be part of every patch test series for food preparation workers.[129] Because of the frequency of irritant reactions to spices, Kanerva et al.[682] recorded only 2+ and 3+ reactions as allergic. Prick testing and radioallergosorbent tests (RASTs) are adjunctive diagnostic measures for type I reactions, although prick testing must be performed with great caution and always with the availability of resuscitation measures, should a severe reaction occur.

Phototoxic reactions, which are often bullous and streaked, have been reported from furocoumarins in figs, parsnips, parsley, celery, and others. In celery, phototoxicity is enhanced by the present of the so-called pink rot fungus (Sclerotinia sclerotiorum), which has long been known to induce photodermatitis in field workers harvesting the vegetable.[82] Ordinary celery may also induce dermatitis, especially following UVA exposure from heavy sunbathing, tanning-salon exposure, and exposure to UVA by grocery clerks at check-out counters.[1112] Photodermatitis, so-called berlock dermatitis, can also be caused by the juice of the rind of the Persian lime Citrus aurantifolia, which is widely grown in south Florida and Mexico.[506] Phototoxic reactions often leave areas of hyperpigmentation, which are disfiguring and long-lasting.

Dermatitis from handling asparagus has been recognized for more than a century. Asparagus officinalis L. is cultivated throughout Europe, Asia Minor, Africa, and North America. White asparagus is produced by growing the plant under a fine silt of dirt, protecting it from sunlight, creating a tender white asparagus especially popular throughout Europe. When the stalks are peeled prior to cooking, the juice runs along the palm and volar wrist of the person holding the stem. Long suspected as containing one or more irritants,[74] investigation has revealed a sulfur-containing growth inhibitor, 1,2,3-trithiane-5-carboxylic acid, which is thought to be the contact sensitizer.[565]

Several reports have appeared of dermatitis from contact with gallate preservatives (propyl, octyl, and dodecyl gallate), which are widely used in foods, beverages, and washing powders.[94, 1232]

Sulfites used to maintain the appearance of freshness were challenged several years ago by the FDA, which proposed they not be allowed on "fresh" potatoes intended to be sold or served unpackaged and unlabeled at retail food establishments or institutions such as hospitals and nursing homes. Sulfite use in salad bars had been previously banned. These agents (usually sodium or potassium metabisulfite) are known to cause allergic-type reactions, including urticaria, itching, dizziness, nausea, diarrhea, dyspnea, and, in rare instances, anaphylaxis and death. According to an FDA report,[399] 1 million persons in the United States were estimated to be type I sulfite sensitive, most of them asthmatics. Contact, delayed-type hypersensitivity to sodium and potassium metabisulfite, although uncommon, has also been reported.[341, 929, 1256, 1262]

Young persons with acne often experience worsening of their condition when working in hot, grease-laden environments, as when "flipping" hamburgers.

Burns frequently occur in restaurant work. Grease burns from deep fryers are common, as when employees spill grease from a fryer while transporting the hot grease to a disposal bin or splatter grease while lowering food into a fryer. Hot grills, other cooking equipment, and boiling hot water and coffee are also responsible for many serious restaurant burns, most of which are preventable.[577]

Irritants

Vegetables and fruit juices (contact urticaria)[74, 599, 602]
Raw fish[518, 519]
Raw meats[381, 602] (benzylpenicilloyl polylysine, immediate reaction[269])
Garlic[74, 90, 105, 321]
Onion[74, 1237]
Leeks, chives, shallots
Spices
Moisture
Sugar
Flour
Heat
Soaps and detergents
Scouring pads

Patch test to standard and vehicle preservative allergens, with special attention to the following.

Standard Allergens

Hjorth[599] describes a battery of test materials for chefs and other kitchen workers.
2-Mercaptobenzothiazole, 1% pet; 0.075 mg/cm^2 (rubber gloves)
Carba mix, 3% pet; 0.25 mg/cm^2 (rubber gloves)
Mercapto mix, 1% pet; 0.075/cm^2 (rubber gloves)
PPD mix (Black rubber mix), 0.6%; 0.075 mg/cm^2 (rubber gloves)
Thiuram mix, 1% pet; 0.025 mg/cm^2 (rubber gloves)
Nickel sulfate, 2.5% pet; 0.2 mg/cm^2 (hand tools)

Additional Allergens

Asparagus juice, 10% pet (or 1,2,3-trithiane-5-carboxylic acid, 1% pet)[565]

Balsam of Peru, 25% pet (crossreacts with flavors)[599]
BHA, 2% pet (antioxidants)
BHT, 2% pet (antioxidants)
Cinnamic aldehyde, 1% pet (flavorings)[1288]
Cashew nutshell oil (nuts used as decoration for cashew nut ice cream)[848]
Cinnamon oil, 0.5% pet (flavoring)
Citrus peel (specific allergen unknown)[556]
Cocobolo wood, 10% pet (knife handles)
East Indian Rosewood (*Dalbergia latifolia* Roxb.) (methoxydalbergions), 1% pet (knife handles)[1002]
Flour (both type I and type IV allergy)[556]
Garlic, 10% aq[556] (The allergen diallyldisulfide is not yet commercially available. Campolmi et al.[196] recommend 0.5% allyl disulfide in vaseline. Mitchell,[902] however, states 10% concentration for patch testing with raw garlic is probably irritant.)
Onion, 10% aq
Chives, leeks, shallots, 10% aq (juice)
Lauryl gallate (also termed *dodecyl gallate*), 0.25% pet (antioxidant)[274]
Propyl gallate, 1% pet (antioxidant)[274]
Sodium metabisulfite, 1% aq (antioxidant for vegetables, especially potatoes and salads)[399]
Sorbic acid, 2% pet (antioxidants)

Spices Reported To Cause Irritant or Allergic Reactions

The following list is adapted from Hausen and Hjorth[556] and Dooms-Goossens et al.[307]

Basil	Mugwort
Bay leaf	Mustard
Capers	Nutmeg, mace
Caraway	Oregano
Cardamom	Paprika
Cayenne, chili pepper	Parsley
Cinnamon	Parsnip
Clove	Pepper
Coriander	Rosemary
Curry	Sage
Dill	Sesame
Fennel	Star anise
Ginger	Tarragon
Laurus nobilis	Thyme
Lovage	Turmeric
Mint, peppermint	

Condiments Used In Indian Cuisine That Most Often Cause Contact Dermatitis[1105]

Turmeric
Asafetida
Mustard seed
Coriander
Cumin
Red chilis

FOREST WORKERS AND LOGGERS

This group of workers includes those who protect, manage, and propagate forest tracts. They gather plants, barks, greens, saps, gums, and related products from the forest; they may operate forest nurseries and grow, harvest, and prepare Christmas trees for shipment and sale. They plant tree seedlings, cut out diseased, weak, or undesirable trees, and prune limbs of young trees using handsaws, powersaws, and pruning tools. They fell trees and clear brush from fire breaks using chainsaws, shovels, and engine-driven or hand pumps. They clear and pile brush, tree limbs, and other debris from roadsides, fire trails, and camp sites using an ax, mattock, or brush hook. Dermatitis from poison ivy/oak is very common among these workers. They also may spray or inject trees, brush, and weeds with herbicides using hand or powered sprayers or a tree injector tool. They also erect signs and fences using posthole diggers, shovels, tampers, or other handtools. In addition, they often clean kitchens, rest rooms, and campsites and other recreational facilities. They are also called on to fight forest fires, and they often plant trees to reforest timber lands.

The most common skin condition among foresters is contact dermatitis, predominantly due to sawdust[890] and sap, but also insect bites, mycotic infections, and staphylococcal and streptococcal infections are frequent.[1139] Tick bites are especially common, which may be associated with the development of Lyme disease. Recent research suggests that tick attachment of long duration, such as more than 72 hours, increases the chances of developing this serious disease.[1152]

Logging is the harvesting of trees. The initial task is cutting the tree down and cutting (bucking) it into logs for maximum product value and easier handling. Fallers, working singly or in pairs, use powersaws to cut down large trees previously marked by a forester. Expert fallers can drop a tree in the exact desired spot without injuring other trees. Buckers then cut off the limbs and saw the trunk into logs. Sometimes small trees are felled with tree harvesters, which are machines mounted on a tractor and operated by a tree shear operator. The next task is "skidding," a method of removing logs from a cutting area. A steel cable is noosed around a log by hooktenders (chockermen) and then attached to a tractor, which drags or skids the log to a landing. A rigging slinger supervises and assists the hooktenders and tractor drivers. In rough terrain where logs must be moved up or down steep slopes or across ravines another method is used: Steel cables are run from a diesel-powered winch through pulleys at the top of a large steel tower and down to the cutting area, which may be hundreds of feet away from the tower. Choke setters noose the end of the cable around a log and a yarder engineer operates the winch to pull the log into the landing. Other methods of moving logs include heavy-duty helicopters and balloons that lift logs and carry them to the loading site.

After the logs reach the landing they are loaded on a truck-trailer and hauled to a mill. A loader engineer operates the machine that picks the logs up and places them on a trailer. A second loader directs the positioning of logs on the trailer. Although trucks are usually used, logs are sometimes carried by railroad cars or are floated down a river.

Most hazards from logging are due to flying and falling objects; rolling logs; chainsaw accidents; slips, trips, and falls; and moving equipment. Sixty-seven percent of injuries in one study were caused by rolling or falling logs.[617] The isolation of logging camps from hospitals and major trauma centers aggravates the hazards. Insect bites, mycotic infections, and infections caused by staphylococci and streptococci are common.[1139] The vibration syndrome is frequent in chainsaw operators, especially in cold weather, when typical episodes of "white fingers" may occur. Cigarette smoking greatly aggravates this condition.[869]

Contact allergic dermatitis from exposure to liverwort (*Frullania*) on the tree bark is common in forest workers and loggers ("woodcutters' eczema"[904]). The eruption often begins around the wrists and spreads up the forearms, also involving the face. The cause is one or more of the sesquiterpene lactones found in various plants. Workers who fell the trees are often affected, but those planting trees can also become sensitized.[509] Hooktenders and others who drag the trees out of the forest with chains are also often affected.[903] On patch testing, reaction to *Frullania* is nearly always present, and most workers also react to alantolactone (0.1% pet); approximately three-fourths may also be positive on testing with D-usnic acid. Most affected workers are forced to leave forest work or change to truck driving or other occupations where there is no exposure to wet vegetation. Mitchell[903] does not recommend pre-employment screening with *Frullania* because of the likelihood of sensitization. Thune[1199] and Thune and Solberg[1200] report that aromatic lichen acids are ultraviolet-absorbing chemicals and thus able to induce photosensitization. Mitchell,[903] however, was unable to confirm this.

Preservatives are necessary to protect timber against fungi and insects. The chemicals in common use are listed later under Additional Allergens.[1169, 1309]

Irritants

Friction
Heat
Wet work
Preservatives
Stains
Parasites
Pesticides
Fungicides
Bark removers (chloracetaldehyde)[1011]
Sawdust
Vibration syndrome in chain saw operators
Caterpillars and moths (in Douglas fir), ants, spiders, snakes

Patch test to standard and vehicle preservative allergens, with special attention to the following.

Standard Allergens

2-Mercaptobenothiazole, 1% pet; 0.075 mg/cm² (rubber)
Carba mix, 3% pet; 0.25 mg/cm² (rubber gloves)

Mercapto mix, 1% pet; 0.075 mg/cm^2 (rubber)
PPD mix (Black rubber mix), 0.6% pet; 0.075 mg/cm^2
(rubber)
Thiuram mix, 1% pet; 0.025 mg/cm^2 (rubber gloves)
Nickel sulfate, 2.5% pet; 0.2 mg/cm^2

Additional Allergens

Atranorin, 0.1% pet[1200]
Frullania (liverwort; see Chapter 31)
Poison oak/ivy
D-usnic acid, 0.1% pet (lichens)[905, 1200]
Alantolactone, 0.1% pet
Atranorin, 0.5% pet
Evernic acid, 0.1% acetone[1200]
Pentachlorophenol, 3% pet (fungicide)
Captafol (Difolatan), 0.1% pet (fungicide)[1169]
Sawdust (e.g., jelutong wood[890, 1139]), 5% or 10% pet
Tributyl tin oxide, 0.01% aq (fungicide)[1309]

FOUNDRY WORKERS

Foundry workers (pattern makers, hand molders, sand mixers, core makers, core oven tenders, core setters, furnace operators, and others) make the metal castings that are essential for thousands of products from missiles to cooking utensils. Nearly all metals can be molded. The most common type of mold is made of sand and clay packed over the face of a pattern, forming a cavity in which the casting is to be made. The unit is enclosed in a mold box, which must be strong enough to resist the pressure of molten metal but sufficiently permeable to permit the escape of air and other gases. The mold is made in two halves, each contained in its own box. The pattern must be designed so that the half-mold can be lifted from the mold material without breaking or tearing its surface. Sometimes the mold is strengthened by oven baking or bonding with synthetic resins.

Approximately three-fourths of foundry workers work in iron and steel foundries and the remainder in plants that cast nonferrous metals, such as aluminum, bronze, copper-based alloys, and zinc. Modern foundries are highly automated, and most have good ventilating systems to reduce heat, fumes, dust, and smoke.

Foundry workers are subject to burns from hot metal and cuts and bruises from handling metal castings. Molten metal burns are often deep and may not be immediately recognized as such by emergency department or industrial physicians. These burns can be very serious and are responsible for much expense and time lost from work.[672] The injury rate in foundries is very high, much higher than in manufacturing. Silicosis has also been reported, as well as asthma from methylene di-*p*-phenylene isocyanate. Carbon monoxide exposure is also a hazard in foundries.

The sand most commonly used in foundry work is silica sand, but zircon, chromite, and chrysolite sand may be used. The sand is mixed with oil (often a linseed oil substitute) and casting clay, bentonite, and various resins in a drier. The resins may be phenol,

urea, or furfural formaldehyde resins, or rosin based, or methylene di-*p*-phenylene isocyanate, and the drier may be cobalt naphthenate. For years hexamethylenetetramine has been used as a hardener for phenolformaldehyde-type resins used in the core molding process. Hayakawa et al.[569] reported a foundry worker with allergic contact dermatitis caused by this hardener.

Chromium in foundry sand has been reported as a cause of hand dermatitis in foundry workers.[629] Burrows[163] reported the amount of hexavalent chromium in foundry sand to be approximately the same amount as contained in concrete and cement.

Powders may be manually added to molten steel, and, when poured into an ingot mold at the high melting point temperatures, the atmosphere can become very dusty, resulting in considerable pruritus with excoriations from sharp-edged particles.[743]

Irritants

Heat
Water (wet work)
Dust
Sand
Soaps and detergents
Resins
Compressed air
Vibration
Solvents
Acids
Lime
Ultraviolet light

Patch test to standard and vehicle preservative allergens, with special attention to the following.

Standard Allergens

Formaldehyde, 2% pet; 0.18 mg/cm^2 (phenolic resins)
Nickel sulfate, 2.5% pet; 0.2 mg/cm^2 (tools)
Cobalt chloride, 1% pet; 0.02 mg/cm^2 (foundry sand, driers)
Potassium dichromate, 0.25% pet; 0.023 mg/cm^2 (foundry sand)
Rosin (colophony), 20% pet; 0.85 mg/cm^2 (foundry sand)

Additional Allergens

Hexamethylenetetramine, 1% pet (coupling agent for phenolic resins)
Methylene di-*p*-phenylene isocyanate (foundry sand resin), 1% pet
Phenol-formaldehyde resin, 10% pet (foundry sand resin)
Diethylthiourea, 1% pet (safety shoes)[410]
Urea formaldehyde resin, 10% pet (foundry sand resin)

FUNERAL DIRECTORS

See Embalmers.

FUR PROCESSORS

The processing of fur varies with the type of fur, but in general the procedure is composed of these steps: (1) cleaning and softening the pelt, (2) removing the fleshy material from the skin (fleshing), (3) stretching, (4) tanning, (5) dyeing, (6) removal of guard hairs by hand or machine, and (7) shaping and sewing into a garment. A final cleaning completes the procedure.

The pelts are received from the trappers with much of the fat and subcutaneous tissue removed, and they usually have already been stretched and air dried. The skins are then soaked for several hours in a salt solution. Remaining particles of flesh and fat are removed with extremely sharp hand or power knives, a process known as *fleshing*. The operator prepares tanning solutions according to formulas and places the pelts first in a revolving drum containing a solution of aluminum potassium sulfate (alum) acidified with hydrochloric or sulfuric acid. The pelts are then dried, and, after as much liquid as possible is removed, they are treated with an oil to soften them prior to dyeing.

Fur dyeing is a very old art, but with the development in the last century of modern dyes and dye techniques, the process has become very sophisticated. The fur is first treated with a mildly alkaline solution and then soaked in a mordant such as ferric sulfate. After soaking in the desired dye, they are rinsed repeatedly and dried by tumbling with sawdust. The dyes used are carefully guarded secrets, but they include the entire gamut of textile dyes. *p*-Phenylenediamine (known as Ursol in the industry) was once a common fur dye, but is rarely used today.

Fur blenders tint and dye furs according to specifications by applying liquid dyes to the tips of guard hair (tipping) or to all surface hair, using a feather or brush to produce lustrous finishes and to accentuate colors and shades. They may spray the dye onto the furs using a spray gun or apply stripes using a feather brush or spray gun. After dyeing, the furs are trimmed and made even, perhaps stretched, and then sewn into the desired garment. Fur farming today is almost entirely occupied with mink production, with a small amount of chinchilla husbandry. Scandinavia, Russia, and the United States are the principal producers.

With the breeding and husbandry of animals in captivity, the risk of transmission of animal diseases to humans has been much reduced. Anthrax is still a possibility, but it is rare today. Numerous irritants are present, including acids, alkalis, alum, chromates, bleaching agents, oils, salt, and the various dyes and mordants. The bales of pelts may be treated with a dusting powder, which can irritate the skin of those unpacking the furs prior to processing.

Irritants

Soaps and detergents (and other cleaning agents)
Solvents (used for cleaning)
Alkalis
Alum
Formic acid
Boric acid
Softening agents (surfactants)
Fats and flesh (rancid or decayed)
Sulfuric acid
Salt
Chrome
Oil
Dust
Ammonia
Lime
Mordants
Dyes
Oxidizing agents

Patch test to standard and vehicle preservative allergens, with special attention to the following.

Standard Allergens

Potassium dichromate, 0.25% pet; 0.023 mg/cm² (tanning agent)
p-Phenylenediamine, 1% pet; 0.090 mg/cm² (rarely used today, but may cross-react with other dyes)
Formaldehyde, 2% aq; 0.18 mg/cm² (tanning agent)

Additional Allergens

p-Aminoazobenzene, 0.25% pet (dyes)
p-Aminophenol, 1% pet (dyes)
Glutaraldehyde, 0.25% pet (tanning agent)

GLAZIERS

Glaziers install glass in window skylights, store fronts, display cases, building fronts, interior walls, ceilings, and table tops. They also install stained glass windows and assemble and install metal-framed glass enclosures for showers. First they mark the pattern on the glass, then cut the glass using glass cutters. Excess glass is broken by hand or with a notched tool. The glass pane is then placed in the sash with a glazier's points, and putty is spread and smoothed around the edges of the panes with a knife to seal the joints. Mirrors or structural glass may be installed using mastic screws or decorative moldings. Glaziers may place a plastic adhesive film over the glass or spray the glass with tinting solutions to prevent light glare. In making stained glass windows, epoxy resin may be used to laminate the pieces of glass, causing dermatitis in some workers.[587]

One of the most important occupational injuries among glaziers occurs from using hydrofluoric acid in etching solutions (see Chapter 1). Aluminum window frames may be cleaned with a blancher containing ammonium bifluoride. Edema of the fingertips and loss of sensation in the fingers, with shedding of the nails, was reported by Pedersen.[985] Glaziers may also use cutting fluids to cool diamond cutting edges. These have skin hazards such as oil folliculitis and eczematous eruptions, including allergic contact dermatitis. Plain soap and water are often used for cooling.

Richter et al.[1028] reported two employees of a glass works with contact allergy to sodium selenite, which is used as a glass coloring agent. Testing was done at 0.1% pet. Arsenic has been employed in the manufacture of crystal. The powder, the exact composition of which is often highly secret, may contain arsenic salts to facilitate the melting of the powder. During mixing, contact dermatitis may occur; testing is done with sodium arsenate 1% aq.[59]

Leucoplakia of the mucous membrane of the oral cavity has been observed in workers in a glass factory ("glass blowers' white patch").[120]

Irritants

Cutting fluids
Etching compounds ("Diamond Ink," a mixture of
   hydrofluoric acid, barium sulfate, and fluoride salts)
Putty
Dusts
Solvents
Detergents
Moisture
Cleaners
Sealants

Patch test to standard and vehicle preservative allergens, with special attention to the following.

Standard Allergens

2-Mercaptobenzothiazole, 1% pet; 0.075 mg/cm^2
   (rubber in mastic)
Cobalt chloride, 1% pet; 0.02 mg/cm^2 (driers, putty)
Mercapto mix, 1% pet; 0.075 mg/cm^2 (rubber, as
   above)
PPD mix (Black rubber mix), 0.6% pet; 0.075 mg/cm^2
   (rubber, as above)
Thiuram mix, 1% pet; 0.025 mg/cm^2 (rubber gloves
   and as above)
Formaldehyde, 2% aq; 0.18 mg/cm^2 (glass cleaners)
Nickel sulfate, 2.5% pet; 0.2 mg/cm^2 (hand tools)
Rosin (colophony), 20% pet; 0.85 mg/cm^2 (adhesives)
Thimerosal, 0.1% pet; 0.0080 mg/cm^2 (preservatives)

Additional Allergens

Ammoniated mercury, 1% pet (mirror silvering)
Dichlorophene, 1% pet (preservative in putty)
N-isopropyl-N'-phenyl-p-phenylenediamine (IPPD),
   0.1% pet (rubber seals)
Phenylmercuric nitrate, 0.05% pet (preservatives)
Polysulfide sealants, 1% pet (Thiokol)[1311]
Sodium selenite, 0.1% pet[1028]
Sodium arsenate, 1% aq[59]

HEALTH CARE WORKERS

This category includes physicians, podiatrists, nurses, respiratory technicians, dialysis workers, physiothera-pists, x-ray technicians, and hospital cleaning persons. Dentists, dental personnel, and veterinarians are discussed in separate sections.

Because the work is well known, a work description is not given. Most dermatitis in health care workers is due to irritation, especially in cleaning personnel.[530, 1137] Those with a history of atopic dermatitis develop more severe hand eczema than do individuals with only atopic mucosal symptoms or persons with no atopic history. Wet work in hospitals greatly increases the chances of developing dermatitis, especially in atopics; nursing staff and kitchen workers/cleaners are at greatest risk.[953]

Contact urticaria to natural rubber latex of rubber gloves has been an increasingly serious problem for health care workers during the last decade or so.[889, 959, 1188, 1189, 1216, 1219] Some cases appear to be IgE mediated,[50, 447, 1218, 1329] but not all.[1189] The conditon is much more common than previously believed; atopy and pre-existing hand dermatitis seem to favor its development.[15, 722] The powder in gloves may enhance the development of contact urticaria by acting as a carrier of the latex allergen.[1203] The reaction to natural latex may be very severe and lead to life-threatening anaphylaxis.[981, 1233] On the other hand, a significant number of those afflicted continue to work with relatively mild symptoms.[1189] Nonlatex gloves must be provided these persons; however, it is important to remember that some gloves considered to be free of natural latex in fact may have a lining of natural latex.[588] Powder-free gloves are less likely to induce this reaction, whereas applying a protective hand cream before donning the gloves *increases* the likelihood of a reaction.[70] So-called hypoallergenic gloves may contain an inside coating of natural latex, which can be added to reduce the greater cost of the synthetic rubber, and its presence may not be noted on the glove package.[588]

The rubber elongation factor (REF) of the tree *Hevea brasiliensis* may be the major allergen in latex. If this complex protein could be removed, the cause of these sometimes life-threatening reactions might also be eliminated.[252]

Ethylene oxide is used widely for sterilization of medical supplies and pharmaceuticals.[772] If the articles sterilized are not sufficiently aerated, severe burns can result from their use. Surgical gowns and drapes,[83] anesthesia masks,[748] and prepacked nitrofurazone dressings[524] have been reported to induce severe burns when not subjected to an aeration phase following sterilization. Furthermore, engineering controls and safe work practices are equally important to reduce exposure to this irritant/carcinogen.[616, 1164] Engineering controls are more effective.[324]

Numerous opportunities exist for development of contact allergic sensitization.[217] Contact delayed hypersensitivity to rubber gloves is very common, usually to the accelerators tetramethylthiuram mono- and disulfide and carbamates.[347] Although probably uncommon, contact delayed allergic sensitization to natural latex itself has been reported.[775, 1312]

Important also are medications and germicidal agents as causes of dermatitis. These include glutaraldehyde in respiratory and dental technicians,[415] formaldehyde,

Kathon CG, imidazolidinyl urea, Euxyl K, Glyoxal (ethandial),[325] and quaternium 15. Airborne glutaraldehyde exposure appeared to be related to episodes of asthma in a respiratory technician.[206] Sensitivity to thimerosal, when due to the thiosalicylic fraction, may result in concomitant sensitivity to piroxicam gel among physiotherapists.[39] Patch test reactions to thimerosal are common and often severe; patients found sensitive to thimerosal probably should be warned about use of piroxicam topically, and perhaps even systemically, in treatment of arthritis. (As of 1996, topical prioxicam is not available in the United States.) Contact allergic dermatitis due to the biocide Parmetol K 40 (identical to Kathon CG), from its use as a germicidal agent in developing tanks, has been reported in a radiology technician.[977]

Contact allergy to topical corticosteroids, often overlooked, is increasingly common. It is more frequent among patients with chronic eczema with coexistent hypersensitivity to ingredients of topical medications.[299, 505] Patch testing should be done with the steroid used by the patient, as well as with tixocortol pivalate and budesonide.[313] Studies have shown that tixocortol pivalate and hydrocortisone contact allergies are associated, and reactions to budesonide can be correlated with reactions to both the acetonide and ester groups of corticosteroids. Therefore, both should probably be used in patch testing to detect corticosteroid sensitivity.

For years sterilization has been done with ultraviolet radiation. The light intensity for bactericidal and fungicidal action has been 254 and 300 to 400 nm ultraviolet.[1331] Usually personnel are not exposed, but if they are, exposure should be limited, especially in fair-skinned persons. Ultraviolet radiation is also used in management of many dermatological disorders. Studies have shown that a hospital staff may receive UVB and UVC (actinic) doses in excess of the recommended maximum permissible limits for occupational exposure, but UVA doses may be well within normal limits.[759] Repeated exposure to ultraviolet radiation may lead to actinic skin changes and the later development of squamous cell, basal cell, and melanocytic carcinomas.

Forty years ago penicillin, sulfonamide drugs, and mercurial antiseptics were common causes of sensitivity, but today these medications are less frequently used topically. Neomycin, streptomycin, and related drugs, as well as isoniazid and chloramphenicol, occasionally induce sensitization.[1007a]

Certain injectable drugs are possible causes of allergic contact dermatitis—thorazine and related drugs administered by psychiatric nurses, for example. The dermatitis first appears on the hand holding the vial while drawing the drug up into a syringe, usually a leaky one. In right-handed individuals, it first appears on the left hand, which results from droplets splashing onto the fingers.[408] Injectable aminophyllin, which contains ethylenediamine, may induce dermatitis in ethylenediamine-sensitive patients.[258, 389] Although the reactions to povidone-iodine cleansing agents are usually irritant, allergic contact dermatitis has been reported.[25, 850]

Dialysis workers are exposed to several irritants and contact allergens, especially formaldehyde and glutaraldehyde.[415] The latter is frequently used as a cold sterilizing solution for endoscopes and other instruments. It is also a component of some x-ray developing fluids. Exposure is greatest when it is poured into tubs and used for manual cleaning and sterilization of endoscopes, with the potential for splashes and inhalation of vapor.[770]

Morgue attendants and tissue technicians are also exposed to formaldehyde and glutaraldehyde. Dermatitis may be induced in highly sensitive persons merely by being present in a room where containers of formaldehyde and glutaraldehyde are left open.

Nurses counting tablets of methenamine may develop dermatitis on the fingertips caused by the release of free formaldehyde from the tablets in the presence of acid sweat. Nurses counting tablets of the antihypertensive captopril may develop contact dermatitis.[319] Nitroglycerine tablets have also been reported to cause contact allergy.[692]

Soaps and detergents are uncommon causes of allergic sensitization. The germicidal agent chlorhexidine is occasionally responsible.[1130] Benzalkonium chloride, a common disinfectant, has been reported as a cause of contact allergic reactions in surgical personnel.[1270] Alcohol-impregnated swabs have been implicated as a cause of dermatitis in a few patients.[1250]

Sensitivity to nitrogen mustard may develop in persons applying topical nitrogen mustard to treat mycosis fungoides. Personnel who apply Sulfamylon (mafenide acetate, α-amino-p-toluenesulfonamide monoacetate) to patients with burned skin may also develop contact allergic dermatitis. On the other hand, silver sulfadiazine (Silvadene) appears to have no contact sensitizing potential.[272, 1227] Rasmussen[1019] found four patients with positive patch tests to a silver sulfadiazine-propylene glycol ointment, but the allergen appeared instead to be the propylene glycol.

Orthopedic surgeons may become sensitized to methyl methylacrylate in bone cement during fixation of prostheses during hip and knee operations. The acrylic monomer readily penetrates rubber gloves.[989] Nurses mixing bone cement during the operations have developed dermatitis.[704] Glutaraldehyde, a potent antiseptic widely used for cold sterilization of medical and dental equipment, is a common contact sensitizer.[415, 666] It readily penetrates rubber gloves.[485, 531] Fisher[387] reported a radiologist and assistant in whom contact allergy developed to glutaraldehyde present in the x-ray developer.

Occupational vitiligo developed in a darkroom assistant in a hospital x-ray department from dipping films with bare hands in a developer containing hydroquinone.[264]

Quinidine sulfate tablets have been reported as an allergic sensitizer in nurses counting tablets.[413, 1274]

Infections of various kinds are a constant threat to medical personnel.[342] The threat of AIDS is a major problem for medical personnel today, as are hepatitis B and C and syphilis. Exposure to aerosol particles as well as penetration and leakage of masks during surgical procedures such as dermabrasion and skin peeling are important sources of infection to consider.[1286] Scabies is an ever-present risk, especially in nursing home personnel, who have close contact in the care of patients.[13]

Cutaneous tuberculosis in recent years has been increasing in frequency; evaluation of PPD-positive workers who received a BCG vaccination previously is difficult. Some of these workers had prior disease, but a considerable number of the positive reactions may be related to the BCG vaccine received in another country.[1114]

Health care workers are at risk for accidental needlesticks, which are a common occurrence, especially during use and clean-up procedures. Most of the needle injuries seem to occur during recapping after use.[628] A proposed solution is to redesign the standard needle cap to include a large-diameter funnel-shaped shield at the mouth of the needle to assist in recapping. Scabies and herpetic infections are also common in medical personnel.[664, 1091] Halothane, a bromine-containing trifluoroethane, has been reported to cause acne in personnel administering anesthetics.[510, 1153]

Chinese medicinal materials are increasingly used today, not only by nontraditional practitioners. Because the ingredients are "natural" substances, many people consider them safe. However, side effects, including hepatic toxicity and renal damage, have been reported, some of them fatal. The most common cutaneous reactions are irritation and allergic contact dermatitis; also increasing in incidence are immediate allergic reactions and, occasionally widespread, systemic contact dermatitis. Topical analgesics and antiinflammatory compounds, especially those containing a fragrance, are the common causes of sensitization.[776]

Irritants

Soaps and detergents
Alcohol
Medications
Ethylene oxide[1131]
Plaster of Paris (*o*-phenylphenate as a cause of contact urticaria[1214])
Water (wet work)
Ultraviolet light
Infrared light

Patch test to standard and vehicle preservative allergens, with special attention to the following.

Standard Allergens

Potassium dichromate, 0.25% pet; 0.023 mg/cm^2 (chromic sutures)
Wool alcohols, 30% pet; 1.00 mg/cm^2 (creams, lotions)
2-Mercaptobenzothiazole, 1% pet; 0.075 mg/cm^2 (rubber)
Neomycin sulfate, 20% pet; 0.23 mg/cm^2 (medications)
Balsam of Peru, 25% pet; 0.80 mg/cm^2 (physiotherapy preparations)
Carba mix, 3% pet; 0.25 mg/cm^2 (rubber)
Mercapto mix, 1% pet; 0.075 mg/cm^2 (rubber)
Ethylenediamine dihydrochloride, 1% pet; 0.05 mg/cm^2 (medications)
Balsam of Peru, 25% pet; 1 mg/cm^2 (physiotherapy preparations)

PPD mix (Black rubber mix), 0.6% pet; 0.075 mg/cm^2 (rubber)
Thiuram mix, 1% pet; 0.025 mg/cm^2 (rubber)
Formaldehyde, 2% aq; 0.18 mg/cm^2 (disinfectants)
Nickel sulfate, 2.5% pet; 0.2 mg/cm^2 (hand tools, skin clips)
Thimerosal, 0.1% pet; 0.0080 mg/cm^2 (Piroxicam gel)[39]

Additional Allergens

Ammoniated mercury, 1% pet (medications)
Bacitracin, 20% pet
Benzocaine, 5% pet
Benzoyl peroxide, 1% pet (catalyst for acrylic bone cement)
Benzylkonium chloride, 0.01% aq (disinfectant)
Chloramphenicol, 2% pet
Chlorhexidine, 0.5% enthanol[969, 1278]
Chlorpromazine, 1% pet
p-Chloro-*m*-xylenol, 2% pet (EKG electrode jelly)
Dichlorophene, 1% pet (germicidal agent in cast materials)
Glutaraldehyde, 0.25% pet (disinfectant, especially in dialysis and endoscopic apparatuses)[415, 485, 531, 666, 770]
Glyoxal (ethandial) (disinfectant), 2% (wt/wt) aq[325]
Latex (ammoniated), 1:10[1311]
Isoniazid, 2.5% aq
Methyl methacrylate monomer, 5% pet (orthopedic bone cement)
Nitroglycerin, 0.5% to 2% pet (tablets and transdermal patches)[692]
Penicillin, 1% pet
Procaine, 1% pet
Streptomycin, 1% pet
Sulfamylon, 5% pet
Tetracaine, 5% pet
4,4'-Thiobis(6-*tert*-butyl-*m*-cresol) (Lowinox 44S36, antioxidant in certain latex gloves), 1% pet[1025]

Corticosteroid Patch Test Series

Tixocortol pivalate, 1% pet (sufficient for screening series)
Budesonide, 1% in ethanol (sufficient for screening series)
Hydrocortisone, 1% pet
Hydrocortisone-17-butyrate, 1% in ethanol
Amcinonide, 1% in ethanol
Fluocortin butyl, 1% in ethanol
Clobetasol propionate, 1% in ethanol
Triamcinolone acetonide, 0.5% in ethanol

HIGHWAY CONSTRUCTION WORKERS

Highway construction involves not only concrete and asphalt paving, but also operation of heavy equipment and earth-moving machinery, welding, and other activities. The use of asphalt involves completely different hazards from those associated with concrete. The asphalt used in paving is a viscous material that must be heated to a fluid consistency before mixing with various aggregates such as stones and gravel. The smoke that rises for a few seconds when the hot mix is being dumped on the surface is composed of carbon monoxide, nitrogen dioxide, sulfur compounds, ozone, aldehydes, and various hydrocarbons. Burns and irritation of the skin and eyes are common, and photosensitivity (phototoxic) reactions frequently follow, as well as hyperpigmentation from the greenish-yellow fumes of the boiling asphalt. Actinic damage is also frequently seen. Rosin, sometimes used in road asphalt, may induce allergic sensitization. Highway construction workers are also exposed to dermatitis-producing plants such as poison ivy/oak, as well as to ticks, fleas, mosquitoes and snakes. Vibration effects from powered hand tools and heavy equipment are common (see sections Air Hammer Operators and Asphalt Workers).

Irritants

Hot asphalt (actinic damage)
Water (wet work)
Lasers
Dusts

Patch test to standard and vehicle preservative allergens, with special attention to the following.

Standard Allergens

Potassium dichromate, 0.25% pet; 0.023 mg/cm^2
  (concrete)
Cobalt dichloride, 1% pet; 0.02 mg/cm^2
2-Mercaptobenzothiazole, 1% pet; 0.075 mg/cm^2
  (rubber)
Epoxy resin, 1% pet; 0.05 mg/cm^2 (resins)
Mercapto mix, 1% pet; 0.075 mg/cm^2 (rubber)
PPD mix (Black rubber mix), 0.6% pet; 0.075 mg/cm^2
  (rubber gaskets, weather seals)
Thiuram mix, 1% pet; 0.025 mg/cm^2 (rubber)
Formaldehyde, 2% aq; 0.18 mg/cm^2 (phenolic resins)
Nickel sulfate, 2.5% pet; 0.2 mg/cm^2 (hand tools)
Rosin (colophony), 20% pet; 0.85 mg/cm^2 (asphalt
  additive)

Additional Allergens

Diethylthiourea, 1% pet (safety shoes)[410]
Coal tar, 5% pet (photosensitization)
Poison ivy/oak and other plants

HISTOLOGY TECHNICIANS

The histology technician usually receives tissues already fixed in formaldehyde, and the technician then dehydrates the tissue by immersion in acetone or alcohol. After a specified period, the specimen is placed in paraffin or imbedded in some other plastic material

until it is ready for processing. Frequently, specimens are frozen with carbon dioxide gas for immediate analysis. Either way, the prepared specimen is inserted into a microtome in which very thin slices are removed and then stained with a variety of stains. The tissue is then mounted on microscope slides and delivered to the pathologist for evaluation. Histology workers (including tissue technologists and medical technologists) also prepare and maintain the reagents, paraffin, stains, and various solutions according to standard formulas.

Mathias and coworkers[866] described a histology technician with hand dermatitis who also had associated symptoms of nausea, diarrhea, and persistent paresthesias of the fingertips. Patch testing to hydroxyethyl methacrylate was positive and reproduced the gastrointestinal symptoms. Vinyl gloves failed to impede the passage of the resin onto the skin.

Because of the considerable exposure to formaldehyde in these workers, the risk of nasal cancer must be considered. Holmstrom and Lund[618] have reported malignant melanoma of the nasal cavity in a histology technician.

Irritants

Formalin
Xylene
Epoxy resin
Nitrocellulose adhesives
Stains
Inks
Cellusolve
Alcohol
Carbon dioxide gas
Acetone
Water (wet work)
Acids (oxalic acid, chromic acid)

Patch test to standard and vehicle preservative allergens, with special attention to the following.

Standard Allergens

2-Mercaptobenzothiazole, 1% pet; 0.075 mg/cm^2
  (rubber)
Carba mix, 3% pet; 0.25 mg/cm^2 (rubber gloves)
Cobalt chloride, 1% pet; 0.02 mg/cm^2 (stains)
p-Phenylenediamine, 1% pet; 0.090 mg/cm^2 (stains)
Epoxy resin, 1% pet; 0.05 mg/cm^2 (adhesives)
Mercapto mix, 1% pet; 0.075 mg/cm^2 (rubber gloves)
PPD mix (Black rubber mix), 0.6% pet; 0.075 mg/cm^2
  (rubber gloves)
Thiuram mix, 1% pet; 0.025 mg/cm^2 (rubber gloves)
Formaldehyde, 2% aq; 0.18 mg/cm^2 (fixative)

Additional Allergens

Congo red, 2% pet (stains)
Glutaraldehyde, 0.25% aq (fixative)[237]
Gold sodium thiomalate, 0.1% pet (gold stains for
  Langerhans' cells)[670]

Hydroxyethyl methacrylate, 5% pet (imbedding plastic)[866]

D-limonene hydroperoxide, 0.5% pet (cleansers, alternative to xylene)[702, 758]

Picric acid, 1% aq (van Gieson's stain)

Sudan III (C.I. No. 26100) (stain), 2% pet

Sudan IV (C.I. No. 26105) (stain), 2% pet

HOUSEWORKERS

Housework comprises a multitude of jobs, most of which are related to food preparation and cleaning. Workers may be supervisors, such as butlers, but usually they are houseworkers or housewives. Soaps and other cleaning agents are well-known irritants. The irritant potential of detergents appears in part to be determined by their content or anionic detergent, as well as by the temperature of the solution.[213] The home is a minifactory that contains some very irritating substances and a few strong sensitizers. For example, some toilet bowl cleaners contain hydrochloric acid in a concentration of 23 to 25%, which is highly irritating to the skin. Drain cleaners often contain alkali, usually sodium hydroxide, in very high and corrosive concentrations. Some laundry products contain sodium fluorosilicate, a corrosive agent. Formaldehyde, in concentrations of 35%, may be present in toilet deodorants. This concentration is very irritating and can be highly sensitizing. In Europe, household bleach may contain sufficient chromate to induce dermatitis.[368, 745] In sampling household bleaches popular in the United States, an amount of hexavalent chromium only slightly greater than the detection limit of 0.1 ppm was found, which is considerably less than the threshold level for dermatitis in sensitized persons.[623] Numerous foods,[556] flavoring, and spices[307] are well known to cause allergic sensitization.

There are very few studies of dermatitis among houseworkers. In a study of 616 housewives between 1970 and 1974, Förg et al.[400] found the highest rate of contact allergy in individuals older than 60 years of age. The most common allergens were the phenylenediamine class of hair dyes, balsam of Peru, and lanolin alcohols. Surprisingly, little nickel allergy was found in this study, probably because ear piercing was less frequently done when this group was young. On the other hand, in 1975 Katz and Samitz[707] reported that household detergents and sweat possessed the capacity to release nickel from stainless steel in kitchen utensils. They also found that a negative spot test (dimethylglyoxime) does not necessarily indicate the "safety" of a nickel alloy.

Andersen[31] reported contact allergy in a cleaner from diethylthiourea present in an acidic detergent, which is unusual as this chemical is usually used as an accelerator in certain (sponge) rubbers, as an anticorrosion agent, and in metal pickling solutions. Cronin[244] found a significant percentage of houseworkers with formaldehyde sensitivity. The most common sources were popular cleaning agents containing formaldehyde and formaldehyde releasers, such as quaternium 15, Bronopol, Euxyl K 400, and imidazolidinyl urea, preservatives

that are also frequently present in hand creams. Because of the nearly universal presence in household products, fragrance is also a common cause of sensitization.[1085]

An often overlooked dermatitis in housekeeping personnel is latex allergy.[1176] These workers almost as a rule have exposure to unlined, high-protein latex gloves and often spend their entire workday wearing the same gloves.

It has been claimed that enzyme-containing washing powders can cause rashes or exacerbation of pre-existing rashes. Investigation and usage over more than three decades have failed to demonstrate allergic sensitization to these substances, which are mixtures of cationic and nonionic surface active agents, with the addition of minor ingredients such as thickening agents, dyes, and perfumes.[1036] A 1985 study of 80 volunteers in Britain found no evidence that the enzyme (alcalase) in a washing powder was responsible for any dermatological problem.[1296] Patch testing, prick testing, and double-blind user testing were performed with negative results.

Sodium hypochlorite is a simple chemical with many uses as a disinfectant and laundering agent in dishwashing and scouring powders, for water purification (swimming pools), and as bleach. There are reports of allergic sensitization to this compound,[353, 512, 968] although this must be quite rare.

Even incense should not be overlooked as a cause of dermatitis in houseworkers. Hayakawa et al.[570] described depigmented contact dermatitis due to incense containing musk ambrette and sandalwood.

Numerous plants and flowers can induce contact dermatitis in houseworkers (see Chapter 31).

Atopics, especially those in whom the disease is active, experience difficulty in many aspects of this work, especially from repeated, heavy contact with soaps, detergents, abrasive cleaning agents, and so forth. In recent years housedust mites have been reported to aggravate this disease. Vincenzi et al.[1268] found positive patch tests to mite extracts in a group of atopic adults and children. Flares of dermatitis are thought to be triggered and aggravated by sensitivity (delayed, type IV) to mite bodies.

Irritants

Soaps and detergents
Abrasives
Polishes and waxes
Window cleaners
Oven cleaners
Toilet bowl cleaners
Disinfectants for hot tubs (bromine)

Patch test to standard and vehicle preservative allergens, with special attention to the following.

Standard Allergens

Potassium dichromate, 0.25% pet; 0.023 mg/cm² (leather; "Javelle water," bleaches)

Wool alcohols, 30% pet; 1.00 mg/cm² (creams, lotions)

2-Mercaptobenzothiazole, 1% pet; 0.075 mg/cm^2 (rubber)

Neomycin sulfate, 20% pet; 0.23 mg/cm^2 (medications)

Carba mix, 3% pet; 0.25 mg/cm^2 (rubber)

Cl + Me-isothiazolinone (Kathon CG), 0.01% aq; 0.0040 mg/cm^2 (germicidal agents, hand creams, and lotions)

Fragrance mix, 8% pet; 0.43 mg/cm^2 (e.g., cleaning agents, polishes)[1085]

Quinoline mix, 0.19 mg/cm^2 (germicidal agents, especially pets)

p-Phenylenediamine, 1% pet; 0.090 mg/cm^2 (dyes)

Balsam of Peru, 25% pet; 0.80 mg/cm^2 (crossreacts with many fragrances)

Paraben mix, 12% pet; 1 mg/cm^2 (creams, lotions)

Epoxy resin, 1% pet; 0.05 mg/cm^2 (adhesives, epoxy "putty")[171]

Mercapto mix, 1% pet; 0.075 mg/cm^2 (rubber)

Ethylenediamine dihydrochloride, 1% pet; 0.05 mg/cm^2 (topical medications)

PPD mix (Black rubber mix), 0.6% pet; 0.075 mg/cm^2 (rubber)

p-tert-Butylphenol–formaldehyde resin, 1% pet; 0.04 mg/cm^2 (leather)

Thiuram mix, 1% pet; 0.025 mg/cm^2 (rubber gloves, herbicides)

Formaldehyde, 2% aq; 0.18 mg/cm^2 (preservatives)

Quaternium 15, 2% pet; 0.1 mg/cm^2 (cosmetics)

Nickel sulfate, 2.5% pet; 0.2 mg/cm^2 (tools, jewelry)

Rosin (colophony), 20% pet; 0.85 mg/cm^2 (cleaning agents)

Additional Allergens

Air fresheners (sprays)

Ammoniated mercury, 1% pet (creams, lotions, disinfectants)

p-Chloro-m-xylenol, 1% pet (medications)

Benzalkonium chloride, 0.01% aq (cleaning solutions)

Bronopol, 0.25% pet (cosmetics)

Camphor, 10% pet (medications, deodorants)

Captan, 0.25% pet (pesticides)

Chlorhexidine digluconate, 0.5% aq

Euxyl K 400, 0.5% pet (cosmetics)

House plants (e.g., chrysthanthemums, *Primula obconica*)

Imidazolidinyl urea, 2% pet (cosmetics)

D-limonene hydroperoxide, 0.5% pet (cleansers)[702]

Pyrethrum, 2% pet (insect repellents)

Medications for household pets (e.g., neomycin, bacitracin, ethylenediamine, sulfa preparations)

Menthol, 1% pet (medications)

Musk ambrette, 5% pet (incense,[570] cosmetics, photosensitizer)

Nonoxynol 9, 2% aq (nonionic surface active agent)[300]

Nitro-p-phenylenediamine, 1% pet (semipermanent hair dyes)

Pine oil, 10% in olive oil (cleaners)

Propylene glycol, 4% aq

Sodium hypochlorite, 0.1% aq (bleaching powders, swimming pool and hot tub disinfectants, scouring agents)

Thiourea, 5% aq (silver polish)[304]

INSULATION WORKERS

Insulation workers paste, wire, tape, or spray insulation onto an appropriate surface. When covering a steam pipe, for example, insulation workers cut a tube of insulation to the necessary length, stretch it open along a cut that runs the length of the tube, and then slip it over the pipe. To secure the insulation they wrap and fasten wire bands around it, tape it, or wrap a cover of tar paper, cloth, plastic, or canvas over it and then sew or staple the cover in place.

When insulating a wall or other flat surface, insulation workers use a hose to spray foam insulation onto a wire mesh. The wire mesh provides a rough surface to which the foam clings and adds strength to the finished wall. When desired, workers apply a final coat for a finished appearance.

In open spaces, such as attics that do not require either wire mesh for adhesion or a final coat for appearance, insulators use a compressor to blow in the insulation. They fill a machine with shredded fiberglass insulation, allow the compressor to force the insulation through a hose, and control the direction and flow of insulation until the required amount is installed.

Fiber glass is a notorious irritant,[195, 225, 391] but, when impregnated with an epoxy or other sensitizing resin, allergic sensitization may occur.[251] Fiberglass and rock wool (from furnace slag) are used for thermal and acoustic insulation, as well as fire protection. The usual dermatitis is caused by mechanical irritation, which is transient and caused mainly by fibers with a diameter exceeding 4.5 μm. Fibers with the smallest diameter are the least irritating, and the largest are more irritating.[1160] Fiberglass and rock wool dust may contain trace amounts of contaminants such as mercury, lead, arsenic, or cadmium, and the mastics used in insulation may sometimes contain rosin acids.

Farkas[359] described fiberglass dermatitis in office workers in a new building where the office ceilings were covered with aluminum boards with circular openings, above which were packets of glass wool in plastic bags that had been partially torn when being laid. In windy weather and in a draught, fragments of glass fiber fell onto the furniture and the employees. Intense itching developed in numerous employees, while others were not affected. Verbeck et al.[1258] also emphasized the intense itching of workers exposed to glass fibers. Atopics are especially affected.

Insulation workers use hand tools, trowels, brushes, scissors, sewing equipment, and stapling guns. They also use powersaws to cut and fit insulating materials. They must wear protective clothing, particularly masks, when removing asbestos, which was once a common form of insulation, but is not used today because of its well-recognized serious health hazards.

Rock wool, or mineral wool, which is frequently used in insulation, is composed of mineral fibers from molten furnace slag. The dust, like glass dust, is vitreous and may contain trace amounts of contaminants such as mercury, lead, arsenic, and cadmium. Mastics used in insulation may contain rosin acids.

Two types of foam insulation have been widely used. The first, urea formaldehyde foam (which is relatively inexpensive and easily installed), is an efficient insulation, but its use has aroused considerable protest in recent years because of possible toxicity caused by the release of free formaldehyde. The second is polyurethane foam, which, unlike urea formaldehyde, is completely cured before construction, and toxicity occurs only during manufacture and curing, not during installation.[537] Other insulation foams in current use include expanded polystyrene bead foam, extruded polystyrene foam, and a phenolic foam.

Irritants

Metal cleaners
Fibrous glass
Asbestos fibers
Rock wool[85]
Dust
Adhesives
Plaster of Paris

Patch test to standard and vehicle preservative allergens, with special attention to the following.

Standard Allergens

Potassium dichromate, 0.25% pet; 0.023 mg/cm^2
  (leather gloves, welding fumes)
2-Mercaptobenzothiazole, 1% pet; 0.075 mg/cm^2
  (rubber)
Epoxy resin, 1% pet; 0.05 mg/cm^2 (adhesives)
Mercapto mix, 1% pet; 0.075 mg/cm^2 (rubber)
PPD mix (Black rubber mix), 0.6% pet; 0.075 mg/cm^2
  (rubber)
Thiuram mix, 1% pet; 0.025 mg/cm^2 (rubber gloves)
Formaldehyde, 2% aq; 0.18 mg/cm^2
Nickel sulfate, 2.5% pet; 0.2 mg/cm^2 (hand tools)
Rosin (colophony), 20% pet; 0.85 mg/cm^2 (soldering
  flux, asphalt-type mastic)
p-tert-Butylphenol–formaldehyde resin, 1% pet; 0.04
  mg/cm^2 (leather)

Additional Allergens

Urea formaldehyde resin, 10% pet (insulation foam)

JEWELERS

The majority of jewelry today is mass-produced by assembly-line methods. Jewelers generally perform only one or two jobs in the manufacturing process, such as making molds to cast jewelry or dies for stamping. The molds for gold rings, for example, are often rubber based, and hot wax is used to make a wax "tree," which is then dipped in plaster. The resulting plaster cast is then slid into a kiln. The wax melts, and liquid gold is injected into the resulting hollow cavity. When the metal has set, the hot cast is immersed in cold water, which shatters the plaster, revealing an exact duplicate of the original wax model. The rings are then pruned, and each ring is ground, buffed with a hand file or emery paper, frosted, and polished.

Jewelers offer many services to their customers. Much of their time is spent repairing jewelry. They may also repair watches and do hand engraving. Some jewelers are qualified gemologists and appraise the quality and value of diamonds and other stones. A few highly skilled jewelers make jewelry by hand, following their own designs or those created by designers. They shape the metal with pliers or hand tools or cast it in molds. Individual parts are soldered to form a finished piece. Designs may be carved in metal, and diamonds or other stones may be mounted.

Jewelers use pliers, files, saws, hammers, torches, soldering irons, and a variety of other small hand tools. They also use polishing compounds, such as jeweler's rouge (red iron oxide, 87%; fat, 13%), for soldering and finishing. Because the work is very detailed, jewelers often wear magnifying glasses.

Radon seeds containing radon 222 in gold jewelry[1134] may cause radiodermatitis and malignancy. Radiation skin changes appear slowly, and initially they may not resemble radiation dermatitis.[1287] The affected skin becomes dry, atrophic, with a mottled appearance. Years later Bowen's disease and squamous cell carcinomas appear in the affected areas,[467] and the latter tend to be more malignant than those resulting from sunlight exposure.

Rhodium, a metal long considered to be free of the potential for inducing contact allergy, was reported to cause contact dermatitis in a goldsmith. Patch testing to 0.1% hexachlororhodiate in water was positive at 96 hours. In the past, rhodium has been used to plate nickel and cobalt, and it was believed sensitization to rhodium did not occur. Bedello et al.[68] emphasize the rarity of this allergy and suggest that the patient's prolonged contact with the metal and with solvents, degreasers, and other chemicals during work made it somewhat more likely for allergic sensitization to occur.

In a study of 2,300 patients for contact dermatitis, Vincenzi et al.[1267] found 171 (7.4%) allergic to palladium, which with rhodium (above) is a member of the VIII group of the periodic table. White gold may contain as much as 20% palladium. All but 2 of the 2,300 patients were also sensitive to nickel sulfate, suggesting crossreactivity between the two metals, which are closely related in group VIII of the periodic table. However, Wahlberg and Boman[1275] have suggested that palladium is a more potent sensitizer than nickel in guinea pigs; nevertheless, many cases of palladium sensitivity cannot be traced. Olivarius and Menné[961] also report that a positive patch test to palladium chloride almost always represents crossreaction with nickel in subjects already nickel sensitive. Testing with a disk of metallic palladium revealed only 3 of 1,307 patients with a positive reaction, except in those in whom there was also a simultaneous reaction either to palladium or nickel.

Gold is now recognized as a more common allergen

than previously realized,[141, 414, 1018, 1073, 1287] although the real frequency is not yet entirely clear. In the past, the material chosen for patch testing was probably inadequate. For years, gold chloride was used, but irritant reactions were common, and it is no longer recommended for testing.[1017] Later, potassium dicyanoaurate and gold leaf were found to induce false-negative reactions. In 1987, Fowler[414] reported that gold sodium thiosulfate was a better test material, more often giving relevant results. Since then most studies have used this compound.

Positive patch test reactions to gold sodium thiosulfate may not appear during the 72 to 96 hour test period; reading solely at day 3, and even at 1 week, is considered insufficient by Bruze et al.,[145] who do not believe late reactions are due to active sensitization from the test, but represent true allergic sensitivity. Bruze et al.[145] also suggest using a higher test concentration than 0.5%. In some gold-sensitized patients the reaction persists for months,[145, 397] often initiating a granulomatous/lymphadenoid cellular reaction on histological examination.[40, 643, 1287]

It must be emphasized, however, that allergic reactions to white gold may also result from its nickel content. "Black dermographism," a discoloration of the skin that occurs from contact with gold jewelry, should not be confused with allergy.

Nickel allergy is an occupational disease in jewelers. For years it was thought that stainless steel did not release sufficient nickel to cause contact dermatitis in nickel-sensitive persons. Recently, however, it has been shown that high-sulfur–containing stainless steel may release sufficient nickel to induce positive patch test reactions in about 14% of nickel-sensitive patients.[545] Even earrings and ear piercing bits designated as "hypoallergenic," as well as some stainless steel and 14-karat gold, may release nickel.[374] Liden et al.[789] reported that nickel interliners under gold, silver, or chromium plating, as well as nickel-silver and some white gold alloys, may induce positive patch test reactions. Besides earrings, bracelets, wrist watches, and buttons containing nickel frequently may cause dermatitis.

The provocation threshold for nickel varies widely between individuals and probably ranges from 0.15 to 1.5 µg. Individual thresholds for reaction also vary, ranging from 118 to 0.47 µg, a 250-fold variation.[333]

Increasingly in recent years jewelry is made from exotic woods. *Dalbergia latifolia* Roxb., also known as East Indian rosewood or Bombay blackwood, may be used for jewelry and jewelry boxes, as well as knife handles, musical instruments, and desk accessories. The heartwood contains sensitizing quinones termed *dalbergiones,* a class of neoflavanoids.[352] Patch testing is positive to the sawdust and the four dalgergiones (R)-4-methoxy-dalbergione, (S)-4-methoxy-dalgbergione (also present in *Dalbergia nigra* All. (Brazilian rosewood), (S)-4′-hydroxy-4-methoxy-dalbergione, and (S)-4,4′-dimethoxy-dalbergione. The test concentration is 1% in petrolatum.[1002]

Also used in bracelets and other jewelry is *Grevillea robusta* A. Cunn. Also known as silver oak, a tree native to Australia, it contains a resorcinol, Grevillol, which is chemically related to the urushiols. Testing

should be done with Grevillol at 0.01% concentration in petrolatum.[611] Testing with the sawdust "as is" may produce irritant reactions.

Irritants

Acid and alkalis (metal cleaners)
Soaps and detergents
Solvents
Metal dust
Molten metal
Abrasives (polishing wheels and emory paper)
Soldering fluxes (zinc chloride)
Metal polishes
Rust removers
Electroplating solutions
Heat
Adhesives (cyanoacrylates)

Patch test to standard and vehicle preservative allergens, with special attention to the following.

Standard Allergens

Potassium dichromate, 0.25% pet; 0.023 mg/cm² (metal)
2-Mercaptobenzothiazole, 1% pet; 0.075 mg/cm² (rubber gloves and molds)
Carba mix, 3% pet; 0.25 mg/cm² (rubber)
Cobalt chloride, 1% pet; 0.02 mg/cm²[2284]
Epoxy resin, 1% pet; 0.05 mg/cm² (adhesives)
Mercapto mix, 1% pet; 0.075 mg/cm² (rubber)
Formaldehyde, 2% aq; 0.18 mg/cm² (cleaners)
Nickel sulfate, 2.5% pet; 0.2 mg/cm² (jewelry)
Rosin (colophony), 20% pet; 0.85 mg/cm² (soldering fluxes)

Additional Allergens

Methyl methacrylate monomer, 5% pet (adhesives)
Aminoethylethanolamine, 1% pet (soldering flux)
Ammoniated mercury, 1% pet (metal)
Beeswax, 30% pet (molds)
Diethylenetriamine, 1% pet (used in ultrasonic baths)[884]
Gold sodium thiosulfate, 0.5% pet[414]
Gold sodium thiomalate, 0.5 to 2%[1287]
Hexachlororhodiate, 0.1% aq (for rhodium)[68]
Hexanediol diacrylate, 0.1% pet (adhesives)
Hydrazine monobromide or sulfate, 1% pet (soldering flux)
Palladium sodium dichloride, 1% pet[961, 1275]
Platinum chloride, 1% aq
Rhodium 50, 1% aq[68, 284]
Triethylenetetramine, 0.5% pet (epoxy catalyst)

LAUNDRY WORKERS

Laundry workers wash, dry, and mend garments and household furnishings such as blankets, curtains, and washable rugs in commercial laundries. They first sort the soiled clothing and examine articles to be laundered for spots, tears, stains, wrinkles, and other defects. They then load machines with the articles, start the machines, and turn valves to admit specified amounts of soap, detergents, water, blueing, and bleach. They may wash delicate fabrics by hand. They also mix solutions, such as bleach, blueing, or starch, and apply them to articles before and after washing to remove color or improve appearance. They also do some spot cleaning of articles before washing to remove heavy stains. Some articles may be sterilized. After washing the articles, laundry workers hang curtains, draperies, or blankets on stretch frames to dry. They pull trousers over heated metal forms to dry and stretch the legs. Blankets may be brushed or fed into a carting machine to raise and fluff the nap.

Lifting the clean, wet articles from the washer and placing them onto dryers and into wringers may cause a considerable amount of irritation due to exposure to the wet fabrics and water, especially in atopics.

"Dhobi itch" is an eczematous contact dermatitis after contact with the residue from the Indian marking nut *(Semecarpus anacardium),* which is used in India and other regions as a laundry mark. The reaction is usually delayed and eczematous, but contact urticaria from this allergen has been reported.[1117]

Irritants

Soaps and detergents (phosphates, alkalis, fluorosilicates)
Water (wet work)
Heat
Bleaches
Disinfectants (peracetic acid and others)
Fabric softeners
Stain removers (oxylates)
Spray starch (urticaria)[880]
Solvents (cleaners)

Patch test to standard and vehicle preservative allergens, with special attention to the following.

Standard Allergens

2-Mercaptobenzothiazole, 1% pet; 0.075 mg/cm^2 (rubber)
Carba mix, 3% pet; 0.25 mg/cm^2 (rubber)
Mercapto mix, 1% pet; 0.075 mg/cm^2 (rubber)
PPD mix (Black rubber mix), 0.6% pet; 0.075 mg/cm^2 (rubber)
Thiuram mix, 1% pet; 0.025 mg/cm^2 (rubber gloves)
Formaldehyde, 2% aq; 0.18 mg/cm^2 (detergent concentrates)
Nickel sulfate, 2.5% pet; 0.2 mg/cm^2 (hand tools, zippers, buttons)

Additional Allergens

Tribromosalicylanilide, 1% pet (commercial cleaners, photosensitizer)

LOCKSMITHS

Locksmiths repair and open locks, make keys, and change lock combinations using hand tools and special equipment. They disassemble locks and repair and replace worn parts. They shorten tumblers using files and insert new and repaired tumblers into locks to change combinations. They cut new or duplicated keys using key-cutting machines. They move lock picks and cylinders to open door locks without keys and open safe locks by listening to lock sounds or by drilling.

Irritants

Rust removers (WD-40)
Lubricants
Solvents
Degreasing compounds

Patch test to standard and vehicle preservative allergens, with special attention to the following.

Standard Allergens

Nickel sulfate, 2.5% pet; 0.2 mg/cm^2 (metal)
Cobalt chloride, 1% pet; 0.02 mg/cm^2

MACHINISTS

Machinists (including tool machine or machine tool operators) set up and operate conventional, special purpose, or numerical control machines and machining centers, including lathes ("turners"), milling machines, jig borers, shapers, and grinders. In addition, almost every factory that uses large amounts of machinery employs machinists to maintain mechanical equipment.

Before they begin work on a part, machinists operating conventional cutting machines consult blueprints or written specifications for the item. They select tools and materials for the job and plan the cutting and finishing operations. They then secure the part on blocks or plates and, using hand tools such as files, scrapers, and wrenches, fit and assemble the part into the machine. They must verify dimensions and alignment with measuring instruments such as micrometers, gauges, and gauge blocks. They also must decide how fast they can feed the metal work piece into the machine and what cooling fluids they should use to keep the metal from overheating and ruining the job. While operating the machine they observe the operation or test it with inspection equipment to diagnose malfunctions. An air hose is used to free the parts of metal chips ("swarf"). In machines without protective shielding, there can be considerable exposure to liquid coolants and lubricants. Dermatitis, when it occurs, may be very persistent[658] and, when allergic, is often caused by biocides in water-based coolants (see below).

Increasingly in recent years, machining has become automated, with highly sophisticated cutting machines that offer considerably less exposure to coolants than in the past, except when changing cutting tools or repairing the machines.

After completing machining operations, machinists use hand files and scrapers to smooth rough metal edges before assembling the finished product with wrenches and screwdrivers.

Today most dermatitis in machinists arises from the irritating properties of soluble coolants. During operation of the older machines, especially, there may be nearly constant skin contact with the coolants. Considerable variation in irritancy exists between various metalworking fluids.[630] In electrodischarge machining, used in precision engineering, a dielectric fluid containing both straight-chain parafinic hydrocarbons and aromatics may cause irritant dermatitis,[479] especially in those with atopic backgrounds. Metal particles in recycled coolants cause abrasive injuries, which are usually rather mild, and occur more often during grinding operations. Gloves can rarely be worn while operating the machines because of the danger of their becoming caught in the machinery. Hand dermatitis is common in metalworkers, and some studies have shown that, once developed, the dermatitis has a poor prognosis, with many workers remaining symptomatic long after exposure to coolants and oils has ceased.[1116]

Allergic sensitization, although less common than irritancy,[1034] may develop from the germicidal agents and corrosion inhibitors, such as o-phenylphenol,[4, 1238] PCMX,[3] Kathon 886 (MCI/MI-methylchloroisothiazolone/methylisothiazolinone),[815, 945] the formaldehyde-releasing agents,[143, 254, 811, 1034] and others. Greases, although widely used throughout industry, are not common allergic sensitizers. However, Freeman[425] reported allergic contact dermatitis to an antioxidant, phenyl-α-napthylamine, in an industrial grease. Patch testing was performed at 5% in petrolatum.

Even when a relevant allergen is found and the machinists avoid contact, some of them continue to experience flares of dermatitis, which are sometimes due to persistent contact with the allergen in other substances, especially hand creams and household products. Underlying atopy may also be responsible for persistence.

Bioban (TM) P 1487 is a common preservative in metal-working fluids. It consists of two active and sensitizing ingredients: 4-(2-nitrobutyl)-morpholine (4-2-M) and 4,4'-(2-ethyl-2-nitrotrimethylene)-dimorpholine (4-2-DM). Of the two, 4-2-DM appears to be the more active sensitizer, and, by lowering the content of 4-2-DM, the risk of sensitization may be reduced.[498] Although Bioban P 1487 is used in water-based metalworking fluids, the preservative is not stable in aqueous solution. Thus the vehicle for patch testing should be petrolatum.[499] Tris-Nitro (2-[hydroxymethyl])-2-nitro-1,3-propanediol) is also a common biocide used in metal-working fluids. Related to bronopol (2-bromo-2-nitropropane 1,3 diol), it may also induce allergic contact dermatitis.[1034]

Contact allergy develops occasionally to metals themselves.[375, 1072] Hexavelent chromium is a well-known allergen.[439] Wass and Wahlberg[1284] have proposed that the mean release of Cr6 from chromated parts should not exceed 0.3 µg/cm², a level that could reduce the risk of chromate allergy in machinists and other workers. Other well-known metallic allergens are nickel, cobalt, and occasionally platinum. Allergic contact sensitization to iron is considered extremely rare. Allergic sensitivity to ferric chloride, 2% aqueous, was reported by Baer[52] in a toolmaker employed in lathe and bench work who had considerable exposure to metallic dust.

The antioxidant tert-butylhydroquinone has been reported to be a contact allergen in a metal worker.[887] Coconut diethanolamine has been found to be a sensitizer in metal-working fluids.[270, 592, 1003] The latter is also found in hand soaps. Alkanolamineborates, used as corrosion inhibitors, may be allergic sensitizers; the sensitizers are not known, but it appears that there are at least two. Because these substances are highly alkaline, an acidic buffer (sodium acetate 0.1N, 50%; acetic acid 0.1N, 50%) should be used as the test vehicle, with a pH below 9.[133, 147]

The numerous bacteria that are found in used cutting fluids (water based or soluble), especially after several days of operation, are frequently blamed for dermatitis. Rycroft[1057] could find no evidence that the indigenous microflora of soluble oil emulsions contribute directly to dermatitis, although the presence of certain bacteria causes the foul odors that stale coolants often have ("Monday morning stink").

"Metal fume fever," also known as "brass or bronze chills," is a syndrome caused by inhalation of excessive concentrations of metallic oxide fumes. The symptoms resemble influenza, with chills, a mild fever, nausea, and vomiting. Feelings of weakness and exhaustion may also be present. The condition rarely lasts more than a day or two. The most frequent cause is exposure to zinc oxide fumes, but other metallic fumes may also be responsible, including antimony, cadmium, cobalt, copper, iron, lead, magnesium, manganese, mercury, nickel, and tin. These symptoms should be differentiated from the more serious condition caused by arsenic exposure.

Cutting fluids may contain varying amounts of nitrites and amines and may also contain N-nitrosamines, which are carcinogenic to animals. Cutting fluids containing nitrosamines, however, were withdrawn from the market in the late 1970s. No increase in cancer mortality was found in a study of 219 grinders working for at least 5 years between the years 1950 and 1966.[652] Roush et al.[1053] found 45 machinists with squamous cell carcinoma of the scrotum and concluded, after statistical analysis, that more than one-half of these cases were related to exposure to cutting oils.

The so-called rusters are individuals whose perspiration leaves a corrosion on metallic objects that they handle, a potentially serious problem with precision instruments and other highly polished metals. Treatment has consisted of application of a solution of 5% glutaraldehyde in water and propantheline bromide (Probanthine) orally. A sometimes more successful treatment consists of occlusive dressings (overnight) with a complex of aluminum chloride hexahydrate in alcohol.[1125]

Barrier creams are often recommended for protection of the skin of machinists. In a 1991 study of cutting oil dermatitis on guinea pig skin, barrier creams did not provide protection against the irritant effects of the cutting fluid, and some actually appeared to exacerbate the irritation.[1991]

Irritants

Abrasives
Acids
Amines
Antifoam agents (silicone derivatives)
Coupling agents (propylene glycol, cresylic acid, triethylene glycol)
Corrosion inhibitors (benzotriazole, hydrazine sulfate, triethanolamine)
Emulsifiers (e.g., tall oil, oleic acid, coconut diethanolamide)
Extreme pressure agents (dipentine, chlorinated paraffins)
Degreasing agents
Solvents (perchlorethylene and systemic scleroderma[1179])
Coolants and cutting oils[41]
Heat
Metal chips
Mineral oils
Greases
Soaps and detergents[466]
Heat

Patch test to standard and vehicle preservative allergens, with special attention to the following.

Standard Allergens

Potassium dichromate, 0.25% pet; 0.023 mg/cm^2 (cutting fluids, rarely)[177]
2-Mercaptobenzothiazole, 1% pet; 0.075 mg/cm^2 (rubber aprons, cutting fluids)[444]
Carba mix, 3% pet; 0.25 mg/cm^2 (biocides, rubber)
Balsam of Peru, 25% pet; 0.80 mg/cm^2[2973]
Cobalt chloride, 1% pet; 0.02 mg/cm^2 (metal parts, especially hand grinding and etching)[375, 1072]
Epoxy resin, 1% pet; 0.05 mg/cm^2 (corrosion inhibitors, free radical stabilizers)[1084]
Formaldehyde, 1.0% aq
Fragrance mix, 16% pet
Mercapto mix, 1% pet; 0.075 mg/cm^2 (rubber)
Ethylenediamine dihydrochloride, 1% pet; 0.05 mg/cm^2 (soluble cutting fluids)[193, 249]
Quaternium 15, 1% pet; 0.1 mg/cm^2 (preservative in barrier and hand creams)
PPD mix (Black rubber mix), 0.6% pet; 0.075 mg/cm^2 (rubber)
Thiuram mix, 1% pet; 0.025 mg/cm^2 (rubber, especially gloves)
Formaldehyde, 2% aq; 0.18 mg/cm^2 (formaldehyde-releasing agents in soluble cutting fluids)
Kathon CG, 0.01% pet; 0.0040 mg/cm^2 (preservative)[281, 815] (also may be listed as Parmetol K 40[977])
Nickel sulfate, 2.5% pet; 0.2 mg/cm^2 (small tools, leaching from machined metals)[323, 1078]
Rosin (colophony), 20% pet; 0.85 mg/cm^2 (cutting fluids)

Thimerosal, 0.1% pet; 0.0080 mg/cm^2 (germicidal agents, merthiolate)

Additional Allergens

Abietic acid, 10% pet (in rosin)[1094]
Alkanolamineborates, 5% in buffer solution[133, 147]
Amerchol L 101, 50% pet
p-Aminoazobenzene, 0.25% pet[1094]
Benzotriazole, 1% pet (low potential for sensitization[876])
Bioban CS 1246, 1% pet[143, 811]
Bioban P 1487, 0.1% pet[254, 498, 1034, 1382]
Bioban CS 1135[811]
Bronopol (2-bromo-2-nitropropane 1,3-diol), 0.25% pet[268, 1034]
p-tert-Butylbenzoic acid, 1% pet
p-tert-Butylcatechol, 1% pet[1094]
tert-Butylhydroquinone, 1% alc (antioxidant[887])
Chloroacetamide, 0.2% pet (tested at 2% pet[752])
n-Methylol chloroacetamide, 0.1% pet (Parmetol K 50)[268, 601]
p-Chloro-m-xylenol, 0.5% pet (cutting fluids)
p-Chloro-m-cresol, 1% pet (germicidal agents)[34]
Cocamide DEA (coconut diethanolamide), 0.5% pet[268, 592, 1003]
Dichlorophene, 1.0% pet (germicidal agent)
2,6-Di-tert-butyl cresol, 2% pet
Diethylthiourea, 1% pet (safety shoes)[410]
Dipentene (Limonene), 1.0% pet
Ethylenediamine dihydrochloride, 1.0% pet
Euxyl K 400, 0.5% pet (hand creams, germicidal agent)
Fluorescein sodium, 1% pet[607, 1034]
Grotan BK (1,3,5-tris[hydroxyethyl]hexahydrotriazine), 1% aq (germicidal agent)[19, 1055, 1248]
Grotan HD2 (see n-methylol chloroacetamide, above)
Grotan K (2-chloro-2-methyl-4-isothiazolin-one), 0.1% pet[1034]
Hexahydro-1,3,5-tris(hydroxyethyhl)triazine, 1.0% aq
Hydrazine sulfate, 1% pet (cutting fluids)
p-tert-Hydroquinone, 1% pet
N-isopropyl-N'-phenyl-p-phenylenediamine (IPPD), 0.1% pet (rubber)
Kathon 886 MW, 0.02% aq[268]
Kathon LP (2-n-octyl-4-isothiazolon-3-one), 0.1% pet
Monoethanolamine (2-amino ethanol), 1% aq[727]
Oleyl alcohol, 6% aq (cutting fluids)[727]
o-Phenylphenol (Dowicide 1), 1% pet (germicidal agents)[4, 1034]
Pine oil, 10% in olive oil (cutting fluids);[384] 5% pet[1034]
Phenylmercuric nitrate, 0.05% pet (cutting fluids)
Preventol D-2 (benzyl hemiformal), 2.0% pet[1034]
Propylene glycol, 5% pet
Proxcel CRL (1,2-benzisothiazolin-3-one), 0.05% alc;[1034] 0.1% pet[18, 19] (0.1% is probably irritant;[211] test concentration under review.)
Rosin, 20% pet
Sodium-2-pyridinethil-1-oxide, 0.1% pet
tert-Butylhydroquinone, 1% pet
Tricresyl phosphate, 5% pet
Sodium omadine, 0.1% pet[1034]

Tribromosalicylanilide, 1% pet (germicidal agent)
Trichlorocarbanilide, 1% pet
Triethanolamine, 2% pet (cutting fluids)[384, 1094]
Tris-nitro (2-[hydroxymethyl]-2-nitro-1,3-propanediol),
    1% pet[268, 1034]

Some Biocides Used in Cutting Oils

The following list is provided by Dr. K. E. Anderson,
Odense, Denmark.

Preventol O extra	o-Phenylphenol
Preventol ON extra	Sodium 2-phenylphenolate
Preventol L	Mixture of phenols, contains pentachlorophenol and chlorocresol
Preventol CMK	Chlorocresol
Preventol GD	2,2'-Methylenebis(4-chlorophenol)
Proxel XL	1,2-Benzisothiazolin-3-one, 20% in aqueous propylene glycol
Proxel HL	1,2-Benzisothiazolin-3-one, 30% in a mixture of morpholine di- and triethanolamine
Cytox 3522	Methylene-bis-thiocyanate 10% in solvent
Preventol D2	Hydroxymethylene and polyhydroxy methylene monobenzyl ether
Forcide 78	1,2,5-tris(Hydroxyethyl) hexahydrotriazine and 1,3,5-tris(ethyl)-hexahydrotriazine 1:1
Grotan BK	1,3,5-tris(Hydroxyethyl) hexahydrotriazine
Grotan OX	N,N-methylene-bis-5-methyloxazolidine

MEDICAL PERSONNEL

This category includes physicians, podiatrists, nurses,
respiratory technicians, dialysis workers, and physiotherapists. Dentists, dental personnel, and veterinarians
are discussed in separate sections.

Because the work is well known and extremely varied, a work description is not given. Most cases of
dermatitis in medical personnel are due to irritation.
Personnel with atopic dermatitis develop more severe
hand eczema than do individuals with only atopic mucosal symptoms or those with no atopic history. Wet
work in a hospital greatly increases the chance of developing dermatitis, particularly in atopics; the nursing
staff and kitchen workers/cleaners are at greatest risk.[953]
Nurses have the highest prevalence of contact hand
dermatitis of almost any other occupation.[1146]

Contact urticaria to rubber gloves is increasingly
common.[521, 1182, 1188, 1189, 1216, 1220, 1327] For example, operating room nurses[749, 1216] and delivery room nurses[1219]
are especially likely to develop symptoms of immediate-type latex allergy, as are medical laboratory technicians.[1075] The housekeeping personnel are also at risk
for latex allergy, especially because they often wear
latex gloves throughout the entire workday.[1176] Glove
powder appears to be a vehicle for the latex antigens,
especially if the powder is airborne, as occurs while
the gloves are donned. It has been postulated that the
combination of the latex and the cornstarch may be
more antigenic than the latex alone.[69] It is important to
remember that the reaction to latex in surgical gloves
can be anaphylactoid and life threatening.[1182, 1217, 1218]
Operating room personnel are especially at risk.[1182]
Atopy is a common associated condition.[63]

The FDA in 1995 required all manufacturers of medical devices that contain natural rubber latex and that
come directly or indirectly in contact with the body to
state on the principal display panel the following: "This
product contains natural rubber latex." If desired, manufacturers may also state the following: "This product
contains natural rubber latex which may cause allergic
reactions in some individuals." The FDA believes the
previously approved term *hypoallergenic* to be misleading. Since October 1988, the FDA has received over
800 adverse reaction reports related to latex-containing
products from a wide array of medical devices.

Delayed contact allergic sensitization to rubber additives, usually thiuram derivatives and the carbamates,
is also common. Even delayed hypersensitivity to basic
natural rubber latex, 1,4-*cis*-polyisoprene, has been reported.[1333]

Allergic sensitivity to medications is frequent. At
one time penicillin, sulfonamide drugs, and mercurial
antiseptics were common causes of sensitivity, but today these medications are rarely used topically. Neomycin, bacitracin, and related drugs are occasionally found
to induce sensitization.[1007a] Bacitracin ointment has been
reported to cause a severe anaphylactic reaction in a
patient when applied to a chronic stasis ulcer. Though
perhaps rare, these reactions can be life threatening.[999]
The cephalosporins were reported to induce contact
allergy in a chemical analyst in a pharmaceutical laboratory and in a nurse preparing cephalosporin solutions.[364]
The sensitizing capacity of topically applied antihistamines has been questioned recently, and further studies
utilizing an enlarged database, animal studies, and more
epidemiological investigations are indicated.[1180]

Certain injectable drugs are possible causes of allergic contact dermatitis—thorazine and related drugs administered by psychiatric nurses, for example. In right-handed persons, the dermatitis first appears on the left
hand from holding the vial while filling a leaking syringe. The right hand is affected by the process of
removing air bubbles prior to injection, which results
in droplets splashing onto the fingers.[408] Injectable
aminophyllin, which contains ethylenediamine, may induce dermatitis in ethylenediamine-sensitive patients,
according to Fisher.[389]

Dialysis workers, as well as morgue attendants and
tissue technicians, are exposed to several irritants and
contact allergens, especially formaldehyde, glutaraldehyde, and rubber allergens. Dermatitis may be induced
in highly sensitive persons merely by being present in
a room where a container of formaldehyde is left open.

Airborne contact dermatitis from metaproterenol (Alupent-R) in a respiratory therapist has been reported[452] and from a bronchodilator, salbutamol (Atrovent-R),[1145] as well as from benzalkonium chloride.[228] Glutaraldehyde, in addition to its use in cold sterilization, is present as a hardener in certain x-ray solutions. Latex rubber gloves are a common source of urticarial reactions in these workers also.[1217]

Topical corticosteroid preparations are possible causes of allergic contact dermatitis in medical personnel, although less common than in patients. Freeman[426] has found corticosteroid contact allergy to be the 15th most common positive patch test among her patients. Testing should be done with the actual preparation used, as well as with a patch test series of corticosteroids (including tixocortal pivalate), as well as the nonsteroidal ingredients in the formulation.[647]

Nurses counting tablets of methenamine may develop dermatitis on the fingertips because the tablets release formaldehyde in the presence of acid sweat. Nurses, physicians, and technicians in dermatology departments may receive doses of ultraviolet radiation in excess of recommended maximum permissible limits for occupational exposure to UVB and UVC.[759]

Inhalation of mercury vapor from a broken thermometer in someone previously sensitized to mercurials may induce an exanthem of the thighs, buttocks, groin, and abdomen, which has been termed the "baboon syndrome." The pattern of the eruption is an inverted triangular or V-shaped erythema on the upper anteromedial thighs.[34, 358, 366, 767, 928]

Soaps and detergents are uncommon causes of allergic sensitization, but, when they are, germicidal agents such as p-chloro-m-xylenol and formaldehyde-releasing germicidal agents are usually responsible. Benzalkonium chloride, a common disinfectant, has been reported to cause contact allergic reactions in surgical personnel,[1270] but this appears to be rare. Alcohol-impregnated swabs have been reported to cause dermatitis.[1250] Chloramine T (sodium p-toluenesulfonchloramide), used as a sterilizer, antiseptic, and disinfectant, has been described to cause contact urticaria[310, 716] and allergic contact dermatitis in a nurse.[798]

Sensitivity to nitrogen mustard may develop in persons applying topical nitrogen mustard to patients' skin in treatment of mycosis fungoides. Those who apply sulfamylon (mafenide acetate, α-amino-p-toluenesulfonamide monoacetate) to burned skin may also develop contact allergic dermatitis. Silver sulfadiazine (Silvadene), on the other hand, appears to have no contact sensitizing potential.[272, 1227]

Orthopedic surgeons may become sensitive to methyl methylacrylate in bone cement used to fix prostheses to bone during operations on the hip and knee joints, for example. The monomer readily penetrates rubber gloves.[989] Plaster casts containing formaldehyde-type resins (melamine formaldehyde resins) may induce contact allergy in orthopedic technicians and nurses applying the wet dressings.[1050]

Infections of various kinds are a constant threat to medical personnel. *Cutaneous tuberculosis* in recent years has been increasing in frequency. The cutaneous manifestations of *AIDS* are a major problem for medical personnel. Scabies and herpetic infections are also common in medical personnel, especially hospital and nursing home attendants.[1091] An outbreak of tropical *rat mite dermatitis* has been reported in laboratory personnel following exposure to asymptomatic laboratory mice infested with the mite that gained access to an animal research building on wild rodents living in crevices near the laboratory rodent caging areas.[419]

Research personnel may also be exposed to a variety of irritants and allergens. Polyacrylamide solutions for electrophoresis, which contain acrylamide and *N,N'*-methylenebisacrylamide, may induce allergic contact dermatitis. The allergens readily penetrate latex and PVC gloves.[309]

The use of topical traditional Chinese medicaments has become more widespread in recent years. Leow et al.[771] have recommended that patients with positive reactions to balsam of Peru and fragrance mix, for example, should avoid most traditional topical Chinese medicaments. Common herbal medications used in the United States are listed later.[1020]

Irritants

Soaps and detergents
Alcohol
Medications
Ethylene oxide
Plaster of paris
Water (wet work)
Ultraviolet light
Infrared light
Plaster cast material

Patch test to standard and vehicle preservative allergens, with special attention to the following.

Standard Allergens

Potassium dichromate, 0.25% pet; 0.023 mg/cm² (chromic sutures)
Wool alcohols, 30% pet; 1.00 mg/cm² (creams, lotions)
2-Mercaptobenzothiazole, 1% pet; 0.075 mg/cm² (rubber)
Balsam of Peru, 25% pet; 0.80 mg/cm² (physiotherapy preparations)
Carba mix, 3% pet; 0.25 mg/cm² (rubber)
Mercapto mix, 1% pet; 0.075 mg/cm² (rubber)
Ethylenediamine dihydrochloride, 1% pet; 0.05 mg/cm² (medications)
Neomycin sulfate, 20% pet; 0.23 mg/cm²
Paraben mix, 12% pet; 1 mg/cm² (medications, creams)
PPD mix (Black rubber mix), 0.6% pet; 0.075 mg/cm² (rubber)
Thiuram mix, 1% pet; 0.025 mg/cm² (rubber)
Thimerosal, 0.1% pet; 0.0080 mg/cm² (eye drops, contact lens solutions, vaccines, eardrops, certain storage solutions)[967, 1323]
Formaldehyde, 2% aq; 0.18 mg/cm² (disinfectants)
Nickel sulfate, 2.5% pet; 0.2 mg/cm² (hand tools, skin clips)

Additional Allergens

Ammoniated mercury, 1% pet (medications)
Bacitracin, 20% pet
Benzocaine, 5% pet
Benzoyl peroxide, 1% pet (catalyst for acrylic bone cement)
Benzylkonium chloride, 0.01% aq (disinfectant)
Captan, 0.25% pet (e.g., germicidal agent in shampoos)
Cephalosporins 1 to 5% aq[364, 402]
Chloramphenicol, 2% pet
Chlorhexidine, 0.5% enthanol
Chlorpromazine, 1% pet
p-Chloro-m-cresol, 1% pet (antimicrobials, especially antifungals)
p-Chloro-m-xylenol, 2% pet (EKG electrode jelly)
Diazolidinyl urea, 1% pet (Germall II) (germicidals)
Dichlorophene, 1% pet (germicidal agent in cast materials)
DMDM hydantoin, 1% pet (antimicrobial, creams, lotions)
Euxyl K 400, 0.5% pet (creams, lotions, ultrasonic gels)[462]
Glutaraldehyde, 0.5% pet (disinfectant, especially in dialysis and endoscopic apparatuses; x-ray developing solutions)[770]
Imidazolidinyl urea 2% (Germall 115) (germicidal agent in creams and lotions)
Isoniazid, 2.5% aq
Lignocaine, 1% aq gel[522]
Melamine-formaldehyde resin, 10% pet (plaster casts[1050])
Methyl methacrylate monomer, 5% pet (orthopedic bone cement)
Penicillin, 1% pet
Procaine, 1% pet
Propylene glycol, 10% aq (EKG electrode gels)[392]
Streptomycin, 1% pet
Sulfamylon, 5% pet
Tetracaine, 5% pet

Herbal Medicines

The following are used in the United States[1020]:

Echinacea (*Echinacea* sp.)
Garlic *(Allium sativum)*
Goldenseal *(Hydrastis canadensis)*
Ginseng *(Panax* sp.)
Gingko *(Ginkgo biloba)*
Saw palmetto *(Serenoa repens)*
Aloe gel *(Aloe barbadensis)*
Ephedra *(Ephedra* sp.)
Eleuthero *(Eleutherococcus senticosus)*
Cranberry *(Vaccinium macrocarpon)*

METAL POLISHERS

Metal polishers remove excess metal and surface defects from various items such as automobile trim and accessory parts and then buff or plate the surfaces using revolving abrasive wheels or belts. The metals most commonly polished are aluminum, brass, bronze, and zinc.

Aluminum, steel, and certain alloys are usually treated with a protective coating to inhibit corrosion, especially during storage, which is often out of doors. These coatings may contain lanolin,[180] a dichromate salt (for anticorrosion), and a dye that shows that the metal has been treated. The dyes vary, but may be an aniline-type dye that can induce allergic contact dermatitis in workers handling the metal.[1012]

Irritants

Cleaners and scale removers
Solvent degreasers
Abrasives
Rust-proofing agents
Alcohols

Patch test to standard and vehicle preservative allergens, with special attention to the following.

Standard Allergens

Potassium dichromate, 0.25% pet; 0.023 mg/cm² (antirust compounds)
2-Mercaptobenzothiazole, 1% pet; 0.075 mg/cm² (rubber)
Carba mix, 3% pet; 0.63 mg/cm² (rubber)
Mercapto mix, 1% pet; 0.075 mg/cm² (rubber)
Nickel sulfate, 2.5% pet; 0.2 mg/cm² (metals)
p-Phenylenediamine, 1% pet; 0.090 mg/cm² (dyes used as indicators)
PPD mix (Black rubber mix), 0.6% pet; 0.075 mg/cm² (rubber, indicator dyes)
Thiuram mix, 1% pet; 0.025 mg/cm² (rubber, gloves)
Wool alcohols (lanolin), 30% pet; 1.00 mg/cm² (protective coatings for metal, especially aluminum)[180]

Additional Allergens

Oil of limonene, 1% pet (solvent degreasers)
Diethylthiourea, 1% pet (scale removers)

MUSICIANS

Skin conditions among musicians are of fairly frequent occurrence. Because almost no musicians are exposed to chemical irritants, with the possible exception of horn players, who polish their instruments with pastes or silver polish containing solvents and string players who use rosin, the dermatology problems of musicians most often occur from various forms of repeated physical trauma, including calluses, folliculitis, paronychia, and secondarily infected minor wounds. Allergic sensitization is rare and occurs occasionally in string players from rosin (colophony) used on bows and strings and in woodwind players from cocobolo or other exotic woods in mouthpieces. Rosin may also be used on the shoes of dancers to prevent slippage on wooden floors.[580] Nickel dermatitis has been reported in a guitarist from nickel guitar strings;[854] changing to 24-karat gold strings prevented a relapse.

Schwartz et al.[1103] described eczematous dermatitis of the lower lip of flute players from sensitivity to the wood of the mouthpiece. Hausen[549] reported a violinist–physician who was sensitive to the wooden chin rest, which was made of Brazilian rosewood (*Dalbergia nigra* All.). This wood has also been reported to cause dermatitis in the lips of a recorder player. Patch testing with S-4'-hydroxy-4-methoxydalbergione at 1% was positive. Violin chin rests made from East Indian rosewood (*Dalbergia latifolia* Roxb.) may also cause dermatitis,[568, 1002] as may ebony (*Diospyros* sp.). Substitution could be chin rests made from boxtree wood (*Boxus sempervirens* L). Bork[97] described a violinist who developed allergic contact dermatitis to *p*-phenylenediamine used to stain an ebony chin rest. Cocobolo wood is a common a source of contact allergy among recorder players.[562] An immediate-type allergic reaction was seen in an atopic saxophonist, who showed a positive scratch test to the reed, which was made of the wood *Arundo donax*.[1235]

Nickel dermatitis in a cellist occurred on the flexor surfaces of the distal phalanges of the second and third fingers of the right hand, at the exact site of contact with very small metallic parts embedded in the bow. The dimethylglyoxime test on the metal was positive.[810]

Propolis (bee glue) has been used for centuries as an ingredient in violin varnish. Stradivari (1644?–1737) used it in the varnish of his stringed instruments.[912] It should be considered as a source of contact allergy not only in makers of stringed instruments but also those who repair them, especially ancient instruments.[566, 663]

"Fiddler's neck" affects violin and viola players.[1045] It consists of an area of lichenification and hyperpigmentation on the left side of the neck just below the mandible, where the instrument is held. Folliculitis, cyst formation, edema,[1165] and scarring may be seen.[746, 1192] A similar condition exists on the chest of cellists. This condition, which is clearly an example of mechanical acne,[124] is more common in players with badly fitting neck rests and/or a faulty technique.[978] Factors such as pressure, friction, rubbing, pinching, sweating, and poor hygiene play a role.[549]

Pianists and harpists are likely to develop paronychia and calluses on the sides or tips of the fingers. Onycholysis and subungual hemorrhages are common in harpists. Callosities are frequent in many instrumentalists and in fact often provide protection against additional trauma. They can thus be considered valid "occupational marks." The callosities are characteristic of the way the musicians grasp and hold their instruments. They are especially common in drummers and other percussionists. A characteristic callosity occurs on the midportion of the upper lip of clarinet and oboe players. A circumscribed atrophy of the upper lips of horn players may occur,[718] as well as ischemia of the lips and tears of the oral mucosa.[756] Hyperhidrosis can be a serious problem in a variety of instrumentalists, especially pianists; the emotional stress of performance contributes to its severity.

Because musicians often share instruments and mouthpieces, herpes labialis is more common among brass players, induced in part by minor trauma while playing and practicing.

Irritants

Rosin (colophony) (string players)
Polishing compounds (horn players)

Patch test to standard and vehicle preservative allergens, with special attention to the following.

Standard Allergens

Nickel sulfate, 2.5%; 0.2 mg/cm^2
Wool alcohols, 30% pet; 1.00 mg/cm^3
Colophony (rosin), 20% pet; 0.85 mg/cm^2
Cobalt dichloride, 1% pet; 0.02 mg/cm^2 (drier in varnishes)
p-Phenylenediamine, 2% pet; 0.090 mg/cm^2 (wood stain[97])

Additional Allergens

Violin and Other Stringed Instruments

Rosin (colophony), 20% pet
Ebony (*Diospyros* sp.)[559]
Rosewood (Brazilian rosewood: *Dalbergia nigra* All.[549])
East Indian rosewood[568] (*Dalbergia latifolia* Roxb; R-4-methoxydalbergione and S-4,4'-dimethoxydalbergione[548, 568])
Macassar ebony (*Diospyros celebia*) (in pegs)
Nickel sulfate, 2.5% pet; 0.2 mg/cm^2[810]
Propolis

Oboe and Other Reed Instruments

Rosewood
Cocobolo *(Dalbergia retusa)*
African blackwood *(Dalbergia melanoxylon)*
Other exotic woods[547]

Horn, Flute, and Harmonicas

Nickel sulfate, 2.5% pet; 0.2 mg/cm^2
Preservatives in polishing compounds

Percussion Instruments

Nickel sulfate, 2.5% pet; 0.2 mg/cm^2

Recorders

East Indian rosewood (*Dalbergia latifolia*)
Brazilian rosewood (*Dalbergia nigra*)
Cocobolo wood (*Dalbergia retusa*)

OFFICE WORKERS

Office work involves a variety of duties, including operating office machines, such as computers, copiers, duplication machines, and typewriters, and filing. Dermatitis is infrequent in this occupation. Considerable time is spent in copying documents, letters, and so forth. The chief method is photocopying, but in certain occupations diazo copying is required.

Allergic contact dermatitis may develop from contact with diazo dye on copy paper. Diazodiethylaniline chloride is commonly used in paper for heliographic copying, especially in architects' offices, and may induce contact allergic dermatitis, with special involvement of the tips of the first three fingers. The chemical is inactivated by UV radiation, and patch testing should be done with unexposed paper. In a case reported by Pambor and Poweleit,[971] however, patch testing with unexposed paper was negative. In addition to the diazo dye, the paper may contain propylene glycol, ethylene glycol 1500, theophilline, aromatic alcohols, dimethylthiourea, and thiourea. The latter two chemicals may also cause allergic contact dermatitis.[678, 1205]

Polymorphous light eruption has been reported from photocopy machines with quartz-halogen lamps, which emit UV light in the spectral range of 300 nm to the visible band. Occasionally a copy machine will give off ozone, which can cause stinging of the eyes, or workers may smell fumes from the solvent (e.g., toluene). If present in the atmosphere in only small amounts, the sole preventive measure necessary is improved ventilation.[954]

Carbonless copy paper (NCR—"no copy required") was introduced in the early 1950s and is almost ubiquitous today. Two types of reactions have been reported from working with this paper. In one type, itching and redness of skin, burning of the eyes, nose, and face, headache, nausea, and hoarseness have been reported.[753, 848, 894] A second type is allergic contact dermatitis caused by the color former p-toluene sulfonate, or Michler's hydrol.[847] Contact urticaria and airway obstruction from this paper have been described.[852] Allergic contact dermatitis caused by diethylenetriamine present in the microcapsules is recorded.[684] Cronin[242] reported four patients sensitive to Proxel used as a preservative in the emulsion of NCR paper.

In contrast, a study of 134 patients in Sweden could establish no specific relationship between urticaria and respiratory complaints and the chemicals used in carbonless copy paper.[653] Results of a questionnaire-based survey conducted in Denmark and the United States suggested that such symptoms may be related to poor ventilation or low humidity, as well as to psychosocial factors, rather than to chemicals in the copy paper.[158] Calnan[183] recommended improved ventilation to eliminate symptoms in many cases. Molhave and Grunnet[909] analyzed more than 42 chemicals degassed from NCR paper and found a large amount of alkanes and alkenes (olefins), which were harmless in the concentrations measured, although at higher concentrations alkanes may produce mild mucosal symptoms.

Rosin is widely used in paper and paper products. Its chief components, abietic acid and dehydroabietic acid, are not especially strong allergens. When oxidzed in contact with atmospheric oxygen, they may become rather potent sensitizers. Paper products manufactured with mechanical pulps, although generally considered environmentally "friendly," are more likely to induce allergic contact dermatitis to rosin.[703] A telefax paper containing colophony was suspected to cause a hand dermatitis in a colophony-sensitive secretary handling telefax papers.[683]

An office clerk with a recurring dermatitis on the palms, dorsa, and sides of fingers was positive on patch testing to crystal violet lactone, one of the color formers in carbonless NCR paper. Positive reactions were found on testing with 0.01% in pet.[1119]

Since 1982 there have been reports of facial rashes from visual display terminal work.[848, 952] The early reports originated from Scandinavian countries, and the eruptions were rosacea-like; subjects with rosacea, acne, and seborrheic dermatitis in one study were over-represented among visual display terminal operators compared with controls.[790, 1277] A relationship to rosacea could not be confirmed in other countries, with the exception of preliminary and inconclusive reports from Britain.[1066] A large study of 353 office workers from 7 companies in 16 locations in Sweden[78] did not show a relationship between visual display terminal users and skin disease, with the possible exception of seborrheic dermatitis, which was suspected to be related more to the nature of the work than to the visual display terminal. Other studies have also confirmed that video display unit work probably does not cause facial skin disease.[76, 200, 733, 785]

Itching in office workers from glass fibers released from newly installed insulation material may occur,[1258] especially if indoor air is recirculated. Fiberglass may be present on chairs made from reinforced fiberglass and cause itching.[320] Air conditioning systems can be responsible for a variety of disorders. Asthma, "humidifier fever," and allergic alveolitis have been related to contaminated humidifiers, especially cold water spray and spinning disk humidifiers.[372] So-called legionnaires' disease is associated with contamination of air conditioning cooling units with a gram-negative bacterium, which has been named Legionella pneumophila.

The "sick building syndrome" is seen in workers in response to sealed, air-conditioned offices and can be associated with a variety of complaints that are often vague and nonspecific: dry skin, headache, lethargy, nasal congestion, dry throat, and so on.[848, 1141] Sometimes the complaints seem to exceed rational limits.[101, 848] Risk factors include atopy, seborrhea, general skin dryness and itchiness, and female gender.[608] Work with carbonless copy paper and photocopiers, working in recently renovated areas, low fresh outdoor air supply provided the workers, presence of unusual odors, and a lack of cleanliness of the premises are also important factors. Psychosocial factors are often found. However, careful investigation of the complaints in each case is vital, especially investigation of any possible pollutant sources, regardless of the presence of obvious psychosocial factors.[608]

A common condition is low humidity occupational

dermatosis, occurring especially in persons with dry, atopic skin. The workers complain of intense, migratory itching, without primary lesions. The relative humidity is usually found to be 35% or below; raising the level to 45% or higher will usually alleviate most of the symptoms.[1061, 1069, 1298] This condition may occur in semiconductor plants where "bunny suits" are worn and where the relative humidity is maintained at low levels. Atopics are more likely to be symptomatic. In 1962, Chernosky[210] described pruritic skin disease in workers exposed for periods of time to refrigerated air conditioning. The condition is frequently misdiagnosed as, for example, neurodermatitis, contact dermatitis, or seborrhea.

Typewriter correction paper containing a phenol formaldehyde maleic anhydride resin (Arochem 455) has been reported to cause allergic contact dermatitis in a secretary/typist.[667] Patch testing with this resin produced a positive reaction.

The plastic of the computer "mouse" has been found to induce contact dermatitis. Patch testing with dimethyl and diethyl phthalate, both plasticizers, at 5% in petrolatum was positive in two patients.[199] Desk accessories made of exotic woods such as East Indian rosewood (*Dalbergia latifolia* Roxb.) may cause allergic contact dermatitis.[1002]

As part of their jobs, office workers often tend fish tanks, which are part of the office decor. Cleaning tropical freshwater aquariums sometimes results in atypical mycobacterial infections due to *Mycobacterium marinum*. The lesions are usually nodular and may ascend the hand and arm in a sporotrichoid pattern.[11, 1266] Treatment with minocycline is usually effective, but must be continued for up to 3 to 4 months.

Irritants

Soaps and detergents
Fiberglass
Papers, especially carbonless paper[178, 817, 848, 894]
Inks
Solvents, especially typewriter cleaners
Ammonia

Patch test to standard and vehicle preservative allergens, with special attention to the following.

Standard Allergens

Potassium dichromate, 0.25% pet; 0.023 mg/cm² (leather)
Wool alcohols, 30% pet; 1.00 mg/cm² (hand creams)
2-Mercaptobenzothiazole, 1% pet; 0.075 mg/cm² (rubber in gloves and finger cots, erasers, rubber bands, sponges)
Paraben mix, 12% pet; 1 mg/cm² (hand creams)
Carba mix, 3% pet; 0.25 mg/cm² (rubber, as above)
Cobalt chloride, 1% pet; 0.02 mg/cm² (driers in inks)
Mercapto mix, 1% pet; 0,075 mg/cm² (rubber, as above)
PPD mix (Black rubber mix), 0.6% pet; 0.075 mg/cm² (rubber, as above)

Thiuram mix, 1% pet; 0.025 mg/cm² (rubber, as above; rubber bands[720])
Formaldehyde, 2% aq; 0.18 mg/cm² (pastes, paper,[378, 431] glues, polishes)
Quaternium 15, 2% pet; 0.1 mg/cm² (hand creams)
Nickel sulfate, 2.5% pet; 0.2 mg/cm² (coins, hand tools, machines, diazo paper, and ?chalk)[1016]
Rosin (colophony), 20% pet; 0.85 mg/cm²[703] (inks, tapes, paper, including telefax[683] and computer paper)
p-tert-Butylphenol–formaldehyde resin, 1% pet; 0.04 mg/cm² (leather)

Additional Allergens

p-Aminoazobenzene, 0.25% pet (diazo dyes in blueprint paper and ball point pen ink)[201]
o-Aminophenol, 1% pet (diazo dyes in blueprint paper and ball point pen ink)
Bronopol, 0.25% pet (hand creams)
Cedar wood (pencils)[173]
Chloro cresol, 1% pet (preservatives in glues, inks)
p-Chloro-*m*-xylenol, 1% pet (hand creams)
Diazodiethylaniline chloride, 1% pet[971]
Diazo copy paper (unexposed), as is
Diazo copy paper (exposed), as is
Diethylenetriamine, 0.5% pet (cross-linking agent in the capsules of NCR paper[684])
Dimethyl (also diethyl) phthalate, 5% pet (plasticizer in computer "mouse")[199]
Euxyl K 400, 0.5% pet (hand creams, cosmetics)
Imidazolidinyl urea, 2% pet (hand creams)
N-Isopropyl-*N'*-phenyl-*p*-phenylenediamine (IPPD), 0.1% pet (rubber fingerstalls)[1040]
East Indian rosewood (*Dalbergia latifolia* Roxb.), 1% pet (desk accessories)[1002]
Methyl salicylate, 2% pet (pastes and glues)
Methyl violet, as is[175]
Nigrosin B, 1% pet (carbon paper)[1862]
PRSMH (*p*-toluenesulfonate of Michler's hydrol), 1% pet (carbonless paper)[847, 848]
Resorcinol, 2% pet (blueprint dye coupler, some photocopy machines)
Resorcinol monobenzoate, 1% pet (UV-light inhibitor in cellulose acetate plastics)
Tektamer 38 (2,3-dibromo-2,4-dicyanobutane), 0.1% pet[862]
Thiourea, 1% pet (copy machine antioxidant for paper—photosensitizer); 0.1% pet[712, 1205, 1230]
Dimethylthiourea, 5% aq[1205]
Tricresyl phosphate, 2% pet (carbon paper)

Also consider ornamental plants and household cleaning materials. Office personnel often keep cosmetics and medications in their desks, as well.

OPTICAL TECHNICIANS

Optical technicians make eyeglasses from specifications received from dispensing opticians, ophthalmologists, and optometrists. Some optical technicians manufacture contact lenses. There are two types of ophthalmic laboratory technicians: (1) surfacer or lens grinder and (2) bench technician or finisher. In large laboratories work is divided into separate operations, but in small laboratories one person may perform both tasks. Starting with standard-sized lens blanks mass produced by large optical firms, surfacers set up and operate machines to grind and polish eyeglass lenses according to prescription specifications. They use precision instruments, such as lensometers and objective lens analyzers, to measure the lenses and make sure they fit the prescription.

In the manufacture of high-quality prescription lenses, diallylglycol carbonate (CR 39) is widely used as a monomer in a polymerization process using a peroxide catalyst. During the formation of the lenses, plastic circular molds are filled with the mixture, and considerable spillage may occur. The monomer is very irritating and produces marked dermatitis on exposed areas such as hands and forearms. An unusual feature is the marked aggravation that occurs on exposure to cold.[160] Most cases are irritant in nature,[160, 747, 801] but patch testing to a concentration of 0.001% induced reaction in an extremely sensitive worker.[102] Lovell et al.[801] suggest useful methods of prevention.

Bench technicians mark and cut lenses and smooth their edges to fit frames. They then assemble the lenses and frame parts into finished glasses. Bench technicians use tools such as lens cutters and glass drills as well as small files, pliers, and other hand tools. They also use automatic edging machines to shape lens edges and precision instruments to detect imperfections.

Bench technicians especially need to wear goggles to protect their eyes. The dermatological hazards are few and consist mostly of irritation from grinding compounds and cleaning solutions and solvents.

Irritants

Resins
Soaps and detergents
Solvents
Grinding compounds
Glass
Dust

Patch test to standard and vehicle preservative allergens, with special attention to the following.

Standard Allergens

2-Mercaptobenzothiazole, 1% pet; 0.075 mg/cm^2 (goggles, gloves)
Carba mix, 3% pet; 0.25 mg/cm^2 (goggles, gloves)
Cobalt chloride, 1% pet; 0.02 mg/cm^2 (metallic parts)
Wool alcohols, 30%; 1.00 mg/cm^2 (lanolin) (polishing compounds)
Mercapto mix, 1% pet; 0.075 mg/cm^2 (goggles, gloves)
Thiuram mix, 1% pet; 0.025 mg/cm^2 (goggles, gloves)
Nickel sulfate, 2.5% pet; 0.2 mg/cm^2 (hand tools)
Rosin (colphony), 20% pet; 0.85 mg/cm^2 (polishing compounds)

Additional Allergens

Resorcinol monobenzoate, 1% pet (UV inhibitor in cellulose acetate plastics)
Turpentine, 10% olive oil (polishing compounds)
CR 39 monomer (diallyglycol carbonate), 0.001% in olive oil;[102] probably most cases are irritant[801]

PAINTERS AND PAPERHANGERS

Painters

Paint contains approximately 33 to 35% resins, 32 to 36% solvents, 15 to 16% pigments, 13 to 14% fillers and extenders, and about 3% additives and modifiers. Oil-based paints incorporate a variety of organic solvents, which inhibit bacterial growth. Water-based paints, of which latex paints are an example, provide a favorable environment for bacteria and thus require biocides.

Painters ordinarily use sandpaper, brushes, or steel wool, as well as paint remover, scrapers, wire brushes, and blow torches to prepare surfaces and remove old paint and varnish. They then fill holes, cracks, and joints with putty, plaster, or other filler. They select premixed paints or mix the paints themselves to match specified colors. The actual painting is done with brushes, spray gun (airbrush), or paint rollers. Electrostatic spraying is also widely used, in which the spraying of objects is performed automatically. Curing may take place in air or ovens. Accidents with spray guns may cause severe penetrating injuries.

Spray painting is widely performed in a variety of different industries. During spray painting there is exposure to solvents, resins, and metals in addition to paint droplets. Downdraft spray-painting booths are safer than those with crossdraft and semidowndraft booths because the worker stands on a grid and a downward draft removes vapors and paint droplets from the breathing zone. Studies have also shown that proper respiratory usage at many shops is lacking: Either the wrong respirator is used, or the mask does not fit or has become clogged with spray droplets, causing the worker to remove the mask in order to breathe.[578]

Painters may produce special effects, such as marbling or tile effects, by applying paint with sponges, cloths, or even the fingers. Stencils may be used, as well as masks, screens, or tape. After completion of a job the painter cleans the brushes, gun, and hose with various solvents or water. Exposure to paint occurs frequently while connecting and disconnecting paint containers and during cleaning equipment. The clothing of painters often becomes heavily contaminated with paint and solvents. Contamination with the antifouling agent tributyl tin oxide, widely used to formulate marine paints, may cause a severe irritant contact dermatitis;[472] the clothing must be discarded because laundering will fail to remove the material.[491] Isothiazolone antifoulants are also used, marketed by Philadelphia-based Rohm and Haas under the trade name Sea-Nine 211, which has been recommended for oceangoing and coastal vessels, ferries, and barges. Sea-Nine 211 is 4,5-

dichloro-2-n-octyl-4-isothiazolin-3-one, which is said to degrade rapidly with a half-life in seawater of 1 day.[1015]

Epoxy resin systems, polyesters, and phenol formaldehyde resins may be used in paints. A trifunctional epoxy compound, triglycidyl isocyanurate (TGIC), for cross-linking polyester pigments on heat activation has been reported to cause airborne contact dermatitis in workers exposed to spray paint. Patch testing at 5% pet or MEK showed strong positive reactions.[300, 958, 1304] Foulds and Koh[404] also reported four paint factory workers with dermatitis from contact allergy to triglycidyl isocyanurate. Patch testing was done at 1% in methyl ethyl ketone. A powder-coat spray painter developed dermatitis of the forehead and wrists and showed positive patch test reactions to triglycidyl isocyanurate at 1% pet.[881]

Water-based paints have, for many applications, replaced oil-based paints because of greater ease of application as well as fewer side effects. Their use has improved the work environment, and also there is less airway irritation.[1303] Since the Clean Air Act of 1990, U.S. paint manufacturers have reduced the use of solvents that emit volatile organic compounds, many of which are precursors of lower atmospheric smog. However, there has been considerable resistance by a number of manufacturers to limit these oil-based compounds. For certain applications, such as cabinets, furniture, and moldings, oil-based paint may be preferred. Oil-based paints do not require in-can preservatives because the organic solvents will not support the growth of bacteria and fungi. However, solvent-based paints tend to be somewhat irritating, but water-based paints, although less irritating, contain biocides that are continuing causes of contact sensitization and dermatitis. Among these are 5-chloro-2-methyl-4-isothiazolin-3-one/2 methyl-4-isothiazolin-3-one (MCI/MI) and 1,2-benzisothiazolin-3-one (BIT), which are currently used in numerous paints, and also in wallpaper adhesives.[949] In antifouling paints for marine applications, mercuric oleate and other mercury compounds, as well as pentachlorophenol may be used. Chloracetamide[615, 1276] and the formaldehyde-releaser 2-(hydroxymethyl-amino) ethanol[1183] are also used. A strong, corrosive irritant found in some paints is tributyl tin oxide, used as a bacteriocide and fungicide. It is highly corrosive to the skin even in low concentrations.[773] Some paints may have up to 10% of this biocide.[472] Another highly irritating bacteriocide and fungicide is tetrachlorophthalonitrile (e.g., chlorothalonil, Daconil, Bravo, Forturf).[398] It is often used for bathrooms and shower stalls because of its antifungal action.[886] It is also used as a wood preservative with which there have been reports of allergic sensitivity.[659]

Another germicide (fungicide) that is both highly corrosive and moderately sensitizing is 2-n-octyl-4-isothiazolin-3-one (Skane M-8, Kathon 4200, Kathon LM). A patch test concentration of 0.05% has been suggested.[865] It was developed specifically to prevent mildew in paint.[1198] The isothiazolinones have been recognized as potential allergic sensitizers for more than two decades.[355, 982]

Dichlofluanid is a fungicide sometimes found in paints, varnishes, and glazing paints. In guinea pig studies it has been found to be a strong sensitizer; Gruvberger et al.[497] reported five painters to be sensitized.

In the manufacture of UV-light–curable acrylic paints, several sensitizing acrylates are used, for example, 1,6-hexanediol diacrylate (HDDA), BIS-GA, and tripropylene glycol diacrylate (TRPGDA), each of which may induce allergic contact dermatitis in painters.[99, 662] Radiation-curable powders are now becoming available; they are based on urethane, polyether, or polyester oligomers with an acrylate terminal group. Because they produce virtually no volatile organic compounds, they are less likely to irritate the skin, which is a possibility with the radiation-curable liquids.[209]

A benzotriazole-based film preservative, Tinuvin 928, is a stabilizer of paint film, protecting it against breakdown under sunlight exposure.

Paperhangers

Prior to hanging the paper, the surface must be prepared. Paperhangers apply sizing, a material that seals the surface and enables the paper to stick better. In redecorating they may have to remove old paper by wetting it with a water-soaked sponge or, if there are many layers, by steaming. Frequently it is necessary for paperhangers also to patch holes with plaster.

After carefully positioning the patterns to match at the ceiling and baseboards, paperhangers measure the area to be covered and cut a length of wallcovering from the roll. They then apply paste to the strip of paper, place it on the wall, and smooth it by hand or with a brush. They cut and fit edges at the ceiling and base and smooth seams between strips with a roller or other special tool, and finally inspect the paper for air bubbles and other imperfections in the work.

Paperhangers have continuous and heavy contact with wallpaper paste and various chemical additives that may cause allergic contact dermatitis. Paperhangers are exposed to the same chemicals as painters, especially biocides in the glues and pastes.

After years of exposure to solvents in painting, there may be an increased risk of developing acute leukemia.[791] The "organic solvent syndrome" is a neuropsychiatric disorder seen in some painters from heavy exposure to solvents.[1253] Alcoholism may also play a role in its development.

Paint removers ("strippers") often contain methylene chloride, a solvent of choice for this purpose for years and for which OSHA has set a lower exposure limit because of the risk of cancer. The chemical is listed as a toxic air contaminant under the Clean Air Act of 1990. Laboratory animal studies and some epidemiological data indicate that it may cause cancer in exposed workers. It also metabolizes in the body to form carbon monoxide, thus reducing the oxygen-carrying capacity of the blood. Therefore, the previous permissible exposure limit (PEL) has been reduced from an 8-hour time-weighted average of 500 ppm to 25 ppm.[534] Other methods of paint stripping include blasting with dry ice, cornstarch pellets, and water.

Irritants

Adhesives and glues

Solvents (e.g., xylene, toluene, benzene, 2-ethoxyethyl acetate heptane, methylene chloride)

Paints (tributyl tin oxide and acetate used as a bactericide and fungicide in paint, especially antifouling paint for marine use)[472]

Paint removers (methylene chloride and others)

Paint strippers

Fibrous glass

Abrasives (wallpaper)

Soaps and detergents

Tributyl tin oxide (antifouling agent and biocide)[491]

Paint brush cleaners

Water (wet work)

Patch test to standard and vehicle preservative allergens, with special attention to the following.

Standard Allergens

Potassium dichromate, 0.25% pet; 0.023 mg/cm² (primer and anticorrosion paints)[9, 337]

2-Mercaptobenzothiazole, 1% pet; 0.075 mg/cm² (rubber)

Balsam of Peru, 20% pet; 0.80 mg/cm² (paint)[134]

Carba mix, 3% pet; 0.25 mg/cm² (rubber gloves)

Cobalt chloride, 1% pet; 0.02 mg/cm² (pigments, driers in paints, and varnishes)

Colophony (rosin), 20% pet; 0.85 mg/cm² (varnishes)

Epoxy resin, 1% pet; 0.05 mg/cm² (paints)

Mercapto mix, 1% pet; 0.075 mg/cm² (rubber)

Ethylenediamine dihydrochloride, 1% pet; 0.05 mg/cm² (stabilizer occasionally found in paints)

Kathon CG (5-chloro-2-methyl-4-isothiazolin-3-one and 2-methyl-4-isothiazolin-3-one), 0.01% aq; 0.0040 mg/cm²[355, 369]

PPD mix (Black rubber mix), 6% pet; 0.075 mg/cm² (rubber)

Thiuram mix, 1% pet; 0.025 mg/cm² (rubber gloves and other rubber articles)

Formaldehyde, 2% aq; 0.18 mg/cm² (preservative)

Nickel sulfate, 2.5% pet; 0.2 mg/cm² (pigments, hand tools)

Rosin (colophony), 20% pet; a leaching agent in antifouling paints

Thimerosal, 0.1% pet; 0.0080 mg/cm² (germicidal agents)

Additional Allergens

Ammoniated mercury, 1% pet

p-Chloro-m-xylenol, 1% pet (preservatives)

Methyl methacrylate monomer, 5% pet[182]

Benzophenone 1, 1% pet (UV-light inhibitor)

1,2-Benzisothiazolin-3-one, 0.1% pet[355]

BIS-GMA (2,2-bis[4-(2 hydroxy-3-methacryloxypropoxy)phenyl]propane), 2% pet[662]

HDDA (1,6-hexanediol diacrylate), 0.1% pet[99, 662]

TPGDA (tripropyleneglycol diacrylate), 0.1% pet[662]

Trimethylolpropane triacrylate (TMPTA), 0.1% pet[214]

p-tert-Butylphenol–formaldehyde resin (paint)[134]

Camphor, 10% pet (plasticizer)

Captan, 0.25% pet (preservative)

Chloracetamide, 0.2% pet (germicidal agent in wallpaper)[369, 615, 1276]

Chlorocresol, 1% pet (germicidal agent)

Chloromethoxy propyl mercuric acetate, 0.1% aq[1183]

Chlorothalonil ((TCPN) (tetrachloroisophthalonitrile), 0.001% or 0.01% acetone or pet (pesticide)[783]

Coal tar, 5% pet

Dibutyl phthalate, 5% pet (plasticizers)

Dichlorophene, 1% pet (germicidal agent)

Dipentene, 10% MEK (solvent in paints)[179]

Dichlofluanid, .1% wt/vol (fungicide in paints and varnishes)[497]

Euxyl K 400, 0.5% pet (germicidal agent in latex paints and emulsions)

Hexamethylene diisocyanate, 0.5% pet (common resin in paint)[600]

Hydroquinone, 1% pet (inhibitor in paint)

2-(Hydroxymethyl)amino ethanol, 5.0% aq (biocide)[1183]

Hydroxyethyl methacrylate, 2% pet (especially auto paints)[802]

Hydroxypropyl acrylate, 1% pet (especially auto paints)[802]

Hydroxypropyl methacrylate, 2% pet (especially auto paints)[802]

Methyl ethyl ketone peroxide, 1% pet (a catalyst for polyester resins)[1167]

N-methylolacrylamide, 0.1% pet (a 2-n-octyl-4-isothiazolin-3-one, 0.05% pet [Skane M-8; Kathon 893][865]

Pentachlorophenol, 1% aq (paint fungicide)

Phenol-formaldehyde resin, 10% pet (adhesives, binder resins)[134]

Urea formadehyde resin, 10% pet (adhesives, binder resins)

Phenylmercuric nitrate, 0.05% pet (germicidal agent)

o-Phenylphenol, 1% pet (germicidal agent)

Polyester resin monomer, 10% pet (polyester paint)

Tricresyl phosphate, 2% pet (plasticizer)

Triglycidyl isocyanurate (TGIC), 1 or 5% pet (epoxy hardener, polyesters)[306, 409, 863, 921,]

Turpentine, 10% in olive oil (solvents)

Paint Pigments That May Be Contact Allergens

Chloro-p-nitraniline red, 2% pet

F4R red, 2% pet

Hansa yellow, 2% pet

Para red, 2% pet

Toluidine red, 2% pet

Other pigments, 2% pet

PAPERMAKERS

Paper is made from either wood or rags, both of which are sources of cellulose fibers with strength and flexibility. Most paper is made from softwoods (coniferous trees) such as spruce, hemlock, and pine or from hardwoods such as poplar and oak. Some is made from synthetic fibers. After logs are transported to a pulp mill, the bark is removed. The chief machine used for this operation is a large revolving cylinder known as a *drum barker.* Logs are fed into this machine from a conveyor belt by a semiskilled worker called a *barker operator.* The machine cleans the bark from the logs by tumbling and removes chips and dirt with a water spray. Next the pulp wood is transferred by conveyor to a chipper machine (operated by a *chipper*), where the wood is cut into chips of desired size. Sometimes entire trees or logs at the site of felling are fed into large mobile harvesters and chippers, thus reducing transportation costs and the amount of wasted wood.

After the logs have been converted to wood chips, they are cooked in a digester by means of heat and chemicals under pressure. The manufacture of wood pulp is accomplished by two chemical methods: a *sulfite process* and a *kraft process.* The sulfite process, introduced during the 1870s, was for many years the leading process. The cooking liquor consists of free sulfur dioxide dissolved in water at a concentration of 4 to 6% with 2 to 3% bisulfite salts. The digestion is usually carried out in a batch process in a pressure vesicle, a steel shell with an acid-resistant lining of ceramic tile set in acid-proof cement or stainless steel. Digesters with capacities of up to 35 tons have been constructed. After the digester has been filled with chips, hot acid is pumped into the unit, completely filling it and replacing the air. Steam is then introduced to heat the chips. At the end of the cooking process, the contents are blown to a blow pit by rapid opening of the bottom valve, the violence of which defibers the cooked chips. A screening process then separates the unwanted particles such as knots, uncooked chips, dirt, bark, fiber bundles, and so forth from the fiber. Sometimes a centrifuge is used for separation. A light-colored pulp is obtained, which then can be used for paper manufacturing.

In the *kraft process* of pulping, discovered in 1884 in Germany, sodium hydroxide and sodium sulfide are the active agents in the pulp-cooking phase of the process. The chief difference between the two processes is in pH; the kraft process is highly alkaline, while the sulfite process is acidic. Also the kraft process is much more efficient and can utilize practically any type of wood. Today it is the chief method of pulp paper manufacture.

To further prepare the pulp for papermaking, it is mixed thoroughly with water and refined in machines operated by skilled workers called *beater engineers.* The mechanical squeezing and pounding of the cellulose fibers permits water to penetrate the structure, causing the fibers to swell, creating flexibility. Beating also increases paper strength. At this point various additives are introduced, such as sizing, fillers, colors, and interfiber bonding agents. It should be pointed out that paper stock at this point is highly flammable and is considered a dangerous fire risk. A typical sizing solution consists of a rosin soap mixed with stock in the amount of 1 to 5% of the fiber. In pulp and surface sizing, an epoxide, 2,3-epoxypropyl trimethyl ammonium chloride, may be used. It is irritating and also a fairly potent allergic sensitizer.[348] Alum (aluminum sulfate) is employed as a coupling agent. Fillers increase smoothness, opacity, and brightness and include clay (kaolin), titanium dioxide, calcium carbonate, zinc oxide, zinc sulfide, and asbestos. Soluble dyes, direct dyes, basic dyes, and other are added to impart color to the final product. Polyacrylamide resins, natural gums, and starch are the most common agents added to enhance or modify the bonding and coherence between the fibers.

The resulting solution is made into paper or paperboard by huge machines, which are of two general types: the fourdrinier machine (the most commonly used) and a cylinder machine used to make special types of paper, such as building and container board. In the fourdrinier machine the pulp solution is poured into a continuously moving and vibrating belt of fine wire or felt screen. As the water drains, millions of pulp fibers adhere to one another, forming a thin, wet sheet of paper. After passing through presses that squeeze out most of the water and through as many as 40 heated cylinders, the newly formed paper passes into a drier. Drying is accomplished by dozens of steam-heated cylinders; the sheet of paper is held in contact with the heated surfaces by means of drier felts composed of impermeable wool, cotton, asbestos, or a combination of these materials. To prevent growth of fungi, slimicides are required in this process.[432, 1064] Widely used in the Scandinavian paper industry is methylene-bis-thiocyanate, which is used in very low concentrations, perhaps accounting for its low rate of sensitization.[650] Nevertheless, Andersen and Hamman[33] found it to possess a strong sensitization potential in guinea pigs. Other slimicides are described by Fregert.[432] Of special importance are mercaptobenzothiazole[891] and organic bromine compounds such as 2'-bromine-4'-hydroxyacetophenone. Kathon CG is also used to some extent.[139, 281] A common algicide is pentachlorophenol, which has been associated with chloracne.[963]

The newly formed rolls of paper then undergo a number of final operations. One procedure is termed *wet converting,* in which paper in roll form is coated, impregnated, and laminated with a thin layer of clay and various resins to make it suitable for particular purposes. The second process is *dry converting,* in which paper in roll form is converted into such items as bags, envelopes, boxes, and small rolls, and packs of sheets. Polyethylene plastic coatings and other resins may be added at this stage. Laminates may be made from sheets of paper impregnated with a phenol formaldehyde resin. A predetermined number of sheets of paper are piled to a desired thickness and then placed under a warm press. The top layers may be coated with a colored substance to imitate certain types of wood, leather, or plastic veneer. Contact sensitivity to the phenol formaldehyde resin may occur during this process.[840]

When rags are used for making paper pulp, they are received at the mill in bales weighing from 400 to 1,200 lbs. After mechanical threshing, the rags are sorted by hand to remove synthetic fibers and foreign materials such as rubber, metal, and paper. After sorting, the rags are then cut up, dusted to remove small particles of foreign materials, and passed over magnetic rolls to remove iron.

The cleaned rags are then cooked in boilers in a liquor containing an alkaline solution of lime and soda ash or caustic soda combined with wetting agents and detergents. Steam is used to heat the boiler under pressure, and the contents are cooked for up to 10 hours. After being cooked, the rags are washed and mechanically beaten, and the process continues then as the wood pulp process.

Modern papermaking is highly automated, using computers and advanced instrumentation. Beta-ray sensors measure the weight of paper, and electromagnetic sensors measure thickness. A computer compares these measurements with program specifications and adjusts the machine to eliminate differences in the paper. Computers have also greatly reduced manual control but have increased monitoring functions for many operators.

Some of the workers in pulp- and papermaking are exposed to hot, humid, and noisy environments, and most of them complain of the disagreeable sulfide odors from chemicals used in the process.

Carbon Paper

Carbon paper is made by coating very lightweight paper stock with a mixture of pigments and a medium. The pigments include carbon black, Prussian blue, and organic dyes such as nigrosine. The medium is composed of a blend of waxes such as carnauba, candelilla, and beeswax as well as mineral and castor oils. Smudge-proof carbon paper is coated with lacquer.

Although carbon paper is often suspected to be a cause of dermatitis, the paper itself is rarely responsible. In 1972, Calnan[186] reported a male civil servant with a recurrent dermatitis of the hands and face from a special carbon paper used on a computer; the responsible chemical was found to be nigrosine. Calnan[178] reviewed the subject of carbon and carbonless paper. Tricresyl phosphate has been reported as a cause of carbon paper dermatitis, as has methyl violet.[175] The use of carbon paper has almost disappeared in recent years because of the wide use of so-called carbonless paper and computers.

Carbonless Paper

Carbonless paper is made by two different methods. In the first, on the underside of the top sheet are microcapsules composed of gum arabic and gelatin and containing a dye and an oil. The capsules are pressure sensitive, releasing their contents under a pressure of approximately 35 psi or higher. The dyes within the capsules are usually crystal violet lactone, methylene blue, and p-toluene sulfonic acid. A dermatitis resulting from Michler's hydrol (tetramethyl-diaminobenzhydrol) used as a dye intermediate, coupled with p-toluene sulfonic acid dye, was reported by Marks[847] in a secretary using a carbonless paper (see Office Workers). A diazonium dye is sometimes used within these capsules.

The second system uses a chemical coating on the surface that receives the print. This material is a mixture of clay, silica gel, starch, casein, and latex. A fungicide is also present.

Dermatitis from carbonless paper usually consists of dryness and fissuring from irritant effects of the paper. Menné et al.[894] could find no causative agent in patients suspected of dermatitis from this type of paper, but many of their patients also had upper respiratory complaints, which seemed directly related to the frequency of use of the paper. Proper ventilation and a high relative humidity may obviate these complaints.

Photocopy Paper

Photocopy paper is a rare cause of allergic contact dermatitis. Photocopy machines employed for copying are based either on infrared methods (thermography) or on the principle of electrostatics (xerography). In the early 1960s, 4-tert-butyl catechol was used as an antioxidant in the Thermofax machines. Harmon and Sarkany[536] described widespread eczema in two office workers. The catechol is related to the rhus antigen, resorcinol, and phloroglucinol and is a contact allergen. Resorcinol and phloroglucinol are used occasionally as couplers in the older diazo-type photocopiers and may cause dermatitis.

Cronin[242] has stated that computer paper may contain rosin and epoxy resin. Jordan and Vourlas[667] found typewriter correction paper to contain a phenol-formaldehyde resin (see Office Workers).

A retrospective cohort study of 3,545 employees in the Finnish pulp and paper industry showed an excess frequency of lung cancer that could not be attributed to cigarette smoking, especially among male board mill workers.[651]

Irritants

Acids[322]
Alkalis[322]
Alum
Ammonia
Bleaching agents (chlorine gas, sodium hydroxide, sodium hypochlorite)
Caustic soda (may cause serious burns)
Disinfectants (peracetic acid and others)
Heat and humidity
Slimicides[281, 432]
Soaps and detergents
Solvents (for glues and adhesives)
Sulfur dioxide
Water (wet work)

Patch test to standard and vehicle preservative allergens, with special attention to the following.

Standard Allergens

Potassium dichromate, 0.25% pet; 0.023 mg/cm² (sulfate pulp)[440]
2-Mercaptobenzothiazole, 1% pet; 0.075 mg/cm² (rubber, slimicides)[432, 891]

Carba mix, 3% pet; 0.25 mg/cm^2 (rubber gloves)
Cobalt chloride, 1% pet; 0.02 mg/cm^2 (pigments)
p-Phenylenediamine, 1% pet; 0.090 mg/cm^2 (dyes)
Wool alcohols (lanolin), 30% pet; 1.00 mg/cm^2
Epoxy resin, 1% pet; 0.05 mg/cm^2
Kathon CG, 0.01% pet; 0.0040 mg/cm^2 (slimicide)[281]
Mercapto mix, 1% pet; 0.075 mg/cm^2 (rubber gloves)
Ethylenediamine dihydrochloride, 1% pet; 0.05 mg/
    cm^2 (slimicides, Proxel used as preservative)[242]
PPD mix (Black rubber mix), 0.6% pet; 0.075 mg/cm^2
    (rubber)
Thiaram mix, 1% pet; 0.025 mg/cm^2 (rubber)
Formaldehyde, 2% aq; 0.18 mg/cm^2 (preservatives)
Nickel sulfate, 2.5% pet; 0.2 mg/cm^2 (tools)
Rosin (colophony), 20% pet; 0.85 mg/cm^2 (sizing)[1305]

Additional Allergens

Methyl methacrylate monomer, 5% pet (and other
    acrylics in resin emulsions)
p-Aminoazobenzene, 0.25% pet (azo dyes)
p-Aminophenol, 1% pet (dyes)
Anthraquinone, 2% pet (catalyst in delignification
    reactions, photosensitizer[114]
Benzophenone, 1% pet (UV inhibitor)
Dichlorophene, 1% pet (germicidal agent for slime
    control)
Epoxypropyl trimethyl ammonium chloride, 0.2% pet
    (added to increase strength of paper and for surface
    sizing)[348, 349]
Hydroquinone, 1% pet (antioxidant)
Kathon CG, 0.01% pet (slimicide)[281, 349]
Phenol-formaldehyde resin, 10% pet (used in plywood
    and adhesives for paper)
Nigrosine, 1% pet[186]
Phenylmercuric nitrate, 0.05% pet (germicidal agent)
o-Phenylphenol, 1% pet (germicidal agent)
Resorcinol-formaldehyde resin, 5% pet (adhesives
    used in plywood and paper)
Sodium metabisulfite, 1% aq (pulping process)
Tricresyl phosphate, 2% pet (carbon paper)

PERFORMING ARTISTS

See also Musicians.

Skin conditions among performing artists are more frequent than is generally realized.[580] Among symphony orchestra players, for example, skin disease is a recurring and significant problem.[1031] A recent study[941] showed that among 41 orchestra players, 18% of string players and 27% of wind and brass players had active skin problems. Performing artists often suppress and disregard their skin disorders in order to continue practicing and performing. However, a paronychia or fissuring of a finger can severely impede a concert pianist,[1136] and even a simple problem such as excessive sweating can cause a musician's fingers to slip from the instrument's keys. Among the most frequent problems are callosities, hyperkeratoses, and cheilitis of the lips in horn and woodwind players; "fiddlers' neck" in violinists; abrasions and blisters in dancers; onycholysis in pianists; and onycholysis and subungual hemorrhages in harpists and ballet dancers. A circumscribed atrophy of the upper lips of horn players may occur.[718]

Allergic contact dermatitis to cosmetics is also seen in performing artists. Comprehensive reviews of reactions to cosmetics and skin care products have been done by DeGroot and White.[282] Fragrance materials are responsible for a very large number of cosmetic reactions. A detailed review of these reactions is given by DeGroot and Frosch.[277]

Callosities are perhaps necessary "occupational marks" in drummers and other percussionists. A characteristic callosity occurs on the midportion of the upper lip of almost all clarinet and oboe players, for example.

"Fiddlers' neck"[1045] is a combination of folliculitis, lichenification, acneiform lesions, and hyperpigmentation occurring inferior to the mandible where the instrument rests and presses against the skin. Violists appear to be more frequently affected, due to the heavier and larger size of the instrument.[1165] Scarring may occasionally result.[746, 1192] This condition, which is an example of mechanical acne,[124] seems to be more common in players with badly fitting neck rests or a faulty technique.[978] Other factors such as pressure, friction, rubbing, pinching, sweating, and sometimes poor hygiene play a role.[549]

Chemical irritation is less common in performing artists, with the exception of the heavy oil-based makeups worn by actors, singers, and television personalities, which aggravate and may even precipitate acne. Allergic sensitization can occur from preservatives in makeup preparations and moisturizers used by actors. Horn players polish their instruments with pastes or silver polish that usually contain potentially irritating solvents.

Allergic sensitization may also occur in string players from rosin (colophony) used on bows and strings and in woodwind players from cocobolo or other exotic woods. Hausen[549] reported a violinist/physician who was sensitive to a wooden chin rest that was made of Brazilian rosewood (Dalbergia nigra All.). Patch testing with S-4'-hydroxy-4-methoxydalbergione, the active ingredient, at 1% was positive. Violin chin rests made from East Indian rosewood (Dalbergia latifolia Roxb.) may also cause dermatitis.[568] Dermatitis of the lips of a recorder player has been reported due to Brazilian rosewood (Dalbergia nigra All.); however, cocobolo wood is a more common source of contact allergy among recorder players[562] and also drummers using drumsticks made of cocobolo wood (Dalbergia grenadillo). Schwartz et al.[1103] describe an eczematous dermatitis of the lower lip of flute players from sensitivity to the wood of the mouthpiece.

Nickel dermatitis in a cellist occurred on the flexor surfaces of the distal phalanges of the second and third fingers of the right hand, at the exact site of contact with very small metallic parts embedded in the bow. The dimethylglyoxime test on the metal was positive.[810]

Propolis (bee glue) has been used for centuries as an ingredient in violin varnish. Stradivari used it in the varnish of his stringed instruments.[912] It should be considered as a source of contact allergy not only in makers but also in those who repair instruments.[566, 567, 663]

Epidemics of scabies are not uncommon in theaters from sharing contaminated costumes.

Irritants

Rosin (colophony) (string players)
Polishing compounds (horn players)

Patch test to standard vehicle preservative allergens and additional allergens, with special attention to the following.

Violin and Other Stringed Instruments

Rosin (colophony), 20% pet
Ebony
Rosewood (Brazilian rosewood: *Dalbergia nigra* All.; East Indian rosewood: *Dalbergia latifolia* Roxb.), R-4-methoxydalbergione, and S-4,4'-dimethoxydalbergione[548, 568]
Macassar ebony *(Diospyros celebia)* (in pegs)
Nickel sulfate, 2.5% pet[810]
Propolis

Oboe and Other Reed Instruments

Rosewood
Cocobolo *(Dalbergia retusa)*
African blackwood *(Dalbergia melanoxylon)*
Other exotic woods[547]

Horn, Flute, and Harmonica

Nickel sulfate, 2.5% pet
Preservatives in polishing compounds

Percussion Instruments

Nickel sulfate, 2.5% pet

Recorder

East Indian rosewood *(Dalbergia latifolia)*
Brazilian rosewood *(Dalbergia nigra)*
Cocobolo wood *(Dalbergia retusa)*

PEST CONTROL WORKERS

Pest controllers use pesticides, sprayers, traps, and other supplies servicing homes, restaurants, food stores, hotels, and other facilities that are infested with rats, mice, or insects. The workers first inspect the facility to determine the extent of infestation. They spray pesticides in and around areas where insects live, such as cabinets and sinks, and set traps and poisonous bait in areas where rats or mice nest and travel. Termite specialists kill termites and also prevent them from reaching wood structures. They usually work in pairs, using poison and constructing barriers, often with cement.

They may remove and rebuild foundations or insulate wood from earth contact with concrete. They also dig around and underneath houses and do general cleanup work. They spray poison directly onto wood structures and into soil through a steel nozzle inserted into the ground.

In addition to the irritants and allergens listed below, pest controllers may come in contact with poison oak/ivy, caterpillars, snakes, spiders, rats, and moths. They may also get burns from wet cement during repairs.

Irritants

Soaps and detergents
Solvents (ethyl acetate, xylene)
Pesticides
Fumigants
Wet cement
Dirt and dust
Plants and woods
Repellents
Rodenticides

Patch test to standard and vehicle preservative allergens, with special attention to the following.

Standard Allergens

Potassium dichromate, 0.25% pet; 0.023 mg/cm² (wet cement)
2-Mercaptobenzothiazole, 1% pet; 0.075 mg/cm² (rubber, rubber face mask)
Carba mix, 3% pet; 0.25 mg/cm² (rubber)
Epoxy resin, 1% pet; 0.05 mg/cm² (adhesive and repairs)
Mercapto mix, 1% pet; 0.075 mg/cm² (rubber, rubber face mask)
PPD mix (Black rubber mix), 0.6% pet; 0.075 mg/cm² (rubber)
Thiuram mix, 1% pet; 0.024 mg/cm² (rubber gloves, face mask of respirator, and control of deer, rabbits, and squirrels)
Formaldehyde, 2% aq; 0.18 mg/cm² (fumigant)
Nickel sulfate, 2.5% pet; 0.2 mg/cm² (tools)
Rosin (colophony), 20% pet; 0.85 mg/cm² (eradication of moles)

Additional Allergens

Ammoniated mercury, 1% pet (mercuric chloride for termite control)
Captan, 0.1% pet (fungicide, also seed treatment)
p-Chlorophenol, 1% (termites)
o-Dichlorobenzene, 1% pet (termites)
Pentachlorophenol, 1% aq (termites)
Pine oil, 10% in olive oil (termites, ticks, fleas, moths, and other insects)

Fumigants, Repellents, and Rodenticides

Acrylonitrile (with carbon tetrachloride: Acritet) (fumigant)

Aluminum phosphide (fumigant)
Aminopyridine (repellent)
Anthraquinone (repellent)[114]
ANTU (rodenticide)
Avitrol (repellent)
Barium carbonate (rodenticide)
Bromodiolone (rodenticide)
2,3,4,5-Bis(2-butylene)tetrahydrofural (repellent)
Calcium cyanide (fumigant, rodenticide)
Carbon disulfide (fumigant)
Carbon tetrachloride (fumigant)
Chlorophacinone (rodenticide)
Chloropicrin (fumigant)
Coumafuryl (repellent)
Cyanogen chloride (fumigant)
Dazomet (fumigant)
DBCP (fumigant)
DDVP (soil fumigant)
Denatonium benzoate (repellent)
Dibromochloropropane (fumigant)
1,2-Dibromoethane (ethylene bromide) (fumigant)
Dibutyl phthalate (repellent)
Dibutyl succinate (repellent)
p-Dichlorobenzene (fumigant)
Dichloropropene (fumigant)
p-Dichlorobenzene (fumigant)
1,3-Dichloropropene (fumigant)
N,N-Diethyl-m-toluamide (repellent)
Di-n-propyl isocinchomerate (repellent)
Ethylene dichloride (fumigant)
Ethylene dibromide (fumigant)
Ethylene oxide (fumigant)
2-Ethyl-1,3-hexanediol (repellent)
Fluoroacetate (repellent)
Fluoroacetamide (repellent)
Formaldehyde (fumigant)
Furfural (fumigant)
Hydrocyanic acid (fumigant)
2-Hydroxyethyl-n-octyl sulfide (repellent)
Magnesium phosphide (fumigant)
Metam-sodium (fumigant)
Methyl bromide (fumigant)
Methyl bromide/chloropicrin mixture (fumigant)
Methyl isothiocyanate (soil fumigant)
Methyl nonyl ketone (repellent)
Methyl phthalate (repellent)
Naphthalene
Paraformaldehyde (fumigant)
Phosphine (fumigant)
2-Pivalyl-1,3-indandione (repellent)
Propylene dichloride (fumigant)
Propylene oxide (fumigant)
Red Squill (rodenticide)
Sodium N-methyldithiocarbamate (metam-sodium)
    (soil fumigant)
Strychnine (repellent)
Sulfuryl fluoride (fumigant)
Tetramethylthiuram disulfide (repellent) (also rubber
    accelerator)
Thallium sulfate (repellent)
Warfarin (repellent, rodenticide)
Zinc phosphide (repellent)

Ziram (zinc dimethyldithiocarbamate) (repellent) (also
    rubber accelerator)

PHARMACISTS

Retail pharmacists do little compounding today. Most of their time is employed in dispensing drugs, record keeping, and providing information to patients. Almost the only contact retail pharmacists have today with allergenic chemicals is when they are required to make up patch testing materials for dermatologists. Pharmacists ordinarily work under satisfactory conditions, although they often are under considerable pressure. Most of their drugs are kept on shelves. Some items are refrigerated, and controlled substances are kept under lock and key.

In Britain, pharmacists dispense pet supplies and pesticides in addition to drugs and cosmetics. They are delivered in bulk bags, and many of them must be packaged before display. The risks of sensitization, particularly for potent sensitizers, can be considerable. Workers in pharmaceutical manufacturing plants may develop immediate allergic reactions to latex in gloves.[1217]

Forty-five factory workers developed contact dermatitis to semisynthetic penicillins during manufacture. Strong positive patch test reactions were found; the dermatitis appeared to be aggravated by highly contaminated dust that impregnated the worker's clothing.[910]

Irritants

Soaps and detergents
Certain medications (particularly when compounding
    materials such as podophyllin, salicylic acid, and
    others)
Safety caps on prescription containers (koebnerizing
    psoriasis[385])

Patch test to standard and vehicle preservative allergens, with special attention to the following.

Standard Allergens

Wool alcohols (lanolin), 30% pet; 1.00 mg/cm²
2-Mercaptobenzothiazole, 1% pet; 0.075 mg/cm²
    (rubber)
Neomycin sulfate, 20% pet; 0.23 mg/cm²
Balsam of Peru, 25% pet; 0.80 mg/cm²
Caine mix, 8% pet; 0.63 mg/cm²
Carbo mix, 3% pet 0.25 mg/cm² (rubber)
Mercapto mix, 1% pet (rubber); 0.075 mg/cm²
    (rubber)
Ethylenediamine dihydrochloride, 1% pet; 0.05 mg/
    cm² (medications)
Fragrance mix, 8% pet; 0.43 mg/cm²
Cl + Me-isothiazolinone (Kathon CG), 0.01% aq;
    0.0040 mg/cm² (germicidals)
Paraben mix, 15% pet; 1 mg/cm² (preservatives)
PPD mix (Black rubber mix), 0.6% pet; 0.075 mg/cm²
    (rubber)

Quaternium 15, 1% pet; 0.1 mg/cm^2
Thiuram mix, 1% pet 0.025 mg/cm^2 (rubber gloves)
Formaldehyde, 2% aq; 0.18 mg/cm^2
Nickel sulfate, 2.5% pet; 0.2 mg/cm^2 (tools)
Thimerosal, 0.1% pet; 0.0080 mg/cm^2

Additional Allergens

Ammoniated mercury, 1% pet
Azathioprine, 0.1% pet[154, 1149]
Bacitracin, 20% pet
Benzalkonium chloride, 0.01% aq
Benzoic acid, 5% pet
Benzoin tincture, 10% alc
Benzyl alcohol, 5% pet
Cetyl alcohol, 30% pet
Chloramphenicol, 2% pet
Chlorocresol, 1% pet
Chlorpromazine, 1% pet
Chlorquinaldol, 5% pet
Corticosteroids[299, 313, 314]
Gentamycin, 20% pet
Hexachlorophene, 1% pet
Hexylresorcinol, 1% pet
Menthol, 1% pet
Methyl salicylate, 2% pet
Paraben mix, 12% pet
Penicillin and relations[721]
Potassium metabisulfite, 1% pet (preservative)
Promethazine[721]
Propylene glycol, 4%
Quinidine sulfate, 0.5% aq[1274]
Resorcinol, 2% pet
Sodium lauryl sulfate, 0.1% aq
Sodium metabisulfite, 5% pet (1%) (antioxidant,
    preservative)[302]
Sorbic acid, 2% pet
Triethanolamine, 1% pet or aq
Vitamin E (DL-a-tocopherol), 10% pet
Vitamin K$_1$ (phytomenadione), 0.1% pet

PHOTOCOPY PAPER WORKERS

See Office Workers and Papermakers.

PHOTOGRAPHERS

In addition to the familiar black-and-white and color photography for home and commercial use, photography includes many industrial categories: aerial and underwater photography, stereoscopic and three-dimensional photography, infrared and ultraviolet photography, radiography, nuclear tract recording, astronomical photography, and microfilming. Photography plays a vital role in lithography and printing, police work, medicine, the construction of electronic microdevices, and many other occupational activities.

Dermatitis in photography arises almost entirely from the process of developing film. In its simplest form, a roll of film is wound around a reel and passed through a succession of processing baths: developers, intermediate rinses, fixing baths, washing, and drying. The resulting negative is then printed in a printing box with a built-in light source. Nearly all photo developing today is with automatic machines. The operator contacts the chemicals only when the machine breaks down or requires periodic cleaning and repairing; however, when the machine breaks down during film processing, there is often no time for the operator to don protective gloves.

Photography is one of the most "chemical" of all industries, and the allergens are numerous.[489, 1126] Black-and-white photography only occasionally induces sensitization; color photography rather frequently does if precautions are not strictly observed. Photographers often prepare their own solutions from formulas available in "cookbooks." Manufacturers advise against skin contact, but many workers disregard warnings and immerse their bare hands and arms in the solutions. Argyria may occur from prolonged contact with silver salts, especially if there is ingestion of photographic film from chewing on it, as in one reported case.[1008] The skin appears to be an excretory organ for silver, as in argyria there is a gradual movement of silver from the general body pool through the dermis into the epidermis. Silver is then released from melanin–silver complexes near the surface of the epidermis as soluble ionic silver.[150] The discoloration is seen only in light-exposed areas. Generalized toxic side effects do not occur.

The prototype of *black-and-white developers* is Metol (methyl-*p*-aminophenol sulfate), also termed Elon, Photol, and Graphol. In combination with hydroquinone, potassium bromide, and sodium sulfite in an alkaline solution at a pH of approximately 8.7, Metol has served as the most important developer since 1895. Dermatitis from this class of developers is not uncommon.[1041]

Color film developers are numerous; most are related to *p*-phenylenediamine and Metol. Lichen planus-like eruptions have been seen following contact with these developers.[104, 110, 149, 197, 448, 481, 714, 843, 1041] Occasionally a worker sensitive to a color developer can work without problems with black-and-white film processing. Dark-skinned workers especially should use caution in working with developers containing hydroquinone because of the possibility of depigmentation. Allergic sensitization to Metol followed by prolonged contact with hydroquinone resulted in widespread vitiligo-like lesions in a black patient treated by the author. The worker was not allergically sensitive to hydroquinone on patch testing. Kersey and Stevenson[714] reported similar depigmentation following an eczematous allergic dermatitis due to a color developer in a man servicing automatic self-photography machines.

After it is developed, exposed film must be fixed. The usual fixing baths contain ammonium or sodium thiosulfate with sodium bisulfite in acid solution. Potassium chromium sulfate may also be present. Sodium bisulfite is a potential, but rare, contact allergen as well as a cause of immediate sensitivity reactions.

Polaroid film is made of polyvinyl chloride with a silver halide coating, in addition to carbon black, zinc

powder, manganese dioxide, and a binder of a polyamide adhesive. Red, blue, and green merocyanine dyes
are present. Between the dye layers (these so-called
space layers are proprietary), titanium dioxide and alkali
are present.[361]

A detailed study of a large number of employees of
the film laboratory was published by Liden.[779] Approximately 20% had occupational dermatoses, of which
one-half were due to allergic sensitization to one or
more photographic chemicals, especially CD-2, CD-3,
CD-4, Metol, and PBA-1. The latter is a chemical
especially used in the development of motion picture
film. PBA stands for Persulfate Bleach Accelerator; it
is an isothiouronium compound with a strong potential
for sensitization.[788] Patch testing should be done at 1%
in pet.[1294] Although PBA-1 may be contaminated with
traces of thiourea, patch testing with thiourea was negative.[782] Comprehensive reviews of occupational dermatoses from photographic chemicals are given by Liden.[781–784]

Irritants

Acids (fixing baths, stabilizers, tray cleaners, and
  "short stop")
Alcohols
Alkalis (developers, film detergent-type cleaners,
  hypoeliminators, activators)
Bleach
Solvents (film cleaners)
Formaldehyde (hardeners, print flattening solutions)
Surfactants (photoresists)
Ammonium persulfate (to remove hypo) (urticarial
  reactions)
Ammonium thiosulfate (fixing agent, for rapid
  development)
Aluminum chloride
Water (wet work)
PBA-1 (accelerator for motion picture film, see
  sensitizers, later)[778, 782]
Lacquers
Phenol (preservative)
Developers (alkalinity; as above, and also Metol and
  dimethylformamide)
Diethylene glycol
Sodium metabisulfite (asthma, anaphylactic
  reactions)[393]
Silver halides

Patch test to standard and vehicle preservative allergens, with special attention to the following.

Standard Allergens

Potassium dichromate, 0.25% pet; 0.023 mg/cm²
  (developers, processing aids, tray cleaners,
  intensifiers, reversal solutions)
2-Mercaptobenzothiazole, 1% pet; 0.075 mg/cm²
  (rubber)
Carba mix, 3% pet; 0.25 mg/cm² (rubber)
Epoxy resin, 1% pet; 0.05 mg/cm² (for "image
  addition")

Ethylenediamine dihydrochloride, 1% pet; 0.05 mg/
  cm² (in certain developers)
Formaldehyde, 2% aq; 0.18 mg/cm² (some developers,
  hardeners, print flattening solutions)
Thiuram mix, 1% pet; 0.025 mg/cm² (rubber gloves)
Nickel sulfate, 2.5% pet; 0.2 mg/cm² (hand tools)

Additional Allergens

Ammoniated mercury, 1% pet (mercuric chloride as
  intensifier in hypo test solution)
p-Aminophenol, 1% pet (developers)
2,4-Diaminophenol (amidol), 2% pet (developer)
1,2,3-Benzotriazole, 0.5% aq (photographic
  restrainer)[54]
Camphor, 10% pet
CD-2, 1% pet (color developer)
CD-3, 1% pet (color developer)
CD-4, 1% pet (color developer)
2,4-Diaminophenol, 2% pet
Dichlorophene, 1% pet (to prevent mildew on
  negatives in storage)[581]
Dimethylhydantoid-formaldehyde resin, 1% in 95% alc
  and pet[315]
Glutaraldehyde, 0.25% aq (print hardener)
Gold sodium thiosulfate, 0.1% pet (for gold, toners)
Hydrazine sulfate, 1% pet (developers)
Hydroquinone, 1% pet (developers)
N-isopropyl-N'-phenyl-p-phenylenediamine (IPPD),
  0.1% pet (rubber)
Metol, 1% pet (4-methyl aminophenol) (black and
  white developer)
Pentachlorophenol, 1% aq (fungicide to preserve
  developers)
Persulfate Bleach Accelerator (PBA-1), 1%
  pet[778,782, 788, 1293]
Phenidone (1-phenyl-3-pyrazolidinone), 1% pet (black-
  and-white developer)
Phloroglucinol, 1% pet
Platinum chloride, 1% pet
Pyrocatechol, 2% pet (developers)
Pyrogallol, 1% pet (tanning developer)
Resorcinol, 2% pet (developers)
Sodium or potassium metabisulfite (reducing agent),
  1% pet

PLASTICS ASSEMBLER, FABRICATOR

"In the five decades since the end of World War II,
plastic has crept unceasingly, and often invisibly, into
our homes, cars, offices, even our bodies—Plastic has
become the defining medium of our Synthetic Century
precisely because it combines the ultimate twentieth-
century characteristics—artificiality, disposability and
synthesis—all rolled into one. The ultimate triumph of
plastic has been the victory of package over product, of
style over substance, of surface over essence."[365] The
"big five" plastics today are polyethylene, polypropylene, polystyrene, polyvinyl chloride, and the styrenics,
supplying resins to manufacturers of packaging films,
pipes, electronics housings, bottles, electrical connec-

tors, among many others. In 1996 consumers worldwide purchased and utilized more than 215 billion pounds of these five most widely used commodity plastics.[1021] The most widely used plastic worldwide is polyethylene.

Plastic workers fabricate, assemble, and repair various plastic products using bonding techniques and materials. They also use hand tools, power tools, and curing ovens. They may cut lines on sheet stock and fiberglass or graphite cloth using template patterns, blueprints, and sketches. They usually mix the ingredients themselves, including the resin, catalyst, fillers, accelerators and colors, according to formulas. The mixing may be done either by hand or, more commonly, by using a power mixer. After curing, they trim, drill, grind, and finish the parts according to specification using various hand tools and power tools. They apply tape, foam, or other types of adhesive to assembly for later bonding in an autoclave. Sometimes a heat gun is used.

Other titles include *assemblers and gluers* of laminated plastics (mix resin and apply to surfaces, and, after curing, remove excess material using hacksaw, mallet, and so forth; they also often solder and buff parts); *casters* (place the part in mold after applying parting agents such as soap, wax, or lacquer to the mold; there is some direct contact with resin and other ingredients when weighting); *hand finishers* (use hand tools and sandpaper); and *knock-out hand workers* (place product in tank of water to loosen the product from a mandrel).

Most cases of contact dermatitis arise from laminating, mixing, and cleaning.[376, 1186] Fiberglass, organic solvents, resins, resin additives, and organic peroxides are common causes of irritant and allergic contact dermatitis. Epoxy resins are especially common causes,[1186] and the diglycidyl ether bisphenol A type (MW 340) is responsible for the majority of cases. Contact allergy to hardeners alone is unusual,[690] although testing should be done with hardeners, especially polyamine hardeners, and with reactive diluents as well.[660] The hardeners actually used by the workers should always be tested.[690]

Most acrylates are fairly potent allergic sensitizers, such as UV radiation-cured acrylate surface coatings.[84, 376, 676, 1029] Active sensitization may even occur from patch testing, especially with ethyl acrylate, 2-hydroxyethyl acrylate, and 2-hydroxypropyl acrylate.[676] Contact urticaria and occupational allergic contact dermatitis have been described from a polyfunctional aziridine hardener used in two-component paints, paint primers, lacquers, and so on.[685] A common adhesive is Locktite, which contains polyethyleneglycol dimethacrylate (PEGMA).[1113] A frequent cause of contact urticaria (and allergic contact dermatitis) in this industry is natural rubber-based gloves.

Resins based on phenol and formaldehyde are common contact allergens. They were the first synthetic thermosetting polymers developed, discovered by Baekeland in 1907. Polymerization is of the condensation type, using an acid catalyst, producing a so-called novolak resin. They are widely used in molded and cast articles, as bonding agents (often as powders), for lamination and impregnating, and for plywood and glass-fiber composites. In a plant where decorative

equipment was made of paper sheets impregnated with these resins, over 9% of workers were found allergically sensitive to the phenolic resins.[135]

Polyurethane chemicals are also widely used in the production of plastics, especially synthetic rubber and other elastomers. In addition to urticaria, asthma, and rhinitis, which are most likely to occur from toluene diisocyanate, several commonly used polyurethanes and their catalysts are potential allergic contact sensitizers. These include 4,4'-diphenylmethane diisocyanate, 1,6-hexamethylene diisocyante, and diaminodiphenylmethane.[351]

The incidence of dermatitis can be reduced when preventive measures are instituted: skin protection at all times, especially the use of impermeable disposable gloves, which should be laminated and multilayered. The risk of sensitization is increased when worker exposure is combined with simultaneous contact with organic solvents or when there is a pre-existing skin condition such as atopic dermatitis.[660] The risk of cancer can be posed by certain organic solvents used in this industry. The PEL of methylene chloride, a solvent long used in plastics processing, has been reduced from 500 to 25 ppm. This widely used solvent has been known to cause cancer in rats and mice, and recent epidemiological data also suggest it may cause cancer in exposed workers.[534] Recent studies suggest that plastics workers have an increased risk for pancreatic cancer, which appears to be associated with exposure to vinyl processing.[287, 1111] Styrene is also an important occupational hazard in this industry, chiefly because of its neurological effects.[923]

Irritants

Acids
Alkalis
Solvents (e.g., methylene chloride, *n*-methyl-2-pyrolidone)

Patch test to standard and vehicle preservative allergens, with special attention to the following:

Standard Allergens

Nickel sulfate, 2.5% pet; 0.2 mg/cm² (tool handles)
Wool alcohols, 30% pet; 1.00 mg/cm² (part agents)
Fragrance mix, 8% pet; 0.43 mg/cm² (protective creams, soaps)
Epoxy resin, 1% pet; 0.05 mg/cm² (resins)
Ethylenediamine dihydrochloride, 1% pet; 0.05 mg/cm²
Cobalt dichloride, 1% pet; 0.02 mg/cm² (metals, driers)
p-tert-Butylphenol–formaldehyde resin, 1% pet; 0.04 mg/cm² (resin)
Cl + Me-isothiazolinone, 0.01% pet; 0.0040 mg/cm² (Kathon CG) (protective creams)
Quaternium 15, 1% pet; 0.1 mg/cm² (protective creams)
Mercaptobenzothiazole, 2% pet; 0.075 mg/cm² (rubber, adhesives)

Formaldehyde, 1% in water; 0.18 mg/cm^2 (plastics, adhesives)

Mercapto mix, 2% pet; 0.075 mg/cm^2 (rubber)

Thiuram mix, 1% pet; 0.025 mg/cm^2 (rubber)

Additional Allergens

Acrylonitrile, 0.1% pet

Methyl methacrylate, 1% pet (w/w)

Ethyl methacrylate, 1%

Triethylenetetramine, 0.5%

Diaminodiphenylmethane, 0.5%

Dimethylaminopropylamine (DMAPA), 1% pet (epoxy catalyst)[681]

Ethylenediamine, 1%

Benzoyl peroxide, 1%

Allyl glycidyl ether, 0.05 to 0.1% in olive oil (reactive diluent for silicone, polyurethane, and epoxy resins)[301]

Benzoyl peroxide, 1% (catalyst)

Cyanoacrylate, 2% pet

Triglycidyl isocyanurate, 1% pet[300, 863, 881, 958]

2,3-Dibromocresylglycidyl ether, 0.01% acetone (flame retardant)[974]

Methylhexahydrophthalic anhydride, 0.5% pet (a phthalic anhydride hardener for epoxy resins)[688]

Methyl methacrylate, 1% pet

Phenol formaldehyde resin, 5%

Dibutyl phthalate, 5%

Epichlorhydrin, 0.3%

Epoxy acrylate, 0.5%[376]

1,6-Hexanediol diacrylate, 0.1%[376]

Triethylene glycol dimethacrylate, 2% pet[376]

Trimethylol propane triacrylate, 0.1% pet[376]

Tripropylene glycol diacrylate, 0.1% pet[376]

2-Hydroxy-2-methyl-1-phenylpropane, 2% pet

2,2-Dimethoxy-1,2-diphenylethane-1-one, 2% pet

1-Hydroxy-cyclohexyl-phenyl-ketone, 2% pet

Polyethyleneglycol dimethacrylate (PEGMA) (adhesive), 1% pet[1113]

Polyfunctional aziridine hardener, 0.5% pet[685]

Toluene-2,4-diisocyanate, 0.1% pet

4,4'-Diphenylmethane diisocyanate, 1% pet

1,6-Hexamethylene diisocyanate, 0.1% pet

Isophoronediamine, 1% pet (epoxy resin hardener)[502]

Diaminodiphenylmethane, 0.5% pet[351]

Unsaturated polyester resin, 0.5 to 10% pet[305, 1185]

Resorcinol, 5% pet

Triethylenetetramine, 0.5% pet

Common Epoxy Hardeners

Diethylenetriamine (DETA)

Isophoronediamine (IPDA)

2,4,6-Tris-(dimethylaminomethyl)phenol (Tris-DMP)

2,2,4-Trimethylhexamethylenediamine (2,2,4-IMD)

2,4,4-Trimethylhexamethylenediamine (2,4,4-IMD)

m-Xyleylenediamine (*m*-XDA)

PLUMBERS AND PIPE FITTERS

Plumbers and pipe fitters install pipe systems that carry water, steam, air, or other liquids or gases. They also maintain, alter, and repair existing piping and install plumbing fixtures, appliances, and heating, air conditioning, and refrigeration equipment. Plumbing and pipe fitting are often a single trade, but some workers specialize.

Most pipes are made of steel, copper, cast iron, or other metals. Others may be plastic or glass or made of other nonmetallic materials. To fit pipes workers may have to measure, bend, cut, and thread pipes and then bolt, braze, solder, screw, or weld them together. Plumbers use pipe cutters, gas or acetylene torches, arc welders, and other welding, soldering, and brazing equipment.

Irritants

Wet work

Soldering flux

Metal cleaners (phosphates, solvents, acids, alkalis)

Abrasive skin cleansers (silica and pumice)

Rust removers (potassium dichromate, solvents, acids such as hydrofluoric acid)

Sewage

Soaps and detergents

Chemical, sewer, cesspool, and drain openers (sodium hydroxide in high concentrations)

Solvents

Greases

Enzymes (drain cleaners)

Hand cleaners (abrasives)

Water (wet work)

Patch test to standard and vehicle preservative allergens, with special attention to the following.

Standard Allergens

Potassium dichromate, 0.25% pet; 0.023 mg/cm^2 (rust removers, leather gloves, boiler cleaners, antirust paints, welding fumes, cement, boiler linings)[1063]

2-Mercaptobenzothiazole, 1% pet; 0.075 mg/cm^2 (rubber, hoses, gaskets)

Carba mix, 3% pet; 0.25 mg/cm^2 (rubber, hoses, gaskets)

Cobalt dichloride, 1% pet; 0.02 mg/cm^2 (drier in caulks)

Epoxy resin, 1% pet; 0.05 mg/cm^2 (adhesives)

Mercapto mix, 1% pet; 0.075 mg/cm^2 (rubber, gaskets)

PPD mix (Black rubber mix), 0.6% pet; 0.075 mg/cm^2 (black insulation rubber)

p-tert-Butylphenol–formaldehyde resin, 1% pet; 0.04 mg/cm^2 (leather)

Thiuram mix, 1% pet; 0.025 mg/cm^2 (rubber gloves, gaskets)

Formaldehyde, 2% aq; 0.18 mg/cm^2 (cleaners)

Nickel sulfate, 2.5% pet; 0.2 mg/cm^2 (hand tools)

Rosin (colophony), 20% pet; 0.85 mg/cm^2 (caulking compounds, soldering fluxes)

Additional Allergens

Dichlorophene, 1% pet (preservative in caulks)

Epichlorohydrin, 0.1% alc (in certain solvent cements)[66]

Hydrazine sulfate, 1% pet (soldering flux)
N-isopropyl-N'-phenyl-p-phenylenediamine (IPPD),
    0.1% pet (rubber seals)
Methyl salicylate, 2% pet (drain and pipe cleaners)
Phenylmercuric nitrate, 0.05% pet (germicidal agent in
    caulks)
Pine oil, 10% in olive oil (drain and pipe cleaners)
Diethylthiourea, 1% pet (safety shoes)[410]

POLICE OFFICERS AND DETECTIVES

Police duties, in addition to policing, arresting, and
investigating, range from clerking to photography, parking enforcement, radio dispatching, inspecting, in-
structing, and driving. The irritants and allergens associated with these duties vary with the type of work
performed.

Police also may work mounted on horses and in
harbor patrols, helicopter patrols, canine corps, mobile
rescue teams, and youth aid services. Detectives are
often plainclothes officers assigned to criminal investigations; others work as experts in chemical and microscopic analysis, firearms identification, and handwriting
and fingerprint identification.

Special problems may arise from the use of tear
gas, or mace (α-chloroacetophenone [CN]). Besides its
strong lacrimating effect, CN is a powerful skin irritant
and potential allergic sensitizer.[450, 769, 994] In direct contact with the skin, CN and CS (o-chlorobenzalmalononi-
trile; see later) cause extreme irritation with erythema
and vesicles. The irritating effect may be enhanced by
the presence of moisture and occlusion. One exposure
may be sufficient to induce sensitization, the first symptoms of which may not appear until 9 or 10 days after
exposure.[401] Patch testing must be done with very dilute
solutions, 0.001% or even less.[769]

CS is widely used as an aerosol in the United States
for riot control. Cutaneous hypersensitivity to this tear
gas was reported over 30 years ago.[814] In 1973,
Shmunes and Taylor[1129] showed 2 of 25 workers manufacturing this chemical to be allergically sensitive, reacting to a concentration of 0.1% CS in olive oil. Like
CN, CS is also a strong skin irritant. Contaminated
uniforms are possible sources of continuing dermatitis.[181, 1129, 1289]

Police in many cities are required to purchase their
own guns and other equipment. Less expensive guns
may have nickel-plated handles or nickel inlaid into
wood. Handcuffs may also be a source of nickel contact. Rubber sensitivity has been reported from a Black
rubber truncheon[106] and from rubber motorcycle handles.[474]

Routine office work consumes a large part of some
police officers' time (see Office Workers).

Because of their greater working time spent out of
doors, law enforcement workers may have a greater
risk for development of actinically caused skin cancer.
Three cases of melanoma among 715 police officers
represented a 14.2-fold increase over the expected normal incidence for this group of employees.[16] In evaluating these persons for worker compensation purposes,

the actual percentage of time of sunlight exposure during employment must be estimated, a difficult task with
imprecise results.

Irritants

Soaps and detergents
Solvents
Riot control agents, especially CS and CN

Patch test to standard and vehicle preservative allergens, with special attention to the following.

Standard Allergens

Potassium dichromate, 0.25% pet; 0.023 mg/cm²
    (leather and photographic chemicals)
2-Mercaptobenzothiazole, 1% pet; 0.075 mg/cm²
    (rubber)
Carba mix, 3% pet; 0.25 mg/cm² (rubber)
Mercapto mix, 1% pet; 0.075 mg/cm² (rubber)
PPD mix (Black rubber mix), 0.6% pet; 0.075 mg/cm²
    (rubber, rubber truncheon,[106] motorcycle handles[474])
Thiuram mix, 1% pet; 0.025 mg/cm² (rubber)
Nickel sulfate, 2.5% pet; 0.2 mg/cm² (metal handles of
    guns and handcuffs)
Rosin (colophony), 20% pet; 0.85 mg/cm² (ink)

Additional Allergens

p-Aminophenol, 1% pet (photographic developers)
CD-2, 1% pet (color photographic developers)
CD-3, 1% pet (color photographic developers)
α-Chloroacetophenone (CN), 0.001% acetone[242, 769]
o-Chlorobenzylidene malonitrile (CS), 0.001% in
    acetone[769]
Gold sodium thiomalate, 0.1% pet (analysis of
    spermatic fluid, alkaloid tests)
Hydroquinone, 1% pet (photographic developers)
Menthol, 1% pet
Metol, 1% pet (photographic developers)
Pyrocatechol, 2% pet (photographic developers)
Resorcinol, 2% pet (photographic developers)

POSTAL WORKERS

Postal clerks sell postage and revenue stamps, post-
cards, and stamped envelopes. They also sell postal
savings certificates and U.S. savings stamps. They fill
out and sell money orders, register and insure mail, and
compute mailing costs for letters and parcels. They
examine mail for correct postage and cancel mail using
a rubber stamp or a canceling machine. Recently the
U.S. Postal Service has accepted credit cards for payment.

Mail sorters separate the mail into groups of letters,
parcel post, magazines, and newspapers and then feed
the letters through canceling machines. Afterwards,
mail handlers take the mail into other workrooms to
sort them according to destination, usually using electronic mail sorting machines.

Among Danish postal workers dermatitis was found to be rare, the incidence being lower than in any other type of Danish union members.[1040] Rubber bands for wrapping small batches of sorted mail are possible sources of allergic sensitization.[720]

Irritants

Paper
Soaps and detergents
Ultraviolet light

Patch test to standard and vehicle preservative allergens, with special attention to the following.

Standard Allergens

2-Mercaptobenzothiazole, 1% pet; 0.075 mg/cm^2 (rubber fingerstalls, rubber bands,[720] stamp moisteners, money counters[344])
Balsam of Peru, 25% pet; 0.80 mg/cm^2 (stamp adhesives)
Carba mix, 3% pet; 0.25 mg/cm^2 (rubber)
Mercapto mix, 1% pet; 0.075 mg/cm^2 (rubber)
PPD mix (Black rubber mix), 0.6% pet (rubber)
Thiuram mix, 1% pet; 0.025 mg/cm^2 (rubber)
Formaldehyde, 2% aq (stamp adhesives)
Nickel sulfate, 2.5% pet; 0.2 mg/cm^2 (hand tools)
Rosin (colophony), 20% pet; 0.85 mg/cm^2 (adhesives)
Thimerosal, 0.1% pet; 0.0080 mg/cm^2 (preservatives)

Additional Allergens

N-isopropyl-*N'*-phenyl-*p*-phenylenediamine (IPPD), 0.1% pet (rubber fingerstalls)[1040]

POTTERY AND PORCELAIN MAKERS

In this occupation workers form, decorate, and finish pottery and porcelain ware. Pottery is either cast in molds or is pressed. In mold casting, the liquid clay is extruded by the pottery machine operator from a mill where the clay mixture is ground and amalgamated (a "pug mill") into plaster molds where it gradually hardens. After several hours, the piece is removed and allowed to dry. In the pressing method, plates and flat pieces are made using a hydraulic press, squeezing the clay around a mold and pushing excess clay around the sides. The piece is then passed to a trim line where the excess and rough edges are removed, and cracks, holes, and pin holes are filled with liquid clay. The piece is then fired and glazed. The glaze, consisting of mixtures of silicates, calcium carbonate, cadmium barium iron, nickel, biocides, and at one time lead compounds, is sprayed on with an air gun. Sometimes the piece is dipped in the glaze. The dipper grasps the piece with tongs or fingers and dips it into a tub or glaze solution. The article is twisted and turned to spread the glaze over its surface, and then the excess is removed by shaking. Using the fingers, glaze may be rubbed over missed, difficult-to-reach areas; or glaze may be poured onto a ceramic tile or the tile held against a roller containing the glaze. With a wire brush, the edges are then cleaned. The glaze must also be removed from the bottom of the piece before firing, which is done in a tunnel kiln, open at both ends. The temperature inside is about 2,000°C, at the exit end about 350°C. The glaze changes color during heating. After cooling, the piece is inspected for rough edges, which may be smoothed with a pumice stone or abrasives on a wet sponge. Larger clay fragments may be removed by a grinding wheel.

Model makers (pattern makers) construct models of particular pieces of ware to be used in casting molds. The model is formed by carving it from plaster of Paris or from clay, or both, and then shaping the material with the hands as it revolves on a spinning table and at the same time removing rough edges with cutting tools. The models may be spray painted and solvents, including turpentine, used for "clean up." A releasing oil is applied to make separation of the plaster model possible. These oils contain preservatives that may be allergenic.[1314]

Because the bare hands are often used in this work, and also from repeated contact with water and various irritants, contact dermatitis is common in the pottery industry. Atopics do poorly in this work.[1147] Seidenari et al.[1106] found dermatitis on the hands in 37% of the workers examined. Smith[1147] and Wilkinson et al.[1314] found the peak age of incidence of dermatitis among workers to be the early 20s.

At one time pneumoconiosis was fairly common in this industry. In recent years, however, the incidence has declined.[207]

Irritants

Wet clay (especially under fingernails)
Glazes
Hydrofluoric acid (etching)
Solvents
Bits and pieces of dried clay

Patch test to standard and vehicle preservative allergens, with special attention to the following.

Standard Allergens

Nickel sulfate, 2.5% pet; 0.2/cm^2 (glaze and clay,[1314] hand tools)
Colophony (rosin), 20% pet; 0.85 mg/cm^2[243]
Balsam of Peru, 25% pet; 0.80 mg/cm^2 (crossreacts with colophony)
Cobalt dichloride, 1% pet; 0.02 mg/cm^2 (wet clay, pottery pigment)[1005]
Epoxy resin, 1% pet; 0.05 mg/cm^2 (to repair defects)[1147]
Potassium dichromate, 0.25% pet; 0.023 mg/cm^2
Thiuram mix, 1% pet; 0.025 mg/cm^2 (rubber squeegees, gloves)

Additional Allergens

Ammoniated mercury, 1% pet
Bioban CS-1246, 1% pet (biocide in releasing oils)[1314]
Gold sodium thiosulfate, 0.5% pet (gilding)
Proxel XL2 (1,2-benzisothiazolin-3-one), 1% aq
   (biocide in releasing oils)[1032]
Turpene peroxides, 0.3% pet (from turpentine) (used
   to clean brushes and machinery, paint solvent)[1147]

PRINTERS

Modern printing is performed primarily by four methods: letterpress (relief), gravure (intaglio), lithography (offset printing or planography), and stencil (screen process).

The oldest method is letterpress, based on the simple method of movable type invented in the 15th century by Johannes Gutenberg and used without important changes until the 20th century. The method consists of transferring ink from a surface containing raised type to paper. Today the presses are of three types: (1) plates or platens, (2) flatbeds, and (3) rotary presses. The platen press has two flat surfaces, the bed and the platen. The type and plates are mounted on the bed and are inked by a roller. The platen carries the paper. The impression is made by pressing the two surfaces together. Platen presses are used today for printing small articles such as stationery, calling cards, envelopes, and gold-leaf stamping. Flatbed presses are horizontal or vertical. The type form sits on a flat bed, which is usually mobile and moves back and forth over inked rollers. The paper is wrapped around an impression cylinder, which exerts pressure on the paper by pressing against the flat bed. Flatbed presses print larger sheets than the platen presses. The most popular letterpress is the rotary press. The curved type form is attached to one cylinder, and the other cylinder provides the pressure. Most newspapers, magazines, and other kinds of commercial work are printed on this type of press.

Letterpress plates are made of zinc, magnesium, copper, or plastic, often plated with nickel or copper for added strength. Each column line is cast in a single slug of lead alloy type on a Linotype machine. In recent years, the use of lead plates has ceased. Most printing is now done with the offset process.

Gravure printing (intaglio) utilizes two cylinders: a larger printing cylinder on which the type is present and a smaller impression cylinder. The paper moves between these rollers. The figures are etched or engraved onto metal plates. A solvent-type ink containing a resin and binder is flooded over the surface of the printing cylinder by an ink roller or spray from an ink "fountain." Excess ink is removed from the nonimage areas of the printing cylinder by a special wiping steel blade called a *doctor*, which moves slowly across the cylinder. The impression cylinder is usually covered with a rubber material that presses the paper into contact with the ink in the minute cells of the printing surface. Considerable solvent is released into the atmosphere, especially with high-speed machines, making enclosure of the inking system necessary. With multicolor printing, rapid drying by heating is required. Color reproduction is good with gravure, and thus this method is widely used for printing magazines, newspaper advertising, inserts, catalogs, and boxes and other containers.

In lithography or offset printing, four cylinders are used. The image-containing portion of the printing holds the ink. The nonimage portion holds water but rejects ink. Both the inking and water (dampening) rolls contact the plate cylinder. The principle of lithography is that water and oil do not mix. The inked image is transferred to a rubber "blanket" cylinder, which then transfers the image onto paper by pressure from the impression cylinder. The rollers prevent adhesion of ink on the nonimage area of the plate. To make the image more receptive to ink, a conditioner may be added, 1-methylquinoxalinum-*p*-toluene sulfonate, for example.[340] Acids, a desensitizing gum (usually gum arabic), isopropyl alcohol, fungicides, and anticorrosion agents are added to the inks. As fungicides, formaldehyde and formaldehyde-releasing agents such as Dowicil-75 have been used. Dichromates, with the exception of strongly skin-sensitizing anticorrosion chemicals, are rarely used in printing today. When potassium dichromate was used extensively, until the late 1970s, it was a fairly frequent cause of allergic contact sensitivity among printers.[992]

Offset printing has grown in importance recently in the United States. With the development of rapid and economical photographic methods of plate making, offset printing has been widely available for many different types of printing. Stencil or screen process (silkscreen) printing is especially useful for printing on fabrics, leather, metal, glass, and ceramics (see Silk-Screening Workers).

Photosensitive Printing Processes

To greatly increase printing speed and decrease or eliminate the need for solvents, photosensitive printing processes were developed. These plastic photographic printing processes have revolutionized the industry since 1960. The first was Dupont's Dycril, a photosensitive plastic bonded to steel, aluminum, or plastic.[820] Next, Eastman Kodak developed a type of relief printing, and then W. R. Grace and Company came out with Letterflex, a urethane process, in the early 1960s. The Letterflex process consists of an aluminum pre-coated sheet, coated with a photopolymer just before use. First the plate is pre-exposed to UV light, and then the negative is applied and re-exposed to UV. The plate is then removed and exposed to an air current, which removes the unreacted photopolymer. The unreacted polymer can be recycled. There is then another re-exposure to UV light to increase the strength of the now elevated parts.

The photochemical used in Letterflex is a mixture of toluene 2,4-diisocyanate and trimethylol propane dialyl ether. The catalyst is dibutylin dilaurate, and the antioxidant is 2,6-di-*tert*-butyl-*p*-methylphenol. A cross-linking agent (pentaerythritol-tetrakis-3-mercaptopropionate) is employed. A benzophenone is added as a UV initiating agent.

Allergic contact dermatitis can result from this mixture. Although the sensitizer is not known, it appears to be the cross-linking agent pentaerythritol-tetrakis-3-mercaptopropionate.[168, 834] Zimmerman[1340] reported three printers with allergic contact dermatitis in a newspaper printing establishment. The workers were sensitive on patch testing to the unreacted polymer and the cross-linking agent. To prevent dermatitis it is important to keep the machines free of unreacted polymer, especially the reverse side of the aluminum plates.

The Nyloprint process consists of a metal carrier sheet with prepolymer, covered with a sheet of protective plastic, which must be removed by the worker, who may accidentally touch the undersurface containing the dermatitis-causing prepolymer. After UV exposure, the unreacted polymer is dissolved with an alcohol solution, and the plate is dried and irradiated one more time to further harden the exposed areas.

The Nyloprint process is chiefly proprietary, but the contact allergen appears to be N,N'-methylene bisacrylamide.[839] Inhibitors are pyrogallol and hydroquinone. Photoinitiators are benzoquinone, benzaldehyde, and acetophenone.[1014, 1201]

For the printing of surfaces of containers such as cans and cartons, and occasionally for printing high-gloss publications such as corporate annual reports, a three-system, UV-light–cured process has been employed in recent years. An acrylated synthetic resin (epoxy or alkyd) is cross-linked with multifunctional acrylic monomer and activated by a chromophore and an intense, continuous UV emission of wavelengths between 300 and 400 nm. The monomers commonly are pentaerythritol triacrylate (PETA), trimethylpropane triacrylate (TMPTA), and hexanediol diacrylate (HDODA). While TMPTA is a well-known sensitizer,[84] it may also contain a hardening agent, a polyfunctional aziridine, which has been reported to cause dermatitis of the hands and face of 13 of 51 workers[457] and in workers applying a top coat floor varnish.[257] Epoxy acrylates, urethane acrylates, and linseed oil acrylates are also used. Nethercott[936–938] and Emmett et al.[335] have reviewed this process and emphasize that patch testing must be done with the epoxy acrylate actually used by the worker. Testing with the epoxy resin present on the standard patch test tray will not suffice; testing must be done with the chemical used by the worker. There is also no crossreactivity to methyl methacrylate monomer.

Water-based polyfunctional aziridines (PFA) may be used as hardeners in printing. Water-soluble printing dyes are mixed with these aziridine hardeners, sometimes by hand using a stick, providing an opportunity for considerable contact. Patch testing with 0.5% PFA hardeners in petrolatum is recommended. Contact urticaria also occurs.[685] Driers include cobalt compounds of which cobalt naphthenate is a well-known sensitizer; cobalt-2-ethylhexoate[691] has also been found to be a sensitizer.

Printing Occupations

The compositor receives the copy and specifications regarding size and style of type, column width, and size of pictures and illustrations.

The linotype machine automatically selects the type, completes the lines, and deposits the completed lines in the galley from which the plates are made. The operator sits at a keyboard and selects the letters and other characters and, after finishing a line, shoves a lever that casts the line and deposits it in the galley. The operator may place pigs of lead alloy on the feed chain to replenish the stock of molten metal. In the hot metal area, all consumption of food and drink should be discouraged, as well as smoking. Biological monitoring for lead should be done at regular intervals.

Monotype keyboard operators also sit at a keyboard and install a band of keys to make sizes and styles of type according to the editor's specifications. The keyboard perforates paper tape, which controls the casting of type. Compressed air is used. The monotype machine was invented in 1885, and today a typesetter at this machine can produce 10,000 to 12,000 pieces of type an hour.

Photosetters operate at a keyboard that photographically prints type material onto photosensitive paper. The operator types the text without concern for column width or hyphenation, producing a magnetic tape. The tape is then fed to a computer, which makes all the adjustments for column width and hyphenation, spitting out a second tape with the text as it will appear in final print. The process can also be done electronically, with the text displayed on a cathode ray tube (CRT) or other screen, where errors can be seen and corrected. The completed and corrected text is placed in a phototype-setting machine, which photographically translates the electronic data into type, which is then ready for printing. The plates are made by photoengraving or by photocomposition.

The camera operator photographs the material to be printed, making a negative. Lithographic artists retouch to lighten or darken certain parts using various dyes and special tools. Strippers cut the film to size and arrange and paste the negatives onto a layout sheet. Platemakers cover the metal plates with photosensitive material or select plates already coated. The layout sheet with the negative in place is placed on top of the metal plate and placed in a vacuum machine where it is exposed to ultraviolet light for the required period of time. The plate is then exposed, washed, and treated with lacquers, developing inks, desensitizing etches, and gum solution; then it is dried and ready for the press. The platemaker may mix solutions, including photosensitizing compounds and counter etches. The chief allergens are diazonium salts and bichromate, although the latter is much less used today than in the past.

Photoengravers make metal printing plates of pictures and copy that cannot be set in type. The picture is mounted on a board and photographed. The negative is laid on the sensitized plate, which has been layered with a photosensitizing chemical. The exposed areas are polymerized when exposed to UV light. The plate is then washed in an appropriate solution to remove the unreactive chemical and etched in an acid bath to eat away the areas to a required depth, permitting the image areas to stand out in relief.

From the metal forms made by the compositor, the stereotyper and the electrotyper make the press plates for use in the printing machines. Electrotype is used chiefly in magazine and book work, while the less durable stereotype is used for newspapers. Electrotypers make a plastic mold, which is then sprayed with a silver nitrate solution and immersed in an electroplating bath to form the final mold. Molten lead is then placed in the shell at the back of the mold, and excess lead is routed with a power machine. Stereotypers operate machines that press the face of the type copy into fiberboard mats. The mat is then placed in a casting machine, which makes a lead plate of the mold. Again the hazard of lead poisoning in these operations is always present.

The press operator's job differs depending on the type of press being used. These workers set up and adjust the press before starting, locking the plates in place and determining the correct alignment of the plate. They often clean and oil the machines and make occasional repairs. The computerized presses now used in many larger establishments require little direct attention. Pressroom workers usually have a significantly higher risk of developing dermatitis than those who work in composing.[1335] Solvents, inks, and rubber gloves are responsible for most cases of dermatitis. Pressroom workers appear to have the highest risk of developing dermatitis, particularly from solvents (Fig. AP–18).[1335]

In the printing industry, latex and neoprene gloves offer little protection from UV-cured acrylate resin systems. Nitrile gloves seem to provide adequate protection under use conditions, provided that they are not re-used within 8 hours.[1030] Printers must use protective clothing when working not only with solvent-borne printing inks but also those that are water based. Protective masks, gloves, and aprons, as well as a no-touch technique, are important. Immediate-type allergic reactions may also occur from contact with polyfunctional aziridine hardeners, including asthma and rhinitis,[46] and these patients should probably not continue in this work.

Irritants

Acids and alkalis (sodium hydroxide solution to clean presses, especially gravure presses)
Gum arabic (antioxidant for metal plates) (may contain

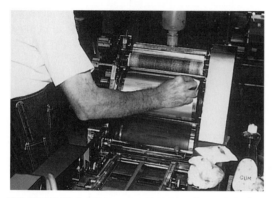

FIGURE AP–18 • Printers operating a small press may be especially exposed to the solvents and inks.

1,2-benzisothiazolin-3-one [Proxcel] as a preservative[423])
Solvents (preservative, cleaners, image remover fluid, blanket cleaning solvents, "blanket wash," ink/glaze removers)
Water (wet work)
Soaps and detergents
Inks
Greases and waxes
Desensitizing solutions
Electrostatic solutions
Electrostatic image remover solutions
Lacquers
Multifunctional acrylates
Surfactants
Ultraviolet light (carbon arc, xenon tubes, or mercury vapor tubes; used also for rapid drying)

Patch test to standard and vehicle preservative allergens, with special attention to the following.

Standard Allergens

Potassium dichromate, 0.25% pet; 0.023 mg/cm^2 (printing plates, fountain solutions)[163, 774, 992, 1076, 1158]
2-Mercaptobenzothiazole, 1% pet; 0.075 mg/cm^2 (rubber gloves, cylinder coverings such as offset roller blanket)
Carba mix, 3% pet; 0.25 mg/cm^2 (rubber gloves, cylinder coatings)
Cobalt chloride, 1% pet; 0.02 mg/cm^2 (driers in inks and varnishes;[691] may be as cobalt tallate, which is rosin-based)
Epoxy resin, 1% pet; 0.090 mg/cm^2 (photopolymer coatings in printing inks)
Kathon CG, 0.01% aq; 0.0040 mg/cm^2 (MCI/MI) (germicidal agent in fountain solutions;[1067] in fountain solutions and hand cleaners; in gum arabic[423])
Mercapto mix, 1% pet; 0.075 mg/cm^2 (rubber, offset roller blanket)
PPD mix (Black rubber mix), 0.6% pet; 0.075 mg/cm^2 (rubber)
Thiuram mix, 1% pet; 0.025 mg/cm^2 (rubber gloves)
Formaldehyde, 2% aq (formaldehyde releasers in fountain solutions and letterpress inks)
Quaternium 15, 2% pet; 0.1 mg/cm^2 (bactericidal agent in fountain solutions)
Nickel sulfate, 2.5% pet; 0.2 mg/cm^2 (electroplating solutions for plates and hand tools)
Rosin (colophony), 20% pet; 0.85 mg/cm^2 (inks, paper)

Additional Allergens

p-Aminoazobenzene, 0.25% pet (diazonium salts in lithography)[222]
p-Aminophenol, 1% pet (photo developers)
Beeswax, 30% pet (waxes)
p-Chloro-m-xylenol, 1% pet (hand cleaners)
Dibutyl phthalate, 5% pet (glues)
Benzoin tincture, 10% alc (polymerization catalysts for polymethacrylate coatings)

Benzophenone, 1% pet (photoinitiators)
Bronopol, 0.25% pet (fountain solutions)[1067]
CD-2, 1% pet (color developers)
CD-3, 1% pet (color developers)
Coal tar, 5% pet (newsprint ink)[636]
Ethoxylated phenol, 1% aq[44]
Hydroquinone, 1% pet (photo developers, printing inks)
1-Methylquinoxalinium-*p*-toluene sulfonate, 1% aq (Instafax Offset Etch, Kodak Ltd.)[340]
Metol, 1% pet (photo developers)
Pine oil, 3% pet (?)
PABA, 5% pet (photoinitiators in UV-cured inks)
Tricresyl phosphate, 2% pet (inks)
Turpentine, 10% olive oil (solvents, rarely used today)

Chemicals for Testing with Multifunctional Acrylics

Benzophenone, 1% pet
Dibutyl phthalate, 5% pet
Epoxy acrylates, 1% pet (as used by worker)
Hexanediol diacrylate (HDODA), 0.1% pet[182]
Hydroxyethyl methacrylate, 1% pet[837]
Napp and Nyloprint WD printing plates[987]
N,N'-methylene-bis-acrylamide, 1% pet[839]
Napp printing plates[984, 987, 1273]
Pentaerythritol triacrylate (PETA), 0.1% pet[330, 335, 936, 938]
Trimethylolpropane triacrylate (TMPTA), 0.1% pet[84, 330, 335, 457, 634, 685, 938]
Urethane acrylate, 0.1% pet (as used by workers)
Linseed oil acrylates, 1%[938]

Possible Allergenic Dyes Used in Printing[408]

Brown Sudan, 2% pet
Chloro-*p*-nitroaniline red, 2% pet
Eosin, 50% pet
Lake Red C, 2% pet
p-Phenylenediamine (PPD), 1% pet
Para red, 2% pet
Toluidine red (Helio red), 2% pet

RADIO AND TELEVISION REPAIRERS

Workers in the television and radio repair profession examine equipment for damaged components or loose or broken connections or wires. Using hand tools, they replace defective components with parts such as condensers, transformers, transistors, and generators. They solder or tighten loose connections and clean and lubricate motor generators. Radio repairers test the equipment for power output, frequency power, losses of antenna and transmission lines, noise level, audio quality, and so forth, using oscilloscopes, radiofrequency, and wattmeters, ammeters, and voltmeters. They may charge batteries. Many hand tools such as pliers, soldering

irons, and wire cutters are used in both types of work. Electronic equipment is also used.

Ammonium bichromate has been used in the manufacture of color television tubes and screens during the process of flow coating to produce cross-linking of the light-sensitive polyvinyl alcohol, enabling fluorescent compounds to adhere to the screen (red, green, and blue).[317] Skin contact is especially likely during weighing of the chromate powder.[17] Stevenson[1166] suggested using the Wood's light to detect fluorescence on the workers' skin, which would indicate contamination with the mixture. Krook[738] have also described contact dermatitis arising from the chromate found in certain magnetic tapes.

Irritants

Solvents
Metal cleaners
Soldering fluxes
Epoxy resins
Soaps and detergents

Patch test to standard and vehicle preservative allergens, with special attention to the following.

Standard Allergens

Potassium dichromate, 0.25% pet; 0.023 mg/cm^2 (metal anticorrosion agents, television screens)
2-Mercaptobenzothiazole, 1% pet; 0.075 mg/cm^2 (rubber connections)
Carba mix, 3% pet; 0.25 mg/cm^2 (rubber)
Epoxy resin, 1% pet; 0.05 mg/cm^2 (adhesives, potting compounds)
Mercapto mix, 1% pet; 0.075 mg/cm^2 (rubber)
PPD mix (Black rubber mix), 0.6% pet; 0.075 mg/cm^2 (rubber)
Thiuram mix, 1% pet; 0.25 mg/cm^2 (rubber gloves)
Formaldehyde, 2% aq; 0.18 mg/cm^2 (metal cleaners)
Nickel sulfate, 2.5% pet; 0.2 mg/cm^2 (hand tools)
Rosin (colophony), 20% pet; 0.85 mg/cm^2 (soldering flux, insulating tape)

Additional Allergens

Hydrazine sulfate, 1% pet (soldering fluxes)
Polyethylene glycol dimethacrylate, 1% pet (rapid-acting adhesives)[867]

RAILROAD SHOP WORKERS

Railroad shop workers include car repairers, who repair and assemble motors of locomotives and street cars; machinists, who do mostly mechanical work on engines, although a few use cutting tools; electricians, who repair and install wiring and also maintain air conditioning and cooling systems in refrigeration cars; sheet-metal workers; boilermakers; and blacksmiths. Every railroad employs its own workers in these categories.

For specific dermatological hazards for these workers, see the corresponding occupational profiles. Other workers include car cleaners, inspectors, janitors, and firefighters.

Operating employees make up about one-third of all railroad workers. This group includes locomotive engineers, conductors, and brake operators. The brake operators play the most important role in making locomotives and cars into trains. Working with engineers under the direction of conductors, they do the physical work involved in adding and removing cars at railroad stations and assembling and disassembling trains at railroad yards. They inspect trains to make sure that all couplers and air hoses are fastened, that the hand brakes on all cars are released, and that the air brakes are functioning correctly. They check moving trains for smoke, sparks, and other signs of sticking brakes, overheated axle bearings, and other faulty equipment. They may make minor repairs to air hoses and couplers. In case of unexpected stops, they set out signals to protect both ends of the train. Conductors are in charge of train and yard crews, and their work is entirely supervisory. Other employees in this group are hostlers, who prepare locomotives for the train crews, and switch tenders, who throw track switches within the railroad yards. Another one-third of railroad employees are station and office employees, who direct train movements and handle the railroads' business affairs. They are mostly professionals, such as managers, accountants, statisticians, and systems analysts. About one-fifth of railroad employees are equipment maintenance workers, who service and repair locomotives and cars. The final group consists of property maintenance workers, who build and repair tracts, tunnels, signal equipment, and so forth.

Among the most skilled employees of the railroad are the engineers, who must have a thorough knowledge of the signal systems, yards, and terminals along the route and be constantly aware of the condition and make up of the train. They operate the throttle, use the air brakes, watch gauges and meters that measure speed, fuel, temperature, and so forth, and constantly watch for signals that indicate track obstructions, other train movements, and speed limits. Before and after each run engineers check locomotives for mechanical problems but rarely make adjustments themselves.

Irritants

Petroleum distillates (the most common cause of dermatitis)[699]
Diesel fuel oil
Diesel lubricating oil
Kerosene and mineral spirits
Trichloroethane and other solvents
Grease
Gasoline
Toluene
Chromates
Soaps and detergents
Dusts

Patch test to standard and vehicle preservative allergens, with special attention to the following.

Standard Allergens

Potassium dichromate, 0.25% pet; 0.023 mg/cm^2 (anticorrosion agent in diesel cooling systems,[1320] largely replaced by other anticorrosion agents)
2-Mercaptobenzothiazole, 1% pet; 0.075 mg/cm^2 (rubber and anticorrosion agent)
Carba mix, 3% pet; 0.25 mg/cm^2 (rubber)
Cobalt dichloride, 1% pet; 0.02 mg/cm^2 (greases)
Epoxy resin, 1% pet; 0.05 mg/cm^2 (adhesives)
Mercapto mix, 1% pet; 0.075 mg/cm^2 (rubber)
PPD mix (Black rubber mix), 0.6% pet; 0.075 mg/cm^2 (rubber)
Thiuram mix, 1% pet; 0.025 mg/cm^2 (rubber)
Formaldehyde, 2% aq; 0.18 mg/cm^2 (germicidal agent)
Nickel sulfate, 2.5% pet; 0.2 mg/cm^2 (hand tools)
Rosin (colophony), 20% pet; 0.85 mg/cm^2 (soldering fluxes)

Additional Allergens

Hydrazine sulfate, 1% pet (soldering fluxes)
N-isopropyl-N'-phenyl-p-phenylenediamine (IPPD), 0.1% pet (rubber gaskets and hoses)
Diethylthiourea, 1% pet (safety shoes)[410]

ROOFERS

The nature of the roofer's work varies with the type of roof and roofing material. Many roofing contractors specialize in either commercial or home roofing.

Flat (commercial) roofs are covered with several layers of material. Roofers first spread a coat of hot tar over the roof's insulation, which they may lay first. They next lay roofing felt—fabric soaked in tar—over the entire surface. The roofers then apply hot tar from a bucket, using a mop to spread it over and under the felt. This seals the seams and makes the surface watertight. Roofers repeat these steps to build up the desired number of layers, ending with a thick layer of tar over the surface. They finally add gravel, which sticks firmly to the top.

Pitched roofs (as on many homes) are often covered with tile, slate, or wooden shingles. When applying asphalt shingles, roofers first lay, cut, and tack 3-foot strips of roofing felt lengthwise over the entire roof. Then, starting from the bottom edge, they nail overlapping rows of asphalt shingles to the roof. They measure and cut the felt and shingles to fit around corners, pipes, and chimneys. Wherever two roof surfaces intersect or where the shingles touch a pipe or chimney, roofers cement or nail flashing (strips of felt or metal) over the joints to make them watertight. Finally, roofers cover exposed nail heads with a cement substance to prevent rust and water leakage. Slate shingles and tiles are installed in a similar manner.

Some roofers also waterproof and damp-proof masonry in concrete walls and floors. To prepare surfaces for waterproofing, they hammer and chisel away rough spots or remove them with a rubber brick before brushing on a coat of liquid waterproofing compound. They also paint or spray surfaces with waterproofing material or nail waterproofing fabric to surfaces.

Roofing has one of the highest rates for work injuries in all industry, almost as high as coal mining. The chief hazard is that of falls, from the roof, through unfinished roofs, or through aged roofs that have disintegrated. Inhalation of asphalt fibers is a significant hazard. Burns from hot pitch and tar are the most common, usually due to faulty methods of adding fresh asphalt to the cooking kettle. In addition, the fumes cause dermatitis, including photosensitivity reactions.[247, 334] Explosions may occur when the fume concentration is too high. Gasoline is often used as a solvent and cleaner. When leaded gasoline is used there is also the hazard of excessive lead exposure, while unleaded gasoline may contain benzene. Tetrahydrofuran is often used to weld sheets of polyvinyl chloride plastic together. This substance is very flammable and irritating to the skin and eyes and also has a narcotic effect.

Photosensitivity due to asphalt and pitch usually begins with intense smarting of the skin and eyes after a latent period of sometimes as much as 2 weeks between first exposure and reactions, during which time tar builds up in the skin to a critical level.[247] The burning and erythema of the skin continue for several days after the last exposure. The reaction is worse in the summer and milder in winter and affects Caucasians almost exclusively. Long wavelengths of sunlight (340 to 400 nm) are causative. Crow et al.[247] stressed the importance of anthracene in the fumes as causative agents and also acridine. To demonstrate the photohazard of coal tar, Emmett et al.[334] instilled coal tar pitch distillate into rabbit conjunctivae, producing marked photophobia and severe keratoconjunctivitis after irradiation with long UV light, but only minimal or mild irritation in its absence.

Tar has been recognized as a cause of occupational skin cancer since the 18th century, when Percivall Pott first described such a relationship in chimney sweeps (see Chapter 8). Menck[893] showed that roofers have a fivefold excess incidence of lung cancer, probably from the heavy exposure to polycyclic aromatic hydrocarbons in tar. Wheeler et al.[1291] found that the carcinogenic compounds in tar may also be absorbed through the skin in sufficient quantities to represent a mutagenic and carcinogenic threat to other organs of the body. In assay studies of the urine of patients with psoriasis, for example, being treated with daily tar baths followed by exposure to UV light, Wheeler and his colleagues[1291] showed significant amounts of mutagenic materials in the urine of these patients, both smokers and nonsmokers.

Irritants

Tar
Pitch
Asphalt
Heat
Ultraviolet light
Solvents
Gasoline
Roofing putty
Adhesives
Asbestos
Sawdust
Insects

Patch test to standard and vehicle preservative allergens, with special attention to the following.

Standard Allergens

Potassium dichromate, 0.25% pet; 0.023 mg/cm² (leather gloves)
2-Mercaptobenzothiazole (MBT), 1% pet; 0.075 mg/cm² (rubber)
Carba mix, 3% pet; 0.25 mg/cm² (rubber)
Mercapto mix, 1% pet; 0.075 mg/cm² (rubber)
PPD mix (Black rubber mix), 0.6% pet; 0.075 mg/cm² (rubber)
Thiuram mix, 1% pet; 0.025 mg/cm² (rubber)
Formaldehyde, 2% aq; 0.18 mg/cm² (resins)
Nickel sulfate, 2.5% pet; 0.2 mg/cm² (hand tools)
Rosin (colophony), 20% pet; 0.85 mg/cm² (tackifier in asphalt)

Additional Allergens

Coal tar, 5% pet (tar, pitch, asphalt)
Diethylthiourea, 1% pet (safety shoes)[410]
Phenol-formaldehyde resin, 10% pet (roof putty, asphalt additive)
Western red cedar, 10% sawdust in pet[547]

SEMICONDUCTOR (ELECTRONICS) WORKERS

The semiconductor (electronics) industry produces many thousands of types of electrical products such as capacitors, switches, transistors, relays, television picture tubes, and amplifiers and other components for computers, tape recorders, phonographs, and military electronic products. This section describes work in manufacturing and assembling electronic components, such as resistors, capacitors, coils, chokes, inductors, printed circuit boards, semiconductors, tubes, transistors, diodes, television antennas, headphones, piezoelectric crystal, and crystal devices. The chief industrial processes are fabrication of semiconductor wafers and printed circuit boards.

Many different jobs exist in production, maintenance, transportation, and service occupations. A large number of these workers are scientists, engineers, and physicists, but those exposed to the greatest skin hazards are the production workers, most of whom are semiskilled in assembly occupations. Although semiconductor manufacturing has generally been considered as a "clean" industry, the potential for dermatitis and other injury is high. In recent years the industry has become automated to a remarkable extent, and the risks have decreased. Approximately one-third of the workforce is in fabrication, where the work involves installing components in parts on circuit boards, panels, and other units using power tools, hand tools, and especially various kinds of soldering and welding equipment. They read directions for the circuitry and terminals. Considerable assembly work is done on microelectronic units using binocular microscopes. Precision welding and soldering equipment is used to make connections in microminiature components in circuit assemblies.

Other workers in this industry are electroplaters and tinners, anodizers, silk-screen printers, etching equipment operators, glassblowers and glass lathe operators, and tool and die makers. Operators of infrared ovens and hydrogen furnaces remove moisture and foreign deposits from ceramic, metal, and glass parts.

Inspectors check incoming parts and components and perform inspections during manufacturing and at the completion of the operation to make certain that everything is working properly.

The working conditions in semiconductor manufacturing are usually very good; the plants tend to be well-lighted, clean, and quiet and are often located in suburban or semirural areas. Assembly line work is monotonous but not strenuous. Dermatitis is uncommon, considering the many irritating and allergenic chemicals used in the industry; this is mainly because closed systems are employed to a very large extent. Skin conditions arising from this industry have decreased in frequency in recent years; contact urticaria from latex gloves and allergic contact dermatitis from the ingredients of rubber gloves cause the greatest number of cases of dermatitis today. Chemical burns are still occasionally seen, however. There have been several reports of erythema multiforme–Stevens-Johnson syndrome associated with exposure to trichloroethylene.[9395, 1000] A scleroderma-like connective tissue disorder similar to vinyl chloride disease was reported in workers exposed to certain organic solvents such as trichloroethylene and perchlorethylene.[1155, 1281, 1334] The central nervous symptoms of solvent toxicity should be recognized by dermatologists. These may appear as varying degrees of inebriation while at work, as well as irritation of the mucous membranes of the eyes and upper respiratory tract.

A widespread, pruritic dermatitis may occur from the *low humidity* in the clean rooms,[1069] where the relative humidity may be as low as 20 to 25%.[1104] Atopics tolerate this environment very poorly not only because of the low relative humidity but also because of the numerous irritants present, especially if there is direct contact with organic solvents. Because of the nature of the work and the many potentially harmful chemicals used in electronics, a minor outbreak of dermatitis may involve a large number of workers.[730, 1298] Often the symptoms are unrelated and minor, but, because of misunderstanding of the work hazards, the symptoms may assume major levels. It is important for physicians to take prompt action to rectify the problems early, remove the cause if present, correct misconceptions on

the part of the workers, and provide reassurance if this is warranted. A team approach is advisable, with the investigation team comprised of environmental engineers, health department personnel, and others. The dermatologist should usually be a central player, in any case. Often early examination by the dermatologist can clarify the nature of the dermatitis and rapidly eliminate the need for more extensive evaluation.

At one time contact allergy to *epoxy resins* was common in this industry. With better engineering controls resulting in almost total elimination of skin exposure to the resins and hardeners, the incidence of dermatitis has markedly diminished in recent years. Airborne dermatitis may sometimes occur when workers remove epoxied parts from curing ovens. Many epoxy resins have a pH close to 13 or 14 and are strong irritants as well as potent sensitizers. In patch testing for resins used in the electronics industry, it is important to test with the resin actually used by the worker, properly diluted to a nonirritating, accepted patch test concentration. A large number of plastics are used in this industry, and it is imperative to learn from the Material Safety Data Sheets exactly which resin a worker is using. The most actively sensitizing epoxy resins are those of lower molecular weight, usually around 350; the most irritating and sensitizing hardeners are the aliphatic amine curing agents (see Chapters 25 and 26).

Hydrofluoric (HF) acid burns have been common in this occupation. HF is used in wafer etching and polishing, as well as in quartz surface cleaning. At one time it was a common cause of burns in this industry, but with nearly completely closed systems being used today, it is only rarely seen. Because concentrations of 15 to 20% afford little or no initial pain when in contact with the skin, the worker may not be aware that contact has taken place, and prolonged exposure may occur. The fluoride ion has the capacity to penetrate deep layers of the skin into the subcutaneous tissue and bone, causing extensive damage. Treatment is outlined by MacKinnon[812, 813] (see also Vance in Chapter 1).

Gallium arsenide is used in replacement of silicon to some extent in the manufacture of wafers for microelectronic components. It is widely used in electronic components of military hardware, as in light-emitting diodes, microwave-integrated circuits, and photovoltaic cells. Although gallium is poorly absorbed, the compound releases a fraction of its arsenic content into biological systems. Trivalent inorganic arsenic is a well-known human carcinogen. Poisoning by arsine gas (arsenic hydride) is an ever-present hazard of this industry, where it is used as a dopant in the manufacture of the semiconductor chips.

A comprehensive review of semiconductor manufacturing is given by Wald and Jones,[1280] and for the glass-fiber–reinforced plastics industry one is given by Tarvainen et al.[1185]

Irritants[732]

Cleaners (acids, alcohols, alkalis, solvents)
Solvents (acetone, freons, xylene, methyl ethyl ketone, methylene chloride, trichloroethylene, and

perchloroethylene—used as cleaners, driers, and
degreasers)
Peroxide catalysts
Soldering fluxes (zinc chloride)
Acids (hydrofluoric, chromic, nitric, sulfuric, and
hydrochloric—many used in etching)
Fiberglass (from printed circuit boards)[731]
Hot air blowers
Oxidizers (hydrogen peroxide, potassium iodide,
iodine, ammonium hydroxide)
Plating chemicals (gold and nickel compounds)
Photoresists (polymeric quaternary ammonium
compounds, esters of polyvinyl alcohols, azide
polymers, acrylics)
Epoxy resins, catalysts, and other resins
Strippers (acids, alkalis, solvents)
Antistatic agents (bis-hydroxyethyl tallow amine)[75]

Patch test to standard and vehicle preservative allergens, with special attention to the following.

Standard Allergens

Potassium (and ammonium dichromate), 0.25% pet;
0.023 mg/cm² (electroplating)
2-Mercaptobenzothiazole, 1% pet; 0.075 mg/cm²
(rubber)
Carba mix, 3% pet; 0.25 mg/cm² (rubber)
Cobalt chloride, 1% pet; 0.02 mg/cm² (magnets)
Epoxy resin, 1% pet; 0.05 mg/cm²
Ethylenediamine hydrochloride, 1% pet; 0.05 mg/cm²
(epoxy catalyst)
PPD mix (Black rubber mix), 0.6% pet; 0.075 mg/cm²
(rubber)
Thiuram mix, 1% pet; 0.0080 mg/cm² (rubber gloves)
Formaldehyde, 2% aq; 0.18 mg/cm² (phenolic resins)
Nickel sulfate, 2.5% pet; 0.2 mg/cm² (hand tools)
Rosin (colophony), 20% pet; 0.85 mg/cm²
(soldering)[557, 777, 864, 1302]

Additional Allergens

Aminoethylethanolamine, 5% pet[471]
Ammoniated mercury, 1% pet (mercury compounds)
Beryllium sulfate, chloride, or nitrate, 0.5% aq[242]
Gold sodium thiosulfate, 0.1% pet (electroplating)
Hydrazine sulfate, 1% pet (soldering flux)
Hydroquinone, 1% pet (photographic developers)
Isophorone diisocyanate, 1% pet
Metol, 1% pet (photographic developer)
Methyl diisocyanate, 1% pet
m-Phenylenediamine, 2% pet
Phthalic anhydride, 1% pet
Ammonium tetrachloroplatinate, 0.25% pet (platinum)
(thermocouples, electrical contacts)
Toluene 2,4-diisocyanate, 1% pet (uncommon allergen)
Diethylenetriamine, 0.5% pet (epoxy catalyst)
Triethylenetetramine, 0.5% pet (epoxy catalyst)
Turpentine, 10% in olive oil

SHEET-METAL WORKERS

Sheet-metal workers fabricate and install ducts for air
conditioning, heating, and ventilating systems; kitchen
walls and counters; and roofing and siding. They also
install roof gutters and downspouts for rainwater drainage and make skylights and vents for industrial buildings. Some workers specialize in either shop work or
on-site installation; others do both.

Shop workers fabricate much of the metal at the
shop. Working from blueprint specifications, they measure, cut, bend, shape, and fasten most of the pieces
that will be used on the job. Tapes and steel rulers are
used for measuring; hand shearers, hacksaws, and
power saws for cutting; and specially designed heavy
steel presses for cutting, bending, and shaping. Once
the metal is measured and cut, workers then bolt, cement, rivet, solder, or weld the seams and joints together
to form ducts, pipes, tubes, and other items. Construction-site workers usually assemble and install pieces
previously fabricated at the shop. They use hammers,
shearers, and drills to make parts by hand. To hold
pieces together they bolt, weld, glue, or solder, or use
specially formed sheet metal for connections.

Irritants

Acids and alkalis
Adhesives
Sharp edges of metal
Cleaning compounds
Soldering flux

Patch test to standard and vehicle preservative allergens, with special attention to the following.

Standard Allergens

Potassium dichromate, 0.25% pet; 0.023 mg/cm²
(anticorrosion agent for sheet metal, especially
galvanized steel)[437, 439, 1062]
Epoxy resin, 1% pet; 0.05 mg/cm² (adhesives)
Nickel sulfate, 2.5% pet; 0.2 mg/cm² (metal)
Rosin (colophony), 20% pet; 0.85 mg/cm² (soldering
flux)
Cobalt chloride, 1% pet; 0.02 mg/cm² (metals, driers
in glues)

Additional Allergens

Hydrazine monobromide, 1% pet (soldering flux)
Diethylthiourea, 1% pet (safety shoes)[410]

SHOE REPAIRERS

Replacing soles and heels is the most common type of
shoe repair. Repairers also may replace insoles, restitch
loose seams, and restyle old shoes by changing heels
and dyeing the upper part of the shoe. Highly skilled
repairers may design, make, and repair orthopedic shoes
according to physicians' prescriptions. Shoe repairers
also mend other leather, rubber, or canvas articles, such
as handbags, luggage, and tents. They also replace zippers, dye handbags, and stretch shoes to conform to the

foot. They occasionally polish shoes and stain new soles and heels to match the shoe color.

A variety of power-operated equipment is used, such as sole stitchers, heel nailing machines, sewing machines, and sanding wheels. Among the hand tools are hammers, knives, awls, nippers, and skivers (a special tool for splitting leather). Hyperkeratosis of the fingertips is frequent in these workers, as well as itching without dermatitis, probably from dust. A review of occupational dermatitis in shoemakers is given by Mancuso et al.[842] In a shoe factory, exposure to solvents, including benzene, which is present as a contaminant in certain solvents such as toluene, may occur to a greater extent than previously appreciated.[700] Leukemia is a well-known result of such exposure in some exposed cases.

Irritants

Solvents
Stains
Dyes
Adhesives and cements (*p-tert*-
   butylphenol–formaldehyde resins and
   cyanoacrylates)
Buffing materials
Polishes

Patch test to standard and vehicle preservative allergens, with special attention to the following.

Standard Allergens

Potassium dichromate, 0.25% pet; 0.023 mg/cm²
   (leather)
Wool alcohols, 30% pet; 1.00 mg/cm² (polish)
2-Mercaptobenzothiazole, 1% pet; 0.075 mg/cm²
   (rubber)
Carba mix, 3% pet; 0.25 mg/cm² (rubber)
Cobalt chloride, 1% pet; 0.02 mg/cm² (driers, stains)
p-Phenylenediamine, 1% pet; 0.090 mg/cm² (dyes)
Epoxy resin, 1% pet; 0.05 mg/cm² (adhesives)
Ethylenediamine dihydrochloride, 1% pet; 0.02 mg/
   cm²[842]
Mercapto mix, 1% pet; 0.075 mg/cm² (rubber)
PPD mix (Black rubber mix), 0.6% pet; 0.075 mg/cm²
   (rubber)
p-tert-Butylphenol–formaldehyde resin, 1% pet; 0.04
   mg/cm² (leather adhesives)[12, 409, 842, 853]
Thiuram mix, 1% pet; 0.025 mg/cm² (rubber)
Formaldehyde, 2% aq; 0.18 mg/cm² (adhesives,
   polishes)
Nickel sulfate, 2.5% pet; 0.2 mg/cm² (hand tools)
Rosin (colophony), 20% pet; 0.85 mg/cm² (cements,
   polishes)

Additional Allergens

Methyl methacrylate, 1% pet
p-Aminoazobenzene, 0.25% pet (dyes)
Beeswax, 20%
Bismark brown, 1% pet (dyes)

Bisphenol A, 1% pet[1159]
p-tert-Butylphenol, 1% pet[188, 832, 842]
Camphor, 10% pet (plasticizers, adhesives)
2-Chloroacetamide, 0.2% pet (leather preservative)[654]
Diaminodiphenyl methane, 0.5% pet[842]
Dibutyl phthalate, 5% pet (plasticizers in cements)
Dichlorophene, 1% pet (preservatives in cements)
Diphenylmethane-4-4'-diisocyanate, 0.1% pet[842]
Disperse Yellow 3, 1% pet
Disperse Red 1, 1% pet
Dibutyl thiourea, 1% pet
Diethylthiourea, 1% pet
Diphenyl thiourea, 2%
Diphenylmethane diisocyanate, 0.1% pet
Ethylbutylthiourea, 1% pet
Glutaraldehyde, 0.25% aq (leather tanning chemical)[666]
Linseed oil, as is[842]
Nigrosine B, 1% pet (polishes)
Nitrocellulose resin, 30%[842]
Phenylmercuric nitrate, 0.01% pet (preservatives,
   polishes)[842]
o-Phenylphenol, 1% pet (preservatives in cements)
Pine oil, 10% in olive oil (polishes)[593]
Toluene diisocyanate, 0.1% pet
Triethylenediamine, 1% pet[842] (in the author's
   experience, 0.5% is less irritating)
Turpentine, 10% in olive oil (polishes)

SILK-SCREENING WORKERS

Silk screening, which is probably better called screen processing or screen printing, is a process whereby colors are withheld from certain surface areas while color is applied to other areas. This is the primary method of printing decals. It is also used to print billboard posters, wallpaper designs, and lettering on bottles, clothing, and other surfaces where other types of printing are impossible. Several occupations are involved: screen maker, stencil maker, squeegee operator, and color mixer.

The printing process involves attaching various types of stencil to a fabric or wire screen stretched across a frame to create a mesh through which ink or paint can flow. The rate of flow is regulated by controlling the amount of pressure that is applied to the mesh. Silk is not used any longer, having been replaced by nylon, dacron, and polyester fabric, which possess very small mesh sizes. When metallic mesh is used, there may be up to 2,000 holes psi. Screen printing is very adaptable, not only for large items, but also for miniature printed circuit boards in the electronics industry. It is widely used in the printing of textiles.

The light sources used in silk screening include carbon arc lamps, mercury vapor lamps, and pulsed xenon lamps. The so-called safe light is a light of long wavelengths that is used for drying that does not at the same time cause polymerization of the light-sensitive materials.

Heavy-duty cleaners are used to clean the screens, and many of these contain solvents, abrasive materials, and enzymes. Solvent exposure may be considerable, especially to mixed solvents, some of which have neurotoxic properties[1299] at high exposure levels, causing significant impairment of tasks involving manual dexterity, visual memory, and mood.

Screen makers build screen frames and/or make photographic stencil plates. They are responsible for the printing quality of the photographic stencil plate and the proper selection of fabric or wire mesh for the screen. They also may operate machinery to produce contact printed films.

Stencil cutters or makers cut stencils by hand. They have knowledge of lettering styles and may cut clean stencils from photographs or rough art with sharp stencil knives. They may also perform other duties, such as planning the printing sequence.

Squeegee operators or screen printers set up patterns commonly called *registers* to determine the exact placement of successive colors. They use a hand squeegee, which spreads the paint or ink over the screen, and position stock using special setup table guides. They also may clear screens and rack their own work. Color mixers match and mix ink and paint colors for the desired tones and shades.

Irritants

Solvents
Toluene
Methyl ethyl ketone
Mineral spirits
Ether
Methylene chloride
Acetic acid
Paints
Photoresist
Ultraviolet light
Soaps and detergents
Water (wet work)
Abrasive cleaners
Degreasers
Forced air (dryers)

Patch test to standard and vehicle preservative allergens, with special attention to the following.

Standard Allergens

Potassium dichromate, 0.25% pet; 0.023 mg/cm^2 (dichromated gelatin)
2-Mercaptobenzothiazole, 1% pet (rubber)
Carba mix, 3% pet; 0.25 mg/cm^2 (rubber)
Cobalt chloride, 1% pet; 0.02 mg/cm^2 (drier in inks)
p-Phenylenediamine, 1% pet; 0.090 mg/cm^2 (pigments)
Epoxy resin, 1% pet; 0.05 mg/cm^2 (adhesives)
Mercapto mix, 1% pet; 0.075 mg/cm^2 (rubber)
PPD mix (Black rubber mix), 0.6% pet; 0.075 mg/cm^2 (rubber)
Thiuram mix, 1% pet; 0.025 mg/cm^2 (rubber)
Formaldehyde, 2% aq; 0.18 mg/cm^2 (inks)
Nickel sulfate, 2.5% pet; 0.2 mg/cm^2 (hand tools)
Rosin (colophony), 20% pet; 0.85 mg/cm^2 (inks)

Additional Allergens

p-Aminoazobenzene, 0.25% pet (dyes, diazo sensitizer)
p-Aminophenol, 1% pet (dyes)
Beeswax, 30% pet (waxes)
Camphor, 10% pet (plasticizer in inks)
CD-2, 1% pet (photographic developer)
CD-3, 1% pet (photographic developer)
Disperse Orange 3, 1% pet (dyes)
Disperse Yellow 3, 1% pet (dyes)
Hydroquinone, 1% pet (photographic developer)
N-isopropyl-N'-phenyl-p-phenylenediamine (IPPD), 0.1% pet (rubber)
Phenol-formaldehyde resin, 10% pet (inks)
Phenylmercuric nitrate, 0.05% pet (preservatives)

SOLDERERS AND BRAZERS

The solderer or solderer-assembler bonds and repairs pieces of metal. First the parts to be joined are clamped together using rules and hand tools and then positioned in a vice. Parts are either dipped in cleaning solution or the solution, which includes a flux, is brushed or sprinkled along the seams. The soldering iron is heated in a gas flame or electric induction coil or by plugging it into an electrical outlet. The tip of the iron is plunged into the cleaning compound and is rubbed into a tin alloy to clean and tin it. The tip is guided along the seam to heat the work piece to bonding temperature. The solderer dips a bar or wire of subsolder in the seam to solder the joint. The work piece may be dipped into molten solder ("tin dip"), or the solder may be placed between seams and the seam heated with iron to sweat them together. The work piece is cleaned with a file, hand brush, or grinder to remove corrosion. Power grinders or hand tools are used. Fumes of the soldering flux must be adequately ventilated.

Soldering fluxes are usually compounds with zinc chloride and hydrochloric acid, but tallow, rosin, and olive oil may also be added. Hydrazine monobromide as well as rosin may be used in the core of soft solder. For silver soldering, borax is a common flux, as are fluorides and chlorides. Fluxes are important to prepare metal surfaces, to prevent oxidation, and to aid in heat transfer. The flux also acts as a wetting agent, permitting the solder to flow more easily. Solder flux rosin usually derives from gum rosin.

Solders themselves, especially those with low melting points, contain bismuth, lead, tin, cadmium, indium, and sometimes mercury. Other combinations are cadmium and zinc, cadmium and tin, or tin and antimony. The most common solder is *plumber's solder*, also called *half and half,* which consists of equal parts of lead and tin and melts at about 360°F. Hard solder (solder with a higher melting point) may contain aluminum, copper, zinc, and tin. The so-called Richards solder is a yellow brass with aluminum and phosphor tin. Nickel solders may be used for nickel-silver soldering. So-called cold solder is used to fill cracks in metals and is a mixture of a metallic powder with adhesives such as epoxy resins. An example is aluminum powder with epoxy, useful because it has little shrinkage.

In the electronics industry soldering is usually done with a lead-zinc alloy. Goh and Ng[482] describe the wave-soldering process to be the most popular soldering technique in the printed circuit board industry. Allergic contact dermatitis from soldering flux is rather common in this industry.[864] Bronchial asthma has been reported in solderers exposed to significant concentrations of rosin (colophony) fumes.[157, 362]

Brazing is performed at temperatures much higher than soldering, between 800°F and 2,150°F, and is used when much stronger joints are required. A common brazing solder is brass (Fig. AP–19). Fluorides, which are especially used for silver and aluminum brazing, are very irritating. Brazing is often done by machine. The chief hazards of brazing are heat, chemicals, and irritating fumes. A heat torch is used, providing the possibility of burns. Infrared from the torch may injure the eyes. When cadmium is present in the alloy, fumes of cadmium oxide may be produced, which are highly toxic. Possible allergens of the brazing process include nickel and chromium.

Irritants

Acids and salts (hydrochloric acid, hydrofluoric acid, zinc chloride)
Metal cleaners
Degreasing agents
Fluxes

Patch test to standard and vehicle preservative allergens, with special attention to the following.

Standard Allergens

Potassium dichromate, 0.25% pet; 0.023 mg/cm² (brazing processes)
Cobalt dichloride, 1% pet; 0.02 mg/cm²
Formaldehyde, 2% aq; 0.18 mg/cm² (metal cleaners)
Nickel sulfate, 2.5% pet; 0.2 mg/cm² (hand tools, brazing processes)

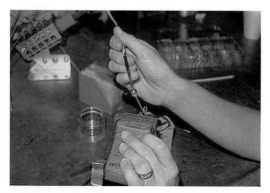

FIGURE AP–19 • Soldering in the electronics industry. The fluxes are somewhat irritating, and some contain fairly potent allergens.

Rosin (colophony), 20% pet; 0.85 mg/cm² (soldering flux)[482, 864, 1302]

Additional Allergens

Amino ethyl ethanolamine, 5% aq (soldering flux)[274, 473]
Hydrazine sulfate, 1% pet (soldering flux, hydrazine monobromide)[1290]

STONEMASONS

Stonemasons, bricklayers, and marble setters work in closely related trades. Stonemasons build stone walls and set stone exteriors and floors. They work with two types of stone: natural cut stone, such as marble, granite, and limestone; and artificial stone made from cement, marble chips, plastics, or other masonry materials. Because stone is expensive, stonemasons work mostly on high-cost buildings such as offices, hotels, and churches. Bricklayers build walls, partitions, fireplaces, and other structures with brick, cinder block, and other masonry materials. They also install firebrick linings in industrial furnaces. Marble setters install marble, which provides decorative and highly durable surfaces. Marble setters, like stonemasons, also work mostly on high-cost buildings. The marble they use is usually cut and polished before it is sent to the job site.

The workers shape the materials prior to setting, using chisels, hammers, and other shaping tools. They spread mortar with trowels and set the stone or other material in place by hand or with a crane. They align the piece with a plumb line and finish joints with a pointing trowel. They also wash the stone at the completion of the job.

Bricklayers, stonemasons, and marble setters primarily use hand tools, including trowels, brick and stone hammers, wooden or rubber mallets, and chisels. For exacting cuts of brick, stone, or marble, they use high-powered electric saws equipped with special cutting blades.

Irritants

Cement and mortar
Water (wet work)
Polishes
Solvents
Oils
Dust
Stains and paints
Lime
Heat
Cold
Vibrating tools

Patch test to standard and vehicle preservative allergens, with special attention to the following.

Standard Allergens

Potassium dichromate, 0.5% pet; 0.023 mg/cm² (cement, mortar)

2-Mercaptobenzothiazole, 1% pet; 0.075 mg/cm^2 (rubber)

Carba mix, 3% pet; 0.63 mg/cm^2 (rubber)

Mercapto mix, 1% pet; 0.075 mg/cm^2 (rubber)

PPD mix (Black rubber mix), 0.6% pet; 0.075 mg/cm^2 (rubber)

Thiuram mix, 1% pet; 0.025 mg/cm^2 (rubber)

Formaldehyde, 2% aq; 0.18 mg/cm^2 (cleaning agents)

Nickel sulfate, 2.5% pet; 0.2 mg/cm^2 (hand tools)

SWIMMING POOL PERSONNEL

These workers clean, adjust, and perform minor repairs on swimming pools and auxiliary equipment. They remove leaves and other debris from the surface of the water using a net. They clean the bottom and sides of the pool using underwater vacuum cleaner hoses, brushes, detergent and acid solutions, and sanders. They inspect and replace loose or damaged tiles. They clean and repair filter systems and adjust and perform minor repairs to heating and pumping equipment using mechanic's hand tools. They add chemicals in prescribed amounts to purify the water and pool. They prepare service reports of materials used and work performed. They also may clean and repair hot tubs.

Contact urticaria has been reported from chlorinated swimming pool water,[934] but brominated water appears to be more commonly associated with dermatitis, especially in hot tubs.[1068] The reaction is generally considered an irritant folliculitis, but Fitzgerald et al.[396] reported positive patch test reactions with Halobrome-R (1-bromo-3-chloro-5,5-dimethylhydantoin) in three patients exposed from swimming in a spa where the disinfectant was used.

Irritants

Acids (sulfuric acid)

Chlorine solutions (sodium hypochlorite)[1239]

Bromine compounds (1-bromo-3-chloro-5,5-dimethylhydantoin)[396, 1068]

Water (wet work)

Sunlight

Acids for cleaning pools

Mortar

Algicides (copper sulfate, quaternary ammonium compounds, organic polyamines, copper chelates, others)

Patch test to standard and vehicle preservative allergens, with special attention to the following.

Standard Allergens

Potassium dichromate, 0.25% pet; 0.023 mg/cm^2 (cement, mortar)

2-Mercaptobenzothiazole, 1% pet; 0.075 mg/cm^2 (rubber)

Carba mix, 3% pet; 0.25 mg/cm^2 (rubber)

Epoxy resin (bisphenol A-epichlorhydrin type), 1% pet; 0.05 mg/cm^2 (sealants)[1301]

Kathon CG, 0.01% aq; 0.0040 mg/cm^2[2281, 1208]

Mercapto mix, 1% pet; 0.075 mg/cm^2 (rubber)

PPD mix (Black rubber mix), 0.6% pet; 0.075 mg/cm^2 (rubber)

Thiuram mix, 1% pet; 0.025 mg/cm^2 (rubber)

Formaldehyde, 2% aq; 0.18 mg/cm^2

Additional Allergens

1-Bromo-3-chloro-5,5-dimethylhydantoin (Di-Halo, Aquabrome,[394] and Halobrome,[396] 0.1% aq

Isophorone diamine, 0.5% pet (epoxy catalyst in sealants)[1301]

Sodium hypochlorite, 1% aq[624, 1239]

Tego G, 0.1% aq (dodecylic aminoethyl glycine hydrochloride)[1226]

TANNERY WORKERS

Tannery work involves considerable exposure to irritants and allergens. After removal from the animal, the hides must be preserved. In countries with dry climatic conditions such as India and parts of Africa, the hides may be dried in the sun. To preserve them for shipment, they may be treated with arsenic, pesticides such as naphthalene and zinc chloride, or chlorophenols. Methods of preserving hides in other regions are dry or brine salting. The cured hides are then sorted and trimmed (Fig. AP–20), soaked in a bath containing such chemicals as caustic soda, sodium sulfide, and various surfactants and wetting agents. The soaked hides are then placed in vats of hydrated lime to soften the epidermis and remove the fat and other subcutaneous tissue. The pieces are cleaned of hair by machine, then fleshed to remove the remaining fatty tissue. They are then bated (which involves neutralization of the alkalinity with buffering salts and proteolytic enzymes) and pickled. Tanning itself is done with vegetable extracts or basic chromium salts, or mixtures of the two, or it is done synthetically with formaldehyde, glutaraldehyde, or other chemicals. Its purpose is to change the hide to a

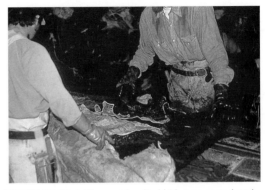

FIGURE AP–20 • The cured, salted hides are sorted and trimmed before the tanning process is begun.

soft, porous, flexible fabric. Following tanning, the skins and hides are dried on wooden racks and are then split to the desired thickness (Fig. AP–21) and perhaps dyed. The leather is lubricated to give it strength and flexibility. The pieces are then dried, perhaps bleached, oiled, and then "stuffed," a process by which waxes, oils, and greases are added to the leather to make it water repellent. Final finishes may be given, such as covering the hide with a hardening substance such as shellac or albumen or, more often, a synthetic resin.

Chrome ulceration of the hands may occur in tanning, although it is much less common today. The irritants are numerous, and some are highly caustic.

Irritants

Acids
Alkalis
Lime
Sodium sulfide
Various salts
Hydrogen sulfide
Ammonia
Trisodium phosphate
Hair
Arsenic sulfide
Ammonium sulfate
Chlorine
Formic acid
Chromic acid (ulcerations of hands and nose, "chrome holes")
Borax
Proteolytic enzymes
Oxalic acid
Formaldehyde
Organic solvents
Dust
Sulfuric acid
Soaps and detergents
Acrolein (may be used in place of glutaraldehyde in tanning; always contains hydroquinone as an inhibitor to prevent polymerization; highly irritating)

Patch test to standard and vehicle preservative allergens, with special attention to the following.

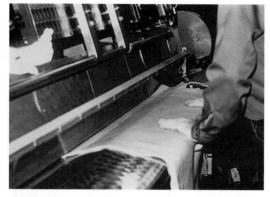

FIGURE AP–21 • A splitting machine is here separating the chrome-tanned hide at the dermal–epidermal junction.

Standard Allergens

Potassium dichromate, 0.25% pet; 0.023 mg/cm^2 (present in leather tanned with basic chromic sulfate)
Wool alcohols, 30% pet; 1.00 mg/cm^2 (finishing agents)
2-Mercaptobenzothiazole, 1% pet; 0.075 mg/cm^2 (rubber)
Carba mix, 3% pet; 0.25 mg/cm^2 (rubber)
p-Phenylenediamine, 1% pet; 0.090 mg/cm^2 (dyes)
Mercapto mix, 1% pet; 0.075 mg/cm^2 (rubber)
PPD mix (Black rubber mix), 0.6% pet; 0.075 mg/cm^2 (rubber)
Thiuram mix, 1% pet; 0.025 mg/cm^2 (rubber)
Formaldehyde, 2% aq; 0.18 mg/cm^2 (tanning agent) (may cause contact urticaria)[579]
Nickel sulfate, 2.5% pet; 0.2 mg/cm^2 (dyes, tools)
Rosin (colophony), 20% pet; 0.85 mg/cm^2 (binder in finishes and glues)
p-tert-Butylphenol–formaldehyde resin, 1% pet; 0.04 mg/cm^2 (finishing plastic) (small amounts of free formaldehyde may be released from this resin)[142, 409]

Additional Allergens

Acrolein, 0.5% alc
p-Aminoazobenzene, 0.25% pet (dyes)
p-Aminophenol, 1% pet (dyes)
Ammoniated mercury, 1% pet (for mercury sensitivity)
Beeswax, 30% pet (dressing and finishing)
Camphor, 10% pet (plasticizer used in finishing and in artificial leather)
p-Chlorophenol, 1% pet (disinfectants)
Dibutyl phthalate, 5% pet (plasticizer)
o-Dichlorobenzene, 1% pet (leather dyes)[1330]
Dichlorophene, 1% pet (insecticide, disinfectant)
1,4-Dioxane, 0.5% aq (solvent in finishing)
Disperse Yellow 3, 1% pet (sheep skin and fur dyeing)
Gold sodium thiomalate, 0.1% pet (gold decorations)
Hydroquinone, 1% pet (inhibitor with acrolein to prevent the latter's polymerization)
Isocyanate resins (catalysts and finishes; see Chapter 25)
Melamine-formaldehyde resins, 10% pet (finishes)
4,4'-Methylenedianiline, 1% pet (isocyanate catalyst)
Methyl methacrylate monomer, 10% pet (adhesives)
Phenylmercuric nitrate, 0.05% pet (removal of fat, disinfectant)
o-Phenylphenol, 1% pet (disinfectant)
Polyester resin monomer, 10% pet (adhesives, shoe soles)
Pyrocatechol, 2% pet (vegetable tanning agents)
Resorcinol, 2% pet (tanning and processing, especially condensed with aromatic bases such as aniline to make synthetic tannins)
Tricresyl phosphate, 2% pet (plasticizer in finishing)
Urea-formaldehyde resin, 10% pet (finishes, retanning)
Zirconium salts, 1% pet (tanning, retanning, pigments)

Vegetable Tannins[187]

The chief source of vegetable tannins are the bark, wood, fruit, leaves, and roots of certain plants.

Bark

Wattle, 1% pet
Mangrove, 1% pet
Oak, 1% pet
Eucalyptus, 1% pet
Hemlock, 1% pet
Pine, 1% pet
Larch, 1% pet
Willow, 1% pet

Fruits

Myrobalans, 1% pet
Valonia, 1% pet
Divi-divi, 1% pet
Tara, 1% pet
Algarrobilla, 1% pet

Wood

Quebracho, 1% pet
Chestnut, 1% pet
Oak, 1% pet
Urunday, 1% pet

Leaves

Sumac, 1% pet
Gambier, 1% pet

Roots

Canaigre, 1% pet
Palmetto, 1% pet

TATTOO ARTISTS

A tattoo artist first shaves the area to be tattooed and then washes it, usually with a germicidal soap. A charcoal-coated stencil is used to draw the design on the skin. An electric needle is then dipped into the color pigment solution and pressed into the skin to insert the pigment. A sterile dressing is usually applied after the work is completed, and needles are ordinarily sterilized in a steam-heated cabinet. Transmission of AIDS and other infections is a constant threat in this work.

Tattoo operators themselves may be tattooed, sometimes heavily so. The cutaneous reactions to tattoo pigments may at times histologically resemble Spiegler-Fendt pseudolymphoma, and awareness of this type of reaction can avoid the erroneous diagnosis of lymphoma.[93] Lichenoid reactions have also been described.[1319] The red pigment in tattoos at one time was mercuric sulfide,[711] which may contain small amounts of cadmium sulfide to attain a brighter color in the skin. The amount of cadmium may be sufficient to induce photoallergic reactions in red tattoos in some persons after sunshine exposure.[484]

Irritants

Soaps and detergents
Solvents

Disinfectants
Pigments
Heat

Patch test to standard and vehicle preservative allergens, with special attention to the following.

Standard Allergens

Potassium dichromate, 0.25% pet; 0.023 mg/cm² (from chrome green, chromic oxide, trivalent chromium compounds; green tattoos)[1191]
Cobalt chloride, 1% pet; 0.02 mg/cm² (cobalt aluminate, light blue color, as in tattoos)[1191]
Wool alcohols, 30% pet; 1.00 mg/cm² (lotions, creams)
Neomycin sulfate, 20% pet; 0.23 mg/cm² (germicidal ointments)
Caine mix, 8% pet; 0.63 mg/cm² (topical anesthetics)
Formaldehyde, 2% aq; 0.18 mg/cm² (disinfectants)
Nickel sulfate, 2.5% pet; 0.2 mg/cm² (hand tools)

Additional Allergens

Ammoniated mercury, 1% pet (pigments)
Bacitracin, 20% pet
Cadmium chloride, 1% aq
p-Chloro-*m*-xylenol, 1% pet (germicidal ointments and creams)

TAXIDERMIST

A taxidermist mounts the skins of animals, birds, and mammals in life-like positions. The taxidermist may remove the skin with special knives, scissors, and pliers, using care to preserve hair and feathers in a natural state. The skin is then preserved in salt, borax, arsenic, or phenol. Alum, mercuric chloride, and zinc chloride may be used as disinfectants and embalming chemicals. Preservative solutions may be rubbed onto the skin. Using a wire foundation and papier mache and adhesive tape, the body contour is built up to give a natural appearance, showing the form and muscles of the specimen. Adhesive tape and modeling clay are used to cover the foundation after which the skin is applied and eyes, teeth, and claws affixed. Feathers and fur are cleaned with gasoline, dressed, and brushed. The specimen may be mounted in a case giving representation of natural surroundings.

In the past, anthrax was a hazard of taxidermy, and it still should be kept in mind when handling specimens from certain countries. Ornithosis from infected birds is another hazard.

Irritants

Arsenicals
Gasoline and other solvents
Phenol
Alum

Zinc chloride
Mercuric chloride
Tannins
Potassium aluminum sulfate

Patch test to standard and vehicle preservative allergens, with special attention to the following.

Standard Allergens

Potassium dichromate, 0.25% pet; 0.023 mg/cm^2
Cobalt dichloride, 1% pet; 0.02 mg/cm^2 (plaster casts)
Formaldehyde, 2% aq; 0.18 mg/cm^2 (preservatives)
Nickel sulfate, 2.5% pet; 0.2 mg/cm^2 (hand tools)
Rosin (colophony), 20% pet; 0.85 mg/cm^2

Additional Allergens

Mercuric chloride, 1% aq (preservatives)

TEXTILE WORKERS

The textile industry today is almost totally mechanized, with sophisticated electronic equipment and computers. Irritant and allergic dermatitis are relatively uncommon and usually are due to dyes and dye manufacture-related chemicals and to resins used for finishes,[350, 831, 948, 1150] although relatively few workers come into direct contact with dyes because of the extensive automation of this industry.[350] The exact identity of many dyes is difficult to determine, as many have a secret chemical composition.[445] Multiple dye sensitization is common and may be attributed to group sensitization usually to azo dyes.[924] Polyesters, acrylics, and nylons are most commonly dyed with disperse dyes of the azo type. Disperse dyes are found on patch testing to be the most frequent sensitizers, especially Disperse Blue 106, Disperse Blue 124, and p-aminophenol, which are derived from p-phenylenediamine, as well as Disperse Brown 1 and Disperse Yellow 3. It should be noted that p-phenylene-diamine is an unreliable detector of textile dye allergy.[859]

The textile process consists of carding the fibers to remove impurities and straighten the fibers; spinning, which thins and elongates the fibers; weaving; dyeing; and finishing. The hazardous dusts are found chiefly during the spinning processes, especially asbestos, where it may be found in asbestos spinning, weaving, and yarn workrooms. Finishing processes include bleaching, glazing to improve the appearance, sizing to increase the body and texture, and preshrinking. During textile finishing processes, the temperature and humidity in work areas may be quite high due to release of steam. A potent allergen used in sizing is 2,3-epoxypropyl trimethyl ammonium chloride, which is also a strong irritant.[348] Burling removes knots and loose threads and any accumulated foreign material. Other processes include scouring and bleaching, which may use sulfur dioxide or hydrogen peroxide. Noise is a constant problem of many of these processes. Fire is also a continuing hazard of this industry.

Mercerization, which is performed on cotton or cotton blends, consists of immersing the fabric under tension in a sodium hydroxide solution, causing permanent swelling of the fibers so that shrinking does not take place in normal washing. Following finishing processes, the fabric is centrifuged and dried by vacuum suction.

Durable press is achieved in one of two ways: (1) precuring, in which the resin is added, the fabric dyed and cured by baking, and heat applied after the garment is constructed; and (2) postcuring, in which the resin is added and the fabric is dried, made into a garment, pressed, and then cured. These finishes are complex formaldehyde-containing resins.[73, 345, 418, 625, 833, 1044, 1097] The screening chemical most likely to detect allergic contact sensitivity to these resins is ethylene urea melamine formaldehyde resin, according to Fowler et al.[418]

Other additives used in textile work include soil-release agents, antistatic compounds; antibacterial-antifungal agents; moth repellents; compounds to make the fabric water repellent, flameproof, fireproof, and fire resistant; and of course many dyes, which can be added at almost any stage.[350, 948] Fire retardants are most commonly bromine based, but also antimony oxide, phosphorus, chlorine, and alumina trihydrate are used. The dyes are numerous and complex, and occasionally cause dermatitis in users. Disperse dyes with azo or anthraquinone structures are, by far, the most common allergens, most likely because they do not cling tightly to the synthetic fiber.[29, 111, 113, 176, 235, 236, 350, 407, 411, 445, 560, 582, 856, 1133, 1171, 1318]

Kathon CG has been reported to cause hand dermatitis in nylon production workers, specifically by the isothiazolinone mixture Grotan TK2. The latter is also used as a preservative in lubricating oil employed in the spinning unit to reduce the electrostatic charge produced by high-speed spinning and to reduce the likelihood of yarn breakage.[1228] Kathon 930 has also been reported to cause allergic contact dermatitis when used as a biocide in finishing agents.[708]

The incidence of dye dermatitis varies throughout the world from 1% to 15.9%, depending on the country, patient sample, and number of dyes in the test series. Disperse dyes appear to be the most frequent cause of allergic contact dermatitis.[98, 541, 543] A minor "epidemic" of contact dermatitis from wearing stretch leggings and other clothes manufactured from black "velvet" fabric was reported by Hausen.[550] The color mixture extracted from this clothing was Disperse Blue 124 and 106, Disperse Red 1, Disperse Yellow 3, and small amounts of Disperse Blue 1 (an anthraquinone dye). These dyes are also used in blouses, skirts, dresses, aerobic outfits, and headbands.[558] The chief constituents of the black "velvet" dye mixture are Disperse Blue 106 and 124, both recognized allergens.[550] Cross-sensitizations between these azo dyes and p-amino compounds are common and can be partially explained on the basis of structural affinities.[1107] Allergens for patch testing have been recommended by Hatch and Maibach.[541, 543] Symptoms of immediate-type respiratory allergy and urticaria appear to be more commonly associated with fur dyes.[350]

Reactive dyes for textiles were introduced in 1956 and are used on both natural and synthetic fibers. The color-forming part of the molecule is usually an azo, anthraquinone, or phthalocyanine derivative. Certain of these dyes can induce allergic contact dermatitis, respiratory disease, and urticaria.[346, 844]

"Mule spinner's disease" is scrotal cancer occurring in cotton textile workers heavily exposed to mineral oils for long periods of time while working on a machine called "the mule."[203] Mineral oils containing polycyclic aromatic hydrocarbons (including 3,4-benzpyrene) are most likely responsible.[80] Lung cancer and nonmalignant respiratory disease appear to be significantly increased in workers in plants processing asbestos, such as chrysotile asbestos (hydrated magnesium silicate),[288–290] the form of asbestos that accounts for 95% of asbestos production in the United States and Canada.

The cost benefit of patch testing with textile finish resins was studied and confirmed by Andersen and Hamann.[30a] Of 428 patients, 15 were found positive to textiles, 10 of whom were positive to finishes. All were also positive to formaldehyde, which the authors consider an accurate screening chemical for textile finish dermatitis. Most investigators, on the other hand, report that patients can be allergic to formaldehyde resins in clothing without also being sensitive to formaldehyde.[418] In a study from North Carolina,[1150] 72 textile workers with dermatitis were evaluated, representing 56 different textile manufacturers. Twenty-nine percent were diagnosed with work-related allergic contact dermatitis and 38% with primarily work-related irritant contact dermatitis. Textile dyes accounted for 46.1% of the total allergic contact dermatitis allergens, textile finishes in 42.3%, and rubber-related allergens in 38.5%. Other allergens included machine oil and epoxy resin. A single case of contact urticaria was included.

A 5-year study of the leather and shoe industry in Germany[729] found 85 patients with occupational contact dermatitis. Common allergens were potassium dichromate, glutaraldehyde, p-aminoazobenzene, p-tert-butylphenol–formaldhyde resin, and mercaptobenzothiazole.

Irritants[541]

Bleaches
Dyes
Finishing agents
Solvents
Lubricating oils with detergents[161]
Sodium hydroxide
Sulfuric acid
Hydrochloric acid
Hydrogen peroxide
Tetrasodium pyrophosphate
Mono-, di-, and triethanolamine
Peracetic acid (bleaching and germicide)
2,3-Epoxypropyl trimethyl ammonium chloride
Sodium perborate
Sodium bisulfate
Calcium hypochlorite
Sodium silicate
Caustic soda
Rough fibers

Zinc nitrate
Ethanol and other alcohols
Various other solvents
Polyethylene and polypropylene glycols (in optical brighteners)
Detergents
Quinones (1,4-benzoquinone, a severe irritant and allergen producing brown staining as well as staining of the cornea)
Antimony compounds (used in dyeing and flameproofing)
Barium compounds
Cerium sulfate (mildew-proofing and dyeing in textile printing)
Chrome compounds (mordants)
Magnesium compounds (for sizing, weighting, dyeing)
Stannous and stannic compounds
Heat (weaving, dyeing)
Steam
Vibration (textile machines)

Patch test to standard and vehicle preservative allergens, with special attention to the following.

Standard Allergens

Potassium dichromate, 0.25% pet; 0.023 mg/cm^2 (mordants and finishing processes)
p-tert-Butylphenol–formaldehyde resin, 1% pet; 0.04 mg/cm^2[142, 438, 1102]
2-Mercaptobenzothiazole, 1% pet; 0.075 mg/cm^2 (elastics and gloves)
Carba mix, 3% pet; 0.25 mg/cm^2 (elastics and gloves)
Epoxy resin, 1% pet; 0.05 mg/cm^2[442]
Ethylenediamine hydrochloride, 1% pet; 0.05 mg/cm^2[153, 1332]
p-Phenylenediamine, 1% pet; 0.090 mg/cm^2 (dyes for fur, leather)[360]
Mercapto mix, 1% pet; 0.075 mg/cm^2 (elastics, gloves)
Kathon CG, 0.01% aq; 0.0040 mg/cm^2[1228]
PPD mix (Black rubber mix), 0.6% pet; 0.075 mg/cm^2 (elastics, gloves)
Formaldehyde, 2% aq; 0.18 mg/cm^2 (resin finishes)
Thiuram mix, 1% pet; 0.025 mg/cm^2 (rosin manufacture)
Nickel sulfate, 2.5% pet; 0.2 mg/cm^2 (hand tools, buttons and other metal clothing objects)[205]

Additional Allergens

p-Aminoazobenzene, 0.25% pet (textile dyes)[42]
Chloracetamide, 0.2% pet (preservative)[1083]
Dimethoxane, 1% olive oil (preservative)[1128]
Dimethyloldihydroxyethylene urea–formaldehyde resin, 10% pet[542]
Dimethylol melamine resin, 10% pet
Dimethylol propylene urea resin, 10% pet
2,3-Epoxypropyl trimethyl ammonium chloride[348]
Ethylene urea melamine formaldehyde resin (Fixpret AC)[418]
Hydrazine sulfate, 1% pet (stain removers)
N-isopropyl-N'-phenyl-p-phenylenediamine (IPPD), 0.1% pet (rubber)

Kathon 930, 0.2% (?) aq (biocide in finishing agents)[708]
Mercaptobenzimidazole, 1% pet[463]
2-Monomethylol phenol, 1% (resin finish)[142]
Pentachlorophenol, 1% pet (fungicide)
Phenol formaldehyde resin, 5% pet[142, 1044]
Phenylmercuric nitrate, 0.05% pet (fungicide)
Tribromosalicylanilide, 2% pet (preservatives)
Tricresyl phosphate, 5% pet (fire proofing)
Urea formaldehyde resin, 10% pet
Tris(2,3-dibromopropyl)phosphate, 5% pet[30] (This substance was used as a fire retardant in clothing but is no longer used because of suspected carcinogenicity. It is still used as a flame retardant in plastics.)

Formaldehyde-Related Resins Used in Clothing Finishes[418]

Dimethylol dihydroxyethylene urea formaldehy resin (Fixapret CPN), 4.5% aq[1150]
Dimethylol propylene urea formaldehyde resin (Fixapret PH), 5% aq
Tetramethylol acetylene diurea formaldhyde resin (Fixapret 140), 5% pet[1150]
Ethylene urea melamine formaldehyde resin (Fixapret AC), 10% pet
Urea formaldehyde resin (Kaurit S), 7% pet
Melamine formaldehyde resin (Kaurit M70), 7% pet
Ethylene urea formaldehyde resin, 1% pet
Phenol formaldehyde resin, 1% pet

Common Sensitizing Clothing Dyes

Acid Yellow 36, 1% pet[28]
p-Aminoazobenzene, 0.25% pet[350, 736]
p-Aminodiphenylamine[350, 859]
Basic Brown 1, 1% pet
Basic Red 46, 2% pet[350, 405] (note: 1% pet[1150])
Bismark Brown, 1% pet[794]
Benzidine, 1% pet[495]
CI Reactive Black 5, 5% pet (may crossreact with p-phenylenediamine[1315])
Diaminodiphenylmethane, 0.5% pet[1240]
p-Dimethylaminoazobenzene, 1% pet (azo dyes)
Disperse Brown 1, 1% pet[859, 924, 1150]
Disperse Orange 1, 1% pet[350, 1150]
Disperse Orange 3, 1% pet[350, 794, 858, 924, 1150]
Disperse Orange 13[350, 924, 1150]
Disperse Yellow 3, 1% pet[73, 350, 794, 859, 1150]
Disperse Yellow 9, 1% pet[73, 350, 794, 1150]
Disperse Yellow 39[73, 794]
Disperse Yellow 64, 1% pet[176]
Disperse Orange 76[360, 794]
Disperse Red 1, 1% pet[73, 350, 794, 858, 1150]
Disperse Red 11, 1% pet[73, 794]
Disperse Red 17, 1% pet[73, 350, 360, 794, 1150]
Disperse Red 153, 1% pet[924]
Disperse Blue 3, 1% pet[73, 350, 794, 1150]
Disperse Blue 7, 1% pet[794]
Disperse Blue 35, 1% pet[73, 350, 1150]
Disperse Blue 85, 1% pet[73, 350, 1150]

Disperse Blue 106, 1% pet[114, 350, 794, 859, 924]
Disperse Blue 124, 1% pet[73, 113, 350, 858, 859, 924, 1150]
Disperse Blue 153, 1% pet[73, 350, 1150]
Disperse Black 1, 1% pet[794]
Disperse Black 2, 1% pet[794]
Disperse Brown 1, 1% pet[73, 350, 924]
Reactive dyes, 1 to 2% pet[346]
Naphthol AS, 5% aq (dye)[29, 571, 717]
o-Nitro-p-phenylenediamine (dyes)[350]

THEATRICAL ARTISTS

Most dermatitis in actors and actresses is related to makeup, hair dyes, hairpieces, artificial noses, and so on. Often various oils, greases, and coloring materials are mixed, either by the actor or actress or by a makeup artist. Cosmetic acne is common among these persons.

Irritants

Acetone (to remove spirit, gum, and collodion)
Adhesives (for beards, mustaches, hairpieces, and rubber prosthetic pieces)
Alcohol (for removing gums)
Collodion
Soaps and detergents

Patch test to standard and vehicle preservative allergens, with special attention to the following.

Standard Allergens

2-Mercaptobenzothiazole, 1% pet; 0.075 mg/cm^2 (e.g., rubber prostheses, noses, warts)
Balsam of Peru, 25% pet; 0.8 mg/cm^2 (cosmetics)
Carba mix, 3% pet; 0.25 mg/cm^2 (rubber)
p-Phenylenediamine, 1% pet; 0.090 mg/cm^2 (hair dyes)
Mercapto mix, 1% pet; 0.075 mg/cm^2 (rubber)
PPD mix (Black rubber mix), 0.6% pet; 0.075 mg/cm^2 (rubber)
Thiuram mix, 1% pet; 0.025 mg/cm^2 (rubber)
Formaldehyde, 2% aq; 0.18/cm^2 (adhesives)
Quaternium 15, 2% pet; 0.1 mg/cm^2 (cosmetics)
Nickel sulfate, 2.5% pet; 0.2 mg/cm^2 (eyelash curlers, other metal objects)
Rosin (colophony), 20% pet; 0.85 mg/cm^2 (adhesives)

Additional Allergens

m-Aminophenol, 1% pet
p-Aminophenol, 1% pet
Benzoin tincture, 10% alc (greasepaint makeup)[609]
Flowers, especially chrysanthemums
Henna, 10 mg/100 cc water[274]
Imidazolidinyl urea, 2% pet (cosmetics)
o-Nitro-p-phenylenediamine, 1% pet (semipermanent hair dyes)
m-Phenylenediamine, 2% pet (hair dyes)
p-Phenyl-p-phenylenediamine, 1% pet

Pyrocatechol, 2% pet
Resorcinol, 2% pet (hair dyes)
Toluene-2,4-diamine, 1% pet (hair dyes)
Toluene-2,5-diamine, 1% pet (hair dyes)

TILE SETTERS

Tile setters attach tile to walls, floors, and ceilings. Terrazzo workers apply a mixture of cement, sand, pigment, and marble chips to floors, stairways, and cabinet fixtures to provide an attractive and long-lasting covering. Tile setters first tack a support of screen-like mesh to the floor, wall, or ceiling. Using a trowel to mix and spread coarse cement onto the screen, they next use a rake-like device to scratch the surface of wet cement. After the cement is dried, they then trowel on a richer coat of cement, which they work back and forth in sweeping motions until it is smooth and even. The tiles are then placed onto the cement and gently tapped on their surface with a small block of wood so that they all rest evenly and flatly. When the cement has set, the tile setters use a rubber trowel to cover the tile and joints with grout, a very fine cement. They then scrape the surface with a squeegee, force grout from the face of the tile into joints, and remove any excess. Before the grout dries, they wash the surface with a damp sponge. Tile setters also sometimes use mastic, which may be rubber based, or plastic adhesives, especially epoxy, as adhesive resins.

The terrazzo worker first prepares an underlying layer of cement, embeds metal or other strips into it to separate colors and to allow for expansion and contraction, and then pours a layer of terrazzo, a mixture of tinted concrete or resin and marble chips, over the base. After it is allowed to dry, it is ground and polished with small hand-controlled machines.

Irritants

Wet cement
Dust
Water (wet work)
Detergents

Patch test to standard and vehicle preservative allergens, with special attention to the following.

Standard Allergens

Potassium dichromate, 0.25% pet; 0.023 mg/cm^2
(cement)
2-Mercaptobenzothiazole, 1% pet; 0.075 mg/cm^2
(rubber)
Carba mix, 3% pet; 0.25 mg/cm^2 (rubber)
Epoxy resin, 1% pet; 0.05 mg/cm^2 (mastic)
Mercapto mix, 1% pet; 0.075 mg/cm^2 (rubber)
PPD mix (Black rubber mix), 0.6% pet; 0.075 mg/cm^2
(rubber)
Thiuram mix, 1% pet; 0.025 mg/cm^2 (rubber)

TOBACCO WORKERS

During cultivation of tobacco, the plants are repeatedly debudded ("topped") using fingers or a small knife. When the leaves have reached a certain size and have turned yellow, they are harvested and cured by a variety of means: in air, sun, or containers through which air is passed. The leaves are then stored or hung for fermentation, which is achieved chemically rather than by bacteria, usually in air-conditioned chambers for up to 10 to 14 days. After aging, moistening, and drying, the leaves are packed in casks and kept for up to 1 to 3 years during the process of fermentation. The tobacco is then packed and shipped for the manufacture of cigarette, pipe, and cigar tobacco. During debudding especially, there may be absorption of sufficient nicotine to induce giddiness, respiratory and gastrointestinal symptoms, and irritant dermatitis on the fingers and hands.

In making cigarettes, a machine operator encases the ground tobacco and additives in a continuous paper roll and cuts cigarettes from the roll. The additives include a large number of vegetable and chemical substances. The operator first places cigarette paper on a spindle and sets a monogram-printing device to print the brand name on the paper at a specified position. The flow of shredded tobacco is regulated by valves to ensure delivery of an exact amount. Ink and glue reservoirs are filled. The operator then starts the machine and observes the process. A separate operator tends a machine that packs and fills the cigarette packages. Both may have contact with tobacco and dust, especially when cleaning the machines. The chief hazard is absorption of nicotine, due essentially to tobacco dust. Cigarette filters have been manufactured from cellulose acetate and triacetate.

Irritants

Moist tobacco leaves

Patch test to standard allergens, with special attention to the following.

Standard Allergens

Fragrance mix, 8% pet; 0.43 mg/cm^2
Nickel sulfate, 2.5% pet; 0.2 mg/cm^2
Epoxy resin, 1% pet; 0.05 mg/cm^2

VETERINARIANS

This category of work includes veterinary medicine, various occupations involved in caring for animals, and animal husbandry (breeders, shearers, dehorners, and so on). Veterinarians are exposed to all of the allergens listed earlier under Health Care Workers. In addition, many of the medications long ago discarded for use in humans are still used in the treatment of animal disease. An example is Donovan's solution, which is a combination of arsenic and mercuric iodides used for chronic skin diseases of horses, cattle, sheep, swine, and dogs. Increasingly veterinarians are engaged in preventive measures against animal disease in animal husbandry, including castration and artificial insemination. Clinical veterinarians are also exposed to all of the biological and physical hazards of other medical personnel, with emphasis on the zoonoses. Many of the topical medications used on animals contain several different antibacterial and antifungal agents, some of which may be sensitizing to humans. Veterinarians are also exposed to ionizing radiation, ethylene oxide, and anesthetic gases. Needlestick injury is an important occupational hazard for veterinarians.[914] Latex allergy is also common in veterinarians and their supporting personnel. Some veterinarians are engaged in research and teaching.

Poison ivy/oak/sumac dermatitis is common in veterinarians and can be very disabling unless recognized. Poison oak plants from a coastal area of the Western United States have higher levels of the allergen urushiol than those from inland sites. There also is an increase in urushiol concentration in the late fall, which may explain why a larger number of cases are seen during the autumn.[459]

In a study of veterinary surgeons, chronic, relapsing irritant dermatitis of the hands was common. Penicillin, neomycin, and streptomycin were frequent causes of contact allergy, as well as rubber chemicals, antiseptics, and local anesthetics. Multiple contact allergies were often found, as were immediate-type contact reactions.[356] Bovine amniotic fluid and blood are among the causes of protein contact dermatitis.[271] With IgE studies, cow hair and dander have been demonstrated in the etiology of eczema in veterinary surgeons, as well as asthma.[1009] Cow dander has been considered the most common cause of occupational contact urticaria in Finland.[695]

Other antibiotics that may induce dermatitis and allergic contact dermatitis in veterinary surgeons are spiramycin,[1255] Penethamate BP, and tylosin.[60, 603, 1255] Allergic contact dermatitis from contact with tylosin during vaccine injection of chicks has been described.[60] Hjorth and Roed-Petersen[603] found protein contact dermatitis as a frequent predisposing factor in development of incapacitating allergic contact dermatitis in veterinary surgeons. Obstetrical work performed without gloves may induce recurring episodes of dermatitis.

Contact urticaria has been reported from dog saliva.[170, 841, 1225]

Atopic allergy to animals is common, not only in commercial veterinarians but also in biomedical laboratory workers, among whom much of the research on occupational animal allergy has been done.[1194]

Irritants

Soaps and detergents
Alkalis (dehorning agents)
Germicidal solutions (sodium hypochlorite)[353]
Animal hair, saliva (contact urticaria[841]), urine, and feces
Medications, including serums and vaccines
Animal feed

Repellents
Rodenticides
Deodorants
Insecticides

Patch test to standard and vehicle preservative allergens, with special attention to the following.

Standard Allergens

Potassium dichromate, 0.25% pet; 0.023 mg/cm² (leather, veterinarian laxatives, and for treatment of cecal coccidiosis in chickens and turkeys)
Wool alcohols, 30% pet; 1.00 mg/cm² (medications)
2-Mercaptobenzothiazole, 1% pet; 0.075 mg/cm² (rubber, insecticides, fungicides)
Balsam of Peru, 25% pet; 0.80 mg/cm² (medications)
Neomycin sulfate, 20% pet; 0.23 mg/cm² (medications)
Caine mix, 8% pet; 0.63 mg/cm² (medications)
Carba mix, 3% pet; 0.25 mg/cm² (rubber and insecticides)
Cobalt dichloride, 1% pet; 0.02 mg/cm² (feed additives)
Mercapto mix, 1% pet; 0.075 mg/cm² (rubber, insecticides, fungicides)
Ethylenediamine dihydrochloride, 1% pet; 0.075 mg/cm² (medications)
PPD mix (Black rubber mix), 6% pet; 0.075 mg/cm² (rubber)
Thiuram mix, 1% pet; 0.025 mg/cm² (rubber)
Formaldehyde, 2% aq; 0.18 mg/cm² (disinfectants, avian inhalant)
Nickel sulfate, 2.5% pet; 0.2 mg/cm² (hand tools)
Rosin (colophony), 20% pet; 0.85 mg/cm² (topical medications)
p-tert-Butylphenol–formaldehyde resin, 1% pet; 0.04 mg/cm² (leather)

Additional Allergens

Ammoniated mercury, 1% pet (medications)
Benzyl penicillin 30% aq[356]
Bronopol, 0.25% pet (medications)[1317]
Camphor, 10% pet (medications)
Captan, 0.25% pet (shampoos)
Chloramine T, 0.5% aq[356]
Chloramphenicol, 2% pet
Chloro cresol, 1% pet (medications)
Chlorpromazine, 1% pet (medications)
Chlorothymol, 1% pet (liniments)
p-Chloro-m-xylenol, 1% pet (liniments)
Cinnamon oil, 0.5% pet (liniments)
Coal tar, 5% pet (medications)
Dichlorophene, 1% pet (fungicide and taeniacide for dogs)
Dihydrostreptomycin, 5% aq[356]
Glutaraldehyde, 0.25% pet (disinfectants)
Hexachlorophene, 1% pet (disinfectant)
Hexylresorcinol, 1% pet (vermifuge)
N-isopropyl-N'-phenyl-p-phenylenediamine (IPPD), 0.1% pet (rubber)

Menthol, 1% pet (medications)
Phenothiazine, 2.5% pet (sheep dip)
Phenylmercuric nitrate, 0.05% pet (medications)
Piperazine, 1% pet (anthemintic, rare sensitizer)[1093]
o-Phenylphenol, 1% pet (disinfectants)
Procaine, 2% pet
Procaine penicillin, 30% aq[356]
Resorcinol, 2% pet (medications)
Rhus plants
Sodium hypochlorite, 0.25% aq[353]
Spiramycin, 10% aq[1255]
Streptomycin, 2.5% aq[356]
Tetracycline, 1% pet[356]
Tylosin, 1% aq (antibiotic)[356] (5% pet[60, 1255])

WELDERS

The three most common ways to permanently join metal parts are electric arc welding, resistance welding, and gas welding. In arc welding, heat is produced by the electric current, usually about 4,000°C at the point of fusion. Molten metal is usually added to the joint. Much arc welding is done by hand with a hand-held electrode holder. Also many welding processes are performed by semiautomatic or fully automatic means. Arc welding is the preferred method for large jobs, such as fabricated work with heavy plates and large shapes or in production lines and general assembly operations where speed is desirable. In resistance welding, heat is created in the metal by resistance to the flow of current through the metal. In gas welding, oxygen or air is mixed with a fuel gas prior to combustion at the nozzle. Between the parts to be joined, a filler metal is used with a lower melting temperature than that of the parts to be joined. A chemical flux is used to prevent oxidation and facilitate adhesion.

"Metal fume fever" is a self-limited syndrome with symptoms resembling a flu-like illness: malaise, myalgia, fevers in the range of 38° to 39°C, and frequently cough, hoarseness, and dyspnea. The condition is often caused by exposure to fumes of welding galvanized metals or melting brass, especially the oxides of zinc, copper, and magnesium.[919] Welders and brass founders are most likely affected, and the condition is known by several names, such as brass chills, smelter shakes, and "Monday morning fever."[87] The condition is easily confused with common respiratory illnesses, but recognition is important to prevent recurrence. Treatment is supportive. Chronic sequelae do not occur.

Silver brazing, one of the most versatile methods of metal joining, is the process of joining metals by heat with a silver alloy filler metal at temperatures about 429°C. In both welding and silver brazing the possibility of cadmium poisoning is present, which can cause acute inhalation symptoms with pulmonary edema and death; from chronic exposure, pulmonary emphysema, a Fanconi-like syndrome, and renal tubular damage can occur. Inhalation by welders of cadmium fumes can be a serious work hazard, which is often unrecognized. The initial symptoms can be confused with the relatively mild condition "metal fume fever." Cadmium is also a human carcinogen, causing lung cancer in smelting and plating workers.

Welders are often highly skilled technicians with extensive knowledge of metals and of the melting points of steel, aluminum, and other commonly used metals. At the journeyman level, the job includes fabrication and repair of machine parts, motors, trailers, and manufacturing plant equipment. Journeymen also repair broken parts, fill holes, cut metal, and increase the sizes of metal parts. Welders clean and degrease work pieces using a wire brush, portable grinder, or chemical bath. After welding they chip or grind off excess material. They also occasionally use flame cutting machines to cut metal plates. In metal cutting the part is first heated by the flame, and a stream of oxygen is directed at the site of cutting, moved along the line to be cut. In gas pressure welding the parts are heated and fused by gas jets under pressure.

Welding fluxes are used for high-temperature welding. A common one is lithium fluoride, which is very potent and highly irritating. Another flux, called *white flux*, is a mixture of sodium nitrate and sodium nitrite, a strong oxidizer and irritant.

Welding rods may be standard metals or special alloys and are often coated with flux. Welding alloys may be aluminum powder with iron oxide, nickel, manganese, or steel. The amount of chromium in the stainless steel in electrode rods used in electric arc welding may be as much as 18%, and during use considerable hexavalent chromium may be released in the welding fumes.[675]

In addition to burns, the most prevalent occupational disease of welders is acute keratoconjunctivitis, which arises from exposure to UV light.[329, 332] Emmett and his colleagues[329, 332] also found localized cutaneous erythema to be frequent in welders, as are small cutaneous scars from burns and lacerations. Spot welding without the proper protection may result in severe facial photodermatitis,[1120] even from a UVC light reflected from a white hood.[146, 591] Burns may occur from the UV light, sparks, or, rarely, from a direct flame.[352] Skin cancer is a potential adverse effect on the skin from welding. Chronic photo-ophthalmia with functional visual disturbances may also occur. Chronic discoid lupus erythematosus is also an occupational disease in welders.[1322, 1326] Allergic contact dermatitis to chromate,[443, 1122, 1342] cobalt, and other metals has been noted. Occupational asthma due to stainless steel welding fumes has also been reported.[715] A relationship between chrome-containing welding fumes and pulmonary carcinoma has been suggested (Fig. AP–22).[37, 1140]

Irritants

Abrasives
Heat
Ultraviolet light
Metal cleaners
Metal particles
Degreasing agents

Patch test to standard and vehicle preservative allergens, with special attention to the following.

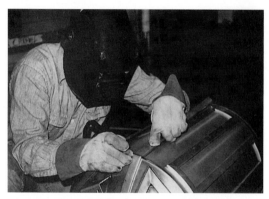

FIGURE AP–22 • Welding fumes may contain, among other compounds, chromate, cobalt, and nickel.

Standard Allergens

Potassium dichromate, 0.25% pet; 0.023 mg/cm^2 (welding fumes)
2-Mercaptobenzothiazole, 1% pet; 0.075 mg/cm^2 (rubber gloves and face masks)
Carba mix, 3% pet; 0.63 mg/cm^2 (rubber)
Cobalt dichloride, 1% pet; 0.02 mg/cm^2 (metals)
Mercapto mix, 1% pet; 0.075 mg/cm^2 (rubber)
PPD mix (Black rubber mix), 0.6% pet; 0.075 mg/cm^2 (rubber)
Thiuram mix, 1% pet; 0.025 mg/cm^2 (rubber)
Formaldehyde, 2% aq; 0.18 mg/cm^2 (metal cleaners)
Nickel sulfate, 2.5% pet; 0.2 mg/cm^2 (metal hand tools; welding fumes)[1089]

Additional Allergens

Glutaraldehyde, 0.25% pet (metal cleaners)
Diethylthiourea, 1% pet (safety shoes)[410]

WINE MAKERS

Viticulture, the growing of wine grapes, involves considerable manual labor. The vines are grafted approximately 3 years after planting, and the plants must be thinned and subdivided at yearly intervals. Large amounts of fertilizers and pesticides are used, especially sulfur and copper sulfate. Much of this work is mechanized.

The process of wine making is relatively simple, but, for large commercial operations, specialized equipment is used. Initially the grapes are crushed in either simple mills or large centrifugal crushers, rollers, and so on. The ancient method of grape crushing by treading on the grapes with bare feet is hardly ever utilized today. The crushed grapes are then transferred to large tanks in which they are then further pressed, separating juice from skins and stems. The *must* (grape juice) is transferred to fermentation containers, which may be made of wood, concrete, stainless steel, or iron lined with epoxy resins or a thin layer of stainless steel. After fermentation, the stems and skins (called *pomace* or *marc*) are transferred from the fermentor to a press. The pomace is flushed with wine from the bottom of the tank. The wine press may be the old crew-type basket press or, more common today, a hydraulic press. After pressing, the wine is withdrawn and passed into storage tanks. Filtering removes impurities and remaining pieces of skin or stem; centrifugal filtering may be employed at this stage. The wine may then be refrigerated and stored at a constant temperature. The yeasts of the genus *Saccharomyces* found in the grapes are essential for fermentation. To prevent growth and competition of undesirable organisms, sulfur dioxide is added before the yeast culture is added. Additives include sodium or potassium metabisulfite, tartaric acid, various tannins, proteolytic enzymes, ascorbic acid, sorbic acid, sorbates, potassium bitartrate, and so on. Salicylic, benzoic, and monochloracetic acids are prohibited in U.S. wines, but in many other states except California it is permitted to add sugar.

Wine normally contains a large number of substances, including carbohydrates, alcohols and related compounds, ketones and aldehydes, acids, various esters, polyphenols and related compounds, nitrogenous compounds, and a small amount of mineral substances.

Irritants

Water (wet work)
Detergents
Enzymes
Ascorbic acid
Tartaric acid
Sulfur dioxide
Tannins
Cold

Patch test to standard and vehicle preservative allergens, with special attention to the following.

Standard Allergens

Mercaptobenzothiazole, 1% pet; 0.075 mg/cm^2 (rubber articles)
Carba mix, 3% pet; 0.25 mg/cm^2 (rubber)
Mercapto mix, 12% pet; 0.075 mg/cm^2 (rubber)
PPD mix (Black rubber mix), 0.6% pet; 0.075 mg/cm^2 (rubber)
Thiuram mix, 1% pet; 0.025 mg/cm^2 (rubber)
Formaldehyde, 2% aq; 0.18 mg/cm^2 (disinfectants)
Nickel sulfate, 2.5% pet; 0.2 mg/cm^2 (tools)

Additional Allergens

Sodium (or potassium) metabisulfite, 1% aq (additive)

WIRE DRAWING OPERATORS

These workers operate machines that draw rods, usually steel, through dies to reduce the diameter to a specified size. The rods usually have a scale covering that must first be removed by one of two methods, mechanical and chemical. In the latter method, hydrochloric and sulfuric acid are most commonly used, but also nitric and phosphoric acids. Next the rods are washed in water to remove excess acid and usually given a "drawing coat" of lime, phosphate, or copper to neutralize acid residues, prevent rust, and provide lubrication. Following thorough drying in ovens, they are passed through drawing machines to reduce their diameter, usually through several dies and blocks. Sometimes the acid cleaning and water washing are repeated. The dies consist of tungsten carbide contained in a steel case. To further reduce friction, lubricants are used, such as soap or various stearates, or solutions of soap, paraffin, or others, giving the wire a bright finish. The reels of wire may be lifted onto a spindle, manually or with a hoist. The ends of wire are sometimes welded together with a welding machine. The diameter is verified with a micrometer, and the physical properties of the wire, such as tensile strength and bend set, may also be measured.

The hazards of dangerous moving parts, such as a broken wire that can whip around and injure workers; fumes; and dust are present. Workers require personal protective equipment such as safety helmets, goggles, face masks, gloves, aprons, and footwear. Periodic evaluation for lead levels in those workers possibly exposed to lead is vital.

Irritants

Acids
Lime
Lubricants
Soaps and detergents

Patch test to standard and vehicle preservative allergens, with special attention to the following.

Standard Allergens

Potassium dichromate, 0.25% pet; 0.023 mg/cm^2
2-Mercaptobenzothiazole, 1% pet; 0.075 mg/cm^2
　(rubber)
Carba mix, 3% pet; 0.25 mg/cm^2 (rubber)
Cobalt chloride, 1% pet; 0.02 mg/cm^2
Ethylenediamine hydrochloride, 1% pet (wire drawing
　lubricants)[874, 1081]
PPD mix (Black rubber mix), 0.6% pet; 0.075 mg/cm^2
　(rubber)
Thiuram mix, 1% pet; 0.0080 mg/cm^2 (rubber)
Formaldehyde, 2% aq; 0.18 mg/cm^2 (phenolic resins)
Nickel sulfate, 2.5% pet; 0.2 mg/cm^2 (hand tools)
Rosin (colophony), 20% pet; 0.85 mg/cm^2
　(soldering)[557, 777, 864, 1302]

References

1. Aberer W, Holub H, Strohal R, Slavicek R. Palladium in dental alloys—The dermatologists' responsibility to warn? *Contact Dermatitis* 1993; 28:163–165.
2. Abrams K, Hogan DJ, Maibach MI. Pesticide-related dermatoses in agricultural workers. State Art Rev Occup Med 1991; 6:463–492.
3. Adams RM. *p*-Chloro-*m*-xylenol in cutting fluids: Two cases of allergic contact dermatitis in machinists. *Contact Dermatitis* 1981; 7:341–342.
4. Adams RM. Allergic contact dermatitis due to *o*-phenylphenol. *Contact Dermatitis* 1981; 7:332.
5. Adams RM. Contact allergic dermatitis due to diethylthiourea in a wetsuit. *Contact Dermatitis* 1982; 8:277–278.
6. Adams RM. Dermatitis in the microelectronics industry. In: LaDou J, ed. The Microelectronics industry. Occupational Medicine. State Art Rev Occup Med 1986; 1:1.
7. Adams RM, Arnau J-MG. Allergic contact dermatitis caused by the sawdust of *Grevillea* A Cunn. *Am J Contact Dermatitis* 1991; 2:192–193.
8. Adams RM, Daily AD, Brancaccio RR, et al. *Alstroemeria*, a new and potent allergen for florists. *Dermatol Clin* 1990; 8:73–76.
9. Adams RM, Fregert S, Gruvberger B, et al. Water solubility of zinc chromate primer paints used as antirust agents. *Contact Dermatitis* 1976; 2:357–358.
10. Adams RM, Manchester RD. Allergic contact dermatitis to Maneb in a housewife. *Contact Dermatitis* 1982; 8:271.
11. Adams RM, Remington JS, Steinberg J, Seibert JS. Tropical fish aquariums: A source of *Mycobacterium marinum* infection resembling sporotrichosis. *JAMA* 1970; 211:457–461.
12. Agatha G, Schubert H. Investigations for allergen identification in contact allergy due to *p*-tert-butylphenolformaldehyde resin. (Translation.) *Dermatol Monatsschr* 1979; 165:337–345.
13. Agathos M. Berufskrankheit scabies. *Dermatosen* 1996; 44:126–128.
14. Agner T, Menné T. Sensitization to acrylates in a dental patient. *Contact Dermatitis* 1994; 30:249–250.
15. Akasawa A, Matsumoto K, Saito H, et al. Incidence of latex allergy in atopic children and hospital workers in Japan. *Arch Allergy Immunol* 1993; 101:177–181.
16. Aldrich TE, Nash R. Occupational clustering of melanoma. Letter to the editor. *Arch Dermatol* 1981; 117:1–2.
17. Ali Salim A. Ammonium dichromate powder in flow coat sector of color TV tube manufacture. *Personal communication*, 1996.
18. Alomar A. Contact dermatitis from benzisothiazolone in cutting oils. *Contact Dermatitis* 1981; 7:155–156.
19. Alomar A, Conde-Salazar L, Romaguera C. Occupational dermatoses from cutting oils. *Contact Dermatitis* 1985; 12:129–138.
20. Alomar A, Smandia JA. Allergic contact dermatitis from Minoxidil. *Contact Dermatitis* 1988; 18:51–52.
21. Alomar A, Vilaltella I. Contact dermatitis to dibutylthiourea in swimming goggles. *Contact Dermatitis* 1985; 13:348–349.
22. Alonso MD, Martin JA, Cuevas M, et al. Occupational protein contact dermatitis from lettuce. *Contact Dermatitis* 1993; 29:109–110.
23. American Dental Association. *Dentist's Desk Reference*, 2nd ed. Chicago: American Dental Association; 1983:71–72.
24. Ancona-Alayon A. Occupational koilonychia from organic solvents. *Contact Dermatitis* 1975; 1:367–369.
25. Ancona A, de la Torre RS, Macotela E. Allergic contact dermatitis from povidone-iodine. *Contact Dermatitis* 1985; 13:66–68.
26. Ancona AA, Monroy F, Fernandez-Diez J. Occupational dermatitis from IPPD in tyres. *Contact Dermatitis* 1982; 8:91–94.

27. Ancona A, Ramos M, Suarez R, et al. Mercury sensitivity in a dentist. *Contact Dermatitis* 1982; 8:218.

28. Ancona A, Serviere L, Trejo A, Monroy F. Dermatitis from an azo-dye in industrial leather protective shoes. *Contact Dermatitis* 1982; 8:220–221.

29. Ancona-Alayon A, Escobar-Marques R, Gonzales-Mendosa A, et al. Occupational pigmented contact dermatitis from Naphthol AS. *Contact Dermatitis* 1976; 2:129–134.

30. Andersen KE. Sensitivity to a flame retardant, tris-(2,3-dibromopropyl)phosphate (Firemaster LVT 23P). *Contact Dermatitis* 1977; 3:297–300.

30a. Andersen KE, Hamann K. Cost benefit of patch testing with textile finish resins. *Contact Dermatitis* 1982; 6:64–67.

31. Andersen KE. Diethylthiourea contact dermatitis from an acidic detergent. *Contact Dermatitis* 1983; 9:146.

32. Andersen KE, Boman A, Hamann K, Wahlberg JE. Guinea pig maximization tests with formaldehyde releasers. *Contact Dermatitis* 1984; 10:257–266.

33. Andersen KE, Hamman K. Is Cytox 3522 (10% methylene-bis-thiocyanate) a human sensitizer? *Contact Dermatitis* 1983; 9:186–189.

34. Andersen KE, Hamann K. How sensitizing is chlorocresol? Allergy tests in guinea pigs versus the clinical experience. *Contact Dermatitis* 1984; 11:11–20.

35. Andersen KE, Hjorth N, Menné T. The baboon syndrome: Systemically induced allergic contact dermatitis. *Contact Dermatitis* 1984; 10:97–100.

36. Angelini G, Rigano L, Foti C, et al. Occupational sensitization to epoxy resin and reactive diluents in marble workers. *Contact Dermatitis* 1996; 35:11–16.

37. Angerer J, Amin W, Heinrich-Ramm R, et al. Occupational chronic exposure to metals. I. Chromium exposure of stainless steel welders—Biological monitoring. *Int Arch Occup Environ Health* 1987; 59:503–512.

38. Apetato M, Marques MSJ. Contact dermatitis caused by sodium metabisulfite. *Contact Dermatitis* 1986; 14:194.

39. Arevalo A, Blancas R, Ancona A. Occupational contact dermatitis from piroxicam. *Am J Contact Dermatitis* 1995; 6:113–114.

40. Armstrong DKB, Walsh MY, Dawson JF. Granulomatous contact dermatitis due to gold earrings. *Br J Dermatol* 1997; 136:776–778.

41. Arndt KA. Cutting fluids and the skin. *Cutis* 1969; 5:143–147.

42. Arnold WP, van Joost T, van der Valk PGM. Adding *p*-aminoazobenzene may increase the sensitivity of the European standard series in detecting contact allergy to dyes, but carries the risk of active sensitization. *Contact Dermatitis* 1995; 33:444.

43. Aronson PJ, Shettler C, Yakes B, et al. Weak patch test reactions at 48 hours can provide an understanding of a work-related dermatitis: A study of epidemic hand dermatitis in industrial clay modellers. *Am J Contact Dermatitis* 1993; 4:163–168.

44. Ashworth J, White IR. Contact allergy to ethoxylated phenol. *Contact Dermatitis* 1991; 24:133–134.

45. Austad J, Kavli G. Phototoxic dermatitis caused by celery infected by *Sclerotinia sclertioum. Contact Dermatitis* 1983; 9:448–451.

46. Autio P, Estlander T, Jolanki R, Keskinen H, Kanerva L. Allergy caused by aziridine hardeners [in Finnish]. *Duodecim* 1993; 109:125–130.

47. Avnstorp C. Chromate eczema in Denmark. *Int J Dermatol* 1984; 23:82.

48. Avnstorp C. Risk factors for cement eczema. *Contact Dermatitis* 1991; 25:81–88.

49. Avnstorp C. Cement eczema. An epidemiological intervention study. *Acta Derm Venereol (Stockh)* 1993; (suppl 179).

50. Axelsson JGK, Johansson SGO, Wrangsjo K. IgE-mediated anaphylactoid reactions to rubber. *Allergy* 1987; 42:46–50.

51. Bach B, Pedersen NB. Contact dermatitis from a wood preservative containing tetrachloroisophthalonitrile. *Contact Dermatitis* 1980; 6:142.

52. Baer RL. Allergic contact sensitization to iron. *J Allergy Clin Immunol* 1973; 51:35–38.

53. Bahmer FA, Koch P. Formaldehyd-induzierte Erythema multiforme-artige Reaktion bei einem Sektionsgehilfen. *Dermatosen* 1994; 42:71–73.

54. Baker H. Contact dermatitis: Triazine film hardener. *Trans St Johns Hosp Dermatol Soc* 1971; 57:243.

55. Bangha E, Elsner P. Occupational contact dermatitis toward sesquiterpene lactones in a florist. *Am J Contact Dermatitis* 1996; 7:188–190.

56. Bangha E, Elsner P. Skin problems in sugar artists. *Br J Dermatol* 1996; 135:772–774.

57. Bang-Pedersen N. Allergy from NAPP. *Contact Dermatitis* 1980; 6:35.

58. Baran RL. Nail damage caused by weed killers and insecticides. *Arch Dermatol* 1974; 110:467.

59. Barbaud A, Mougeolle JM, Schmutz JL. Contact hypersensitivity to arsenic in a crystal factory worker. *Contact Dermatitis* 1995; 33:272–273.

60. Barbera E, de la Cuadra J. Occupational airborne allergic contact dermatitis from tylosin. *Contact Dermatitis* 1989; 20:308–309.

61. Bauer M, Rabens SF. Cutaneous manifestations of trichloroethylene toxicity. *Arch Dermatol* 1974; 110:886–890.

62. Bauer M, Rabens SF. Trichloroethylene toxicity. *Int J Dermatol* 1977; 16:113–116.

63. Beaudouin E, Pupil P, Jacson F, et al. Allergie professionaelle au latex. *Rev Fr Allergol* 1990; 30:157–161.

64. Beck HI, Nissen BK. Type I and type IV allergy to specific chicken organs. *Contact Dermatitis* 1982; 8:217–218.

65. Beck MH, Hausen BM, Dave VK. Allergic contact dermatitis from *Macherium scleroxylum*, Tul (Pao ferro) in a joinery shop. *Clin Exp Dermatol* 1984; 9:159–166.

66. Beck MH, King CM. Allergic contact dermatitis to epichlorhydrin in a solvent cement. *Contact Dermatitis* 1983; 9:315.

67. Becker TM. Herpes gladiatorum: A growing problem in sports medicine. *Cutis* 1992; 50:150–152.

68. Bedello PG, Goitre M, Roncarolo G, et al. Contact dermatitis to rhodium. *Contact Dermatitis* 1987; 17:111–112.

69. Beezhold D, Beck WC. Surgical glove powders bind latex antigens. *Arch Surg* 1992; 127:1354–1357.

70. Beezhold DH, Kostyal DA, Wiseman J. The transfer of protein allergens from latex gloves: A study of influencing factors. *J Assoc Operating Room Nurses* 1994; 59:605–613.

71. Behrens RH, Dukes DCD. Fatal methyl bromide poisoning. *Br J Ind Med* 1986; 43:561–562.

72. Belsito DV. Contact dermatitis to ethyl-cyanoacrylate–containing glue. *Contact Dermatitis* 1987; 17:234–236.

73. Belsito DV. Textile dermatitis. *Am J Contact Dermatitis* 1993; 4:249–252.

74. Benezra C, Ducombs G, Sell Y, Foussereau J. *Alstroemeria*. In: Decker BC, ed. *Plant Contact Dermatitis*. Toronto: CV Mosby; 1985:236–237.

75. Bennett DE, Mathias CGY, Susten AS, et al. Dermatitis from plastic tote boxes impregnated with an antistatic agent. *J Occup Med* 1988; 30:252–255.

76. Berg M, Liden S, Axelson O. Facial skin complaints and work at visual display units. An epidemiologic study of office employees. *J Am Acad Dermatol* 1990; 22:621–625.

77. Bergfeld WF. Dermatologic problems in athletes. *Dermatol Clin* 1984; 2:653–660.

78. Bergqvist U, Wahlberg JE. Skin symptoms and disease during work with visual display terminals. *Contact Dermatitis* 1994; 30:197–204.

79. Berkley SF, Hightower MS, Beier RC, et al. Dermatitis in grocery workers associated with high natural concentrations of furanocoumarins in celery. *Ann Intern Med* 1986; 105:351–355.

80. Bingham E, Horton W, Tye R. The carcinogenic potency of certain oils. *Arch Environ Health* 1965; 10:449–451.

81. Bird H. Development of Garrod's pads in the fingers of a professional violinist. *Ann Rheum Dis* 1987; 46:169–170.

82. Birmingham DJ. Occupational dermatitis on the farm and in industry. *Arch Environ Health* 1961; 3:46–48.

83. Biro L, Fisher AA, Price E. Ethylene oxide burns, a hospital outbreak involving 19 women. *Arch Dermatol* 1974; 110:924–925.

84. Bjorkner B, Dahlquist I, Fregert S. Allergic contact dermatitis from acrylates in ultraviolet curing inks. *Contact Dermatitis* 1980; 6:405–409.

85. Björnberg A, Lowhagen GB. Patch test reactions to rockwool. *Contact Dermatitis* 1975; 1:242.

86. Blair A, Decoufle P, Grauman D. Causes of death among laundry and dry cleaning workers. *Am J Public Health* 1979; 69:508–511.

87. Blanc P, Boushey HA. The lung in metal fume fever. *Semin Respir Med* 1993; 14:212–225.

88. Blanco C, Carrillo T, Castillo R, et al. Latex allergy: Clinical features and cross-reactivity with fruits. *Ann Allergy* 1994; 73:309–314.

89. Bleicher JN, Blinn DL, Massop D. Hand infections in dental personnel. *Plast Reconstr Surg* 1987; 80:420–422.

90. Bleumink E, Doeglas HMG, Klokke AH, et al. Allergic contact dermatitis to garlic. *Br J Dermatol* 1972; 87:6–9.

91. Bleumink E, Mitchell JC, Nater JP. Allergic contact dermatitis from wood *(Thuja plicata)*. *Br J Dermatol* 1973; 88:499–504.

92. Blondeel A. Contact allergy to vitamin A. *Contact Dermatitis* 1984; 11:191–192.

93. Blumental G, Okun MR, Ponitch JA. Pseudolymphomatous reaction to tattoos. *J Am Acad Dermatol* 1982; 6:485–488.

94. Bojs G, Nicklasson B, Svensson A. Allergic contact dermatitis to propyl gallate. *Contact Dermatitis* 1987; 17:294–298.

95. Boonk WJ. Dermatologic hazards from hidden contacts with penicillin. *Dermatosen* 1981; 29:131–135.

96. Boose K, Christopher SE. Beitrage zur Epidermiologie der Wargen. *Hautarzt* 1964; 15:80–86.

97. Bork K. Allergic contact dermatitis on a violinist's neck from para-phenylenediamine in a chin rest stain. *Contact Dermatitis* 1993; 28:250–251.

98. Borrego L, Ortiz-Frutos J. Textile dye dermatitis: Spanish experience. (Letter to the editor.) *J Am Acad Dermatol* 1996; 34:715–716.

99. Botella-Estrada R, Mora E, de la Cuadra J. Hexanediol diacrylate sensitization after accidental occupational exposure. *Contact Dermatitis* 1992; 26:50–51.

100. Bowman KF, Barbery RT, Swango LJ, et al. Cutaneous form of bovine papular stomatitis in man. *JAMA* 1981; 246:2813–2818.

101. Boxer PA. Occupational mass psychogenic illness. *J Occup Med* 1985; 27:867–872.

102. Boyle J, Peachey RDG. Allergic contact dermatitis from diallyglycol carbonate monomer. *Contact Dermatitis* 1985; 13:186–203.

103. Brancaccio RR, Chamales MH. Contact dermatitis and depigmentation produced by the herbicide Carbyne. *Contact Dermatitis* 1977; 3:108–109.

104. Brancaccio RR, Cockerell CJ, Belsito D, et al. Allergic contact dermatitis from color film developers: Clinical and histologic features. *J Am Acad Dermatol* 1993; 28:827–830.

105. Brandao FM. Dermatite de contacto pelo alho. *Trab Soc Port Dermatol Venereol Ano* 1977; XXXV:27.

106. Brandao FM. Occupational contact dermatitis from rubber antioxidants. *Contact Dermatitis* 1978; 4:246.

107. Brandao FM. Release of nickel by permanent wave liquids, shown by the dimethylglyoxime test. *Contact Dermatitis* 1979; 5:406.

108. Brandao FM. Contact dermatitis to ethoxyquin. *Contact Dermatitis* 1983; 9:240.

109. Brandao FM. Occupational allergy to lavender oil. *Contact Dermatitis* 1986; 15:249–250.

110. Brandao FM. Colour developers and lichen planus. *Contact Dermatitis* 1986; 15:253.

111. Brandao FM, Altermatt C, Pecegueiro M, et al. Contact dermatitis to Disperse Blue 106. *Contact Dermatitis* 1985; 13:80–84.

112. Brandao FM, Cardoso JPM. Contact dermatitis to CD4. *Contact Dermatitis* 1985; 12:48–62.

113. Brandao FM, Hausen BM. Cross reaction between Disperse Blue dyes 106 and 124. *Contact Dermatitis* 1987; 16:289–290.

114. Brandao FM, Valente A. Photodermatitis from anthraquinone. *Contact Dermatitis* 1988; 18:171–172.

115. Brasch J. Allergic contact dermatitis from 4-chloro-7-nitrobenzofurazan. *Contact Dermatitis* 1991; 25:121–124.

116. Brown M, Hebert AA. Insect repellents: An overview. *J Am Acad Dermatol* 1997; 36:243–249.

117. Brown R. Simultaneous hypersensitivity to 3 topical corticosteroids. *Contact Dermatitis* 1982; 8:339–340.

118. Brown R. Contact sensitivity to difolatan (Captafol). *Contact Dermatitis* 1984; 10:181–182.

119. Brubaker MM. Urticarial reactions to ammonium persulfate. *Arch Dermatol* 1972; 106:413–414.

120. Bruins WW, Stalder K. Symptome beruflich bedingter Erkrankungen und berufsbedingter Stigmata der Mundhöle. *Dermatosen* 1996; 44:135–137.

121. Brun R. Kontaktekzema auf Laurylgallat und *p*-hydroxybenzoesaureester. *Berufsdermatosen* 1964; 12:281–284.

122. Brun R. Eczema de contact a un antioxidant de la margarine (gallate) et changement de metier. *Dermatologica* 1970; 140:390–394.

123. Brun R. Contact dermatitis to orangewood in a manicurist. *Contact Dermatitis* 1978; 4:315.

124. Brun P, Baran R. Geigerknoten. *Ann Derm Venereol* 1984; 111:241.

125. Brun R, Jadassohn W, Paillard R. Epicutaneous test with immediate type reactions to ammonium persulfate. *Dermatologia* 1960; 133:89–98.

126. Bruynzeel D. Allergic contact dermatitis to hydrangea. *Contact Dermatitis* 1986; 14:128.

127. Bruynzeel DP, de Boer EM, Brouwer EJ, et al. Dermatitis in bulb growers. *Contact Dermatitis* 1993; 29:11–15.

128. Bruynzeel DP, Hannipman G, van Ketel WG. Irritant contact dermatitis and chrome-passivated metal. *Contact Dermatitis* 1988; 19:175–179.

129. Bruynzeel DP, Prevoo RLMA. Patch tests with some spices. *Dermatol Clin* 1990; 8:85–87.

130. Bruynzeel DP, Tafelkruijer J, Wilks MF. Contact dermatitis due to a new fungicide used in the tulip bulb industry. *Contact Dermatitis* 1995; 33:8–11.

131. Bruynzeel DP, van Ketel WG. Contact dermatitis due to chlorthalonil in floriculture. *Contact Dermatitis* 1986; 14:67–68.

132. Bruynzeel DP, Verburgh CA. Occupational dermatitis from isothiazolinones in diesel oil. *Contact Dermatitis* 1996; 34:64–65.

133. Bruze M. Use of buffer solutions for patch testing. *Contact Dermatitis* 1984; 10:267–269.

134. Bruze M. A nonrelevant contact allergy to balsam of Peru as an indication of a relevant contact allergy to phenol-formaldehyde resin. *Am J Contact Dermatol* 1994; 5:162–164.

135. Bruze M, Almgren G. Occupational dermatoses in workers exposed to resins based on phenol and formaldehyde. *Contact Dermatitis* 1988; 19:272–277.

136. Bruze M, Bjorkner B, Hellstrom A-C. Occupational dermatoses in nursery workers. *Am J Contact Dermatitis* 1996; 7:100–103.

137. Bruze M, Bjorkner B, Lepoittevin J-P. Occupational allergic contact dermatitis from ethyl cyanoacrylate. *Contact Dermatitis* 1995; 32:156–159.

138. Bruze M, Boman A, Bergqvist-Karlsson A, et al. Contact allergy to a cyclohexanone resin in humans and guinea pigs. *Contact Dermatitis* 1988; 18:46–49.

139. Bruze M, Dahlquist I, Gruvberger B. Chemical burns and allergic contact dermatitis due to Kathon WT. *Am J Contact Dermatol* 1989; 1:91–93.

140. Bruze M, Edenholm M, Engstrom K, Svensson G. Occupational dermatoses in a Swedish aircraft plant. *Contact Dermatitis* 1996; 34:336–340.

141. Bruze M, Edman B, Bjorkner B, Moller H. Clinical relevance of contact allergy to gold sodium thiosulfate. *J Am Acad Dermatol* 1994; 31:579–583.

142. Bruze M, Fregert S, Zimerson E. Contact allergy to phenol-formaldehyde resins. *Contact Dermatitis* 1985; 12:81–86.

143. Bruze M, Gruvberger B. Contact allergy to Bioban CS 1246 in humans and guinea pigs. *Am J Contact Dermatol* 1994; 5:88–89.

144. Bruze M, Gruvberger B, Agrup G. Sensitization studies in the guinea pig with the active ingredients of Euxyl K 400. *Contact Dermatitis* 1988; 18:37–39.

145. Bruze M, Hedman H, Bjorkner B, Möller H. The development and course of test reactions to gold sodium thiosulfate. *Contact Dermatitis* 1995; 33:386–391.

146. Bruze M, Hindsen M, Trulsson L. Dermatitis with an unusual explanation in a welder. *Acta Derm Venereol (Stockh)* 1994; 74:380–382.

147. Bruze M, Hradil E, Eriksohn I-L, et al. Occupational allergic contact dermatitis from alkanolamineborates in metalworking fluids. *Contact Dermatitis* 1995; 32:24–27.

148. Buckley DB. Skin burns due to wet cement. *Contact Dermatitis* 1982; 8:407–409.

149. Buckley WR. Lichenoid eruptions following contact dermatitis. *Arch Dermatol* 1958; 78:454–457.

150. Buckley WR, Terhaar CJ. The skin as an excretory organ in argyria. *Trans St Johns Hosp Dermatol Soc* 1973; 59:39–44.

151. Budda U, Schwanitz HJ. Kontaktdermatiden bei Auszubildenden des Friseaurhandwerks in Niedersachsen. *Dermatosen* 1991; 39:41–48.

152. Bunney MH. Contact dermatitis in beekeepers due to propolis (bee glue). *Br J Dermatol* 1968; 80:17–23.

153. Burckhardt W, Kaufmann J, Brenn H. Ekzem durch Aethylendiamin in der Kunstfaserindustrie. *Dermatologica (Basel)* 1970; 141:154.

154. Burden A, Beck M. Contact hypersensitivity to azathioprine. *Contact Dermatitis* 1992; 27:329–330.

155. Burdick KH. Dermatitis involving the dentists' hands. *JAMA* 1961; 160:643.

156. Burge PS, Harries MG, O'Brien IM, et al. Evidence for specific hypersensitivity in occupational asthma due to small molecular weight chemicals and an organic (locust) allergen. In: *International Proceedings on the Mast Cell: Its Role in Health and Disease.* Tunbridge Wells, England: Pitman; 1979:301–308.

157. Burge PS, Harries MG, O'Brien I, et al. Bronchial provocation studies in workers exposed to the fumes of electronic soldering fluxes. *Clin Allergy* 1980; 10:137–149.

158. Buring JE, Hennekens CH. Carbonless copy paper: A review of published epidemiologic studies. *J Occup Med* 1991; 33:486–495.

159. Burrows D. Contact dermatitis in animal feed mill workers. *Br J Dermatol* 1975; 92:167–170.

160. Burrows D. Contact dermatitis in lens makers due to diallyglycol carbonate. *Contact Dermatitis* 1977; 3:342–343.

161. Burrows D. Contact dermatitis to machine oil in hosiery workers. *Contact Dermatitis* 1980; 6:10.

162. Burrows D. Chromium dermatitis in tyre fitter. *Contact Dermatitis* 1981; 7:55–56.

163. Burrows D. *Chromium: Metabolism and Toxicity.* Boca Raton, Fla: CRC Press, Inc.; 1983:154.

164. Burrows D, Calnan CD. Cement dermatitis II. Clinical aspects. *Trans St Johns Hosp Dermatol Soc* 1965; 51:27–39.

165. Burrows D, Cooke MA. Trivalent chromium plating. *Contact Dermatitis* 1980; 6:222.

166. Burrows D, Irvine J. Contact dermatitis to hexylresorcinol. *Contact Dermatitis* 1980; 6:222.

167. Burry JN. Contact dermatitis from agricultural fungicide in South Australia. *Contact Dermatitis* 1976; 2:289.

168. Calas E, Castelain PY, LaPointe HR, et al. Allergic contact dermatitis to a photopolymerizable resin used in printing. *Contact Dermatitis* 1977; 3:186–194.

169. Calnan CD. Cement dermatitis. *J Occup Med* 1960; 2:15–22.

170. Calnan CD. Allergy to dog saliva. *Contact Dermatitis Newslett* 1968; 3:41.

171. Calnan CD. Epoxy resin putty. *Contact Dermatitis Newslett* 1969; 5:89.

172. Calnan CD. Lichenoid dermatitis from isopropylaminodiphenylamine. *Contact Dermatitis Newslett* 1971; 10:237.

173. Calnan CD. Dermatitis from cedar wood pencils. *Trans St Johns Hosp Dermatol Soc* 1972; 58:43–47.

174. Calnan CD. Malt flour dermatitis. *Contact Dermatitis Newslett* 1973; 14:390.

175. Calnan CD. Methyl violet in carbon paper. *Contact Dermatitis Newslett* 1974; 15:426.

176. Calnan CD. Textile dye Disperse Yellow 64. *Contact Dermatitis* 1977; 3:209–210.

177. Calnan CD. Chromate dermatitis from soluble oil. *Contact Dermatitis* 1978; 4:378.

178. Calnan CD. Carbon and carbonless copy paper. *Acta Derm Venereol* 1979; 59(suppl 85):27–32.

179. Calnan CD. Allergy to dipentene in a paint thinner. *Contact Dermatitis* 1979; 5:123–124.

180. Calnan CD. Lanolin in protective metal coatings. *Contact Dermatitis* 1979; 5:267–268.

181. Calnan CD. Chloracetophenone (CS) dermatitis. *Contact Dermatitis* 1979; 5:195.

182. Calnan CD. Acrylates in industry. *Contact Dermatitis* 1980; 6:53–54.

183. Calnan CD. Unsolved problems in occupational dermatology. *Br J Dermatol* 1981; 105(suppl 21):3–6.

184. Calnan CD. Monotertiary butyl hydroquinone in lipstick. *Contact Dermatitis* 1981; 7:280–281.

185. Calnan CD, Bandmann HJ, Cronin E, et al. Hand dermatitis in housewives. *Br J Dermatol* 1970; 82:543–548.

186. Calnan CD, Connor BL. Carbon paper dermatitis due to nigrosine. *Berufsdermatosen* 1972; 20:248–254.

187. Calnan CD, Cronin E. Vegetable tans in leather. *Contact Dermatitis* 1978; 4:295–296.

188. Calnan CD, Harman RRM. Sensitivity to para-tertiary-butylphenol. *Trans St Johns Hosp Dermatol Soc* 1959; 43:27–32.

189. Calnan CD, Hill RN. Allergy to diphenyloxazole. *Contact Dermatitis* 1979; 5:269–270.

190. Calnan CD, Schuster S. Reactions to ammonium persulfate. *Arch Dermatol* 1963; 88:812–815.

191. Calnan CD, Stevenson CJ. Studies in contact dermatitis XV: Dental materials. *Trans St Johns Hosp Dermatol Soc* 1963; 49:9–26.

192. Camarasa JG. Contact eczema from cow saliva. *Contact Dermatitis* 1986; 15:117.

193. Camarasa JMG, Alomar A. Ethylenediamine sensitivity in metallurgic industries. *Contact Dermatitis* 1978; 4:178.

194. Camarasa JG, Barnadas M. Occupational dermatosis by vitamin K_3 sodium bisulphite. *Contact Dermatitis* 1982; 8:268.

195. Camarasa JMG, Moreno A. Fiberglass dermatitis. *Contact Dermatitis* 1984; 10:43.

196. Campolmi P, Lombardi P, Lotti T, Sertoli A. Immediate and delayed sensitization to garlic. *Contact Dermatitis* 1982; 8:352–353.

197. Canizares O. Lichen planus-like eruption caused by color developer. *Arch Dermatol* 1959; 80:81–86.

198. Caplan RM. Cutaneous hazards posed by agricultural chemicals. *J Iowa Med Soc* 1969; 59:295–299.

199. Capon F, Cambie MP, Clinard F, et al. Occupational contact dermatitis caused by computer mice. *Contact Dermatitis* 1996; 35:57–58.

200. Carmichael AJ, Roberts DL. Visual display units and facial rashes. *Contact Dermatitis* 1992; 26:63–64.

201. Castelain P-Y. Eczema des mains a episodes multiples par sensibilisation a l'aminoazotoluene. *Bull Soc Fr Dermatol* 1967; 74:561.

202. Castelain P-Y, Com J, Castelain M. Occupational dermatitis in the aircraft industry: 35 years of progress. *Contact Dermatitis* 1992; 27:311–316.

203. Castiglione RM Jr, Selikowitz SM, Dimond RL. Mule spinner's disease. *Arch Dermatol* 1985; 121:370–372.

204. Catalano PM. Substances in coins and paper money of the United States. *Contact Dermatitis Newslett* 1972; 12:307.

205. Cavelier C, Foussereau J, Massin M. Nickel allergy: Analysis of metal clothing objects and patch testing to metal samples. *Contact Dermatitis* 1985; 12:65–75.

206. Chan-Yeung M, McMurren T, Cantonio-Begley F, et al. Occupational asthma in a technologist exposed to glutaraldehyde. *J Allergy Clin Immunol* 1993; 91:974–978.

207. Chatterjee AK. Pneumoconiosis in pottery workers and its trends in North Staffordshire from the point of view of the medical boarding centre (respiratory diseases). Stoke-on-Trent. *Ann Occup Hyg* 1989; 33:369–374.

208. *Chemical and Engineering News* October 14, 1996:66.

209. *Chemical and Engineering News* December 16, 1996:28.

210. Chernosky ME. Pruritic skin disease and summer air conditioning. *JAMA* 1962; 179:1005–1010.

211. Chew A-L, Maibach HI. 1,2-Benzisothiazolin-3-one (Proxel-R): Irritant or allergen? *Contact Dermatitis* 1997; 36:131–136.

212. Chieregato C, Vincenzi C, Guerra L, et al. Occupational airborne contact dermatitis from *Machaerium scleroxylon* (Santos rosewood). *Contact Dermatitis* 1993; 29:164–165.

213. Clarys P, Manou I, Barel AO. Influence of temperature on irritation in the hand/forearm immersion test. *Contact Dermatitis* 1997; 36:240–243.

214. Cofield BG, Storrs FJ, Strawn CB. Contact allergy to aziridine paint hardener. *Arch Dermatol* 1985; 121:373–376.

215. Coggon D, Acheson ED. Do phenoxy herbicides cause cancer in man? *Lancet* May 8, 1982:1057–1059.

216. Cohen SR. Dermatologic hazards in the poultry industry. *J Occup Med* 1987; 16:94–97.

217. Cohen SR. Skin diseases in health care workers. *Occup Med State Art Rev* 1987; 2:565–580.

218. Cohen SR, Davis DM, Kramkowski RS. Nasal lesions in electroplate workers. *Cutis* 1974; 13:558–568.

219. Cole GW, Stone O, Gates D, Culver D. Chloracne from pentachlorophenol-preserved wood. *Contact Dermatitis* 1986; 15:164–168.

220. Conde-Salazar L, Baz M, Guimaraens D, et al. Contact dermatitis in hairdressers: Patch test results in 379 hairdressers (1980–1993). *Am J Contact Dermatitis* 1995; 6:19–23.

221. Conde-Salazar L, Garcia DA, Rafensperger F, Hausen BM. Contact allergy to the Brazilian rosewood substitute *Macherium scleroxylum* Tul (Pao ferro). *Contact Dermatitis* 1980; 6:246–250.

222. Conde-Salazar L, Gonzalez M, Guimaraens D, Meza B. Allergy contact dermatitis from newpaper ink. *Am J Contact Dermatitis* 1991; 2:245–246.

223. Conde-Salazar L, Guimaraens D, Romero L. Occupational contact dermatitis from cytosine arabinoside synthesis. *Contact Dermatitis* 1984; 10:44–45.

224. Conde-Salazar L, Guimaraens D, Romero LV. Occupational allergic contact dermatitis from anaerobic acrylic sealants. *Contact Dermatitis* 1988; 18:129–132.

225. Conde-Salazar L, Guimaraens D, Romero LV, et al. Occupational dermatitis from glass fiber. *Contact Dermatitis* 1985; 13:195–196.

226. Conde-Salazar L, Romero L, Guimaraens D. Allergic contact dermatitis from diazo paper. *Contact Dermatitis* 1982; 8:210–211.

227. Conde-Salazar L, Romero LV, Guimaraens D, et al. Fistula y tricogranuloma interdigital de los peluqueros. *Gaceta Dermatol* 1982; 3:205–209.

228. Corazza M, Virgili A. Airborne allergic contact dermatitis from benzalkonium chloride. *Contact Dermatitis* 1993; 28:195–196.

229. Corbett JF, Menkart J. Hair coloring. *Cutis* 1973; 12:190–197.

230. Couperus M. Discussion. *Arch Dermatol* 1973; 107:768.

231. Cox NH, Mustchin CP. Prolonged spontaneous and alcohol-induced flushing due to the solvent dimethylformamide. *Contact Dermatitis* 1991; 24:69–70.

232. Crijns MB, Boom BW, van der Schroeff JG. Allergic contact dermatitis to a diazonium compound in copy paper. *Contact Dermatitis* 1987; 16:112–113.

233. Crisi G, Belsito DV. Contact urticaria from latex in a patient with immediate hypersensitivity to banana, avocado and peach. *Contact Dermatitis* 1993; 28:247–248.

234. Cronin E. Lanolin dermatitis. *Br J Dermatol* 1966; 78:167.

235. Cronin E. Studies in contact dermatitis, XIX: Nylon stocking dyes. *Trans St Johns Hosp Dermatol Soc* 1968; 54:165.

236. Cronin E. Studies in contact dermatitis XVIII. Dyes in

clothing. *Trans St Johns Hosp Dermatol Soc* 1968; 54:156–164.

237. Cronin E. Sensitivity to glutaraldehyde. *Contact Dermatitis Newslett* 1968; 3:3.

238. Cronin E. Sensitivity to tulip and *Alstroemeria*. *Contact Dermatitis Newslett* 1972; 11:286.

239. Cronin E. Impregum (dental impression material). *Contact Dermatitis Newslett* 1973; 13:362.

240. Cronin E. Immediate-type hypersensitivity to henna. *Contact Dermatitis* 1979; 5:198–199.

241. Cronin E. Contact dermatitis from barley dust. *Contact Dermatitis* 1979; 5:196.

242. Cronin E. *Contact Dermatitis*. Edinburgh: Churchill-Livingston; 1980.

243. Cronin E. Dermatitis of the hands in caterers. *Contact Dermatitis* 1987; 17:265–269.

244. Cronin E. Formaldehyde is a significant allergen in women with hand eczema. *Contact Dermatitis* 1991; 25:276–282.

245. Cronin E, Calnan CD. Rosewood knife handle. *Contact Dermatitis* 1975; 1:121.

246. Crow KD. Dermatitis in cable joiners. *Contact Dermatitis Newslett* 1968; 2:10.

247. Crow KD, Alexander E, Buck WHL, et al. Photosensitivity due to pitch. *Br J Dermatol* 1961; 73:220–232.

248. Crow KD, Harman RRM, Holden H. Amine flux sensitization on dermatitis in electricity cable joiners. *Br J Dermatol* 1968; 80:701–710.

249. Crow KD, Peachey RDG, Adams JE. Coolant oil dermatitis due to ethylenediamine. *Contact Dermatitis* 1978; 4:359–361.

250. Curley RK, Macfarlane AW, King CM. Contact dermatitis to 2-phenyl tetralone tosylhydrazone. *Contact Dermatitis* 1986; 14:257–258.

251. Cuypers JMC, Bleumick E, Nater JP. Dermatologische Aspekte der Glasfaserfabrikation. *Dermatosen* 1975; 23:143–154.

252. Czuppon AB, Chen Z, Rennert S, et al. The rubber elongation factor of rubber trees *(Hevea brasiliensis)* is the major allergen in latex. *J Allergy Clin Immunol* 1993; 92:633–635.

253. Dahl MGC. Patch test concentrations of Grotan BK. *Br J Dermatol* 1981; 104:607.

254. Dahlquist I. Contact allergy to the cutting oil preservatives Bioban CS-1246 and P-1487. *Contact Dermatitis* 1984; 10:46–47.

255. Dahlquist I, Fregert S. Contact allergy to the epoxy hardener isophoronediamine (IPD). *Contact Dermatitis* 1979; 5:120–121.

256. Dahlquist I, Fregert S, Gruvberger B. Release of nickel from plated utensils in permanent wave liquids. *Contact Dermatitis* 1979; 5:52–53.

257. Dahlquist I, Fregert S, Trulson L. Contact allergy to trimethylolpropane triacrylate (TMPTA) in an aziridine plastic hardener. *Contact Dermatitis* 1983; 9:122–124.

258. Dal Monte A, de Benedictis E, Laffi G. Occupational dermatitis from ethylenediamine hydrochloride. *Contact Dermatitis* 1987; 17:254.

259. Dannaker CJ. Allergic sensitization to a non-Bisphenol A epoxy of the cycloaliphatic class. *J Occup Med* 1988; 30:641–643.

260. Dannaker CJ. Long-term prognosis in occupational chromate allergy: An attempted 18-year follow-up study. *Contact Dermatitis* 1989; 21:59.

261. Dannaker CJ, Maibach HI, O'Malley M. Contact urticaria and anaphylaxis to the fungicide chlorothalonil. *Cutis* 1993; 52:312–315.

262. Dannaker CJ, White IR. Cutaneous allergy to mustard in a salad maker. *Contact Dermatitis* 1987; 16:212–214.

263. Das M, Misra MP. Acne and folliculitis due to diesel oil. *Contact Dermatitis* 1988; 18:120–121.

264. Das M, Tandon A. Occupational vitiligo. *Contact Dermatitis* 1988; 18:184–185.

265. Davies MG. Contact allergy to dicyclohexyl-carbodiimide. *Contact Dermatitis* 1983; 9:318.

266. Dawber R. Occupational koilonychia. *Br J Dermatol* 1974; 91(suppl 10):11.

267. Dawe RS, Green CM, MacLeod TM, Ferguson J. Daisy, dandelion and thistle contact allergy in the photosensitivity dermatitis and actinic reticuloid syndrome. *Contact Dermatitis* 1996; 35:109–110.

268. de Boer EM. *Occupational Dermatitis by Metalworking Fluids*. Thesis. Amsterdam: Vrije Universiteit; 1989.

269. de Boer EM, van Ketel WG. Occupational dermatitis caused by snackbar meat products. *Contact Dermatitis* 1984; 11:322.

270. de Boer EM, Van Ketel WG, Bruynzeel DP. Dermatoses in metal workers II. Allergic contact dermatitis. *Contact Dermatitis* 1989; 20:280–286.

271. Degreef H, Bourgeois M, Naert C, et al. Protein contact dermatitis with positive RAST caused by bovine blood and amniotic fluid. *Contact Dermatitis* 1984; 11:129–130.

272. Degreef H, Dooms-Goossens A. Patch testing with silver sulfadiazine cream. *Contact Dermatitis* 1985; 12:33–37.

273. Degreef H, Hendrickx I, Dooms-Goossens A. Allergic contact dermatitis to Minoxidil. *Contact Dermatitis* 1985; 13:194–195.

274. DeGroot AC. Patch testing: Test Concentrations and Vehicles for 2800 Allergens. Amsterdam: Elsevier; 1986:23.

275. DeGroot AC, Bos JD, Jagtman BA, et al. Contact allergy to preservatives (II). *Contact Dermatitis* 1986; 15:218–222.

276. DeGroot AC, Bruynzeel DP, Jagtman BA, et al. Contact allergy to diazolidinyl urea (Germall II). *Contact Dermatitis* 1988; 18:202–205.

277. DeGroot AC, Frosch PJ. Adverse reactions to fragrances. A clinical review. *Contact Dermatitis* 1997; 36:57–86.

278. DeGroot AC, Paul AJ, de Cock JM, et al. Methyldibromoglutaronitrile is an important contact allergen in the Netherlands. *Contact Dermatitis* 1996; 34:118–120.

279. DeGroot AC, van der Walle HB, Weyland JW. Contact allergy to cocamidopropyl betaine. *Contact Dermatitis* 1995; 33:419–422.

280. DeGroot AC, van Joost T, Bols JD. Patch test reactivity to DMDM hydantoin. Relationship to formaldehyde allergy. *Contact Dermatitis* 1988; 18:197–210.

281. DeGroot AC, Weyland JW. Kathon CG: A review. *J Am Acad Dermatol* 1988; 18:350–358.

282. DeGroot AC, White IR: Cosmetics and skin care products. In: Rycroft RJ, Menne T, Frosch PG, eds: *Textbook of Contact Dermatitis,* 2nd ed. Berlin: Springer-Verlag; 1995:461–476.

283. Dejobert Y, Parmin P, Thomas P, et al. Multiple azo dye sensitization revealed by the wearing of a black "velvet" body. *Contact Dermatitis* 1995; 33:276–277.

284. De La Cuadra J, Grau-Massanes M. Occupational contact dermatitis from rhodium and cobalt. *Contact Dermatitis* 1991; 25:182–184.

285. DeLeo VA, Suarez SM, Maso MJ. Photoallergic contact dermatitis. *Arch Dermatol* 1992; 128:1513–1518.

286. Delgado J, Castillo R, Quiralte J, et al. Contact urticaria in a child from raw potato. *Contact Dermatitis* 1996; 35:179–180.

287. Dell L, Teta MJ. Mortality among workers at a plastics

manufacturing and research and development facility: 1948–1988. *Am J Ind Med* 1995; 28:373–384.

288. Dement JM, Brown DP. Cohort mortality and case-control studies of white male chrysotile asbestos textile workers. *J Occup Med Toxicol* 1993; 2:355–363.

289. Dement JM, Harris RL, Symons MJ, Shy CM. Exposures and mortality among chrysotile asbestos workers. Part I: Exposure estimates. *Am J Ind Med* 1983; 4:399–419.

290. Dement JM, Harris RL, Symons MJ, Shy CM. Exposures and mortality among chrysotile asbestos workers. Part II: Mortality. *Am J Ind Med* 1983; 4:421–433.

291. Demers PA, Boffetta P, Kogevinas M, et al. Pooled reanalysis of cancer mortality among five cohorts of workers in wood-related industries. *Scand J Work Environ Health* 1995; 21:179–190.

292. Dempsey KJ. Hypersensitivity to Sta-Lok and Loctite anaerobic sealants. *J Am Acad Dermatol* 1982; 7:779–784.

293. de Peauter M, de Lerq M, et al. An epidemiological survey of virus warts of the hands among butchers. *Br J Dermatol* 1977; 96:427–431.

294. Derrick E, Darley C. Contact dermatitis to nasturtium. *Br J Dermatol* 1997; 136:290–291.

295. Deschamps D, Garnier R, Savoye J, et al. Allergic and irritant contact dermatitis from diethyl-B-choroethylamine. *Contact Dermatitis* 1988; 18:103–104.

296. Diamond SP, Wiener SG, Marks JG Jr. Allergic contact dermatitis to nasturtium. *Dermatol Clin* 1990; 8:77–80.

297. Dinis A, Brandao M, Faria A. Occupational contact dermatitis from vitamin K3 sodium bisulphite. *Contact Dermatitis* 1988; 18:170–171.

298. Diogenes MJN, Morais SM, Carvalho FF. Contact dermatitis among cashew nut workers. *Contact Dermatitis* 1996; 35:114–115.

299. Dooms-Goossens A. Identification of undetected corticosteroid allergy. *Contact Dermatitis* 1988; 18:124–125.

300. Dooms-Goossens A, Bedert R, Vandaele M, Degreef H. Airborne contact dermatitis due to triglycidylisocyanurate. *Contact Dermatitis* 1989; 21:202–203.

301. Dooms-Goossens A, Bruze M, Buysse L, et al. Contact allergy to allyl glycidyl ether present as an impurity in 3-glycidyloxypropyltrimethoxysilane, a fixing additive in silicone and polyurethane resins. *Contact Dermatitis* 1995; 33:17–19.

302. Dooms-Goossens A, de Alam AG, Degreef H, Kochuyt A. Local anesthetic intolerance due to metabisulfite. *Contact Dermatitis* 1989; 20:124–126.

303. Dooms-Goossens A, de Boulle K, Snauwaert J. Sensitization to 3,4,6-trichloropyridazine. *Contact Dermatitis* 1986; 14:64–65.

304. Dooms-Goossens A, Debusschere K, Morren M, et al. Silver polish: Another source of contact dermatitis reactions to thiourea. *Contact Dermatitis* 1988; 19:133–135.

305. Dooms-Goossens A, De Jonge G. Letter to the editor. *Contact Dermatitis* 1985; 12:238.

306. Dooms-Goossens A, Deveylder H, de Alam AG, et al. Contact sensitivity to nonoxynols as a cause of intolerance to antiseptic preparations. *J Am Acad Dermatol* 1989; 21:723–727.

307. Dooms-Goossens A, Dubelloy R, Degreef H. Contact and systemic contact-type dermatitis to spices. *Dermatol Clin* 1990; 8:89–93.

308. Dooms-Goossens A, Dupre K, Borghijs A, et al. Zinc rincinoleate: Sensitizer in deodorants. *Contact Dermatitis* 1987; 16:292–294.

309. Dooms-Goossens A, Garmyn M, Degreef H. Contact allergy to acrylamide. *Contact Dermatitis* 1991; 24:71–72.

310. Dooms-Goossens A, Gevers D, Mertens A, et al. Allergic contact urticaria due to chloramine. *Contact Dermatitis* 1983; 9:319–320.

311. Dooms-Goossens A, Holvoet C, Degreef H. 2(*p*-Carboxyphenol)-4,5-diphenylimidazole: A new sensitizing agent in photo-processing. *Contact Dermatitis* 1978; 4:373.

312. Dooms-Goossens A, Matura M, Drieghe J, Degreef H. Contact allergy to imidazoles used as antimycotic agents. *Contact Dermatitis* 1995; 33:73–77.

313. Dooms-Goossens A, Morren M. Results of routine patch testing with corticosteroid series in 2073 patients. *Contact Dermatitis* 1992; 26:182–191.

314. Dooms-Goossens A, Vanhee J, Vanderheyden D, et al. Allergic contact dermatitis to topical corticosteroids: Clobetasol propionate and clobetasol buyrate. *Contact Dermatitis* 1983; 9:470–478.

315. Downham TF, Birmingham DJ. Contact dermatitis to photographic print coating liquid. *Cutis* 1980; 25:421–423.

316. Drake TE, Maibach HI. Allergic contact dermatitis and stomatitis caused by a cinnamic aldehyde-flavored toothpaste. *Arch Dermatol* 1976; 112:202–203.

317. Duncalf B, Dunn AS: Light sensitized cross linking of polyvinyl alcohol by chromium compounds. *J Appl Polymer Sci* 1964; 8:1763.

318. Dunkel FG, Elsner P, Pevny I, Burg G. Olaquindox-induced photoallergic contact dermatitis and persistent light reaction. *Am J Contact Dermatitis* 1990; 1:235–239.

319. Dziuk M, Gall H, Sterry W. Kontaktdermatitis auf den ACE-Hemmer Captopril. *Dermatosen* 1994; 42:159–161.

320. Eby CS, Jetton RL. School desk dermatitis. *Arch Dermatol* 1972; 105:890.

321. Edelstein AJ. Dermatitis caused by garlic. *Arch Dermatol* 1950; 61:111.

322. Efskind J. Prevalence of occupational eczema in a woodpulp factory. *Contact Dermatitis* 1980; 6:77–78.

323. Einarsson O, Kylin B, Lindstedt G, Wahlberg JE. Chromium, cobalt and nickel in used cutting fluids. *Contact Dermatitis* 1975; 1:182–183.

324. Elliott LJ, Ringenburg VL, Morelli-Schroth P, et al. Ethylene oxide exposures in hospitals. *Appl Ind Hyg* 1988; 3:141–145.

325. Elsner P, Pevny I, Burg G. Occupational contact dermatitis due to glyoxal in health care workers. *Am J Contact Dermatitis* 1990; 1:250–253.

326. Emmett EA. Contact dermatitis from poly-functional acrylic monomers. *Contact Dermatitis* 1977; 3:245–248.

327. Emmett EA, Bingham EM, Barkley W. A carcinogenic bioassay of certain roofing materials. *Am J Ind Med* 1981; 2:59–64.

328. Emmett EA, Buncher RC, Suskind RB, et al. Skin and eye disease among arc welder and those exposed to welding operations. *J Occup Med* 1981; 23:85–90.

329. Emmett EA, Horstman SW. Factors influencing the output of ultraviolet radiation during welding. *J Occup Med* 1976; 18:41–44.

330. Emmett EA, Kominsky JR. Allergic contact dermatitis from ultraviolet cured inks. *J Occup Med* 1977; 19:113–115.

331. Emmett EA, Maroni M, Schmith JM, et al. Studies of transformer repair workers exposed to PCBs: I. Study design, PCB concentrations, questionaire and clinical examination results. *Am J Ind Med* 1988; 13:415–427.

332. Emmett EA, Maroni M, Schmith JM, et al. Skin and eye disease among arc welders and those exposed to welding operations. *J Occup Med* 1981; 23:85–90.

333. Emmett EA, Risby TH, Jiang L, et al. Allergic contact dermatitis to nickel: Bioavailability from consumer products and provocation threshold. *J Am Acad Dermatol* 1988; 19:314–322.

334. Emmett EA, Stetzer L, Taphorn B. Phototoxic keratoconjunctivitis from coaltar pitch volatiles. *Science* 1977; 198:841–842.

335. Emmett EA, Taphorn BR, Kominsky JR. Phototoxicity occurring during the manufacture of ultraviolet-cured ink. *Arch Dermatol* 1977; 113:770–775.

336. Ena P, Cerri R, Dessi G, et al. Phototoxicity due to *Cachrys libanotis. Contact Dermatitis* 1991; 24:1–5.

337. Engel HO, Calnan CD. Chromate dermatitis from paint. *Br J Ind Med* 1963; 20:192–198.

338. English JSC, Lovell CR, Rycroft RJG. Contact dermatitis from dibutyl maleate. *Contact Dermatitis* 1985; 13:337–338.

339. English JSC, Rycroft RJG, Calnan CD. Allergic contact dermatitis from aminotriazole. *Contact Dermatitis* 1986; 14:255–256.

340. English JSC, White IR, Rycroft RJG. Sensitization by 1-methylquinoxalinium-*p*-toluene sulfonate. *Contact Dermatitis* 1986; 14:261–262.

341. Epstein E. Sodium bisulfite. *Contact Dermatol Newslett* 1970; 7:155.

342. Epstein JB, et al. Infectious diseases in outpatient practice. *J Can Dent Assoc* 1987; 53:767–772.

343. Epstein S. Occupational dermatoses among farmers. *Postgrad Med* 1961; 30:1–10.

344. Eriksson G, Ostlund E. Rubber band note counters as the cause of eczema among employees at the Swedish post office. *Acta Derm Venereol (Stockh)* 1968; 48:212–214.

345. Eskelson YD, Goodman LS. Contact dermatitis from "Scotchgard," a stain repellant for fabrics *JAMA* 1963; 183:136.

346. Estlander T. Allergic dermatoses and respiratory diseases from reactive dyes. *Contact Dermatitis* 1988; 18:290–297.

347. Estlander T, Jolanki R, Kanerva L. Dermatitis and urticaria from rubber and plastic gloves. *Contact Dermatitis* 1986; 14:20–25.

348. Estlander T, Jolanki R, Kanerva L. Occupational dermatitis to 2,3-epoxypropyl trimethyl ammonium chloride. *Contact Dermatitis* 1986; 14:49–52.

349. Estlander T, Jolanki R, Kanerva L. Occupational allergic contact dermatitis from 2,3-epoxypropyl trimethyl ammonium chloride (EPTMAC) and Kathon LX in a starch modification factory. *Contact Dermatitis* 1997; 36:191–194.

350. Estlander T, Kanerva L, Jolanki R. Occupational allergic dermatoses from textile, leather, and fur dyes. *Am J Contact Dermatitis* 1990; 1:13–20.

351. Estlander T, Keskinene H, Jolanki R, Kanerva L. Occupational dermatitis from exposure to polyurethane chemicals. *Contact Dermatitis* 1992; 27:161–165.

352. Eun HC, Kim KC, Cha CW. Occupational burns. *Contact Dermatitis* 1984; 10:20–22.

353. Eun HC, Lee AY, Lee YS. Sodium hypochlorite dermatitis. *Contact Dermatitis* 1984; 11:45.

354. Eyton WB, Ollis WD, Sutherland IO, et al. Dalbergiones: A new group of natural products. *Proc Chem Soc* 1962; 6:301–302.

355. Ezzelarab M, Hansson C, Wallengren J. Occupational allergy caused by 1,2-benzisothiazolin-3-one in water-based paints and glues. *Am J Contact Dermatitis* 1994; 5:165–167.

356. Falk ES, Hektoen H, Thune PO. Skin and respiratory tract symptoms in veterinary surgeons. *Contact Dermatitis* 1985; 12:274–278.

357. Fancalanci S, Giorgini S, Gola M, Sertoi A. Occupational dermatitis in a butcher. *Contact Dermatitis* 1984; 11:320–321.

358. Faria A, de Freitas C. Systemic contact dermatitis due to mercury. *Contact Dermatitis* 1992; 27:110–111.

359. Farkas J. Fiberglass dermatitis in employees of a project-office in a new building. *Contact Dermatitis* 1983; 9:79.

360. Farli M, Gasperini M, Giorgini S, Sertoli A. Clothing dermatitis. *Contact Dermatitis* 1986; 14:316.

361. Fast film, powerful battery improve Polaroid. *Chem Eng News*, June 22, 1981, pp 52–54.

362. Fawcett IW, Newman TAJ, Pepys J. Asthma due to inhaled chemical agents—Fumes from "Multicore" soldering flux and colophony rosin. *Clin Allergy* 1976; 6:577–585.

363. Feder HM Jr, Witaker DL, Hoss DM. The truth about erythema migrans. [Editorial.] *Arch Dermatol* 1997; 133:93–94.

364. Felipe P, Silva RL, Soares A, et al. Occupational allergic contact dermatitis from cephalosporins. *Contact Dermatitis* 1996; 34:226.

365. Fenichell S. *Plastic: The Making of a Synthetic Century.* New York: Harper-Business; 1996.

366. Fernandez L, Maquiera E, Garcia-Abujeta JL, et al. Baboon syndrome due to mercury sensitivity. *Contact Dermatitis* 1995; 33:56–57.

367. Fernandez de Corres L, Leansizbarrutia I, Munoz D. Contact sensitivity to *Anthemis* plants. In: Frosch PJ, Dooms-Goossens A, Lachapelle JM, et al., eds. *Current Topics in Contact Dermatitis.* Berlin: Springer-Verlag; 1989:141–145.

368. Feuerman EJ. Chromates as the cause of contact dermatitis in housewives. *Dermatologica* 1971; 143:292.

369. Finkbeiner H, Kleinhans D. Airborne allergic contact dermatitis caused by preservatives in home-decorating paints. *Contact Dermatitis* 1994; 31:275–276.

370. Finkel ML, Finkel DJ. Warts among meat handlers. *Arch Dermatol* 1984; 120:1314–1315.

371. Finkelstein E, Afek U, Gross E, et al: An outbreak of phytophotodermatitis caused by celery. *Int J Dermatol* 1994; 33:116–118.

372. Finnegan MJ. Air-conditioning and disease. *Practitioner* 1987; 231:482–485.

373. Fischer T. Contact allergy to choline choride. *Contact Dermatitis* 1984; 10:316–317.

374. Fischer T, Fregert S, Gruvberger B, et al. Nickel release from ear-piercing bits and earrings. *Contact Dermatitis* 1984; 10:39–41.

375. Fischer T, Rystedt I. Cobalt allergy in hard metal workers. *Contact Dermatitis* 1983; 9:115–121.

376. Fischer T, Nylander L, Rosen G. Dermatologic risk to workers in the UV-radiation wood surface-coating industry. *Am J Contact Dermatitis* 1994; 5:201–206.

377. Fisher AA. Allergic sensitization of the skin and oral mucosa to acrylic denture materials. *JAMA* 1954; 156:238.

378. Fisher AA. *Contact Dermatitis,* 2nd ed. Philadelphia: Lea & Febiger; 1973.

379. Fisher AA. Metallic gold: The cause of a persistent allergic "dermal" contact dermatitis. *Cutis* 1974; 14:177–180.

380. Fisher AA. Patch tests with perfume ingredients. *Contact Dermatitis* 1975; 1:166–168.

381. Fisher AA. Allergic occupational hand dermatitis due to calf's liver: An urticarial "immediate" type hypersensitivity. *Cutis* 1977; 19:561–565.

382. Fisher AA. Propylene glycol dermatitis. *Cutis* 1978; 21:166–178.

383. Fisher AA. *Atlas of Aquatic Dermatology.* New York: Grune & Stratton, 1978.

384. Fisher AA. Allergic contact dermatitis of the hands due to industrial oils and fluids. *Cutis* 1979; 23:131–242.

385. Fisher AA. Occupational palmar psoriasis due to safety prescription container caps. *Contact Dermatitis* 1979; 5:56.

386. Fisher AA. Cement burns resulting in necrotic ulcers due to kneeling. *Cutis* 1979; 23:272.

387. Fisher AA. Glutaraldehyde reactions among radiologists. *Cutis* 1981; 28:113.

388. Fisher AA. Hand dermatitis—A "baker's dozen." Current contact news. *Cutis* 1982; 29:214–221.

389. Fisher AA. Contact dermatitis in medical and surgical personnel. In: Maibach HI, Gellin GA, eds. *Occupational and Industrial Dermatology.* Chicago: Yearbook Medical Publishers; 1982:224.

390. Fisher AA. Allergic contact urticaria to raw beef: Histopatholgoy of the specific wheal reaction at the scratch test site. *Contact Dermatitis* 1982; 8:425–426.

391. Fisher AA. Fiberglass vs mineral wool (Rockwool) dermatitis. *Cutis* 1982; 29:412–513.

392. Fisher AA. *Contact Dermatitis,* 3rd ed. Philadelphia: Lea & Febiger; 1986:248.

393. Fisher AA. Reactions to sulfites in foods: Delayed eczematous and immediate urticarial, anaphylactoid, and asthmatic reactions. Part III. *Cutis* 1989; 44:187–190.

394. Fisher AA. Contact dermatitis from brominated water, Query in Ask Alex. *Am J Contact Dermatitis* 1992; 3:110.

395. Fisher AA, Dooms-Goossens A. Persulfate hair bleach reactions. *Arch Dermatol* 1976; 112:1407–1409.

396. Fitzgerald DA, Wilkinson SM, Bhaggoe R, et al. Spa pool dermatitis. *Contact Dermatitis* 1995; 33:53.

397. Flannigan SA, Tucker SB. Variation in cutaneous sensation between synthetic pyrethroid insecticides. *Contact Dermatitis* 1985; 13:140–147.

398. Flannigan SA, Tucker SB, Calderon V. Irritant dermatitis from tetrachloroisophthalonitrile. *Contact Dermatitis* 1986; 14:258–259.

399. Food and Drug Administration. Sulfiting agents on potatoes. *JAMA* 1988; 259:794.

400. Förg T, Burg G, Zirbs S. Häufigheitsanalytische Untersuchungen allergischer Kontaktekzeme bei Hausfrauen. *Dermatosen* 1982; 30:48–51.

401. Forstrom L, Hannuksela M, Kiistala R. Allergic contact dermatitis from tear gas (CN). In: *Proceedings of the International Congress of Dermatology.* Mexico City: Excerpta Medica, 1976:357–358.

402. Foti C, Bonamonte D, Trenti R, et al. Occupational contact allergy to cephalosporins. *Contact Dermatitis* 1997; 36:104–105.

403. Foulds IS, Koh D. Dermatitis from metalworking fluids. *Clin Exp Dermatol* 1990; 15:157–162.

404. Foulds IS, Koh D: Allergic contact dermatitis from resin hardeners during the manufacture of thermosetting coating paints. *Contact Dermatitis* 1992; 26:87–90.

405. Foussereau J. Contact dermatitis to Basic Red 46. *Contact Dermatitis* 1986; 15:106.

406. Foussereau J. An epidemiological study of contact allergy to 5-chloro-3-methyl isothiazolone/3-methyl isothiazolone in Strasbourg. *Contact Dermatitis* 1990; 22:68–70.

407. Foussereau J, Benezra C. *Les Eczemas Allergiques Professionals.* Paris: Masson et Cie, 1970.

408. Foussereau J, Benezra C, Maibach HI. *Occupational Contact Dermatitis: Clinical and Chemical Aspects.* Philadelphia: W.B. Saunders Co., 1982.

409. Foussereau J, Cavelier C, Selig D. Occupational eczema from para-tertiary butylphenol formaldehyde resins: A review of the sensitizing resins. *Contact Dermatitis* 1976; 2:254–258.

410. Foussereau J, Muslmani M, Cavelier C, et al. Contact allergy to safety shoes. *Contact Dermatitis* 1986; 14:233–236.

411. Foussereau J, Tanahaski Y, Grosshans E et al. Allergic eczema from Disperse Yellow 3 in nylon stockings and socks. *Trans St Johns Hosp Dermatol Soc* 1972; 58:75.

412. Fowler JF Jr. Occupational dermatitis to Honduran mahogany. *Contact Dermatitis* 1985; 13:336–337.

413. Fowler JF Jr. Allergic contact dermatitis to quinidine. *Contact Dermatitis* 1985; 13:280–281.

414. Fowler JF Jr. Selection of patch test materials for gold allergy. *Contact Dermatitis* 1987; 17:23–25.

415. Fowler JF Jr. Allergic contact dermatitis from glutaraldehyde exposure. *J Occup Med* 1989; 31:852–853.

416. Fowler JF Jr. Cocamidopropyl betaine: The significance of positive patch test results in twelve patients. *Cutis* 1993; 52:281–284.

417. Fowler JF Jr. Gold. In: Rietschel FL, Fowler JF Jr., eds. *Fisher's Contact Dermatitis,* 4th ed. Baltimore: Williams & Wilkins; 1995:843.

418. Fowler JF Jr., Skinner SM, Belsito DV. Allergic contact dermatitis from formaldehyde resins in permanent press clothing: An underdiagnosed cause of generalized dermatitis. *J Am Acad Dermatol* 1992; 27:962–968.

419. Fox JG. Outbreak of tropical rat mite dermatitis in laboratory personnel. *Arch Dermatol* 1982; 118:676–678.

420. Francalanci S, Gola M, Giorgini S, et al. Occupational photocontact dermatitis from Olaquinox. *Contact Dermatitis* 1986; 15:112–114.

421. Fransway AF. The problem of preservation in the 1990s: I. Statement of the problem, solution(s) of the industry, and the current use of formaldehyde and formaldehyde-releasing biocides. II: Formaldehyde and formaldehyde-releasing biocides: Incidences of cross-reactivity and the significance of the positive presponse to formaldehyde. III: Agents with preservative function independent of formaldehyde release. *Am J Contact Dermatitis* 1991; 2:6–23, 78–88, 145–174.

422. Freeman K, Hubbard HC, Warin AP. Strimmer rash. *Contact Dermatitis* 1984; 10:117–118.

423. Freeman S. Allergic contact dermatitis due to 1,2-benzisothiazolin-3-one in gum arabic. *Contact Dermatitis* 1984; 11:146–149.

424. Freeman S. Fragrance and nickel: Old allergens in new guises. *Am J Contact Dermatitis* 1990; 1:47–52.

425. Freeman S. Allergic contact dermatitis due to an industrial grease caused by the antioxident phenyl-alpha-naphthylamine. *Am J Contact Dermatitis* 1991; 2:117–118.

426. Freeman S. Corticosteroid allergy. *Contact Dermatitis* 1995; 33:240–242.

427. Freeman S, Lee M-S, Gudmundsen K. Adverse contact reactions to sculptured acrylic nails: 4 case reports and a literature review. *Contact Dermatitis* 1995; 33:381–385.

428. Freeman S, Rosen RH. Urticarial contact dermatitis in food handlers. *Med J Aust* 1991; 155:91–94.

429. Fregert S. Contact dermatitis due to chromate in foundry sand. *Acta Derma venereol* 1963; 43:477.

430. Fregert S. Allergic contact dermatitis from dioxane in a solvent for cleaning metal parts. *Contact Dermatitis* 1974; 15:438.

431. Fregert S. Allergic contact dermatitis from formaldehyde in paper. *Contact Dermatitis Newslett* 1974; 15:459.

432. Fregert S. Registration of chemicals in industries. Slimi-

cides in the paper–pulp industry. *Contact Dermatitis* 1976; 2:358–359.

433. Fregert S. Allergic contact dermatitis from ethylacrylate in a window sealant. *Contact Dermatitis* 1978; 4:56.

434. Fregert S. Chromium valencies and cement dermatitis. *Br J Dermatol* 1981; 105(suppl 21):7–9.

435. Fregert S. Construction work. In: Maibach HI, ed. *Occupational and Industrial Dermatology,* 2nd ed. Chicago: Year Book Medical Publishers, Inc.; 1987:404.

436. Fregert S, Gruvberger B. Chemical properties of cement. *Berufsdermatosen* 1972; 20:238–248.

437. Fregert S, Gruvberger B. Chromate dermatitis from oil emulsion contaminated from zinc-galvanized iron plate. *Contact Dermatitis* 1976; 2:121.

438. Fregert S, Gruvberger B, Goransson K, et al. Allergic contact dermatitis from chromate in military textiles. *Contact Dermatitis* 1978; 4:223–224.

439. Fregert S, Gruvberger B, Heijer A. Chromium dermatitis from galvanized sheets. *Berufsdermatosen* 1970; 18:254–260.

440. Fregert S, Gruvberger B, Heijer A. Sensitization to chromium and cobalt in processing of sulphate pulp. *Acta Derm Venereol* 1972; 52:221–224.

441. Fregert S, Gustafsson K, Trulsson L. Contact allergy to *N*-hydroxyphthalimide. *Contact Dermatitis* 1983; 9:84–85.

442. Fregert S, Orsmark K. Allergic contact dermatitis due to epoxy resin in textile labels. *Contact Dermatitis* 1984; 11:131–132.

443. Fregert S, Ovrum P. Chromate in welding fumes with special reference to contact dermatitis. *Acta Derm Venerol* 1963; 43:119–124.

444. Fregert S, Skog E. Allergic contact dermatitis from mercaptobenzothiazole in cutting oil. *Acta Derm Venereol* 1962; 42:235–238.

445. Fregert S, Trulsson L. Difficulties in tracing sensitizing textile dyes. *Contact Dermatitis* 1978; 4:174.

446. Frosch PJ, Burrows D, Camarasa JG, et al. Allergic reactions to a hairdressers' series: Results from 9 European centres. *Contact Dermatitis* 1993; 28:180–183.

447. Frosch PJ, Wahl R, Bahmer FA, Maasch HJ. Contact urticaria to rubber gloves is IgE-mediated. *Contact Dermatitis* 1986; 14:241–245.

448. Fry L. Skin disease from color developers. *Br J Dermatol* 1965; 77:456–461.

449. Fuchs T, Enders F, Przybilla B, et al. Contact allergy to Euxyl K 400. *Dermatosen,* 1991; 39:151–153.

450. Fuchs T, Ippen H. Kontaktallergie auf CN- und CS-Tränengas. *Dermatosen* 1986; 34:12–14.

451. Fullerton A, Gammelgaard B, Avstrorp C, Menné T. Chromium content in human skin after in vitro application of ordinary cement and ferrous-sulphate–reduced cement. *Contact Dermatitis* 1993; 29:133–137.

452. Fung MA, Geisse JK, Maibach HI. Airborne contact dermatitis from metaproterenol in a respiratory therapist. *Contact Dermatitis* 1996; 35:317–318.

453. Gall H. Allergien auf zahnärztliche Werkstoffe und Dentalpharmaka. *Hautarzt* 1983; 34:326.

454. Gallagher W. Hockey dermatitis traced to glass. *Physicians Sportsmed* 1979; 7:17–18.

455. Gamsky TE, McCurdy SA, Wiggins P, et al. Epidemiology of dermatitis among California farm workers. *J Occup Med* 1992; 34:304–310.

456. Gan SL, Goh CL, Lee CS, et al. Occupational dermatosis among sanders in the furniture industry. *Contact Dermatitis* 1987; 17:237–240.

457. Garabrant DH. Dermatitis from aziridine hardener in printing ink. *Contact Dermatitis* 1985; 12:209–212.

458. Garcia J, Armisen A. Cement dermatitis with isolated cobalt sensitivity. *Contact Dermatitis* 1985; 12:52.

459. Gartner BL, Wasser C, Rodriguez E, Epstein WL. Seasonal variation of urushiol content in poison oak leaves. *Am J Contact Dermatitis* 1993; 4:33–36.

460. Gauchia R, Rodriguez-Serna M, Silvestre JF, et al: Allergic contact dermatitis from streoptomycin in a cattle breeder. *Contact Dermatitis* 1996; 35:374–375.

461. Gebhardt M, Geier J. Evaluation of patch test results with denture material series. *Contact Dermatitis* 1996; 34:191–195.

462. Gebhardt M, Stuhlert A, Knopf B. Allergic contact dermatis due to Euxyl K 400 in an ultrasonic gel. *Contact Dermatitis* 1993; 29:272.

463. Geier J, Pilz B, Frosch PJ, et al. Contact allergy due to 2-mercaptobenzimidazole. *Dermatosen* 1994; 42:190–193.

464. Geier J, Schnuch A. A comparison of contact allergies among construction and nonconstruction workers attending contact dermatitis clinics in Germany. *Am J Contact Dermatitis* 1995; 6:86–94.

465. Geiser JD. Sensitization factors in cement eczema. *Schweiz Med Wochenschr* 1968; 98:1193–1195.

466. Gellin GA. Cutting fluids and skin disorders. *Ind Med* 1970; 39:38–40.

467. Gerwig T, Winer MN. Radioactive jewelry as cause of cutaneous tumor. *JAMA* 1968; 205:595–596.

468. Gibbs RC. Tennis toe. *Arch Dermatol* 1973; 107:918.

469. Gleich GJ, Welsh PW, Yuninger JW, et al. Allergy to tobacco: An occupational hazard. *N Engl J Med* 1980; 302:617–619.

470. Goette DK. Raccoon-like periorbital leukoderma from contact with swim goggles. *Contact Dermatitis* 1984; 10:129–131.

471. Goh CL. Occupational dermatitis from soldering flux among workers in the electronics industry. *Contact Dermatitis* 1985; 13:85–90.

472. Goh CL. Irritant dermatitis from tri-*N*-butyl tin oxide in paint. *Contact Dermatitis* 1985; 12:161–163.

473. Goh CL. Occupational dermatitis from soldering flux among workers in the electronics industry. *Contact Dermatitis* 1985; 13:85–90.

474. Goh CL. Hand dermatitis from a rubber motorcycle handle. *Contact Dermatitis* 1987; 16:40–41.

475. Goh CL. Occupational dermatitis from gold plating. *Contact Dermatitis* 1988; 18:122–123.

476. Goh CL. Occupational allergic contact dermatitis from Rengas wood. *Contact Dermatitis* 1988; 18:300.

477. Goh CL. Cutting oil dermatitis on guinea pig skin. *Contact Dermatitis* 1991; 24:16–21, 81–85.

478. Goh CL, Gan SL, Ngui SJ. Occupational dermatitis in a prefabrication construction factory. *Contact Dermatitis* 1986; 15:235–240.

479. Goh CL, Ho SF. Contact dermatitis from dielectric fluids in electrodischarge machining. *Contact Dermatitis* 1993; 28:134–138.

480. Goh CL, Kwok SF, Gan SL. Cobalt and nickel content of Asian cements. *Contact Dermatitis* 1986; 15:169–172.

481. Goh CL, Kwok SF, Rajan VS. Cross sensitivity in colour developers. *Contact Dermatitis* 1984; 10:280–285.

482. Goh CL, Ng SK. Airborne contact dermatitis to colophony in soldering flux. *Contact Dermatitis* 1987; 17:89–91.

483. Goh CL, Ng SK. Allergic contact dermatitis to *Curcuma longa* (turmeric). *Contact Dermatitis* 1987; 17:186.

484. Goldstein N. Mercury-cadmium sensivity in tattoos. *Ann Intern Med* 1967; 67:984–989.

485. Goncalo S, Brandao FM, Pecegueiro M, et al. Occupational contact dermatitis to glutaraldehyde. *Contact Dermatitis* 1984; 10:183–184.

486. Göransson K. Allergic contact dermatitis to an epoxy hardener: Dodecyl-succinic anhydride. *Contact Dermatitis* 1977; 3:277–278.

487. Göransson K. Occupational contact urticaria to fresh cow and pig blood in slaughtermen. *Contact Dermatitis* 1981; 7:281–282.

488. Göransson K. Contact urticaria to fish. *Contact Dermatitis* 1981; 7:282–283.

489. Gordon M. Darkroom diseases and how to combat them. *J Soc Health* 1987; 3:102–103.

490. Goulden V, Wilkinson SM. Occupational allergic contact dermatitis from epoxy resin on chipboard. *Contact Dermatitis* 1996; 35:262–263.

491. Grace CT, Ng SK, Cheong LL. Recurrent irritant contact dermatitis due to tributylin on work clothes. *Contact Dermatitis* 1991; 25:250–251.

492. Grattan CEH, Harman RRM, Tan RSH. Milk recorder dermatitis. *Contact Dermatitis* 1986; 14:217–220.

493. Greig DE. Another isothiazolinone source. *Contact Dermatitis* 1991; 25:201–202.

494. Grimalt F, Romaguera C. *Dermatitis de Contacto.* Valencia: Editorial Fontalba; 1980:477.

495. Grimalt F, Romaguera C. Cutaneous sensitivity to benzidine. *Dermatosen* 1981; 29:95–97.

496. Gronka PA, Bobkoskie RL, Tomchick GJ, et al. Mercury vapor exposures in dental offices. *J Am Dent Assoc* 1970; 81:923–925.

497. Gruvberger B, Bjorkner B, Bruze M. Contact allergy to dichlofluanid in humans and guinea pigs. *Am J Contact Dermatitis* 1995; 6:221–224.

498. Gruvberger B, Bruze M. Contact allergy to 4-(2-nitrobutyl)-morpholine and 4,4′-(2-ethyl-2-nitrotrimethylene)-dimorpholine as active ingredients of a preservative recommended for metalworking fluids in the guinea pig. *Dermatosen* 1995; 43:126–128.

499. Gruvberger B, Bruze M, Zimerson E. Contact allergy to the active ingredients of Bioban P 1487. *Contact Dermatitis* 1996; 35:141–145.

500. Guerra L, Bardazzi F, Tosti A. Contact dermatitis in hairdressers' clients. *Contact Dermatitis* 1992; 26:108–111.

501. Guerra L, Tosti A, Bardazzi F, et al. Contact dermatitis in hairdressers: The Italian experience. *Contact Dermatitis* 1992; 26:101–107.

502. Guerra L, Vincenzi C, Bardazzi F, Tosti A. Contact sensitization due to isophoronediamine. *Contact Dermatitis* 1992; 27:52–53.

503. Guidetti MS, Vincenzi C, Guerra L, Tosti A. Contact dermatitis due to oleyl alcohol. *Contact Dermatitis* 1994; 31:260–261.

504. Guidotti S, Wright WE, Peters JM. Multiple myeloma in cosmetologists. *Am J Ind Med* 1982; 3:169–171.

505. Guin JD. Contact sensitivity to topical corticosteroids. *J Am Acad Dermatol* 1984; 10:773–782.

506. Guin JD. Foods. In: *Practical Contact Dermatitis.* New York; McGraw-Hill, Inc.; 1995; 534.

507. Guin JD. Balsam of Peru. In: *Practical Contact Dermatitis.* New York; McGraw-Hill, Inc.; 1995; 265–270.

508. Guin JD. Patch testing to plants; Some practical aspects of what has become an esoteric area of contact dermatitis. *Am J Contact Dermatitis* 1995; 6:232–235.

509. Guin JD, Schosser RH, Rosenberg EW. *Magnolia grandiflora* dermatitis. *Dermatol Clin* 1990; 8:81–84.

510. Guldager H. Halothane allergy as cause of acne. *Lancet* 1987; 1:1211–1212.

511. Gupta BN, Mathur AK, Agarwal C, et al. Contact sensitivity to henna. *Contact Dermatitis* 1986; 15:303–304.

512. Habets JMW, Geursen-Reitsma AM, Stolz E, et al. Sensitization to sodium hypochlorite causing hand dermatitis. *Contact Dermatitis* 1986; 15:140–142.

513. Hackel H, Miller K, Elsner P, et al. Unusual combined sensitization to palladium and other metals. *Contact Dermatitis* 1991; 24:131–132.

514. Hadfield E. Tumours of the nose and sinuses in relation to woodworkers. *J Laryngol Otol* 1969; 83:417–420.

515. Haenen C, de Moor A, Dooms-Goossens A. Contact dermatitis caused by the insecticides omethoate and dimethoate. *Contact Dermatitis* 1996; 35:54–55.

516. Halbert AR, Gebauer KA, Wall ML. Prognosis of occupational chromate dermatitis. *Contact Dermatitis* 1992; 27:214–219.

517. Halkier-Sorensen L. Occupational skin diseases. *Contact Dermatitis* (suppl 1), 1996; 35.

518. Halkier-Sorensen L, Heickendorff L, Dalsgaard I, et al. Skin symptoms among workers in the fish processing industry are caused by high molecular weight compounds. *Contact Dermatitis* 1991; 24:94–100.

519. Halkier-Sorensen L, Thestrup-Pedersen K. Skin irritancy from fish is related to its postmortem age. *Contact Dermatitis* 1989; 21:172–178.

520. Hall AF. Occupational dermatitis among aircraft workers. *JAMA* 1944; 125:179.

521. Hamann CP. Natural rubber latex protein sensitivity in review. *Am J Contact Dermatitis* 1993; 4:4–21.

522. Handfield-Jones SE, Cronin E. Contact sensitivity to lignocaine. *Clin Exp Dermatol* 1993; 18:342–343.

523. Handley J, Burrows D. Dermatitis from hexavalent chromate in the accelerator of an epoxy sealant (PR1422) used in the aircraft industry. *Contact Dermatitis* 1994; 30:193–196.

524. Hanifin JM. Ethylene oxide dermatitis. *JAMA* 1971; 217:213.

525. Hannuksela M. Rapid increase in contact allergy to Kathon CG in Finland. *Contact Dermatitis* 1986; 15:211–214.

526. Hannuksela M, Hassi J. Hairdressers hand dermatoses. *Dermatosen* 1980; 28:149–151.

527. Hannuksela M, Lahti A. Immediate reaction to fruit and vegetables. *Contact Dermatitis* 1977; 3:79–84.

528. Hannuksela M, Suhonen R, Karvonen J. Caustic ulcers caused by cement. *Br J Dermatol* 1976; 95:547–549.

529. Hansbrough JF, Zapata-Sirvent R, Dominic W, et al. Hydrocarbon contact injuries. *J Trauma* 1985; 25:250–252.

530. Hansen KS. Occupational dermatoses in hospital cleaning women. *Contact Dermatitis* 1983; 9:343–351.

531. Hansen KS. Glutaraldehyde occupational dermatitis. *Contact Dermatitis* 1983; 9:81–82.

532. Hansen KS, Petersen HO. Protein contact dermatitis in slaughterhouse workers. *Contact Dermatitis* 1989; 21:221–224.

533. Hanson D. EPA told to name inert pesticide components. *Chem Eng News* October 28, 1996.

534. Hanson D. Methylene exposure sharply limited. *Chem Eng News* January 13, 1997.

535. Hansson C, Ezzelarab M, Sterner O. Isolation and structural determination of two new haptens in an aziridine hardener. *Am J Contact Dermatitis* 1994; 5:216–220.

536. Harman RRM, Sarkany I. Copy paper dermatitis. *Trans St Johns Hosp Dermatol Soc* 1960; 44:37.

537. Harris JC, Rumack BH, Aldrich FD. Toxicology of urea formaldehyde and polyurethane foam insulation. *JAMA* 1981; 245:243–246.

538. Harrison R, Letz G, Pasternak G, et al. Fulminant hepatic failure after occupational exposure to 2-nitropropane. *Ann Intern Med* 1987; 107:466–468.

539. Hata M, Sasaki E. Ota M, et al. Allergic contact dermatitis from curcumin (turmeric). *Contact Dermatitis* 1997; 36:107–108.

540. Hatch KL, Maibach HI. Textile fiber dermatitis. *Contact Dermatitis* 1985; 12:1–11.
541. Hatch KL, Maibach HI. Textile dye dermatitis. A review. *J Am Acad Dermatol* 1985; 12:1079–1092.
542. Hatch KL, Maibach HI. Textile chemical finish dermatitis. *Contact Dermatitis* 1986; 14:1–13.
543. Hatch KL, Maibach HI. Textile dye dermatitis. *J Am Acad Dermatol* 1995; 32:631–639.
544. Hatch KL, Maibach HI. Textile dermatitis: An update. I. Resins, additives and fibers. *Contact Dermatitis* 1995; 32:319–326.
545. Haudrechy P, Foussereau J, Mantout B, Baroux B. Nickel release from nickel-plated metals and stainless steels. *Contact Dermatitis* 1994; 31:249–255.
546. Hausen BM. A simple method for extracting crude sesquiterpene lactones from Compositae plants for skin tests, chemical investigations and sensitizing experiments in guinea pigs. *Contact Dermatitis* 1977; 3:58–60.
547. Hausen B. *Woods Injurious to Human Health: A Manual.* Berlin: Walter de Gruyter; 1981.
548. Hausen BM. Palisanderholz-Allergie durch Armreifen und Blockflöte. *Dermatosen* 1982; 30:189–192.
549. Hausen BM. Chin rest allergy in a violinist. *Contact Dermatitis* 1985; 12:178–179.
550. Hausen BM. Contact allergy to Disperse Blue 106 and Blue 124 in black "velvet" clothes. *Contact Dermatitis* 1993; 28:169–173.
551. Hausen BM. The sensitizing potency of Euxyl K 400 and its components 1,2-dibromo-2,4-dicyanobutane and 2-phenoxyethanol. *Contact Dermatitis* 1993; 28:149–153.
552. Hausen BM. A 6-year experience with Compositae mix. *Am J Contact Dermatitis* 1996; 7:94–99.
553. Hausen BM, Bröhan J, König WA, et al. Allergic and irritant contact dermatitis from falcarinol and didehydrofalcarinol in common ivy (*Hedera helix* L.) *Contact Dermatitis* 1987; 17:1–9.
554. Hausen BM, Emde L, Marks V. An investigation of the allergenic constituents of *Cladonia stellaris* (Opiz) Pous & Vezda ("silver moss," "reindeer moss" or "reindeer lichen." *Contact Dermatitis* 1993; 28:70–76.
555. Hausen BM, Heesch B, Kiel U. Studies on the sensitizing capacity of imidazole derivatives. *Am J Contact Dermatitis* 1990; 1:25–33.
556. Hausen BM, Hjorth N. Skin reactions to topical food exposure. In: Storrs F, ed. *Dermatologic Clinics*, vol 2. Philadelphia: W.B. Saunders, Co.; 1984:567–578.
557. Hausen BM, Kuhlwein A, Schulz KH. Kolophonium und Verwendung von Kolophonium und Kolophonium-modifizierten Produkten. *Dermatosen* 1982; 30:107–115, 145–152.
558. Hausen BM, Kulenkemp D, Börries M. Kontakallergie auf blaue Dispersionsfarbstoffe in schwarzen "Samt'leggins." *Akt Derm* 1991; 17:337–340.
559. Hausen BM, Mau HH. Kontaktallergie durch einen Geigen-Kinnhalter aus Palisander. *Dermatosen Beruf Umwelt* 1979; 27:18–20.
560. Hausen BM, Menezes Brandao F. Disperse Blue 106, a strong sensitizer. *Contact Dermatitis* 1986; 5:102–103.
561. Hausen BM, Milbrodt M, Koenig WA. The allergens of nail polish I. Allergenic constituents of common nail polish and toluenesulfonamide-formaldehyde resin (TS-F-R). *Contact Dermatitis* 1995; 33:157–164.
562. Hausen BM, Munster G. Cocobolo-Holz, ein vergessenes Ekzematogen? Neuere Erkenntnisse über das Hauptallergen des Cocobolo-Holzes (*Dalbergia* sp.). *Dermatosen* 1983; 31:110–117.
563. Hausen BM, Shoji A. Orchid allergy. *Arch Dermatol* 1984; 120:1206–1209.
564. Hausen BM, Spring O. Sunflower allergy: On the constituents of the trichomes of *Helianthus annuus* L. (Compositae). *Contact Dermatitis* 1989; 20:326–334.
565. Hausen BM, Wolf C. 1,2,3-Trithiane-5-carboxylic acid, a first contact allergen from *Asparagus officinalis* (Liliaceae). *Am J Contact Dermatitis* 1996; 7:41–46.
566. Hausen BM, Wollenweber E, Senff H, Post B. Propolis allergy (1) Origin, properties, usage and literature review. *Contact Dermatitis* 1987; 17:163–170.
567. Hausen BM, Wollenweber E, Senff H, Post B. Propolis allergy II. The sensitizing properties of 1,1-dimethylallyl caffeic acid ester. *Contact Dermatitis* 1987; 17:171–177.
568. Haustein U-F. Violin chin rest eczema due to east-Indian rosewood. (*Dalbergia latifolia* R.xb). *Contact Dermatitis* 1982; 8:77–78.
569. Hayakawa R, Arima Y, Hirose O, et al. Allergic contact dermatitis due to hexamethylenetetramine in core molding. *Contact Dermatitis* 1988; 18:226–228.
570. Hayakawa R, Matsunage K, Arima Y. Depigmented contact dermatitis due to incense. *Contact Dermatitis* 1987; 16:272–274.
571. Hayakawa R, Matsunaga K, Kojima S, et al. Naphthol AS as a cause of pigmented contact dermatitis. *Contact Dermatitis* 1985; 13:20–25.
572. Hayes RB, Blair A, Stewart PA, et al. Mortality of U.S. embalmers and funeral directors. *Am J Ind Med* 1990; 18:641–652.
573. Heacock HJ, Rivers JK. Occupational diseases of hairdressers. *Can J Public Health* 1986; 77:109–113.
574. Hearn CED, Keir W. Nail damage in spray operators exposed to Paraquat. *Br J Ind Med* 1971; 28:399–403.
575. Heidenheim M, Jemec GBE. Occupational allergic contact dermatitis from vitamin A acetate. *Contact Dermatitis* 1995; 33:439.
576. Heine A, Fox G. Bäckerekzem durch Chromverbindung in Mehlen. *Dermatosen* 1980; 28:113–115.
577. Heinzman M, Thoreson S, McKenzie L, et al. Occupational burns among restaurant workers: Colorado and Minnesota. *Arch Dermatol* 1994; 130:699–701.
578. Heitbrink WA, Wallace ME, Bryant CJ. Control of paint overspray in autobody repair shops. *Am Ind Hyg Assoc J* 1995; 56:1023–1032.
579. Helander I. Contact urticaria from leather containing formaldehyde. *Arch Dermatol* 1977; 113:1443.
580. Helm TN, Taylor JS, Adams RM, et al. Skin problems of performing artists. *Am J Contact Dermatol* 1993; 4:27–32.
581. Henn RW, Olivares IA. Tropical storage of processed negatives. *Photographic Sci Eng* 1960; 4:229.
582. Herve-Bazin B, Foussereau J, Cavelier C. L'eczema allergique au support de pigments textiles. *Dermatosen* 1977; 25:113–117.
583. Herve-Bazin B, Foussereau J, Cavelier C. Allergy to diphenylamine from an industrial grease. *Contact Dermatitis* 1986; 14:116.
584. Herzheimer H. Skin sensitivity to flour of bakers' apprentices: Final report of long-term investigation. *Acta Allergol* 1973; 28:42–49.
585. Herzog J. Milton S. Hershey Medical Center, PA, Report presented at the American Academy of Dermatology Annual Meeting, San Antonio, Texas, December 1987.
586. Herzog J, Dunne J, Aber R, et al. Milk tester dermatitis. *J Am Acad Dermatol* 1988; 19:503–508.
587. Heskel NS. Epoxy resin dermatitis in a stained glass window maker. *Contact Dermatitis* 1988; 18:182–183.
588. Hesse A. Letter to the editor re allergic contact dermatitis to natural latex. *J Am Acad Dermatol* 1992; 27:651.

589. Hesse A, Peters K-P, Hornstein OP. Anaphylactic reaction to unexpected latex in a polychloroprene glove. *Contact Dermatitis* 1992; 27:336–337.

590. Hileman B. Bisphenol A: Regulatory, scientific puzzle. *Chem Eng News* March 24, 1997:37–39.

591. Hindsen M, Bruze M, Trulsson L. Harlequin dermatitis. *Contact Dermatitis* 1990; 23:283.

592. Hindson C, Lawlor F. Coconut diethanolamide in a hydraulic mining oil. *Contact Dermatitis* 1983; 9:168.

593. Hindson TC. Contact allergy to a-pinene in boot polish. *Contact Dermatol Newslett* 1969; 6:116.

594. Hindson TC. *o*-Nitro-*p*-phenylenediamine in hair dye: An unusual dental hazard. *Contact Dermatitis* 1975; 1:333.

595. Hippke WE, Barth J. Ein Beitrag zur Problematik der Chromsäureverätzung. *Dermatosen* 1994; 42:156–158.

596. Hjerpe L. Chromate dermatitis at an engine assembly department. *Contact Dermatitis* 1986; 14:66–67.

597. Hjorth N. *Eczematous Allergy to Balsams, Allied Perfumes, and Flavoring Agents.* Copenhagen: Munksgaard; 1961.

598. Hjorth N. Primula dermatitis: Sources of errors in patch-testing and patch test sensitization. *Trans St Johns Hosp Dermatol Soc* 1966; 52:207–219.

599. Hjorth N. Battery for testing of chefs and other kitchen workers. *Contact Dermatitis* 1975; 1:63.

600. Hjorth N. Dermatitis from trimethyl hexamethylene diisocyanate. *Contact Dermatitis* 1975; 1:59.

601. Hjorth N. *N*-methylol-chloroacetamide: A sensitizer in coolant oils and cosmetics. *Contact Dermatitis* 1979; 5:330–342.

602. Hjorth N, Roed-Petersen J. Occupational protein contact dermatitis in food handlers. *Contact Dermatitis* 1976; 2:28–42.

603. Hjorth N, Roed-Petersen J. Allergic contact dermatitis in veterinary surgeons. *Contact Dermatitis* 1980; 6:27–29.

604. Hjorth N, Weismann K. Occupational dermatitis in chefs and sandwich makers. *Contact Dermatitis* 1972; 11:301.

605. Hjorth N, Weismann K. Occupational dermatitis among veterinary surgeons caused by spiramycin, tylosin and penethamate. *Acta Derm Venereol* 1973; 53:229–232.

606. Ho VC, Mitchell JC. Allergic contact dermatitis from rubber boots. *Contact Dermatitis* 1985; 12:110–111.

607. Hodgson G. Cutaneous hazards of lubricants. *Ind Med* 1970; 39:41–46.

608. Hodgson M. Sick building syndrome. *Occup Med* 1995; 10:167–175.

609. Hoffman TE, Adams RM. Contact dermatitis to benzoin in greasepaint makeup. *Contact Dermatitis* 1978; 4:379–380.

610. Hoffman TE, Adams RM. Allergic contact dermatitis to dicyclohexylcarbodiimide in chemists. *J Am Acad Dermatol* 1989; 21:436–437.

611. Hoffman TE, Hausen BM, Adams RM. Allergic contact dermatitis to "silver oak" wooden arm bracelets. *J Am Acad Dermatol* 1985; 13:778–779.

612. Hogan DJ. Subungual trichogranuloma in a hairdresser. *Cutis* 1988; 42:105–106.

613. Hogan DJ, Dosman JA, Li KYR, et al. Questionaire survey of pruritus and rash in grain elevator workers. *Contact Dermatitis* 1986; 14:170–175.

614. Hogan DJ, Lane PR. Allergic contact dermatitis due to a herbicide (barban). *Can Med Assoc J* 1985; 132:387–389.

615. Högberg M, Wahlberg JE. Health screening for occupational dermatoses in house painters. *Contact Dermatitis* 1980; 6:100–106.

616. Hogstedt C, Arginer L, Gustavsson A. Epidemiologic support for ethylene oxide as a cancer causing agent. *JAMA* 1986; 255:1575–1578.

617. Holman RG. The epidemiology of logging injuries in the Northwest. *J Trauma* 1987; 27:1044–1049.

618. Holmstrom M, Lund VJ. Malignant melanomas of the nasal cavity after occupational exposure to formaldehyde. *Br J Ind Med* 1991; 48:9–11.

619. Holness CL, Nethercott JR. Health status of funeral service workers exposed to formaldehyde. *Arch Environ Health* 1989; 44:222–228.

620. Holness DL, Nethercott JR. Dermatitis in hairdressers. *Dermatol Clin* 1990; 8:119–126.

621. Holness DL, Nethercott JR. Epicutaneous testing results in hairdressers. *Am J Contact Dermatitis* 1990; 1:224–234.

622. Horvath EP Jr. Arsenic exposure. Letter to the Editor. *JAMA* 1985; 253:634.

623. Hostynek JJ, Maibach HI. Chromium in US household bleach. *Contact Dermatitis* 1988; 18:206–209.

624. Hostynek JJ, Patrick E, Younger B, Maibach HI. Hypochlorite sensitivity in man. *Contact Dermatitis* 1989; 20:32–37.

625. Høvding G. Contact eczema due to formaldehyde in resin finished textiles. *Acta Derm Venereol* 1961; 41:194–200.

626. Høvding G. *Cement Eczema and Chromium Allergy: An Epidemiological Investigation.* Bergen: University of Bergen; 1970 [thesis].

627. Hradil E, hersle K, Nordin P, Faergemann J. An epidemic of tinea corporis caused by *Trichophyton tonsurans* among wrestlers in Sweden. *Acta Derm Venerol* (Stockh) 1995; 75:305–306.

628. Huber K, Sumner W. Recapping the accidental needlestick problem. *Am J Infect Control* 1987; 15:127–130.

629. Hudson LD. Phototoxic reaction triggered by a new dental instrument. Letter to the editor. *J Am Acad Dermatol* 1987; 17:508.

630. Hüner A, Fartasch M, Hornstein OP, et al. The irritant effect of different metalworking fluids. *Contact Dermatitis* 1994; 31:220–225.

631. Hunter D. *The Diseases of Occupation.* London: English University Press; 1974:304.

632. Huriez C, Martin P, Lefebre M. Sensitivity to dichromate in a milk analysis laboratory. *Contact Dermatitis* 1975; 1:247–248.

633. IBM develops laser electroplating method. *Chem Eng News* October 29, 1979.

634. Ibbotson SH, Lawrence CM. Allergic contact dermatitis from aziridine crosslinker cx100. *Contact Dermatitis* 1994; 30:306–307.

635. Iliev D, Elsner P. Allergic contact dermatitis from the fungicide Rondo-M (R) and the insecticide Alfacron. *Contact Dermatitis* 1997; 36:31–35.

636. Illchyshyn A, Cartwright PH, Smith AG. Contact sensitivity to newsprint: A rare manifestation of coal tar allergy. *Contact Dermatitis* 1987; 17:52–53.

637. Illuminati R, Russo R, Guerra L, et al. Occupational airborne contact dermatitis in a florist. *Contact Dermatitis* 1988; 18:246.

638. Imbus HR, Dyson WL. A review of nasal cancer in furniture manufacturing and woodworking in North Carolina, the United States, and other countries. *J Occup Med* 1987; 29:734–740.

639. Ippen H. Hautschäden in der metalverarbeitenden Industrie. *Dermatosen* 1978; 26:25–28.

640. Ippen H. Bestandteile moderner Haarfarben. *Dermatosen* 1987; 35:157–161.

641. Ippen H. Phytophotodermatitis durch "Rasentrimmer" ("Strimmer rash"). *Dermatosen* 1990; 38:190–192.

642. Irvine C, Reynolds A, Finlay AY. Erythema multiforme-

like reaction to "rosewood." *Contact Dermatitis* 1988; 19:224–225.

643. Iwatsuki K, Tagami H, Moriguchi T, Yamada M. Lymphadenoid structure induced by gold hypersensitivity. *Arch Dermatol* 1982; 118:608–611.

644. Jacobs M-C, Rycroft RJG. Contact dermatitis and asthma from sodium metabisulfite in a photographic technician. *Contact Dermatitis* 1995; 33:65–66.

645. Jacobs M-C, Rycroft RJG. Allergic contact dermatitis from cyanoacrylate? *Contact Dermatitis* 1995; 33:71.

646. Jäger H, Pelloni E. Tests epicutanes aux bichromates, positifs dans l'eczema au ciment. *Dermatologica* 1950; 100:207.

647. Jagodzinski LJ, Taylor JS, Oriba H. Allergic contact dermatitis from topical corticosteroid preparations. *Am J Contact Dermatitis* 1995; 6:67–74.

648. Jakubowski M, Trojanowska B, Kowalska G, et al. Occupational exposure to cadmium and kidney dysfunction. *Int Arch Occup Environ Health* 1987; 59:567–577.

649. Jakush J. AIDS: The disease and its implications for dentistry. *J Am Dent Assoc* 1987; 115:395–403.

650. Jäppinen P, Eskelinen A. Patch tests with methyene-bis-thiocyanate in paper mill workers. *Contact Dermatitis* 1987; 16:233.

651. Jäppinen P, Hakulinen T, Pukkala E, et al. Cancer incidence of workers in the Finnish pulp and paper industry. *Scand J Work Environ Health* 1987; 13:197–202.

652. Järvholm B, Laveniuis B, Sällsten G. Cancer morbidity in workers exposed to cutting fluids containing nitrites and amines. *Br J Ind Med* 1986; 43:563–565.

653. Jeansson I, Lofstrom A, Lidblom A. Complaints relating to the handling of carbonless copy paper in Sweden. *Am Ind Hyg Assoc J* 1984; 45:1324–1327.

654. Jelen G, Cavelier C, Protois JP, Foussereau J. A new allergen responsible for shoe allergy: Chloroacetamide. *Contact Dermatitis* 1989; 21:110–111.

655. Jirasek L. Dermatologic hazards in electron microscopy laboratories. *Cesk Dermatol* 60:371, 1985 [as reviewed in *Dermatosen* 1987; 35:29–30].

656. Johansen JD, Rastogi SC, Menne T. Contact allergy to popular perfumes; assessed by patch test, use test and chemical analysis. *Br J Dermatol* 1996; 135:419–422.

657. Johnson DR, Mathias CGT. Case report: A dentist with allergic contact dermatitis caused by ethylene glycol dimethacrylate. *Am J Contact Dermatitis* 1993; 4:90–92.

658. Johnson ML, Wilson HTH. Oil dermatitis: An enquiry into its prognosis. *Br J Ind Med* 1971; 28:122–125.

659. Johnsson M, Buhagen M, Leira HL, Solvang S. Fungicide-induced contact dermatitis. *Contact Dermatitis* 1983; 9:285–288.

660. Jolanki R. Occupational skin diseases from epoxy compounds: Epoxy resin compounds, epoxy acrylates and 2,3-epoxypropyl trimethyl ammonium chloride. *Acta Derm Venereol* 1991(suppl 159):1–80.

661. Jolanki R, Alanko K, Pfaffli, et al. Occupational allergic contact dermatitis from 5-chloro-1-methyl-4-nitroimid-azole. *Contact Dermatitis* 1997; 36:53–54.

662. Jolanki R, Kanerva L, Estlander T. Occupational allergic contact dermatitis caused by epoxy diacrylate in ultraviolet-light cured paint, and bisphenol A in dental composite resin. *Contact Dermatitis* 1995; 33:94–99.

663. Jolly VG. Propolis varnish for violins. *Bee World* 1978; 59:158–161.

664. Jones JG. Herpetic whitlow: An infectious occupational hazard. *J Occup Med* 1985; 27:725–728.

665. Jordan WP Jr. Resorcinol monobenzoate, steering wheels, Peruvian balsam. *Arch Dermatol* 1973; 108:278.

666. Jordan WP Jr., Dahl MV, Albert HL. Contact dermatitis from glutaraldehyde. *Arch Dermatol* 1972; 105:94–95.

667. Jordan WP Jr., Vourlas M. Contact dermatitis from typewriter correction paper. *Cutis* 1975; 15:594.

668. Joselow MM, Ruiz R, Goldwater LJ, et al. Absorption and excretion of mercury in man. XV. Occupational exposure among dentists. *Arch Environ Health* 1968; 17:39–43.

669. Joseph HL, Gifford H. Barbers' interdigital pilonidal sinuses. *Arch Dermatol* 1954; 70:616–624.

670. Juhlin L, Shelley WB. New staining techniques for the Langerhans cell. *Acta Derm Venereol* 1977; 57:289–296.

671. Jung H-D, Rothe A, Heise H. Zur Epikutantestung mit Pflanzenschutz und Schädlingsbekämpfungsmitteln (Pestiziden). *Dermatosen* 1987; 35:43–51.

672. Kahn AM, McCrady-Kahn VL. Molten metal burns. *West J Med* 1981; 135:78–80.

673. Kahn G, Phanuphak P, Claman HN. Propyl gallate: Contact sensitization and orally-induced tolerance. *Arch Dermatol* 1974; 109:506–509.

674. Kanerva L. Occupational IgE-mediated protein contact dermatitis from pork in a slaughterman. *Contact Dermatitis* 1996; 34:301–302.

675. Kanerva L, Aitio A. Dermatotoxicological aspects of metallic chromium. *Eur J Dermatol* 1997; 7:79–84.

676. Kanerva L, Estlander T, Jolanki R. Double active sensitization caused by acrylics. *Am J Contact Dermatitis* 1992; 3:23–26.

677. Kanerva L, Estlander T, Jolanki R. Occupational allergic contact dermatitis from nickel in bartender's metallic measuring cup. *Am J Contact Dermatitis* 1993; 4:39–41.

678. Kanerva L, Estlander T, Jolanki R. Occupational allergic contact dermatitis caused by thiourea compounds. *Contact Dermatitis* 1994; 31:242–248.

679. Kanerva L, Estlander T, Jolanki R. Occupational allergic contact dermatitis caused by ylang-ylang oil. *Contact Dermatitis* 1995; 33:198–199.

680. Kanerva L, Estlander T, Jolanki R. Allergic patch test reactions caused by the rubber chemical cyclohexyl thiophthalimide. *Contact Dermatitis* 1996; 34:23–26.

681. Kanerva L, Estlander T, Jolanki R. Occupational allergic contact dermatitis from 3-dimethylaminopropylamine in shampoos. *Contact Dermatitis* 1996; 35:122.

682. Kanerva L, Estlander T, Jolanki R. Occupational allergic contact dermatitis from spices. *Contact Dermatitis* 1996; 35:157–162.

683. Kanerva L, Estlander T, Jolanki R, et al. Contact dermatitis from telefax paper. *Contact Dermatitis* 1992b; 27:12–15.

684. Kanerva L, Estlander T, Jolanki R, et al. Occupational allergic contact dermatitis caused by diethylenetriamine in carbonless copy paper. *Contact Dermatitis* 1993; 29:147–151.

685. Kanerva L, Estlander T, Jolanki R, Tarvainen K. Occupational allergic contact dermatitis and contact urticaria caused by polyfunctional aziridine hardener. *Contact Dermatitis* 1995; 33:304–309.

686. Kanerva L, Estlander T, Jolanki R, Tarvainen K. Statistics on allergic patch test reactions caused by acrylate compounds, including data on ethyl methacrylate. *Am J Contact Dermatitis* 1995; 6:75–77.

687. Kanerva L, Estlander T, Tarvainen K, Jolanki R. Active sensitization caused by Elecampane *(Inula helenium).* *Am J Contact Dermatitis* 1994; 5:30–33.

688. Kanerva L, Hyry H, Jolanki R, et al. Delayed and immediate allergy caused by methylhexahydrophthalic anhydride. *Contact Dermatitis* 1997; 36:34–38.

689. Kanerva L, Jolanki R, Estlander OD. Occupational dermatitis due to an epoxy acrylate. *Contact Dermatitis* 1986; 14:80–84.

690. Kanerva L, Jolanki R, Estlander T. Allergic contact

dermatitis from epoxy resin hardeners. *Am J Contact Dermatitis* 1991; 2:89–97.

691. Kanerva L, Jolanki R, Estlander T. Offset printer's occupational allergic contact dermatitis caused by cobalt-2-ethylhexoate. *Contact Dermatitis* 1996; 34:67–68.

692. Kanerva L, Laine R, Jolanki R, et al. Occupational allergic contact dermatitis caused by nitroglycerin. *Contact Dermatitis* 1991; 24:356–362.

693. Kanerva L, Lauerma A, Estlander T, et al. Occupational allergic contact dermatitis caused by photobonded sculptured nails and a review of (meth)acrylates in nail cosmetics. *Am J Contact Dermatitis* 1996; 7:109–115.

694. Kanerva L, Lauerma A, Jolanki R, Estlander T. Methyl acrylate: A new sensitizer in nail lacquer. *Contact Dermatitis* 1995; 33:203–204.

695. Kanerva L, Susitaival P. Cow dander: The most common cause of occupational contact urticaria in Finland. *Contact Dermatitis* 1996; 35:309–310.

696. Kanerva L, Toikkanen J, Jolanki R, et al. Statistical data on occupational contact urticaria. *Contact Dermatitis* 1996; 35:229–233.

697. Kanerva L, Turjanmaa K, Estlander T, Jolanki R. Occupational allergic contact dermatitis caused by 2-hydroxyethyl methacrylate (2-HEMA) in a new dentin adhesive. *Am J Contact Dermatitis* 1991; 2:24–30.

698. Kantor GR, Taylor JS, Ratz JL, et al. Acute allergic contact dermatitis from diazolidinyl urea (Germall II) in a hair gel. *J Am Acad Dermatol* 1985; 13:116–119.

699. Kaplan I, Zeligman I: Occupational dermatitis of railroad workers. *Arch Dermatol* 1962; 85:95–102.

700. Karacic V, Skender L, Prpic-Majic D. Occupational exposure to benzene in the shoe industry. *Am J Ind Med* 1987; 12:531–536.

701. Karlberg A-T. Is unmodified rosin (colophony) the best screening material for rosin allergy? *Am J Contact Dermatitis* 1990:189–194.

702. Karlberg A-T, Dooms-Goossens A. Contact allergy to oxidized D-limonene among dermatitis patients. *Contact Dermatitis* 1997; 36:201–206.

703. Karlberg A-T, Gäfvert E, Liden C. Environmentally friendly paper may increase risk of hand eczema in rosin-sensitive persons. *J Am Acad Dermatol* 1995; 33:427–432.

704. Kassis V, Vedel P, Darre E. Contact dermatitis to methyl methacrylate. *Contact Dermatitis* 1984; 11:26–28.

705. Katsambas A, Nicolaidou E. Cutaneous malignant melanoma and sun exposure. *Arch Dermatol* 1996; 132:444–450.

706. Katsarou A, Koufou B, Takou K, et al. Patch test results in hairdressers with contact dermatitis in Greece (1985–1994). *Contact Dermatitis* 1995; 33:347–361.

707. Katz SA, Samitz MH. Leaching of nickel from stainless steel consumer commodities. *Acta Derm Venereol (Stockh)* 1975; 55:113–115.

708. Kawai K, Nakagawa M, Sasaki Y, Kawai K. Occupational contact dermatitis from Kathon 930. *Contact Dermatitis* 1993; 28:117–118.

709. Kawamura T, Fukuda S, Ohtake N, et al. Lichen planus–like contact dermatitis due to methacrylic acid esters. *Br J Dermatol* 1996; 134:358–360.

710. Keckes K, Brown PM. Hexahydro-1,3,5-tris(2-hydroxyethyl)triazine, a new bacteriocidal agent as a cause of allergic contact dermatitis. *Contact Dermatitis* 1976; 2:92–98.

711. Keiller FES, Warin RP. Mercury dermatitis in a tattoo; treated with dimercaprol. *BMJ* 1957; 1:687.

712. Kellett JK, Beck MH, Auckland G. Contact sensitivity to thiourea in photocopy paper. *Contact Dermatitis* 1984; 11:124.

713. Kerre S, Devos LO, Verhoeve L, et al. Contact allergy to diethylthiourea in a wet suit. *Contact Dermatitis* 1996; 35:176–177.

714. Kersey P, Stevenson CJ. Vitiligo and occupational exposure to hydroquinone from servicing self-photographing machines. *Contact Dermatitis* 1981; 7:285–286.

715. Keskinen H, Kalliomaki PL, Alanko K. Occupational asthma due to stainless steel welding fumes. *Clin Allergy* 1980; 10:151–159.

716. Key M. Some unusual allergic reactions in industry. *Arch Dermatol* 1961; 83:57–60.

717. Kieć-Swierczynska M. Occupational contact dermatitis in the workers employed in production of Texas textiles. *Dermatosen* 1982; 30:41–43.

718. Kieć-Swierczynska M, Polakowska B. Haut-Muskel-Atrophie bei Musikern. *Prezegl Dermatol* 1986; 73:290 [reviewed in *Dermatosen*].

719. Kirschner EM. Boomers' quest for agelessness. *Chem Eng News* March 3, 1997:19.

720. Kirton V, Wilkinson DS. Rubber band dermatitis in post office sorters. *Contact Dermatitis Newslett* 1972; 11:257–260.

721. Kleine-Natrop HE, Richter G. Arbeitsdermatosen in der pharmazeutischen Industrie. *Dermatosen* 1980; 28:8–10.

722. Kleinhans D. Contact urticaria to rubber gloves. *Contact Dermatitis* 1984; 10:124–125.

723. Knight TE, Boll P, Epstein WL, Prasad AK. Resorcinols and catechols: A clinical study of cross-sensitivity. *Am J Contact Dermatitis* 1996; 7:138–145.

724. Knight TE, Hausen BM. Koa wood (*Acacia koa*) dermatitis. *Am J Contact Dermatitis* 1992; 3:30–32.

725. Knight TE, Hausen BM. Melaleuca oil (tea tree oil) dermatitis. *J Am Acad Dermatol* 1994; 30:423–427.

726. Knight TE, Whitesell CD. *Grevillea robusta* (silver oak) dermatitis. *Am J Contact Dermatitis* 1992; 3:145–149.

727. Koch P. Occupational allergic contact dermatitis from oleyl alcohol and monoethanolamine in a metalworking fluid. *Contact Dermatitis* 1995; 33:273.

728. Koch P. Occupational allergic contact dermatitis and airborne contact dermatitis from 6 fungicides in a vineyard worker. Cross reactions between fungicides of the dithiocarbamate group. *Contact Dermatitis* 1996; 34:324–329.

729. Koch P, Nickolaus G, Geier J. Kontaktallergien bei Lederherstellern, Lederverarbeitern und in der Schuhindustrie. *Dermatosen* 1996; 44:257–262.

730. Koh D. An outbreak of occupational dermatosis in an electronics store. *Contact Dermatitis* 1995; 32:327–330.

731. Koh D, Aw TC, Foulds IS. Fiberglass dermatitis from printed circuit boards. *Am J Ind Med* 1992; 21:193–198.

732. Koh D, Foulds IS, Aw TC. Dermatological hazards in the electronics industry. *Contact Dermatitis* 1990; 22:1–7.

733. Koh D, Goh CI, Jeyaratnam J, et al. Dermatologic complaints among visual display unit operators and office workers. Letter to the Editor. *Am J Contact Dermatitis* 1991; 2:136–137.

734. Kokelj F, Patussi V, Basei R, et al. Contact dermatitis to Loctite 221 and 270. *Contact Dermatitis* 1987; 17:51.

735. Koppula SV, Fellman JH, Storrs FJ. Screening allergens for acrylate dermatitis associated with artificial nails. *Am J Contact Dermatitis* 1995; 6:78–85.

736. Kozuka T, Tashiro M, Sano S, et al. Pigmented contact dermatitis from azo dyes. *Contact Dermatitis* 1980; 6:330–336.

737. Krook B, Fregert S, Gruvberger B. Chromate and cobalt eczema due to magnetic tapes. *Contact Dermatitis* 1977; 3:60–61.

738. Krook G. Occupational dermatitis from *Lactuca sativa*

(lettuce) and *Cichorium* (endive). *Contact Dermatitis* 1977; 3:27–36.

739. Kulenkamp D, Hausen BM, Schulz K-H. Kontaktallergie durch neurartige, zahnartlich verwendete Abduckmaterialien. *Hautartz* 1977; 28:353–358.

740. Kullavanijaya P, Ophaswongse S. A study of dermatitis in the lacquerware industry. *Contact Dermatitis* 1997; 36:244–246.

741. Kumar A, Freeman S. Photoallergic contact dermatitis in a pig farmer caused by olaquindox. *Contact Dermatitis* 1996; 35:249–250.

742. Kwangsukstith C, Maibach HI. Contact urticaria from polyurethane-membrane hypoallergenic gloves. *Contact Dermatitis* 1995; 33:200–201.

743. LaChapelle JM. Occupational airborne irritant contact dermatitis to slag. *Contact Dermatitis* 1984; 10:315–316.

744. LaChapelle JM. Occupational allergic contact dermatitis to povidone-iodine. *Contact Dermatitis* 1984; 11:189–190.

745. LaChapelle JM, Lauwerys R, Tennstedt D, et al. Eau de Javel and prevention of chromate allergy in France. *Contact Dermatitis* 1980; 6:107–110.

746. LaChapelle JM, Tennstedt D, Cromphaut P. Pseudofolliculitis of the beard and "fiddler's neck." *Contact Dermatitis* 1984; 10:247.

747. Lacroix M, Burkel J, Foussereau JE, et al. Irritant dermatitis from diallyglycol carbonate monomer in the optical industry. *Contact Dermatitis* 1976; 2:183–195.

748. LaDage LH. Facial irritation from ethylene oxide sterilization of anesthesia masks. *Plast Reconstr Surg* 1970; 45:179.

749. Lagiere F, Vervloet D, Lhermet I, et al. Prevalence of latex allergy in operating room nurses. *J Allergy Clin Immunol* 1992; 90:319–322.

750. Lahti A. Contact urticaria and respiratory symptoms from tulips and lilies. *Contact Dermatitis* 1986; 14:317–318.

751. Lahti A, Hannuksela M. Hypersensitivity to apple and carrot can be reliably detected with fresh material. *Allergy* 1978; 33:143–146.

752. Lama L, Vanni D, Barone M, et al. Occupational dermatitis to chloroacetamide. *Contact Dermatitis* 1986; 15:243.

753. LaMarte FP, Merchant JA, Casule TB. Acute systemic reactions to carbonless copy paper associated with histamine release. *JAMA* 1988; 260:242–243.

754. Lamb JH, Lain ES. Occurrence of contact dermatitis from oil soluble gasoline dyes. *J Invest Dermatol* 1951; 17:141–146.

755. Lamminpaa A, Estlander T, Jolanki R, Kanerva L. Occupational allergic contact dermatitis caused by decorative plants. *Contact Dermatitis* 1996; 34:330–335.

756. Landeck E. Lippenlesionen bei Blechblasinstrumentalisten. *Derm Mschr* 1974; 160: 762–765.

757. Lange CE, Jühe S, Stein G, et al. Scleroderma in persons handling pesticides. *Int Arch Arbeitsmed* 1974; 32:1–3.

758. Langman JM. D-Limonene: Is it a safe, effective alternative to xylene? *J Histotechnol* 1995; 18:131–137.

759. Larko O, Diffey BL. Occupational exposure to ultraviolet radiation in dermatology departments. *Br J Dermatol* 1986; 114:479–484.

760. Larko O, Lindstedt G, Lundberg P-A, et al. Biochemical and clinical studies in a case of contact urticaria to potato. *Contact Dermatitis* 1983; 9:108–114.

761. Larsen W, Nakayama H, Lindberg M, et al. Fragrance contact dermatitis: A worldwide multicenter investigation (part 1). *Am J Contact Dermatitis* 1996; 7:77–83.

762. Larsen WG. Detection of allergic dermatitis to fragrances. *Acta Derm Venereol (Stockh)* 1987; 134:83–86.

763. Larsen WG, Maibach HI. Fragrance contact allergy. *Semin Dermatol* 1982; 1:85–90.

764. Laurell H. Contact allergy to tertiary-butyl-catechol. *Contact Dermatitis* 1984; 10:115.

765. Lear JT, Heagerty HM, Tan BB, et al. Transient re-emergence of oil of turpentine allergy in the pottery industry. *Contact Dermatitis* 1996; 35:169–172.

766. Leavell UW, Philips IA. Milker's nodules. *Arch Dermatol* 1975; 111:1307–1311.

767. Le Coz C, Boos V, Cribier B, et al. An unusual case of mercurial baboon syndrome. *Contact Dermatitis* 1996; 35:112.

768. Lee HS, Goh CL. Occupational dermatosis among chrome platers. *Contact Dermatitis* 1988; 18:89–93.

769. Leenutaphong V, Goerz G. Allergic contact dermatitis from chloroacetophenone (tear gas). *Contact Dermatitis* 1989; 20:316.

770. Leinster P, Baum JM, Baxter PJ. An assessment of exposure to glutaraldehyde in hospitals: Typical exposure levels and recommended control measures. *Br J Ind Med* 1993; 50:107–111.

771. Leow Y-H, Ng S-K, Wong W-K, Goh C-L. Contact allergic potential of topical traditional Chinese medicaments in Singapore. *Am J Contact Dermatitis* 1995; 6:4–8.

772. Lerman L, Ribak J, Skulsky M, et al. An outbreak of irritant contact dermatitis from ethylene oxide among pharmaceutical workers. *Contact Dermatitis* 1995; 33:280–281.

773. Lewis PG, Emmett EA. Irritant dermatitis from tri-butyl tin oxide and contact allergy from chlorocresol. *Contact Dermatitis* 1987; 17:129–132.

774. Levin HM, Brunner MJ, Rattner H. Lithographer's dermatitis. *JAMA* 1959; 169:566–569.

775. Lezuan A, Marcos C, Martin JA. Contact dermatitis from natural latex. *Contact Dermatitis* 1992; 27:334–335.

776. Li L-F. A clinical and patch test study of contact dermatitis from traditional Chinese medicinal materials. *Contact Dermatitis* 1995; 33:392–395.

777. Liden C. Patch testing with soldering fluxes. *Contact Dermatitis* 1984; 10:119–120.

778. Liden C. Contact allergy to the photographic chemical PBA-1. *Contact Dermatitis* 1984; 11:256.

779. Liden C. Occupational dermatoses at a film laboratory. *Contact Dermatitis* 1984; 10:77–87.

780. Liden C. Lichen planus in relation to occupational and non-occupational exposure to chemicals. *Br J Dermatol* 1986; 115:23–31.

781. Liden C. *Occupational Dermatoses from Photographic Chemicals.* Stockholm: Arbets Miljo Institutet; 1988.

782. Liden C. Persulfate Bleach Accelerator—A potent contact allergy in film laboratories: Chemical identification, purity studies, and patch testing. *Am J Contact Dermatol* 1990; 1:21–24.

783. Liden C. Facial dermatitis caused by chlorothalonil in a paint. *Contact Dermatitis* 1990; 22:206–211.

784. Liden C. Occupational dermatoses from photographic chemicals. *Acta Derm Venereol (suppl)* 1990; 141:1–37.

785. Liden C. Contact allergy: A cause of facial dermatitis among visual display unit operators. *Am J Contact Dermatitis* 1990; 1:171–176.

786. Liden C. Cold-impregnated aluminum. A new source of nickel exposure. *Contact Dermatitis* 1994; 31:22–24.

787. Liden C, Berg M, Farm G, Wrangsjo K. Nail varnish allergy with far-reaching consequences. *Br J Dermatol* 1993; 128:57–62.

788. Liden C, Boman A, Hagelthorn G. Flare-up reactions from a chemical used in the film industry. *Contact Dermatitis* 1982; 8:136–137.

789. Liden C, Menne T, Burrows D. Nickel-containing alloys and platings and their ability to cause dermatitis. *Br J Dermatol* 1996; 134:193–198.

790. Liden C, Wahlberg JE. Does visual display terminal work provoke rosacea? *Contact Dermatitis* 1985; 13:235–241.

791. Lindquist R, Nilsson B, Eklund G, et al. Increased risk of developing acute leukemia after employment as a painter. *Cancer* 1987; 60:1378–1384.

792. Lintum JCA, Nater J. Contact dermatitis caused by rubber chemicals in dairy workers. *Dermatosen* 1973; 21:16–22.

793. Lips R, Rast H, Elsner P. Outcome of job change in patients with occupational chromate dermatitis. *Contact Dermatitis* 1996; 34:268–271.

794. Lisboa C, Antonia M, Azenha A. Contact dermatitis from textile dyes. *Contact Dermatitis* 1994; 31:9–10.

795. Lisi P, Caraffini S, Assalve D. Irritation and sensitization potential of pesticides. *Contact Dermatitis* 1987; 17:212–218.

796. Lodi A, Mancini LL, Pozzi M, et al. Occupational airborne allergic contact dermatitis in parquet layers. *Contact Dermatitis* 1993; 29:281–282.

797. Lohiya GS, Lohiya S. Lead poisoning in a radiator repairer. *West J Med* 1995; 162:160–164.

798. Lombardi P, Gola M, Acciae MC, Sertoli A. Unusual occupational allergic contact dermatitis in a nurse. *Contact Dermatitis* 1989; 20:302–303.

799. Lonkar A, Mitchell JC, Calnan CD. Allergic contact dermatitis from *Parthenium hyterophorus*. *Trans St Johns Hosp Dermatol Soc* 1974; 60:43–49.

800. Lovell CR, Rycroft RJG. Contact urticaria from winged bean *(Psophocarpus tetragonolobus)*. *Contact Dermatitis* 1984; 10:314–315.

801. Lovell CR, Rycroft RJG, Vale PT. Irritant contact dermatitis from diallyl glycol carbonate monomer and its prevention. *Contact Dermatitis* 1988; 18:288–286.

802. Lovell CR, Rycroft RJG, Williams DMJ, et al. Contact dermatitis from the irritancy (immediate and delayed) and allergenicity of hydroxypropyl acrylate. *Contact Dermatitis* 1985; 12:117–118.

803. Lübbe D von. Professionelle dinitrochlorbenzol Kontaktdermatitis. *Dermatosen* 1993; 41:19–24.

804. Lucas A. Sensitivity reactions after using chromium reported in an artist. *Dermatol Times* Jan 1983:21.

805. Lück H, Jentsch G. Chromium dermatitis caused by epoxy resin. *Contact Dermatitis* 1988; 19:154–155.

806. Lyde DM. The present status of trivalent chromium plating. *Product Finishing* 1978; 31:9–14.

807. Lyle WH, Spence TWM, McKinneley, et al. Dimethylformamide and alcohol intolerance. *Br J Ind Med* 1979; 36:63–66.

808. Lynde CW, Mitchell JC. Patch test results in 66 hairdressers 1973–81. *Contact Dermatitis* 1982; 8:302–307.

809. MacAulay JC. Orchid allergy. *Contact Dermatitis* 1987; 17:112–113.

810. Machackova J, Pock L. Occupational nickel dermatitis in a cellist. *Contact Dermatitis* 1986; 15:41–42.

811. Mackey SA, Marks JG Jr. Dermatitis in machinists: A retrospective study. *Am J Contact Dermatitis* 1993; 4:22–26.

812. MacKinnon MA. Treatment of hydrofluoric acid burns. *J Occup Med* 1986; 28:804.

813. MacKinnon MA. Hydrofluoric acid burns. In: Taylor JS, ed. *Occupational Dermatoses*. Vol. 6. Philadelphia: W.B. Saunders, Co.; 1988:67–74.

814. Madden JF. Cutaneous hypersensitivity to tear gas (chloroacetophenone). *Arch Dermatol* 1951; 63:133.

815. Madden S, Thiboutot DM, Marks JG Jr. Occupationally induced allergic contact dermatitis to methylchloroisothiazolinone/methylisothiazolinone among machinists. *J Am Acad Dermatol* 1994; 30:272–274.

816. Magnusson B. Sensitizing effect of eurgenol/colophony in surgical dressing. *Contact Dermatitis Newslett* 1974; 15:454–455.

817. Magnusson B. Irritation of the skin and mucous membranes by NCR paper. *Contact Dermatitis Newslett* 1974; 15:450.

818. Magnusson B, Koch G, Nyquist G. Contact allergy to medicaments and materials used in dentistry. *Odontol Revy* 1971; 22(II):275–289.

819. Magnusson B, Koch G, Nyquist G. Contact allergy to medicaments and materials used in dentistry. *Odontol Revy* 1973; 24(IV):109–114.

820. Magnusson B, Mobacken H. Allergic contact dermatitis from acrylic (Dycril) printing plates in a printing plant. *Dermatosen* 1972; 20:138–142.

821. Magnusson B, Mobacken H. Contact allergy to a selfhardening acrylic sealer for assembling metal parts. *Dermatosen* 1972; 20:198–199.

822. Magnusson B, Wilkinson DS. Cinnamic aldehyde in toothpaste. 1. Clinical aspects and patch tests. *Contact Dermatitis* 1975; 1:70–76.

823. Mahajan VK, Sharma VK, Kaur I, Chakrabarti A. Contact dermatitis in agricultural workers: Role of common crops, fodder and weeds. *Contact Dermatitis* 1996; 35:373–374.

824. Maibach H. Scuba diver facial dermatitis: Allergic contact dermatitis to *N*-isopropyl-*N*-phenylparaphenylenediamine. *Contact Dermatitis* 1975; 1:330.

825. Maibach H. Immediate hypersensitivity in hand dermatitis. Role of food-contact dermatitis. *Arch Dermatol* 1976; 112:1289–1291.

826. Maibach HI. Irritation, sensitization, photoirritation and photosensitization assays with a glyphosate herbicide. *Contact Dermatitis* 1986; 15:152–156.

827. Maibach HI, Gellin GA, eds. *Occupational and Industrial Dermatology*. Chicago: Yearbook Medical Publishers; 1982:224.

828. Maizlish N, et al. Mortality among California highway workers. *Am J Ind Med* 1988; 13:363–379.

829. Majoie IML, Bruynzeel DP. Occupational immediate-type hypersensitivity to henna in a hairdresser. *Am J Contact Dermatitis* 1996; 7:38–40.

830. Majoie IML, von Blomberg BME, Bruynzeel DP. Development of hand eczema in junior hairdressers: An 8-year follow-up study. *Contact Dermatitis* 1996; 34:243–247.

831. Malten KE. Eczema in a cotton-printing mill. *Acta Derm Venereol (Stockh)* 1957; 2:353.

832. Malten KE. Occupational eczema due to para-tertiarybutylphenol in a shoe adhesive. *Dermatologica* 1958; 117:103–109.

833. Malten KE. Textile finish contact hypersensitivity. *Arch Dermatol* 1964; 89:215–221.

834. Malten KE. Contact sensitization to Letterflex urethane photoprepolymer mixture used in printing. *Contact Dermatitis* 1977; 3:115–121.

835. Malten KE. 4,4'-Diisocyanatodicyclohexyl methane (Hylene W): A strong contact sensitizer. *Contact Dermatitis* 1977; 3:344–346.

836. Malten KE. Four bakers showing positive patch tests to a number of fragrance materials which can be used in flavors. *Acta Derm Venereol (Stockh)* 1979; 59 (suppl 85):117–121.

837. Malten KE, Bende WJM. 2-Hydroxy-ethylmethacrylate and di- and tetraethylene glycol dimethacrylate. *Contact Dermatitis* 1979; 5:214–220.

838. Malten KE, den Arend JACJ, Wiggers RE. Delayed irritation: Hexanediol diacrylate and butanediol diacrylate. *Contact Dermatitis* 1979; 5:178–184.

839. Malten KE, Meer-Roosen CH, Seutter E. Nyloprint-sensitive patients react to *N,N'*-methylene bis acrylamide. *Contact Dermatitis* 1978; 4:214–222.

840. Malten KE, Seutter E. Phenolformaldehyde resin in paper. *Contact Dermatitis* 1984; 11:127–128.

841. Mancuso G, Berdondini RM. Contact urticaria from dog saliva. *Contact Dermatitis* 1992; 26:133.

842. Mancuso G, Reggiani M, Berdondini RM. Occupational dermatitis in shoemakers. *Contact Dermatitis* 1996; 34:17–22.

843. Mandel EH. Lichen planus–like eruption caused by color developer. *Arch Dermatol* 1960; 81:516–519.

844. Manzini BM, Motolese A, Conti A, et al. Sensitization to reactive textile dyes in patients with contact dermatitis. *Contact Dermatitis* 1996; 34:172–175.

845. Marcussen PV. Occupational nickel dermatitis: Rise in incidence and prevention. *Acta Derm Venereol* (Stockh) 1957; 2:289–295.

846. Marks J, DeMelfi T, McCarthy A, et al. Dermatitis from cashew nuts. *J Am Acad Dermatol* 1984; 10:627–631.

847. Marks JG Jr. Allergic contact dermatitis from carbonless carbon paper. *JAMA* 1981; 245:2331–2332.

848. Marks JG. Dermatologic problems of office workers. In: Taylor JS, ed. *Dermatologic Clinics.* Philadelphia: W.B. Saunders, Co.; 1988:75–79.

849. Marks JG Jr. Allergic contact dermatitis to *Alstroemeria. Arch Dermatol* 1988; 124:914–915.

850. Marks JG Jr. Allergic contact dermatitis to povidone-iodine. *J Am Acad Dermatol* 1982; 6:473–475.

851. Marks JG Jr., Rainey CM, Rainey MA, et al. Dermatoses among poultry workers. "Chicken poison disease." *J Am Acad Dermatol* 1983; 9:852–857.

852. Marks JG, Traulei JJ, Zwillich CW, et al. Contact urticaria and airway obstruction from carbonless copy paper. *JAMA* 1984; 252:1038–1040.

853. Marques C, Goncalo M, Goncalo S. Sensitivity to para-tertiary-butylphenol–formaldehyde resin in Portugal. *Contact Dermatitis* 1994; 30:300–301.

854. Marshman G, Kennedy CTC. Guitar-string dermatitis. *Contact Dermatitis* 1992; 26:134.

855. Martins C, Goncalo M, Goncalo S. Allergic contact dermatitis from dipentene in wax polish. *Contact Dermatitis* 1995; 33:126–127.

856. Marzulli FN, Maibach HI. Antimicrobials: Experimental contact sensitization in man. *J Soc Cosmet Chemists* 1973; 24:399–421.

857. Massmanian A, Cavero FV, Bosca AR, et al. Contact dermatitis from variegated ivy (*Hedera helix* subsp. *canariensis* Willd.). *Contact Dermatitis* 1988; 18:247–248.

858. Massone L, Anonide A, Isola V, Borghi S. Two cases of multiple azo dye sensitization. *Contact Dermatitis* 1991; 24:60–61.

859. Mathelier-Fusage P, Aissaoui M, Chabane MH, et al. Chronic generalized eczema caused by multiple dye sensitization. *Am J Contact Dermatitis* 1996; 7:224–225.

860. Mathew SN, Melton AL Jr. Wagner WO. Latex hypersensitivity: A case study. *Ann Allergy* 1993; 70:483–486.

861. Mathias CGT. Contact dermatitis from cyanide plating solutions. *Arch Dermatol* 1982; 118:420–422.

862. Mathias CGT. Contact dermatitis to a new biocide (Tektamer 38) used in a paste glue formulation. *Contact Dermatitis* 1983; 9:418–435.

863. Mathias CGT. Allergic contact dermatitis from tryglycidyl isocyanurate in polyester paint pigments. *Contact Dermatitis* 1988; 19:67–68.

864. Mathias CGT, Adams RM. Allergic contact dermatitis from rosin used as soldering flux. *J Am Acad Dermatol* 1984; 10:454–456.

865. Mathias CGT, Andersen KE, Hamann K. Allergic contact dermatitis from 2-*n*-octyl 4-isothiazolin-3-one, a paint mildewcide. *Contact Dermatitis* 1983; 9:507–509.

866. Mathias CGT, Caldwell TM, Maibach HI. Contact dermatitis and GI symptoms from hydroxyethylmethacrylate. *Br J Dermatol* 1979; 100:447–449.

867. Mathias CGT, Maibach HI. Allergic contact dermatitis from anaerobic acrylic sealants. *Arch Dermatol* 1984; 120:1202–1205.

868. Mathias CGT, Morrison JH. Occupational skin diseases, United States: Results from the Bureau of Labor Statistics Annual Survey of Occupational Injuries and Illnesses, 1973 through 1984. *Arch Dermatol* 1988; 124:1519–1524.

869. Matikainen E, Leinonen H, Juntunen J, et al. The effect of exposure to high and low frequency hand-arm vibration on finger systolic pressure. *Eur J Appl Physiol* 1987; 56:440–443.

870. Matsunaga K, Hosokawa K, Suzuki M, et al. Occupational allergic contact dermatitis in beauticians. *Contact Dermatitis* 1988; 18:94–96.

871. Matsunaga K, Hayakawa R, Yoshimura K, et al. Patch-test–positive reactions to Solvent Red 23 in hairdressers. *Contact Dermatitis* 1990; 23:266.

872. Matsushita S, Kanekura T, Saruwatari K, Kanzaki T. Photoallergic contact dermatitis due to Daconil. *Contact Dermatitis* 1996; 35:115–116.

873. Matsushita T, Nomura S, Wakatsuki T. Epidemiology of contact dermatitis from pesticides in Japan. *Contact Dermatitis* 1980; 6:255–259.

874. Matthieu L, Weyler J, Deckers I, et al. Occupational contact sensitization to ethylenediamine in a wire-drawing factory. *Contact Dermatitis* 1993; 29:39–51.

875. Matura M, Poesen N, de Moor A, et al. Glycidyl methacrylate and ethoxyethyl acrylate: New allergens in emulsions used to impregnate paper and textile materials. *Contact Dermatitis* 1995; 33:123–124.

876. Maurer T, Meier F. Sensitization potential of benzotriazole. *Contact Dermatitis* 1984; 10:163–165.

877. Mazini BM, Donini M, Motolese A, Seidenari S. A study of 5 newly patch-tested reactive textile dyes. *Contact Dermatitis* 1996; 35:313.

878. McCunney RJ. Diverse manifestations of trichloroethylene. *Br J Ind Med* 1988; 45:122–126.

879. McCunney RJ, et al. Occupational illness in the arts. *Am Fam Phys* 1987; 36:145–153.

880. McDaniel WR, Marks JG. Contact urticaria due to sensitivity to spray starch. *Arch Dermatol* 1979; 115:628.

881. McFadden JP, Rycroft RJG. Occupational contact dermatitis from triglycidyl isocyanurate in a powder paint sprayer. *Contact Dermatitis* 1993; 28:251.

882. McGeown G. Cement burns of the hand. *Contact Dermatitis* 1984; 10:246.

883. McLaughlin JK, et al. Malignant melanoma in the printing industry. *Am J Ind Med* 1988; 13:301–304.

884. Meding B. Allergic contact dermatitis from diethylenetriamine in a goldsmith workshop. *Contact Dermatitis* 1982; 8:142.

885. Meding B. Immediate hypersensitivity to mustard and rape. *Contact Dermatitis* 1985; 13:121–122.

886. Meding B. Contact dermatitis from tetrachloroisophthalonitrile in paint. *Contact Dermatitis* 1986; 15:187.

887. Meding B. Occupational contact dermatitis from ter-

tiary-butylhydroquinone (TBHQ) in a cutting fluid. *Contact Dermatitis* 1996; 34:224.

888. Meding B, Ahman M, Karlberg A-T. Skin symptoms and contact allergy in woodwork teachers. *Contact Dermatitis* 1996; 34:185–190.

889. Meding B, Fregert S. Contact urticaria from natural latex gloves. *Contact Dermatitis* 1984; 10:52–53.

890. Meding B, Karlberg A-T, Ahman M. Wood dust from jelutong *(Dyera costulata)* causes contact allergy. *Contact Dermatitis* 1996; 34:349–353.

891. Meding B, Toren K, Karlberg A-T, et al. Evaluation of skin symptoms among workers at a Swedish paper mill. *Am J Ind Med* 1993; 23:721–728.

892. Melli MC, Giorgini S, Sertoli A. Occupational dermatitis in a bee keeper. *Contact Dermatitis* 1983; 9:427–428.

893. Menck HR. Occupational differences in rate of lung cancer. *J Occup Med* 1976; 18:797–801.

894. Menné T, Asnaes G, Hjorth N. Skin and mucous membrane problems from "no carbon required" paper. *Contact Dermatitis* 1981; 7:72–76.

895. Menné T. Nickel allergy. Thesis. Gentofte Hospital Hellerup, Copenhagen, Denmark, 1983.

896. Menter P, Harrison W, Woodin WG. Patch testing of coolant fractions. *J Occup Med* 1975; 17:565–568.

897. Milković-Kraus S, Macan J. Can pre-employment patch testing help to prevent occupational contact allergy? *Contact Dermatitis* 1996; 35:226–228.

898. Miller EG. Prevalence of mercury hypersensitivity in dental students. *J Prosth Dent* 1987; 58:235–237.

899. Miller MM, Goldberg HS, Wilkerson WG. Allergic contact dermatitis to 1,4-bis(isopropylamino) anthraquinone. *Arch Dermatol* 1978; 114:1793–1794.

900. Mitchell J, Rook A. *Botanical Dermatology.* Vancouver BC: Greengrass; 1979:699.

901. Mitchell JC. Contact sensitivity to *Tulipa* and *Alstroemeria.* *Contact Dermatitis Newslett* 1974; 16:506.

902. Mitchell JC. Contact sensitivity to garlic *(Allium).* *Contact Dermatitis* 1980; 6:356–357.

903. Mitchell JC. Industrial aspects of 112 cases of allergic contact dermatitis from *Frullania* in British Columbia during a 10 year period. *Contact Dermatitis* 1981; 7:268–269.

904. Mitchell JC. *Frullania* (liverwort) phytodermatitis (woodcutter's eczema). *Clin Dermatol* 1986; 4:62–64.

905. Mitchell JC, Armitage JS. Dermatitis venenata from lichens. *Arch Environ Health* 1965; 11:701–709.

906. Mitchell JC, Maibach HI. Difficulties to investigate dermatitis from plants. A practical approach to office-based diagnosis. *Dermatosen* 1996; 44:29–33.

907. Mitchell JNS. Plant dermatitis. In Cronin E, ed. *Contact Dermatitis.* Edinburgh: Churchill-Livingstone; 1980:518.

908. MMWR. Case control study of HIV seroconversion in health-care workers after percutaneous exposure to HIV-infected blood—France, United Kingdom, and United States. *MMWR* 1995; 44:929–933.

909. Molhave L, Grunnet K. Headspace analysis of gases and vapors emitted by carbonless paper. *Contact Dermatitis* 1981; 7:76.

910. Møller NE, Nielsen B, von Wurden K. Contact dermatitis to semisynthetic penicillins in factory workers. *Contact Dermatitis* 1986; 14:307–311.

911. Moneret-Vautrin D-A, Beaudouin E, Widmer S, et al. Prospective study of risk factors in natural rubber latex hypersensitivity. *J Allergy Clin Immunol* 1993; 92:668–677.

912. Monti M, Berti E, Carminati G, et al. Occupational and cosmetic dermatitis from propolis. *Contact Dermatitis* 1983; 2:161.

913. Monti M, Berti E, Cavicchini S, et al. Unusual cutaneous reaction after a gold chloride patch test. *Contact Dermatitis* 1983; 9:150–151.

914. Moore RM Jr., Davis YM, Kaczmarek RG. An overview of occupational hazards among veterinarians, with particular reference to pregnant women. *Am Ind Hyg Assoc J* 1993; 54:113–120.

915. Morgan JWW, Orsler RJ, Wilkinson DS. Dermatitis due to wood dusts of *Khaya anthotheca* and *Machaerium scleroxylon.* *Br J Ind Med* 1968; 25:119–125.

916. Moroni P, Tomasini M. Contact leukoderma induced by occupational contact with fibre-glass and polyester resins with quinones and tertiary butylcatechol. *Dermatosen* 1992; 40:195–197.

917. Morren M-A, Janssens V, Dooms-Goosens A, et al. α-Amylase, a flour additive: An important cause of protein contact dermatitis in bakers. *J Am Acad Dermatol* 1993; 29:723–728.

918. Morrison LH, Storrs FJ. Persistence of an allergen in hair after glyceryl monothioglycolate–containing permanent wave solutions. *J Am Acad Dermatol* 1988; 19:52–59.

919. Mueller EJ, Seger D. Metal fume fever—A review. *J Emerg Med* 1985; 2:271–274.

920. Munro-Ashman D, Munro DD, Hughes TH. Contact dermatitis from palladium. *St Johns Hosp Dermatol Soc* 1969; 55:196–197.

921. Munroe CS, Lawrence CM. Occupational contact dermatitis from triglycidyl isocyanurate in a powder paint factory. *Contact Dermatitis* 1992; 26:59.

922. Mürer AJL, Poulsen OM, Tuchsen F, Roed-Petersen J. Rapid increase in skin problems among dental technician trainees working with acrylates. *Contact Dermatitis* 1995; 33:106–111.

923. Mutti A, et al. Exposure–effect and exposure–response relationships between occupational exposure to styrene and neuropsychological functions. *Am J Ind Med* 1984; 5:275–286.

924. Nakagawa M, Kawai K, Kawai K. Multiple azo disperse dye sensitization mainly due to group sensitizations to azo dyes. *Contact Dermatitis* 1996; 34:6–11.

925. Nakamura T. Tobacco dermatitis in Japanese harvesters. *Contact Dermatitis* 1984; 10:310.

926. Nakayama H. Hypersensitivity to palladium is linked to oral lichen planus. *Dermatol News* February 1982.

927. Nakayama H, Harada R, Toda M. Pigmented cosmetic dermatitis. *Int J Dermatol* 1976; 15:673–675.

928. Nakayama H, Niki F, Shono M, Hada S. Mercury exanthem. *Contact Dermatitis* 1983; 9:411–417.

929. Nater JP. Allergic contact dermatitis due to potassium metabilsulfite in developers. *Dermatolgica* 1968; 136:477–478.

930. Nater JP, de Groot AC. *Unwanted Effects of Cosmetics and Drugs Used in Dermatology*, 2nd ed. Amsterdam: Elsevier; 1985.

931. Nater JP, Gooskens VH. Occupational dermatosis due to a soil fumigant. *Contact Dermatitis* 1976; 2:227–229.

932. Nater JP, Terpstra H, Bleumink E. Allergic contact sensitization to the fungicide Maneb. *Contact Dermatitis* 1979; 5:24–26.

933. Natow AJ. Henna. 1986; *Cutis* 37:21.

934. Neering H. Contact urticaria from chlorinated swimming pool water. *Contact Dermatitis* 1977; 3:279.

935. Neldner KH. Contact dermatitis from animal feed additives. *Arch Dermatol* 1972; 106:722–723.

936. Nethercott JR. Skin problems associated with multifunctional acrylic monomers in ultraviolet curing inks. *Br J Dermatol* 1978; 98:541–552.

937. Nethercott JR. Allergic contact dermatitis due to an epoxy acrylate. *Br J Dermatol* 1981; 104:697–703.

938. Nethercott JR. Dermatitis in the printing industry. *Dermatol Clin* 1988; 6:61–66.

939. Nethercott JR, Albers J, Guirguis S, et al. Erythema multiforme exudativum linked to the manufacture of printed circuit boards. *Contact Dermatitis* 1982; 8:314–322.

940. Nethercott JR, Holness DL, Page E. Occupational contact dermatitis due to glutaraldehyde in health care workers. *Contact Dermatitis* 1988; 18:193–196.

941. Nethercott JR, Holness DZ. Dermatologic problems of musicians. *J Am Acad Dermatol* 1991; 25:870.

942. Nethercott JR, Jakubovic HR, Pilger C, et al. Allergic contact dermatitis due to urethane acrylate in ultraviolet-cured inks. *Br J Ind Med* 1983; 40:241–250.

943. Nethercott JR, MacPherson M, Choi BCK, et al. Contact dermatitis in hairdressers. *Contact Dermatitis* 1986; 14:73–79.

944. Nethercott JR, Nosal R. Contact dermatitis in printing tradesmen. *Contact Dermatitis* 1986; 14:280–287.

945. Nethercott JR, Rothman N, Holness DL, et al. Health problems in metal workers exposed to a coolant oil containing Kathon 886 MW. *Am J Contact Dermatitis* 1990; 1:94–99.

946. Newhouse M, McEvoy D, Rosenthal D. Percutaneous Paraquat absorption. *Arch Dermatol* 1978; 114:1516–1519.

947. Newhouse ML. Epidemiology of skin disease in an automobile factory. *Br J Ind Med* 1964; 21:287–293.

948. Newhouse ML. Dermatitis in a clothing factory. *Contact Dermatitis Newslett* 1974; 16:478–480.

949. Nielsen H. Occupational exposure to isothiazolinones. *Contact Dermatitis* 1994; 31:18–21.

950. Niinimäki A, Hassi J. An outbreak of epoxy dermatitis in insulation workers at an electric power station. *Dermatosen* 1983; 31:23–25.

951. Niklasson B, Bjorkner B, Hansen L. Occupational contact dermatitis from antitumor agent intermediates. *Contact Dermatitis* 1990; 22:233–234.

952. Nilsen A. Facial rash in visual display unit operators. *Contact Dermatitis* 1982; 8:25–28.

953. Nilsson E, Mikaelsson B, Andersson S. Atopy, occupation and domestic work as risk factors for hand eczema in hospital workers. *Contact Dermatitis* 1985; 13:216–223.

954. NIOSH. Health Hazard Report 80–6–667. Washington, DC: U.S. Department of Health, Education and Welfare, Public Health Service; October 15, 1979.

955. NIOSH. 2,3,7,8-Tetrachlorodibenzo-*p*-dioxin (TCDD, "dioxin"). *Curr Intelligence Bull* 40, January 23, 1984.

956. NIOSH. Cadmium. *Curr Intelligence Bull* 42, September 27, 1984.

957. Nishioka K, Murata M, Ishikawa T, et al. Contact dermatitis due to rubber boots worn by Japanese farmers, with special attention to 6-ethoxy-2,2,4-trimethyl-1,2-dihydroquinoline (ETMDQ) sensitivity. *Contact Dermatitis* 1996; 35:241–245.

958. Nishioka K, Ogasawara M, Asagami C. Occupational contact allergy to triglycidyl isocyanurate (TGIC, Tepic). *Contact Dermatitis* 1988; 19:379–380.

959. Nutter AF. Contact urticaria to rubber. *Br J Dermatol* 1979; 101:597–598.

960. Okuno T. Measurement of ultraviolet radiation from welding arcs. *Ind Health* 1987; 25:147–165.

961. Olivarius F de Fine, Menné T. Contact dermatitis from metallic palladium in patients reacting to palladium chloride. *Contact Dermatitis* 1992; 27:71–73.

962. O'Malley MA, Barba R. Bullous dermatitis in field workers associated with exposure to mayweed. *Am J Contact Dermatitis* 1990; 1:34–42.

963. O'Malley MA, Carpenter AV, Sweeney MH, et al. Chloracne associated with employment in the production of pentachlorophenol. *Am J Ind Med* 1990; 17:411–421.

964. O'Malley MA, Rodriguez P, Adams RM. Pilot study for evaluation of contact dermatitis in California nursery workers. Submitted for publication.

965. O'Reilly FM, Murphy GM. Occupational contact dermatitis in a beautician. *Contact Dermatitis* 1996; 35:47–48.

966. Orth G, Jablonska S, Favre M, et al. Identification of papillomaviruses in butcher's warts. *J Invest Dermatol* 1981; 76:97–102.

967. Osawa J, et al. A probable role for vaccines containing thimerosal in thimerosal hypersensitivity. *Contact Dermatitis* 1991; 24:178–182.

968. Osmundsen PE. Contact dermatitis due to sodium hypochlorite. *Contact Dermatitis* 1978; 4:177–178.

969. Osmundsen PE. Contact dermatitis to chlorhexidine. *Contact Dermatitis* 1982; 8:81–83.

970. Pambor M. Contact dermatitis due to ammonium bisulfite in a bleaching cream. *Contact Dermatitis* 1996; 35:48–49.

971. Pambor M, Poweleit H. Allergic contact dermatitis due to diazo copy paper. *Contact Dermatitis* 1992; 26:131–132.

972. Panconesi E, Sertoli A, Fabbri P, et al. Anaphylactic shock from mustard after ingestion of pizza. *Contact Dermatitis* 1980; 6:294–295.

973. Panconesi E, Sertoli A, Spallanzani P, et al. Balsam of Peru sensitivity from a perfumed cutting fluid in a laser factory. *Contact Dermatitis* 1980; 6:197.

974. Parslew R, King CM, Evans S. Primary sensitization to a single accidental exposure to a flame retardant and subsequent allergic contact dermatitis. *Contact Dermatitis* 1995; 33:286.

975. Pasricha JS, Gupta R, Panjwani S. Contact dermatitis to henna *(Lawsonia) Contact Dermatitis* 1980; 6:288–289.

976. Paulsen E, Andersen KE, Hausen BM. Compositae dermatitis in a Danish dermatology department in one year (1). Results of routine patch testing with the sesquiterpene lactone mix supplemented with aimed patch testing with extracts and sesquiterpene lactones of the Compositae plants. *Contact Dermatitis* 1993; 29:6–10.

977. Pazzaglia M, Vincenzi C, Gasparri F, Tosti A. Occupational hypersensitivity to isothiazolinone derivatives in a radiology technician. *Contact Dermatitis* 1996; 34:143.

978. Peachey RDG, Matthews CNA. "Fiddler's neck." *Br J Dermatol* 1978; 98:669–674.

979. Pecegueiro M. Airborne contact dermatitis to tobacco. *Contact Dermatitis* 1987; 17:50–51.

980. Pecegueiro M. Contact dermatitis due to nickel in fertilizers. *Contact Dermatitis* 1990; 22:114–115.

981. Pecquet C, Leynadier F, Dry J. Contact urticaria and anaphylaxis to natural latex. *J Am Acad Dermatol* 1990; 22:631–633.

982. Pedersen NB. Occupational allergy from 1,2-benzisothiazolin-3-one and other preservatives in plastic emulsions. *Contact Dermatitis* 1976; 2:340–342.

983. Pedersen NB. Topical treatment of a "ruster" (correspondence). *Br J Dermatol* 1977; 96:332.

984. Pedersen NB. Allergy from NAPP. *Contact Dermatitis* 1980; 6:35.

985. Pedersen NB. Edema of fingers from hydrogen fluoride containing aluminium blancher. *Contact Dermatitis* 1980; 6:41.

986. Pedersen NB, Fregert S. Occupational allergic contact dermatitis from chloracetamide in glue. *Contact Dermatitis* 1976; 2:122–123.

987. Pedersen NB, Senning A, Nielsen A. Different sensitizing acrylic monomers in Napp printing plates. *Contact Dermatitis* 1983; 9:459–464.

988. Pedersen NB, Thormann J, Senning A. Occupational contact allergy to bis-(4-chlorophenyl)-methyl chloride. *Contact Dermatitis* 1980; 6:56.

989. Pegum J, Medhurst FA. Contact dermatitis from penetration of rubber gloves by acrylic monomer. *BMJ* 1971; 2:141–143.

990. Pelmear PL, Roos JO, Maehle WM. Occupationally-induced scleroderma. *J Occup Med* 1992; 34:20–25.

991. Peltonen L, Wickström G, Vaahtoranta M. Occupational dermatoses in the food industry. *Dermatosen* 1985; 33:166–169.

992. Peltonen L, Fraki J. Prevalence of dichromate sensitivity. *Contact Dermatitis* 1983; 9:190–194.

993. Penagos H, Jimenez V, Fallas V, et al. Chlorothalonil, a possible cause of erythema dyschromicum perstans (ashy dermatitis). *Contact Dermatitis* 1996; 35:214–218.

994. Pennys NS, Israel RM, Indgin SM. Contact dermatitis due to 1-chloroacetophenone and chemical mace. *N Engl J Med* 1969; 281:413–415.

995. Perone VB, Moffitt AE, Possick PA, et al. The chromium cobalt and nickel contents of American cement and their relationship to cement dermatitis. *Am Ind Hyg Assoc J* 1974; 35:301–306.

996. Perrenoud D, Homberger HP, Augerset PC, et al. An epidemic outbreak of papular and follicular contact dermatitis to tocopheryl linoleate in cosmetics. *Dermatology* 1994; 189:225–233.

997. Peters K-P, Frosch PJ, Uter W, et al. Typ IV-allergien auf Friseurberufsstoffe. *Dermatosen* 1994; 42:50–57.

998. Peuter M de Clerq, Minette A, Lachapelle JM. An epidemiological survey of virus warts of the hands among butchers. *Br J Dermatol* 1977; 96:427–431.

999. Phillips TJ, Rogers GS, Kanj LF. Bacitracin anaphylaxis. *J Geriatr Dermatol* 1995; 3:83–85.

1000. Phoon WH, Magdalene OY, Chan V, et al. Stevens-Johnson syndrome associated with occupational exposure to trichloroethylene. *Contact Dermatitis* 1984; 10:270–276.

1001. Pigatto PD, Riva F, Altomare GF, et al. Short-term anaphylactic antibodies in contact urticaria and generalized anaphylaxis to apple. *Contact Dermatitis* 1983; 9:511.

1002. Piletta PA, Hausen BM, Pasche-Koo F, et al. Allergic contact dermatitis to East-Indian rosewood (*Dalbergia latifolia* Roxb.). *J Am Acad Dermatol* 1996; 34:298–300.

1003. Pinola A, Estlander T, Jolanki R, et al. Occupational allergic contact dermatitis due to coconut diethanolamide (cocamide DEA). *Contact Dermatitis* 1993; 29:262–265.

1004. Pirila V. On occupational diseases of the skin among paint factory workers, painters, polishers and varnishers in Finland. *Acta Derm Venereol* (Stockh) 1947; (suppl 16):1–163.

1005. Pirila V. Sensitization to cobalt in pottery workers. *Acta Derm Venereol (Stockh)* 1953; 33:193–198.

1006. Pirila V. Über Kobaltallergie bei Porzellanarbeitern. *Hautartz* 1964; 15:491–493.

1007. Pirila V, Kajanne H. Sensitization to cobalt and nickel in cement eczema. *Acta Derm Venereol* 1965; 45:14.

1007a. Pirila V, Pirila C. Sensitization to the neomycin group of antibiotics. *Acta Derm Venereol* 1966; 46:489–496.

1008. Plack W, Belliti R. Generalized argyria after chewing photographic film. *Oral Surg* 1980; 49:504.

1009. Prahl P, Roed-Petersen J. Type I allergy from cows in veterinary surgeons. *Contact Dermatitis* 1979; 5:33–38.

1010. Price VH. Double-blind, placebo-controlled evaluation of topical minoxidil in extensive alopecia areata. *J Am Acad Dermatol* 1987; 16:730–736.

1011. Proctor NH, Hughes JP, Fischman ML. Chemical Hazards in the Workplace, 2nd ed. Philadelphia: J.B. Lippincott, 1988:132.

1012. Prout J. Allergic dermatitis due to aniline dye additive. *Proc R Soc Med* 1973; 66:261.

1013. Puig L, Alomar A, Randazzo L, Cuatrecases M. Erythema multiformlike reaction caused by topical application of *Thuja* essential oil. *Am J Contact Dermatitis* 1994; 5:94–97.

1014. Pye RJ, Peachey RDG. Contact dermatitis due to Nyloprint. *Contact Dermatitis* 1976; 2:144–146.

1015. Raber L. Green chemistry challenge. *Chem Eng News* July 15, 1996.

1016. Raith L, Jaeger K. The nickel content of chalk—cause of contact dermatitis? *Contact Dermatitis* 1986; 14:61–71.

1017. Raith L, Prater E, Becker S. Kontaktdermatitis durch Kaliumgoldzyanid. *Dermatol Monatschr* 1980; 166:382–388.

1018. Rapson WS. Skin contact with gold and gold alloys. *Contact Dermatitis* 1974; 13:56–65.

1019. Rasmussen I. Patch test reactions to Flamazine. *Contact Dermatitis* 1984; 11:133–134.

1020. Rawls R. Europe's strong herbal brew. *Chem Eng News* September 23, 1996.

1021. Reich MS. Plastics makers remold industry. *Chem Eng News* May 26, 1997:14–16.

1022. Reid CM, Rycroft RJG. Allergic contact dermatitis from multiple sources of MCI/MI biocide and formaldehyde in a printer. *Contact Dermatitis* 1993; 28:252–253.

1023. Reid CM, van Grutten M, Rycroft RJG. Allergic contact dermatitis from ethylbutylthiourea in neoprene. *Contact Dermatitis* 1993; 28:193.

1024. Reuveni H, Yagupaky P. Diethyltoluamide-containing insect repellent. *Arch Dermatol* 1982; 118:582–583.

1025. Rich P, Belozer ML, Norris P, Storrs FJ. Allergic contact dermatitis to two antioxidants in latex gloves: 4,4′-Thiobis(6-*tert*-butyl-meta-cresol) (Lowinox 44S36) and butylhydroxyanisole: Allergen alternatives for glove-allergic patients. *J Am Acad Dermatol* 1991; 24:37–43.

1026. Richards TB, Gamble JF, Castellan RM, Mathias CGT. Knuckel pads in live-chicken hangers. *Contact Dermatitis* 1987; 17:13–16.

1027. Richter G. Arbeitsdermatologische und epidemiologische Aspekte der Sensibilisierung gegen das Gummi-Alterungsschutzmittel *N*-phenyl-*N*-isopropyl-*p*-phenylendiamin. *Dermatosen* 1995; 43:262–265.

1028. Richter G, Heidelbach U, Heidenbluth I. Allergische Kontaktekzeme durch Selenit. *Dermatosen* 1987; 35:162–164.

1029. Rietschel RL. Contact allergens in ultraviolet-cured acrylic resin systems. *Occup Med State Art Rev* 1986; 1:301–306.

1030. Rietschel RL, Huggins R, Levy N, et al. In vivo and in vitro testing of gloves for protection against UV-curable acrylate resin systems. *Contact Dermatitis* 1984; 11:279–282.

1031. Rimmer S, Spielvogel RL. Dermatologic problems of musicians. *J Am Acad Dermatol* 1990; 22:657–663.

1032. Roberts DL, Messenger AG, Summerly R. Occupational dermatitis due to 1,2-benzisothiazolin-3-one in the pottery industry. *Contact Dermatitis* 1981; 7:145–147.

1033. Roberts JL, Hanifin JM. Athletic shoe dermatitis. Contact allergy to ethyl butyl thiourea. *JAMA* 1979; 241:275–276.

1034. Robertson MH, Storrs FJ. Allergic contact dermatitis in two machinists. *Arch Dermatol* 1982; 118:997–1002.

1035. Rock WP. Fissure sealants: Results of a 3-year clinical trial using an ultraviolet sensitive resin. *Br Dent J* 1977; 142:16–18.

1036. Rodriguez A, Echechipia S, Alvarez M, et al. Occupational contact dermatitis from vitamin B$_{12}$. *Contact Dermatitis* 1994; 31:271.

1037. Rodriguez C, Daskaleros PA, Sauers LJ. Effects of fabric softeners on the skin. *Dermatosen* 1994; 42:58–61.

1038. Roed-Petersen J. Frequency of sensitivity to Grotan BK in Denmark. *Contact Dermatitis* 1977; 3:212–213.

1039. Roed-Petersen J, Hjorth N. Contact dermatitis from antioxidants. Hidden sensitizers in topical medications and foods. *Br J Dermatol* 1976; 94:233–241.

1040. Roed-Petersen J, Hjorth N, Jordan WP, et al. Postal sorter's rubber fingerstall dermatitis. *Contact Dermatitis* 1977; 3:143–147.

1041. Roed-Petersen J, Menné T. Allergic contact dermatitis and lichen planus from black-and-white photographic developing. *Cutis* 1976; 18:699–705.

1042. Roed-Petersen J, Menné T, Mann Nielsen K, Hjorth N. Is it possible to work with pao ferro (*Machaerium scleroxylum* Tul.)? *Arch Dermatol Res* 1987; 279(suppl 8):810–812.

1043. Romaguera C, Grimalt F, Conde-Salazar L. Occupational dermatitis from vitamin K$_3$ sodium bisulphite. *Contact Dermatitis* 1980; 6:355–356.

1044. Romaguera C, Grimalt F, Lecha M. Occupational purpuric textile dermatitis from formaldehyde resins. *Contact Dermatitis* 1981; 7:152–153.

1045. Ronchese F. *Occupational Marks and Other Physical Signs.* New York: Grune & Stratton; 1948:124.

1046. Rook A. *Alsteroemeria* causing contact dermatitis in a florist also allergic to tulips. *Contact Dermatitis Newslett* 1970; 7:166.

1047. Rook A. Dermatitis from *Alstroemeria*: Altered clinical pattern and probably increasing incidence. *Contact Dermatitis* 1981; 7:355–356.

1048. Rosen RH, Freeman S. Prognosis of occupational contact dermatitis in New South Wales, Australia. *Contact Dermatitis* 1993; 29:88–93.

1049. Rosenzweig R, Scher R. Nail cosmetics: Adverse reactions. *Am J Contact Dermatitis* 1993;4:71–77.

1050. Ross JS, Rycroft RJG, Cronin E. Melamine-formaldehyde contact dermatitis in orthopedic practice. *Contact Dermatitis* 1992; 26:203–204.

1051. Rossmoore HW. Antimicrobial agents for water-based metalworking fluids. *J Occup Med* 1981; 23:247–254.

1052. Rothe A, Heine A, Rebohle E. Wacholderbeeröl als Berufsallergen für Haut und Atemtbrakt. *Berufsdermatosen* 1973; 21:11–16.

1053. Roush GC, Kelly JO, Meigs JW, et al. Scrotal carcinoma in Connecticut metal workers. *Am J Epidemiol* 1982; 116:76–85.

1054. Rustemeyer T, Frosch PJ. Occupational skin diseases in dental laboratory technicians. (I). Clinical picture and causative factors. *Contact Dermatitis* 1996; 34:125–133.

1055. Rycroft RJG. Is Grotan BK a contact sensitizer? *Br J Dermatol* 1978; 99:346–347.

1056. Rycroft RJG. Acute ulcerative contact dermatitis from ready-mixed cement. *Clin Exp Dermatol* 1980; 5:245–247.

1057. Rycroft RJG. Bacteria and soluble oil dermatitis. *Contact Dermatitis* 1980; 6:7–9.

1058. Rycroft RJG. Occupational contact sensitization to 2,6-dichloropurine. *Contact Dermatitis* 1981; 7:349–350.

1059. Rycroft RJG. Allergic contact dermatitis from laboratory synthesis of 4-bromomethyl-6,8-dimethyl-2(IH)-quinolone. *Contact Dermatitis* 1981; 7:39–42.

1060. Rycroft RJG. Allergic contact dermatitis from a novel diamino intermediate, 5[(2-aminoethyl)thiomethyl]-N,N-dimethyl-2-furanmethanamine, in laboratory synthesis. *Contact Dermatitis* 1983; 9:456–458.

1061. Rycroft RJG. Low humidity occupational dermatoses. *Dermatol Clin* 1984; 2:553.

1062. Rycroft RJG, Calnan CD. Relapse of chromate dermatitis from sheet metal. *Contact Dermatitis* 1977; 3:177–180.

1063. Rycroft RJG, Calnan CD. Chromate dermatitis from a boiler lining. *Contact Dermatitis* 1977; 3:198–200.

1064. Rycroft RJG, Calnan CD. Dermatitis from slimicides in a paper mill. *Contact Dermatitis* 1980; 6:435–439.

1065. Rycroft RJG, Calnan CD. *Alstroemeria* dermatitis. *Contact Dermatitis* 1981; 7:284.

1066. Rycroft RJG, Calnan CD. Facial rashes among visual display unit operators. In Pearce BG, ed. *Health Hazards of VDTs?* Chichester: John Wiley & Sons; 1984:17–23.

1067. Rycroft RJG, Neild VS. Allergic contact dermatitis from MCI/MI biocide in a printer. *Contact Dermatitis* 1992; 26:142.

1068. Rycroft RJG, Penny PT. Dermatoses associated with brominated swimming pools. *BMJ* 1983; 287:462.

1069. Rycroft RJG, Smith WDL. Low humidity occupational dermatoses. *Contact Dermatitis* 1980; 6:488–492.

1070. Rycroft RJG, Smith NP, Stok ET, et al. Investigation of suspected contact sensitivity to tobacco in cigarette and cigar factory employees. *Contact Dermatitis* 1981; 7:32–38.

1071. Rystedt I. Work-related hand eczema in atopics. *Contact Dermatitis* 1985; 12:164–171.

1072. Rystedt I, Fischer T. Relationship between nickel and cobalt sensitization in hard metal workers. *Contact Dermatitis* 1983; 9:195–200.

1073. Sabroe RA, Sharp LA, Peachey RDG. Contact allergy to gold sodium thiosulfate. *Contact Dermatitis* 1996; 34:345–348.

1074. Sainio E-L, Kanerva L. Contact allergens in toothpastes and a review of their hypersensitivity. *Contact Dermatitis* 1995; 33:100–105.

1075. Salkie ML. The prevalence of atopy and hypersensitivity to latex in medical laboratory technologists. *Arch Pathol Lab Med* 1993; 117:897–899.

1076. Samitz M, Shrager J. Dermatitis prevention in printing and lithography industries. *Arch Dermatol* 1966; 94:307–309.

1077. Samitz MH. Dermatological hazards. The poultry industry. *Ind Med* 1947; 16:94–97.

1078. Samitz MH, Katz SA. Skin hazards from nickel and chromium salts in association with cutting oil operations. *Contact Dermatitis* 1975; 1:158–160.

1078a. Samitz MH, Mori P, Long CF. Dermatological hazards in the cigar industry. *Ind Med Surg* 1949; 18:434–439.

1078b. Samitz MH, Shmunes E. Occupational dermatoses in dentists and allied personnel. *Cutis* 1969; 5:180–184.

1079. Samman PD, Johnston ENM. Nail damage associated with handling of Paraquat and Diquat. *BMJ* 1969; 1:818–819.

1080. Sangro y Torres PD. Tobacco industry. In Parmeggiani L, ed. *Encyclopedia of Occupational Health and Safety*, 3rd ed. Geneva: International Labor Office; 1983:2182–2184.

1081. Sasseville D, Al-Khenaizan S. Occupational contact dermatitis from ethylenediamine in a wire-drawing lubricant. *Contact Dermatitis* 1997; 36:228–229.

1082. Sasseville D, Balbul A, Kwong P, Yu K. Contact sensitization to pyridine derivatives. *Contact Dermatitis* 1996; 35:100–101.

1083. Savage J. Chloracetamide in nylon spin finish. *Contact Dermatitis* 1978; 4:179.

1084. Scerri L, Dalziel KL. Occupational contact sensitization to the stabilized chlorinated paraffin fraction in neat cutting oil. *Am J Contact Dermatitis* 1996; 35–37.

1085. Scheinman PL. Allergic contact dermatitis to fragrance: A review. *Am J Contact Dermatitis* 1996; 7:65–76.

1086. Schittenhelm A, Stockinger W. Uber die Idiosynkrasie gegen Nickel (Nickelkrätze) under ihre Beziehung zur Anaphylaxie. *Zeitschrift Ges Exp Med* 1925; 45:58–74.

1087. Schmidt H. Contact urticaria to teak with systemic effects. *Contact Dermatitis* 1978; 4:176–177.

1088. Schmidt RJ, Kingston T. Chrysanthemum dermatitis in South Wales: Diagnosis by patch testing with feverfew *(Tanacetum parthenium)* extract. *Contact Dermatitis* 1985; 13:120–121.

1089. Schmitt AF, Murphy TD. Assessment of worker exposure to hexavalent chromium and inorganic nickel during stainless steel welding processes. *Proc 2nd Chromates Symp Ind Health Found Pittsburgh* 1981:259–266.

1090. Schneider HG. Schwefelallergie. *Hautarzt* 1978; 29: 340–342.

1091. Schneider WJ. Considerations regarding infection during hospital employment. *J Occup Med* 1982; 24:53–57.

1092. Schnuch A, Geier J. Kontaktallergene bei Dentalberufen. *Dermatosen* 1994; 42:253–255.

1093. Schnuch A, Geier J. Kontaktallergie gegen Piperazin. *Dermatosen* 1995; 43:185–186.

1094. Schnuch A, Geier J. Aktuelle sensibilisierungshäufigkeiten bei der DKG-Testreihe "Metallverarbeitung." *Dermatosen* 1996; 44:34–36.

1095. Schonning L. Sensitizing properties of *p*-amino-diphenylamine. *Acta Derm Venereol (Stockh)*1969; 49:501–502.

1096. Schorr WF. Formaldehyde in shampoos and toiletries. *Contact Dermatitis Newslett* 1971; 5:220.

1097. Schorr WF, Keran E, Plotka E. Formaldehyde allergy: The quantitative analysis of American clothing for free formaldehyde and its relevance in clinical practice. *Arch Dermatol* 1974; 110:73–76.

1098. Schubert H. Allergic contact dermatitis due to propachlor. *Dermatol Monatschr* 1979; 165:495–498.

1099. Schubert H, Prater E. Nickel allergy in hairdressers (Letter to the Editor). *Contact Dermatitis* 1982; 8:414–415.

1100. Schubert H, von Wurbach G, Prater E, et al. Kontaktdermatitis auf Metham-Natrium. *Dermatosen* 1993; 41:28–33.

1101. Schuman SH, Dobson RL, Fingar JR. Dyrene dermatitis. *Lancet* 1980; 2:1252.

1102. Scutt RWB. Chrome sensitivity associated with tropical footwear in the Royal Navy. *Br J Dermatol* 1966; 78:337–343.

1103. Schwartz L, Tulipan L, Birmingham DJ. *Occupational Diseases of the Skin*, 3rd ed. Philadelphia: Lea & Febiger; 1957:886.

1104. Schwarz G, Rakoski J. Spezielle dermatologische Probleme bei der Arbeit in Reinräumen. *Dermatosen* 1987; 35:98–99.

1105. Seetharam KA, Pasricha JS. Condiments and contact dermatitis of the finger-tips. *Indian J Dermatol Venereol Leprol* 1987; 53:325–328.

1106. Seidenari S, Danese P, Di Nardo A, et al. Contact sensitization among ceramics workers. *Contact Dermatitis* 1990; 22:45–49.

1107. Seidenari S, Mantovani L, Mazini BM, Pignatti M. Cross-sensitization between azo dyes and para-amino compounds. *Contact Dermatitis* 1997; 36:91–96.

1108. Seidenari S, Manzini BM, Danese P. Contact sensitization to textile dyes: Description of 100 subjects. *Contact Dermatitis* 1991; 24:253–258.

1109. Seidenari S, Manzini BM, Schiavi ME, Motolese A. Prevalence of contact allergy to non-disperse azo dyes for natural fibers: A study in 1814 consecutive patients. *Contact Dermatitis* 1995; 33:118–122.

1110. Seite-Bellezza D, el Sayed F, Bazex J. Contact urticaria from cinnamic aldehyde and benzaldehyde in a confectioner. *Contact Dermatitis* 1994; 31:272–273.

1111. Selenaskas S, Tata MJ, Vitale JN. Pancreatic cancer among workers processing synthetic resins. *Am J Ind Med* 1995; 28:385–398.

1112. Seligman PJ, Mathias CG, Malley MA, et al. Phototoxic bullae among celery harvesters. *Arch Dermatol* 1987; 123:1478–1482.

1113. Senff H, Köllner A, Kunze J. Allergisches Kontaktekzem auf polyethyleneglycoldimethacrylat. *Dermatosen* 1992; 40:24–26.

1114. Sepkowitz KA, Fella P, Rivera P, et al. Prevalence of PPD positivity among new employees at a hospital in New York City. *Infect Control Hosp Epidemiol* 1995; 16:344–347.

1115. Sequeira JH. A case of bullous eruption caused by Mayweed. *Lancet* 1921; 2:560.

1116. Shah M, Lewis FM, Gawkrodger DJ. Prognosis of occupational hand dermatitis in metalworkers. *Contact Dermatitis* 1996; 34:27–30.

1117. Shankar DSK. Contact urticaria induced by *Semecarpus anacardium*. *Contact Dermatitis* 1992; 26:200.

1118. Sharp DS, Eskensazi B, Harrison R, et al. Delayed health hazards of pesticide exposure. *Annu Rev Public Health* 1986; 7:441–471.

1119. Shehade SA, Beck MH, Chalmers RJG. Allergic contact dermatitis to crystal violet (lactone) in carbonless copy paper. *Contact Dermatitis* 1987; 17:310–326.

1120. Shehade SA, Roberts PJ, Diffey BL, et al. Photodermatitis due to spot welding. *Br J Dermatol* 1987; 117:117–119.

1121. Shelley ED, Shelley WB. Chronic dermatitis simulating small-plaque parapsoriasis due to cyanoacrylate adhesive used on fingernails. *JAMA* 1984; 252:2455–2456.

1122. Shelley WB. Chromium in welding fumes as cause of eczematous hand eruption. *JAMA* 1964; 189:772–773.

1123. Shelley WB. Golf course dermatitis due to thiram fungicide. *JAMA* 1964; 188:415–417.

1124. Shelley WB, Epstein E. Contact sensitivity to gold as a chronic papular eruption. *Arch Dermatol* 1963; 87:388.

1125. Shelley WB, Hurley HJ. Studies on topical control of axillary hyperhidrosis. *Acta Derm Venereol* (Stockh) 1975; 55:241.

1126. Shemesh A, Ackerman N. Medical hazards of photography. *Ind Med Surg* 1964; 33:807–812.

1127. Sherertz EF. Clothing dermatitis: Practical aspects for the clinician. *Am J Contact Dermatitis* 1992; 3:55–64.

1128. Shmunes E, Kempton RJ. Allergic contact dermatitis to dimethoxane in a spin finish. *Contact Dermatitis* 1980; 6:421–424.

1129. Shmunes E, Taylor JS. Industrial contact dermatitis: Effect of the riot control agent ortho-chlorobenylidene malononitrile. *Arch Dermatol* 1973; 107:212–216.

1130. Shoji A. Contact dermatitis from chlorhexidine. *Contact Dermatitis* 1983; 9:156.

1131. Shupack JL, Andersen SR, Romano SJ. Human skin reactions to ethylene oxide. *J Lab Clin Med* 1981; 98:723–729.

1132. Silverman S Jr. Infectious disease control and the dental office: AIDs and other transmissible diseases. *Int Dent J* 1987; 37:108–113.

1133. Sim-Davies D. Studies in contact dermatitis XXIV. Dyes in trousers. *Trans St Johns Hosp Dermatol Soc* 1972; 58:251–260.

1134. Simon H, Harley G. Skin reactions from gold jewelry contaminated with radon. *JAMA* 1967; 200:254–255.

1135. Simpson JR. Contact dermatitis due to dicyclohexylcarbodiimide. *Contact Dermatitis* 1979; 5:333.

1136. Singer K. *Diseases of the Musical Profession: A Systematic Presentation of Their Causes, Symptoms and Methods of Treatment* [translated from the German by Vladimir Lakond]. New York: Areenberg, 1932:129.

1137. Singgih SR, Lantinga H, Nater JP, et al. Occupational hand dermatoses in hospital cleaning personnel. *Contact Dermatitis* 1986; 14:14–19.

1138. Sinha SM, Pasricha JS, Sharma RC, et al. Vegetables responsible for contact dermatitis of the hands. *Arch Dermatol* 1977; 113:776–779.

1139. Siregar RS. Occupational dermatoses among foresters. *Contact Dermatitis* 1975; 1:33–37.

1140. Sjogren B, Gustavsson A, Hedstrom L. Mortality in two cohorts of welders exposed to high and low levels of hexavalent chromium. *Scand J Work Environ Health* 1987; 13:247–251.

1141. Skov P, Valbjorn O, Pedersen BV. Influence of personal characteristics, job-related factors and psychosocial factors on the sick building syndrome. *Scand J Work Environ Health* 1989; 15:286–295.

1142. Slob A, Jekel B, De Jong B, et al. On the occurrence of tuliposides in the liliflorae. *Phytochemistry* 1975; 14:1997–2005.

1143. Slovak AJM. Contact dermatitis due to benzisothiazolone in a works analytical team. *Contact Dermatitis* 1980; 6:187–190.

1144. Slovak AJM, Payne AR. Delayed dermal burns caused by dimethyl acetylenedicarboxylate. *Contact Dermatitis* 1984; 11:29–30.

1145. Smeenk G, Burgers GJA, Teunissen PC. Contact dermatitis from salbutamol. *Contact Dermatitis* 1994; 31:123.

1146. Smit HA, Burdorf A, Coenraads PJ. Prevalence of hand dermatitis in different occupations. *Int J Epidemiol* 1993; 22:288–293.

1147. Smith AG. Skin disease in the pottery industry. *Ann Occup Hyg* 1983; 33:365–368.

1148. Sneid P. Dermatoses on the farm. *Indiana Med* 1955; 24:117–118.

1149. Soni B, Sherertz E. Allergic contact dermatitis from azathioprine. *Am J Contact Dermatitis* 1996; 7:116–117.

1150. Soni B, Sheretz E. Contact dermatitis in the textile industry. A review of 72 patients. *Am J Contact Dermatitis* 1996; 7:226–230.

1151. Sonnex TS, Rycroft RJG. Allergic contact dermatitis from othobenzyl parachlorophenol in a drinking glass cleaner. *Contact Dermatitis* 1986; 14:247.

1152. Sood SK, Salzman MB, Johnson BA, et al. Duration of tick attachment as a predictor of the risk of Lyme disease in an area in which Lyme disease is endemic. *J Infect Dis* 1997; 175:996–999.

1153. Soper LE, Vitez TS, Weinberg D. Metabolism of halogenated anaesthetic agents as a possible cause of acneiform eruptions. *Anaesth Analg* 1973; 52:125–127.

1154. Sosman AJ, Schlueter DO, Fink JN, et al. Hypersensitivity to wood dust. *N Engl J Med* 1969; 281:977–980.

1155. Sparrow GP. A connective tissue disorder similar to vinyl chloride disease in a patient exposed to perchloroethylene. *Clin Dermatol* 1977; 2:17–22.

1156. Spinelli JJ, Gallagher RP, Band PR, et al. Multiple myeloma, leukemia, and cancer of the ovary in cosmetologists and hairdressers. *Am J Ind Med* 1984; 6:97–102.

1157. Spott DA, Shelley WB. Exanthem due to contact allergen (Benzoin) absorbed through skin. *JAMA* 1970; 214:1881–1882.

1158. Spruit D, Malten KE. Occupational cobalt and chromium dermatitis in an offset printing factory. *Dermatologica* 1975; 151:34–42.

1159. Srinivas CR, Devadiga R, Aroor AR. Footwear dermatitis due to bisphenol A. *Contact Dermatitis* 1989; 20:150–151.

1160. Stam-Westerveld EB, Coenraads PJ, van der Valk PGM, et al. Rubbing test responses of the skin to man-made mineral fibres of different diameters. *Contact Dermatitis* 1994; 31:1–4.

1161. Starr JC, Yunginger J, Brahser GW. Immediate type I asthmatic response to henna following occupational exposure in hairdressers. *Ann Allergy* 1982; 48:98–99.

1162. State of the Workplace 1988; 2:4–5.

1163. Steciuk A, Dompmartin A, Saussey J, et al. Pustular contact dermatitis from fluorine in an antirust solution. *Contact Dermatitis* 1997; 36:276–277.

1164. Steenland K, Stayner L, Greif A, et al. Mortality among workers exposed to ethylene oxide. *N Engl J Med* 1991; 324:1402–1407.

1165. Stern JB. The edema of fiddler's neck. *J Am Acad Dermatol* 1979; 1:538–540.

1166. Stevenson CJ. Fluorescence as a clue to contamination in TV workers. *Contact Dermatitis* 1975; 1:242.

1167. Stewart L, Beck MH. Contact sensitivity to methyl ethyl ketone peroxide in a paint sprayer. *Contact Dermatitis* 1992; 26:52–53.

1168. Stingeni L, Lapomarda V, Lisi P. Occupational hand dermatitis in hospital environments. *Contact Dermatitis* 1995; 33:172–176.

1169. Stoke JCJ. Captafol dermatitis in the timber industry. *Contact Dermatitis* 1979; 5:284–292.

1170. Storrs FJ. Permanent wave contact dermatitis: Contact allergy to glyceryl monothioglycolate. *J Am Acad Dermatol* 1984; 11:74–85.

1171. Storrs FJ. Dermatitis from clothing and shoes. In: Fisher AA, ed. *Contact Dermatitis*, 3rd ed. Philadelphia: Lea & Febiger; 1986:283–337.

1172. Stransky L, Usunov P. Occupationally induced rat mite dermatitis *(Ornithonyssus bacoti). Dermatosen* 1992; 40:73–74.

1173. Straube M, Uter W, Schwanitz HJ. Occupational allergic contact dermatitis from thiolactic acid contained in "ester-free" permanent-waving solutions. *Contact Dermatitis* 1996; 34:229–230.

1174. Susitaival P, Hannuksela M. The 12-year prognosis of hand dermatosis in 896 Finnish farmers. *Contact Dermatitis* 1995; 32:233–237.

1175. Suskind RR, Hertzberg VS. Human health effects of 2,4,5 T and its toxic contamination. *JAMA* 1984; 251:2372–2380.

1176. Sussman GL, Lem D, Liss G, et al. Latex allergy in housekeeping personnel. *Ann Allergy Asthma Immunol* 1995; 74:415–418.

1177. Suzuki Y, Ohkido M. Contact dermatitis from hydrazine derivatives. *Contact Dermatitis* 1979; 5:113–114.

1178. Symington I, Cross JD, Dale IM, et al. Mercury poisoning in dentists. *J Soc Occup Med* 1980; 30:37–39.

1179. Szeimies R-M, Lissner A, Meurer M. Perchlorethylen-induzierte systemische Sklerodermie. *Dermatosen* 1992; 40:66–69.

1180. Szolar-Platzer C, Maibach HI. Allergic contact dermatitis to topically applied anithistamines. *Dermatosen* 1996; 44:205–212.

1181. Tacke J, Schmidt A, Fartasch M, Diepgen TL. Occupational contact dermatitis in bakers, confectioners and cooks. *Contact Dermatitis* 1995; 33:112–117.

1182. Tan BB, Lear JT, Watts J, et al. Perioperative collapse: Prevalence of latex allergy in patients sensitive to anaesthetic agents. *Contact Dermatitis* 1997; 36:47–50.

1183. Tanaka S, Lucas JB. Dermatitis in paperhangers. *Contact Dermatitis* 1984; 10:54–55.

1184. Tandon R, Aarts B. Chromium, nickel and cobalt contents of some Australian cements. *Contact Dermatitis* 1993; 28:201–205.

1185. Tarvainen K, Jolanki R, Forsman-Gronholm L, et al. Exposure, skin protection and occupational skin disease in the glass-fibre–reinforced plastics industry. *Contact Dermatitis* 1993; 29:119–127.

1186. Tarvainen K, Kanerva L, Jolanki R, Estlander T. Occupational dermatoses from the manufacture of plastic composite products. *Am J Contact Dermatitis* 1995; 6:95–104.

1187. Taylor JS. Contact dermatitis from goggles. Paper presented at the Annual Meeting of the American Academy of Dermatology, Washington, DC, 1984.

1188. Taylor JS. Latex allergy. *Am J Contact Dermatitis* 1993; 4:114–117.

1189. Taylor JS, Praditsuwan P. Latex allergy. Review of 44 cases including outcome and frequent association with allergic hand eczema. *Arch Dermatol* 1996; 132:265–271.

1190. Taylor SWC. A prevalence study of virus warts on the hands in a poultry processing and packing station. *J Soc Occup Med* 1980; 30:20–23.

1191. Tazelaar DJ. Hypersensitivity to chromium in a light-blue tattoo. *Dermatologica* 1970; 141:282–287.

1192. Tennstedt D, Cromphout P, Dooms-Goosens A, et al. Dermatoses of the neck affecting violin and viola players (fiddler's neck and contact dermatitis). *Dermatosen* 1979; 27:165–169.

1193. Tennstedt D, Dumont-Fruytier M, Lachapelle JM. Occupational allergic contact dermatitis to virginiamycin, an antibiotic used as a food additive for pigs and poultry. *Contact Dermatitis* 1978; 4:133–134.

1194. Terr AI. The atopic worker. *Clin Rev Allergy* 1986; 4:267–288.

1195. Textiles in the seventies. *Chem Eng News* April 20, 1970:65–73.

1196. Themido R, Brandao F. Contact allergy to thiurams. *Contact Dermatitis* 1984; 10:251.

1197. Thiboutot DM, Hamory BH, Marks JG Jr. Dermatoses among floral shop workers. *J Am Acad Dermatol* 1990; 22:54–58.

1198. Thormann J. Contact dermatitis to a new fungicide, 2-*n*-octyl-4-isothiazolin-3-one. *Contact Dermatitis* 1982; 8:204.

1199. Thune P. Contact allergy due to lichens in patients with a history of photosensitivity. *Contact Dermatitis* 1977; 3:267–272.

1200. Thune PO, Solberg YJ. Photosensitivity and allergy to aromatic lichen acids, Compositae oleoresins and other plant substances. *Contact Dermatitis* 1980; 6:64–71, 81–87.

1201. Tilsley DA. Contact and photo-dermatitis from Nyloprint. *Contact Dermatitis* 1975; 1:334–335.

1202. Tobler M, Freiburghaus AU. A glove with exceptional protective features minimizes the risks of working with hazardous chemicals. *Contact Dermatitis* 1992; 26:299–303.

1203. Tomazic VJ, Shampaine EL, Lamanna A, et al. Cornstarch powder on latex products is an allergen carrier. *J Allergy Clin Immunol* 1994; 93:751–758.

1204. Tomb RR, Lepoittevin J-P, Durepaire F, et al. Ectopic contact dermatitis from ethyl cyanoacrylate instant adhesives. *Contact Dermatitis* 1993; 28:206–208.

1205. Torres V, Campos Lopes J, Lobo L, et al. Occupational contact dermatitis to thiourea and dimethylthiourea from diazo copy paper. *Am J Contact Dermatitis* 1992; 3:37–39.

1206. Tosti A, Bardazzi F, Valeri F, et al. Contact dermatitis from butylated hydroxyanisole. *Contact Dermatitis* 1987; 17:257–258.

1207. Tosti A, Guerra L, Vincenzi C, et al. Contact sensitization caused by toluene sulfonamide-formaldehyde resin in women who use nail cosmetics. *Am J Contact Dermatitis* 1993; 4:150–153.

1208. Tosti A, Manuzzi P, de Padova MP. Contact dermatitis to Kathon CG. *Contact Dermatitis* 1986; 14:326–327.

1209. Tosti A, Melino M, Veronesi S. Contact urticaria to tobacco. *Contact Dermatitis* 1987; 16:225–226.

1210. Tosti A, Peluso AM, Varotti C. Skin burns due to transit-mixed Portland cement. *Contact Dermatitis* 1989; 21:58.

1211. Towers GHN, Mitchell JC. The current status of the weed *Parthenium hysterophorus* L. As a cause of allergic contact dermatitis. *Contact Dermatitis* 1983; 9:465–469.

1212. Treudler R, Tebbe B, Orfanos CE. Coexistence of type I and type IV sensitization in occupational coffee allergy. *Contact Dermatitis* 1997; 36:109.

1213. Trivalent chromium is basis of plating process. *Chem Eng News* June 23, 1975:16–17.

1214. Tuer WF, James WD, Summer RJ. Contact urticaria to *o*-phenylphenate. *Ann Allerg* 1986; 56:19–21.

1215. Tuomi A-L, Rasanen L. Contact allergy to tylosin and cobalt in a pig-farmer. *Contact Dermatitis* 1995; 33:285.

1216. Turjanmaa K. Incidence of immediate allergy to latex gloves in hospital personnel. *Contact Dermatitis* 1987; 17:270–275.

1217. Turjanmaa K. Update on occupational natural rubber latex allergy. *Dermatol Clin Occup Dermatoses* 1994; 12:561–567.

1218. Turjanmaa K, Reunala I, Tuimala R, et al. Severe IgE-mediated allergy to surgical gloves. *Proceedings of the Fifteenth Nordic Congress of Allergology. Allergy* 1984; 39(suppl 2):Abstract No. 35.

1219. Turjanmaa K, Reunala T, Tuimala R, et al. Allergy to latex gloves: Unusual complication during delivery. *BMJ* 1988; 297:1029.

1220. Turk K, Rietschel RL. Effect of processing cement to concrete on hexavalent chromium levels. *Contact Dermatitis* 1993; 28:209–211.

1221. Tuskes PM, Tilton MA, Greff RM. Ammonia exposures in blue-line printers in Houston, Texas. *Appl Ind Hyg* 1988; 3:155–157.

1222. Urbach F. Reply to Hudson L. *J Am Acad Dermatol* 1987; 17:508–509.

1223. Vader JP, Minder CE. Die Sterblichkeit an Krebsen der Nasen- und Nasennebenhölen bei Schweizer Schreinern. *Schweiz Med Wochenschr* 1987; 117:481–486.

1224. Vale PT. Prevention of phytophotodermatitis from celery. *Contact Dermatitis* 1993; 29:108.

1225. Valsecchi R, Cainelli T. Contact urticaria from dog saliva. *Contact Dermatitis* 1989; 20:62.

1226. Valsecchi R, Cassina GP, Migliori M, et al. Tego dermatitis. *Contact Dermatitis* 1985; 12:230.

1227. Valsecchi R, Foiadelli L, Cainelli T. Is silver sulfadiazine a sensitizer? *Contact Dermatitis* 1986; 15:45–46.

1228. Valsecchi R, Leghissa P, Piazzolla S, et al. Occupational dermatitis from isothiazolinones in nylon production. *Dermatology* 1993; 187:109–111.

1229. van den Akker TW, Roesyanto-Mahadi ID, van Toorenenbergen AW, et al. Contact allergy to spices. *Contact Dermatitis* 1990; 22:267–272.

1230. van der Leun JC, de Kreek EJ, Leeuwen MD, et al. Photosensitivity owing to thiourea. *Arch Dermatol* 1977; 113:1611.

1231. van der Mark S. Contact urticaria from horse saliva. *Contact Dermatitis* 1983; 9:145.

1232. van der Meeren HLM. Dodecyl gallate, permitted in food, is a strong sensitizer. *Contact Dermatitis* 1987; 16:260–262.

1233. van der Meeren HLM, van Erp PEJ. Life-threatening contact urticaria from glove powder. *Contact Dermatitis* 1986; 14:190–191.

1234. van der Walle HB, Brunsveld VM. Dermatitis in hairdressers (1). The experience of the past 4 years. *Contact Dermatitis* 1994; 30:217–221.

1235. van der Wegen-Keijser MH, Bruynzeel DP. Allergy to cane reed in a saxophonist. *Contact Dermatitis* 1991; 25:268.

1236. van Groeningen G, Nater JP. Reactions to dental impression materials. *Contact Dermatitis* 1975; 1:373–376.

1237. van Hecke E. Contact allergy to onion. *Contact Dermatitis* 1977; 3:167–168.

1238. van Hecke E. Contact sensitivity to *o*-phenylphenol in a coolant. *Contact Dermatitis* 1986; 15:46.

1239. van Joost T, Habets JMW, Stolz E, et al. Sodium hypochlorite sensitization. *Contact Dermatitis* 1987; 16:114.

1240. van Joost T, Heule F, De Boer J. Sensitization to methylenedianiline and para-structures. *Contact Dermatitis* 1987; 16:246–248.

1241. van Joost T, Naafs B, van Ketel WG. Sensitization to benomyl and related pesticides. *Contact Dermatitis* 1983; 9:153–154.

1242. van Ketel WG. Contact dermatitis from hydrazine derivative in stain remover: Cross sensitization to apresoline and isoniazide. *Acta Derm Venereol (Stockh)* 1964; 44:49–53.

1243. van Ketel WG. Dermatitis from an aftershave. *Contact Dermatitis* 1978; 4:117.

1244. van Ketel WG. Contact dermatitis from propylene oxide. *Contact Dermatitis* 1979; 5:191–192.

1245. van Ketel WG. Skin eruptions caused by vegetables and fruit including pears. *Contact Dermatitis* 1982; 8:352.

1246. van Ketel WG. Allergy to benzylamine and benzyl-1-amino-3-chloro-2-hydroxypropane. *Contact Dermatitis* 1984; 11:186–187.

1247. van Ketel WG, van Diggelen MW. A farmer with allergy to cows. *Contact Dermatitis* 1982; 8:279.

1248. van Ketel WG, Kisch LS. The problem of the sensitizing capacity of some grotans used as bacteriocides in cooling oils. *Dermatosen* 1983; 31:118–121.

1249. van Ketel WG, Nieboer C. Allergy topalladium in dental alloys. *Contact Dermatitis* 1981; 7:331–357.

1250. van Ketel WG, Tan-Lim KN. Contact dermatitis from ethanol. *Contact Dermatitis* 1975; 1:7–10.

1251. van Loon LA, van Elsas PW, van Joost T, et al. Test battery for metal allergy in dentistry. *Contact Dermatitis* 1986; 14:158–161.

1252. van Putten PB, Coenraads PJ, Nater JP. Hand dermatoses and contact allergic reactions in construction workers exposed to epoxy resins. *Contact Dermatitis* 1984; 10:146–150.

1253. van Vliet C, Swaen GMH, Slangen JJM, et al. The organic solvent syndrome. A comparison of cases with neuropsychiatric disorders among painters and construction workers. *Int Arch Occup Environ Health* 1987; 59:493–501.

1254. Veien N, Hattel T, Justesen O, Norholm A. Causes of eczema in food industry. *Dermatosen* 1983; 31:84–86.

1255. Veien NK, Hattel T, Justesen O, et al. Occupational contact dermatitis due to spiramycin and/or tylosin among farmers. *Contact Dermatitis* 1980; 6:410–413.

1256. Vena GA, Foti C, Angelini G. Sulfite contact allergy. *Contact Dermatitis* 1994; 31:172–175.

1257. Veraldi S, Benelli C, Pigatto PD. Occupational allergic contact dermatitis from minoxidil. *Contact Dermatitis* 1992; 26:211–212.

1258. Verbeck SJA, Buise-van Unnik EMM, Malten KE. Itching in office workers from glass fibres. *Contact Dermatitis* 1981; 7:354.

1259. Verbov J. Tylosin dermatitis. *Contact Dermatitis* 1983; 9:325–326.

1260. Verspijck Mijnssen GAW. Preliminary report on a case of contact dermatitis due to ozalid and radex copy papers. *Dermatologica* 1964; 128:93.

1261. Verspijck Mijnssen GAW. Dermatitis from Ozalid and Radex copy paper. *Contact Dermatitis Newslett* 1967; 1:13–14.

1262. Vestergaard L, Andersen KE. Allergic contact dermatitis from sodium metabisulfite in topical preparation. *Am J Contact Dermatitis* 1995; 6:174–175.

1263. Vickers HR, Edwards DH. Cement burns. *Contact Dermatitis* 1976; 2:73–78.

1264. Vilaplana J, Azon A, Romaguera C, Lecha M. Phototoxic contact dermatitis with toxic hepatitis due to the percutaneous absorption of paraquat. *Contact Dermatitis* 1993; 29:163–164.

1265. Vilaplana J, Romaguera C. Captan, a rare contact sensitizer in hairdressing. *Contact Dermatitis* 1993; 29:107.

1266. Vincenzi C, Bardazzi F, Tosti A, et al. Fish tank granuloma: Report of a case. *Cutis* 1992; 49:275–276.

1267. Vincenzi C, Tosti A, Guerra L, et al. Contact dermatitis to palladium: A study of 2,300 patients. *Am J Contact Dermatitis* 1995; 6:110–112.

1268. Vincenzi C, Trevisi P, Guerra L, et al. Patch testing with whole dust mite bodies in atopic dermatitis. *Am J Contact Dermatitis* 1994; 5:213–215.

1269. von Odia SG, Purschel WC, Vocks E, et al. Noxen und Irritantien im Beruf. *Dermatosen* 1994; 42:179–183.

1270. Wahlberg JE. Two cases of hypersensitivity to quaternary ammonium compounds. *Acta Derm Venereol (Stockh)* 1962; 42:230–234.

1271. Wahlberg JE. Nickel allergy and atopy in hairdressers. *Contact Dermatitis* 1975; 1:161–165.

1272. Wahlberg JE. Nickel allergy in hairdressers (Letter to the Editor). *Contact Dermatitis* 1981; 7:358–359.

1273. Wahlberg JE. Contact sensitivity to NAPP printing plates secondary to a relapsing hand dermatitis. *Contact Dermatitis* 1983; 9:239.

1274. Wahlberg JE, Boman A. Contact sensitivity to quinidine sulfate from occupational exposure. *Contact Dermatitis* 1981; 7:27–31.

1275. Wahlberg JE, Boman AS. Cross-reactivity to palladium and nickel studied in the guinea pig. *Acta Derm Venereol* (Stockh) 1992; 72:95–97.

1276. Wahlberg JE, Högberg M, Skare L. Chloracetamide allergy in house painters. *Contact Dermatitis* 1978; 4:116–117.

1277. Wahlberg JE, Liden C. Is the skin affected by work at visual display terminals? In: Taylor JS, ed. *Occupational Dermatoses*. Philadelphia: W.B. Saunders, Co; 1988:81–85.

1278. Wahlberg JE, Wannesten G. Hypersensitivity and photosensitivity to chlorhexidine. *Dermatologica* 1971; 143:376–379.

1279. Wahlberg JE, Wrangsjo K. Is cobalt naphthenate an allergen? *Contact Dermatitis* 1985; 12:225.

1280. Wald PH, Jones JR. Semiconductor manufacturing: An introduction to processes and hazards. *Am J Ind Med* 1987; 11:203–221.

1281. Walder BK. Do solvents cause scleroderma? *Int J Dermatol* 1983; 22:157–158.

1282. Wall LM, Oakes D, Rycroft RJG. Virus warts in meat handlers. *Contact Dermatitis* 1981; 7:259–267.

1283. Warshaw EM, Zug KA. Sesquiterpene lactone allergy. *Am J Contact Dermatitis* 1996; 7:1–23.

1284. Wass U, Wahlberg JE. Chromate steel and contact allergy. *Contact Dermatitis* 1991; 24:114–118.

1285. Wassilew SW von. Berufstypische Viruserkrankungen der Haut. *Dermatosen* 1995; 43:179–183.

1286. Weber A, Willeke K, Marchioni R, et al. Aerosol penetration and leakage characteristics of masks used in the health care industry. *Am J Infect Control* 1993; 21:167–173.

1287. Webster CG, Burnett JW. Gold dermatitis. *Cutis* 1994; 54:25–28.

1288. Weibel H, et al. Cross sensitization patterns in guinea pigs between cinnamaldehyde and cinnamyl alcohol and cinnamic acid. *Acta Derm Venereol* (Stockh) 1989; 69:302–307.

1289. Weigand DA. Cutaneous reaction to the riot control agent CS. *Military Med* 1969; 134:437–440.

1290. Wheeler CE Jr, Penn SR, Cawley E. Dermatitis from hydrazine hydrobromide solder flux. *Arch Dermatol* 1965; 91:235–239.

1291. Wheeler LA, Saperstein MD, Lowe NJ. Mutagenicity of urine from psoriatic patients undergoing treatment with coal tar and ultraviolet light. *J Invest Dermatol* 1981; 77:181–185.

1292. White GP Jr, Mathias CGT, Davin JS. Dermatitis in workers exposed to antimony in a melting process. *J Occup Med* 1993; 35:392–395.

1293. White IR, Calnan CD. Contact urticaria to fruit and birch sensitivity. *Contact Dermatitis* 1983; 9:164–165.

1294. White IR, Catchpole HE, Rycroft RJG. Rashes amongst persulphate workers. *Contact Dermatitis* 1982; 8:168–172.

1295. White IR, Cronin E. Irritant contact urticaria to diethyl-fumarate. *Contact Dermatitis* 1984; 10:315.

1296. White IR, Lewis J, Alami AE. Possible adverse reactions to an enzyme-containing washing powder. *Contact Dermatitis* 1985; 13:175–179.

1297. White IR, MacDonald DM. Dicyclohexyl carbodiimide sensitivity. *Contact Dermatitis* 1979; 5:275–276.

1298. White IR, Rycroft RJG. Low humidity occupational dermatosis—An epidemic. *Contact Dermatitis* 1982; 8:287–290.

1299. White RF, Proctor SP, Echeverria D, et al. Neurobehavioral effects of acute and chronic mixed-solvent exposure in the screen printing industry. *Am J Ind Med* 1995; 28:221–231.

1300. White WC, Vickers HR. Diethylthiourea as a cause of dermatitis in a car factory. *Br J Ind Med* 1970; 27:167–169.

1301. Whitfeld MJ, Rivers JK. Erythema multiforme after contact dermatitis in response to an epoxy sealant. *J Am Acad Dermatol* 1991; 25:386–388.

1302. Widstrom L. Contact allergy to colophony in soldering flux. *Contact Dermatitis* 1983; 9:205–207.

1303. Wieslander G, Norback D, Edling C. Occupational exposure to water based paint and symptoms from the skin and eyes. *Occup Environ Med* 1994; 51:181–186.

1304. Wigger-Alberti W, Hofmann M, Elsner P. Contact dermatitis caused by triglycidyl isocyanurate. *Am J Contact Dermatitis* 1997; 8:106–107.

1305. Wikstrom K. Allergic contact dermatitis caused by paper. *Acta Derm Venereol (Stockh)* 1969; 49:547–551.

1306. Wilkinson DS. Sensitivity to *N*-isopropyl-*N′*-phenyl-*p*-phenylenediamine. *Contact Dermatitis Newslett* 1968; 3:42.

1307. Wilkinson DS. Sulphur sensitivity. *Contact Dermatitis* 1975; 1:58.

1308. Wilkinson DS. Careers advice to youth with atopic dermatitis. *Contact Dermatitis* 1975; 1:11–12.

1309. Wilkinson DS. Timber preservatives. *Contact Dermatitis* 1979; 5:278–279.

1310. Wilkinson DS, Hambly EM. Prognosis of hand eczema in hairdressing apprentices. *Contact Dermatitis* 1978; 4:63.

1311. Wilkinson SM, Beck MH. Allergic contact dermatitis from sealants containing polysulphide polymers (Thiokol (R). *Contact Dermatitis* 1993; 29:273–274.

1312. Wilkinson SM, Beck MH. Allergic contact dermatitis from latex rubber. *Br J Dermatol* 1996; 134:910–914.

1313. Wilkinson SM, Cartwright PH, Armitage J, English JSC. Allergic contact dermatitis from 1,6-diisocyanato-hexane in an antipill finish. *Contact Dermatitis* 1991; 25:94–96.

1314. Wilkinson SM, Heagerty AHM, English JSC. Hand dermatitis in the pottery industry. *Contact Dermatitis* 1992; 26:91–94.

1315. Wilkinson SM, McGechaen K. Occupational allergic contact dermatitis from reactive dyes. *Contact Dermatitis* 1996; 35:376.

1316. Wills JH. Nasal carcinoma in woodworkers: A review. *J Occup Med* 1982; 24:526–530.

1317. Wilson CL, Powell SM. Bronopol as allergen for veterinarians. *Contact Dermatitis* 1990; 23:42.

1318. Wilson HTH, Cronin E. Dermatitis from dyed uniforms. *Br J Dermatol* 1971; 85:67–69.

1319. Winkelmann RA. Lichenoid delayed tattoo reactions. *J Cutan Pathol* 1979; 6:59–65.

1320. Winston JR, Walsh EN. Chromate dermatitis in railroad employees working with diesel locomotives. *JAMA* 1951; 147:1133–1134.

1321. Wolf H. Nasenkrebs bei Holzarbeitern. *Dermatosen* 1984; 32:191.

1322. Wong NL, Greene I. Cutaneous lupus erythematosus in a welder. *Am J Contact Dermatitis* 1990; 1:180–182.

1323. Wong WK, Tan C, Ng SK, Goh CL. Thimerosal allergy and its relevance in Singapore. *Contact Dermatitis* 1992; 26:195–196.

1324. Wood WS, Fulton R. Allergic contact dermatitis from ethoxyquin in apple packers. *Contact Dermatitis Newslett* 1972; 11:295.

1325. Woods B. Contact dermatitis from Santos rosewood. *Contact Dermatitis* 1987; 17:249–250.

1325a. World Health Organization. Environmental Health Criteria. Mercury. WHO, Geneva, 1976.

1326. Wozniak KD. Chronic discoid lupus erythematosus as occupational disease in a welder. *Dermatosen* 1971; 19:187–196.

1327. Wrangsjo K. Latex allergy in medical, dental, and laboratory personnel: A follow-up study. *Am J Contact Dermatitis* 1994; 5:194–200.

1328. Wrangsjo K, Martensson A, Widstrom L, et al. Contact dermatitis from Bioban P 1487. *Contact Dermatitis* 1986; 14:182–183.

1329. Wrangsjo K, Mellstrom G, Axelsson G. Discomfort from rubber gloves indicating contact urticaria. *Contact Dermatitis* 1986; 15:79–84.

1330. Wright RC. Dermatitis from *o*-dichlorobenzene in a leather dye. *Contact Dermatitis* 1979; 5:124–125.

1331. Wulf HC. Work in ultraviolet radiation. *Contact Dermatitis* 1980; 6:72–76.

1332. Wüthrich B. Berufsekzem durch Aethylenediamin in der Kunstfaser-Industrie. *Dermatosen* 1972; 4:200–203.

1333. Wyss M, Elsner P, Wuthrich B, Burg G. Allergic contact dermatitis from natural latex without contact urticaria. *Contact Dermatitis* 1993; 28:154–156.

1334. Yamakage A, Ishikawa H. Generalized morphea-like

scleroderma occurring in people exposed to organic solvents. *Dermatologica* 1982; 165:186–193.

1335. Yates B, Kelsey K, Seitz T, et al. Occupational skin disease in newspaper pressroom workers. *J Occup Med* 1991; 33:711–717.

1336. Young E. Allergic reactions among bakers. *Dermatologica* 1974; 148:39–46.

1337. Zachariae COC, Agner T, Menné T. Chromium allergy in consecutive patients in a country where ferrous sulfate has been added to cement since 1981. *Contact Dermatitis* 1996; 35:83–85.

1338. Zenarola P, Lomuto M. Protein contact dermatitis with positive RAST in a slaughterman. *Contact Dermatitis* 1991; 24:134–1354.

1339. Zerboni R, Tarantini G, Muratori S. Virus warts in a meat-processing factory. *Dermatosen* 1994; 42:237–240.

1340. Zimmerman EH. Letterflex in printers. *Dermatol News* June 8, 1981:1, 11.

1341. Zschunke E, Folesky M. Some effects of dicyclohexylcarbodiimide on human skin. *Contact Dermatitis* 1975; 1:188.

1342. Zugerman C. Chromium in welding fumes. *Contact Dermatitis* 1982; 8:69–70.

Index

Note: Page numbers in *italics* refer to illustrations;
page numbers followed by t refer to tables.